EUROPEAN
MasterCourse in
Paediatrics

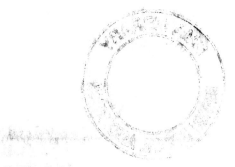

Commissioning Editor: Pauline Graham
Development Editor: Fiona Conn
Project Manager: Glenys Norquay
Design Direction: Stewart Larking
Illustration Manager: Merlyn Harvey
Illustrator: Cactus

EUROPEAN
MasterCourse in Paediatrics

Editors in Chief

Alfred Tenore
MD BA

Professor and Chair, Paediatrics
University of Udine School of Medicine
Udine, Italy

Malcolm Levene
MD FRCPCH FRCP FMedSc

Professor of Paediatrics and Child Health
University of Leeds
Leeds General Infirmary
Leeds, UK

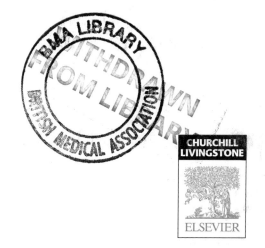

CHURCHILL LIVINGSTONE

ELSEVIER

EDINBURGH LONDON NEW YORK OXFORD PHILADELPHIA ST LOUIS SYDNEY TORONTO 2011

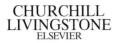

First edition 2011

Adapted from *MRCPCH MasterCourse, Volumes 1 and 2*, first edition published 2007 by Churchill Livingstone, © 2007 Royal College of Paediatrics and Child Health

ISBN 978-0-7020-4063-4

British Library Cataloguing in Publication Data
A catalogue record for this book is available from the British Library

Library of Congress Cataloging in Publication Data
A catalog record for this book is available from the Library of Congress

Notices
Knowledge and best practice in this field are constantly changing. As new research and experience broaden our understanding, changes in research methods, professional practices, or medical treatment may become necessary.

Practitioners and researchers must always rely on their own experience and knowledge in evaluating and using any information, methods, compounds, or experiments described herein. In using such information or methods they should be mindful of their own safety and the safety of others, including parties for whom they have a professional responsibility.

With respect to any drug or pharmaceutical products identified, readers are advised to check the most current information provided (i) on procedures featured or (ii) by the manufacturer of each product to be administered, to verify the recommended dose or formula, the method and duration of administration, and contraindications. It is the responsibility of practitioners, relying on their own experience and knowledge of their patients, to make diagnoses, to determine dosages and the best treatment for each individual patient, and to take all appropriate safety precautions.

To the fullest extent of the law, neither the Publisher nor the authors, contributors, or editors, assume any liability for any injury and/or damage to persons or property as a matter of products liability, negligence or otherwise, or from any use or operation of any methods, products, instructions, or ideas contained in the material herein.

ELSEVIER your source for books, journals and multimedia in the health sciences

www.elsevierhealth.com

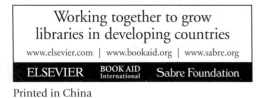

Working together to grow libraries in developing countries

www.elsevier.com | www.bookaid.org | www.sabre.org

ELSEVIER   BOOK AID International   Sabre Foundation

The publisher's policy is to use paper manufactured from sustainable forests

Printed in China

Preface

The formation of the European Union (EU) has had many political and economical consequences — such as disappearing borders, free movement between countries and the use of one currency. However, alongside these advantages many potential problems have evolved, especially in the field of medicine.

With the provision of free access for European medical specialists to the European job market, diplomas and certificates of qualification in medicine in all member countries have been mutually recognized. The EU directives enforcing this are based on the assumption that the quality of training is comparable throughout Europe, but although the EU has produced a strong stimulus for European harmonization and standardization of training in medical specialties, the EU principle of subsidiarity means that the regulation of training standards, assessment and qualifications has been delegated to national authorities and to date, no document produced at the European level has effective legal power over medical curricula or training programmes. National authorities may (but do not have to) comply with recommendations for harmonization and standardization and so paediatric training programmes in Europe, at this moment, are not comparable in quality or content. European medical umbrella organizations (such as the UEMS through its paediatric section, the European Academy of Paediatrics) therefore have as their primary objective to harmonize training programs in all member countries and to set standards for quality control of training centres, training programs and trainees.

The idea of adapting the MasterCourse of the Royal College of Paediatrics and Child Health for the European Community, to produce a more broadly applicable European MasterCourse in Paediatrics, came out of this desire for harmonization. The intent is to create a comprehensive teaching programme both for paediatric trainees who need to fulfil the knowledge-based requirements of the three-year Common Trunk portion of paediatric training across Europe and for non-paediatric physicians taking care of children in order to give them the essential information required to give high-quality, appropriate care.

The *European MasterCourse in Paediatrics* is not a traditional textbook of paediatrics. The conceptual framework of this book is based on case-based learning and therefore, a more interactive product, designed to stimulate learning and produce a learner who will engage the problems they will face in their professional life with initiative and enthusiasm.

Each chapter heading gives both its contents and 'learning objectives'. Most of the chapters contain Problem-orientated Topic boxes, clinical vignettes that can be used both as an introduction, putting each section in a clinically relevant context, and as a tool for self-assessment. In addition the book is well illustrated with many photographs, colourful drawings and summary boxes.

As elegantly expressed by Professor Sir David Hall in his foreword to the original *MRCPCH MasterCourse*, the intent of the book was to amalgamate the biological and social sciences with essential clinical practice in a way that would be relevant to any doctor practicing paediatrics, whether in the primary care setting or in the hospital as a paediatric generalist or specialist. Basic science has been used as effectively as possible to illustrate paediatric problems and disorders.

The book tries to bring primary care paediatrics and specialist paediatrics closer together and to define the body of knowledge and skills that need to be attained by all physicians in order to meet the demands of today's paediatric clinical practice.

Children represent our future. It is the firm conviction of the EAP that we need to safeguard that future by appropriately training doctors who will guarantee, to the best of their capabilities, the health and well-being of our children regardless of where they live. The *European MasterCourse in Paediatrics* is a first step towards the harmonization of the Common Trunk portion of paediatric training throughout Europe.

In conclusion we would like to thank, first of all, the RCPCH, Malcolm Levene and the numerous UK contributors firstly for creating the original version of the *MasterCourse* but above all for allowing the 'Europeanization' of their superb work. Secondly, we would like to thank all of the contributors who represent the European Academy of Paediatrics for their revisions, updates and 'Europeanization' of the chapters. A special thank you goes to Adamos Hadjipanayis and Diego van Esso, as module editors. Last, but not least, we would like to thank the staff at Elsevier, Pauline Graham (Commissioning Editor), Fiona Conn (Development Editor) and Glenys Norquay (Project Manager) for their invaluable help, guidance and, above all, patience.

On behalf of the European Academy of Paediatrics,

Alfred Tenore, MD
Vice President

How to use this book and DVD

Thank you for purchasing *European MasterCourse in Paediatrics*. We hope that this book will be an important asset to your preparation as a paediatrician, as well as help you pass any paediatric examination you will encounter. But above all we hope that it will be instrumental in making you adopt a style of working which will stay with you for lifelong learning.

Book

The written material is grouped into eight modules. Modules 1 to 5 are directed towards the toolkit of skills and knowledge that you will require to become proficient in the care of children, both in the community and in hospital. Modules 6 to 8 contain material relevant to career paediatricians and those working mainly in a hospital setting.

Children rarely present with a diagnosis but much more commonly present with a symptom or abnormal sign. Clinical material is initially presented as a 'Problem-orientated topic' (POT). Each POT contains a short clinical vignette followed by a number of questions. We recommend that you read the POT and think about the answers to each of the questions before reading on. This will allow you to gauge your level of knowledge and understanding at an early stage of your learning. At the end of each POT the answer to each question is provided and the disorders are discussed.

DVD

A numbered DVD icon points to where supporting video clips are provided on the separate DVD to aid learning. These may illustrate a disorder, clinical sign or show a competency that you will be expected to know. An index of icons describing the contents of each clip is supplied on page ix.

We hope that you enjoy using *MasterCourse* and, of course, we hope you enjoy working with children in your professional life and that what you learn from the *MasterCourse* package provides you with life-long skills used for the benefit of children.

Good Luck.

Index of DVD clips

Module editors

Mitch Blair
MBBS BSc MSc FRCP FRCPCH FRIPH MILT
Consultant Reader in Paediatrics and Child Public Health, Imperial College
(Northwick Park Campus), London, UK

Jonathan Darling
MB ChB MD FRCPCH
Senior Lecturer in Paediatrics and Child Health, St James's University Hospital, Leeds, UK

Diego van Esso
MD
Primary Care Paediatrician, Health Care Center Pare Claret, Catalan Institute of
Health, Barcelona, Spain

Adamos Hadjipanayis
MD PhD
Paediatrician, Larnaca Hospital, Cyprus

Michael A. Hall
MB ChB FRCPCH FRCP DCH
Consultant Neonatologist and Paediatrician, Honorary Senior Clinical Lecturer,
University of Southampton Princess Anne Hospital and Southampton General Hospital,
Southampton, UK

Henry L. Halliday
MD FRCP FRCPE
Honorary Professor of Child Health and Consultant Neonatologist, Regional Neonatal
Unit, Royal Maternity Hospital, Belfast, UK

Malcolm Levene
MD FRCPCH FRCP FMedSc
Professor of Paediatrics and Child Health, University of Leeds, Leeds General Infirmary,
Leeds, UK

Mary Rudolf
MB BS BSc DCH FRCPCH FAAP
Professor of Child Health and Consultant Paediatrician, University of Leeds, Leeds, UK

Alfred Tenore

MD BA

Professor and Chairman of Paediatrics, University of Udine School of Medicine, Udine, Italy

Martin Ward Platt

MB ChB MD FRCP FRCPCH

Consultant Paediatrician, Newcastle upon Tyne Hospitals NHS Trust; Reader in Neonatal and Paediatric Medicine, Newcastle University, Newcastle, UK

DVD Editor

S. Andrew Spencer

BM BS BMedSci MRCP DM FRCPCH

Consultant Paediatrician, University Hospital North Staffordshire; Honorary Reader in Neonatal Medicine, Keele University, North Staffordshire, UK

Module editors

Contributors

Noura Faital Al-Aufi
MB ChB DCH Dip Arab Board Peds
Consultant Paediatrician, Maternity and Children's Hospital, Jeddah, Saudi Arabia

Huda Al-Hussamy
MB BS DCH Dip Arab Board Peds
Consultant Paediatrician, Maternity and Children's Hosptial, Jeddah, Saudi Arabia

Sabah Alvi
MB ChB MD MRCP MRCPCH
Consultant in Paediatric and Adolescent Endocrinology, Department of Paediatric and
Adolescent Endocrinology, Leeds Teaching Hospitals NHS Trust, Leeds, UK

Mario Angi
MD
Aggregate Professor of Ophthalmology, Department of Neurosciences, Padua
University, Italy

Paul Arundel
MB BS MRCPCH DCH
Clinical Lecturer in Child Health, University of Sheffield, Sheffield, UK

Per Ashorn
MD PhD DTM
Professor of International Health, University of Tampere Medical School, Tampere,
Finland

Inês Azevedo
MD PhD
Professor of Paediatrics, Hospital de S. João, Porto, Portugal

Shimon Barak
MD PhD
Senior Physician, Neonatology Department, Tel Aviv Sourasky Medical Center, Israel

Carine E. de Beaufort
MD PhD
Consultant Paediatric Endocrinology and Diabetes, DECCP, Clinique
Pédiatrique/CHL, Luxembourg

Julie-Clare Becher
MB ChB MD MRCPCH
Higher Specialist Trainee in Neonatology, Department of Neonatology, Simpson Centre for Reproductive Health, Royal Infirmary of Edinburgh, Edinburgh, UK

Ravindra Bhat
MB BS MD MRCPCH
Specialist Registrar, Neonatal Unit, St George's Hospital NHS Trust, London, UK

Mark Bradbury
MB BS
Consultant Paediatric Nephrologist, Central Manchester and Manchester Children's University Hospital, NHS Trust, Manchester, UK

David Branski
MD
Dr Israel J. and Dena B. Zimmerman Professor of Pediatrics, Hadassah University Hospitals, Jerusalem, Israel

Susan Bunn
MB ChB MRCPCH MD
Consultant Paediatric Gastroenterologist, Newcastle upon Tyne Hospitals NHS Foundation Trust, Newcastle upon Tyne, UK

David M. Burge
FRCS FRCPCH
Consultant Paediatric Surgeon, Southampton General Hospital, Southampton, UK

Alan Cade
MB ChB DCH MRCP FRCPCH
Consultant Respiratory Paediatrician, Derriford Hospital, Plymouth, UK

Frank Casey
MD FRCP MRCPCH BSc
Consultant Paediatric Cardiologist, Royal Belfast Hospital for Sick Children, Belfast; Honorary Senior Lecturer, Department of Child Health, Queen's University, Belfast, UK

Ekaterine Chkhartishvili
MD PhD
Professor, Paediatric Allergist, Children's Clinical Hospital, Tbilisi, Georgia

Imti Choonara
MD FRCPCH
Professor in Child Health, University of Nottingham, Derbyshire Children's Hospital, UK

Julia Clark
BMedSci BM BS DCH FRCPCH
Consultant in Paediatric Immunology and Infectious Diseases, Newcastle upon Tyne Hospitals NHS Foundation Trust, Newcastle upon Tyne, UK

Angus J. Clarke
DM FRCP FRCPCH
Professor and Honorary Consultant in Clinical Genetics, Cardiff University, University Hospital of Wales, Cardiff, UK

Julia Colomer Revuelta
MD
Professor of Medicine (Pediatrics), University of Valencia, Spain

Anthony Costello
MA FRCP FRCPCH
Professor of International Child Health; Director of International Perinatal Care Unit, Institute of Child Health, London, UK

Sir Alan Craft
MD FRCPCH FRCP FMedSci
Professor of Child Health, University of Newcastle upon Tyne, Newcastle upon Tyne, UK

Rachel Crowther
MB BChir MSc MFPH DipLATHE
Consultant in Public Health Medicine, South East Public Health Observatory, UK

Jonathan Darling
MB ChB MD FRCPCH
Senior Lecturer in Paediatrics and Child Health, St James's University Hospital, Leeds, UK

Mark Davies
MA MB BCh MRCP
Specialist Registrar in Medical Genetics, Institute of Medical Genetics, University Hospital of Wales, Cardiff, UK

Melanie Drewett
RCN RSCN MSc
Clinical Nurse Specialist, Neonatal Surgery, Neonatal Surgical Service, Department of Neonatal Medicine and Surgery, Princess Anne Hospital, Coxford Road, Southampton, UK

Melanie Epstein
MBBCh MRCPCh Dip Psych
Department of Community Paediatrics, St James's University Hospital, Leeds, UK

Diego van Esso
MD
Primary Care Paediatrician, Health Care Center Pare Claret, Catalan Institute of Health, Barcelona, Spain

David Evans
BM BCh MA MRCP FRCPCH
Consultant Neonatologist, Southmead Hospital, Bristol, UK

Gun Forsander
MD PhD
Consultant Pediatrician, Head of Department of Diabetes, The Queen Silvia Children's Hospital, Sahlgrenska University Hospital, Gothenburg, Sweden

Simon Frazer
MB ChB MRCPCH
Consultant Paediatrician, Bradford Teaching Hospitals Foundation Trust, Bradford, UK

Susan M. Gentle
FRCPCH
Consultant Paediatrician, Ryegate Children's Centre, Sheffield Children's NHS Trust, Sheffield, UK

Brian Grant
MD MRCPCH
Specialist Registrar in Paediatric Cardiology, Department of Paediatric Cardiology, Royal Belfast Hospital for Children, Belfast, UK

Anne Greenough
MD FRCP FRCPCH DCH
Professor of Neonatology and Clinical Respiratory Physiology, Guy's, King's and St Thomas School of Medicine, King's College, London, UK

Adamos Hadjipanayis
MD PhD
Paediatrician, Larnaca Hospital, Cyprus

John Hain
MB ChB BSc MRCGP DFFP Dip Derm
General Practitioner and Approved GP Trainer for the Yorkshire Deanery, Yorkshire, UK

Richard Hain
MB BS MSc MD MRCP FRCPCH DipPalMed
Senior Lecturer/Honorary Consultant in Paediatric Palliative Medicine, Department of Child Health, Cardiff School of Medicine, University Hospital of Wales, Cardiff, UK

Ragnar Hanas
MD PhD
Senior Consultant in Pediatric Diabetology and Endocrinology, Department of Pediatrics, Uddevalla Hospital, Uddevalla, Sweden

Valerie Harpin
FRCP FRCPCH MD
Consultant Paediatrician (Neurodisability), Ryegate Children's Centre, Sheffield Children's NHS Trust, Sheffield, UK

Carl J. Harvey
BMedSc MBChB MRCPCH
Specialist Registrar, Birmingham Heartlands Hospital, Birmingham, UK

Breda Hayes
MB BCh NUI MRCPCH
Neonatology Registrar, Rotunda Hospital, Dublin, Eire

Chris J. Hendriksz
MB ChB MSc MRCPCH
Consultant in Clinical Inherited Metabolic Disorders, Birmingham Children's Hospital, Birmingham, UK

Therese Hesketh
MRCPCH MFPHM MPH PhD
Senior Lecturer in International Child Health, Institute of Child Health, University College London, London, UK

Stephen Hodges
MB ChB FRCP FRCPCH DCH
Consultant Paediatric Gastroenterologist, Newcastle upon Tyne Hospitals NHS
Foundation Trust, Newcastle upon Tyne, UK

Wolf-Rüdiger Horn
MD
Paediatrician, Gernsbach, Germany

Delyth Howard
MB BChir MRCP MSc
Consultant Community Paediatrician, Great Ormond Street NHS Trust and Islington
Primary Care Trust, London, UK

Peter Hoyer
MD
Professor of Paediatrics, Director and Chair, University Children's Hospital Essen,
University Duisburg-Essen, Germany

Elke Jaeger-Roman
MD
Primary Care Paediatrician, Berlin, Germany

Alison Kelly
MB ChB MRCPCH
Consultant Community Paediatrics, Yorkhill Hospitals, Glasgow, UK

Neil Kennedy
BSc MB ChB MRCPCH MRCP DTMH
Senior Lecturer in Child Health, Queen's University, Belfast; Consultant Paediatrician,
Royal Belfast Hospital for Sick Children, Belfast, UK

Nigel Kennedy
MB BS FRCP FRCPCH DCH DRCOG
General Practitioner, Aylesbury; Hospital Practitioner, Paediatrics, Stoke Mandeville
Hospital, Aylesbury, UK

Hojka G. Kumperscak
MD PhD
Assistant of Medicine, Department of Paediatrics, University of Maribor, Maribor, Slovenia

Heather Lambert
PhD FRCP FRCPCH
Consultant Paediatric Nephrologist, Newcastle upon Tyne Hospitals NHS Foundation
Trust, Newcastle upon Tyne, UK

Malcolm Levene
MD FRCPCH FRCP FMedSc
Professor of Paediatrics and Child Health, University of Leeds, Leeds General Infirmary,
Leeds, UK

Vernon Long
FRCOphth
Consultant Ophthalmologist, St James' University Hospital, Leeds, UK

José Manuel de Azevedo Lopes dos Santos
MD
Director of Mother, Child and Adolescent Department, Hospital Pedro Hispano, Matosinhos, Portugal

Raisa H.K. Lounamaa
MD PhD MSc MRCPCH
Paediatrician, Porvoo Hospital and Jorvi Hospital, Helsinki University Central Hospital (HUCH), Helsinki, Finland

Niamh Lynch
MB BCh BAO MRCPI(Paeds)
Specialist Registrar in Paediatrics, Our Lady's Hospital, Dublin, Eire

Florence McDonagh
MB BCh BAO LRCPSI(Irel)DipCommunityPaed MSc FRCPCH
Consultant Community Paediatrician Audiology, St Mary's Hospital, Leeds, UK

Aidan MacFarlane
MB BChir FRCP FRCPCH FFPH
Independent International Consultant in Child and Adolescent Health, Oxford, UK

Neil McIntosh
DSc(Med) FRCP FRCPE FRCPCH
Professor of Child Life and Health, University of Edinburgh; Honorary Consultant Paediatrician, Lothian University Hospitals NHS Trust, Edinburgh, UK

Marta Macedoni-Luksic
MD PhD
Assistant Professor of Medicine, Medical Faculty, University of Ljubljana, Medvode, Slovenia

Sachin Mannikar
MB BS MD MRCPCH
Specialist Registrar in Paediatrics, Queen Elizabeth Hospital, Gateshead, Tyne and Wear, UK

Michael J. Marsh
MB BS MRCP FRCPCH
Director of Paediatric Intensive Care Unit, Southampton General Hospital, Southampton, UK

Thomas G. Matthews
MD FRCPI FAAP DCH
Professor, Children's University Hospital, Dublin, Eire

Jean-Christophe Mercier
MD
Professor of Paediatrics, Université Paris, France

Zsofia Meszner
MD PhD
General Director to the National Institute of Child Health, Budapest, Hungary

Francis B. Mimouni
MD FAAP FACN
Professor of Pediatrics, the Sackler School of Medicine, Tel Aviv, Israel
Chief of Staff, the Wilf Children's Hospital at Shaare Zedek Medical Center, and the
Hebrew University of Jerusalem Medical School, Jerusalem, Israel

Neena Modi
MB ChB MD FRCP FRCPCH
Professor of Neonatal Medicine, Faculty of Medicine, Imperial College, London;
Honorary Consultant in Neonatal Paediatrics, Chelsea and Westminster Hospital,
Hammersmith and Queen Charlotte Hospitals, London, UK

Eleanor J. Molloy
MB BCh BAO PhD FRCPI FRCPCH FJFICM
Consultant Neonatologist , National Maternity Hospital and Our Lady's Children's
Hospital and Clinical Senior Lecturer in Neonatology, University College Dublin

Colin Morgan
MD MRCP FRCPCH
Consultant Neonatologist, Liverpool Women's Hospital, Liverpool, UK

Matthew Murray
MA MB BChir MRCPCH DCH
Clinical Research Fellow in Paediatric Oncology, Addenbrooke's Hospital,
Cambridge, UK

David Neubauer
MD PhD
Professor of Paediatrics, University of Ljubljana, Ljubljana, Slovenia

Alfred J. Nicholson
FCRCPCH FRCPI
Professor of Paediatrics, RCSI Medical School, Children's University Hospital,
Dublin, Ireland

James C. Nicholson
DM MA MB BChir MRCP FRCPCH
Consultant Paediatric Oncologist, Addenbrooke's Hospital, Cambridge, UK

Paola Nicolaides
MB CHB MRCP FRCPCH
Senior Paediatric Neurology Consultant, Epilepsy Specialist, Director of Clinical Services,
The Cyprus Paediatric Neurology Institute (CING),Visiting Scientist Status,The Cyprus
Institute of Neurology and Genetics (CING), Cyprus

Agostino Nocerino
MD PhD
Consultant Paediatric Haematologist, Clinica Pediatrica, Azienda Ospedaliero
Universitaria Udine, University of Udine

Steven J. Novek
MD FAAP MRCPCH
Director of Pediatrics, US Army Health Center, Vicenza, Italy; Consultant Pediatrician,
Ospedale Civile San Bortolo, Vicenza, Italy

Bernadette S. O'Connor
MB MRCPCH
Senior Paediatric Registrar and Research Fellow, Royal Belfast Hospital for Sick Children, Belfast, UK

Mary O'Sullivan
MB BCh BAO MSc DCH FRCPCH
Consultant Community Paediatrician, Audiology, St Mary's Hospital, Leeds, UK

Eva Orzan
MD
Consultant in Pediatric Audiology, University Hospital of Padova, Italy

David Osrin
MRCPCH
Clinical Research Fellow, International Perinatal Care Unit, Institute of Child Health, University College London, London, UK

Lars Palm
MD PhD
Consultant in Paediatrics and Paediatric Neurology, Malmö University Hospital, Malmö, Sweden

Fernand M. Pauly
MD PhD
Practicien Associé, Chargé de cours, University of Strasbourg, Strasbourg, France

Ed Peile
MB BS EdD FRCP FRCGP FRCPCH MRCS DCH DRCOG
Professor, Associate Dean (Teaching), Head of Institute of Clinical Education, Medical Teaching Centre, Warwick Medical School, The University of Warwick, Coventry, UK

Giorgio Perilongo
MD
Professor and Chair, Department of Pediatrics, University Hospital of Padua, Padua, Italy

Alison Pike
MD DCH MRCP FRCPCH
Consultant Neonatologist, Southmead Hospital, Bristol, UK

Jose Ramet
MD PhD
Professor of Medicine, UZA, Medical Faculty, University of Antwerp, Belgium

Janet M. Rennie
MD FRCP FRCPCH DCH
Consultant and Senior Lecturer in Neonatal Medicine, Elizabeth Garrett Anderson Obstetric Hospitals, University College London Hospitals, London, UK

Edward Michael Richards
MA BM BCh DM MRCP FRCPath
Consultant Paediatric Haematologist and Honorary Senior Lecturer, Leeds Teaching Hospitals Trust, Leeds, UK

Stefan Riedl
MD
Consultant Paediatric Endocrinologist, St Anna Children's Hospital, Vienna, Austria

Gillian Robinson
MB ChB MRCP(Paeds) MMedSc
Consultant Paediatrician, Leeds PCT, Leeds, UK

Mary Rudolf
MB BS BSc DCH FRCPCH FAAP
Professor of Child Health and Consultant Paediatrician, University of Leeds, Leeds, UK

Odilija Rudzeviciene
MD PhD
Associate Professor of Paediatrics, Vilnius University, Vilnius, Lithuania

Martin Samuels
MB BS BSc MD FRCP FRCPCH
Consultant Paediatrician, University Hospital of North Staffordshire; Senior Lecturer in Paediatrics, Keele University, UK

Saikat Santra
MB BChir BA MRCPCH
Specialist Registrar, Worcester Royal Hospital, Worcester, UK

Pieter J. J. Sauer
MD PhD
Professor of Pediatrics, University of Groningen, Groningen, The Netherlands

Rotraud K. Saurenmann
MD
Head of Pediatric Rheumatology, University Children's Hospital Zurich, Switzerland

Arnab K. Seal
MD DCH FRCPCH
Consultant Paediatrician, Leeds General Infirmary, Leeds, UK

Neela Shabde
FRCP FRCPCH DCH DCCH
Consultant Paediatrician/Clinical Director of Children's Services, Northumbria Healthcare Trust, UK

Michael D. Shields
MF FRCP FRCPCH
Senior Lecturer in Child Health, Queen's University of Belfast and Royal Belfast Hospital for Sick Children, Belfast, UK

Kathleen Skinner
MB ChB MRCP MRCPCH MPH
Specialist Registrar in Public Health, Oxford City PCT, Oxford, UK

Flemming Skovby
MD DMSci FAAP
Professor of Paediatrics and Clinical Genetics, University of Copenhagen, Copenhagen, Denmark

Constantinos J. Stefanidis
MD PhD
Pediatric Nephrologist, P. & A. Kyriakou Children's Hospital, Athens, Greece

Tom Stiris
MD PhD
Senior Consultant in Neonatology, Oslo University Hospital, Oslo, Norway

Giorgio Tamburlini
MD PhD
Director, Centro per la Salute del Bambino, Trieste, Italy

Alfred Tenore
MD BA
Professor and Chair, Paediatrics, University of Udine School of Medicine, Udine, Italy

Ragbir Thethy
MBChB MRCPI MSc
Consultant Paediatrician, St James's University Hospital, Leeds, UK

Marta Thió
MD
Consultant Neonatologist, Hospital Sant Joan de Déu, University of Barcelona, Barcelona, Spain

Amanda J. Thomas
MB BS DCH MMedSci MA FRCPCH
Consultant Community Paediatrician, East Leeds Primary Care Trust, Leeds, UK

Andrew Tomkins
MB BS FRCP FRCPCH FFPHM FMedSci
Head, Centre for International Child Health, Institute of Child Health, University College, London, UK

Stefano del Torso
MD
Primary Care Pediatrician, Padova Italy

Sabita Uthaya
MBBS MD MRCP FRCPCH
Consultant and Honorary Senior Lecturer in Neonatal Medicine, Chelsea and Westminster Hospital, Imperial College, London, UK

Arunas Valiulis
MD PhD
Vilnius City University Hospital, Vilnius, Lithuania

Julian L. Verbov
MD FRCP FRCPCH CBiol FSB FLS
Honorary Professor of Dermatology, University of Liverpool,
Consultant Paediatric Dermatologist, Royal Liverpool Children's Hospital NHS
Foundation Trust, Liverpool, UK

Richard B. Warren
BSc(Hons) MBChB(Hons) MRCP PhD
Senior Lecturer and Honorary Consultant Dermatologist, The Dermatology Centre, The
University of Manchester Salford Royal Foundation Hospital, Salford, Manchester, UK

David W. Webb
MB BCh BAO MD MRCP(Edin)(Lon) FRCPI FRCPCH
Consultant Paediatric Neurologist, Our Lady's Hospital for Sick Children, Dublin, Eire

Linda Wolfson
RM ADM/DPSM BSc
Mid Infant Feeding Specialist, Queen Mother's Maternity Hospital, Yorkhill Hospitals,
Glasgow

Charlotte M. Wright
BMedSci BM BCH MSc MD FRCPCH FRCP
Professor of Community Child Health, Glasgow University, Yorkhill Children's Hospital,
Glasgow, UK

Maximilian Zach
MD
Professor of Paediatrics, Klinische Abteilung für Pädiatrische Pulmonologie und
Allergologie, Graz, Austria

List of abbreviations

AABR	(automated) auditory brainstem responses
AAP	American Academy of Pediatrics
ABC	airway, breathing, circulation
ABPA	allergic bronchopulmonary aspergillosis
ABR	auditory brainstem response
AC	air conduction
ACE	angiotensin-converting enzyme
ACPC	Area Child Protection Committee
ACTH	adrenocorticotrophic hormone
AD	autosomal dominant
ADEM	acute disseminating encephalomyelitis
ADH	antidiuretic hormone
ADHD	attention deficit hyperactivity disorder
ADPKD	autosomal dominant polycystic kidney disease
ADR	adverse drug reaction
AFP	alpha-fetoprotein
AGA	antigliadin antibody
AIDS	acquired immune deficiency syndrome
ALCL	anaplastic large cell lymphoma
ALI	acute lung injury
ALL	acute lymphoblastic leukaemia
ALP	alkaline phosphate
ALSG	Advanced Life Support Group
ALT	alanine aminotransferase
ALTE	apparent life-threatening event
ANA	antinuclear antibodies
ANCA	antineutrophil cytoplasmic antibody
ANF	antinuclear factor
ANP	atrial natriuretic peptide
AOM	acute otitis media
AP	antero-posterior
APC	antigen-presenting cell
APLS	advanced paediatric life support
APTT	activated partial thromboplastin time
AR	autosomal recessive
ARDS	acute respiratory distress syndrome
ARF	acute renal failure
ARI	acute respiratory infection
ARPKD	autosomal recessive polycystic kidney disease
ART	antiretroviral therapy

ASD	atrial septal defect
ASOT	antistreptolysin O titre
AST	aspartate aminotransferase
ATN	acute tubular necrosis
ATP	adenosine triphosphate
AVP	arginine vasopressin
AV(SD)	atrioventricular (septal defect)
AXR	abdominal X-ray
AZT	zidovudine
BAL	bronchoalveolar lavage
BBB	blood–brain barrier
BC	bone conduction
BCG	bacille Calmette–Guérin
BDR	bronchodilator responsiveness
BG	blood glucose
BHR	bronchial hyper-reactivity
BMA	British Medical Association
BMI	body mass index
BMT	bone marrow transplant
BNF	British National Formulary
BP	blood pressure
BPD	bronchpulmonary dysplasia
BSER	brainstem evoked response
BSPED	British Society for Paediatric Endocrinology and Diabetes
BTS	British Thoracic Society
CAH	congenital adrenal hyperplasia
CAKUT	congenital anomalies of the kidney and urinary tract
CAMHS	Child and Adolescent Mental Health Services
CBC	complete blood count
CBD	common bile duct
CBF	cerebral blood flow
CBT	cognitive behavioural therapy
CCAM	congenital cystic adenomatoid malformation
CCK	cholecystokinin
CD	conduct disorder
CDC	children in difficult circumstances, Centers for Disease Control,
CDD	control of diarrhoeal disease
CDH	congenital diaphragmatic hernia
cDNA	complementary DNA
CEDC	children in especially difficult circumstances
CF	cystic fibrosis
CFAM	cerebral function activity monitor
CFM	cerebral function monitor
CFS	chronic fatigue syndrome
CFTR	cystic fibrosis transmembrane regulator
CGD	chronic granulomatous disorder
CGH	comparative genomic hybridization
CGMP	cyclic guanosine monophosphate
CHT	congenital hypothyroidism
CHD	congenital heart disease
CHEOPS	Children's Hospital of Eastern Ontario Pain Scale
CHT	congenital hypothyroidism
CI	confidence interval
CJD	Creutzfeldt–Jakob disease
CK	creatine kinase

CLO	Campylobacter-like organism
CML	chronic myeloid leukaemia
CMV	cytomegalovirus
CNS	central nervous system
CNSD	chronic non-specific diarrhoea
CNSP	children in need of special protection
CO	cardiac output
CONS	coagulase-negative streptococci
CP	cerebral palsy
CPAP	continuous positive airway pressure
CPCC	Child Protection Case Conference
CpG	cytidine-phosphate-guanosine
CPP	cerebral perfusion pressure
CPR	cardiopulmonary resuscitation
CRF	chronic renal failure
CRH	corticotrophin-releasing hormone
CRP	C-reactive protein
CRT	capillary refill time
CSC	children in special circumstances
CSF	cerebrospinal fluid
CSOM	chronic suppurative otitis media
CT	computed tomography
CTG	cardiotochograph
CTZ	chemoreceptor trigger zone
CVA	cough variant asthma
CVC	central venous catheter
CVID	common variable immune deficiency
CVL	central venous line
CVS	chorionic villus sampling
CXR	chest X-ray
CYP	cytochrome P450
DCD	developmental coordination disorder
DCH	Diploma of Child Health
DDH	developmental dysplasia of the hip
DEXA	dual-energy X-ray absorptiometry
DFES	Department for Education and Skills
DGP	deamidated gliadin peptides
DHEA(S)	dihydroepiandrosterone (sulfate)
DHR	dihydroflavonol-4-reductase
DHS	Demographic and Health Survey
DI	diabetes insipidus
DIC	disseminated intravascular coagulation
DIDMOAD	diabetes insipidus, diabetes mellitus, optic atrophy, deafness
DJ	duodenojejunal
DKA	diabetic ketoacidosis
DLA	Disability Living Allowance
DMSA	demercaptosuccinic acid
DNA	deoxyribonucleic acid
DOT(S)	directly observed therapy
DPPC	dipalmitoyl phosphatidylcholine
DSM	Diagnostic and Statistical Manual of Mental Disorders
DTaP/IPV/Hib	diphtheria, tetanus, acellular pertussis, polio and Hib
DU	duodenal ulcer

DVLA	Driver and Vehicle Licensing Authority
EAP	European Academy of Paediatrics
EB	epidermolysis bullosa
EBM	evidence-based medicine
EBV	Epstein–Barr virus
EC	European country
ECF	extracellular fluid
ECG	electrocardiography
ECMO	extra-corporeal membranous oxygenation
EDD	expected delivery date
EEG	electroencephalography
EHEC	enterohaemorrhagic E. coli
ELISA	enzyme-linked immunosorbence assay
EMA	endomysial antibody
EMG	electromyography
EN	erythema nodosum
ENMR	early neonatal mortality rate
ENT	ear, nose and throat
EOAE	evoked oto-acoustic emissions
EPI	Expanded Programme on Immunization
ESR	erythrocyte sedimentation rate
ETEC	enterotoxigenic *Escherichia coli*
EVD	extraventricular drain
FAB	French, American, British
FBC	full blood count
FDG	flurodeoxyglucose
FEV_1	forced expiratory volume in 1 second
FII	factitious or induced illness
FIL	feedback inhibitor
FISH	fluorescent in situ hybridization
FLACC	faces, legs, activity, cry and consolability
FRC	forced residual capacity
FSGS	focal and segmental glomerulosclerosis
FSH	follicle-stimulating hormone
FTT	failure to thrive
FVC	forced vital capacity
FXTAS	fragile X-associated tremor/ataxia syndrome
G6PD	glucose-6-phosphate dehydrogenase
GABA	gamma-aminobutyric acid
GABHS	group A β-haemolytic streptococci
GAD	glutamic acid decarboxylase
GALT	gut-associated lymphoid tissue
GAS	group A streptococci
GBM	glomerular basement membrane
GBS	group B streptococci
GCS	Glasgow Coma Scale/Score
G-CSF	granulocyte colony stimulating factor
GET	graded exercise therapy
GFAP	glial fibrillary acidic protein
GFR	glomerular filtration rate
GGT	gamma-glutamyl transferase
GH(D)	growth hormone (deficiency)
GHIS	growth hormone insensitivity syndrome
GHRH	growth hormone-releasing hormone
GI	gastrointestinal

GMC	General Medical Council
GMH	germinal matrix haemorrhage
GnRH	gonadotrophin-releasing hormone
GOR(D)	gastro-oesophageal reflux (disease)
GP	general practitioner
GRF	growth hormone releasing factor
GTP	guanine triphosphate
GTT	glucose tolerance test
GU	gastric ulcer
GUM	genitourinary medicine
GvHD	graft versus host disease
HAART	highly active antiretroviral therapy
HAV	hepatitis A virus
HbCO	carboxyhaemoglobin
HBsAg	hepatitis B surface antigen
HBV	hepatitis B virus
HBV	hepatitis B vaccine
hCG	human chorionic gonadotrophin
HCOM	hypertrophic obstructive cardiomyopathy
HCV	hepatitis C virus
HD	Hirschsprung's disease; high-dose
HDN	haemolytic disease of the newborn
HDR	hypoparathyroidism, deafness and renal dysplasia
HELPP	haemolysis, elevated liver enzymes and low platelets
HFJV	high-frequency jet ventilation
HFOV	high-frequency oscillatory ventilation
hGH	human growth hormone
HHV	human herpes virus
HiB	Haemophilus influenzae type B
HIE	hypoxic–ischaemic encephalopathy
HIV	human immunodeﬁciency virus
HKD	hyper kinetic disorder
HLA	human leucocyte antigen
HMA	homovanillic acid
HMO	Health Maintenance Organization
HMSN	hereditary motor sensory neurophathies
HPI	haemorrhagic periventricular infarction
HPV	human papillomavirus
HSP	Henoch–Schönlein purpura
HSV	herpes simplex virus
HTA	Health Technology Assessment
HUS	haemolytic uraemic syndrome
HVA	homovanillic acid
ICAM	intercellular adhesion molecule
ICD–10	International Statistical Classification of Diseases — 10th revision
ICF	International Classification of Functioning and Disability, intracellular fluid
ICH	intracranial haemorrhage
ICIDH	International Classification of Impairments, Disabilities and Handicaps
ICP	intracranial pressure
ICU	intensive care unit
IDT	infant distraction test
IEM	inborn error of metabolism
IFN	interferon

IGF	insulin-like growth factor
IL	interleukin
ILO	International Labour Organization
i.m.	intramuscular
IMCI	Integrated Management of Childhood Illness
IMD	Index of Multiple Deprivation
IMPS	injury minimization and prevention
IMR	infant mortality rate
INR	international normalized ratio
INSI	International Life Sciences Institute
IPEC	International Programme for the Elimination of Child Labour
IPL	intraparenchymal lesion
IPPV	intermittent positive pressure ventilation
IPV	inactivated polio vaccine
IQ	intelligence quotient
IRT	immunoreactive trypsinogen
ISKDC	International Study of Kidney Disease in Children
i.t.	intrathecal
ITP	idiopathic thrombocytopenic purpura
IUGR	intrauterine growth retardation
i.v.	intravenous
IVH	intraventricular haemorrhage
JE	Japanese encephalitis
JIA	juvenile idiopathic arthritis
JVP	jugular venous pressure
KD	Kawasaki disease
KSADS	Kiddie Schedule for Affective Disorders and Schizophrenia
LA	left atrium
LABA	long-acting bronchodilator
LDH	lactate dehydrogenase
LGA	large for gestational age
LH(RH)	luteinizing hormone (releasing hormone)
LIP	lymphocytic interstitial pneumonitis
LKM	liver, kidney, microsomal (antibodies)
LNMR	late neonatal mortality rate
LOC	loss of consciousness
LOS	lower oesophageal sphincter
LP	lumbar puncture
LRTI	lower respiratory tract infection
LSCB	Local Safeguarding Children Board
LV	left ventricle
LVH	left ventricular hypertrophy
MAG3	mercaptoacetyltriglycine
MAP	mean arterial pressure
MAS	meconium aspiration syndrome
MCAD(D)	medium chain acyl CoA dehydrogenase (deficiency)
MCH	mean cell haemoglobin
MCUG	micturating cystourethrogram
MCV	mean cell volume
MD	muscular dystrophy
MDI	multiple daily injections
MDR-TB	multidrug-resistant tuberculosis
MEE	middle ear effusions
MELAS	mitochondrial encephalomyopathy with lactic acidosis and stroke-like episodes

MERRF	myoclonic epilepsy and ragged red fibres
MHC	major histocompatibility complex
mIBG	meta-iodobenzylguanidine imaging
MIF	migratory inhibition factor
MIP	macrophage inflammatory protein
MMR	measles/mumps/rubella vaccination
MODY	maturity-onset diabetes of the young
6-MP	6-mercaptopurine
MPGN	membranoproliferative glomerulonephritis
MRA	magnetic resonance angiography
MRCPCH	Membership of the Royal College of Paediatrics and Child Health
MRD	minimal residual disease
MRI	magnetic resonance imaging
mRNA	messenger RNA
MRSA	meticillin-resistant *Staphylococcus aureus*
MRV	magnetic resonance venography
MSH	melanocyte-stimulating hormone
MSU	midstream urine
MTB	Mycobacterium tuberculosis
MTCT	mother-to-child transmission
MTX	methotrexate
NAHI	non-accidental head injury
NAI	non-accidental injury
NAITP	neonatal alloimmune thrombocytopenia
NBT	nitro-blue tetrazolium
NDI	nephrogenic diabetes insipidus
NEC	necrotizing enterocolitis
NGT	nasogastric tube
NHL	non-Hodgkin's lymphoma
NHS	National Health Service
NHSP	newborn hearing screening programme
NIBP	non-invasive blood pressure
NICE	National Institute for Clinical Excellence
NICU	neonatal intensive care unit
NIH	NIH National Institutes of Health
NK	natural killer
NMR	neonatal mortality rate
NNTB	number needed to treat for benefit
NO	nitric oxide
NOFTT	non-organic failure to thrive
NPA	nasopharyngeal aspirate
NPH	neutral protamine hagedorn
NPV	negative predictive value
NPY	neuropeptide Y
NSAID	non-steroidal anti-inflammatory drug
NSE	non-specific enolase
NSF	National Service Framework
NSPCC	National Society for Prevention of Cruelty to Children
NT	nuchal translucency
NTD	neural tube defect
OA	oesophageal atresia
OAE	oto-acoustic emissions
OFTT	organic failure to thrive
OCD	obsessive–compulsive disorder
ODD	oppositional/defiant disorder

OGTT	oral glucose tolerance test
OHC	outer hair cell
OM(E)	otitis media (with effusion)
OMIM	Online Mendelian Inheritance in Man
ONS	Office for National Statistics
OPCS–4	Office of Population, Censuses and Surveys' Classification of Surgical Operations and Procedures — 4th revision
ORS/T	oral rehydration solution/therapy
OPV	oral polio vaccine
OSAS	obstructive sleep apnoea syndrome
OT	occupational therapy
OVC	orphans and vulnerable children (made vulnerable through HIV)
PA	pulmonary artery; postero-anterior
PAF	platelet-activating factor
PALS	paediatric advanced life support
PAN	polyarteritis nodosa
PAPP-A	pregnancy-associated plasma protein-A
PAS	Patient Administration System
PBSCT	peripheral blood stem cell transplants
PC	phosphatidylcholine
PCA	post-conceptual age
PCP	Pneumocystis carinii (jirovecii) pneumonia; primary care physician
PCR	polymerase chain reaction
PCT	Primary Care Trust
PCV	packed cell volume
PCWP	pulmonary capillary wedge pressure
PDA	patent ductus arteriosus
PDD-NOS	Pervasive developmental disorder — not otherwise specific
PEEP	positive end-expiratory pressure
PEFR	peak expiratory flow rate
PET	positron emission tomography
PFT	pulmonary function testing
PG	prostaglandin; phosphatidylglycerol
PHCT	primary healthcare team
PHI	persistent hyperinsulinism of infancy
PICU	paediatric intensive care unit
PIE	pulmonary interstitial emphysema
PIP	peak inspiratory pressure
PIVKA	proteins produced in vitamin K absence
PKU	phenylketonuria
PMA	post-menstrual age
PML	polymorphonuclear leucocyte
PMR	perinatal mortality rate
PMTCT	perinatal mother-to-child transmission
PN	parenteral nutrition
PNET	primitive neuroectodermal tumour
PNMR	post-neonatal mortality rate
PPH	primary pulmonary hypertension
PPHN	persistent pulmonary hypertension of the newborn
PPI	proton pump inhibitor
PPV	positive predictive value; patent processus vaginalis
PRL	prolactin
PSGN	post-streptococcal glomerulonephritis
PT	prothrombin time
PTH	parathyroid hormone

PTU	propylthiouracil
PTV	patient-triggered ventilation
PUO	pyrexia of unknown origin
PVL	periventricular leukomalacia
PVR	pulmonary vascular resistance
PVS	pulmonary valve stenosis
PWS	Prader–Willi syndrome
QALY	quality-adjusted life year
QS	quiet sleep
RA	right atrium
RAAS	renin–angiotensin–aldosterone system
RAST	radioallergosorbence testing
RCP	Royal College of Physicians
RCPCH	Royal College of Paediatrics and Child Health
RCT	randomized controlled trial
RDS	respiratory distress syndrome
REM	rapid eye movement
RF	rheumatoid factor
RMS	rhabdomyosarcoma
RNA	ribonucleic acid
RNS	repetitive nerve stimulation
ROP	retinopathy of prematurity
RP	retinitis pigmentosa
RRT	renal replacement therapy
RSV	respiratory syncytial virus
RTA	road traffic accident
RV	right ventricle; residual volume
RVOT	right ventricular outfl ow tract
SALT	speech and language therapy
SAM	severe acute malnutrition
SBR	stillbirth rate
SCBU	special baby care unit
SCID	severe combined immunodeficiency disease
SD	standard deviation
SEN	special education needs
SENCO	special educational needs coordinator
SFD	somatoform disorder
SGA	small for gestational age
SHO	senior house officer
SIDS	sudden infant death syndrome
SIGN	Scottish Intercollegiate Guideline Network
SIMV	synchronous intermittent mandatory ventilation
SIOP	International Society of Paediatric Oncology
SIP	spontaneous isolated intestinal perforation
SIRS	systemic inflammatory response syndrome
SLE	systemic lupus erythematosus
SLT	speech and language therapist
SM	severe malnutrition
SNHL	sensorineural hearing loss
SNP	single nucleotide polymorphism
SP	surfactant protein
SPA	suprapubic aspiration
SPF	sun protection factor
SRSV	small round structured virus
SSNS	steroid-sensitive nephrotic syndrome

SSPE	subacute sclerosing panencephalitis
SSRI	selective serotonin reuptake inhibitor
STBI	severe traumatic brain injury
STD/I	sexually transmitted disease/infection
SUDI	sudden unexplained death in infancy
SVT	supraventricular tachycardia
T_3	tri-iodothyronine
T_4	thyroxine
TB	tuberculosis
TBG	thyroid-binding globulin
TBI	total body irradiation
^{99}TC	technetium-99
TCA	tricyclic antidepressant
TCR	T-cell receptor
TDM	therapeutic drug monitoring
TGF	transforming growth factor
Ti	inspiratory time
TLC	total lung capacity
TNF-α	tumour necrosis factor-alpha
TOF	tracheo-oesophageal fistula; tetralogy of Fallot
TORCH	toxoplasmosis, rubella, cytomegalovirus, herpes simplex
TPN	total parenteral nutrition
TPPPS	Toddler–Preschooler Post-operative Pain Scale
TRALI	transfusion-associated lung injury
TRH	thyrotrophin-releasing hormone
tRNA	transfer RNA
TS	tuberous sclerosis
TSH	thyroid-stimulating hormone
TSS	toxic shock syndrome
tTG	tissue transglutaminase
TTN	transient tachypnoea of the newborn
TTP	thrombotic thrombocytopenic purpura
TTTS	twin-to-twin transfusion syndrome
U5MR	under-5 mortality rate
UDPGT	uridine diphosphate glucuronyl transferase
UE	unconjugated oestriol
U&Es	urea and electrolytes
UKCCSG	UK Children's Cancer Study Group
UNAIDS	Joint United Nations Programme on HIV/AIDS
UNCRC	United Nations Convention on the Rights of the Child
UNHS	universal newborn hearing screening
UNICEF	United Nations Children's Fund
URTI	upper respiratory tract infection
US	ultrasonography
UTI	urinary tract infection
V	volume of distribution
VAPP	vaccine-associated paralytic polio
vCJD	variant Creutzfeld–Jakob disease
VRA	visual reinforcement audiometry
VSD	ventricular septal defect
VT	ventricular tachycardia
WAGR	Wilms tumor, aniridia, gonadoblastoma/genitourinary abnormalities, mental retardation
WHO	World Health Organization
XLR	X-linked recessive
ZIG	zoster immunoglobulin

Contents

Please note: Authors are ordered alphabetically.

Contents

*Edited by Jonathan Darling,
Diego van Esso, Adamos Hadjipanayis*

Normal children and child health

MODULE ONE

Alan Craft   Odilija Rudzeviciene   Arunas Valiulis

Child health in a changing society and the role of the paediatrician

LEARNING OUTCOMES

By the end of this chapter you should know and understand the following principles concerning paediatrics and child health:

- The duties of a paediatrician
- The need for changes to the service in light of social, environmental, economic and disease changes
- The major causes of mortality and morbidity in childhood
- The skills required to be a good paediatric practitioner
- The necessary competencies for paediatric practice.

MODULE ONE

Introduction

The United Nations Convention on the Rights of the Child defines a 'child' as 'every human being below the age of eighteen years'. Children are a nation's most important asset and their health and welfare must be safeguarded. A recent report emphasized the need to commit to support children in order to:

- Be healthy
- Stay safe
- Enjoy and achieve
- Make a positive contribution
- Achieve economic wellbeing.

Paediatricians play a crucial role in achieving these aims, where necessary working with other healthcare professionals, social workers and teachers.

Paediatrics is not just about the recognition and treatment of illness in babies and children. It also encompasses child health, which covers all aspects of growth and development and the prevention of disease. At the end of childhood, paediatricians must ensure a smooth transition of care to adult services, especially for those with chronic conditions.

Paediatrics and child health include every aspect of life from birth (and often before) up to adulthood. Paediatricians are usually responsible for children up to the age of 18 years, although in some European countries paediatricians take care of young adults with rare chronic diseases over this age limit.

Paediatrics covers everyone from a totally dependent newborn baby to a fully independent adult, and from a 24-week-gestation baby weighing less than 500 g to an obese teenager of 150 kg or more.

Every facet of paediatrics is coloured by the fact that a child is growing and developing in both a physical and an emotional sense. More than in any other aspect of medicine, the needs of the family and carers have to be considered in everything that is done.

There is increasing evidence that factors operating in fetal life, infancy and childhood are important determinants of adult health.

Paediatrics and child health are about ensuring optimum health during a critical period of life and, by so doing, putting the young adult on the road to a healthy future.

What is a paediatrician?

He or she is someone who is medically qualified and who commits himself or herself to a career of working with children. Paediatrics covers a huge spectrum of different areas so it is difficult to say that there is a typical paediatrician profile. The specialty includes everything from neonatal and paediatric intensive care, where very sick children have to be managed, rapid decisions have to be made and the outcomes are often uncertain, to areas such as neurodisability, where different skills are required to manage a chronic condition and outcomes may not be seen for many years. There is also the public health role of disease prevention and the planning and evaluation of services.

So are there any particular attributes necessary to be a paediatrician? A liking for children is obviously a prerequisite, along with an ability to communicate with children and their families.

The need for triadic consultations, e.g. taking a history from a child as well as a parent or carer, makes paediatricians unusual but not unique.

The Royal College of Paediatrics and Child Health (RCPCH) has a statement indicating the duties of a paediatrician and this gives a good summary of the very wide roles that should be played (Box 1.1).

The paediatrician must be aware of the United Nations Convention on the Rights of the Child (1989), to which virtually every country in the world has signed up. This embodies the right of every child to:

- Equality regardless of race, religion, nationality or sex
- Special protection for full physical, intellectual, moral, spiritual and social development in a healthy and normal manner
- A name and nationality
- Adequate nutrition, housing and medical services
- Special care if handicapped
- Love, understanding and protection
- Free education, play and recreation
- Priority for relief in times of disaster
- Protection against all forms of neglect, cruelty and exploitation

---

BOX 1.1 Duties of a paediatrician

- Paediatricians should commit themselves to practise in accordance with the Objects of the College and the UN Convention on the Rights of the Child
- Paediatricians have a responsibility to safeguard the reputation of paediatrics through their personal clinical practice and through participation in continuing professional development, enabling them to maintain and enhance their knowledge, skills and competence for effective clinical practice to meet the needs of children
- Paediatricians should recognize the limitations of their skills and seek advice and support when this would be in the best interests of the child
- Paediatricians should espouse paediatric research and promote interchange between medical science and clinical practice as it affects the life and health of children
- Paediatricians should pay due regard to the domestic, sociological, environmental and genetic dimensions of the health of children
- Paediatricians, whatever their specialty interest, should understand their particular responsibilities for the holistic and life-long health of children who come under their care; each contact is an opportunity for health promotion and disease prevention
- Paediatricians should serve as clinicians to the individual child while contributing to public health medicine
- Paediatricians should be aware of current medical and political affairs affecting the lives and health of children
- Paediatricians should serve as advocates for the health needs of children locally, nationally and internationally
- Paediatricians should see themselves as ambassadors for children and for the specialty of paediatrics
- Above all, paediatricians should be courteous and compassionate in all their professional dealings with children, their parents and other carers, placing the child's best interests at the centre of all clinical considerations

---

- Protection from any form of discrimination, and the right to be brought up in a spirit of universal brotherhood, peace and tolerance.

Paediatrics is changing

In the early part of the 20th century infection was the major cause of both morbidity and mortality. There was a clear link between infection and social circumstances. Improvements in housing and the environment began the trend for improvements to the health of the population and this was accelerated by the introduction of both immunization to prevent infections and antibiotics to treat them. The first day of life is the time when children are most vulnerable but improvements in antenatal and neonatal care have done much to minimize the dangers present at this time.

There are many indicators used to monitor the health of populations and those applied to children are often a good measure of the health and health services of the total population. The key measures are:

- *Perinatal mortality*: stillbirths plus first week deaths per 1000 total births
- *Infant mortality rate (IMR)*: deaths in the first year per 1000 live births
- *Under-5 mortality*: deaths in the first 5 years of life per 1000 live births.

There has been a steady fall in all of these indicators over the last 100 years and both babies and children are now very healthy. However, this is not universal. Although economically advantaged countries have IMRs in single figures, economically less well-off countries, for example in sub-Saharan Africa, still have levels of over 200. More worrying is the fact that, for some of the least well-off countries, indicators of health are getting worse. It is also interesting to note that there can be substantial differences within individual countries according to social class and other factors.

So, in spite of children getting healthier, demands for health services are increasing. The reasons for this paradox are complex. Parents are much less experienced than previously as they have usually grown up in small families with few siblings. Parental and grandparent support used to be readily available from relatives who were experienced. In addition, the 'nuclear' family is now no longer the closed unit of the past. A great deal more can be done for those who are ill and more is expected. Finally, parents are better educated but because of this they are more worried and concerned about ill health.

Causes of morbidity and mortality

The causes and rates of deaths and loss of health in children vary widely across Europe. In general, Eastern countries have higher morbidity and mortality from respiratory and infectious diseases, and external causes (injuries and poisoning). Children's disease patterns in Western countries include proportionately more noncommunicable diseases, such as asthma and allergies, diabetes, obesity and neuropsychiatric disorders. Vaccine preventable diseases remain a worry across Europe.

Table 1.1 Major causes of death in children (WHO, 2005)

Causes	Deaths per 100 000
All causes	102.4
Respiratory diseases	17.9
Congenital malformations	17.0
Infectious and parasitic diseases	5.9
Cancer	3.9
Cardiovascular diseases	2.2
External causes	15.1
Other diseases	40.4

Mortality

Death is the childhood health outcome that is most difficult to accept. The major causes of death in Europe are given in Table 1.1; whereas, Table 1.2 gives the ranking of the major causes of death at various age intervals up to 19 years.

Diseases of the respiratory system are the main cause of death in children aged 0–14 years. After respiratory diseases, congenital anomalies still cause very high mortality in most countries, although occurring mostly in children under 5. In most countries, death rates from injuries and poisoning in older teenagers are 3–5 times higher than those found in the 10–14-year age group.

Morbidity

Primary care remains the first port of call for most children with an acute problem. In many European countries paediatricians are responsible for both primary and secondary-tertiary outpatient care. In others, primary care is delivered by family doctors or general practitioners. Systems vary between countries. The average number of consultations in the first 4 years of life is 6 per year, falling to 2.5 in the 5–14 age group. Boys are slightly more likely to consult than girls (ratio 1.1:1).

Common causes of consultation are non-infectious respiratory problems and acute infections, most commonly of the respiratory tract, ear, eyes and skin.

Outpatient care

In all, 1 in 5 children attends a hospital each year, either in accident and emergency or in the outpatient department. Major reasons for attendance are accidents, respiratory disorders, and neonatal, developmental and disability problems. In addition, 1 in 300 children will attend a child and adolescent mental health unit.

Inpatient care

In all, 1 in 8 children is admitted to hospital between the ages of 0 and 4 years and 1 in 16 between 5 and

Table 1.2 **Ranking of the major causes of death at various periods of life**

Rank	0–1 years	1–4 years	5–9 years	10–14 years	15–19 years
1st	**Congenital anomalies**	**Non-intentional accidents**	Non-intentional accidents	Non-intentional accidents	Non-intentional accidents
2nd	**Prematurity & IUGR**	Congenital anomalies	Malignant neoplasms	Malignant neoplasms	Homicides
3rd	**SIDS**	**Malignant neoplasms**	Congenital anomalies	**Suicides**	Suicides
4th	**RDS**	**Cardiac diseases**	**Homicides**	Homicides	Malignant neoplasms
5th	**From maternal complications**		Cardiac diseases	Congenital anomalies	Cardiac diseases

Bold font denotes first mention of cause.

15 years. Many children are now admitted to hospital for relatively short periods. Over the last 50 years the total number of children admitted to hospital has increased whilst the total length of stay has gone down dramatically. Most of these children are acutely unwell and probably have an infection. A short period of admission to hospital, or day case observation, allows the child to be assessed and discharged home to recover once serious problems have been excluded. The major causes of admission to hospital, including during the neonatal period, are:

- Perinatal conditions   17%
- Disorders of the respiratory system   14%
- Disorders of the ear   11%
- Injuries and poisoning   10%
- Ill-defined symptoms, e.g. abdominal pain   9%
- Disorders of the digestive system   7%.

Influences on child health

Maternal factors

Disease in the mother can directly affect the newborn baby. Examples of this are maternal diabetes (a baby may be born preterm with a disproportionately high birth weight) and thyroid disease (babies of thyrotoxic mothers may also have such symptoms in the newborn period). Drugs, e.g. antiepileptics, given to mothers during pregnancy can directly affect the fetus and newborn. Maternal influences are covered in Chapter 8.

Influence of fetal and infant life on adult life

Over the last few years increasing evidence has emerged of the effect of fetal and infant factors in adult disease. This was first described by Professor David Barker from Southampton UK and in 1995, the British Medical Journal named this the Barker Hypothesis. This states:

Under-nutrition in utero programmes foetal metabolism to produce a 'thrifty' phenotype. Thus babies who are small at birth are liable to become adults with increased susceptibility to hypertension, cardiovascular disease, central obesity, impaired glucose tolerance.

Barker has found a correlation between birth weight and other measures of fetal nutrition and the subsequent development of cardiovascular disease, hypertension and diabetes in later life. There seems little doubt that the Barker effect does exist but it remains to be shown what the total contribution is to adult disease. It is likely that adult lifestyle, e.g. tobacco smoking, lack of exercise and poor diet leading to obesity, is a greater and more easily remediable influence.

Gender

At all ages boys have a higher death rate than girls. This is particularly true as boys get older, when the difference is largely due to increased danger from accidents.

Behavioural factors

According to the WHO Health Behaviour in School-aged Children study, behavioural factors play an increasing role in the lives of teenagers. Smoking is a habit that is usually established during the teenage years; some 80% of adult smokers started before the age of 18. Weekly smokers comprise 11–57% of boys and 12–67% of girls aged 15. Alcohol is a regular feature in the lives of many European adolescents. Almost 30% of 15-year-olds report regular drinking. Young people in many countries appear to start drinking at an earlier age than previously. Rates of teenage pregnancy vary across Europe, with Eastern countries in general experiencing higher rates than Western ones. The rates in most Western European countries range between 13 and 25 pregnancies per 1000 girls aged 15–19 years.

Social factors

The socioeconomic status, usually measured by social class, is a powerful predictor of most aspects of child health and illness; for example, in the neonatal period there is a clear association between birth weight, neonatal outcome and social class. In the first year of life, sudden unexplained death in infancy (SUDI) is strongly influenced by social and environmental factors; the risk is of the order of 1 in 200 for high-risk families but 1 in 8500 for those of low risk. For the rest of childhood there is a clear association between social class and most causes of morbidity and mortality, including admission to hospital.

Skills needed for paediatric practice

All paediatricians need to have the basic medical skills as outlined in the General Medical Council's booklet on 'Good Medical Practice'. The principles apply to all doctors but have been amplified for paediatricians by the RCPCH in its publication, 'Good Medical Practice in Paediatrics and Child Health' (http://www.rcpch.ac.uk/doc.aspx?id_Resource=1621). This again expands on the principles outlined in Box 1.1. The importance of working in teams and of recognizing the skills and contribution of other professionals must be acknowledged. All doctors must maintain professional etiquette and the particular needs of children and families need to be considered. A general principle in all medical practice is the need to communicate with patients and in paediatric practice this needs to involve both child and family. Children's level of understanding develops with age and also with stage of development, and the latter in particular must be assessed in order to ascertain an appropriate level of communication.

There are particular ethical and legal issues that need to be considered in the practice of paediatrics and these are covered in Chapter 11. Some of the most difficult areas are around issues of confidentiality and those relating to child protection have been summarized in the RCPCH document, 'Responsibility of Doctors in Child Protection Cases with Regard to Confidentiality' (see also Chs 21 and 36).

There have been significant changes in the way that medicine is practised compared to just 25 years ago. Medicine is now so complex that no doctor can expect to know everything in his or her particular field of expertise, let alone outside of it. Medical students are taught in a different way, so that they learn and understand the principles of medicine and how to find out about those areas where they are uncertain. The shorter time periods available for postgraduate training, along with this rapid expansion of knowledge, make the newly qualified paediatrician less experienced than in the past. It is important therefore not to work in isolation, to be part of a team, and not to be afraid to ask for a second opinion.

The environment in which we work has also changed and, partly because of greater public expectation, there is a greater tendency to complain when things have not gone the way that might have been expected. All doctors — and paediatricians are no exception — have to be prepared for complaints and must know how to handle them. Good communication is the key both to preventing complaints and to dealing with them well. Clear explanations of the aims and limitations of treatment and what is likely to be the outcome in a particular situation will do much to produce realistic expectations. If something does go wrong, then honesty and a clear explanation are important. The most important factor for patients and parents when adverse outcomes have occurred is to know what the reasons are and that every step has been taken to try to prevent the same outcome for future patients.

A career working with children is hugely rewarding and there can be no greater pleasure than to have an adult, whom you treated as a child, come into your consulting room and tell you about their life achievements and show you their own offspring.

Paediatric competencies

The Accreditation Council on Graduate Medical Education (ACGME) requires that all trainees be assessed on the six competencies listed below. The list of specific skills found within each competency category was developed by the project team for the APA Educational Guidelines for Paediatric Training programmes. Kittredge D, Baldwin CD, Bar-on ME, Beach PS, Trimm RF (Eds) (2004). APA Educational Guidelines for Pediatric Residency. Academic Pediatric Association Website. Available online: http://www.academicpeds.org/egwebnew/index.cfm. [Accessed 10/03/2010]. Project to develop this website was funded by the Josiah Macy, Jr. Foundation 2002–2005.

Patient Care. Provide family-centred patient care that is development- and age-appropriate, compassionate, and effective for the treatment of health problems and the promotion of health.
- Use a logical and appropriate clinical approach to the care of patients [with condition/in setting], applying principles of evidence-based decision-making and problem-solving.
- Provide sensitive support to patients and their families [with condition/in setting].
- Provide effective preventive health care and anticipatory guidance to patients and families [with condition/in setting].

Medical Knowledge. Understand the scope of established and evolving biomedical, clinical, epidemiological and social-behavioural knowledge needed by a paediatrician; demonstrate the ability to acquire, critically interpret and apply this knowledge in patient care.

- Demonstrate a commitment to acquiring the knowledge needed for care of children [with condition/in setting].
- Know and/or access medical information efficiently, evaluate it critically, and apply it appropriately to the care of patients [with condition/in setting].

Interpersonal Skills and Communication. Demonstrate interpersonal and communication skills that result in information exchange and partnering with patients, their families and professional associates.

- Provide effective patient education, including reassurance, for conditions common to [condition/setting].
- Communicate effectively with physicians, other health professionals, and health-related agencies to create and sustain information exchange and teamwork for patient care.
- Develop effective strategies for teaching students, colleagues and other professionals.
- Maintain accurate, legible, timely and legally appropriate medical records in this clinical setting.

Practice-based Learning and Improvement. Demonstrate knowledge, skills and attitudes needed for continuous self-assessment, using scientific methods and evidence to investigate, evaluate, and improve one's patient care practice.

- Identify standardized guidelines for diagnosis and treatment of conditions common to [condition/setting], and adapt them to the individual needs of specific patients.
- Work with health care team members to assess, coordinate, and improve patient care for patients [with condition/in setting].

- Establish an individual learning plan, systematically organize relevant information resources for future reference, and plan for continuing acquisition of knowledge and skills.

Professionalism. Demonstrate a commitment to carrying out professional responsibilities, adherence to ethical principles and sensitivity to diversity.

- Demonstrate personal accountability to the wellbeing of patients (e.g. following up on lab results, writing comprehensive notes, and seeking answers to patient care questions).
- Demonstrate a commitment to professional behavior in interactions with staff and professional colleagues.

Adhere to ethical and legal principles, and be sensitive to diversity.

Systems-based Practice. Understand how to practise high-quality health care and advocate for patients within the context of the healthcare system.

- Identify key aspects of healthcare systems (e.g. public and private insurance) as they apply to patients [with condition/in setting], such as the role of the primary care provider and consultant in decision-making, referral and coordination of care.
- Demonstrate sensitivity to the costs of clinical care for patients [with condition/in setting], and take steps to minimize costs without compromising quality.
- Recognize and advocate for families who need assistance to deal with system complexities, such as lack of insurance, multiple medication refills, multiple appointments with long transport times, or inconvenient hours of service.
- Recognize one's limits and those of the system; take steps to avoid medical errors.

Delyth Howard   Rotraud K. Saurenmann

CHAPTER

2

Child development and developmental problems

LEARNING OUTCOMES

By the end of this chapter you should:
- Understand prenatal brain development
- Know the factors influencing a child's development
- Understand the process of normal development
- Know how to assess development in a child under 5 years of age
- Know the common patterns of developmental abnormality.

You should also take this opportunity to ensure that:
- You are able to perform a developmental assessment on a child under the age of 5 years
- You know how to perform basic assessment of hearing and vision
- You can recognize common patterns of developmental delay
- You know when to refer on for detailed developmental assessment.

MODULE ONE

Introduction

A knowledge of child development is integral to all of our work as paediatricians. It influences how we interact with our patients and how we manage their medical conditions. In addition, we need to be able to assess and diagnose developmental problems.

Basic science: the development of the nervous system

Prenatal development is an important factor in postnatal developmental issues. The developing brain is vulnerable to a range of influences.

16 days	Neural plate forms from ectoderm
18 days	Neural groove
22 days	Neural tube
27 days	Neural tube closed, brain and spinal cord differentiation begins
4 weeks	Triencephalon: three-vesicle stage of brain development
6 weeks	Five-vesicle stage, with differentiation of cerebral hemispheres
From 4–9 months	Histogenesis, cell differentiation into neurons and supporting cells
	Cell proliferation and neuronal migration
Near term	Myelination

Table 2.1 Malformations and timings

Stage	Normal development	Failure
Stage 1 (weeks 3–4)	Formation and closure of spinal cord	Anencephaly Encephalocele Chiari malformation Spina bifida
Stage 2 (weeks 5–10)	Formation of brain segments	Holoprosencephaly Corpus callosum agenesis Dandy–Walker syndrome
Stage 3 (2–5 months)	Neuronal migration and cellular differentiation	Heterotopias Polymicrogyria Agyria-pachygyria Lissencephaly
Stage 4 (5–15 months)	Myelination	Developmental delay Dysmyelinating disease

Prenatal brain development (Box 2.1)

1st trimester

Differentiation of the nervous system starts with the development of the neural plate from the ectoderm, 16 days after conception. This plate, which stretches along the entire back of the embryo, lengthens and starts folding up, forming a groove at around 18 days. The neural groove then begins fusing shut into a tube at around 22 days post-conception. By 27 days, the neural tube is fully closed and has begun its transformation into the brain (cephalic portion) and spinal cord (caudal portion). Neural crests give rise to the peripheral nervous system. The brain undergoes further differentiation, but the spinal cord retains the tubular structure.

Defects in formation of the neural tube lead to major brain or spinal cord defects, often lethal. Incomplete closure (dysraphism), occurring in the first 3–4 weeks of gestation, may give rise to anencephaly, encephaloceles or spina bifida (Ch. 28). At 4 weeks the brain structures are differentiated into three vesicles: forebrain (prosencephalon), midbrain (mesencephalon) and hindbrain (rhombencephalon). From 4 to 6 weeks further development of the forebrain takes place, with differentiation of the cerebral hemispheres. The next stage in brain development is histogenesis, with cells differentiating into neurons or glial cells. Neuronal proliferation begins at 2 months of gestation.

Neurological activity in the fetus is manifest by 6 weeks' gestation, with spontaneous arching of the body. Reflex limb movements follow at 8 weeks, with more complex coordinated movements by 10 weeks (hiccuping, yawning, thumb sucking).

2nd trimester

Neuronal proliferation continues. Neuronal migration spans a period between 4 and 9 months of gestation. Disorders in neuronal proliferation, migration and maturation result in a variety of brain malformations (Ch. 28). These include lissencephaly, schizencephaly and agenesis of the corpus callosum. These are generally associated with psychomotor delay and seizures. Microcephaly (p. 257) may be a manifestation of abnormal neuronal proliferation or migration.

The second trimester marks the onset of more neurological activity in the form of critical reflexes: continuous breathing movements and coordinated sucking and swallowing reflexes. These abilities are controlled by the brainstem. The brainstem is largely mature by the end of the second trimester, which is when babies first become able to survive outside the womb. The grasp reflex is evident by 17 weeks, with the Moro reflex seen from 25 weeks.

3rd trimester

By the 6th month, nearly all the neurons needed for life are present. Last to mature is the cerebral cortex. Myelination begins near term.

In the last trimester, fetuses are capable of simple forms of learning, like habituating (decreasing their startle response) to a repeated auditory stimulus, such as a loud clap just outside the mother's abdomen.

Brain malformations may result from exogenous and endogenous causes (Table 2.1). Exogenous causes may be nutritional, radiological, viral, chemical, medications or ischaemic. Endogenous causes are genetic.

Postnatal brain development

The nervous system continues to undergo further development and maturation for some time after birth. By birth, only the lower portions of the nervous system (the spinal cord and brainstem) are very well developed, whereas the higher regions (the limbic system and cerebral cortex) are still rather primitive. Although all of the neurons in the cortex are produced before birth, they are poorly connected. In contrast to the brainstem and spinal cord, the cerebral cortex produces most of its synaptic connections after birth. Synapses are formed at a very rapid rate during the early months of life, achieving maximum density between 6 and 12 months after birth. The infant's brain forms and retains synapses that are frequently used. Synapses decrease due to disuse or natural attrition (apoptosis). Early experiences are thus vital to the formation and retention of synapses. By 2 years of age, a child's cerebral cortex contains well over 100 trillion synapses.

Myelination continues throughout childhood and possibly onwards in adulthood. The timing of myelination depends on the area of the brain in question.

Factors influencing development

There are many influences on a child's development (Box 2.2). These influences interact to produce the picture we see in the child. Genes and environment interact at every step of brain development. Generally speaking, genes are responsible for:
- The basic wiring plan
- Forming neurons and connections between different brain regions.

BOX 2.2 Factors influencing development

Prenatal
- Toxins: infections, drugs, alcohol
- Ischaemia
- Nutrition
- Genetic: chromosomal disorders, single gene defects

Pre- or postnatal?
- Parental IQ: IQ may be partially genetically determined, but parental IQ may also influence parenting

Postnatal
- Social environment
- Personality
- Emotional factors: interaction with caregivers
- Cultural factors
- Nutrition
- Parenting
- Physical health

Experience is responsible for fine-tuning those connections. It is usually not possible to separate out the most significant influences on an individual's development: the 'nature versus nurture' debate.

Normal development

Normal development follows a recognized sequence in most children. Children have to acquire certain skills before being able to move on to the next skill (for example, the development of head control is a prerequisite for sitting). Previous mass observations of children have given us the typical sequence of acquiring developmental skills, as well as the range of expected ages for key developmental skills (known as 'milestones'). It is on these that we base our decisions about whether a child is developing normally. There are, of course, significant variations within the 'normal' range.

During your career, you will build up your own personal knowledge of normal development from interacting with hundreds of children. Nothing can replace this experience, but before you have built up this memory bank, you will need a foundation from which to start. Tables of developmental milestones can provide some guidance on expected developmental skills at certain ages. It is never possible to provide an exhaustive list of milestones. You must also be aware that suggested ages for certain skills may vary between authors. As you gain experience, you will get a feel for what is usual at each age. Nevertheless, it is helpful to learn some key milestones, as well as the normal sequence of skill development, which is perhaps more important.

Typically developing children may show slight variations in their skill levels in different areas of development. For example, they may be slightly more advanced in their gross motor skills and relatively less advanced in their speech and language skills, or vice versa.

Categories of development

Developmental skills can be grouped into the following four categories. These categories are not mutually exclusive, and some skills may span categories:
- *Fine motor and vision*: hand skills, including drawing, puzzles
- *Speech, language and hearing*: communication skills, including receptive and expressive language, and non-verbal communication
- *Gross motor*: large movements, including sitting, walking, running, going upstairs
- *Social behaviour and play*: including feeding, toileting, dressing and social relationships.

In school-aged children different types of tests (intelligence tests, language tests) are used to assess the development of skills relative to an age-matched normal population (Ch. 29).

Fine motor and vision

A child's visual abilities are developing and changing along with other areas of development. During the first year of life, babies progress from only being able to focus on objects very close by, to rapidly developing distance vision. From a few months of age, visual abilities are being integrated with hand skills in reaching for objects. Subsequently infants develop the ability to focus on rapidly moving objects and to judge distances. Between 1 and 2, children will develop their visual interest in simple pictures, in addition to recognizing real objects. Refinement of hand skills continues, with development in grasp and control. Children often do not have a clear hand preference until around 3 years of age, with 90% demonstrating a clear preference by age 4.

Speech, language and hearing

Prelingual (1st year)

Babies in their first year are learning about communication, and have a variety of communication strategies before they develop language. Newborns are already able to mimic the facial expressions of adults. Conversational exchanges occur, with babies learning about turn-taking in reciprocal vocalization. Vocalizations are shaped by the language babies hear. Humans have an inherent capacity to learn any language, but our speech sound system is shaped during the first year of life. Vocalizations start as open vowel sounds. Next comes double-syllable babble. Vocalizations become more expressive, varying in pitch and volume. Social communication is an important aspect. Babies use eye contact and facial expressions as part of their communication. Receptive language develops in advance of expressive language. Babies learn to recognize their own name. They develop situational awareness (e.g. when their coat is put on, they become excited about going out) before understanding single words in context. An understanding of an object's use (definition by use) develops prior to understanding object names.

Early lingual (1–2 years)

Receptive language or comprehension of single words begins in this phase. Initially a child can point to named familiar objects. This might include pointing to named body parts on themselves. The ability to recognize those same objects in photographs or pictures develops later.

Expressive language may start as sound labels (for example, 'mmm' at mealtimes, or animal noises). Single words come next. Single words may be used for a variety of purposes: to comment or label or to request. Next comes the ability to join two words together to create novel phrases (e.g. 'mummy car'). Common phrases do not count as joining words together (e.g. 'all fall down').

Non-verbal communication is an important part of this stage of development. Children will use gestures to communicate, particularly pointing to request or to show objects of interest.

Gross motor

Gross motor development proceeds in a cephalo-caudal direction. Typically developing children will all proceed along the same sequence of skill acquisition. Head, neck and trunk control is a vital prerequisite for sitting. Walking is usually achieved by moving through prone into four-point kneeling and then crawling. These actions develop prior to standing and walking. However, some children show a disordered pattern of motor development, which can be considered a normal variant. These are children who bottom-shuffle. They typically prefer the sitting to the prone position. They eventually get up and walk, but often have not crawled. Walking is often delayed in these children, who otherwise develop normally.

Social behaviour and play

Social interactions are of vital importance for the normal development of a child. Eye contact, non-verbal and verbal communication, recognition and interaction with familiar persons, self-recognition and adequate response to the social context of a situation are features of social behaviour development. Paediatricians are often very aware of the different stages of social behaviour in infants and children, from the skilful interactions required when trying to examine children of different ages. As in all other areas of development there is also a wide normal range in the social behaviour of children.

The hallmark of autism disorders is an impairment of social skills. It most often presents as part of a global developmental delay. In some children only social functioning is impaired, with normal or even high skills in other areas (Asperger syndrome) (see Ch. 29).

The strongest hint of abnormal social development is an inability to establish non-verbal communication, especially eye contact. The Checklist for Autism in Toddlers (CHAT) was developed to recognize autism in 18-month-old children (Box 2.3).

Developmental milestones

Centiles can be used to define the range of normal for each milestone, in a similar way to those used for growth or puberty. Often the median age or 50th centile is quoted (as here), which is the age by which 50% of children have achieved the skill in question. Sometimes it can be more useful to know the 95th centile (e.g. 18 months for walking), since if a skill has not been achieved by this age, it is very likely to be of concern. Below is a list of milestones, but this is by no means exhaustive and is intended as a guide only. You can find lists in many texts, often with slight variations in the age quoted.

Fine motor and vision

• Watches own hands in finger play	3 months
• Fixes and follows object through 90 degrees laterally	3 months
• Grasps objects	4 months
• Passes toy from one hand to the other	6 months
• Inferior pincer grasp	9 months
• Looks for falling toys	9 months
• Bangs bricks together in imitation	12 months
• Refined pincer grasp	12 months
• Builds tower of two bricks	15 months
• Builds tower of three bricks	18 months
• To and fro scribble on paper	18 months
• Builds tower of six or seven bricks	2 years
• Circular scribble	2 years
• Builds train of bricks	$2^{1}/_2$ years
• Copies vertical line and circle	3 years
• Builds tower of nine bricks	3 years
• Copies three-brick bridge	$3^{1}/_2$ years
• Copies cross	4 years
• Draws a person with head, body and legs	4 years
• Builds six-brick steps	4 years
• Copies square	$4^{1}/_2$ years

Speech, language and hearing

• Vocalizes when spoken to	3 months
• Babbles in repetitive strings of double-syllable babble	9 months
• Knows and turns to own name	12 months
• Uses 2–6 recognizable words	15 months
• Points to familiar objects when requested	15 months
• Joins two words together	2 years
• Understands commands with two key words	2 years
• Vocabulary of 200 words	2$\frac{1}{2}$ years
• Understands commands with three key words	3 years
• Talks in short sentences	3 years
• Asks 'what?' and 'who?' questions	3 years
• Able to tell long stories	4 years
• Asks 'why?', 'when?' and 'how?' questions	4 years
• Counts up to 20 by rote	4 years

Gross motor

• Lifts head and chest up, supporting self on forearms in prone	3 months
• Little or no head lag on pull-to-sit	3 months
• Rolls front to back (and usually back to front)	6 months
• Sits independently	8 months
• Crawls	10 months
• Walks independently	13 months
• Squats to pick up object	18 months
• Runs	2 years
• Walks upstairs holding on, two feet to a step	2 years
• Jumps with two feet together	2$\frac{1}{2}$ years
• Kicks a ball	2$\frac{1}{2}$ years
• Stands on one foot momentarily	3 years
• Walks upstairs adult fashion (one foot to a step)	3 years
• Pedals tricycle	3 years
• Hops	4 years

Social behaviour and play

• Smiles	6 weeks
• Responds with pleasure to friendly handling	3 months
• Stranger awareness	9 months
• Enjoys peek-a-boo	9 months
• Is interested in mirror image	9 months
• Helps with dressing	12 months
• Waves bye-bye	12 months
• Takes off socks, hat	18 months
• Spoon-feeds self	18 months
• Recognizes self in mirror	2 years
• Speaks of self as 'I'	2 years
• Plays alongside other children	2 years
• Eats with fork and spoon	3 years
• Helps adult around house	3 years
• Joins in make-believe play with peers	3 years
• Can dress and undress, except for laces	4 years
• 'Theory of mind' (recognizes that other persons may have different perceptions)	4 years

Developmental assessment

Developmental assessment is a vital skill for any paediatrician. When conducting a developmental assessment, you are aiming to answer several questions:
• Is the child's development normal for his or her age?
• If not, in which ways and to what degree is it abnormal?
• What is the diagnosis?
• What might be the cause(s)?
• What needs to be done?

Screening assessment

In many situations you might be seeking to answer only the first of these questions. This would be the case, for instance, if a developmental assessment were being conducted as part of child health surveillance. For this purpose, you would present the child with a number of tasks that you would expect him or her to be able to do at that age, and see whether he or she could achieve them. You would not be seeking to find out exactly what the child is able to do in each developmental area, but simply establishing whether he or she can perform a set range of age-appropriate tasks. If the child does not demonstrate the age-appropriate skills, you would refer him or her on for further evaluation. The Denver developmental screening test (DDST, 1967) was revised and updated in 1997 (the Denver II). It is an example of a structured assessment tool designed to monitor the development of infants and pre-school children and to identify children with developmental problems. It is not intended as a detailed diagnostic developmental assessment (http://www.denverii.com/home.html).

Detailed assessment

The aim of a detailed developmental assessment is to discover the child's precise skill level in each area of development.

Informal assessment

This type of assessment should be one of every paediatrician's skills as it is commonly used in clinical practice. A range of appropriate toys are used, although without a formal scoring system. Using your knowledge of normal development, it is possible to ascertain an approximate developmental age that the child has reached. It is important to realize that, even in typically developing children, there may be differences in age-equivalent scores in each area of development. It would be meaningless to give an overall developmental age when there is significant variation between different areas of development.

Formal assessment

There are a number of standardized assessments that can be used, such as the Griffiths Mental Development Scales (0–8 years; Box 2.4), the Bayley Scales of Infant Development (0–42 months) and the Schedule of Growing Skills (0–5 years). Some standardized assessments require attendance on a training course.

Why is it important·to make a diagnosis?

Different developmental difficulties will have differing implications for the child's future. Therefore defining the developmental diagnosis is important. A diagnosis of specific language impairment has very different implications from a diagnosis of autism.

As in other aspects of medicine, diagnosis is important for several reasons:

- *Prognosis*. Diagnosis enables you to give more information about prognosis, based on other children with the same disorder.

Box 2.4 Griffiths Mental Development Scales

- Developmental assessment tool for children aged 0–8 years
- Two separate modules: 0–2 years and 2–8 years
- Assesses development in six areas:
    Locomotor
    Personal/social
    Hearing and speech
    Fine motor
    Performance
    Practical reasoning
- Gives a score for each area of development (age equivalent)
- Overall developmental quotient is calculated from summary of individual scores

---

- *Intervention*. Diagnosis will inform the most appropriate interventions.
- *Genetic*. Many conditions have a genetic basis, which will be particularly important for families with, or planning, other children.

A developmental diagnosis alone does not tell you what the cause is and, vice versa, to know the cause of a developmental delay will not be enough to decide on the necessary interventions needed for an individual child.

Principles of developmental assessment

General

- Explain to carer you do not expect child to be able to do all the tasks you set.
- Use a systematic/structured approach, completing one area of development before moving on to next.
- Use simple, clear language appropriate to child's age level.
- Unless you are assessing language and understanding, use visual/gestural clues to show child what you want him/her to do.
- Assess skills directly where possible, rather than asking carer about them.
- Do not assess 'irrelevant' areas, i.e. tasks that will not give you developmental information or tasks for which you do not know the age-equivalent.
- Keep pace going; do not leave long gaps between tasks or child may get bored and lose interest.
- Keep it fun; give lots of praise and encouragement.
- Observe children carefully throughout, even when you are not directly testing them; they may spontaneously demonstrate skills that will give you more information.
- Observe quality of how child performs a skill, not just whether he/she can do it; this includes looking at both hands for fine motor skills.

Structure

- Start with tasks you expect child to be able to do quite easily (i.e. below child's age level).
- If they cannot manage these, go down to simpler/younger tasks.
- Work up gradually, increasing age level of tasks in sequence until child can no longer do tasks.
- Save gross motor assessment till last (unless asked to do this specifically), as child is likely to get excited/not want to sit down afterwards.

Positioning and equipment

- Limit number of toys out at any one time.
- Use toys provided. Ask for specific items if you need them.
- Put yourself and child in optimal position to get best out of him/her (especially if this is fine motor or speech and language assessment):
    < 18 months: seated on carer's lap at table opposite you (*not* on floor)
    2–5 years: seated at small table opposite you.

Suggested assessment schema

This schema presents a bare minimum of tasks for estimating a child's developmental skills. Tasks should be presented in increasing order of difficulty. You will develop your own order of assessment, but this is suggested as a framework to get you started.

Infant

Equipment

- 3-cm cubes
- Brightly coloured small toy
- Small object (e.g. raisin)
- Cup
- Cloth
- Paper and pencils
- Familiar objects (cup, sock, shoe, brush)
- Mat/blanket on floor

Fine motor and vision

- Ask if there are any concerns about infant's vision.
- Gain infant's visual attention with toy and move through visual fields, looking at fixation and following.
- Offer small toy, looking at reach and grasp, in-hand manipulation, transferring etc.
- Offer one cube to one hand then other hand.
- Offer second cube with child holding first.
- Demonstrate banging two cubes together to see if child imitates you.
- Demonstrate placing one cube on top of another to see if child imitates you.
- Offer third cube.
- Partially hide cube or toy under cloth to see if infant finds it.
- Totally hide cube or toy under cloth to see if infant finds it.
- Hide cube or toy under cup to see if infant finds it.
- Place raisin on table in front of infant (each hand). (N.B. Remove raisin quickly from infant's hand before it is eaten.)

- For older infants, offer pencil/crayon and paper.
- Visual assessment:
    Observed visual behaviour
    Detection of small objects
    Preferential looking acuity system (e.g. Keeler cards).

Speech, language and hearing

- Ask if there are any concerns about infant's hearing.
- Listen throughout assessment for any vocalizations.
- Observe non-verbal communication, including facial expressions, eye contact, gestures.
- Imitate vocalizations back to infant.
- Talk in double-syllable babble to see if infant copies.
- Call infant's name to look for response.
- Clap hands and encourage infant to imitate.
- Wave bye-bye and encourage infant to imitate.
- Offer familiar objects (sock, cup, brush) to look for definition by use.
- Assess understanding of simple instructions ('Give it to Mummy').
- Use limited number of familiar objects to look for single word recognition ('Where's the cup?').
- Hearing assessment:
    Otoacoustic emission and auditory brainstem responses (ABR) testing at birth
    Distraction testing from 7 months (see Ch. 32 for details).

Gross motor

- Lie infant supine on mat.
- Encourage infant to roll.
- Pull to sit.
- Place in sitting position.
- Pull to stand or to bear weight on feet.
- Observe and support stepping/walking.
- Downward parachute.
- Hold in ventral suspension or place in prone position.
- Forward parachute.

Social behaviour and play

- Observe throughout.
- Smile and interact with infant and watch responsiveness.
- Ask about self-feeding etc.

Toddler

Equipment

- Small table and chairs
- 3-cm cubes (at least 12)
- Paper and pencils
- Range of real objects (cup, spoon, brush etc.)

Fig. 2.1 tables:

Age (yrs)	Shape that can be copied (drawn without seeing how it is done)
2	vertical line
3	circle
4	cross
4.5	square
5	triangle

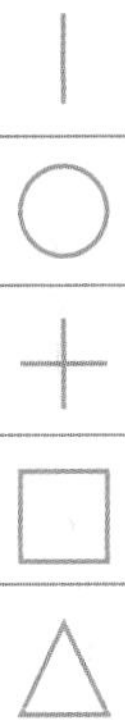

A

Age (yrs)	Tower of bricks (number of bricks in a tower)	Shape with bricks
1.5	3	
2	6	
2.5	8	Train
3	9	Bridge
4		Steps

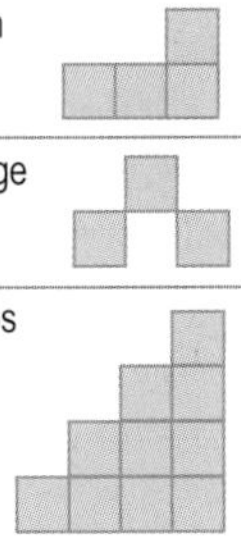

B

Fig. 2.1 (A) Shapes that can be drawn at different ages; **(B)** shapes that can be made with bricks at different ages

- Doll or teddy
- Picture book
- Miniature toys
- Beads or puzzle
- Ball
- Stairs

Fine motor and vision (Fig. 2.1)
- Offer 3-cm cubes; encourage tower building.
- Build three-brick bridge for child to copy/imitate.
- Build train for child to copy/imitate.
- Build six-brick steps for child to copy/imitate.
- Offer paper and pencils; observe spontaneous drawing.
- Draw shapes for child to copy: horizontal and vertical line, circle, cross, square, triangle.
- Ask child to draw picture of a person (e.g. 'Draw Mummy').
- Look at manipulation/coordination using beads or puzzles.
- Visual assessment:
  Preferential looking acuity measure (e.g. Cardiff acuity test)
  Letter matching acuity systems (e.g. Sonksen–Silver, Sheridan–Gardiner)
  Lang stereoscopy chart.

Speech, language and hearing
- Lay out a number of objects/toys to test single word understanding.
- Increase complexity of questions gradually, to check two-word level of understanding, then three-word level, then prepositions, adjectives, verbs (e.g. 'Where's the duck?', then later 'Give me the spoon and the doll', 'Put the spoon in the cup and give me the car', 'Where's the big pencil?', 'Put the car under the table', 'Make teddy kick the ball' etc.).
- Listen for expressive language throughout.
- Observe non-verbal communication, including facial expressions, eye contact, gestures.
- Use picture book to gain sample of expressive language ('What can you see?').
- Hearing assessment:
  Performance/conditioning test — child is conditioned to 'perform' in some way when he or she hears a sound; this is done as a game, e.g. place brick in basket.
  Speech discrimination test (e.g. McCormick toy test) — child is asked to choose a named toy from a set of toys composed of pairs with similar names (e.g. 'tree' and 'key').

Gross motor
- Observe walking
- Place object on floor for child to pick up
- Running
- Jump with two feet together
- Stand on one leg
- Climbs up and down stairs
- Hop
- Kick a ball

Social behaviour and play
- Observe throughout, looking particularly at social interaction and eye contact.
- Ask about self-help skill.
- Ask about play with peers.

Developmental problems

Delay or disorder?

A child's development can be abnormal in many ways. Delayed development simply means that a child is acquiring skills at a later age than the norm. Development can be delayed in just one area (for example, speech and language delay), or in two or more areas — commonly called global developmental delay.

Children with global developmental delay may present initially with delay in one area of development, but on further assessment it becomes clear that they have more general delay. Disordered development means an unusual pattern or sequence of development. The term also suggests that the problem is due to an underlying developmental disorder, and the child is unlikely to 'catch up'.

Any child presenting with delayed development in one area needs careful evaluation of the rest of his or her development. Delay in one area can be the initial presenting feature of global developmental delay (Ch. 18).

Common patterns of developmental delay and their causes

Speech and language delay

Speech and language delay is the most common pre-school developmental problem, occurring in 5–10% of all children. It is more common in boys. This is discussed fully in Chapter 29.

You should understand the difference between speech delay (difficulties with speech sound production), expressive language delay (difficulties in choosing or using appropriate words to convey meaning) and receptive language delay (problems with understanding language). Children with developmental language delay or specific language impairment typically have difficulties in both receptive and expressive language. Usually understanding (receptive language) is in advance of expression.

Tongue tie is not an adequate reason for speech delay, and operative treatment is not indicated unless tongue movements are severely limited.

Delay in gross motor skills

Delay in gross motor skills may typically present with delayed sitting and poor head control, or with delay in walking. The upper limit of the normal age of walking is 18 months.

Possible causes of delayed sitting/poor head and trunk control include:
- Central neurological (brain) disorders, such as cerebral palsy, brain malformations
- Neuromuscular conditions, such as spinal muscular atrophy
- Severe global developmental delay (severe learning difficulties), which may sometimes present initially with delayed gross motor skills.

Possible causes of delayed walking include:
- Central neurological disorders, such as cerebral palsy, particularly of diplegic distribution
- Neuromuscular problems, such as Duchenne muscular dystrophy
- Spinal problems
- Orthopaedic problems, such as developmental dysplasia of the hip
- Global developmental delay.

Bottom-shuffling, a normal variant, is usually associated with a later average age of acquiring independent walking. Children who bottom-shuffle typically do not crawl, dislike the prone position, and are reluctant to take weight through their feet, adopting the 'sitting on air' position when held under their arms. Although it is a normal variant and often seen in several members of the same family, bottom-shuffling can also be associated with pathological underlying causes, such as cerebral palsy; therefore careful clinical examination is warranted.

Global developmental delay

Global developmental delay simply means delay in two or more areas of development. Many children presenting with global developmental delay are subsequently found to have significant learning difficulties (previously termed 'mental retardation'). Where the cause is environmental/social or secondary to ill health, children may 'catch up' with time and appropriate input/stimulation.

Possible causes of global developmental delay include:
- Environmental/psychosocial issues: lack of experience, deprivation, poor parenting, ill health
- Any condition causing learning difficulties, such as chromosomal disorders or syndromes or illnesses of the central nervous system.

http://www.guideline.gov/summary/summary.
aspx?view_id=1&doc_id=4106

National Guideline Clearinghouse.
Practice parameter: evaluation of the child with global
developmental delay: report of the Quality Standards
Subcommittee of the American Academy of Neurology
and The Practice Committee of the Child Neurology
Society.

Further reading

Quality Standards Subcommittee of the American Academy
   of Neurology and the Committee of the Child Neurology
   Society 2003 Practice parameter: evaluation of the child with
   global developmental delay. Neurology 60(3):367–380
Sheridan M, Frost M, Sharma A 1997 From birth to five years:
   children's developmental progress. Routledge, London

Melanie Epstein   Rotraud K. Saurenmann

3

Psychological and emotional development

LEARNING OUTCOMES

By the end of this chapter you should:

- Know how early experiences affect brain development
- Be familiar with the stages of cognitive development
- Understand the links between the attachment system and attachment behaviours
- Know the differences between secure and insecure attachment styles
- Understand some of the long-term effects of trauma and neglect in the first few years.

MODULE ONE

Introduction

No variables have more far-reaching effects on personality development than a child's experiences within the family. As humans, with a long period of helplessness and vulnerability after birth, we rely on adult care longer than any other species. Our physical and psychological security is inextricably linked, and depends on our connections with other people. These connections are sought and maintained because our brains are particularly sensitive to social relationships and the need for psychological security. The key to this is the attachment bond.

Emotional development

The attachment to a newborn is built on prior relationships with an imaginary child, and with the developing fetus that has been part of the parents' world for 9 months. During pregnancy the developing neurobiological structure of the brain follows the genetic blueprint, barring adverse environmental circumstances such as intrauterine infection or teratogens, in particular maternal ingestion of alcohol or other drugs. After birth, brain development becomes experience-dependent. Newborn babies are genetically 'pre-programmed' to seek out and adapt to the relationship that they have with their parents. Interactions with the environment during sensitive periods are necessary for the brain to mature. The capacity of the developing brain to alter its neurobiological structure (neuroplasticity) in response to the environment is an adaptive mechanism that has evolved out of the process of natural selection. This allows the child to adjust to the infinite possibilities created within a family in interaction with the wider culture.

At birth, there are about 100 million neurons, which are not yet part of functional networks. Synaptogenesis occurs predominantly in the first 3 years, and by the age of 2 there is the same number of synapses as in an adult. Brain development is a refining process of strengthening certain synapses and eliminating redundant synapses in a selective way, depending on experience and interactions with caregivers. A popular neuroscientific soundbite is 'Neurons that fire together, wire together'.

Stages of cognitive development

Optimal cognitive development is best achieved when attachment needs are met. Jean Piaget (1896–1980) identified four stages in cognitive development, as shown in Table 3.1.

The attachment bond

The essential task of the first year of life is the creation of a secure attachment bond between the infant and caregiver. This depends on the mother or primary caregiver's pattern of response to the infant's physical and emotional needs. Winnicott saw healthy development as starting with the 'good-enough' mother, who through following her maternal instincts helps the baby learn to express needs and feelings without being overwhelmed by them. She synchronizes and responds to the emotional rhythms of the baby. She is adept at handling negative reactions, and her inevitable failures, in a constructive healing way. In the presence of good-enough parenting, we learn to regulate our emotional reactions and tolerate gradually increasing amounts of frustration. Winnicott distinguished this sort of parent from a 'perfect' mother who satisfies all the needs of the infant on the spot, thus preventing him or her from developing. The responses to cues from the infant are built into an internal model of what the infant expects from the carer. This forms a foundation for future relationships. By the end of the first year, the infant's behaviour is purposeful and based on specific expectations. This is because he has aggregated his past experiences with the caregiver, and

these are becoming 'hard-wired'. Attachment is not just a set of behaviours or a psychological construct; it forms the substrate of the developing brain. Neuroscientific research has demonstrated the synaptic circuitry and anatomical locations. If children grow up with dominant experiences of separation, distress, fear and rage, they will go down a pathogenic developmental pathway, not just psychologically but neurologically. Attachment experiences form the neurodevelopmental framework out of which we emerge, and are important in cortical, prefrontal system and limbic system development. They later form the basis for personality development.

The brain is at its most plastic for the first 2 years after birth. This is the reason for the current emphasis on early prevention and intervention in policy and practice. The older the child becomes, then the harder it can be to 'rewire' certain areas of the brain. Research on children adopted from Romanian orphanages suggests that the sensitive period for developing attachments ends at about 3 years of age. A child who has experienced abuse or neglect as an infant may unwittingly continue with patterns of responses that are engraved in the mind, even if circumstances change. Other relationships later in life can be crucial: for example, relationships with adoptive parents, a relationship with a supportive partner or a therapeutic relationship. The ability to attribute meaning to experience also helps to mitigate the effects of past experience. The best predictor of the pattern of attachment that will later emerge between a mother and her 12-month-old baby is the way the mother currently talks about her own mother and her experiences of being mothered as a girl. How she reflects on and interprets those experiences now is more important than the actual attachment circumstances at the time.

The biological function of the attachment system

The attachment system was first described by the British psychiatrist, John Bowlby. It operates as a homeostatic system with the goal of emotional regulation. It is activated by anxiety and distress, and deactivated by a subjective feeling of security. It operates analogously to other biological homeostatic mechanisms: for example, systems for thermoregulation. The biological function has been thought to be protection from predators. A feature of the attachment system is the *intensity* of the emotion that accompanies it. If all goes well, there is joy and security associated with being protected, comforted and understood. If threatened, there is jealousy, anxiety and anger. If broken, as occurs with loss, there is grief and depression.

Table 3.1 Stages in cognitive development according to Jean Piaget

Stage	Description	Play	Example
Sensorimotor (infancy)	Intelligence is demonstrated through a baby's interactions with the environment and with the carer. These may be sensory (hearing, seeing, touch), motor (grasping, pulling) or expressions of feeling Knowledge of the world is limited (but developing) because it is based on physical interactions/experiences. Children acquire object permanence at about 7 months of age. Physical development (mobility) allows the child to begin developing new intellectual abilities. Some symbolic (language) abilities are developed at the end of this stage	'Practice play' to obtain mastery	A rattle *is* its colour when looked at, its texture when touched or sucked on, its sound when shaken; the baby demonstrates pleasure or another response, and may attempt to reach out to the rattle. Before object permanence develops, the rattle ceases to exist when out of sight
Preoperational (toddler and early childhood)	Intelligence is demonstrated through the use of symbols, language use matures, and memory and imagination are developed The child's world is concrete and absolute; things are as they seem. The child is influenced more by how things look than by principles of logic. This includes the belief that inanimate objects are alive Children tend to observe the world from their point of view (egocentrism)	Symbolic (make-believe play)	Sara (age 3 years 9 months) speaking of a car in the garage: 'The car's gone to bye-byes. It doesn't go out because of the rain'
Concrete operational (primary school and early adolescence)	In this stage (characterized by seven types of conservation: number, length, liquid, mass, weight, area, volume), intelligence is demonstrated through logical and systematic manipulation of symbols related to concrete objects Egocentric thought diminishes, and the child is more able to conceptualize the world from another's viewpoint. This is linked to the child's emotional development	With rules. As thinking becomes more logical, rules are incorporated. These become more sophisticated as children go through their development	If an 8-year-old child is asked, 'If Leon is taller than Lara and Lara is taller than Simon, who is taller, Leon or Simon?,' he or she will need to use real objects, e.g. dolls, to solve the problem. He will not be able to solve this in his head before the age of about 11
Formal operational (adolescence and adulthood)	Intelligence is demonstrated through the logical use of symbols related to abstract concepts. Ideas can now be manipulated, rather than just objects Adolescents can think hypothetically about a situation that they have not experienced before, or even one that nobody has ever experienced before	With rules	Einstein developed the seeds of his theory of relativity when he was about 16. He imagined himself as a particle of light travelling away from a planet at the speed of light and then looking back, thinking how it would appear

Attachment behaviour

Attachment behaviour is any behaviour designed to bring children into a close protective relationship with their attachment figures when they experience anxiety (Fig. 3.1). This brings feelings of security associated with being protected, comforted and understood. Having this 'secure base' enables children to feel safe to explore. For most children, their primary attachment figure is usually their mother or main carer. Children may also have a small but limited number of attachment relationships with other family members, or other adults such as a teacher.

There are three broad types of attachment behaviour:
1. Signalling behaviours (smiling, vocalizing, laughter) that bring the mother to the child for social interaction
2. Behaviours that bring the mother to the child to give comfort (e.g. to stop the child crying)
3. Behaviours that take the child to the mother.

Fig. 3.1 Attachment behaviour: the importance of early experiences

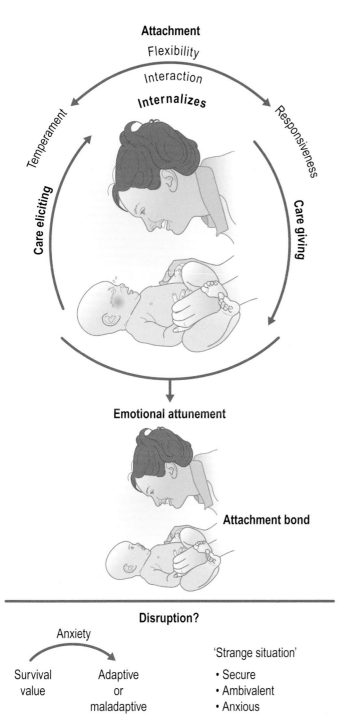

Fig. 3.1 Attachment behaviour: the importance of early experiences

Separation from the mother in distance or time increases anxiety. This activates the attachment system. Attachment behaviours ideally help bring the mother back. When this occurs, the anxiety and behaviours diminish. The attachment system is also activated by:

- Pain
- Tiredness
- Frightening experiences
- Inaccessibility of the primary caretaker: this could be real or apparent, physical or psychological.

By the age of 3, there is less need for direct proximity to the attachment figure, and the child is starting to develop 'a secure base' inside.

When attachment behaviour is activated, a child is unable to engage in other important developmental experiences such as exploration, play and other social interactions. When persistent over time, this will have adverse consequences for social and cognitive development.

There are four styles of attachment behaviour (Table 3.2):

Table 3.2 **Styles of attachment behaviour**

Attachment style	Parenting	Child's behaviour
Secure	Consistently responsive	Approaches carers directly and positively Learns sense of trust; deals better with stress
Avoidant	Consistently unresponsive	Denies or stops communicating distress Leads to low self-esteem and later aggression
Ambivalent	Inconsistently responsive	Maximizes distress Lack of exploration
Disorganized	Cause of the distress*	No strategy can bring comfort or care

* This may occur when parents are abusive, are emotionally unreachable (major unresolved issues from the past, depressed, psychotic, heavy drug or alcohol users) or fail to protect the child. There is no coherent strategy that children can use to reduce anxiety. Children may then *freeze*, either physically or psychologically.

1. Secure attachment
2. Avoidant attachment
3. Ambivalent or inconsistent attachment
4. Incoherent or disorganized attachment.

Around 70% of children develop a secure attachment. Secure attachment with at least one adult is a necessary precondition for the development of resilience (p. 216).

If the normal routes to proximity and security are unsuccessful, children have to either develop psychological strategies that attempt to minimize anxiety (defences), or try to find alternative creative ways to secure the attachment figure psychologically. For example, if parents only respond to negative behaviour rather than to a child's expressions of sad feelings, a child might learn to hit out when he feels sad or insecure. He will then get some emotional security, but at the expense of 'burying' his real feelings.

Insecure attachment is a risk factor that will interact with other risks present in the emotional and physical environment of the growing child (Fig. 3.2).

Attachment behaviour is seen throughout the lifespan and is a key part of our psychological make-up. Parents experiencing a threat to their security associated with ill health in their child may respond with apparently undue anxiety or anger. In this context, it is helpful to consider the parents' emotional state as a normal expression of their attachment behaviour. In this case, the paediatrician is being asked to take the role of the good-enough parent in helping to regulate the parental distress.

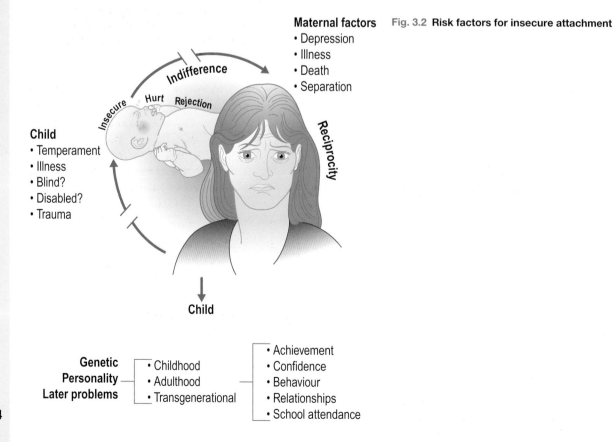

Fig. 3.2 **Risk factors for insecure attachment**

The effect of trauma and neglect

Abuse and neglect in the first years of life have a particularly pervasive impact (see also Chs 21 and 36).

Disorganized attachment, frequently the result of maltreatment, becomes in itself a major risk factor that, in the 'wrong' circumstances, can disrupt many different areas of development. It is predictive of the development of behavioural problems at preschool and school age in both high-risk and normal samples.

Disorganized attachment in infancy has been linked to a number of severe mental health problems in adulthood. Other early attachment experiences are also linked with adult psychopathology. Loss predicts multiple disorders, including depression, anxiety and antisocial personality disorder.

The roots of violence

Delinquent, antisocial and violent behaviour, frequently associated with no sense of either empathy or remorse, has been traced back to being on the receiving end of abuse and neglect during the first 2 years of life. Violence 'is the manifestation of attachment behaviour gone wrong'

The development of a secure attachment relationship protects against later aggression and violence in three ways:
1. Through learning empathy (the ability to be mindful of another's mind, and thus mind how you treat them)
2. Through learning self-control
3. Through learning to modulate feelings, particularly those that are destructive, and the ability to self-soothe.

The context of the attachment relationship

The parent–baby relationship is always located in a wider context, within which are found both risk and protective factors. These can harm the baby directly (e.g. pollution, unhealthy housing) but mostly they are titrated into the relationship via their effects on the parents' functioning, since they dictate the baby's immediate experiences. Box 3.1 summarizes the risk factors that affect parent–child relationships.

Conclusion

Successful parenting is a principal key to this and the next generation. As paediatricians we have the

---

BOX 3.1 Risk factors affecting the parent–child relationship

Child
- Prematurity or congenital abnormalities
- Difficult temperament
- Early problems making a baby difficult and less rewarding
- Language delay, coordination problems, physical or sensory disabilities
- Significant illness

Parents
- Lack of ability to attune to baby
- Lack of interaction or maltreatment
- Mental health problem or background of abuse, neglect or loss
- Addiction (this may be associated with the baby having cognitive/developmental/behavioural difficulties associated with addiction during pregnancy. Addiction is also an attachment-related disorder and may predispose to attachment difficulties in the baby)
- Family dysfunction
- Domestic violence
- Single teenage mother without support

Environment
- Poverty is a major risk factor. There is a high prevalence of depression, attachment difficulties and post-traumatic stress among mothers living in poverty. Associated poor nutrition has effects on the child in utero and during later development

---

privileged role of being offered a window to this part of people's lives. It is important to remember to support and help parents in this role at every opportunity, as well as to know when to intervene when a child is being harmed by inappropriate or dangerous parenting. Whilst our foremost duty is always to the child, the balance between protecting the parent–child attachment and protecting the child poses professional challenges at times for us all.

 http://www.aimh.org.uk

Association for Infant Mental Health UK; follow links to 'The Importance of the Early Years and Evidence-Based Practice'

 http://www.zerotothree.org

Comprehensive interactive resource for parents and professionals on normal development 0–3 years

Shimon Barak   Alison Kelly   Francis B. Mimouni
Linda Wolfson   Charlotte M. Wright

CHAPTER

4

Nutrition, infant feeding and weaning

LEARNING OUTCOMES

By the end of this chapter you should:

- Understand the physiology and mechanics of breastfeeding and how this can best be supported
- Understand the characteristics of infant formula and its role as a breast-milk substitute
- Know how nutrient requirements change through early life to adulthood and how they relate to growth and maturation
- Know how dietary intake varies with the developmental stage of the child in order to fulfil those requirements
- Understand how nutritional status can be most effectively assessed in childhood.

Introduction

Nutrition is the process of intake, assimilation and utilization of nutrients essential to support life, sustain metabolism, provide fuel for activity and supply the basic building blocks for growth and tissue repair. Food has to be ingested, digested and absorbed and adequate neonatal nutrition depends both on the quantity and quality of the food intake and the functional integrity and capacity of the gastrointestinal tract. The quantitative requirement for energy, water, fat, protein, carbohydrate, vitamins and minerals is determined by a delicate equilibrium between supply and demand. But not all can be measured in grams and calories. Eating satisfies physical requirements but nourishment also meets social, psychological and emotional needs. This chapter will consider how the balance of supply and demand is achieved at different stages and how it may be upset. It will consider the change in nutrient requirements through childhood, reflecting the varying pace of growth and changing activity levels, from the immobile but rapidly growing infant to the more active but slower-growing child. In parallel it will consider the variability of dietary intake in relation to the developmental stage of the child in order to fulfil those requirements. Finally it will consider methods by which the nutritional status of children can be effectively assessed, from the simple measure of weight and estimates of dietary intake to the more complex measures of body composition and energy expenditure.

Pregnancy and fetal nutrition

The growth of an individual begins in utero, and maternal health and nutrition can impact on the nutritional status of the fetus in a number of ways. Nowadays pregnancy is regarded as a complex tripartite inter-relationship (maternal, placental, and fetal) reflecting and influenced by both the increased maternal requirements and the needs of an ever-growing developing fetus. The energy cost of a normal preg-

MODULE ONE

nancy is around 50 000 kilocalories with an average maternal weight gain of around 12.5 kg. This necessitates the daily intake of an additional 300 kilocalories and 15 grams of protein as well as 250 milligrams of calcium, 30 milligrams of iron and 400 micrograms of folate, an essential cofactor for DNA synthesis which when supplemented before conception reduces the risk of neural tube defects.

Low maternal weight gain in pregnancy correlates with lower infant birth weight and increased perinatal mortality, but maternal under-nutrition as a *cause* of low weight gain is only seen in conditions of extreme starvation, because of the fetus's preferential access to maternal nutrients. The placenta is a highly active organ metabolically, producing hormones essential for maintenance of pregnancy and growth factors. Additionally active transport mechanisms deliver nutrients from the maternal circulation to the fetus.

Fetal life is the period of most rapid growth and change in body proportion and composition. During early life, the fetal water content is high, and there is a predominance of extracellular ions such as sodium and chloride. With organogenesis and increasing cell mass the content of intracellular ions, such as potassium, increases. During the third trimester the fetus triples in weight and doubles in length, and this period is associated with accretion of minerals such as calcium and iron. Protein stores increase and fat deposition occurs prior to birth. Therefore, infants of malnourished mothers or those born prematurely will have low nutrient stores and their growth and development during the first months of life may be at risk.

Intrauterine growth restriction

Limitation of the fetal growth potential is analogous to weight faltering in the infant. A newborn can be defined as 'Small for Gestational Age' (SGA) if their birthweight is below the 5th or 10th centile for age and 'Very Small for Gestational Age' (VSGA) if below 1–3rd centile, but the exact weight this represents will vary depending on the growth chart used. The causes of both can be either intrinsic or environmental. Infants that have not reached their growth potential due to pathological growth impairment account for approximately 30% of cases whereas babies that are constitutionally small account for the remaining 70%. Ultrasound evaluation usually correlates with this difference and shows two distinct patterns of growth restriction. *Symmetrical* growth retardation is usually related to intrinsic characteristics or pathologies, commences early and results in low weight, length and head circumference. *Asymmetric* retardation, characterized by late flattening of the growth curve and low weight but relative sparing of length and head

circumference, is more likely to result from placental insufficiency, caused by maternal hypertension, preeclampsia or, commonly, smoking. Rapid catch-up growth usually occurs in early infancy.

Infancy

The average term baby is born weighing 2.5 to 4 kg and measuring 47 to 52 cm and having sufficient stores of energy and nutrients to deal with the transition from being a fetus under constant placental nutrient supply to becoming an infant on intermittent oral feeds. Infants require three times more energy per kilogram than adults, reflecting both higher metabolic requirements and energy requirements for growth, particularly the brain. The infant also lays down considerable fat stores to supply rapid growth during the first year, and later on, as the requirements for growth diminish, to supply rising activity levels.

The benefits of breastfeeding and hazards of breast-milk substitutes

Breast milk is the sole and essential food for newborn infants. Fresh human milk is a live, complex substance providing both nutrition and immune protection and no substitute can completely replicate its physiological role (Box 4.1). Recent studies have demonstrated the association of formula feeding with increased morbidity in the UK and excess infant mortality in the USA. Breast milk is particularly important for low birth weight and sick infants where it has been associated with reduced mortality from necrotising enterocolitis and better cognitive function. The protective effect of breast milk is greatest in the early weeks of life, but continues throughout the first year. For this reason, the use of breast-milk substitutes remains, even in Europe, an important cause of preventable morbidity and mortality in infancy. Although increased promotion of breastfeeding has resulted in a substantial improvement in breastfeeding rates, in some parts of Europe a fifth of infants still never receive any breast milk, with only a minority receiving any breast milk beyond the age of 6 months.

In 1981, to overcome a lack of professional support and the effects of marketing of formula, the World Health Organization (WHO) launched the 'International Code of Marketing of Breast milk Substitutes' to protect and promote breastfeeding and to ensure the proper use of breast-milk substitutes. In 1989 the WHO and UNICEF published the 'Ten Steps to Successful Breastfeeding' to establish effective breastfeeding practices amongst professionals. Mothers who deliver in hospitals and communities where the

BOX 4.1 What is in breast milk?

- Water, sugars (7%), fat (4%) and protein (1.3%)
- Enzymes that aid digestion (e.g. lipase) and may also be bactericidal (e.g. lysozyme)
- Hormones, including insulin, thyroid stimulating hormone and growth hormone. Epidermal growth factor helps the gut to mature and become more resistant to pathogens
- Immunoglobulins: antibodies against previous maternal infections and secretory IgA, which coats the lining of the gut as well as the entero/bronchomammary pathway
- Living white cells to engulf/destroy bacteria and viral fragments: thought to trigger the baby's immune response
- Transfer factors to help absorption of nutrients from milk: e.g. lactoferrin, which assists with iron absorption, also 'mopping up' excess iron and making it unavailable to bacteria, thus rendering the gut less conducive to bacterial growth (e.g. *E. coli*, *Giardia lamblia* and *Entamoeba histolytica*)
- Bifidus factor: facilitates the growth of *Lactobacillus bifidus*, which creates an acidic environment (low pH) and inhibits bacterial growth
- Oligosaccharides: simple carbohydrates that prevent pathogens adhering to the gut wall
- Anti-inflammatory molecules: dampen down the inflammatory response of the gut to pathogens. This may be a key factor reducing morbidity in necrotizing enterocolitis

BOX 4.2 Key factors in establishing breastfeeding on maternity units

- Skin-to-skin contact
- Rooming in
- Feeding on demand, not to the clock, for as long as the baby wants
- Good positioning and correct attachment at the breast
- Skilled support when needed

'Ten Steps' have been implemented are more likely to breastfeed successfully (Box 4.2). A further step was the 'Baby-Friendly Hospital Initiative', launched in 1991, by UNICEF and the WHO to ensure all maternity units, whether free standing or in a hospital, become centres of breastfeeding support.

Establishing breastfeeding

For breastfeeding to be established successfully, the mother needs to produce enough milk but the baby

BOX 4.3 The physiology of lactation

The endocrine control of lactation

The anterior pituitary gland secretes prolactin, directing the acini cells to produce milk and priming the prolactin receptor sites for future milk production. Prolactin levels stay high after a feed and stimulate the breast to produce milk for the next feed. Levels are higher at night and therefore night feeding is good for milk production. Inadequate stimulation may lead to sites shutting down and reduced milk capacity.

The hormone oxytocin assists milk ejection. The posterior pituitary secretes oxytocin, causing the myoepithelial cells around the alveoli to contract and leading to the 'let-down' or 'milk ejection' reflex. Milk collected in the alveoli flows along the ducts to the lactiferous sinuses. Oxytocin opens the ducts and helps the milk to flow easily.

The autocrine control of lactation

After the early weeks, milk production is controlled more locally within the breast. The feedback inhibitor (FIL) is a protein within the milk, which enables the breasts to work independently. FIL protects the breast from the harmful effects of being too full; conversely, frequent suckling or expression causes the inhibitor in milk to fall, so that the breast makes more milk. If the baby prefers one breast, this breast will make more milk.

must also remove it frequently and effectively (Box 4.3).

Many breastfeeding problems have their roots in the newborn period when breastfeeding is being established. Ideally this should start with skin-to-skin contact at birth, leading to the first feed when the baby is ready. For lactation to be successful, mothers must learn to recognize signs of hunger, respond to the baby's needs and feed on demand, i.e. as long and as often as the baby wants.

The expected pattern of feeding changes at different stages and varies between babies but frequent feeds and using both breasts at each feed during the early weeks encourages maximal milk production. After the milk supply is established, the breasts may be alternated at successive feedings.

However, babies may sometimes need to be wakened for a feed when the mother's breasts are overfull, or the baby's demands are so infrequent that the breasts are under-stimulated.

On the maternity unit, babies should normally stay with their mother ('roomed in') at all times, except when the mother's or baby's condition prevents this. Of all of the 'ten steps', there is the strongest link between rooming in and successful breastfeeding.

Correct   Incorrect

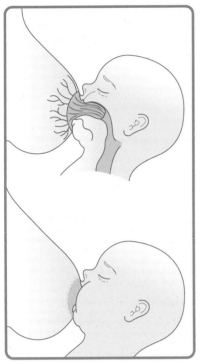 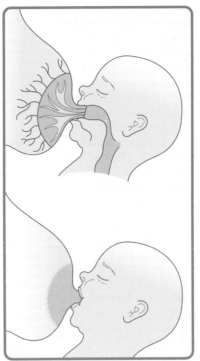

Fig. 4.1 Signs that a baby is correctly attached at the breast.
The baby has a wide gaping mouth. Generally, more of the areola should be seen above the baby's mouth than below. The baby's lower lip will be flared out against the breast and the chin will be directly in contact with the breast. The baby's neck will be slightly extended. The jaw muscles work rhythmically and this movement can be seen extending to the ears. If the cheeks are being sucked in, the baby is not correctly attached. The baby sucks deeply with pauses, rather than continually.

Positioning and attachment at the breast

For a breast to produce milk, it must be emptied frequently and effectively otherwise it will not be stimulated sufficiently to refill. Therefore establishing correct attachment is essential (Fig. 4.1). Babies remove milk by compressing the lactiferous sinuses in the breast, creating a vacuum between the mouth and breast. The breast response of ejection or 'let down' will only occur when the baby can correctly attach and coordinate suckling. Correct positioning also plays a crucial role in the prevention of sore nipples. Each mother will have individual preferences, abilities and needs, but the principles are as follows:

- *The baby's head and body should be in a straight line (without restricting the baby's head from slightly extending backwards).* Babies cannot suckle or swallow easily if their head is twisted or bent, and will not open their mouth or put their tongue forward widely if their head is unable to tilt back.
- *The baby's mouth should face the breast, with the top lip opposite the nipple.* The maternal nipple points to the baby's nostrils, and the head is slightly extended backwards, allowing the baby's chin to come to the breast in advance of his nose.
- *The mother should hold the baby's body close to hers.* The angle at which she holds the baby, directly facing her chest or angled under her breasts, depends on the size and shape of her breasts and the direction her nipples point.

- *The position should be sustainable.* If the baby is newborn, the mother should support his or her whole body, and not just the head and shoulders.

The role of the doctor in maintaining breastfeeding

For most women, normal lactation is possible: milk insufficiency occurs in only 0.2% of mammals. Despite this, many mothers still fail to establish effective feeding and breastfeeding cessation most often occurs in the first few days. While this may partly reflect the lack of a breastfeeding culture, mothers are too easily undermined by conflicting professional information and a lack of support. Effective support for breastfeeding requires a basic understanding of the physiology of lactation, effective newborn feeding behaviour and confidence in normal neonatal adaptation (Boxes 4.3 and 4.4), as well as a practical understanding of the mechanics of feeding. Women most commonly give up breastfeeding very early due to a perception that they are 'failing' at it. They may have sore nipples and breasts or difficulties getting the baby to attach effectively or at all; if so, the baby may be fretful and apparently unsatisfied by feeds. Nursing and medical staff can also inadvertently induce a sense of failure by excessive concern about weight gain or blood sugar levels, or by separation of mother and baby for medical procedures. Confidence in breastfeeding is severely undermined if supplementary

Metabolic adaptation

At birth, the baby must adapt to the abrupt cessation of placental nutrition and to the introduction of milk feeds. In the healthy full-term infant, changes after birth in hormones and enzymes allow energy-providing fuels such as glucose and fat to be released from body stores. Fat is broken down in the liver, forming ketone bodies that are important alternative fuels to glucose, particularly in the first 2–3 postnatal days until feeding is established. Healthy term babies can sustain themselves for several days until demand feeding is established. Some groups of infants (e.g. low-birth weight infants, infants of diabetic mothers) are at risk of failure of metabolic adaptation, resulting in low levels of glucose and fatty fuels in the blood.

Osmoregulation

Most newborn babies lose weight as they excrete surplus interstitial fluid. Colostrum is the ideal way to provide nutrients in concentrated form, allowing the baby to make this adjustment easily. The amount of breast milk available at a feed gradually increases, provided feeding is frequent. Using biochemical means to assess fluid balance can be misleading, as during this period of adaptation later norms may not apply and small rises in sodium and urea may be without significance or consequence. During early infancy fluid requirements are high, due to higher obligatory losses from the skin and respiratory and renal tracts, and this makes the infant susceptible to dehydration, but breastfeeding provides sufficient fluids and does not need to be supplemented in the healthy infant.

formula milk feeds are recommended, particularly in the first days. Doctors should encourage a policy of non-supplementation in maternity units, wherever possible. Neonatal procedures and policies should be designed to ensure minimal interruptions to feeding. Doctors should familiarize themselves with common problems that may arise and what practical interventions can be tried. Supplementation may appear to solve a short-term problem by removing the immediate perceived risk of underfeeding. However, this may lead to permanent cessation of breastfeeding and its protective benefits, exposing the child to more substantial long-term risks; it may also deter breastfeeding of subsequent children.

Common feeding problems in the neonatal period

To assess if nutrition is adequate a full history should be taken including the number of meals, the interval between them, the output of stool and urine, the baby's mood and his daily schedule. If formula fed, the daily quantity should be noted. If breastfed the physician should seek signs and proof that effective lactation has been established, sometimes with the assistance of a feeding advisor or breastfeeding counsellor. Weighing can be a reliable parameter if measurements are correctly recorded on accurate scales.

Delay in establishing feeding

Some babies may initially be too sleepy to attach and suck at the breast. This is not uncommon and over-medicalized management can lead to unnecessary breast-feeding cessation, since it rarely reflects underlying illness or metabolic disturbance. The mother may have had sedatives in labour or have been separated from her baby and missed feeding cues. Breast milk may need to be expressed by hand (at least eight times in 24 hours) to stimulate lactation and keep the mother motivated. Babies who are still unwilling to feed after 48 hours should be examined carefully and investigated if indicated. If alternative feeding is needed, this should consist of expressed breast milk, given by cup, unless the baby is unwell. Tubes are rarely necessary and bottle teats may interfere with the normal imprinting of correct attachment.

Excessive early weight loss

Newborns lose 4–7% of their birth weight with the nadir around 48–72 hours and regain their birth weight usually by the age of 10–14 days. Greater weight loss is seen in relatively large infants, while growth-retarded infants commonly show none. Standard growth charts (apart from the new WHO charts) do not allow for neonatal loss and thus are unreliable in the first weeks. Where weight loss is greater than 10% at any stage, the baby should be fully examined and feeding assessed, but there is rarely a need for supplementation with formula or IV fluids, unless the baby is unwell or has severe hypernatraemia.

With most babies, the feeding technique can be improved or expressed breast milk can be given. This is preferred to formula, as breast milk has the lowest renal solute load and is more easily digested; therefore, larger volumes can be given safely. It also encourages continued breast stimulation and effective milk removal.

Overfeeding and regurgitation

Regurgitation of small amounts of swallowed food during or shortly after meals is very common and as a rule needs no investigation. It can be avoided by proper handling of the infant during meals and eructation of swallowed air towards the end of each meal. On the other hand vomiting, defined as the almost complete emptying of the stomach, may be associated with underlying pathologies and should always be investigated, in particular if the colour of the vomitus is green. The most common cause of regurgitations is overfeeding, mostly seen in formula-fed infants, the result of excessive meals or concentrated food. In many cases the reason is failure on behalf of the parents to recognize the infant's food cues and misinterpretation of his crying as being hungry.

Hypoglycaemia

Hypoglycaemia should be identified and treated in sick, symptomatic or high-risk infants. Concerns may arise in the slow-to-feed or sleepy breastfed baby, but generally speaking, healthy term babies are unlikely to have problems and usually supportive breastfeeding measures and supervision are all that is required. Hypoglycaemia in the high-risk or sick neonate is discussed in Chapter 47.

Jaundice (see also Ch. 47)

Physiological jaundice of the newborn can be more pronounced if feeding is delayed or restricted.

Formula feeding

Types of formula milks and their preparation

If a mother needs or chooses to use a formula milk, it should be one that meets with the Codex Alimentarius of the joint FAO/WHO food programme, which sets standards and recommendations for all formula milks. Recently, a European commission has updated these recommendations and hopefully in the future the Commission Directive 2006/141/EC and Council Directive 92/52/EEC will represent a unified European standard for all infant formulae. Currently, all formulae recommended for general use are made from modified cow's milk.

For infants up to the age of 1 year of life parents should choose a whey-based infant formula ('first' milk). Casein-dominant formulas ('second' milks) are nearer to cow's milk and less physiologically similar to breast milk. Parents may use them after the 1st birthday but may at this stage also switch to commercial cow's milk. Formula milk can be purchased in a 'ready to feed' form or dried for reconstitution with boiled, cooled water. Each feed should be made fresh and not stored, to reduce the risk of contamination. Formula-fed premature and sick babies should be fed initially on sterilized 'ready to feed' milks. All equipment used in the preparation and feeding should be washed thoroughly and sterilized.

Other breast milk substitutes

Current recommendations are to avoid intake of unmodified bovine and goat milk before the age of 1 year, particularly low-fat or skim milks.

Soya milk formulae raise many potential problems, particularly in relation to their phyto-oestrogen content and their use of dextrin maltose in place of lactose and should not be recommended without sound medical reasons. Hypoallergenic formulae should be used for allergy only after a detailed medical and dietetic assessment. Powder milk, concentrated milk, rice milk and other 'white' liquid solutions do not meet the nutritional requirements of infants and parents should be advised that they are unsuitable and potentially unsafe.

Complementary feeding

Both human milk from a mother on a sufficient and balanced diet and commercial infant formulae supply all the necessary nutrients for thriving in the first half year of life. An exception must be made for vitamin D and fluoride (see later). Human milk or commercial formula should also remain the main nutrient sources in the second half-year and an important component of the diet until the age of 2 years. Around the age of 6 months complementary solid foods should be started to ensure adequate intake of proteins and nutrients.

This process, called 'weaning', has been the subject of debate, especially concerning the optimal timing to begin it. If started too early, solid foods may stress the immature gut, kidneys and immune system and reduce breast milk intake, lessening its immune protective effects. Starting too late may result in under nutrition and food refusal. Solid foods require a range of new skills that need to be learnt by infants with the help and encouragement of their caretakers. The skills needed and the types of foods that allow their acquisition are shown in Table 4.1, along with the sorts of problem that may present at different stages.

The toddler diet

Problem-orientated topic:

feeding problems in a toddler

Martyna, a 2-year-old girl, has been found to be iron-deficient and mum describes her as always being a bad feeder, particularly since solids were introduced. Now she eats 'nothing', though she will drink large amounts of milk.

Continued overleaf

Table 4.1 **Complementary feeding stages and associated problems**

Age range	Skills to be acquired	Food types used	Common problems	Solutions
4–6 months	Form a bolus of food and pass it to the back of the mouth so that it can be swallowed without choking	First-stage foods: smooth bland cereal purées, gradually thickened over time	Chokes when fed	May be too young: if under 6 months, suggest waiting Adjust consistency of purée and start with very small amounts
6 months	Become accustomed to new flavours and smells	Addition of puréed fruit or vegetables to feeds	Refuses new flavours and foods	Most infants require repeated exposures to new tastes before accepting them
6–9 months	Chew lumpy foods	Second-stage foods: coarse purées and sloppy foods with lumps	Gags on lumps	Avoid foods with discrete lumps: offer progressively thickened purées of even consistency
6–12 months	Bite and chew solid foods Finger feeding	Solid foods that can be easily softened in the mouth, e.g. potato, pasta	Refuses to be fed from spoon Won't chew solids	Offer dry finger foods suitable for self-feeding: bread, fruit, biscuits, processed meat Avoid very resistant foods Keep offering solids and avoid excessive milk intake

Table 4.2 **Nutrient contents per 50 g of typical infant and toddler food**

Type of food	Energy (kJ)	Fat (g)	Carbohydrate (g)	Protein (g)	Vitamin C (mg)	Iron (mg)
Breast milk	145	2.1	3.6	0.65	2	0.04
Puréed carrot	46	0.20	2.2	0.3	1	0.2
Small banana, mashed	202	0.15	11.6	0.6	5.5	0.15
Mashed potato with margarine	219	2.2	7.8	0.9	2.5	0.2
Mince beef, stewed	870	13.5	0	21.8	0	2.2
Chicken, boiled	384	3.7	0	14.6	0	0.6
Sugared cereal + milk, $^1/_2$ bowl	271	4.6	11.3	1.8	0.4	0.7
Toast and butter, 2 slices	439	6.0	11.4	1.9	0	0.4
Fromage frais, $^2/_3$ small pot	276	2.9	2.7	2.7	0	0.04
Apple slices	76	0.05	4.5	10.2	7	0.05
Digestive biscuits, 3	890	9.4	30.9	2.8	0	1.4

Q1. What should a child be eating at this age and what is the usual main source of iron?

Q2. How will you assess her nutritional status?

Q1. What should a child be eating at this age and what is the usual main source of iron?

During the second year of life the rate of growth slows, but children become increasingly mobile and activity levels rise. Overall nutrient needs per kilogram are slightly less than in the first year of life, but are still around double adult requirements. From the age of 1 year, children should progress to the family diet including all the main food groups. Energy requirements remain high, so that starchy, high-fat foods are often preferred, while fruit and vegetables, which are low-energy, are rejected (Table 4.2). It is important to continue to offer small amounts of these and other new foods to establish familiarity, but it is unrealistic to expect most toddlers to eat large amounts. After the age of 2 years a child can eat the same diet as the rest of the family. A varied diet is recommended, one that supplies all known required nutrients and emphasizes the intake of grains, fruits, and vegetables, restrict dietary fat to a third of the total daily energy intake and limit saturated fatty acids to not more than a third of total fat intake.

Red meat is an important source of haem iron and one which is easily absorbed; solid meat can be challenging for toddlers, but minced and processed meats are popular. Milk remains an important part of the diet, supplying both energy and calcium and toddlers should have two portions of dairy products per day. Follow-on formula milks (which provide additional vitamins and minerals) are only necessary if the solid diet is limited. Occasionally, when very large volumes of milk are consumed and lead to refusal of solid food, the volume or frequency of milk feeds may need to be restricted to stimulate appetite. Drinks should be given from a cup from 1 year of age.

Vitamins and minerals

Vitamin and mineral deficiencies, except for iron, are rare in healthy infants but may occur in higher-risk groups, such as premature babies. Being fortified, breakfast cereals, bread and margarine are important sources of various vitamins and micronutrients, as are citrus fruit juices. If the diet range is poor, vitamin supplements should be given. Supplemental vitamin D drops are recommended from early infancy and even from birth as, in spite of sunshine exposure, deficiency may occur in high-risk groups where there has been maternal deficiency or late introduction of complementary feeding and in infants of South Asian origin because of their pigmentation and relative low intake of routinely fortified foods. Vitamin K is routinely given at birth to prevent haemorrhagic disease of the newborn.

With increasing age, the pace of growth continues to slow. By the age of 5, children should ideally be eating the same range of family foods as their elder siblings and parents, and usual healthy eating guidelines should apply. Food consumed should be less energy-dense than in the early years and consumption of lower-fat, higher-fibre foods should be encouraged (Box 4.5). As eating habits develop, a healthy eating pattern should be adopted, with plenty of fruit and vegetables and sparing amounts of high-fat and high-sugar foods.

Q2. How will you assess her nutritional status?

Although it seems logical to assess nutritional status by measuring what is eaten, this in fact supplies very limited useful information. There are two reasons: firstly, each individual's nutrient requirements vary, depending on many factors, few of which can be accurately estimated; secondly, dietary assessment is intrinsically inaccurate. Thus dietary assessment cannot be safely used to diagnose nutritional insufficiency, although food diaries can provide helpful information about the range and type of foods eaten and the meal pattern, and may act as a guide to dietary advice once a problem has been identified (Fig. 4.2). In contrast, measurements of weight, height and the calculation of body mass index (BMI = weight/height^2), provide essential, objective

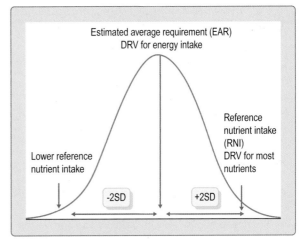

Dietary reference values (DRV)
- These are the reference ideal nutrient requirements set for adults and for different ages of children
- Calculated from amount of nutrients eaten by healthy normally growing individuals
- Values are designed to avoid inadequacy in the diet

Estimated average requirement (EAR)
- The mean value of the requirement for a group of individuals (this is assumed to follow a normal distribution curve)
- Intakes of this amount should be sufficient for 50% of the population

Reference nutrient intake (RNI)
- Intakes two standard deviations (SDs) above the EAR
- Should be sufficient for almost all the population

Lower reference nutrient intake (LRNI)
- Intakes two SDs below the EAR
- Intakes below this level are inadequate for most of the population

Recommended requirements
- Defined as the RNI for most nutrients, where consumption of excess is not harmful
- EAR used for energy, since excess energy intake above average requirements leads to obesity
- DRVs can be used in food labelling or to assess intake and guide dietary prescription

Fig. 4.2 How nutrient requirements are calculated

information about nutrient balance, particularly if used in combination (Table 4.3).

In infancy, moderate deviations in weight are common, but falls through two intercentile spaces (1.3 SD) are rarer, though the exact percentage doing so will depend on the growth chart used and the starting centile. Very small infants (<3rd centile) usually show catch-up growth in the early weeks and any drop away is unusual, but very large infants (>97th) may show falls of up to 3 intercentile spaces (compared to WHO charts). Obtaining accurate height (and length) measurements in the preschool years is intrinsically difficult, so that apparent decelerations are most commonly due to measurement error. After

In recognition of the contribution of diet to cardiovascular diseases, cancer and the rising problem of obesity, policies are being developed throughout Europe to improve the health of its citizens through encouraging healthier eating. Recommendations include:

- Educational campaigns aimed at salt reduction and obesity awareness
- Simplification of food labelling to allow consumers to make healthier choices
- Review of the advertising and promotion of unhealthy food and drink products to children
- Continuation of work with industry to improve the nutritional content of processed foods (e.g. salt and sugar reduction in breakfast cereals)
- Implementing programmes which provide disadvantaged pregnant women and mothers with access to fresh fruit, vegetables and milk
- Healthy schools initiative, e.g. provision of free fruit to 4–6-year-olds

the age of 5 (and before puberty) variations in height of more than one centile space occur in less than 5% of children.

A full assessment should always involve calculating BMI and plotting this on a centile chart, since BMI values vary greatly through childhood. Anthropometry cannot distinguish between different body compartments; thus a muscular athletic child with a low fat mass could have a high BMI, while a child with cerebral palsy with a very low muscle mass could have a low BMI but a high fat mass. However, the current gold standard measure of body composition, using stable isotopes, is expensive and not generally available. Less direct measures, which may prove useful in future, are not yet adequately standardized for routine use in childhood. In practice, in the assessment of obesity, a high BMI (> 98th centile) equates closely with high adiposity.

Energy expenditure can also be measured accurately in a research setting using stable isotopes, but there are currently no standard methods for field or clinical use, although accelerometers are providing interesting research data.

Table 4.3 Strengths and limitations of different nutritional assessment methods

	Method	Strengths	Limitations
Dietary assessment	24-hour recall, 3–7-day diary or weighed record	Allows targeted dietary advice	Individual requirements vary greatly Portion size uncertain in unweighed records Diet during recording period may not be representative, particularly weighed records Exact nutrient content of foods vary
Anthropometry			
Weight	Naked weight on electronic scale	Summary of overall growth, particularly in infancy Serial measures can identify changes in nutritional status Easy to measure accurately	Cannot distinguish between bone, fat and muscle mass
Height	Standing or lying, without shoes on rigid measure or stadiometer	Indicator of stunting if used serially, or related to parental height Easy to measure	Most variation in height not nutritionally determined Inaccurate in preschool children
Weight for height (BMI)	Weight (kg)/height (m²)	Indicator of both wasting and overweight Allows variations in weight to be interpreted in growing child	Cannot distinguish between fat and muscle mass Gives no measure of growth over time Large intrinsic measurement error
Body composition			
Stable isotopes	Deuterium-labelled water given by mouth and concentration in urine measured by mass spectrometry	Gold standard method, highly accurate	Usually unavailable except for extreme cases as is expensive and labour intensive
Dual-energy X-ray absorptiometry (DXA)	Absorption of low-dose X-ray estimates bone and muscle mass	Provides fairly robust, accurate estimates	Costly equipment, not portable Normal range for children not well delineated
Bioelectrical impedance	Conduction of current through limbs and body used to estimate non-fat mass	Portable, cheap, reliable	Current childhood formulae not robust Normal range for children not well delineated

Assessment of micronutrient status presents different challenges. Serum levels usually only partly reflect whole body content, particularly where the nutrient is stored, as with iron, or in a deficiency state where the nutrient may be cleared from plasma very quickly. Signs of frank deficiency may be distinctive but are rare and, ideally, insufficiency should be identified before they occur. The markers and diagnostic criteria for the most common childhood deficiency states, iron deficiency and rickets, are described in later sections.

Religious and cultural dietary restrictions

Families may have special dietary practices or exclusions that reflect a religious or other affiliation. These will vary between apparently similar ethnic groups (e.g. Sikh as opposed to Muslim Punjabis), and within a religious group depending on their degree of adherence (e.g. ultra-orthodox as opposed to reform Jews). Most Muslim and Jewish families will avoid all pork and any non-halal or non-kosher meat respectively, leading sometimes to the false impression that they are vegetarian.

Families who do describe themselves as vegetarian may range from avoidance only of meat (but not fish) to those who avoid all meat, fish, eggs and dairy products. Other families may exclude particular foods due to personal beliefs about the risks associated with them.

Thus it is essential to ask all families about their usual diet and any possible exclusions, and not to make assumptions. In practice dietary variations that lead to nutrient deficiency are usually extreme and rarely religiously determined, with diets that exclude dairy products (an important source of energy) most likely to lead to problems.

Further reading

Committee on Medical Aspects of Food 1994 Annex IV to Weaning and the weaning diet, Report 45. HMSO, London

Department of Health 2005 Dietary reference values for food energy and nutrients for the United Kingdom: Report on Health and Social Subjects. HMSO, London Report 41

Garrow JS, James W, Ralph A 2000. Human Nutrition and Dietetics. 10th ed. Edinburgh: Churchill Livingstone.

Michaelson K, Weaver LT, Branca F, Robertson A 2000 Feeding and nutrition of infants and young children. Copenhagen: World Health Organization; Report nr 87. Available from: http://www.euro.who.int/document/WS_115_2000FE.pdf

Morgan Jane B, Dickerson JWT (eds) 2003 Nutrition in early life. Wiley, Chichester

Wright C, Lakshman R, Emmett P, Ong KK 2008 Implications of adopting the WHO 2006 Child Growth Standard in the UK: two prospective cohort studies. Arch Dis Child 93(7):566–9

Wright CM 2002 The use and interpretation of growth charts. Current Paediatrics 12:279–282

*Edited by Jonathan Darling,
Diego van Esso, Adamos Hadjipanayis*

Toolkit for child health and disease

MODULE TWO

Mark Bradbury   Alan Cade   Alfred J. Nicholson

CHAPTER

History-taking and physical examination

MODULE TWO

LEARNING OUTCOMES

By the end of this chapter you should:

● Be able to take a paediatric history
● Be able to conduct an age-specific general examination of children
● Be able to examine each organ system in detail
● Be able to recognize common and important paediatric conditions and syndromes
● Be able to recognize the pathognomonic features of the more common conditions in childhood
● Know the normal range of physiological parameters in children.

Introduction

The skills of history-taking and physical examination in children are an essential part of your paediatric toolkit. Interacting with children can be rewarding and fun, but it can initially appear daunting. You need to develop and hone these skills through constant practice.

Rather than blindly asking the same questions and performing the same examination sequence by rote in every consultation, you need to develop a logical and strategic approach focused around the child's problem.

5

At the outset of any consultation, you establish the nature of the child's presenting problem(s) and construct a hypothesis of what might be the most likely cause, along with other possible causes. This initial broad differential diagnosis is then modified as you proceed through the history and examination. Throughout the process, you are seeking evidence for and against your various differentials, and this mental list may continually be reordered as you acquire new information. You thus adapt your clinical approach to what you find as you go along, as well as to the individual circumstances of the child and family. Professional examinations look for this thoughtful and logical approach.

At the end of the process, you need to make sense of what you have discovered, construct a problem list and management plan, and communicate with the child and family about these. These aspects are covered later in this module (pp. 61 and 65).

Remember that the process of history-taking and examination can be powerfully therapeutic in its own right through the way you interact with the child and family. Attention to detail, careful listening, treating people with empathy, sensitivity and respect, clear explanations and finding time for questions can all make a difference.

History-taking

In order to formulate a diagnosis and an effective management plan for a child who is ill, it is important to have an appreciation of the problems which the child is presenting with and the context in which they are arising. The foundation for this formulation is a thorough history. An effective history-taking interview utilizes communication skills (active listening, good questioning and observing non-verbal communication) in a structured information-gathering process. The greater the history-taker's skill, the more accurate the differential diagnoses and the greater benefit to the patient.

The objectives of a history-taking interview include:

- Developing an appreciation of the presenting difficulties, their severity and the impact on the child and family
- Reaching a diagnosis or differential diagnosis, including an understanding of what factors may have triggered, exacerbated or maintained the presenting problem
- Consideration of the strengths of the family and child and whether they are able and motivated to work at resolving the presenting complaint, and what opportunities the healthcare team have to support the child and family
- Understanding what expectations, ideas and concerns the child and family have about the illness and its treatment.

Communication skills and the interview process

The initial communication during a history-taking interview offers the opportunity of establishing a good rapport at the same time as demonstrating professional competence and a respect for confidentiality. One of the challenges is the need to communicate relative to the child's age; this especially applies to adolescents. Good communication skills and practice at the interview process enable treatment to begin as soon as the family has entered the room.

With older children and teenagers it is good practice to take the story in their words first, then to repeat the questions to the parent(s). Unfortunately some parents interrupt, trying to be helpful, and at times it is necessary to conduct the interview with parent and child separately. With younger children, always have age-appropriate play materials on hand to entertain and relax the child and siblings. Gaining the child's interest and confidence can have a positive effect when it comes to the physical examination. It will also help parents to answer questions if they do not have to distract or comfort their child.

A simple ABCD approach can be used to plan the interview process:

- Accepting
- Broadening
- Clarifying
- Deepening.

Accepting

Accepting describes the strategy used at the opening of the interview. The factors to consider are:

- Greeting the child and each parent. It is worth asking at this stage how each of the adults and other children present are related to the child. This avoids the very embarrassing situation of mistaking an older parent for a grandparent or younger parent for a sibling later in the interview.
- Establishing a warm friendly atmosphere.
- Establishing rapport to help the child feel comfortable with you.
- Trying to maintain privacy and reduce distractions, switching off mobile phones and adjusting emergency bleeps to the vibrate setting.
- Sustaining eye contact and avoiding getting buried in a set of notes.
- Asking a simple question to prompt the presenting complaint and listening carefully to the reply.
- Observing the child–parent interaction during this early stage.

Often we cannot change the physical environment in which the interview takes place, but try to avoid the barrier of a desk, arranging the chairs in a less formal but practical configuration.

Broadening

At this point in the interview, open questions are useful:

- How?
- What?
- Why?
- When?
- Where?
- Who?

These allow the parent or child to do the majority of talking, again in their own words, about the presenting problems. Do not 'lead the witness'; use open-ended questions. Avoid jargon or more complicated medical words, and define terms that may be misunderstood. After this stage of the history, a broader understanding of the problem exists but specific details are often required, leading to the next stage.

Clarifying

With a long or complicated history, it is often helpful to summarize it and tell it back to the history-giver to check for errors. Important details regarding the presenting complaint may not have been mentioned spontaneously, and can be asked about using more direct, closed-style questions and often saving time. The additional information needed in the other sections of the history may be obtained using the same style of questions.

Deepening

This describes the questions that probe deeper into areas of concern, ideas and expectations, trying to uncover:

- Any hidden agendas
- Self-blame felt by the parents in relation to things they may have done or not done
- The extent of any frightening experiences of the illness for the parents and child
- Any unarticulated fears of death or bad outcomes.

This phase also presents an opportunity to ask about the impact of the illness on family life.

Using rather vague general questions and statements — for example, 'Other parents I have spoken to have said how worrying it was that…,' — and then pausing for a response is a method of deepening the interview.

How long should it take to elicit a history?

If you are presented with a child who is acutely ill with severe asthma or major trauma, take a short focused history, enquiring about the current problems, past medical history, and drug and allergy history only. This can be completed in minutes, not delaying the start of treatment. When the situation is under control, a more complete history can then be taken. This contrasts with a complex history in the outpatient department that may require 30 minutes or longer to complete.

Taking notes during the interview

It is often helpful to limit yourself to writing down a few important details during the history. This will help avoid long pauses for writing, improves eye contact and allows you to observe non-verbal communication. When writing in the medical notes, ensure your entry is **timed** and **dated**, and that you clearly identify yourself. If for any reason you wish to keep notes of the history for your own files, then it would be good practice to anonymize the history and keep it in a secure folder to protect confidentiality.

Organizing the content of the interview

A systematic method of organizing the content of a history-taking interview into separate sections is outlined below:

1. General information
2. Presenting complaint and history of the presenting complaint
3. Past medical history
4. Pregnancy and birth history
5. Feeding and dietary history
6. Growth
7. Developmental history
8. Medications and allergies
9. Immunizations
10. Family history
11. Social history
12. Review of systems.

This structure is familiar from adult history-taking but adds extra sections specifically relevant to children.

1. General information

Note the date, time and location of the interview. Ask or check identifying data, including name, age and birth date, gender, race and referral source. Record the name of the adult giving the history, and his or her relationship to the child. Note who else is present, and record when an interpreter is being used.

2. Presenting complaint and history of the presenting complaint

The presenting complaint should be the focal point of the history. Spend time first itemizing and then detailing the presenting symptoms. Record the main complaint in the informant's or the patient's own words, and the history of the presenting complaints in chronological order. Questions should include:

- Description?
- Recent examples, focusing on main factors, context and exacerbating and relieving factors?
- When did it start?
- Frequency?
- Severity?
- Change of symptoms over time?
- What effects do these symptoms have?
- What help was sought previously and how helpful was this?
- What ideas and concerns about the causation of the symptoms do the child and the family have?
- Are there any other associated symptoms?

At the end of this section one should be able to generate a differential diagnosis.

3. Past medical history

This is a detailed list of the child's previous illnesses, visits to casualty departments, times in hospital and operations. It is worth noting whether these problems are ongoing/active or resolved/inactive.

4. Pregnancy and birth history

Factors important in this section include:

- Health and age of mother in pregnancy
- Antenatal scans and tests
- Length of gestation
- Type of delivery
- Birth weight
- Condition of the baby at delivery
- Any immediate health problems after birth
- Any health problems in the first few weeks of life.

If there were problems prior to, during or after delivery, then more detailed questioning in these areas will be required.

5. Feeding and dietary history (Ch. 4)

Ask whether the baby was breast- or bottle-fed, and how well the baby took to feeding after birth. If the infant has been bottle-fed, enquire about the type of formula milk used and the amount taken during a 24-hour period. Any vomiting, regurgitation, colic, diarrhoea or other gastrointestinal problems should be noted. Ask at what age the child was started on solid food and if supplementation with vitamins was

- When presenting or analysing measurements of a continuous variable (such as height), it is sometimes helpful to group subjects into several equal groups.
- Growth charts often display the cutoff values that split the data such that there is 1% of the observations in each group. These cutoff points are called *centiles*, and there are 99 of them (the middle one also being called the median and the 25th and 75th centiles also representing quartiles).
- If the physiological variable is normally distributed (e.g. height), the centiles can be related to the standard deviation (SD). The growth charts in common use display the centiles that correspond to the intervals two-thirds of a standard deviation from the mean:

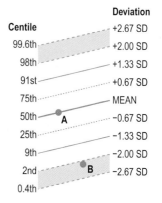

- A child whose height falls on the 50th centile (A) is average for his/her age.
- A child whose height falls just below the 2nd centile (B) is well below average for his/her age, such that he/she is in the bottom 2% of the population. To help parents' understanding, it may be useful to say, 'If a class of 100 pupils were asked to line up, such that the tallest was at one end and the shortest at the other, your son/daughter would be standing next to the shortest pupil.'

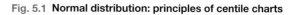

Fig. 5.1 Normal distribution: principles of centile charts

given. For an older child, ask about the range of foods eaten and some examples of meals and snacks from the last few weeks.

6. Growth (Ch. 22)

Parents may have brought along the parent-held child record to the interview. This contains details and plots of previous weights and lengths/heights (Fig. 5.1) that will allow assessment of the child's physical growth. For older children and teenagers, it is important to ask about the onset of puberty.

Be familiar with the parent-held record. These do vary between EU countries but the basic parameters are the same. You may find it useful to refer to such a record when you are taking a history, particularly with regard to growth and immunization.

7. Developmental history (Ch. 2)

The developmental history needs to be appropriate to the child's age. For younger children, questions about milestones in gross motor skills and locomotion, fine motor skills and vision, hearing and speech, and social development are appropriate. In older children, details about school performance are more appropriate.

8. Medication and allergies

List the child's current medications accurately, including dosage and frequency, and (if possible) when they were commenced. Highlight any specific drug allergies or sensitivities. These also need to be recorded in a specific location in the medical records.

9. Immunizations (Ch. 16)

Ask about and make a list of the child's immunizations. If any have been omitted, enquire about the reasons. If parents are unsure, then the parent-held child record may contain helpful information. Many areas of the European Union have a computerized immunization record that can be checked at a later date, if required.

10. Family history

Record family structure and draw a genetic family tree, including parents, siblings and grandparents with their ages, health or cause of death (p. 89). A question such as 'Are you and your partner related?' is a helpful way to detail consanguinity. A positive family history may link to shared genes, infections or environment.

11. Social history

Ask about who makes up the household. Details about the size and type of accommodation may be helpful. Occupation of the parents and whether they smoke are covered in this section. Major or psychiatric illness affecting parents can be clarified at this stage. It is worth asking whether there are any financial problems and what benefits the family are currently receiving. It may be relevant to know if the family has any pets. Further details about the child's school, school work and school friends, as well as any problems at school such as bullying or teasing, can also be checked out at this stage.

This can be a difficult and sensitive area. It can be helpful to practise some clear questions that you can ask in an unembarrassed way.

12. Review of systems

This section serves as a checklist for any information that may have been omitted up to this point in the history. The questions that are relevant to the presenting complaint are best asked earlier in the history when clarifying the further details relating to the presenting complaint. Enquiries concerning each system can be introduced with a question such as 'Are there any symptoms relating to your/his/her...?':

- Head (e.g. injuries, headache)
- Eyes (e.g. loss of vision, squint, discharge, redness, puffiness, injuries, glasses)
- Ears (e.g. difficulty with hearing, pain, discharge, ear infections, surgery/grommets)
- Nose (e.g. discharge, difficulty in breathing through the nose, nose bleeds)
- Throat (e.g. sore throat or tongue, difficulty in swallowing)
- Neck (e.g. swollen glands, masses, stiffness, symmetry)
- Breasts (e.g. lumps, pain, early puberty)
- Chest (e.g. shortness of breath, exercise tolerance, cough, wheezing, haemoptysis, pain in chest, noisy breathing/stridor)
- Heart (e.g. collapse, murmurs, sweating, poor feeding in infants)
- Gastrointestinal system (e.g. reduced appetite, nausea, vomiting with relation to feeding, amount, colour, blood- or bile-stained, projectile, bowel movements with number and character, abdominal pain or distension, jaundice)
- Genitourinary system (e.g. dysuria, haematuria, frequency, oliguria, urinary stream, wetting day or night, urethral or vaginal discharge)
- Extremities (e.g. weakness, deformities, difficulty in moving limbs or in walking, joint pains and swelling, muscle pains or cramps)
- Neurological system (e.g. headaches, fainting, dizziness, clumsiness, seizures, numbness, tremors)
- Skin (e.g. rashes, hives, itching, colour change, hair and nail growth, easy bruising or bleeding)
- Mood and behaviour (e.g. usual mood, nervousness, tension, possible substance abuse).

When you have completed the history, it should be possible to develop a problem list. This will include physical, genetic, developmental, emotional, cognitive, educational, family and social components. With this information a detailed physical examination can be performed and a differential diagnosis developed (Ch. 6).

Principles of the physical examination

Examination of children of different ages presents unique challenges. Without sensitivity to the child's perspective, the examination will be difficult and incomplete. You need to adapt the set routines used in adults to the age, mood, level of understanding and state of health of the child (Box 5.1).

Be both structured and opportunistic, checking on completion that you have not missed any important

- Always wash your hands
- Introduce yourself to the patient and carer
- Do not take the child away from the environment that he or she is comfortable with
- Involve the parent/carer
- Allow time for children to get used to you before placing a hand/stethoscope on them
- Use visual clues to build up a picture of the child's problems, e.g. crutches, helmet, ankle foot orthoses, inhalers, medications
- Do not hurt the child; ask the child/carer if there is any pain or discomfort prior to commencing your examination

signs. If faced with an uncooperative child you may have to return later, although this is obviously not possible in clinical examinations. When presenting your examination findings, concentrate on the relevant system or systems examination, the vital signs, growth as percentiles and developmental assessment.

Preparation and approach

You will learn much about a child and his or her state of health simply by observation. The child's interaction with environment, carer, siblings (if present) and yourself will give you important clues about developmental progress, physical and mental abilities, and desire to be examined. There may be clear visual clues to an underlying problem:

- The presence of spectacles/hearing aids
- The school-age child wearing nappies: physical and developmental problems
- The presence of central cyanosis/dyspnoea at rest: cardiovascular, respiratory and neurological causes
- Nasogastric tubes in situ: eating disorders, swallowing difficulties, gastrointestinal disease
- The nutritional and pubertal state of the child
- Dysmorphic features
- The presence of a rash: psoriasis, dermatomyositis, eczema, erythema nodosum
- The physical characteristics of a parent: achondroplasia, myotonic dystrophy, neurofibromatosis.

At the outset you may well have a clear idea of what you might find and what in particular you need to look for. However, a general physical examination is always advisable, except for when you are directed otherwise in clinical examinations. Do not forget that a child may have co-morbidities.

The general examination

Be confident and take control. Do not ask young children whether you can examine them, because if they say 'no' you must then go against their wishes. Adequate exposure whilst retaining modesty will ensure nothing is missed. Both the environment and your hands should be warm. Get down to the child's level and talk in an age-appropriate manner. Avoid technical terms and unrealistic requests (e.g. 'Take deep breaths' to a 2-year-old). Continue to talk to children whilst examining them, encourage and praise them, and thank them afterwards.

A full and thorough examination of a child, including ears, throat and perineum (if appropriate), should take no more than 3 minutes. This will not include a detailed system or developmental examination but these should be carried out if concerns are raised through either the history or the general examination. The general examination includes assessment of puberty and nutrition.

Growth and nutrition (see Ch. 22)

Accurate measurement of length in a non-walking infant requires two people and a horizontal rigid stadiometer. Height is measured without shoes on and weight in only light clothing, e.g. underwear. Head circumference is the maximum achievable distance around the head in the occipito-frontal plane and should be measured using a non-stretch tape measure! For more detailed assessment of nutritional status, measure mid-arm circumference and skinfold thickness, but this is not routinely necessary. Isolated growth parameters mean little and should be interpreted in the context of previous recordings and position on centile charts.

Child protection concerns (see Ch. 21)

Occasionally such concerns arise during the examination. Observe the following:

- State of dress, hygiene and dentition
- Behaviour: 'frozen watchfulness', fear of strangers, unwillingness to undress
- Relationship with carer: fear, obedience, lack of respect
- Nutritional state: failure to thrive
- Thorough examination, including frenulum, fundi and all of the skin
- Perineal examination — this may be best left to a more experienced colleague to avoid repeated examinations.

Your documentation should be accurate and complete, and should include relevant verbatim statements from carers and child, and any discussions with carers. Confronting the carer with your concerns may again be best left to a colleague with greater experience of child protection matters, when your suspicions have been verified.

Cardiovascular examination

The heart is the principal focus of the cardiovascular examination. However, since infants and children do not always cooperate, organize to perform a complete examination, but be flexible and do what can be done when the opportunity arises. Allow the child to handle the stethoscope and possibly to listen to the parent's heart, a manoeuvre which often helps to minimize anxiety in young patients.

Approach to CVS examination should focus on:

- general condition of the child
- presence/absence of dysmorphic features
- evidence or not of central cyanosis
- evidence or not of congestive heart failure (hepatomegaly, tachycardia or tachypnoea).

General inspection and visual clues

Look for visual clues first: supplemental oxygen, wheelchair, medication, TED stockings, a parent's appearance (Marfan or Holt–Oram syndrome). Children with cardiac disease may have developmental delay because of their underlying syndrome or because of the heart disease itself. If delay is present, you should comment on this at the outset, and although in an examination you may not have time to do a detailed developmental assessment, you should offer to do this. Similarly, mention the state of a child's dentition (risk of endocarditis).

Look for dysmorphic or other features consistent with an underlying specific cardiac lesion:

- *Down syndrome*: atrioventricular septal defect, Fallot tetralogy, atrial septal defect, ventricular septal defect
- *Alagille syndrome*: jaundice, pulmonary stenosis
- *Turner syndrome*: short stature, coarctation, aortic stenosis, bicuspid aortic valve
- *Williams syndrome*: peripheral pulmonary artery stenosis, pulmonary or aortic stenosis.

Does the child have any cardiorespiratory distress at rest (or feeding)? Is there peripheral or central cyanosis? Demonstrate whether the child has finger clubbing (cyanotic heart disease — right-to-left shunt), splinter haemorrhages (infective endocarditis or just trauma!), and comment on the colour and temperature of the hands.

Peripheries

Feel the brachial pulse in all ages for rhythm, character and volume, and measure the heart rate over at least 15 seconds. Heart rate will increase during inspiration

Table 5.1 Age-appropriate heart rate

Age (years)	Heart rate (beats per minute)
< 1	110–160
1–2	100–150
2–5	95–140
5–12	80–120
> 12	60–100

as venous return increases. Normal values for age-specific heart rates are found in Table 5.1. (Beware if the child is on β-blockers.) Assess the pulse (rate, rhythm and character) and see if the pulse volume is equal between left and right and then assess for any radio-femoral delay. Measure the blood pressure with an age-appropriate BP cuff. Examine the head and neck looking for central cyanosis, jugular venous pulse (if over 4 years old) and palpate for a suprasternal thrill (indicates valvular aortic stenosis). Palpation of the femoral pulses is mandatory but can be left until examination of the abdomen (hepatomegaly — heart failure, splenomegaly — infective endocarditis), provided it is not forgotten.

Specific inspection

Expose the chest wherever possible. Look for evidence of asymmetry and surgical scars:

- *Left lateral thoracotomy*: coarctation repair, left Blalock–Taussig shunt, patent ductus arteriosus (PDA) ligation, pulmonary artery (PA) banding
- *Right lateral thoracotomy*: right Blalock–Taussig shunt, tracheo-oesophageal repair
- *Central sternotomy*: reconstructive surgery, valvular surgery
- *Submammary*: atrial septal defect repair in girls
- *Infraclavicular*: pacemaker insertion.

Palpation

Localize the apex beat (normally mid-clavicular line, 4–5th intercostal space). Displacement of the apex is seen in left ventricular hypertrophy and dilated cardiomyopathy. Do not forget to place one hand on either side of the chest to ensure the apex beat is on the left side and to exclude dextrocardia. Feel for thrills and heaves. Palpate for a suprasternal thrill (indicates valvular aortic stenosis). If you can feel a thrill you will be able to hear a murmur very easily.

Auscultation

Auscultate the precordium (do this opportunistically earlier in the examination if the child is likely to become uncooperative). Listen in the four areas (Fig. 5.2) and be clear by the end of auscultation

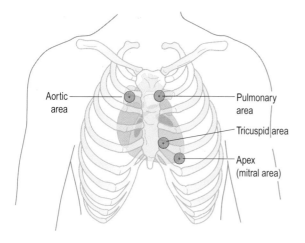

Aortic area

Pulmonary area

Tricuspid area

Apex (mitral area)

Fig. 5.2 Surface anatomy of auscultation points for the four heart valves

Table 5.2 Age-appropriate systolic blood pressure

Age (years)	Systolic blood pressure (mmHg)
< 1	70–90
1–2	80–95
2–5	80–100
5–12	90–110
> 12	100–120

what the characteristics of the heart sounds are, and whether any additional heart sounds are systolic, diastolic or pansystolic; early or late in the cardiac cycle; radiating to anywhere; and pathological or not.

Radiation may be detected in:

- *Aortic stenosis*: neck (thrill may be palpable in the suprasternal notch)
- *PDA and coarctation*: interscapular region of the back.

Splitting of the second heart sound is normal and may be exaggerated during inspiration. Fixed splitting is heard in atrioventricular septal defects.

Extras

To complete the examination of the cardiovascular system, listen to the lung bases (pulmonary oedema in left heart failure), look for peripheral oedema (right heart failure), and measure the blood pressure. This must be done using an appropriately sized sphygmomanometer cuff (to cover two-thirds of the upper arm) on the right arm (unless a four-limb recording is indicated: for example, in coarctation or interrupted arch). Normal values are difficult to remember but as a general rule the systolic blood pressure should be less than 115 mmHg in the under-10s (Table 5.2). A simple formula to use for calculating normal values for systolic blood pressure is:

Systolic blood pressure = 80 + (age in years × 2)

Centile charts exist for age-appropriate means and normal ranges for systolic blood pressure.

Presentation of findings during examination of the cardiac system must concentrate on positive signs rather than compiling a long list of negative or normal ones.

Respiratory examination

As for cardiac examinations, opportunism should be employed to auscultate the chest of a potentially uncooperative child, provided no other part of the examination is compromised or missed. There are three essential questions in the respiratory examination:

- Are there signs of respiratory distress?
- Is clubbing evident?
- Are there features of chronic chest hyperinflation?

General inspection and visual clues

Clues to aid diagnosis include sputum pots (productive cough suggestive of bronchiectasis), inhalers, spacer device and peak flow meter (asthma), suction catheters and machine (ineffective cough due to underlying neuromuscular disease) and non-invasive ventilation equipment (neuromuscular disease). Graduates of neonatal units who have bronchopulmonary dysplasia requiring supplemental oxygen often help with exams. Pointers to prematurity include scaphocephaly, glasses, evidence of previous line insertions and PDA surgery.

Be vigilant throughout to pick up further clues. A child's weak voice may indicate a vocal cord palsy (?any surgical evidence of previous cardiac surgery and damage to a recurrent laryngeal nerve), or an inability to generate enough airflow through the vocal cords secondary to underlying lung or neuromuscular disease.

The nature of a chronic cough can be helpful:

- *Moist*: lower respiratory tract infection (LRTI) or bronchiectasis
- *Barking*: laryngotracheobronchitis or psychogenic
- *Paroxysmal*: whooping cough.

Stridor is indicative of upper and large airway narrowing, and the level is suggested by whether it is expiratory (below the thoracic inlet) or inspiratory (above the thoracic inlet). Duration and variability (persistent/intermittent) give clues to causation.

Peripheries and specific inspection

After looking for finger clubbing and noting whether the child has peripheral or central cyanosis, expose the chest fully where possible and comment on chest shape if abnormal. Note any hyper-expansion, asymmetry, pectus excavatum and carinatum, Harrison sulci, kyphosis or scoliosis. Look for evidence of previous surgery (chest drains, lobectomy, tracheostomy). The

Table 5.3 Age-appropriate respiratory rates

Age (years)	Respiratory rate (breaths per minute)
< 1	30–40
1–2	25–35
2–5	25–30
5–12	20–25
> 12	15–20

Table 5.4 Interpretation of percussion notes

Percussion note	Interpretation
Resonant	Normal
Hyper-resonant	Pneumothorax
Dull	Consolidation
Stony dull	Pleural fluid

Table 5.5 Interpretation of breath sounds

Breath sounds	Interpretation
Vesicular	Normal
Absent breath sounds	Pleural effusion
Decreased breath sounds	Collapse
Bronchial breathing	Consolidation

Table 5.6 Signs of disease in abdominal examination

Condition	Signs to look for
Cystic fibrosis	Portal hypertension
Alagille syndrome	Liver disease
Inflammatory bowel disease	Colectomy, enterostomies, malnutrition, perianal fissuring
Wilson disease	Liver disease
Nephrotic syndrome	Scrotal oedema, ascites
Prematurity	Umbilical and inguinal herniae
Hereditary spherocytosis	Splenomegaly and jaundice
Thalassaemia	Splenomegaly ± hepatomegaly
Sickle cell disease	Splenomegaly up to school age → autosplenectomy

presence of axillary and cervical lymphadenopathy may be relevant.

 Children with respiratory distress may feature in the video section of the clinical exam. Note the nature, pattern and rate of respiration. Normal respiratory rates are given in Table 5.3. Assess the work of breathing by checking for suprasternal, intercostal and subcostal recession (and abdominal breathing in the under-1s). Nasal flaring and use of accessory muscles may be present. Prolongation of either component of the breathing cycle should be noted.

Palpation and percussion (Table 5.4)

Check the position of the apex beat and the trachea (for mediastinal shift).

Percussion of the chest can be frightening to the younger child so explanation is necessary. Do not forget to percuss (and auscultate) in the axillae. Percuss the right chest to find the upper border of the liver (dull note). Identify which intercostal space this is and assess whether the liver is pushed down.

Auscultation (Table 5.5)

Assess air entry and breath sounds. Additional noises include fine and coarse crepitations, inspiratory and expiratory wheezes, transmitted upper airway noises and pleural rub.

Chest wall expansion and tactile vocal fremitus are difficult in the younger child, but worth trying in a cooperative school-age child.

Extras

Palpate and percuss for the liver to assess hyper-expansion further. Normally the edge of the liver may just be palpable, and dullness to percussion may extend up to the nipple line. In hyper-expansion, this area of dullness will be shifted down and the liver more easily palpated.

Finally, in school-age children, measure peak expiratory flow rate (PEFR). This should be undertaken on three occasions whilst the child is standing, taking the best recording. There has been a recent change in the peak flow meters used in the UK, which now give slightly different values to the commonly used mini-Wright meters (Ch. 41).

http://www.peakflow.com

A useful way of calculating expected peak flow based on height of the child is:

Predicted PEFR (litres/min) = (height (cm) × 5) − 450

Abdominal examination

This is often done badly in clinical examinations. Signs are misinterpreted and children who have nothing wrong with them are 'diagnosed' as having a non-existent pathology. Examination can be difficult because young children do not like to be lain down, and older children find it difficult to relax their anterior abdominal wall musculature. Older children tend to have less subcutaneous fat than the average adult and so it is easier to feel a normal liver edge or slightly loaded descending colon.

General inspection and visual clues

Although an enormous variety of conditions will have intra-abdominal manifestations in childhood, there are a number that lend themselves very well to paediatric examinations (Table 5.6).

Many of these have extra-intestinal stigmata that may direct you towards a diagnosis before examining the abdomen. Some haematological conditions that result in abdominal organomegaly occur in certain races. For example:

- *Caucasian*: hereditary spherocytosis
- *Mediterranean*: thalassaemia
- *Afro-Caribbean*: sickle cell disease.

Assess basic nutritional status, and plot height and weight (offer to do this as a matter of course in clinical examinations). Look at the face for skin colour, evidence of dysmorphism, and features of chronic liver disease including jaundice, bruising, spider naevi and xanthelasma. Jaundice is clinically detectable when the serum bilirubin rises above 35 μmol/l. It can be subtle, even at much higher levels and particularly in artificial lighting, and is most easily seen in the sclera.

Peripheries

Look at the hands for evidence of liver disease, including palmar erythema, koilonychia and leuconychia. Clubbing is found in inflammatory bowel disease. Examine the mouth for dentition, ulceration (Crohn and Behçet disease), lip swelling (Crohn disease) and lip pigmentation (Peutz–Jeghers disease).

Specific inspection

If modesty allows, expose the child's abdomen fully and lay the child flat on the bed or parent's lap. Look for spider naevi in the distribution of the superior vena cava. Note any abdominal distension and look for scars, especially in the groin and flank where they can be difficult to see. Diabetes may lead to a number of physical features, including lipoatrophy and multiple injection sites.

Palpation

18 Prior to palpating the abdomen, ensure that the child does not have any pain or tenderness. This can be checked by asking the child to draw the abdomen in and then out — 'make yourself as thin and as fat as possible.' This will not only demonstrate the level of likely discomfort the child is in, but may also reveal larger abdominal masses if the child does not have a lot of subcutaneous fat.

Perform light then deep palpation of all four quadrants of the abdomen, without unnecessary prodding and without causing discomfort (if possible). At completion, you should be able to describe the size, texture and consistency of the liver, spleen and kidneys, if palpable, and any other masses, e.g. bladder, colon, transplanted kidneys. A palpable spleen is abnormal except in the young infant. Differentiate between a normal-sized liver pushed down by over-inflated lungs and hepatomegaly (see above).

Percussion and auscultation

19 Percussion for evidence of ascites should normally be rapid; it does not require the demonstration of shifting dullness or a fluid thrill if there is no abdominal distension or oedema when the child is in the supine position, and no other reason to suspect ascites. Auscultation over the liver, spleen and renal arteries may rarely detect bruits. Listen for bowel sounds if obstruction is suspected.

Extras

20 21 Get the child to sit up and look at the back for evidence of spina bifida, Henoch–Schönlein purpura and striae. In the clinical situation it may be appropriate and necessary to examine the perineum fully. In young boys, early diagnosis of undescended testes can prevent future infertility. Testes may retract due to cold hands. In a chubby baby it can be very difficult to palpate the testes but with perseverance and a relaxed infant it should be possible to clarify the situation. For infants an assessment of the hips to exclude developmental dysplasia of the hips is necessary (p. 79).

To complete the examination, urinalysis should be requested. A variety of 'multistix' exist, the best of which include measurement of nitrites and leucocytes. A urine sample that contains both leucocytes and nitrites gives a sensitivity and specificity of 95% and 60–70% respectively for a urinary tract infection.

Neurological examination

22 ## Limbs and gait (Tables 5.7 and 5.8)

This is an examination that can be enjoyable for the child, and hopefully for you as well. The child should have as little clothing on as possible besides underwear. Look for:

- Asymmetry (unless both arms or legs are abnormal)
- Contractures
- Posture
- Muscle mass
- Involuntary movements
- Fasciculations
- Scars
- Skin abnormalities.

Assess the child's gait if able to walk. Ask the child to walk a reasonable distance looking for a hemiplegic

Table 5.7 Joint movement innervations

Joint	Movement	Root value
Shoulder	Abduction	C5
	Adduction	C5–C8
Elbow	Flexion	C5, C6
	Extension	C7, C8
Hand	Flexion	C8, T1
	Extension	C6–C8
Hip	Flexion	L1–L3
	Extension	L5, S1
Knee	Flexion	S1
	Extension	L3, L4
Ankle	Dorsiflexion	L4, L5
	Plantar flexion	S1, S2

Table 5.8 Muscle power grading

Grade	Power
0	No movement
1	Flicker of contraction
2	Movement if gravity removed
3	Movement against gravity but not resistance
4	Movement against resistance
5	Normal power

Table 5.9 Reflex nerve innervations

Reflexes	Root value
Ankle	S1, S2
Knee	L3, L4
Biceps/supinator	C5, C6
Triceps	C7, C8

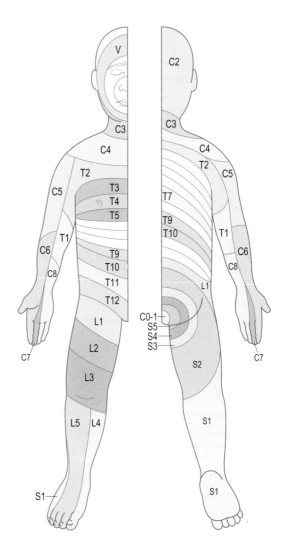

Fig. 5.3 Dermatome distribution

gait, a wide-based cerebellar gait or a waddling gait associated with a proximal myopathy.

Then check tone, power, coordination, sensation, reflexes (Table 5.9) and for clonus. Much of this can be tested by getting the child to walk normally, walk on their toes, walk on their heels, walk heel to toe (over 3 years), hop, jump, run, squat and rise, and climb steps for the lower limb examination. If a child can do all of these with no apparent difficulty, it is unlikely that you will find any abnormality on further testing.

Tone is assessed by moving the limb around the joint in an unpredictable manner. Coordination has already been assessed by walking heel to toe and climbing steps etc., but can be more formally assessed by the finger-to-nose and heel-along-the-shin manoeuvres. Sensation is assessed by means of a piece of cotton wool touched lightly on to the skin, working in a systematic order through the dermatomes (Fig. 5.3).

It would be unusual in the exam to have to proceed to assessing abnormalities of pain (spinothalamic tracts), vibration and proprioception (posterior columns).

However, you should be proficient in these skills for your clinical practice.

Assess the child's gait if able to walk. Ask the child to walk a reasonable distance looking for a hemiplegic gait, a wide-based cerebellar gait or a waddling gait associated with a proximal myopathy; then proceed with the following manoeuvres:

- *Gower's sign.* Lay the child supine and ask him or her to stand. A child with proximal muscle weakness will first turn prone and then 'walk up' the legs with the hands.
- *Trendelenburg's test.* Ask the child to stand on one leg. The pelvis should rise on the side of the elevated leg. If not, this indicates a problem between the femur and pelvis on the weight-bearing side.
- *Fogg's test.* Ask the child to walk on the outsides and then the insides of the feet and observe the associated arm and hand movements; a subtle hemiplegic arm may adopt the typical posture (flexion at the elbow and wrist).

Tremors and abnormal movement disorders

Abnormal limb movements can be confusing, but if described and interpreted correctly, can lead to precise localization of brain pathology.

Tremors

- *Essential tremor*: present only on initiation of movement and maintenance of posture. This is a common condition of adulthood that is inherited in an autosomal dominant fashion and can present in childhood. Other causes include thyrotoxicosis, phaeochromocytoma and Wilson disease.
- *Intention tremor*: seen at the end of movements, due to cerebellar disease including Wilson disease.
- *Static tremor*: seen at rest and disappears on movement. Occurs in Wilson, Parkinson and Huntington disease.

Movement disorders

- *Myoclonus*: brief, sudden muscle contractions. Seen in seizure disorders, metabolic disorders, brain infections, brain injury and degenerative conditions.
- *Chorea*: random rapid movements, seen most commonly in cerebral palsy, Sydenham chorea, Wilson and Huntington disease. Due to damage to the corpus striatum.
- *Athetosis*: slow writhing movements, seen in cerebral palsy and Wilson disease. Due to damage to the putamen.
- *Dystonia*: sustained disturbed muscle contraction causing abnormal posturing. Seen with certain drugs (anticonvulsants), trauma, infections, and vascular, metabolic and degenerative pathologies.
- *Hemiballismus*: random gross proximal limb flailing due to contralateral subthalamic brain damage.
- *Tic*: spasmodic stereotypic involuntary repetitive movements, typically of the facial muscles. Gilles de la Tourette is an inherited form with associated vocal tics, obsessive–compulsive behaviour and attention deficit hyperactivity disorder (ADHD).

Cranial nerves (Table 5.10)

Cranial nerve examination is straightforward in compliant, cooperative children. It is important to be clear about what you want of them. If necessary, demonstrate on yourself. For the younger child, improvisation is required, but with imaginative use of toys most cranial nerves can be assessed.

Table 5.10 Cranial nerve functions

Cranial nerve	Function
I Olfactory nerve	Smell
II Optic nerve	Visual acuity Visual fields Fundoscopy
III Oculomotor nerve	Efferent fibres to superior, inferior and medial recti, inferior oblique and levator palpebrae superioris muscles Parasympathetic supply to pupil
IV Trochlear nerve	Efferent fibres to superior oblique muscle
V Trigeminal nerve	Motor: muscles of mastication Sensory: to the face. Ophthalmic, maxillary and mandibular divisions. Corneal sensation
VI Abducens nerve	Efferent fibres to lateral rectus muscle
VII Facial nerve	Motor: muscles of facial expression Sensory: taste to anterior $2/3$ of tongue
VIII Vestibulocochlear nerve	Hearing, balance and posture
IX Glossopharyngeal nerve	Motor: stylopharyngeus muscle Sensory: tonsillar fossa and pharynx, taste to posterior $1/3$ of tongue
X Vagus nerve	Motor: pharynx and larynx Sensory: larynx
XI Accessory nerve	Trapezius and sternomastoid muscles
XII Hypoglossal nerve	Movements of the tongue

Visual acuity

With older children who can read or recognize pictures, ask them to hold a reading/picture book and to read or point out small objects on the page. The distance they hold the book from their face will give you an indication as to whether they are hypermetropic or myopic. Whilst they are reading, cover one of their eyes and then the other to check for binocular vision. With the infant and toddler, get the child to fix and follow a light or small object and to pick a small object from your open palm. Formalized testing of visual acuity (e.g. using a Snellen chart or Stycar matching letters) should be done at 6 metres if requested.

Visual fields

In the older child, test as for adults by confrontation, moving a wiggling finger in from the peripheries and comparing against your own visual field. With younger children, try bringing objects like a brightly coloured ball on a string into view from behind, or ask when a toy starts to move. Test with both the child's eyes open and then individually if possible.

Pupillary reaction

Shine a torch at one eye twice and then the other twice, looking initially for a direct light reflex and then a consensual reflex.

Fundoscopy

This is probably best left to the end of the examination, certainly in the younger child. There are likely to be only limited conditions or abnormalities on fundoscopic examination, and familiarization with these by means of picture atlases or attendance at paediatric ophthalmology clinics is worth while. These conditions include coloboma, aniridia, false eye, cataract, optic atrophy, papilloedema and retinitis pigmentosa.

Eye movements (III, IV and VI)

It is important to ask children whether they have diplopia at any point during testing. Ask the child to follow an object or your finger through the letter 'H' manoeuvre, finishing off by bringing your finger or the object close towards the child's face to test accommodation. Look for nystagmus throughout testing. A third nerve palsy will give a unilateral ptosis, fixed dilated pupil and an eye that looks down and out. Fourth nerve palsies cause diplopia when looking down and in, causing particular difficulty with walking downstairs.

Fifth nerve

Ask the child to open and close the mouth without and then against resistance, move the jaw sideways against resistance, and clench the teeth to assess the muscles of mastication (masseters, pterygoids and temporalis). Complete the motor component of the nerve by trying to elicit a jaw jerk. Assess sensation using cotton wool on the face, testing all three branches of the nerve. The corneal reflex should not be tested in the exam setting, but mention it.

Seventh nerve

25 Test the muscles of facial expression by asking children to raise their eyebrows, screw their eyes up tight, blow their cheeks out and show you their teeth (or smile). Preservation of normal muscle movement in the upper face and forehead with a facial palsy is indicative of an upper motor neuron defect due to bilateral innervation. Taste testing is not undertaken routinely.

Eighth nerve

Ask about hearing difficulties in any child, and in the older infant (7–9 months) be prepared to perform a hearing distraction test. The Rinne and Weber tests are done to try to elucidate the nature of a hearing loss, i.e. conductive or sensorineural. For the Weber test, place the vibrating tuning fork on the child's forehead and ask in which ear it is heard loudest. For conductive hearing loss it is loudest in the affected ear, and for a sensorineural defect it is loudest in the normal ear. For the Rinne test, place a vibrating tuning fork close to the child's ear and then on the ipsilateral mastoid process. For conductive hearing loss, bone conduction is better than air conduction, but the opposite is true if hearing is normal.

Ninth to twelfth nerves

The ninth and tenth cranial nerves can be assessed together. Observe the child swallowing and talking, look inside the mouth, and ask the child to say 'aah' if old enough for you to look at palatal movement. The gag reflex has a sensory component (IX) and a motor component (X), but is not normally tested. The eleventh nerve is easily tested by asking the child to turn the head sideways and to shrug the shoulders against resistance. Finally, inspect the tongue both inside the mouth and on protrusion. The tongue will protrude to the side of weakness.

Eye and squint examination

This has largely been covered in the assessment of the 26 cranial nerves. However, the eye examination is not complete without looking for the presence of a squint (strabismus).

There are five questions that need answering:
- Is there a squint or not?
- Is it convergent or divergent?
- Is it latent or manifest?
- Is it intermittent or permanent?
- Is it paralytic or not?

Start by direct observation of any obvious abnormality of the eye, size, shape, the cornea, sclera, iris or pupil. Hold a light source approximately 30 cm from the face and look for symmetry of the light source reflected from the pupils. Asymmetry would suggest a manifest squint that you will clarify by means of the cover/uncover test. Sit with your eyes at the same level as the child. Ensure that the child is looking at your face and cover one of his or her eyes with a hand or piece of card. If there is a manifest squint of the uncovered eye, there will be movement of that eye as it takes up fixation on your face (because the good eye is covered). When you uncover the good eye, it should take up fixation again unless the squint is alternating (i.e. involving both eyes). If there is no manifest squint, then cover one eye and look for movement of the eye as you uncover it. If there is movement, then there is a latent squint of this eye, induced by it losing fixation on your face when it is covered. Repeat the test on the other eye.

Cerebellar function

27 Signs of cerebellar disease include truncal ataxia, dysarthric speech, horizontal nystagmus, intention tremor, dysdiadokinesia and dysmetria (inability to coordinate accurate movements, resulting in overshooting the mark). Introduce yourself to the child and encourage him or her to speak. Cerebellar disease may produce stuttering dysarthria. Have the child walk in a straight line, heel to toe if old enough. A child with a unilateral cerebellar lesion may stumble towards the side of the lesion. Undertake the finger–nose test. You will detect an intention tremor and past-pointing with disease. Test for dysdiadokinesia but bear in mind that young children without pathology find this manoeuvre difficult. Finally, ask the child to perform the heel-to-shin manoeuvre.

Examination of the joints

28 Expose the joints proximal and distal to any affected joint(s), together with the corresponding contralateral joint for comparison. Inspect the joints for symmetry, swelling, deformity, scarring, erythema and wasting of adjacent musculature.

Ask about joint pain before palpating the affected joint for alteration in skin temperature, tenderness, swelling or synovial thickening. Movement in the first instance should be active, putting the joint through the full range of anticipated movement. Only if there is limitation should you go on to passive movement, but do not hurt the child unnecessarily. Measure limb circumference at the same place on both limbs for objective assessment of muscle mass. Finally, assess function by asking the child to undertake everyday actions. For example, if assessing hand function, ask the child to shake hands with you, hold a knife and fork, write his or her name, and touch the thumb to each finger pad of the same hand.

Examination of the skin

Examine the skin every time you review a child. This should be straightforward because it is simply a description of what you see. However, the plethora of terms and descriptions can be confusing. The more common ones are listed in Table 5.11.

Where modesty and environment allow, examine all the skin, and the hair, nails and mucous membranes

Table 5.11 Terms used to describe skin lesions

Term	Description
Macule	Area of discoloration or textural change, any size, not raised, e.g. vitiligo, freckle
Papule	Small (< 5 mm), solid, raised lesion, e.g. lichen planus, xanthoma
Nodule	Large (> 5 mm), raised lesion, e.g. dermatofibroma
Petechiae	Haemorrhage in the skin (< 2 mm), non-blanching
Purpura	Haemorrhage in the skin (2–10 mm), non-blanching
Ecchymosis	Large bruise, non-blanching
Vesicle	Small blister (< 5 mm), elevated, fluid-filled
Bulla	Large blister (> 5 mm), elevated, fluid-filled
Wheal	Transient, compressible papule or plaque due to dermal oedema
Pustule	Elevated blister, pus-filled
Lichenification	Thickened skin, accentuated skin creases

in good natural light. Describe the site, distribution, appearance, size and texture of the rash or lesions identified.

Site and distribution

- Localized or widespread
- Symmetrical or asymmetrical
- Centripetal or centrifugal distribution
- Area of the body: limbs, trunk, scalp, palms and soles
- Pattern: flexures, extensor surfaces, sun-exposed areas, nappy area.

Appearance

- Pattern of lesions: linear, grouped, annular or demonstrating the Koebner phenomenon
- Monomorphic (all lesions of similar appearance) or pleomorphic, e.g. chickenpox
- Colour
- Size
- Shape: regular or irregular, discoid, linear
- Characteristics: macular, papular, vesicular etc.
- Borders: clear or ill-defined, any surrounding changes.

Texture

29
30
- Macular or raised lesion
- Blanching or not
- ?Nikolsky sign: separation of layers of the epidermis on slight shear pressure.

Hair

Again, description is all that is necessary and a number of terms can be used:

- Hypertrichosis: excessive hair growth in a non-androgenic pattern
- Hirsute: excessive male-pattern hair growth
- Alopecia: absence of hair:
  - Alopecia areata/totalis/universalis
  - Telogen effluvium (diffuse hair loss: for example, after illness)
  - Trichotillomania (due to the child pulling at the hair)
  - Infection, e.g. ringworm.

Describe the site, distribution (localized or diffuse) and appearance of hair changes, and comment on the scalp.

Nails

Check fingernails and toenails for:

- Pitting: psoriasis, eczema, lichen planus
- Leuconychia: hypoalbuminaemia
- Koilonychia: iron deficiency
- Thickened, discolored nails: fungal infection
- Clubbing
- Beau lines: transverse lines/grooves due to temporary arrest in growth associated with severe systemic illness.

Mucous membranes

Describe any changes you see, which may include ulceration, inflammation and pigmentation.

On completion of a full skin examination, it may be necessary to go on to the examination of other organ systems, depending upon clinical symptoms and signs.

N.B. Areas of skin depigmentation may only be visualized under ultraviolet light using the Woods lamp.

Examination of the neck

31 Thyroid disease is uncommon in children but the examination of a child's neck is commonly requested in paediatric exams. Typically there may be nothing to find, apart from some shotty cervical lymphadenopathy of little consequence (Fig. 5.4).

Goitre

32 With hyper- or hypothyroidism there will typically be evidence of disease beyond the examination of the neck. Shake the child by the hand, looking for

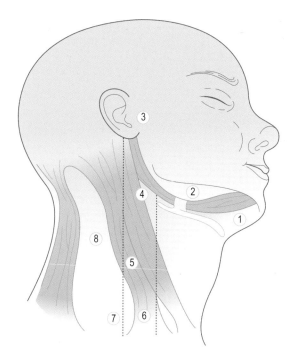

Fig. 5.4 Anatomy of the cervical lymph nodes.
(1) Submental; (2) submandibular; (3) parotid; (4) upper cervical, above the level of the hyoid bone and along the internal jugular chain; (5) middle cervical, between the level of the hyoid bone and cricoid cartilage, and along the internal jugular chain; (6) lower cervical, below the level of the cricoid cartilage and along the internal jugular chain; (7) supraclavicular fossa; (8) posterior triangle (also known as the accessory chain).

evidence of a tremor and feeling for skin temperature (hypothyroidism — cool, hyperthyroidism — warm). Ask the child's name to assess voice quality (deep, hoarse voice — hypothyroidism) and address to assess mental sluggishness. Inspect from the front, looking for eye disease, facial coarsening, hair thinning/thickening, previous surgery and goitre. Describe any swelling in terms of symmetry, size, shape, and whether there are overlying skin changes. Ask the child to take a drink to ensure that the thyroid gland moves with swallowing. Move around to the back of the sitting child to palpate the thyroid gland, making a point of looking down on the child from above to assess whether exophthalmos exists. Palpate the thyroid gland gently, as it can be tender if inflamed. Come back around the front to feel for tracheal deviation and percuss over the manubrium for dullness, both of which signify retrosternal extension of the goitre. Auscultate over the thyroid gland for the presence of a bruit.

Pubertal assessment (Figs 5.5 and 5.6)

This is part of the normal examination, but be sensitive and respect modesty. It is important to recognize pre-

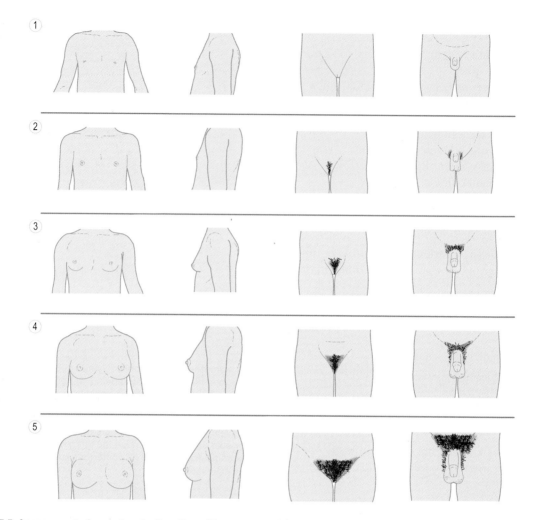

Fig. 5.5 **Assessment of sexual maturity ratings (Tanner stages) for the development of breasts, pubic hair and male genitalia. Stages are from 1 (pre-pubertal) to 5 (adult).**

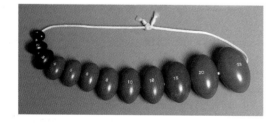

Fig. 5.6 **Orchidometer**

cocious puberty, which is the onset of pubertal changes before 8 years in girls and 9 years in boys.

Testicular size is measured with an orchidometer, and varies from 1–3 ml (prepubertal) to an average adult testicular volume of 20 ml.

Examination of the ear, nose and throat

Examination of the ears and throat, and to a lesser extent the nose, is a standard part of the assessment of every child. In the older child, it is straightforward. For the infant and toddler, leave it until last because, to ensure adequate and safe assessment, the child needs to be held tightly on a parent's lap, and he or she may object to this. Correct positioning is key (Fig. 5.7). Gently pull the pinna backwards and upwards to straighten the external auditory canal and visualize the tympanic membrane. Brace with fingers against the cheek. For the mouth, turn the child to face you and gently depress the tongue, with a tongue depressor if required, to visualize the pharynx, taking note of the dentition, gums and buccal mucosa.

Do not examine the throat of a child with signs of significant respiratory obstruction, as this may precipitate complete obstruction.

Dysmorphology (Fig. 5.8)

It is difficult to learn this from a textbook. Avoid the pitfall of stating that a child is dysmorphic when in fact the child simply looks like other family members

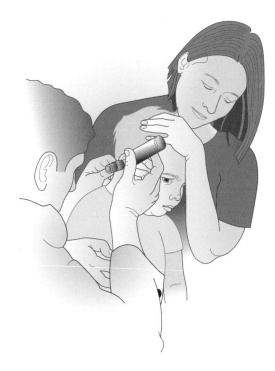

Fig. 5.7 **Technique for ear examination in infants**

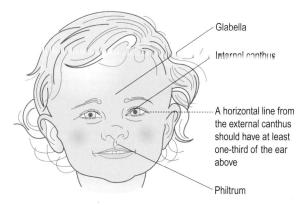

Glabella

Internal canthus

A horizontal line from the external canthus should have at least one-third of the ear above

Philtrum

Fig. 5.8 **A normal face**

who are all normal! Examine the whole child, and avoid 'spot' diagnoses based only on the face.

Whilst asking some questions, such as name, address and school (to assess developmental progress), look at stature and body proportions. Measure height and lower segment length (pubic symphysis to the floor) to calculate the upper segment to lower segment ratio. Measure weight, head circumference and arm span. The latter should approximately equal height (± 4 cm). Look for limb asymmetry, limb shortening, and hand and digit abnormalities. Ask the child to make a fist to see if there is a short fourth metacarpal (pseudohypoparathyroidism) or if the thumb can extend beyond the ulnar border

of the hand (Marfan syndrome). Look at the trunk for evidence of skin abnormalities (ash leaf macules, neurofibromas, café au lait spots) and kyphoscoliosis. Briefly assess pubertal status. Now it is useful to move on to the head and face, by which time the possibilities for diagnosis will have been honed considerably.

Measure head circumference and assess the shape of head and face (triangular in Russell–Silver syndrome, frontal bossing in achondroplasia, mid-facial crowding in Down syndrome). Describe the features of the hair, eyes, nose, mouth, palate, ears, teeth and chin. A number of terms are used in dysmorphology and ease the description of abnormality:

- Hypertelorism: distance between the internal canthi > length of the eye
- Slant of the palpebral fissures:
  - Normal: horizontal or upward-slanting with an angle < 10°
  - Upward-slanting: angle > 10°
  - Downward-slanting: external canthus lower than the internal canthus
- Synophyrs: meeting of the eyebrows in the midline.

It may not be possible by the end of the examination to give a certain diagnosis. However, provided the dysmorphic features have been described correctly, they can be entered into an electronic database to obtain a differential diagnosis.

Summary

The breadth and depth of the physical examination of children is entirely dependent upon the clinical situation and the willingness of the child. For the general practitioner or senior house officer/foundation doctor in paediatrics who is seeing a hot, fractious child with a likely upper respiratory tract infection, a brief but thorough 'top-to-toe' examination, including in particular the lungs, skin, ears, nose and throat, together with a measure of the body temperature and hydration status, may be all that is required. Provided you are dealing with a compliant child, this may take no more than 3–5 minutes. Clearly, any untoward finding or sign that does not fit with the likely diagnosis warrants further, more detailed examination. Because the examination can never be entirely thorough in an uncooperative child, the full examination may have to be undertaken at a different time, should the situation allow this. However, as long as the limited extent of the examination is made clear in the notes, this is acceptable. The chance of a failed or incomplete examination will be minimized by following the principles set out in this chapter.

Ragbir Thethy   Stefano del Torso

Diagnosis and management

LEARNING OUTCOMES

By the end of this chapter you should:

- Understand an approach to differential diagnosis
- Know how to select and interpret diagnostic tests
- Be able to draw up a management plan and co-manage a patient in collaboration with subspecialists
- Understand the importance of family involvement
- Understand psychosocial factors.

Introduction

Reaching a diagnosis is what, as doctors, we all aim for, so that the appropriate treatment can be instituted. The process is not as easy as it first seems, especially for those starting out in paediatrics. This chapter aims to show you the different steps that are required to achieve a differential diagnosis, then a definitive diagnosis, and then an approach to management.

A child does not come into clinic or accident and emergency department with a label or letter saying, 'I have …. Please give me the following treatment…'. Rather, by using a number of processes, the differential diagnosis is arrived at, followed by the final diagnosis.

The process involves the use of:

- A good history and examination
- Reaching a diagnosis or differential diagnosis

- Investigations
- Management planning.

All of these are interlinked (Fig. 6.1).

History and examination

The ability to take a good history and conduct a thorough examination is the cornerstone of being a good doctor. These aspects have been discussed earlier (Ch. 5). The primary care paediatrician is in the unique situation of possessing information which has been accumulated through a long-term trusting relationship obtained from multiple well and ill visits (continuity of care). Once the history has been obtained, 90% of the diagnosis should have been reached, so findings on examination should not come as a surprise. The ability to take a good history is dependent on the doctor being able to communicate with the parent/carer and the child. Use an interpreter

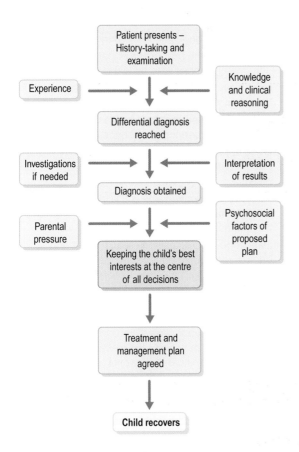

Fig. 6.1 Diagnosis and management

if necessary. Your examination findings are crucial to confirming your thoughts as to what may be wrong with your patient.

Reaching a diagnosis or differential diagnosis

Putting your findings from the history and examination together into a differential diagnosis depends on your knowledge base, clinical reasoning skills and use of other sources of help. These enable you to make sense of the clinical information and to formulate a diagnosis or differential diagnosis that then guides further investigation and management.

Knowledge and pattern recognition

Knowledge will stem from the training you received at medical school, tutorials, reading and experience. In fact, the majority of your knowledge will be from the patients you have seen; it is, in essence, pattern recognition. Obviously, at the beginning of your career, the number of patients you have seen will be small, and therefore your 'data bank' will not be extensive and your knowledge will mainly be that obtained from bookwork and teaching sessions. However, as you progress and see more patients,

then your 'personal knowledge bank' will increase, and there will be more and more pattern recognition. This is how your consultant may impress you by arriving at a diagnosis on just hearing the history. It is because he or she has seen patients with a similar condition before. The experienced clinician may be more concerned to rule out rarer causes of common presentations based on small variations from the usual pattern. For example, a senior house officer might see a child with a stiff neck and might diagnose the child as having a muscle strain causing torticollis. However, the consultant might want further investigations for other causes such as a malignant tumour. To increase your knowledge, follow up each patient you see with reading to reinforce what you have learnt.

Tutorials, ward rounds, teaching sessions and bedside teaching all aim to increase your knowledge base. Then, when you meet a patient with the same or a similar constellation of symptoms, you will be able to recognize the pattern and make a reasonable stab at a diagnosis. Pattern recognition through experience is essential to becoming a good doctor.

Clinical reasoning

To complement your knowledge base, you need sound clinical reasoning skills. When the clinical information does not fit a pattern you recognize, or contains puzzling elements, you need to go back to first principles and consider what clinical and pathological processes might be involved. This is why an understanding of the basic science behind symptoms, signs and disease processes is emphasized in professional exams, and also in this course. A helpful starting point is to list all the major categories of pathological processes (sometimes called the 'surgical sieve'), and for each in turn consider whether there is any way it could explain some or all of the symptoms and signs. Look for the best clinical 'handles' — features that will best enable you to get to grips with what is going on. Symptoms and signs that are *generally unusual* in the patients that you see are most likely to help you.

Once you have your list of differential diagnoses, you need to add your best estimates of the prevalence of the various conditions you think of. 'Common things are common', and so odd presentations are more likely to be unusual manifestations of a common disease than a rare one. Finally, bear in mind the 'rule of parsimony', by which you seek the fewest number of diagnoses (a single one, if possible) to explain all the clinical features. If you have to invoke multiple unrelated pathologies all occurring coincidentally to explain the patient's illness, beware! You are probably missing something. Look hard for a unifying diagnosis. Once you have been through this process, write down your list of differential diagnoses in order of likelihood, briefly citing the key features that support each one. This discipline helps to clarify your thoughts, and if noted in the clinical record, allows others to follow your reasoning easily with regard to further investigation and management.

Other sources of help in diagnosis

Books and journals

Do not be too embarrassed to look things up — you are not expected to know everything! Ideally, the clinical areas that you work in should provide access to a reasonable range of up-to-date texts and journals, along with Internet access to Medline or an equivalent and to electronic journals. Pubmed is a free service provided by the US National Library of Medicine, which provides access to Medline and links to full-text articles. Read the clinical descriptions of conditions on your differential list with which you are less familiar.

> http://www.ncbi.nlm.nih.gov/
> Pubmed

Colleagues

Discussion of interesting and puzzling cases with colleagues is an excellent way to broaden your knowledge, improve your diagnostic skills and help you make difficult diagnoses. Do this informally on the wards and in clinics, as well as more formally at clinical meetings. Discussion groups and forums on the Internet are another way of doing this, but take care to follow General Medical Council guidance on confidentiality, avoid using information that is identifiable to a patient, and only participate in groups run by trustworthy professional organizations. Paediatric forums are available at http://www.doctors. net.uk, and the RCPCH has its own discussion list.

> http://www.doctors.net.uk

Computer-based diagnostic aids

A number of computer-based systems have been developed to assist in diagnosis. These are likely to become more widely available and more sophisticated, and you should check whether there are any in your local area. Some hospital trusts subscribe to 'Isabel', which suggests a checklist of likely diagnoses based on clinical features and age. There are some excellent, though costly, dysmorphology databases (e.g. the London Medical Databases) that can assist in the diagnosis of syndromes.

> http://www.isabelhealthcare.com
> Isabel

BOX 6.1 Test characteristics

- *Sensitivity* is the proportion of patients with confirmed disease who have a positive test result
- *Specificity* is the proportion of patients without the disease who have a negative test result
- *Accuracy* is the percentage of tests that correctly identify the presence or absence of disease
- *Positive predictive value* is the probability that a patient with a positive test result actually has the disease
- *Negative predictive value* is the probability that a patient with a negative test result does not have the disease.
- *Likelihood ratio* is a good measure of a test's usefulness, and in effect combines sensitivity and specificity. The *pre-test probability* is the chance that the person has the disease before the test is done, and this will partly depend on prevalence of the disease in your population, and partly on your clinical findings. The likelihood ratio tells you how likely the test is to alter this probability significantly: for example, by making the diagnosis nearly certain or extremely unlikely. When a test's likelihood ratio is 1, this means it will not alter the pre-test probability at all, and therefore means the test is not clinically useful. High likelihood ratios (e.g. above 10) and low likelihood ratios (e.g. below 0.1) usually indicate clinically useful tests. To calculate the likelihood ratio, the true positive rate (i.e. the proportion of patients with the disease who have a positive test) is divided by the false positive rate (i.e. the proportion of patients without the disease who have a positive test)

> http://www.lmdatabases.com
> London Medical Databases

Investigation

Deciding whether to use a test

Use an evidence-based approach wherever possible (Box 6.1 and see also Ch. 13). Consider the questions below before ordering any test.

Is the test any good?

For the particular question you are asking (e.g. does the patient have disease X?), what are the characteristics of the test (Box 6.1)? It helps to have an idea of the prevalence of the condition you are considering in the population you see, since this influences how well a test performs. In general, the rarer the condition, the worse a test will perform.

Will the test help to make (or rule out) a diagnosis?

Consider how sure you are of the diagnosis, based on the information you already have from the history, examination and other investigations. This is the pre-test probability. If you are already very sure, there may be little point doing the test, particularly if its likelihood ratio is near 1. If you do not know the likelihood ratio, think in these terms: 'If I get a very strongly positive result, how much surer will I be that this patient has the disease or not?' Similarly, what will be the effect of a negative result, or one that is somewhere in the middle? If a test is quite likely to make a difference to how sure you are, then it is likely to be worth doing, provided it is not too costly (see below).

Will the result of this test change the patient's treatment or management?

If you really think that the test result is unlikely to change the patient's treatment or management, you should think twice about doing the test. The patients and parents may benefit from simply knowing what the diagnosis is, and of course this can be a significant benefit in its own right, but appropriate explanation of the possibilities may be all that is needed.

Is there any contraindication to doing the test?

Some tests are contraindicated in certain situations. For example, lumbar puncture should not be performed when a child has suspected raised intracranial pressure or fluctuating consciousness level.

How costly is the test?

This includes cost to the patient and parents, in terms of distress, inconvenience and transport; cost to the medical team, in terms of time taken to arrange and perform the test; and cost of materials and processing. If it is costly in any of these ways, then think twice before doing it and carefully consider any alternatives. In many countries tests such as C-reactive protein, throat swabs, urine analysis etc. can also be performed in the office of the primary care paediatrician, thus reducing inconvenience to the family and waiting time for results.

 http://www.cebm.net/likelihood_ratios.asp

Oxford Centre for Evidence-Based Medicine site, giving more information and examples

'Might-as-well' testing

When you have success with a technically difficult venepuncture, there is a temptation to send off extra tests because you feel you 'might as well' while you are in the vein. You reason that you will spare the child further distress, because you are less likely to have to come back and do further blood tests. *This is not good practice.* For many tests, you are more likely to get false negative results if you do them without clinical indication, since the prevalence of the condition being tested for will be lower and so the test performs less well. If the upper and lower boundaries of normal are placed at +2 and −2 standard deviations from the mean, as is common practice, then for a normal distribution this will encompass only 95% of tests. Thus, if you do 100 tests in healthy individuals, on average you can expect 5 to be abnormal. You have not helped the child if you have to repeat a test that was not indicated in the first place.

Key investigations

Some common investigations are reviewed here. See later in this module (Ch. 12) for further information on practical procedures and investigations.

X-rays

The main risk is increased exposure to radiation. The radiation dose from a chest X-ray is about the same as the average person receives from background radiation in 10 days. An abdominal X-ray is equivalent in radiation dose to 75 chest X-rays. If you request an X-ray, then you also need to be able to read and interpret its significance, at least acutely. Take advantage of every opportunity to review X-rays with radiologists, in review meetings or informally, in order to improve your skills. A chest X-ray may show up an infection that is otherwise undetectable apart from an increase in respiratory rate, particularly in young children.

Blood tests

Some of the basic tests are listed here.

Blood culture
This is the gold standard for diagnosing a bacteraemia and should be taken prior to any antibiotic therapy. The result of this investigation will influence your choice of antibiotic.

Full blood count (FBC)
In acute paediatrics, an increased white cell count usually indicates infection. An increase in lymphocytes suggests viral infection, while a neutrophilia points towards a bacterial cause. The white cell count is also raised in times of stress, e.g. after a convulsion.

Low haemoglobin indicates anaemia. The red cell size (mean cell volume, MCV) and the mean haemoglobin concentration (MCH) will give an indication as to the cause of the anaemia. If these are low (i.e. microcytosis and hypochromia, respectively), this suggests iron deficiency (or more rarely, β-thalassaemia trait). A macrocytosis is seen in vitamin B_{12} and folate deficiency.

If the haemoglobin, white cell count and platelet counts are low, this indicates a pancytopenia and implies bone marrow failure, e.g. due to leukaemia.

Urea and electrolytes (U&Es) and creatinine

These are useful in cases of dehydration, the urea and creatinine rising with increasing levels. The creatinine also gives an indication of renal function. Derangements of sodium and potassium may give diagnostic clues, and if significant, may need urgent action.

C-reactive protein (CRP)

This is a non-specific indicator of inflammation. The higher the value, the more likely that the patient is suffering from a significant illness. Remember that there is a lag of about 12 hours before the CRP starts to rise, so do not be reassured by a normal CRP if the duration of illness is less than this. In acutely febrile children, a CRP of above 80 mg/l is reasonably specific and sensitive for bacterial sepsis.

Blood glucose

A blood glucose level under 2.6 mmol/l indicates hypoglycaemia and needs immediate treatment and further investigation to establish the cause. If determined by 'BM stix', then ensure that a true laboratory glucose measurement is taken to confirm this; consider saving and freezing plasma for later metabolic testing if the hypoglycaemia is confirmed. It can be much harder to make a diagnosis if this opportunity is lost. The causes of hypoglycaemia are discussed in Chapter 35.

Lumbar puncture (LP)

This is required in all children under 3 months old who attend with pyrexia of over 38°C; it should also be considered in any infant in whom there is a fever with no focus (Ch. 43). Know the contraindications to lumbar puncture (p. 120). Cerebrospinal fluid (CSF) is sent for:

- *Microscopy and culture.* The white cell count will give an indication of meningitis/encephalitis (normal polymorph count $< 1 \times mm^3$).
- *Gram staining.* If anything is seen on Gram staining, then the child definitely has a bacterial infection and will need intravenous medication. It will also give an idea as to what the organism is.
- *Biochemistry and protein.* An elevated protein content (> 1000 mg/l) indicates a bacterial

infection. A protein content between 400 and 1000 mg/l is usually associated with viral meningitis, as long as the CSF glucose is normal.
- *Glucose testing.* The level is normally the same as the serum glucose, or at least two-thirds of it. A level much lower than this is associated with a bacterial infection. Do not forget to send a blood sample at the same time as the LP to check this.

Urine

A urine sample is often helpful.

Urinary tract infection (UTI)

This can present in a child who is non-specifically unwell, or with symptoms such as diarrhoea and vomiting, or just a temperature. A clean-catch urine is ideal. A normal dipstick test for protein, blood, leucocytes and nitrites will effectively rule out infection, but if any of these is positive or there is high index of suspicion, urine should be sent for microscopy, culture and sensitivity. An increased number of white cells might be an indication that the child has a urinary tract infection. Culture will confirm this and is the gold standard. Antibiotics can then be rationalized, according to reported sensitivities. A urinary tract infection is diagnosed if there is a pure growth of $> 10^5$ organisms/ml in the presence of pyuria (> 50 white cells per high-power field). Mixed growth, lack of pyuria, or lower numbers of organisms may all indicate a contaminated sample, and a repeat should be arranged.

Metabolic defect

Obtaining the first-passed urine in children with a low blood sugar is mandatory. The urine sample is used to rule out or diagnose metabolic defects (see also Ch. 34). If, as is often the case, the child is admitted or only passes this first urine out of hours, then the urine can be frozen until the next working day. Urine testing for metabolic screening should be considered in any acutely ill child.

Other tests

These will depend on the previous results obtained and the underlying problem.

Management

Once you have reached a diagnosis or differential diagnosis, you need to devise a plan of action. This plan may well be discharge but, even then, you have to take into account whether it is safe for the child to go home. Is the child safe from the illness, and indeed from the carer if there are child protection concerns?

Problem lists

Use of a problem list is a helpful way of ensuring that you address all the issues, particularly in more complex cases, and indeed in clinical examinations! Succinctly list all of the child's problems and then, for each, outline how you plan to deal with it, either through further investigation, initiation of treatment, reassurance or explanation, or referral to other services. Do not forget to find out how each is impacting on the child and family, and ascertain which they see as most important. If your view of what is most important is different, you will need to take time to discuss why, but it is important that you address the family's main concerns.

Management plan

Whatever the decision as to where the child is to be looked after, consider the following:

- Are any investigations required? If so, which ones and why?
- Does the child need any medications? If so, which ones?
- How will the medication be given? Oral, intravenous, per rectum?

For illnesses that follow a predictable course, a management plan can be applied that is specific for that disease. For example, for bronchiolitis, the following criteria could be assessed:

- O_2 saturations > 92%?
- Feeding OK?
- Little respiratory distress?
- Old enough to cope?
- No other coexisting morbidity?

If the answer to these questions is 'yes', then the child can probably be discharged home with the carer. However, there may be other factors specific to the patient that mean it is not appropriate for him or her to go home, e.g. anxious parents, prematurity etc. Therefore, each management plan needs to be adapted to the individual patient. 'One size does not fit all.'

To be able to implement a treatment package, parents must be on board and should be kept informed of their child's condition from the beginning. To obtain this level of parental cooperation, you need excellent communication skills (Ch. 7). In the majority of cases, parents care about their child and are extremely worried. They want to know what is wrong. You need to allay unnecessary fears and understand the parents' expectations. Then you should explain the investigation and management steps clearly and empathetically, including the reasons they are being taken and what they will involve. Conversely, when no test or treatment is required, explaining this to parents can be hard if they have come along with an expectation that their child needs some form of treatment. For example, a child may have a pyrexia and the carer seeks medical attention. The child is found to have an inflamed tympanic membrane. The carer is informed of this diagnosis. As the child has an infection, the carer expects antibiotics to be prescribed. However, the recognized treatment for otitis media is pain relief and temperature control with paracetamol and ibuprofen. The doctor has to explain that the infection is usually caused by a virus, how best to treat it, and the fact that antibiotics are not required since any benefits are outweighed by risk of side-effects. This conversation must be conducted with diplomacy and tact but also, most importantly, with empathy.

Such conversations with parents and children need to be conducted in a language that they are fluent in, via an interpreter if necessary. Lord Lamming's review into the death of Victoria Climbié recommended that a sick child must not act as a translator between parents and doctor. An interpreter should be an independent person skilled in translating medical terms, who the carer trusts, and who appreciates the need for confidentiality. If an interpreter is not available within the hospital setting, then one can be obtained via telephone translator services. These services are available 24 hours a day and are usually able to put you through within minutes to someone, somewhere, who speaks the same language as the carers. This is particularly useful in areas where a large number of languages is spoken, e.g. in parts of London where there are reported to be over 100 different languages and dialects. Check local arrangements each time you start a new job.

Any management plan should consider successful models of co-management and collaborative care between primary care paediatricians or family doctors and subspecialists, in particular for patients with chronic diseases.

Psychosocial factors

Being ill is an unpleasant experience for anyone but for a child it is particularly distressing. Children are unable to articulate their feelings and worries. There are strangers talking to their carers, who may themselves seem anxious, upset and disempowered. The child has to undergo a range of experiences that vary from the strange to the embarrassing and the downright unpleasant. Children have little say in what does or does not happen to them. The process of history-taking, examination and investigation can be a frightening experience for the child, if performed without sensitivity to the child's needs and feelings. Each investigation or procedure involves further psychological stress. Consider carefully whether each one is necessary.

BOX 6.2 Summary of diagnosis and management: an example

> *Lukas, who is 6 years old, is a child whom you are seeing in your office for the first time because he wets the bed most nights.*

You are to take a history from Lukas's mother and prepare a problem list and management plan.

Phase 1: Take the history

Follow the ABCD approach outlined in Chapter 5, taking time for introductions. Find out what the problems are, using open and then closed questions to clarify. Make sure that you know which are most important to Lukas and his family and why, as well as their impact on him and the family. Find out about any treatment already tried, the child's response to it, and what he and his parents thought of it. Complete the rest of the history in a logical focused manner. Be empathetic and avoid rushing.

Phase 2: Checking and closing

If you have not already done so, summarize the key points back to Lukas's mother to make sure that you have understood correctly. Explain that you are going to spend a short time thinking things through, but you may want to ask a few more questions.

Phase 3: Diagnosis or differential diagnosis, problem list and management plan

Spend the next few minutes writing a brief summary and then listing the problems in approximate order of priority, including key points relating to each, and your main diagnoses (and differentials where relevant). At this stage, you may wish to ask Lukas's mother a few more questions that come to mind as you 'process' the history in this way.

Summary

Lukas is a 6-year-old boy whose main problem is daytime wetting; this occurs randomly through the day, including when he is at school but especially when he is engrossed in activities. The wetting is accompanied by mild urgency and frequency. He also has primary nocturnal enuresis, and there is a background of mild but longstanding constipation.

Problem list

Problem	Comment
1. Daytime wetting with mild detrusor instability Differential: emotional upset, UTI	Although not mentioned by the mother in her request for the visit, this is the biggest problem for both Lukas and his parents. There is very mild urgency and frequency. Wetting tends to happen when he is engrossed in activity. He has not had any UTIs or any treatment. There are no particular triggers such as bullying; he is happy at school
2. Functional primary nocturnal enuresis	There is a strong family history. The parents are taking a low-key approach and the problem does not trouble Lukas much at the moment. He wears pull-ups at night. He has occasional dry nights (approximately once per week). He has had no treatment. He has never been reliably dry
3. Mild constipation	Although mild at present, it has been more significant in the past. It started 2 years ago. His mother gives him some lactulose once a week or so. His diet lacks fibre and fluid

Management plan

Problem	Investigation and management
1. Daytime wetting with mild detrusor instability	Dipstick urine to rule out infection and glycosuria Daytime reminder alarm set to go off every 90 minutes at first with a star chart. Ask the mother to phone you in 2 weeks and plan to see Lukas in 3–4 weeks. General behavioural advice about avoiding punishment and rewarding desired behaviour Consider a trial of oxybutinin later, but this is unlikely to be necessary

BOX 6.2 Summary of diagnosis and management: an example (*cont'd*)

Management plan

Problem	Investigation and management
2. Functional primary nocturnal enuresis	Dipstick urine (as above)
	General advice and reassurance
	No other action for now since it is better to focus on either the daytime or the night-time wetting, and it is the daytime that is the priority for the family
	Return to this later once the daytime wetting has resolved; consider starting a chart or possibly an enuresis alarm once he is 7 years old
3. Mild constipation	General advice to improve dietary fibre and increase fluid intake
	Start a small regular dose of lactulose 2.5–5 ml b.d., since it is important to avoid constipation while working on the daytime wetting

This approach helps you generate a clear and useful summary of the problems and a logical management plan. Note that a pitfall in this case would be to focus on the nocturnal enuresis while ignoring (or relegating to low priority) the daytime wetting. There are, of course, a number of ways in which Lukas's problems could be addressed. You need to focus on a sensible and logical approach that takes all the key problems into account and allow yourself time to organize your thoughts clearly.

Admitting a child on to a hospital ward is a decision that must not be taken lightly. It must be a last resort, in view of the inherent risks and problems with admission, which include hospital-acquired infections. The majority of patients on general paediatric wards have infectious illnesses, e.g. viral gastroenteritis, viral upper respiratory tract infections and impetigo. Most hospitals have had to close wards to admissions to control infectious outbreaks such as norovirus (Norwalk) gastroenteritis. Infection control is hard enough on adult wards but can be even more challenging on paediatric wards, where children are more likely to ignore restrictions. Those in isolation soon become bored and lonely, wishing to leave the cubicle and mix with other children on the ward. Then there are also psychosocial factors for the child and the family. Being admitted to hospital can be a traumatic time for child, parents and siblings.

For the child

The hospital stay can be an episode of separation for the child and for the parent who cannot stay with him or her. It was only as recently as the 1950s and 1960s that attitudes to the admission of children changed and the importance of parental presence and involvement was appreciated. Seminal films by the Robertsons played an important role, documenting the adverse impact of separation from parents on children. These remain highly recommended viewing for anyone embarking on a paediatric career (for example, *Laura Goes to Hospital*). Children are seen to go through phases of protest, despair and denial during hospitalization and, on their return home, they exhibit greater behavioural problems.

For the family

Not only is it traumatic for the child when he or she is admitted to hospital, but it can also be a traumatic and stressful time for the family. Parents often feel anxiety, fear and self-blame. A parent is expected to stay with the child during his or her stay in the hospital. This can add to the burden on parents. They have to arrange care for any other children they may have, which can be particularly difficult for single-parent families. They often have to sleep in suboptimal conditions (at best, they can expect a Z-bed next to their child; at worst, a chair next to the bed). Facilities for washing may be limited, and parent rooms are not always provided. Even when these are available, many parents choose not to stay overnight with their child or are unable to do so. In 1959, the Platt report advocated greater parental participation within hospital. In 1991, the Department of Health adopted this as official policy. Parental involvement in a child's hospital care carries a cost. This is partly financial — travelling, subsistence and loss of earnings — but it is also social, in arranging care for siblings. It leads to a loss of privacy and autonomy in family relationships. There is also the personal distress parents suffer from witnessing their child or other children in pain.

Summary

Box 6.2 summarizes the process of diagnosis and management.

Making a diagnosis, then deciding what investigations to conduct and what treatment to institute, are not as

MODULE TWO

clear-cut as they may first seem. After obtaining a good history and conducting an appropriate examination, you need to combine the results of these with the knowledge you have obtained from books, tutorials and experience and with your clinical reasoning skills, in order to arrive at a differential diagnosis. After the patient has been subjected to the appropriate investigations (if needed), these are analysed and a diagnosis is obtained. From these results a treatment and management plan, tailored to the needs of the patient and carer, is established. To arrive at this final point, a good rapport must be developed between doctor, parents and child. The core value of primary care is the long-term trusting relationship between the child, the parents and the provider. Parents and child must be kept fully informed in a language they can understand, which may well require the use of an interpreter. Throughout this whole process, both carer and child must be 'on board' with the treatment and management plan instituted.

John Hain   Richard Hain   Alfred J. Nicholson

Communication skills

LEARNING OBJECTIVES

By the end of this chapter you should:

- Understand how to communicate with families, particularly with respect to breaking bad news
- Be able to review best practice in communicating with colleagues, including the writing of referral letters.

Communication with patients and families

The main challenge of paediatric interviews is to interact effectively with children and their parents, balancing everyone's different factual and emotional needs. The medical care of children is perhaps unique in the extent to which it relies on collaboration with the family. When considering a treatment plan for children, paediatricians take it for granted that the child's parents will always be available to the child, that they will usually have the child's best interests at heart, and that they will be able to work alongside medical and nursing staff. In effect, parents are expected to be colleagues with the paediatric team. Paediatricians must also spend time talking to the child patient in order to establish a rapport that will help the child feel comfortable, that will enable the paediatrician to understand the child's views of the problem so that appropriate information may be furnished to make the child cope better with his ideas and worries.

If this collegiate relationship is going to work safely and effectively, it is essential that families feel both confident and competent. It is the aim of communication with patients and their families to facilitate this, both by imparting information and by encouraging confidence. In many conditions, particularly those that persist for many years, families will come to see themselves as experts not only in their individual child, but also their child's condition. At the time of diagnosis, however, it is important to be able to impart not only facts, but also an understanding of them, in an effective manner.

Factors that can make this more difficult include prior understandings (and misunderstandings), emotional coping mechanisms such as denial, and simple differences in the way information is given and received, such as vocabulary. It can be complicated by difficulty in remembering information. Devices for helping memory, such as audio recordings, diagrams or hand-written notes, are all important.

In this chapter we consider ways of reducing misunderstanding, and of optimizing the transfer of information and understanding, not only from doctor to family but also from family to doctor.

The most common communication scenario is one where the doctor is expected to impart news or information (Box 7.1). It is often the situation in which doctors presume they feel most comfortable. There are always communication needs beyond simple information transfer, however, many of which the doctor will be unaware of but which will inevitably complicate the discussion if they are not acknowledged.

In general, in any communication, the doctor has two responsibilities to the family and patient. The first, and the simplest, is the passing on of the information

An 8-year-old boy, Juris, attends children's accident and emergency with a week's history of tiredness, pallor and easy bruising. Today he had a prolonged epistaxis.

On examination, in addition to bruises over his legs and pallor, there is hepatomegaly, splenomegaly and widespread lymphadenopathy. A full blood count reveals haemoglobin of 6.8 g/dl, white cell count of 1.2×10^9/l and platelets at 9×10^9/l. The diagnosis of leukaemia is strongly suspected.

Before reading on, take a moment to consider your response to the following questions:

- What information do you need to give Juris's mother?
- How will you find out how much she understands?
- Why is it important that she should understand?
- What fears do you think she might already have?
- What do you think will make it difficult for her to understand?
- What techniques can you use to explain things more clearly?

that the doctor holds and the family needs. This needs to be done clearly and honestly.

The second, more nebulous but often more important, is to ensure that the family feels 'valued' by the professional. There is a power imbalance inherent in the relationship between doctor and patient since the doctor has the knowledge and is in his or her own environment. One of the goals of good communication exchange is to redress this imbalance.

This is more than good manners; families or patients who feel that their concerns have not been understood or taken seriously are less likely to work well in the team. Empathy — not only a capacity to understand something of what they are going through, but also an ability to communicate back to the family that you have understood — is a highly effective way to ensure this sense of being valued.

With this in mind, the process of giving news or information can be considered in five stages.

1. Set the scene

A really important skill is flexibility. The hallmark of good communication with children is the adaptation of communication skills to suit the individual child, which considers their age, their emotional response, their state of health and the needs of their parents. Communications should take place in an environment that is conducive to the exchange of information. This needs planning. Of course, this is not always

possible and communication may at times have to be impromptu, but this should usually be avoided — if necessary, by arranging a discussion at a specified later time.

Families may find discussions with doctors quite intimidating and will need positive encouragement to volunteer information. The aim of setting the scene is to provide a physical and temporal space in which communication is facilitated.

Physical space

- *Privacy*. This helps families feel comfortable enough to discuss important issues.
- *Quiet room*. One should be reserved for the purpose (and the door shut).
- *Comfortable furnishings*. Sofas/armchairs are preferable to institutional chairs, allowing professionals and family to be on the same physical level.

Temporal space

- *Unhurried atmosphere*. It is important for families to feel that the doctor has put some time aside specifically for them. Creating this 'space in time' is, paradoxically, time-saving, allowing more efficient information exchange so discussions can be shorter without sacrificing effectiveness.
- *Minimize interruption*. Switch off mobile phones and bleeps or hand them to someone outside the room. This sends the message to the family that, for this period of time, its concerns are the most important.
- *Avoid consulting a watch* during the discussion. This gives an impression of hurry.

Remove barriers

Make a positive effort to remove barriers to avoid unintentionally discouraging contributions from family members:

- *No desk* should separate you from the family.
- *Eye contact* on same level emphasizes equality rather than a power differential. Posture and position, facial expression, pace and tone of voice are all vital in creating rapport.
- *Do not stand* while the family sits, or sit in a higher chair.
- *Maintain eye contact*. This is difficult when breaking bad news, but important. Loss of eye contact gives a sense that information is being withheld, or that you are not being entirely truthful. It can be hard to dispel this misconception once it has taken root.

Have the facts straight

- *Recognize the importance* attached by families to discussions with doctors.

- *Communicate results accurately.* Have the relevant printed reports in front of you, and if uncertain, admit this, rather than discuss a half-remembered result.

Who else should be there?

- *Both parents.* For discussions of any significance, this is ideal but not always possible. Their presence enables mutual support and minimizes the risk of misunderstanding. Alternatively, arrange a second interview to cover the same ground, or make an audio recording for the spouse.
- A *member of the nursing staff*, especially one from the ward to which the child has been (or will be) admitted. This also helps the family identify another person to whom they can turn for information, once they have had time to digest the conversation. The underlying message that you are part of a team can be reassuring for families when everything else seems disturbing and new.
- *Child*, often ideal but not always possible or appropriate.

2. Alignment

It is tempting to start the discussion with what we want to say, but this would be like aiming a gunshot without first looking at the target. Instead, establish what the family already knows or understands by inviting them to talk first. Alignment essentially means understanding what things look like from the family's perspective. Aim to understand the following:

- *What they have already been told.* Many families will have considered leukaemia, perhaps because it has been mentioned as a possibility by the referring physician. Others will have no idea that this is a possibility, while some will be afraid to mention their fear of it.
- *Any prior experience and its impact.* Leukaemia in childhood is cured in around 75% of cases. Most families who have considered it as a possibility will extrapolate from their own knowledge of cancers, which are usually in adults and carry a much worse prognosis. What started as a discussion to 'break bad news' can become an opportunity to reassure. People look for explanations for illness, and in their absence will often assume that inheritance, upbringing and/or contagion might be a factor.
- *What they understand.* Even those with no prior experience usually have preconceptions that may be unhelpful, particularly regarding the implications of the diagnosis and prognosis. Many families assume a diagnosis of leukaemia is universally fatal, or at least always causes long-

term damage, or that a bone marrow transplant (often thought to involve surgery like a solid-organ transplant) will be necessary.
- *What vocabulary they use.* Note how the family uses language. Which words are used and which are avoided? The term 'tumour' (which can be benign or malignant) is usually synonymous with 'cancer' to lay people. Some families studiously avoid using the term 'cancer' or 'leukaemia', preferring instead 'tumour of the blood'. If this is the phrase that the family already understands and which accommodates their coping mechanism, forcing them to use a more precise term may jeopardize both their understanding and their coping. Unnecessary corrections are discourteous and emphasize the power imbalance between doctor and patient.

Tools that assist alignment

Open questions

These encourage a person to define the agenda of the discussion by allowing them free rein to decide how to interpret the question. There are different ways of doing this; a good one is to start by saying, 'We haven't met before, so it would help me if you could summarize for me what has happened up until now.' The family can interpret the question in whatever way it chooses. Such an approach can often be dramatically revealing, such as the response, 'Well, it all started when we moved near some power cables after my husband left us four years ago.'

Closed questions

These are often considered less helpful, as their object is to narrow down the discussion and focus on specific issues. Carelessly used, their effect can be to restrict discussions to what the doctor wants to talk about, rather than what the family needs to hear. Nevertheless, closed questions can be crucial. Consider, for example, the importance of an answer to the question, 'Has anyone in your family suffered from leukaemia?' Discussions with no closed questions can be poorly focused and unsatisfactory.

Summarizing and checking

Since the purpose of the alignment phase is to gain an understanding of the perspective of patient and family, it is important to confirm that your understanding is accurate. This can be done, for example, by using the formula, 'From what you have said, it seems that you already suspect/understand/are worried about etc....' Families can then correct you or confirm your summary. The family then knows that you have listened, and you gain a better sense of their information needs.

3. Imparting information

Although it is important that families feel listened to, this is rarely enough. The family has to trust you and to understand the information you give accurately, since competent collaboration is necessary in patient care. Both level and pace need to be appropriate.

Appropriate level

What information does the family need to deal with the immediate situation, and to allay its major fears and anxieties? At the time of diagnosis of leukaemia, for example, it is important that the family should understand the nature of the disease, the immediate tests that are required and the significance of their results. Families will commonly ask about increasingly remote possibilities, and there is a balance between providing answers and avoiding an unhelpful discussion of things that are very unlikely to happen. Too much information makes it harder to take in what is really important. It can be helpful to make a further appointment at a specific date and time, once further results are available. This avoids a sense of premature closure.

Often, questions raised at the initial interview will reveal more general concerns that need to be addressed. For example, detailed questions about the side-effects of chemotherapy before leukaemia has been confirmed, let alone classified, may indicate a concern that, even if the child is cured, he or she will be left with long-term damage. Whilst addressing the specific detail of different chemotherapy protocols may not be appropriate, reassurance that most cancer survivors are healthy usually is.

There is often surprisingly little difference in the understanding of practical care between families with a high level of education and those without. What is often needed, however, is for the same concepts to be explained in different ways. The danger here is of sounding either patronizing or incomprehensibly technical. One way of minimizing the risk of either extreme is to avoid using jargon words, preferring instead the terms chosen by the family themselves. Most families will need more or less the same amount of information, irrespective of their educational level.

Appropriate pace

The rate at which people can assimilate information depends on many uncertain factors. These include prior understanding and what has already been explained. A useful way of ensuring that information is being given at the appropriate rate is to use summaries. These serve to reiterate what has been said, to punctuate the discussion and provide a pause, and also provide a chance to invite questions. A typical summary would be something like this:

So, we've talked about the two different sorts of leukaemia, lymphoid and myeloid, and the fact that they are treated quite differently and that lymphoid is, on the whole, easier to treat than myeloid. We've also spoken about the fact that before we can know which it is, we will need to do a bone marrow examination, and we talked a little bit about what that will involve and in particular the fact that he will be asleep when it is done. Is there anything you would like to ask about those things before we go on?

Written materials

These can be valuable adjuncts to communication. Drawings can help to clarify what is being said; if complex, practise them beforehand. Good-quality written materials to take away can provide ongoing information that can be accessed at an appropriate pace and without pressure. However, written material should not usually be given without an opportunity for discussion with a knowledgeable person. It is difficult for any process of alignment to take place before printed materials are read, so that families may find themselves presented with a series of words that are unfamiliar but carry a message of dire news they are not yet prepared to hear. Poor written information may be positively harmful, but there are many printed resources of great quality.

Written materials also give an opportunity for families to access their own reference resources outside the meeting in order to clarify or expand on what has been written. The Internet is a mixed blessing in facilitating the development of expertise among families. Much of what is published on the Net is strongly held opinion rather than fact. Nevertheless, there are some extremely valuable resources. It is best to acknowledge that families may want to search for the topic on the Internet, provide three or four reputable websites, and invite them to bring anything else they discover back for further discussion.

4. Checking

Once all the information has been imparted, ask the family if they have had enough information, if their concerns have been addressed, and if they have any further questions. Summarizing is again useful at this point.

Reassure families that they will not be thought stupid if they do ask a question: 'No one expects you to remember everything first time and we are perfectly happy for you to ask again. If I am not here, my nursing colleagues will be around and will usually be able to answer your questions.' This also empowers and supports your nursing colleagues as sources of expert information in their own right. Avoid inviting questions in a way that actively discourages them: 'You don't have any questions, do you?' Generally, families need positive encouragement to ask.

If checking reveals that some issues have not been understood as well as you had thought, go back over the information again. This may need to be done many times. Rarely, it may be necessary to guillotine the discussion: for example, if it becomes clear that the family is simply unable to take in the information at that time.

5. Future plans

Do not let the family feel they are being abandoned at the end of the interview. Most families will feel reassured and more secure, simply knowing that there are plans for further conversations. Introduce other members of the team and refer to them during the conversations, so that families recognize yours is not the only expert voice. Assurances such as 'The nurses who work on this ward are very familiar with children with leukaemia and are always available to answer questions while you are here' can be both encouraging for families and supportive for colleagues. It may be helpful to add that if your colleagues are not sure of the answer, they will know whom else to ask; this allows staff to involve senior members of the team without feeling they have lost face in doing so.

For children who are to be discharged home, the contact may be the primary care team or a nursing outreach team. Provide a contact phone number if at all possible.

Families will appreciate knowing that there will be a second opportunity to discuss things with the person who has initially given them the information. This could be either on the ward (set a time and day) or as an outpatient. Remember that these appointments will be of enormous significance to families, so should not be undertaken lightly. For example, if it is not possible to be sure of the exact time when the next meeting should take place, it is better to say 'I will be there some time on Tuesday afternoon but can't say exactly when', rather than giving a spurious appointment time and then not being able to attend. Families understand that doctors' lives are busy and often unpredictable, and that they may not be able to give an exact time.

Finally, ensure that the plans for meeting again are acceptable to the family. This is particularly important if the child is being discharged since, if the plans are impractical for the family, the child will simply default and be lost to follow-up. So, once again, the conversation should finish by summarizing what has been said and inviting questions.

> **BOX 7.2 Goals of communication with the family**
>
> To enable the family of a child or young person to become competent colleagues in his/her medical care through:
> - Imparting factual information and understanding:
>   - To an appropriate level
>   - At an appropriate pace
>   - Using appropriate language
> - Imparting a sense of participation in the team through:
>   - Seeking their perspective
>   - Empathic acknowledgement (implied and overt) of their concerns
>   - Soliciting their views in decision-making

Summary (Box 7.2)

The discussion of bad news begins with a process of finding out how the situation is seen by the patient and the family (alignment). This is followed by a period when the doctor gives information at a pace, level and amount that the family can assimilate accurately and easily. Check for understanding during the discussion and on completion, and repeat the information if necessary. Finally, make future plans, including arrangements for a follow-up meeting. This should allow the twin purposes of communication with families — the passage of information and establishment of a sense of being 'valued' — to be achieved.

Communication with colleagues

Colleagues, too, need to be treated with courtesy and respect. This is more than simple etiquette; it is essential to good communication and therefore impacts directly on patient care. Brusqueness or rudeness irritates, closing the door to further discussion. Courtesy helps avoid positions becoming entrenched, and instead encourages exchange of professional views.

For situations in which important patient data is to be passed on to colleagues, a combination of verbal and written communication is ideal. Verbal communication is the most effective means of exploring, explaining or clarifying a difficult clinical situation. A verbal handover, for example, allows information about patients to be passed on but, compared with a written handover, can more easily communicate less concrete aspects: relative urgency, non-specific worries, a condition that is improving or worsening, or other diagnostic possibilities that have been considered.

Written information is best when data needs to be stored for easy and repeated access by different professionals.

- Date and sign all entries (name legible)
- Include role (e.g. 'Paeds SHO') and contact bleep/extension number
- Structure with brief summaries of the following:
  - Problem list (existing and new)
  - Important medications (e.g. 'Ribavirin day 4')
  - History and examination findings
  - Status that day (e.g. 'Generally better, but some respiratory problems remain, cause unclear, nasopharyngeal aspirate awaited')
  - Plans (bullet-point list).
- This is sometimes known as the 'SOAP' system: subjective (i.e. what others and the patient tell you), objective (i.e. what you find on examination), analysis (i.e. how you interpret the situation) and finally plan.

Writing in the notes is usually done by a junior member of the team, and is often seen as a chore. As the only permanent record of most of the clinical decisions, it is imperative that entries in medical notes are well written, accurate and legible (Box 7.3).

In outpatients, the main record of an appointment is the letter to the primary care physician (PCP). This is usually more easily legible than hospital notes, as it is typed, and provides a valuable cumulative narrative over months, years or even decades. Family doctor letters are typically written by diverse doctors, of all levels of seniority, many of whom will have moved on from the team at the time their letter is read. Letters need to be clearly and systematically written, and the SOAP system works well. Keep letters to less than one side of paper where possible. The two most important elements are a problem list or introductory paragraph summarizing the issues, and a closing paragraph detailing the plan. This should include further possibilities (e.g. 'If tramadol is ineffective or poorly tolerated, we should consider introducing a small dose of morphine').

It is perhaps ironic that, for paediatricians, the main role of a family doctor letter is often seen as that of providing a record for other members of the paediatric team rather than for the family doctor. Such a letter may not be enough if you are asking the PCP to become actively involved in the child's follow-up care in the community. PCPs receive a huge number of letters each day, more than they can read in detail, and it is difficult to identify in this deluge those that are for action, rather than simply for information. Even when you are not asking the PCP to undertake a specific task, it is the primary care team who will usually renew the prescriptions you have started. They are in the position of needing to write up the medications you

have prescribed, on patients they may not have seen for some time. If a child is to be managed safely by collaboration between hospital and primary care teams, the PCP needs to have information presented in a way that is clear, accurate and quickly assimilated. You can readily derive a set of 'do's and don'ts' of writing to PCPs, simply by imagining yourself in the position of the PCP who has to read the letter.

Do's and don'ts of writing to PCPs

1. Do ask the patient which PCP should receive the letter

Usually, every patient is registered with a PCP or with a practice. Ask the patient or parent who is the PCP, or reply to the referring PCP. A PCP tends to read a letter bearing his or her name more thoroughly. The same applies to addressing the letter to the current registering practice.

2. Do begin the letter with a statement of the diagnosis

Where available, a diagnosis (or diagnoses) should be stated at the beginning of the letter. PCP notes are usually computer-based and use a diagnostic code for diseases, such as the Read code. Where there is a locally agreed disease coding system, including the relevant code in the PCP/clinic letter is helpful, particularly for new diagnoses.

3. Do keep it short and well organized

A short letter is more likely to be read thoroughly. There is potential conflict between the two roles of the clinic letter: a record for hospital notes on the one hand, and communication with the PCP on the other. A particular bugbear for PCPs is having the contents of their own referral letter regurgitated in a clinic letter. These details do need to be recorded among the outpatient letters, but this is really only necessary on the first visit. Reiteration on subsequent occasions is unnecessary and results in a letter that is turgid and difficult to read, for primary care and hospital teams alike. To enable PCPs easily to skip what they already know, one solution is to preface this paragraph with 'to summarize the background' and/or to use subheadings (e.g. 'PCP action') to draw attention to the relevant sections.

4. Do not use specialty-specific jargon

Avoid terminology or abbreviations seldom used outside paediatrics. PCPs should not need a dictionary of paediatrics to translate your letter! Courtesy, as well as the interests of effective communication, demands that you use a professional vocabulary you have in common. Even among paediatricians, some abbreviations are ambiguous; for example, a patient who needs a 'PEG' may end up with a gastrostomy, laxatives or a form of asparaginase chemotherapy.

5. Do write a management plan

This facilitates effective and efficient collaboration between professionals, both between primary and hospital teams and within them. A management plan along the lines of 'If X fails, I would recommend Y or Z' allows others to see what your long-term strategy is. It also allows the primary care team to continue your management plan without the child needing to wait until the next visit. Include a clear plan for follow-up, whether for primary or secondary care.

6. Do give clear, consistent and constructive messages to the family

Where a specific 'PCP action' is recommended, spell out what has been said to the patient. If a PCP reads that he or she should be altering medication, this will be translated into a change on the patient's prescription list. The PCP needs to know whether the patient/parent has been told the prescription will be ready, whether they are expecting the PCP to call first to let them know it is ready, or whether the prescription is contingent on follow-up investigations/examinations etc. Care of the child is through collaboration with the primary care team, and it is important that their working relationship with the family is not jeopardized by unclear or undermining messages from the hospital.

It is rarely appropriate to collude with families who castigate their PCP. Apart from anything else, families with this habit will probably be representing the hospital team in a similarly critical light in parallel discussions with the PCP. It often appears that some agreement is required with the observation, 'I kept telling them that there was something wrong but they wouldn't listen.' The need for families is usually for their anger to be acknowledged and understood, rather than encouraged and fuelled. Most feel more anxious and uncertain if professionals indulge in uninformed criticism of one another. It is better to acknowledge the importance of the issue with an empathic 'That must have been frustrating' or even 'I can see that made you angry'. Such an acknowledgement is true, helpful and supportive irrespective of the actual circumstances, but does not imply that you agree that the PCP (to whose care they will soon return) is incompetent. Once their anger is expressed and understood, families will often not feel the need to mention it again, and the collaborative relationship between family and professionals in primary care and hospital teams is unscathed.

8. Do draw attention to changes in prescription

Any change in medication should be typed in bold, listed before the body of the letter, or highlighted at the time the letter is signed. An exhaustive and up-to-date medication list is useful, but can be misleading unless strictly accurate. Patients may be under several different consultants, so your knowledge of their medication list may be incomplete. Remember that after the first month of a hospital prescription, what the patient will actually be prescribed, and will therefore be able to take, depends upon what is entered on to the PCP's computer.

9. Don't always wait for the letter to go through the mail

Even if you dictate a clinic letter the moment you have seen the patient (as is ideal), there will usually be a delay of around a week while it is typed, signed, posted, and finally received and read. If the PCP may need to know the outcome of the clinic appointment sooner, fax your letter, or better still, contact the PCP by telephone. Most receptionists will quickly recognize the need to put another doctor through. A useful phrase is 'I need to speak directly to Dr X about a patient of ours'. State at the outset whether the urgency is such that the PCP should be interrupted during a consultation. If urgent and the PCP is out on visits, ask for a mobile telephone number. Messages are less satisfactory; you will have no way of knowing whether or not they have got to their recipient. If you have the address, email is the obvious solution, but is still beset by fears about confidentiality.

Summary

Like patients, professional colleagues are part of a collegiate relationship which, in order to function smoothly, demands communication that is sensitive and affirming. Underlying the practical suggestions above is the principle that people should feel they are valued as part of a team supporting and caring for the child. Information exchange should be not just accurate, but also accessible and easily assimilated. Whilst this can be challenging, particularly when communicating with colleagues outside the hospital, it is an essential part of clinical care. It is not simply an issue of politeness, or professional courtesy and etiquette; children's safety depends on it.

CHAPTER 8

Colin Morgan   Tom Stiris

Evaluation of the newborn

LEARNING OUTCOMES

By the end of this chapter you should:
- Be able to assess the newborn infant competently by history and examination
- Be able to manage/refer minor congenital abnormalities appropriately
- Be able to offer appropriate advice regarding feeding the newborn infant
- Be able to describe the screening programmes in place for newborn infants.

You should be able to recognize:
- Major congenital abnormalities and their clinical significance
- The features of innocent cardiac murmurs
- The features of serious congenital heart disease presenting on the postnatal ward; you should also understand the immediate management pathway.

Introduction

The principles outlined in Chapter 5 also apply to the newborn, but this chapter deals with special considerations.

Evaluation of the acutely unwell newborn infant is covered in the neonatology chapters (Chapters 45–48). All newborn infants are assessed and evaluated by midwifery and/or medical professionals in the first few days. This includes a formal assessment within the first 24–48 hours, as well as providing routine postnatal care. This contact with healthcare professionals mostly provides reassurance to parents that their infant is healthy and that minor abnormalities (which can create much parental anxiety) are not of clinical importance. However, in a minority of cases, this assessment identifies a problem or an infant at risk. For example, a thorough history may identify healthy infants at risk of medical problems, prompting screening for infection, hypoglycaemia or jaundice, or parental social problems requiring multidisciplinary support or intervention before discharge. A careful routine examination may reveal previously unsuspected but clinically important abnormalities, such as congenital heart disease.

History

A thorough history should include all available detail in the following areas.

Maternal history (Table 8.1)
- Age
- Social background/occupation

Table 8.1 Maternal disease that affects the neonate

Maternal disease	Neonatal effects
Diabetes	Increased risk congenital abnormalities Macrosomia Hypoglycaemia Increased risk of surfactant-deficient lung disease

Maternal antibodies
  Graves disease
  Systemic lupus erythematosus (SLE)
  Myasthenia gravis
	
	Neonatal thyrotoxicosis
	Complete heart block, haemolysis, thrombocytopenia
	Congenital myasthenia gravis

Chronic maternal disease, e.g. Crohn disease, chronic renal failure	Intrauterine growth retardation

- Medical problems and chronic maternal disease
- Medical treatment and drugs
- Recreational drugs/alcohol/smoking.

Family history

- Father's age/occupation
- Family history of genetic conditions and congenital abnormalities
- Previous pregnancies: dates and outcomes
- Health of siblings.

This pregnancy

- Medical conditions that have complicated the pregnancy, e.g. diabetes, depression, steroid therapy
- Pregnancy-related complications, e.g. pre-eclampsia, hyperemesis, cholestatic jaundice
- Maternal/medical expected delivery date (EDD) and any discrepancy
- Routine screening tests, e.g. ultrasound scan, haematology and infection status at booking
- Non-routine tests (why performed), e.g. additional/specialist ultrasound scans
- Special diagnostic procedures, e.g. amniocentesis.

Labour and delivery

- Maternal health during labour (including length of labour)
- Evidence of fetal distress:
  - Reduced fetal movements
  - Cardiotochograph (CTG) abnormalities
  - Low arterial and venous cord pH (especially < 7.0)
  - Fresh meconium-stained liquor
- Infection risk (most neonatal services have a protocol to assess risk factors for neonatal sepsis

with thresholds for performing a septic screen and treating with intravenous antibiotics):
  - Prolonged and/or preterm rupture of the membranes
  - Maternal pyrexia, chorioamnionitis
  - Maternal group B streptococcal colonization (or previous infected infant)
  - Intrapartum antibiotics given < 4 hours before delivery
- Drugs/anaesthesia given
- Mode of delivery.

Infant history

- Condition at birth with details of any resuscitation
- Age, sex and gestational age
- Progress since birth, including feeding history
- Any concerns from parents or nursing/midwifery staff
- Any antenatal plans for investigation/treatment of infant, e.g. risk of haemolytic disease, hepatitis B vaccine required.

Examination

Many of the key points of the examination are available as video clips, and these are summarized in Figure 8.1.

Conventionally, examination of the newborn progresses from head to toe. It should take about 5–10 minutes, depending on the experience of the examiner and the compliance of the infant. Prepare to adapt the sequence to take advantage of settled periods (to auscultate the heart) and leave more distressing parts (e.g. examining the hips) to the end. To start the examination, the infant should be undressed down to the nappy. Observe the infant first, assessing colour, respiratory effort and any spontaneous movements. Response to handling should be noted throughout the examination. Measure the occipito-frontal head circumference with a non-distendable tape measure (occiput to brow 1 cm above the nasal bridge). Plot head circumference and weight on a centile chart, correcting for gestation.

Head and neck

- Note head shape and presence of moulding.
- Identify evidence of swelling/trauma/bleeding:
  - Caput succedaneum (oedema of presenting part)
  - Cephalohaematoma (bleeding under periosteum)
  - Subaponeurotic haemorrhage (bleeding into subaponeurotic space)

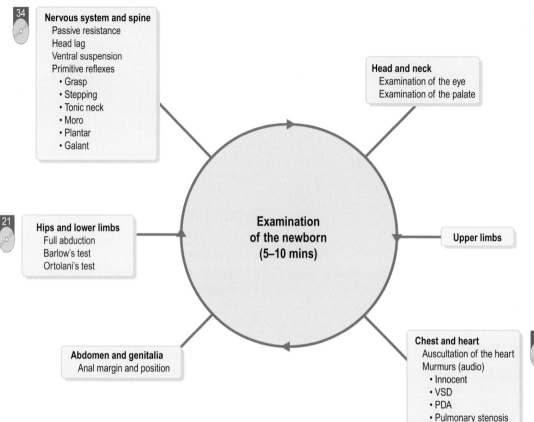

Fig. 8.1 Summary of newborn examination.
(VSD = ventricular septal defect; PDA = patent ductus arteriosus.)

- – Marks from scalp electrodes, fetal blood sampling and instrumental delivery.
- • Feel anterior and posterior fontanelles:
  - – Normal range for anterior fontanelle 0.5–5 cm
  - – Check skull sutures lines
  - – Check for increased tension.
- • Observe facial appearance:
  - – Note any birthmarks, malformations and asymmetry
  - – In newborn (obligate nose-breathers), pass nasogastric tube if any doubt about patency.
- • Assess size, shape and position of ears:
  - – Ensure external auditory meatus patent
  - – Note any pre-auricular pits, skin tags or accessory auricles.
- • Assess size, dimensions, slant and position of eyes, and note:
  - – Pupil size and reactivity
  - – Eye movements, particularly presence of paralytic squint or nystagmus
  - – Iris colour, shape and any defects
  - – Evidence of corneal and lens opacities, using direct inspection/red reflex

- – Evidence of conjunctival inflammation/ haemorrhage
- – Any discharge from eye.
- • Assess size and asymmetry of mouth.
- • Examine for cleft lip and palate, including soft palate.
- • Assess shape, asymmetry and any swellings in neck.

Tips on clinical examination (Table 8.2)

Eyes
- • A bright light (shone from the side) will reveal some cataracts and corneal opacities.
- • Using the ophthalmoscope at 15–20 cm to identify the red retinal reflex will reveal most other lens and corneal opacities.
- • Fundoscopy is not routine and often requires a mydriatic.

Palate
- • Use a bright light (not an ophthalmoscope).
- • The palate is best examined spontaneously (e.g. during crying).

Table 8.2 Common and important abnormalities of the head and neck in the newborn

Abnormality	Comments
Skull	
Cephalohaematoma	Common. Subperiosteal bleeding, so does not cross skull suture lines (cf. caput succedaneum)
Subaponeurotic haemorrhage	Rare. Massive bleeding into potentially large subaponeurotic space can cause sudden collapse
Bulging fontanelle	Common in crying infant. More rarely a sign of raised intracranial pressure (e.g. hydrocephalus, meningitis)
Skull sutures	
Widened	Common in first 48 hours. More rarely indicates hydrocephalus
Overlapping	Common in association with moulding in first 48 hours
Raised	Rare. Suggests craniosynostosis
Skull fractures	Rare. Associated with prolonged labour and/or difficult deliveries. Depressed fractures can be hidden under superficial swelling
Face	
Facial nerve palsy	Uncommon
Birth marks	
Stork mark	Common. On neck and forehead. Fades
Port wine stain	Uncommon. May be associated with intracranial calcification (Sturge–Weber syndrome, rare)
Ears	
Low-set	See Figure 5.8 (p. 55) for description
Malformed	Common feature of many syndromes, from Down syndrome to branchial arch anomalies
Eyes	
Hyper-/hypotelorism	See Figure 5.8 (p. 55) for description
Slanted palpebral fissures	Down syndrome
Microphthalmia	Rare
Conjunctival haemorrhage	Common following delivery
Ptosis	Uncommon. Usually congenital (may be unilateral)
Coloboma (defect in iris)	Rare. Usually involves retina. May be isolated or part of syndrome (e.g. CHARGE — *c*oloboma, *h*eart defects, *a*tresia of choanae, *r*etarded growth, *g*enital hypoplasia, *e*ar anomalies)
Cataract	Uncommon. Usually inherited (autosomal dominant) but intrauterine rubella an important cause
Mouth	
Normal variants	Epstein pearls (small white swellings along palate)
	Ranula (salivary duct cystic swelling in floor of mouth)
	Incisor teeth (usually need removal)
	Short lingual frenulum (tongue tie: rarely requires surgery)
Cleft lip/palate	Consider presence of other congenital anomalies/syndromes
Micrognathia	Uncommon. Can cause feeding or breathing difficulties, may have associated cleft palate (Pierre Robin sequence)
Neck	
Webbed	Turner syndrome
Short	Klippel–Feil syndrome
Redundant skin	Down syndrome
Lumps and swellings	
Midline	Thyroid, thyroglossal cyst, thymic cyst, epidermoid cyst
Lateral	Cystic hygroma, branchial cyst, sternomastoid tumour (not usually present in first 2 weeks)

- Palpate the palate (using the pulp of your finger) to identify submucous clefts.
- A tongue depressor may be required to visualize the soft palate.

Upper limbs

Carefully observe for abnormality and asymmetry in:
- Bones (e.g. absent radius and associated thumb abnormalities)
- Joints (e.g. contractures or limited range of movement)
- Muscles and muscle bulk
- Posture and spontaneous movement (e.g. brachial plexus injuries)
- Fingers and thumbs:
  - Polydactyly (extra digits)
  - Syndactyly (fused/webbed digits)
  - Clinodactyly (shortened/flexed digits)
- Palmar creases:
  - Unilateral single (4% normal population)
  - Bilateral single (1% normal population).

Note any limb deformity, such as partial or complete amputations (suggestive of amniotic band injuries).

unilateral upper limb weakness

Mathis is a 4.8 kg male infant born following a prolonged labour. It is noticed at 6 hours that the right arm appears floppy and is held at the infant's side, with little spontaneous movement except in the hand.

Q1. How are brachial plexus injuries assessed?

Q2. What is the management plan for these injuries?

Q1. How are brachial plexus injuries assessed?

Weakness and flaccidity in one limb are highly suggestive of brachial plexus injury. It is important to exclude a fractured clavicle or humerus (they may coexist with brachial plexus injury). It is also important to look for other evidence of asymmetrical neurology, particularly in the lower limb, as this may suggest hemiplegia rather than lower motor neuron injury.

Even if the whole limb is flaccid at birth, there is often partial recovery over 48 hours, leaving the classical upper nerve root injury (C5, 6 ± 7) of Erb palsy. The arm is internally rotated and pronated, with no abduction at the shoulder or flexion at the elbow. Occasionally, the damage extends to all the nerve roots. Rarely there is an isolated lower nerve root palsy (C8, T1), resulting in a weak claw hand (Klumpke palsy).

Q2. What is the management plan for these injuries?

Early physiotherapy and regular reassessment are required. Infants who do not show good recovery within 3 months require specialist referral.

Heart and chest

Chest

Most useful signs are obtained by observation rather than auscultation:
- Colour
- Shape and asymmetry:
  - Whole chest (e.g. scoliosis)
  - Clavicles and ribs (e.g. swelling/deformity of a fractured clavicle)
  - Muscles (e.g. absent pectoralis major in Poland sequence)

- Respiratory pattern (periodic breathing is normal)
- Respiratory rate (normal 40–60 breaths/min)
- Respiratory distress:
  - Use of accessory muscles
  - Intercostal, subcostal and suprasternal recession
  - Tachypnoea
  - Grunting
  - Stridor
- Auscultate each lung in three areas (apex, axilla and bases).

Heart

Auscultate the heart:
- Pulmonary area (and over left clavicle)
- Aortic area
- Lower left sternal edge
- Apex.

  If a murmur is detected:
- Check for radiation (back, carotids and left clavicular area)
- Palpate for presence of a thrill.

  Palpate the peripheral pulses:
- Radial or brachial
- Femoral (can be included during abdominal examination).

an innocent murmur

Lucas, an apparently healthy, term male infant weighing 3.34 kg and born by spontaneous vaginal delivery, is noted to have a soft systolic murmur at 28 hours. There are no other clinical findings of note. The baby is feeding well and the parents are desperate to take the baby home.

Q1. How is the distinction made between innocent and pathological murmur?

Q2. What causes an innocent murmur?

Q3. What investigations are necessary?

Q4. What advice would you give to the parents?

Q1. How is the distinction between innocent and pathological murmur made?

Murmurs have to have specific characteristics to be described as innocent (Box 8.1). It is important to

Q1. What cardiovascular signs suggest serious congenital heart disease?

Q2. How are duct-dependent lesions investigated and managed?

Q3. What are the important differential diagnoses?

Q4. How should asymptomatic pathological murmurs be managed?

remember that serious congenital heart disease can present without a murmur.

Q2. What causes an innocent murmur?

Innocent murmurs are often attributed to a short delay in normal closure of the ductus arteriosus. There is little evidence to confirm this, and many innocent murmurs are likely to result from blood flow in the pulmonary artery branches and to disappear before 6 months.

Q3. What investigations are necessary?

There is no evidence that chest X-ray or electro-cardiography (ECG) contributes to the diagnosis if the clinical findings suggest an innocent murmur. In most centres, echocardiography for all these cases is not feasible, and if infants remain well without symptoms or signs, then they can be discharged with a follow-up clinical assessment. If the murmur persists, then echocardiography is indicated (Chs 40 and 46).

Q4. What advice would you give to the parents?

It is important to reassure parents that the clinical evidence points to a structurally normal heart. Before discharge, simple advice about recognizing when a baby is unwell as well as the specific symptoms of cardiac failure, colour changes and dusky spells, is required. There needs to be a clear plan for reassessment of the murmur.

Problem-orientated topic:

a cyanosed and breathless baby

Ethan, a 3.5 kg male term infant delivered vaginally, is noted to be 'dusky' at 6 hours of age and slow to feed. The infant has a respiratory rate of 70 breaths/min and a pansystolic murmur is clearly audible over the whole precordium. There is a 2 cm liver edge and the peripheral pulses, including femorals, are normal.

Q1. What cardiovascular signs suggest serious congenital heart disease?

Many congenital heart lesions (especially those that are complex or lethal) are diagnosed antenatally. However, a significant proportion (up to 20%) are still not detected before birth. Some of these will present with a pathological murmur identified during the newborn examination. However, the absence of a murmur does not exclude serious congenital heart disease. It is particularly important to identify congenital heart disease that has a duct-dependent pulmonary or systemic circulation. These infants may appear extremely well in the first few hours (or occasionally days) of life while the duct remains open. This means that they may present on the postnatal wards or as part of the routine evaluation of the newborn.

Lesions with a duct-dependent pulmonary circulation usually present with cyanosis (Ch. 46). This may be subtle or intermittent before becoming progressive, depending on the degree of pulmonary outflow obstruction. With transposition of the great arteries, an open duct is often essential to ensure mixing of the two circulations. Symptoms, and therefore presentation, may be delayed by additional mixing at ventricular level because of a ventricular septal defect (VSD, as in the case above).

A lesion with a duct-dependent systemic circulation presents with progressive collapse of the systemic circulation. Thus peripheral perfusion becomes poor and the peripheral pulses weak. Isolated weak femoral pulses are suggestive of coarctation of the aorta. Four-limb blood pressure and oxygen saturation differences may add to the clinical picture, but can be normal.

Duct-dependent lesions (particularly left-sided outflow obstruction) can also present with heart failure, which in the newborn presents as respiratory distress. Non-duct-dependent lesions can also present with heart failure in the early neonatal period, although these are uncommon (arrhythmias, myocardial disease or a large atrioventricular septal defect, AVSD).

Q2. How are duct-dependent lesions investigated and managed?

Chest X-ray (oligaemic/congested lung fields, cardiomegaly) and ECG (ventricular hypertrophy) may help narrow the differential diagnoses. However, urgent definitive diagnosis is required in duct-dependent lesions, and this means cardiological assessment and echocardiography (Ch. 46). The cardiological advice will include a plan for starting a prostaglandin infusion. If the infant is unwell or deteriorating, then a low-dose prostaglandin infusion should be started immediately.

Q3. What are the important differential diagnoses?

Lesions with a duct-dependent pulmonary circulation need to be differentiated from respiratory causes of cyanosis and persistent pulmonary hypertension of the newborn. Lesions with a duct-dependent systemic circulation can be indistinguishable from other causes of collapse/shock, including sepsis and hypovolaemia.

Q4. How should asymptomatic pathological murmurs be managed?

ECG and chest X-ray may help with the diagnosis of the congenital heart lesion in cases of pathological murmur, but definite diagnosis will require a plan for echocardiography and cardiological assessment. This can be done on an outpatient basis, provided there are no other cardiovascular signs (including abnormalities on ECG and chest X-ray) and the infant is healthy and feeding well. Weight gain is difficult to interpret in the first few days of life (normally there is some weight loss), but excessive gain in the first few days is suspicious.

As with innocent murmurs, parents should be advised of the symptoms and signs to look out for.

Abdomen and genitalia

20
38
39
0

Ask about:
- Vomiting (particularly if the vomit is bile-stained)
- Passage of meconium
- Passing urine (and quality of stream in boys).

Observe for:
- Asymmetry
- Abnormal pigmentation (especially genitalia)
- Umbilical flare and peri-umbilical infection
- Abdominal distension.

Palpate for:
- Organomegaly:
  - Liver edge, normally palpable up to 2 cm
  - Spleen tip, often palpable up to 1 cm
  - Kidneys, can be palpated if posterior abdominal wall supported by fingertips of your other hand: assess asymmetry and enlargement
  - Palpable bladder
  - Other masses
- Herniae in inguinal canal/scrotum.

Examine the anus with the infant in the supine position and hips flexed, checking:
- Position
- Patency
- Anal margin.

Examine the genitalia in males:
- Assessment of size of penis (measured from symphysis pubis):
  - Micropenis (< 2.5 cm), suggesting hypopituitarism
- Position of meatus (epispadias/hypospadias; glandular/penile/perineal)
- Palpation of testes, noting:
  - Whether undescended or ectopic
  - Any swelling or asymmetry (e.g. hydrocele)
  - Hard testicle (e.g. congenital torsion)
- Features suggesting ambiguity or virilization.

Examine the genitalia in females:
- Size of clitoris
- Partial/complete labial fusion
- Presence of vaginal discharge (clear mucus and bloody discharges normal)
- Features suggesting ambiguity or virilization.

Problem-orientated topic:

undescended testicles

Simon, a male term infant weighing 4.2 kg, is born following elective caesarean section for breech presentation. A postnatal check at 24 hours reveals bilateral undescended testicles with no palpable gonads, although the genitalia appear otherwise normal. The infant is otherwise healthy.

Q1. What is the care pathway for undescended testicles?

Q2. What diagnosis is it important to consider in this case?

Q3. How would this diagnosis be excluded?

Q1. What is the care pathway for undescended testicles?

Careful confirmation of bilateral undescended testes is required. This means carefully examining the sites for ectopic testes (usually above the external inguinal ring but including the anterior aspect of the thigh), as well as palpating along the pathway of normal testicular descent (including the groin and internal and external inguinal rings). Do not confuse retractile with undescended testicles.

Most infants just require observation in the first year to establish whether delayed descent finally occurs. This can be done during routine child health surveillance (e.g. at 6-week and 8-month checks), following a neonatal discharge letter to the primary care physician. Surgical management is discussed in Chapter 48.

Q2. What diagnosis is it important to consider in this case?

If there are no palpable gonads, it is essential to consider the possibility that this is a virilized female infant with congenital adrenal hyperplasia. It is important to examine the infant for other signs of virilization, especially hyperpigmentation. Female virilization includes normal scrotum and male phallus (without palpable gonads) at the extreme end of the spectrum.

Q3. How would this diagnosis be excluded?

As there are no other signs of virilization in this infant, a male infant with bilateral undescended testes is the most likely diagnosis. If there is other evidence of virilization, the case should be discussed with a paediatric endocrinologist. The investigation of an infant with ambiguous genitalia is discussed in Chapter 35.

Hips and lower limbs

Hips

Clinical examination of the hips forms a critical part of the examination of the newborn infant. It is an effective screening process for developmental dysplasia of the hip (DDH, formerly congenital dislocation of the hip). However, the sensitivity of the test is highly dependent on the clinical experience of the examiner, with up to 50% of cases missed in some case series. Even in experienced hands, it is estimated that 10–15% of cases may not be detectable at birth.

The purpose of the examination is to classify infants into three categories:

- Normal hips
- Normal hips but requiring ultrasound screening because of a high-risk history:
  - Family history of DDH
  - Breech presentation
  - Other joint deformities such as contractures or talipes equinovarus
  - Clicky hip
- Abnormal hip/hips (requiring orthopaedic assessment):
  - Dislocatable (Barlow's test positive)
  - Dislocated but reducible (Ortolani's test positive)
  - Dislocated and irreducible (reduced abduction).

The examination should be performed on a firm surface with a comforted infant and the nappy removed. The examination often upsets the infant:

- Inspect the legs/groins for asymmetry/deformity, with the infant's hips and knees extended.
- Abduct the hips, testing for limited abduction.
- Perform Barlow's test (reducing a dislocated hip).
- Perform Ortolani's test (dislocating an unstable hip).

Lower limbs

Most lower limb deformities are positional and reflect the posture of the infant in utero. Careful assessment of the range of movement is required before diagnosing a permanent deformity. For example, 'positional talipes' is very common and can be corrected by dorsiflexion and eversion of the foot. This is not possible in true talipes equinovarus, where the combined bony and connective tissue abnormality restricts the full range of movement.

Carefully observe for abnormality and asymmetry in:

- Bones (isolated bone abnormalities very rare)
- Joints (e.g. contractures or limited range of movement)
- Muscles and muscle bulk
- Posture and spontaneous movement
- Toes:
  - Polydactyly (extra digits)
  - Syndactyly (fused/webbed digits)
  - Overlapping toes (common and of no significance).

Note any limb deformity, such as partial or complete amputations (suggestive of amniotic band injuries). The important lower limb deformities are described in Table 8.3.

Table 8.3 Lower limb deformities (all associated with developmental dysplasia of the hip)

Lower limb deformity	Comments
Talipes equinovarus	Common (1:1000). M:F > 2:1. Bilateral 50% Fixed foot held adducted, supinated and plantarflexed (equinus)
Calcaneovalgus	Spectrum of severity (20% mild, 12% very severe) Common Lax ankle with flexible foot dorsiflexed in valgus (foot may touch lower leg) Benign, usually requires physiotherapy only
Metatarsus adductus	Common. Usually bilateral Flexible deformity with forefoot curved medially and toes pointing inwards Nearly always self-correcting
Congenital vertical talus (rocker bottom foot)	Rare. 85% associated chromosome or spinal abnormalities Fixed foot, with forefoot dorsiflexed and abducted, heel in valgus and equinus. Usually requires surgical intervention

---

Problem-orientated topic:

talipes ● ● ● ● ●

Noah, a male term infant weighing 4.2 kg, is born following planned caesarean section for maternal diabetes. The pregnancy was generally unremarkable, except for late polyhydramnios and right-sided talipes equinovarus. A postnatal check at 24 hours confirms bilateral talipes equinovarus, more marked on the right, but no other findings. The infant was fed early and has had no feeding problems or difficulties maintaining a normal blood glucose.

Q1. What is the care pathway for talipes equinovarus?

Q2. What other diagnoses is it important to consider in this case?

Q3. What investigations are required?

Q1. What is the care pathway for talipes equinovarus?

Clinical assessment needs to establish that the deformity is either fixed or only partially correctable. Urgent orthopaedic referral is then indicated. Physiotherapy is initiated for partly flexible deformities, with early plaster casts for severe fixed deformities.

Q2. What other diagnoses is it important to consider in this case?

The combination of polyhydramnios and bilateral talipes equinovarus should alert the paediatrician to the possibility of neuromuscular disease. A history of poor fetal movements, hypotonia and/or poor feeding would increase the likelihood of such an abnormality. However, polyhydramnios is common in diabetic mothers and this infant has an excellent feeding history with no evidence of hypotonia, making neuromuscular disease very unlikely.

Q3. What investigations are required?

All foot deformities are associated with developmental dysplasia of the hip (Table 8.3) and so require ultrasound screening of the hip.

Spine and nervous system

You will already have learned a great deal about the infant's nervous system by observing and handling the infant in the earlier part of the examination.

Lay the infant supine and review any asymmetry previously observed, especially in posture or spontaneous movements. Look for evidence of generalized hypotonia, adducted shoulders or fully abducted hips (frog-like posture).

Test resistance to passive movements by applying gentle traction to each arm, testing muscle power and tone, and repeating for the lower limbs. Gently lift the head by applying traction to both arms, testing for the degree of head lag.

Turn the infant prone, look at posture (limbs should be flexed) and observe the spine and any asymmetry. Now hold the infant in ventral suspension (hand under chest), assessing tone in the trunk, neck and limbs and the appearance of the spine. Hypotonia is suggested by an upside-down U posture, with little flexion of the limbs and no extension of the head, neck or spine. Palpate along the length of the spine for defects and asymmetry. Look for patches of pigmentation, hair or swellings, especially if in the midline. Examine any clefts or pits and determine whether the base can be visualized.

Table 8.4 Primitive reflexes

Reflex	Description (response to)
Grasp	Pressure in the palm or sole
Rooting	Stroking the cheek
Stepping	Lowering on a hard surface (held upright)
Tonic neck	Head being turned to one side (symmetrical start position)
Moro	Dropping head a few cm (symmetrical start position)
Plantar	Stroking sole of foot
Galant	Stroking down one side of the spine (held prone)

It is not usually necessary to elicit the primitive reflexes during a routine examination of the newborn. However, they can be useful in confirming abnormal neurological findings, especially asymmetry (Table 8.4).

Problem-orientated topic:

the jittery infant

Elise is a 2.5 kg female infant born by emergency caesarean section for fetal distress. She was born in reasonable condition, although she needed a couple of inflation breaths before starting to breathe. You are called at 18 hours because of jittery movements. The baby is feeding well and the pre-feed blood sugar is 2.6 mmol/l. The jittery movements have stopped and nothing unusual is found on clinical examination, but you are called again at 36 hours with a history of more jittery movements intermittently over the preceding 4 hours. The last blood sugar measurement was 3.9 mmol/l.

Q1. What are jittery movements?

Q2. Are there any investigations you would perform?

Q1. What are jittery movements?

Up to half of normal newborn infants demonstrate jittery movements. Clearly, it is essential to be able to distinguish them from abnormal movements with a neurological cause, particularly convulsions (Table 8.5).

The history of the pregnancy, labour and delivery must be reviewed carefully for evidence of hypoxic–ischaemic injury, infection and congenital abnormality. The timing, severity and progression of episodes are also important.

Assess the effects of episodes on feeding or lethargy/ irritability in the infant. If the history suggests fits or there are neurological signs on clinical examination, then immediate investigation is required.

Q2. Are there any investigations you would perform?

Jittery movements rarely require investigation, although it is important to exclude hypoglycaemia (essential in high-risk infants). If the movements are particularly frequent or persistent, then it is reasonable to exclude hypocalcaemia (rare, but Asian infants are at higher risk) and hypomagnesaemia. Being called back to the same infant, particularly if the parent and/or midwife are experienced, usually merits a period of observation if you have not seen the movements yourself. This has to be balanced with the problems of separation from the parents. However, direct observation of abnormal movements, together with heart rate and saturation monitoring during episodes, usually removes any doubts about diagnosis in difficult cases.

Problem-orientated topic:

the floppy infant

Ella, a 3.43 kg female infant, is born in good condition following an uncomplicated pregnancy and labour. On the labour ward, 2 hours after birth, it is noted that she remains markedly hypotonic, although pink and alert with her eyes open. The midwife describes the breathing as regular, although not 'normal' in nature, and there are some unusual movements of the tongue.

Q1. What are the causes of neonatal hypotonia?

Q2. What further important features of the history and examination do you require to make a diagnosis?

Q3. How would you investigate this case?

Q1. What are the causes of neonatal hypotonia?

There are two key questions to answer when classifying neonatal hypotonia:

- Does the infant have an associated encephalopathy?
- Is there generalized muscle weakness?

Table 8.5 Comparison of jitteriness and convulsions

Feature	Jitteriness	Convulsions
Nature of movement	'Symmetrical' tremor (both phases of the tremor are of equal length)	'Asymmetrical' tremor (e.g. fast and slow phases of a tonic–clonic seizure)
Frequency	5 Hz	< 1 Hz
Stimulation	Aggravates tremor	No effect
Restraint/flexion	Stops tremor	No effect
Facial involvement	None	Sometimes involves eyes, lips or tongue
Autonomic signs	None	Apnoea, tachycardia
Neurological signs	None	Occasionally present

Neonatal encephalopathy is described in Chapter 47. Hypoxia–ischaemic brain injury is the most common cause of neonatal hypotonia in this group, but congenital malformations of the central nervous system (CNS), antenatal brain injury (e.g. congenital infection) and metabolic disease are also important. In those infants without encephalopathy the causes are classified as described below.

Hypotonia without significant weakness (neurological)

- Intellectual impairment
- Cerebral palsy
- Down syndrome
- Prader–Willi syndrome.

Hypotonia without significant weakness (non-neurological)

- Acute infection or any severe neonatal illness
- Prematurity
- Severe growth failure
- Ligamentous laxity (e.g. Ehlers–Danlos syndrome)
- Metabolic/endocrine (e.g. hypercalcaemia, hypothyroidism).

Hypotonia with muscle weakness

- Spinal cord:
    Trauma (birth injury)
    Congenital/vascular malformation
    Spinal muscular atrophy (anterior horn cells)
- Neuromuscular junction:
    Myasthenia gravis
- Muscle:
    Congenital myotonic dystrophy
    Congenital muscular dystrophies
    Congenital myopathies
- Unknown: benign congenital hypotonia.

Q2. What further important features of the history and examination do you require to make a diagnosis?

You need to see a maternal/family history of neuro-muscular conditions, and a specific history of reduced fetal movements or polyhydramnios during pregnancy. Clinical examination should focus on the observation of posture, spontaneous movement, respiratory pattern, presence of muscle fasciculation, particularly of the tongue, and the assessment of muscle weakness. The clinical history suggests the severe form of spinal muscular atrophy (SMA type I; Werdnig–Hoffmann disease, Ch. 44). The muscle weakness in these infants presents with characteristic 'jug handle' upper limb posture and a frog-like lower limb posture with a paucity of spontaneous movements, and with visible muscle fasciculations. The weak intercostal muscles lead to exaggerated diaphragmatic respiratory effort. The facial muscles are characteristically preserved.

Q3. How would you investigate this case?

Electromyography (EMG) will show fibrillation potentials at rest. Genetic analysis will confirm whether the infant is homozygous for the deletion of SMN1 on chromosome 5 in 98% of cases. This is discussed on page 97.

Skin

Jaundice

Neonatal jaundice is covered in Chapter 47. More than half of newborn infants have clinically detectable jaundice, and so recognizing physiological jaundice is an essential part of evaluating the newborn.

Problem-orientated topic:

the jaundiced infant

Aya is a 3.94 kg female infant born at 37+5 weeks' gestation in good condition following a forceps delivery and a prolonged labour. She is slow to establish breastfeeding, passes meconium at 24 hours, and is noted to be mildly jaundiced on day 2. This is felt to be

Continued overleaf

clinically significant by day 3 (serum bilirubin 230 mmol/l) and rises further by day 4 (serum bilirubin 270 mmol/l). Thereafter, the jaundice gradually resolves, requiring no treatment.

Q1. Is this physiological jaundice?

Q2. How would you investigate this case?

Q1. Is this physiological jaundice?

The timing of onset and peak are consistent with physiological jaundice. The peak level is higher than that typical of physiological jaundice but there are a number of exacerbating factors in this case. The gestation, although term, is more likely to result in relative liver enzyme immaturity. The instrumental delivery and prolonged labour are likely to have increased bruising. Significant bruising or haemorrhage will increase red cell breakdown. Delayed passage of meconium, breastfeeding and poor intake are also exacerbating factors.

Q2. How would you investigate this case?

Investigations should be kept to a minimum if physiological jaundice is suspected. Confirmation that the hyperbilirubinaemia is unconjugated is usually sufficient. A blood group and Coombs test are appropriate if the jaundice seems too rapid in onset for physiological jaundice. The possibility of infection should always be considered.

Common neonatal skin lesions

The presence of birthmarks often provokes parental anxiety, and the nomenclature of such lesions can cause confusion, resulting in inappropriate advice (Table 8.6). There are a number of common neonatal rashes that are transient and benign, but which need to be distinguished from more serious conditions, particularly infections (Table 8.7).

Feeding advice and feeding problems

Human milk is the preferred milk for term infants, but many mothers discontinue breastfeeding. The reasons for this are discussed in Chapter 4. The paediatrician has an important role in supporting breastfeeding mothers in difficulty. As well as the medical implications of poor milk intake (dehydration and hypoglycaemia),

Table 8.6 Birthmarks

Term	Description
Pigmented	
Congenital melanocytic naevi	Raised, irregular, well demarcated, brown/blue/black, often hairy
	Giant lesions have a significant risk of malignancy
	Large lesions may be associated with CNS malformations
	Medium–large lesions over the spine may be associated with spinal abnormalities
Mongolian blue spot	Flat, irregular, poorly defined margin, blue/grey
	80% are found in Asian/black infants, 10% in Caucasian
	Usually over lumbo-sacral area, can be very large
	Fade during childhood
Vascular	
Haemangiomas (includes lesions described as strawberry, capillary and/or cavernous haemangioma)	Haemangiomas are proliferative vascular tumours
	They may grow rapidly after birth and during infancy, but then begin to resolve spontaneously
	They can obstruct airways, eyes or other vital structures
	Lesions over the face may be associated with CNS abnormalities
	Lesions over the lower spine may be associated with spinal, urogenital or rectal abnormalities
Vascular malformations	These are permanent, non-proliferative structural abnormalities, categorized according to the vascular structure involved
Capillary malformation (includes port wine stain, naevus flammeus and Sturge–Weber syndrome)	Abnormal dilated mature capillaries. Most commonly on face (can be anywhere). Responds to laser therapy in infancy
	Sturge–Weber syndrome: association between facial capillary malformation (involves 1st division of trigeminal nerve) and ipsilateral brain vascular malformation
Venous malformation	Bluish raised lump, demonstrates venous filling and emptying
Lymphatic malformation (cystic hygroma, lymphangioma)	Macrocystic, skin-covered deep lesions. Can be detected antenatally; large cervical lesions can obstruct neonatal airway
Arteriovenous malformation	Skin-coloured lump that may have a bruit. Often part of a mixed malformation
Mixed malformation	Complex lesions involving multiple vascular components can occur. Rarely the lesion may involve limb hypertrophy (e.g. Klippel–Trenaunay syndrome)

Table 8.7 Pustular/vesicular rashes in the newborn

Rash	Description
Sterile pustules/vesicles	
Toxic erythema of the newborn	Very common. Usually appears within 48 hours. On any part of body, especially trunk and face
Transient neonatal pustular dermatosis	Common. Usually appears within 24 hours. Usually on trunk and buttocks
Eosinophilic pustulosis	Relatively rare. Late neonatal period. Usually on scalp
Neonatal acne (neonatal cephalic pustulosis)	Common. First few weeks. Usually on cheeks
Infective pustules/vesicles	
Varicella	Neonatal infection, usually severe with widespread rash. Present at birth
Herpes simplex	Rash erupts at 5–8 days. Usually on presenting part (scalp) but can be localized to any area
Staphylococcal infection	Can present as pustules, bullous impetigo or scalded skin syndrome. Umbilicus important site of origin
Candida	Usually erythematous red scaly rash in nappy area. Satellite lesions can appear pustular

poor infant feeding is an important clinical sign of infant wellbeing. It is a non-specific sign of illness (e.g. infection, cardiorespiratory or neuromuscular disease) or abnormality (e.g. Down syndrome, CNS malformation), and does not automatically imply a gastrointestinal problem. The paediatrician asked to assess a breastfed infant that is feeding poorly needs to establish whether this is due to difficulties in lactation/breastfeeding technique or neonatal illness/abnormality.

Although it is tempting in this situation to recommend complementary or supplementary feeds, these can further undermine maternal confidence and interfere with the successful latching on of the infant. Complementary or supplementary feeds can be formula or expressed breast milk and may be given from bottle, cup or even spoon/syringe. If complementary or supplementary feeds are deemed necessary, then expressed breast milk is the preferred option. There is clear evidence that the technique involved when an infant feeds from a teat is different from that required for the infant to latch on and breastfeed. Cup feeding, therefore, offers a theoretical advantage over bottle-feeding in avoiding 'nipple confusion'. Although cup feeding is recommended practice, particularly in preterm infants, the evidence base remains relatively weak.

The duty of the paediatrician, confronted with an infant that is feeding poorly, is to evaluate the infant carefully and establish that he or she is healthy with no abnormalities. Recommended intakes for term infants start at 30–60 ml/kg/day in the first 24 hours and increase by 30 ml/kg/day until 150–180 ml/kg/day. This is easy to establish in the bottle-feeding infant but requires more clinical judgment in the case of the breastfed infant. Breastfeeding mothers should be reassured if the infant appears well and given close support to continue establishing lactation. Complementary or supplementary feeds should be avoided unless the infant is high-risk (see below) or there is clinical evidence of poor intake. This includes:

- Signs of dehydration
- Hypernatraemia
- Hypoglycaemia
- Significant jaundice
- Initial weight loss > 10%
- Failure to gain any weight in first 7 days.

Sometimes lack of milk is clear from infant behaviour: persistent hunger, frequent feeding, repeatedly unsettled soon after a feed, and/or persistent crying. In these circumstances, supplementary feeding may give mothers time to rest, restore morale, and break the cycle of difficult feeding and a fractious infant.

Other newborn feeding difficulties include vomiting and choking episodes. Possetting (frequent but insignificant amounts of regurgitated milk) is normal in newborn infants. Larger vomits can be a non-specific sign of ill health, especially infection or an airway/respiratory problem. Careful assessment of the gastrointestinal system is required, from the mouth (to exclude a soft palate) to the anus (to exclude atresia). Bile-stained (green) vomit and/or abdominal distension suggest bowel obstruction and require immediate surgical assessment. Choking or dusky episodes, clearly related to a feed, are also common as isolated episodes. If the infant appears well and there are no findings on clinical examination, the parents can be reassured. However, a second episode or clinical suspicion of infection, respiratory symptoms/signs or abnormal movements requires admission, observation and investigation.

Problem-orientated topic:

an infant at risk of developing hypoglycaemia

Louise is a 4.2 kg female infant born in good condition at 38 weeks, following planned caesarean section. The mother has had well-controlled insulin-dependent diabetes throughout pregnancy. The infant is noted to have some grunting and tachypnoea initially,

Continued overleaf

but these settle in less than an hour. The infant is tried at the breast in the first hour, but the combination of the mother's post-operative condition (spinal anaesthetic) and the infant's reluctance to feed means that this is not very successful. The blood sugar at 2 hours is 2.2 mmol/l.

Q1. What infants are at risk of developing hypoglycaemia on the labour/postnatal ward?

Q2. How should this infant be managed?

Q1. What infants are at risk of developing hypoglycaemia on the labour/ postnatal ward?

Infants at risk of hypoglycaemia include:

- Infants who are born preterm
- Those of low birth weight (< 2.5 kg)
- Infants of diabetic mothers
- Those with perinatal asphyxia
- Any infant with an evolving illness
- Those with a congenital abnormality affecting feeding (e.g. cleft palate, Down syndrome).

Some infants who are at risk of hypoglycaemia are admitted to the neonatal intensive care unit (NICU) because of the severity of the underlying problem. However, many are well enough to stay with their mothers on the postnatal ward and here their progress requires careful monitoring.

Q2. How should this infant be managed?

It is important to feed high-risk infants early, although ensuring that this is successful is sometimes difficult. Maternal and infant factors can cause delay. This infant requires a supplementary feed to allow maternal post-operative recovery and successful initiation of lactation. The volume can be gradually increased to 75 ml/kg/day (if tolerated) and 2-hourly feeds given in the first few hours. Blood glucose measurements should be taken within 4 hours, sooner if there are feeding difficulties, as in this case. Repeat pre-feed measurements should be performed at least 4-hourly until blood glucose stabilizes above 2.7 mmol/l. Bedside testing is appropriate for monitoring the trend in blood sugar, but at least one laboratory test should be performed to confirm hypoglycaemia.

Infants of diabetic mothers can be slow to establish feeds, so exacerbating the risk of hypoglycaemia. If a combination of lactation support, breast and complementary feeds does not maintain the blood glucose above 2.5mmol/l,

then nasogastric tube (NGT) feeding, hourly feeds and ultimately intravenous dextrose infusion need to be considered. Transitional care facilities (if available) enable mother and the NGT-fed infant to be kept together.

Newborn screening

Routine clinical examination of the newborn in the first 24–48 hours can be considered a form of screening, particularly for DDH. However, its effectiveness as a screening tool is still a matter for debate, and newborn screening is a term usually reserved for the newborn blood spot screening programme and, more recently, the newborn hearing screening programme.

Newborn blood spot screening

Newborn blood spot screenings have been implemented in most European countries. In many countries more than 99% of all newborns are screened between 5 and 8 days of life. The need to support the necessary multidisciplinary collaboration and extend the screening programme has led to the creation of National Screening Programme Centres in many countries that are responsible for delineating clear policies, standards and quality assurance programmes. (p. 168).

Phenylketonuria (Ch. 34)

This was the first condition to undergo newborn screening and comes very close to fulfilling the ideal standards for a screening programme. The incidence is 1:10000. Infants are initially healthy but slowly develop irreversible neurological damage during infancy due to phenylalanine neurotoxicity. This can be prevented by an exclusion diet, if this is started in the first 2–3 weeks. The screening originally took the form of a microbiological assay but now involves direct measurement of phenylalanine levels. If a phenylalanine concentration of > 240 μmol/l is confirmed on repeat testing, then referral to a specialist phenylketonuria team, comprising consultant, dietician and specialist nurse, is indicated.

Congenital hypothyroidism (Ch. 35)

The incidence is 1:3500. As in phenylketonuria, infants initially appear healthy, symptoms and signs appear gradually, and neurological damage is irreversible. The treatment is thyroxine replacement therapy. The screening process measures thyroid-stimulating hormone (TSH), with levels >20mU/l indicating a positive result and <10 mU/l a negative one. Borderline results are repeated. Some national screening programmes (notably in the USA) measure T_4 and TSH to avoid missing the rare possibility of secondary hypothyroidism.

Sickle cell disease and thalassaemia (Ch. 42)

The newborn blood spot screening programme in some countries includes sickle cell screening. In many countries where this has been introduced, there exists an antenatal screening programme offering sickle cell and thalassaemia screening to women as an integral part of early antenatal care. In some countries the form of screening will depend on the local prevalence of the condition, with high-risk areas offering universal screening, and low-risk areas offering targeted screening using an antenatal questionnaire based on ethnic origin.

Cystic fibrosis (Ch. 41)

Biochemical screening for cystic fibrosis, using a method to detect raised levels of immunoreactive trypsinogen (IRT), may be offered as part of the screening programme.

Other inborn errors of metabolism (Ch. 34)

Tandem mass spectrometry now allows broad metabolic screening programmes detecting disorders of fatty acid or amino acid metabolism. Many centres around the world offer such a programme.

Newborn hearing screening (Ch. 32)

Congenital bilateral hearing impairment affects about 1:1000 infants. Neonatal screening can be achieved using transient evoked oto-acoustic emissions. Failures can be retested with automated threshold brainstem evoked responses. This has now become part of the newborn examination before discharge in many centres. In some European countries there are special centres outside the hospital where all newborns are referred for screening in the first 2 weeks of life.

Angus J. Clarke   Mark Davies   Flemming Skovby

CHAPTER

9

Clinical genetics

LEARNING OUTCOMES

By the end of this chapter you should:
- Be able to recognize features suggestive of a genetic disease
- Be able to obtain a family history and draw a pedigree.
- Understand the basic science that underpins genetics
- Understand the potential advantages and difficulties of genetic testing, as well as the long-term implications
- Understand when to refer to the clinical genetics department and what genetic counselling involves.

MODULE TWO

Clinical pointers to genetic disorders

In a genetic disease the fundamental pathological problem is with the genetic material, at the level of either chromosomes or deoxyribonucleic acid (DNA). Some genetic diseases form part of the recognized differential diagnoses for relatively common presenting problems, e.g. Prader–Willi syndrome in a hypotonic child, while others are recognized by their distinctive features, e.g. the dysmorphic features of Down syndrome.

The following features should alert you to the possibility of a genetic condition, even when the precise diagnosis is not initially apparent:

- Multiple problems in the same individual, including:
  - Congenital abnormalities
  - Growth problems (e.g. short stature, microcephaly)
  - Neurodevelopmental problems, including developmental delay or cognitive impairment, regression, seizures and focal neurological signs
  - Unusual tumours (Ch. 50), the presence of multiple tumours in an individual, or more cancers in the family history than would be expected from chance alone
- Multiple individuals in the same family being affected by the same problem(s), such as those listed above.

The history and examination in genetic disorders

There are some areas in the diagnostic process that are of particular significance in genetic conditions, in addition to the history of the presenting complaint, the past medical history and the drug history. When the presenting features do not suggest a limited differential diagnosis, then the subsequent history and examination need to be wide-ranging (Table 9.1).

The physical examination may need to be equally comprehensive, depending on the circumstances. Use of a checklist can help to ensure a systematic record of physical features (Fig. 9.1).

Many genetic conditions are associated with growth abnormalities, particularly short stature, so plot height, weight and head circumference on centile charts. Serial plots are important. Some genetic diseases, e.g. Down

Table 9.1 **Key points in the history and examination of genetic disorders**

Areas within the history	Key points
Antenatal	Infections or skin rashes, exposure to teratogens (such as alcohol or anti-epileptic medication) Intrauterine growth restriction or other complication
Obstetric	Gestational age Birth weight Complications during delivery
Development	Developmental progress Evidence of regression
Family	Construct a pedigree. An adequate family history can be essential for diagnosis of a genetic condition and in determining risk to family members

Height _____ Weight _____ Head circumference _____

Head appearance _____
   Eyes _____
   Ears _____
   Nose _____
   Palpebral fissure _____
   Mouth _____
   Teeth _____
Neck _____
Chest wall _____
   Nipples _____
   Heart _____
   Lungs _____
Abdominal wall _____
Genitalia _____
Anus _____
Spine _____
Arms _____
Hands _____
   Fingers _____
   Fingernails _____
   Palmar creases _____
Legs _____
Feet _____
   Toes _____
   Toenails _____
Skin _____
Hair _____

Fig. 9.1 **A checklist for the recording of physical features**

syndrome and achondroplasia, have condition-specific growth charts.

Clinical photographs are useful when discussing cases with colleagues or reviewing the natural history in the future.

It is not uncommon for parents of an affected child to have mild features of a condition, of which they have been completely unaware. Examination of family members may give clues to the diagnosis, affect the estimated risk of recurrence and have health implications for those found to have a hitherto unrecognized genetic condition.

A number of concepts are relevant when interpreting family histories and the examination of family members:

- *Penetrance* refers to the proportion of individuals possessing a disease-causing alteration who show some evidence of the condition, even if this is mild. The penetrance may vary with age. If a genetic alteration is completely penetrant, all individuals who carry the alteration will show evidence of the condition; if only a proportion manifest the condition, the genetic alteration is said to be incompletely penetrant

- *Expression* refers to the degree to which an individual is affected. Sometimes, even within a family, different individuals with the same underlying alteration may be affected by greatly varying degrees of severity and by different features of the condition.

If an affected child presents with an autosomal dominant condition, but both parents are apparently unaffected and blood tests do not show the relevant mutation in either of them, then two possibilities must be considered:

1. A new mutation may have occurred in the child
2. One of the parents carries the mutation in a proportion of their germ cells and perhaps in other tissues too, but not in their leucocytes.

A person who carries a mutation in a proportion of their cells is said to be mosaic for the mutation. Germinal mosaicism is when the mutation affects a proportion of germ-line cells. People with mosaicism can be severely affected or may have no detectable manifestations of a

Skill: pedigree construction

Drawing a family tree or pedigree is a key skill in genetics. A pedigree synthesizes a large amount of genetic information and presents it in a clear manner that can aid interpretation. Possible mechanisms of inheritance or links between conditions in family members can be clarified, allowing the differential diagnosis to be refined. Understanding the position of a person in the family tree is also essential for risk estimation.

A pedigree should encompass at least three generations and be drawn using conventional symbols (Fig. 9.2). Start with the person you are seeing (known as the consultand) and place that person on the pedigree sheet, positioning him or her according to anticipated place in the family structure. The person through whom the family was brought to attention, or 'ascertained', is known as the proband and should be marked with an arrow. The pedigree should be structured into tiers, with every member of a generation being on the same tier.

When drawing a pedigree it is good practice to:

- Ask about miscarriages, abortions, stillbirths and infant deaths
- Take details about both sides of the family
- Ask about consanguinity, specifically but tactfully
- Record dates of birth rather than ages.

The degree of information required about each family member will vary depending on the nature of condition, the person's position within a family and whether he or she is potentially affected or not. Obtaining a family history, like taking the history of a presenting complaint, should be focused and driven by clear ideas of what information is required and what use is going to be made of that information, bearing in mind that the information required may often be wide-ranging.

Pedigrees can be complicated, particularly in large families or where there is multiple consanguinity. Whilst accuracy is more important than aesthetics, one of the skills of pedigree drawing is to maintain clarity of presentation in such complex families. Even the most experienced pedigree drawer will sometimes have to redraw a pedigree taken in a clinic, particularly when a suddenly remembered uncle with multiple offspring has to be introduced, at the last minute, into what was until then a model of pedigree design.

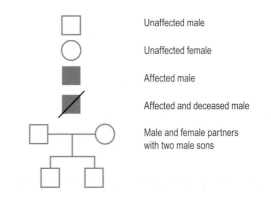

Fig. 9.2 **Symbols used in pedigrees**

condition. Even those with no signs of being affected may have a high risk of the condition recurring in future children, if a high proportion of germ-line cells carry the mutation. If the child of someone who is mosaic inherits the mutation, that child will carry the mutation in every cell in the body and is, therefore, likely to be more severely affected than the parent.

Clinical genetics and genetic counselling

When a referral is made for a clinical genetics assessment, the family may be addressed on more than one level. While a clinical genetic consultation will sometimes have a very clinical or technical focus, with the clinician attempting to understand the cause of a disease or transmitting detailed information about this to the family, at other times it may address deep emotional issues or family strategies for coping with the difficult practical problems of life with disease or disability. It is hoped that this range of issues will be dealt with in an integrated, holistic manner that is experienced by the family as supportive. Clinical genetics services often take pride in being led by their clients; it is therefore difficult to produce standardized measures of outcomes or effectiveness, because the goals differ from one consultation and family to the next.

One of the key tasks of genetic counselling is providing information. However, this process must begin by listening to find out what the concerns and questions of the clients are. (People attending a genetic counselling clinic are generally referred to as clients rather than patients to avoid the implication that they are suffering from a disease when often they are not.) The information sought may encompass diagnosis, likely prognosis and management of the condition, inheritance, risks that other relatives, including future children, may be affected, and options available to deal with these risks.

It is important to establish the diagnosis as clearly as possible. This can involve taking a history and examining affected individuals, performing investigations, obtaining a family history and reviewing the notes of other family members. If the counsellor is unfamiliar with the condition, it may be necessary to seek out information from the medical literature or from colleagues. A risk estimation can be calculated, based on knowledge of the condition and its inheritance, and the position of the clients within their family.

The information sought by the clients must then be communicated to them, in a manner sensitive to their ability to understand it. If clients are then faced with decisions, e.g. regarding prenatal or predictive testing, they can be offered support in the decision-making process. One approach is to discuss the various scenarios that could arise and to encourage them to consider their anticipated responses to the different scenarios and also the possible responses of their partner, family and others. The clients should feel supported, whatever their decision. Once decisions have been made, it may be necessary to make the practical arrangements required to implement them.

One of the long-standing tenets of genetic counselling is that the process should be non-directive, i.e. that a person should not be led to make particular decisions but be helped to make decisions that seem most appropriate from their perspective. This reflects the importance attached to autonomy in the current view of medical ethics.

However, the context in which genetic counselling takes place makes it reasonable to ask if truly non-directive counselling is possible. Choices and beliefs will be clouded by the options made available and by perceived societal values, and the counsellor is not immune from these influences. It is not always necessary to try to maintain a position of strict neutrality when presenting options. For example, when a person is undergoing presymptomatic testing for a condition for which an effective medical intervention is available, then it may be appropriate for the counsellor to favour testing whilst allowing the client to make his or her own informed decision.

Genetic testing

A genetic test can be considered to be any investigation that may reveal evidence of genetic disease. However, genetic testing is generally considered to refer to investigations where DNA or chromosomes are directly analysed, or where a specific genetic condition is tested for by another means (such as abdominal ultrasound for polycystic kidney disease or serum creatine kinase for Xp21 muscular dystrophy).

Types of genetic test include:
- *Diagnostic genetic test.* A person with signs or symptoms of a genetic disease is tested to confirm or exclude the diagnosis
- *Predictive or presymptomatic test.* This establishes whether an otherwise healthy person carries a genetic alteration that may lead to a particular genetic disease in the future.

This distinction is particularly important in children. Genetic investigations are often essential in establishing the diagnosis in a sick child. Genetic testing of healthy (so far unaffected) children may also be warranted in those at increased risk of a condition likely to develop in childhood. Otherwise, uncertainty over a child's risk may lead to serious distress within a family, with over-interpretation of minor problems. If a condition can be prevented or ameliorated by treatment, then genetic testing will be worth while. However, it is not always beneficial to carry out presymptomatic testing in children, particularly for adult-onset conditions for which no treatment is available. Children tested for Huntington disease lose their opportunity to decide for themselves whether to be tested as adults (bearing in mind that only 15–20% of adults at risk of Huntington disease decide to be tested). Adults retain control of the confidentiality over a test result and how this information is used, whilst this control is generally forfeited when a child is tested. Knowledge of the test result could lead to emotional and social problems in the child, altering both relationships within a family and expectation for the future in a variety of areas such as education, employment and relationships.

The nature of genetic disorders, our incomplete understanding of their complexities and the limitations of the techniques used to carry out genetic testing mean that care must be taken when interpreting test results and explaining their implications to children and their families.

For many types of genetic analysis, a negative test result must be interpreted with caution in case it is a false negative, i.e. a genetic abnormality is actually present but was not detected by the test.

The pathological significance of a detected genetic alteration may be unclear. For example, a missense mutation may not always lead to an alteration in a protein's function and may not lead to disease. Even when a person is shown to carry a genetic alteration known to cause disease, it can be difficult to predict just how the person will be affected because expression may be highly variable, even if the gene is fully penetrant.

When performing genetic testing, it is important to be aware that the diagnosis of a genetic disease will not only have implications for the affected individual but may have ramifications for other family members, who may be at risk of being affected or of being carriers for the condition.

Screening (see also Ch. 15)

Genetic screening involves testing apparently unaffected individuals in order to detect unrecognized genetic disease, its precursors or carrier status, when there is no particular reason to suspect that the individual is at increased risk compared to other members of the group being targeted for screening. Screening programmes may include the whole population or large subgroups, e.g. all pregnant women or all newborn babies (Box 9.1).

Screening programmes can be evaluated against well-recognized criteria (Box 9.2). Screening programmes for

---

BOX 9.1 Conditions screened for in newborn babies in Europe

In most countries
- Phenylketonuria
- Congenital hypothyroidism

In some countries
- Cystic fibrosis
- Sickle cell disease
- Medium-chain acyl-coA dehydrogenase (MCAD) deficiency and other inborn errors of metabolism

For a complete listing of neonatal screening programmes in Europe, see Tables 9.4 and 9.5.

BOX 9.2 Abbreviated criteria for a screening programme*

- The condition being screened for is an important health problem despite optimal use of treatments and of other attempts to make an early diagnosis
- Early intervention before affected individuals would otherwise present leads to improved outcome
- The screening test is simple, safe and precise
- The test is acceptable to those screened and to health professionals
- The test is introduced with adequate resources, monitoring and management

* Adapted from National Screening Committee.

---

genetic conditions do not always fulfil these criteria, as with newborn screening for Duchenne muscular dystrophy. Screening for this condition has been advocated on the basis that it enables families to make informed reproductive decisions in the future and spares them from the distress of an often delayed and protracted diagnostic process.

There are four major categories of population genetic screening programme:
1. *Newborn screening* — as for phenylketonuria and congenital hypothyroidism
2. *Antenatal screening* — the use of maternal blood samples and fetal ultrasound screening to identify those pregnancies in which the fetus has a structural malformation or a chromosomal anomaly
3. *Carrier screening* — which may take place in the antenatal clinic or elsewhere
4. *Disease susceptibility screening* — as with cholesterol screening for evidence of familial hyperlipidaemia or DNA-based screening for haemochromatosis.

The word 'screening' has three other related meanings in this context:

- 'Cascade screening' — the relatives of those carrying a genetic disorder are approached to see if they wish to be tested for that condition
- A search for mutations within a gene may be described as 'screening' of the gene — this use is probably best avoided
- The ongoing monitoring of a patient at risk of complications from the family's condition.

Whenever we use the word 'screening', we should strive to keep its meaning clear.

Prenatal testing and the selective termination of pregnancies

Prenatal testing is offered for some but not all genetic conditions. Factors that influence this provision include the severity of the condition, the effectiveness of treatment available and the accuracy of the prenatal test. When prenatal testing is available, then in any individual case several factors need to be taken into account, including the genetic risk to that pregnancy, the couple's wish to proceed with testing and their attitude to the risks involved and to a possible termination of pregnancy. Given the risk to the fetus associated with invasive diagnostic procedures, some consider it unethical to carry them out if the couple would continue with the pregnancy anyway; others accept that parents may wish to prepare themselves for an affected child. It is important to note that promoting the termination of affected pregnancies is not the primary goal of prenatal testing; it is rather to promote informed reproductive decisions and to reduce suffering in those affected by genetic conditions.

Commonly used techniques available for prenatal diagnosis and screening

Maternal serum screening is used to look for evidence of neural tube defects and trisomy 21 (p. 167). Neural tube defects result in elevated serum alpha-fetoprotein levels. Risk of trisomy 21 is assessed using combinations of alpha-fetoprotein, oestriol human chorionic gonadotrophin, inhibin or pregnancy-associated plasma protein-A (PAPP-A). Alpha-fetoprotein, PAPP-A and oestriol are reduced in trisomy 21 pregnancies; human chorionic gonadotrophin and inhibin are raised.

Ultrasound is similarly non-invasive. It can detect a wide range of abnormalities. Some of these, termed 'soft markers', indicate abnormality only in a proportion of cases, e.g. nuchal oedema, which is associated with trisomy 21. A 'fetal anomaly scan' is usually made available to women at 18–20 weeks' gestation, and ultrasound assessment of nuchal translucency is increasingly being performed in the first trimester to identify pregnancies at risk of chromosomal aneuploidy.

Amniocentesis involves the aspiration of amniotic fluid that contains a suspension of cells of fetal origin. It is usually performed at 15–16 weeks and is associated with a 0.5–1% risk of miscarriage. Once obtained, the sample is centrifuged; the supernatant can be used for alpha-fetoprotein estimation and the cells are cultured. Biochemical, molecular and chromosomal studies can be carried out on these cells. The time delay before a result is available depends on the particular test, and is partly due to the time needed to culture sufficient cells. Typically, chromosomal analysis now takes < 10 days.

Chorionic villus sampling (CVS) involves obtaining a sample of the fetal-derived chorionic villus by ultrasound-guided transabdominal aspiration. The procedure can be carried out from ~11 weeks and carries a 1–2% risk of miscarriage. Direct chromosomal analysis of uncultured chorionic villus cells often allows a provisional result to be obtained in 24 hours but detailed chromosomal analysis requires cultured cells. Most DNA and biochemical studies can be performed on uncultured cells.

Counselling issues in genetic laboratory prenatal diagnosis

When counselling a woman or couple regarding prenatal testing, it is important to discuss a number of issues:

- The nature of the condition being tested for
- The risks of the fetus having the condition
- The different options of testing available, including the risks of the procedures
- The fact that results may not be obtained, or may be ambiguous or unexpected
- How the information gained from testing may alter their plans with regard to continuing the pregnancy.

Basic science

DNA

Genetic information is encoded by molecules of DNA, which is a polymer made up of nucleotide units. Each nucleotide consists of a deoxyribose sugar molecule, a phosphate group and a nitrogenous base. There are four different types of base:

- Adenine and guanine (which are based on purine rings)
- Thymine and cytosine (which are based on pyridimine rings).

Two linear but antiparallel and complementary strands of DNA wrap around each other, giving rise to an interlocked double helix. The sugar and phosphate groups form the linear backbone of the strands with the bases projecting inwards towards their partners, forming hydrogen bonds with the complementary base in the opposing strand. Adenine bonds with thymine and guanine with cytosine.

RNA

Ribonucleic acid (RNA) differs from DNA in that it is single-stranded, uracil is found in place of thymine, and the sugar group is ribose. RNA has a number of functions in the cell, including:
- Transfer of information from chromosome to ribosome during protein synthesis
- Bringing the appropriate amino acids to the ribosomes during protein synthesis
- Catalytic activities
- Structural role in macromolecules, such as ribosomes
- Control of gene expression.

Genes

A gene is a unit of DNA containing information that determines the composition of an RNA molecule and is most often translated into protein.

Genotype and phenotype

The genotype refers to a specific version of a gene (alleles at a particular position or locus) or more widely to the genetic constitution of an individual organism. The phenotype refers to the observable characteristics or clinical features arising from a particular genotype.

Genes and the environment

The phenotype arises as a result of an interaction between the genotype and the environment from conception and throughout life. This interaction can account for the phenotypic variation sometimes seen between individuals with the same mutation in a given gene. For some phenotypic features the genetic influence is predominant; for others there is a much larger environmental influence.

A phenocopy is an environmentally induced phenotype that mimics the phenotype produced by a mutation.

For example, autosomal recessive tubular dysgenesis, which is characterized by fetal anuria, perinatal death, skull ossification defects and absent or scarce renal proximal tubules, is caused by mutations in genes encoding components of the renin–angiotensin system. A similar phenotype results from in utero exposure to angiotensin-converting enzyme (ACE) inhibitors or angiotensin II receptor antagonists.

From gene to protein

Protein synthesis requires a number of steps.

Transcription

An RNA copy of one strand of the gene sequence (used as a template) is synthesized by the enzyme, RNA polymerase. The raw transcript is then edited to produce the messenger RNA (mRNA) molecule. Each nucleotide in the mRNA is complementary to one in the DNA template.

Post-transcriptional processing

Most mammalian genes consist of exons, which are units of coding sequence, and introns, the intervening non-coding sequences. The initial transcript is edited to splice out the introns from the RNA and the exons are ligated together.

Translation

Protein synthesis occurs at cytoplasmic structures called ribosomes (consisting of ribosomal RNA and proteins). At the ribosome the mRNA forms a template for the synthesis of a specific sequence of amino acids, giving rise to a polypeptide chain. This process is mediated by transfer RNA (tRNA). A transfer RNA bound to a specific amino acid recognizes a sequence of three bases (termed a codon) in the mRNA. This correlation between codons and amino acids is the basis of the genetic code. There are 20 essential amino acids but, as there are four different types of base, there are 64 possible combinations of three bases. Some of the codons represent stop signals that terminate protein synthesis. Some amino acids are coded for by more than one triplet.

Post-translational modification

Many proteins undergo some form of post-translational modification, e.g. cleavage of the polypeptide chain or addition of sugar groups.

Chromosomes

Chromosomes consist of DNA and proteins with structural or functional roles. Most human cells are diploid; they contain two copies of the genome. There are 22 pairs of autosomal chromosomes and one pair of sex chromosomes, giving a total of 46 chromosomes per somatic (i.e. non-germ line) cell. The normal male karyotype is 46,XY and the normal female karyotype is 46,XX.

Chromosomes are identified under a microscope by their size, by their pattern of banding when stained, and by the position of a region known as the centromere that plays a key role in cell division. The centromere divides chromosomes into short (termed p) and long (termed q) arms. If the centromere is located centrally, the chromosomes are designated metacentric; if it is located peripherally, the chromosome is acrocentric.

The end of each chromosome arm is termed the telomere. This is a specialized structure thought to play an important role in maintaining the integrity of chromosomes. The chromosomal regions adjacent to telomeres, the subtelomeric regions, are particularly gene-rich.

Mitosis and meiosis

There are two different types of cell division: mitosis and meiosis. During the interphase before cell division, there is a round of DNA synthesis leading to duplication of the genome. Each replicated chromosome consists of two sister chromatids, joined at the centromere. Mitosis is the mechanism by which most cells replicate and results in the production of two genetically identical daughter cells, both with a diploid genome. During mitosis there is one cell division, with sister chromatids being split and partitioned into the daughter cells. Meiosis is the type of cell division that gives rise to spermatogonia and öogonia. This involves two successive cell divisions, giving rise to daughter cells with a haploid genome, i.e. only one copy of each chromosome. In the parent cell, one copy of each chromosome was maternally derived, the other paternally derived. As the daughter cells only contain one copy of each chromosome (either the original paternally or maternally derived chromosome), they are not genetically identical. Further genetic diversity results from the exchange of material between homologous chromosome pairs during meiosis.

Chromosomal abnormalities and mutations

A mutation is both the process of alteration of DNA and the altered DNA sequence that results. Mutations range from structural chromosome changes that are visible microscopically to single nucleotide alterations. Mutations may result in disease (pathogenic mutations) or not (non-pathogenic mutations).

A polymorphism is traditionally said to exist when there are at least two variants at a site (at least two alleles at a locus), with the least common variant accounting for at least 1% of the alleles in the population. A polymorphism generally does not result in overt disease, although it may influence factors such as susceptibility to disease or risk of side-effects from a drug. A single nucleotide polymorphism (SNP) is an alteration of a single nucleotide.

Chromosomal abnormalities

These can be classified as either numerical or structural.

Numerical abnormalities (Fig. 9.3)

- *Polyploidy* is the presence of additional sets of 23 chromosomes, e.g. triploidy
- *Aneuploidy* is the presence or absence of one or more individual chromosomes
- *Trisomy* is the presence of three copies of a chromosome, e.g. trisomy 21 in Down syndrome. Box 9.3 shows early clinical findings in trisomies
- *Monosomy* is the presence of only one member of the relevant chromosome pair, e.g. monosomy X in Turner syndrome.

Structural abnormalities (Fig. 9.4)

- *A translocation* involves the transfer of material from one chromosome to another. A balanced translocation results in no loss of genetic material. A reciprocal translocation involves breaks in two

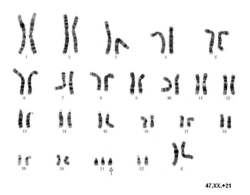

47,XX,+21

Fig. 9.3 Karyotype showing trisomy 21

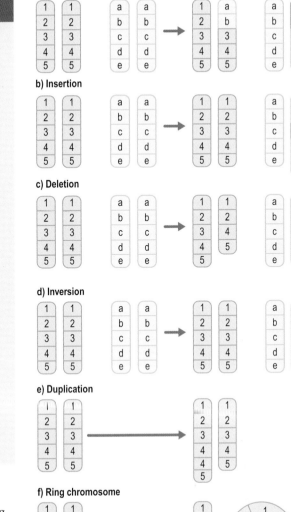

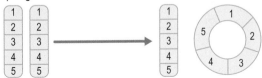

Fig. 9.4 **Chromosome rearrangements**

chromosomes and exchange between them, giving rise to two derivative chromosomes. A Robertsonian translocation arises from breaks at or close to the centromeres of acrocentric chromosomes, leading to the fusion of two acrocentric chromosomes and the loss of their short arm sequences

- *An insertion* is the insertion of a chromosomal segment into another position on a chromosome
- A *deletion* is loss of part of a chromosome
- A *duplication* is the duplication of part of a chromosome
- An *inversion* involves the position of a segment of chromosome being rotated by 180°
- A *ring chromosome* arises when a break occurs in both arms of a chromosome and the two ends then join to form a ring.

Sex chromosome abnormalities

Turner syndrome (p. 245)

There is loss of part or all of one of the sex chromosomes. About 50% of affected individuals have the karyotype 45,X; the remainder have a variety of abnormalities of one of the sex chromosomes. (About 5–10% will have some Y chromosome material.)

Klinefelter syndrome

People affected by Klinefelter syndrome have an additional X chromosome (47,XXY) or occasionally 46,XX chromosomes, with one X carrying the *SRY* gene.

Clinical features include:

- Infertility
- Hypogonadism
- Tall stature

- Gynaecomastia
- Normal cognitive function usually (but can have learning and psychological difficulties).

Submicroscopic mutations

These can be classified as:

- *Substitutions*: the replacement of one nucleotide by another
- *Insertions*: the addition of one or more nucleotide
- *Deletions*: the loss of one or more nucleotide.

Additionally, mutations in the coding regions of genes can be classified depending on their effect on the amino acid sequence:

- *Synonymous mutations*: these do not alter the polypeptide sequence, e.g. the conversion of one codon to another coding for the same amino acid
- *Non-synonymous mutations*: these do lead to an alteration in the polypeptide sequence. There are different types of non-synonymous mutation:
  - *Missense mutations* are single-base pair changes that result in the substitution of one amino acid for another
  - *Nonsense mutations* are changes that result in the formation of a stop codon and lead to premature termination of protein synthesis
  - *Frameshift mutations* are insertions or deletions of nucleotides that are not a multiple of three. This shifts the reading frame, leading to totally different codons downstream from the mutation, usually arriving before very far at a nonsense triplet and therefore to chain termination.

Patterns of inheritance

Autosomal dominant

The disorder is expressed either largely or completely in the heterozygote. All offspring of an affected person will have a 50% chance of inheriting the mutation, giving rise to vertical transmission in a pedigree. Variable expression and incomplete penetrance can complicate recognition of autosomal dominant inheritance. Examples of autosomal dominant conditions are given in Box 9.4.

Autosomal recessive

The disorder is expressed largely or completely in the affected homozygote. Often this presents as an isolated case within a pedigree or as affected siblings. Where both

---

BOX 9.4 Examples of autosomal dominant conditions

- Achondroplasia
- Facioscapulohumeral dystrophy
- Hereditary elliptocytosis
- Hereditary spherocytosis
- Huntington disease
- Marfan syndrome
- Myotonic dystrophy
- Neurofibromatosis types 1 and 2
- Noonan syndrome
- Tuberous sclerosis complex
- von Willebrand disease

BOX 9.5 Examples of autosomal recessive conditions

- Alpha$_1$-antitrypsin deficiency
- Ataxia telangiectasia
- Beta-thalassaemia
- Congenital adrenal hyperplasia
- Cystic fibrosis
- Fanconi anaemia
- Galactosaemia
- Glycogen storage disorders
- Haemochromatosis
- Homocystinuria
- Mucopolysaccharidoses (except Hunter syndrome)
- Oculocutaneous albinism
- Phenylketonuria
- Sickle cell disease
- Spinal muscular atrophy
- Wilson disease
- Zellweger syndrome

---

parents are carriers, each of their offspring has a 25% risk of being homozygous and a 50% risk of being a heterozygous carrier. Examples of autosomal recessive disorders are given in Box 9.5.

Sex-linked (X chromosome) disease

These conditions result from mutations in a gene carried on the X chromosome. Males will usually be affected, as they will only have one copy of the gene. In females one of the X chromosomes is inactivated. This occurs at around day 15 of gestation. Which X

- Becker muscular dystrophy
- Duchenne muscular dystrophy
- Fabry disease
- Glucose-6-phosphate dehydrogenase deficiency
- Haemophilias A and B
- Hunter syndrome (mucopolysaccharidosis type II)
- Hypohidrotic ectodermal dysplasia
- Incontinentia pigmenti (usually in females only)
- Lesch–Nyhan syndrome
- Ocular albinism
- Rett syndrome (very largely restricted to females)
- Wiskott–Aldrich syndrome

Table 9.2 Repeat lengths and expression in fragile X syndrome

Repeat length	Category
5–44	Normal
45–54	Intermediate
55–200	Premutation
> 200	Full mutation

chromosome is inactivated is a random event, but once inactivated, the X chromosome remains inactivated in all daughter cells. Not all the genes on an inactivated X chromosome are silent; some are expressed (which is why XO women exhibit the Turner phenotype). Female carriers of sex-linked conditions are usually unaffected but may show some features of the disease, depending upon the pattern of X chromosome inactivation in the woman's tissues and the biology of the gene product. A woman will tend to manifest such conditions rather less severely than an affected male. Features of this sex-linked form of inheritance are:

- There is no male-to-male transmission
- All daughters of an affected male will be carriers
- The risk to sons of women who are carriers is 50%
- The risk that daughters of female carriers will themselves be carriers is 50%.

There has been a tendency to separate X chromosome gene disorders into X-linked recessive, which tend not to manifest much in females, and X-linked dominant, in which females are commonly affected and males may be so severely affected as to die in utero or in infancy (X-linked dominant, male-lethal). This demarcation is useful in looking at patterns of inheritance in a family, but is not very helpful in understanding how some women but not others come to show signs of the condition. Examples of X-linked disorders are given in Box 9.6.

Duchenne muscular dystrophy (Ch. 28)

This condition results from mutations in the dystrophin gene on Xp21. About 65% of mutations are deletions of one or more exons in the *DMD* gene, with another 5% or so being duplications and most of the rest being point mutations.

Female carriers of DMD mutations can develop problems such as muscle weakness (20%) and dilated cardiomyopathy (8%). About 50% have a raised serum creatine kinase. Rarely, females can have a more severe phenotype like that of affected males, due to chromosomal arrangement involving the *DMD* locus, non-random inactivation of the X chromosome due to problems with the inactivation process, or because they have coexistent Turner syndrome.

Trinucleotide repeat disorders

Trinucleotide repeats are sequences in which a set of three nucleotides is repeated a variable number of times within a gene. Several disorders are associated with the abnormal expansion of trinucleotide repeats. Generally, the severity of the phenotype in these conditions is related to the number of repeats. The number of repeats can increase in successive generations, giving rise to the phenomenon of anticipation where there is an earlier age of onset and/or more severe manifestations in succeeding generations.

Important trinucleotide repeat disorders in paediatrics include the congenital form of myotonic dystrophy, the juvenile-onset form of Huntington disease, Friedreich ataxia and fragile X syndrome.

Fragile X syndrome

Fragile X (Ch. 29) is a common cause of cognitive impairment. It is associated with abnormal tri-nucleotide repeats in the *FMR1* gene. The size of the repeat and the sex of the affected person influence the phenotype (Table 9.2).

The repeat length of a premutation allele can increase during transmission, so the child of a premutation carrier could have a full mutation.

Males with a premutation do not have childhood cognitive impairment but can develop late-onset ataxia/tremor and cognitive deficits: fragile X-associated tremor/ataxia syndrome (FXTAS). Males with a full mutation have cognitive impairment (often moderate, but varies from mild to severe), a distinctive facial appearance (large head, prominent ears and chin) and post-pubertally large testes.

Females with a premutation are at risk of premature ovarian failure and, to a lesser degree than premutation males, late-onset ataxia. Females with a full mutation can exhibit the same physical and cognitive features as full mutation males but usually to a lesser extent.

Problem-orientated topic:

genetic counselling ● ● ● ● ●

Nikolai, a 4-year-old boy, has moderate cognitive impairment. You have received a report from the laboratory, which says he has a full mutation in FMR1, the gene responsible for fragile X syndrome. When you see the parents to give the result, they ask about the risk of this condition recurring in future pregnancies. The boy's mother, who is in her mid-30s, says they have been trying to conceive for the past 2 years without success. When reviewing the family history, you note that Nikolai's maternal grandfather developed a tremor and unsteady gait in later life that was attributed to Parkinson disease.

Q1. What do you tell the parents about the risk of this recurring in another pregnancy?

Q2. Does this diagnosis have health implications for other family members?

Q1. What do you tell the parents about the risk of this recurring in another pregnancy?

There are a number of different possible explanations for this family history that have different implications for the risk to future offspring. It is possible that Nikolai's mother carries a full mutation but is unaffected or, more likely, is a premutation carrier. If she carries a full mutation, there will be a 50% risk of transmitting the mutated allele to each future child. If she is a premutation carrier, the risk of having an affected child depends on the premutation size in her and the sex of the child. For a repeat of 60–69, the risk that a son will be severely affected will be around 10%; for a repeat of 90–99, that risk will be around 47%.

Analysis of the FMR1 gene in Nikolai's mother would help to establish the likely risk for future pregnancies.

Q2. Does this diagnosis have health implications for other family members?

Other family members, who may not have any cognitive problems, may be at risk of having affected offspring, of FXTAS or of premature ovarian failure, and should be counselled accordingly.

Mitochondrial disorders

Each mitochondrion in a cell contains a circular DNA molecule that encodes components of the respiratory chain, ribosomal RNA and tRNA. The mitochondrial DNA is compact, contains little repetitive DNA and has no introns. The genetic code of mitochondrial DNA differs from nuclear DNA using some different amino acid codons.

Mitochondrial disorders can result from mutations in mitochondrial DNA or in nuclear genes coding for proteins that are transported into mitochondria. The nuclear gene abnormalities are inherited in an autosomal dominant or autosomal recessive manner. Mitochondrial DNA mutations are transmitted by maternal inheritance, i.e. they are passed down from mother to child but not from father to child. In most people all mitochondria contain identical copies of the mitochondrial genome at birth (i.e. are homoplastic), but in those with mitochondrial disorders there may be a variable mix of mitochondria with normal (wild-type) and mutated DNA within each cell (heteroplasmy).

Some affected individuals display a cluster of features suggestive of a particular syndrome (Table 9.3 and Box 9.7). However, many display symptoms that do not fit into a specific pattern.

Table 9.3 **Examples of some mitochondrial disorders**

Disorder	Primary features
Mitochondrial encephalomyopathy with lactic acidosis and stroke-like episodes (MELAS)	Stroke-like episodes, seizures, dementia, lactic acidosis
Leber hereditary optic neuropathy	Subacute painless visual loss, cardiac pre-excitation
Leigh syndrome (not always caused by mutations in mitochondrial DNA)	Subacute relapsing encephalopathy, cerebellar and brainstem signs

Where clinical features are suggestive of a particular mitochondrial syndrome, then specific clinical investigations can be used to define the phenotype and diagnostic testing of specific genes can be performed. A family history can be invaluable in suggesting the pattern of inheritance and the diagnosis. When a mitochondrial disorder is suspected but the diagnosis is not so clear, the following can be helpful: blood and/ or cerebrospinal fluid lactate levels; genetic testing on blood for homoplasmic mutations; muscle biopsy (for histological/histochemical evidence of mitochondrial disease and for DNA analysis for heteroplasmic deletions); neuroimaging; and cardiac assessment.

Imprinting

For most autosomal genes, both alleles are expressed in a cell. However, for some genes only one allele is expressed, while the other is switched off. Whether an allele is expressed or not is determined by the sex of the parent that contributed it. This phenomenon is termed 'imprinting' (Fig. 9.5). In a maternally imprinted gene the maternally derived allele is inactivated. In a paternally imprinted gene the paternally derived allele is inactivated. Examples of conditions associated with imprinted genes are:

- Prader–Willi syndrome (PWS)
- Angelman syndrome
- Beckwith–Wiedemann syndrome
- Silver–Russell syndrome (some cases only).

PWS is caused by a lack of *paternal* contribution at 15q11–13. This can arise:

- By deletion of this region in the paternally derived chromosome 15
- By uniparental disomy (where both copies of a chromosome are derived from one parent)

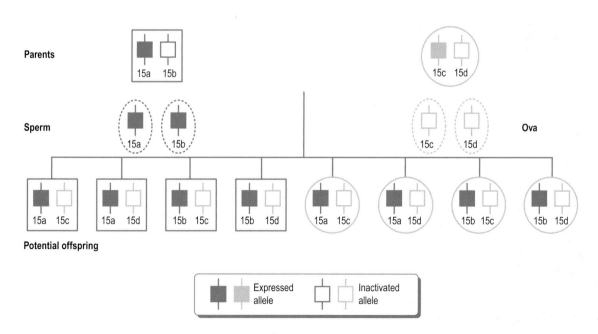

Fig. 9.5 The inheritance of a maternally imprinted gene.
Father represented in blue, mother in mauve. In the parents, only the paternally derived copies are expressed. In the ova, imprinting inactivates all maternally derived copies of the allele.

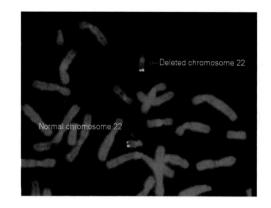

Fig. 9.6 Fluorescent in situ hybridization (FISH) with probes that hybridize to regions of chromosome 22.
The region that the red probe binds to has been deleted in one chromosome 22.

— in this case, two copies of maternally derived chromosome 15
- Very uncommonly, by an imprinting centre mutation.

Angelman syndrome, in which the degree of cognitive and motor problems is rather greater than for PWS, is caused by a lack of *maternal* contribution at part of 15q11–13 that is paternally imprinted. There are often deletions in the same chromosomal region as for PWS or, occasionally, paternal uniparental disomy for chromosome 15, or point mutations in the *UBE3A* gene or in the imprinting control region.

Applications of DNA technology

Examining chromosomes, stained to demonstrate their characteristic bands, under a microscope remains a mainstay of genetic diagnosis. However, techniques are available to demonstrate chromosomal abnormalities too small to be seen by this technique. Fluorescent in situ hybridization (FISH) involves the use of a fluorescently labelled probe to bind to a specific DNA sequence (Fig. 9.6). If that sequence is present in both copies of a chromosome, then under fluorescent microscopy the probe can be visualized binding to both. If it is absent in one copy, the probe will only bind to the chromosome homologue retaining the target sequence.

In the subtelomeric regions, which are gene-rich, small rearrangements can have profound phenotypic consequences. A number of techniques can be used to look for such subtelomeric rearrangements. One of the most commonly applied is multiprobe FISH, in which fluorescently labelled telomere-specific probes for all chromosomes are used. Subtelomeric rearrangements have been found to account for approximately 6% of

cases of mental retardation. Thus, analysis of the subtelomeric region has become an important second-line investigation in affected individuals when conventional cytogenetic techniques have revealed apparently normal chromosomes.

Comparative genomic hybridization (CGH) can be used to look at submicroscopic abnormalities along the length of chromosomes. Different colour fluorescent markers are used to label the patient's DNA (green) and reference DNA (red). These are then applied to a slide covered with normal human chromosomes and allowed to hybridize. The amount of green and red fluorescence is then compared, and will be 1:1 throughout if the patient's DNA is normal. More green means the patient has extra DNA in that area (because more copies of green-labelled patient DNA have 'stuck'). More red indicates that the patient is missing DNA in that area.

Several techniques are available to look for mutations at the DNA level. There is a trade-off between cost in resources needed for a given technique and accuracy. Because of this, one approach is to screen the gene in question using a high-throughput technique and to confirm any abnormalities detected using a resource-intensive but more accurate method. An alternative, useful for genes in which a small number of different mutations account for most cases, is to use the resource-intensive but more accurate methods just to look for those mutations and not to screen the rest of the gene.

Recombinant DNA technology

Recombinant DNA can be defined as DNA molecules constructed outside living cells by joining natural or synthetic DNA segments to DNA molecules that can replicate in living cells, or the molecules that result from their replication.

Recombinant DNA techniques can be used to isolate, characterize or alter genes and to insert genes into cells, allowing their product to be studied or commercially utilized.

Gene cloning refers to the production of multiple identical copies of a gene. One strategy for cloning a mammalian gene is to introduce that gene into bacteria. This strategy requires a number of steps:
1. Prepare complementary DNA (cDNA) from mRNA extracted from the mammalian cells. The total complement of mRNA represents all the genes that are transcribed. The mRNA does not contain any intronic material, as this has been spliced out. Complementary DNA can be prepared from the mRNA using a reverse transcriptase
2. Amplify the cDNA of the target gene by polymerase chain reaction (PCR)

3. Insert the target gene into a cloning vector, a DNA molecule that carries the foreign DNA into a host cell where the vector with the inserted gene can replicate. A typical vector is a bacterial plasmid that has been constructed to carry a selectable marker, e.g. a gene that confirms resistance to an antibiotic

4. Insert the plasmid into bacterial cells. Culturing the bacteria in media containing the antibiotic to which the plasmid confers resistance will select the bacteria that have taken up the plasmid, as only these will grow.

The successfully transformed bacteria, those that contain the plasmid with the target gene, will express the gene product and can be easily grown in the laboratory or, if necessary, on an industrial scale to provide supplies of biomolecules too complex to synthesize commercially using conventional chemical techniques, such as human factor 8 or insulin.

Table 9.4 List of metabolic disorders or abnormalities amenable to newborn screening by acylcarnitine and amino acid profile analyses with ESI-MS/MS. Disorders screened for by identical metabolites are described in one line. (From Bodamer OA et al. Extended newborn screening in Europe 2007. J Inherit Metab Dis (2007) 30:439–444.)

Group of disorders	Disorder	Abbreviation
Defects in amino acid degradation and the urea cycle	Phenylketonuria, hyperphenylalaninemia*	PKU/HPA
	Maple syrup urine disease	MSUD
	Tyrosinaemia type I	TyrI
	Homocystinuria (CBS deficiency)	Homocyst
	Citrullinaemia type I (II)	Cit
	Argininosuccinate lyase deficiency	ASL
	Arginase deficiency	ArginaseD
Defects in organic acid degradation	Glutaric aciduria type I	GA I
	Isovaleric aciduria	IVA
	2-Methylbutyryl-CoA dehydrogenase deficiency*,**	MBD
	Methylmalonic aciduria, propionic aciduria	MMA, PA
	3-Methylcrotonyl-CoA-carboxylase deficiency*	3-MCCD
	2-Methyl-3-hydroxybutyryl-CoA dehydrogenase deficiency*, **	MHBD
	Multiple acyl-CoA dehydrogenase deficiency	MADD
	Malonic aciduria	MA
	3-Methylglutaconic aciduria type I*	MGA I
	Holocarboxylase synthetase deficiency	HCSD
Defects of the carnitine cycle, fatty acid oxidation and ketone body synthesis	Carnitine palmitoyltransferase I deficiency	CPT ID
	Carnitine palmitoyltransferase II deficiency	CPT IID
	Carnitine-acylcarnitine translocase deficiency	CACT
	Systemic carnitine transporter deficiency	CTD
	Medium-chain acyl-CoA dehydrogenase deficiency	MCADD
	Long-chain 3-hydroxyacyl-CoA dehydrogenase deficiency	LCHADD
	Mitochondrial trifunctional protein deficiency	mTFP
	Very long-chain acyl-CoA dehydrogenase deficiency	VLCADD
	β-Ketothiolase deficiency	KT
	3-Hydroxy-3-methylglutaryl-CoA lyase deficiency	HMG-CoA LD
	Short-chain acyl-CoA dehydrogenase deficiency*	SCAD
	Isobutyrl-CoA dehydrogenase deficiency*,**	IBCDD
Other disorders	Guanidinoacetate methyltransferase deficiency	GAMTD

* Indicates a biochemical condition with undefined or without clinical significance (non-diseases).
** probably not detected owing to only slightly elevated or normal metabolite concentrations in the neonatal period.

Table 9.5 Comparison of European Countries (***excluding Scotland) regarding number of screening centres, total population (year 2001*), screened infants (year 2003**) and metabolic disorders included in MS/MS screening; see Table 9.4 for abbreviations. The numbers for screening centres, total population and screened infants are partially based on a questionnaire that was initiated by ISNS in 2003. Details can be found on www.isns-neoscreening.org. (From Bodamer OA et al. Extended newborn screening in Europe 2007. J Inherit Metab Dis (2007) 30:439–444.)

Country	No of centres	Population* (millions)	Number of infants screened** (average sample number/ screening laboratory)	Disorders included in extended screening by MS/MS
Austria (including South Tyrol, Italy)	1	8.18	77186 (77186)	PKU, MSUD, Tyrl, Cit, ASLD, Homocyst, MCADD, LCHADD, VLCADD, CPT ID CPT IID/CACT, CTD, KTD, HMG-CoA LD, MMA, PA, IVA, GA I, 3-MCCD
Belgium	6	10.29	105335 (17555)	PKU, MSUD, Tyrl, MCADD, LCHADD, VLCADD, CPT ID CPT IID/CACT, CTD, KTD, HMG-CoA LD, MMA, PA, IVA, GA I, 3-MCCD
Bulgaria	1	7.55	63190	None
Croatia	1	4.43	No information	None
Czech Republic	4	10.25	93685 (23421)	None
Denmark	1	5.38	66657 (66657)	PKU, MSUD, Cit, ASLD, ArginaseD, MCADD, LCHADD, VLCADD, CPT ID CPT IID/CACT, CTD, KTD, HMG-CoA LD, MMA, PA, IVA, GA I, 3-MCCD (pilot study, not 100% population coverage)
Finland	40	5.19	56000 (1400)	None
France	22	59.94	764212 (34737)	None
Germany	13	83.43	725125 (60427)	PKU, MSUD, MCADD, LCHADD, VLCADD, CPT ID, CPT IID/CACT, IVA, GA I
Great Britain***	20	54.78	625749 (32287)	MCADD (pilot project, not 100% population coverage)
Hungary	4	10.05	approx. 100000 (25000)	None
Iceland	1	0.308	4000 (4000)	None
Ireland	1	3.92	62000 (62000)	None
Italy	22	57.74	566169 (25734)	No information
Netherlands	5	16.14	200635 (40127)	PKU, MSUD, Homocyst, Tyrl, MCADD, LCHADD, VLCADD, HMG-CoA LyaseD, IVA, GA I, 3-MCCD
Norway	1	4.54	56846 (56846)	None
Poland	8	38.62	352152 (44019)	PKU, MSUD, Tyrl, MCADD, LCHADD, VLCADD, CPT ID, CPT IID/CACT, CTD, IVA, GA I; one centre screens for 30% of population
Portugal	1	10.10	112557 (112557)	PKU, MSUD, MCADD, LCHADD, VLCADD, CPT ID, CPT IID/CACT, IVA, GA I, GAMTD
Romania	No information	22.28	No information	None
Serbia	1	10.50	57354 (57354)	None
Slovakia	1	5.43	No information	None
Slovenia	1	1.94	14000 (14000)	None
Spain	20	40.11	441297 (22064)	PKU, MSUD, MCADD, LCHADD, VLCADD, CPT ID, CPT IID/CACT, IVA, GA I; one centre screens <10% of population)
Switzerland	1	7.32	74450 (74450)	PKU, MCADD
Total	**176**	**478418**	**4618599**	

Imti Choonara Jose Ramet

CHAPTER

10

Pharmacology and therapeutics

LEARNING OUTCOMES

By the end of this chapter you should:

- Know and understand the principles of pharmacokinetics in children
- Know and understand the major pathways of drug metabolism in paediatric patients of different ages
- Know and understand some of the major adverse drug reactions that have occurred in paediatric patients
- Know and understand the mechanisms by which adverse drug reactions may occur in paediatric patients
- Know how to prescribe medicines safely
- Be aware of the most frequent types of medication error associated with drug prescribing for children
- Know and understand the principles of the use of antimicrobials
- Know how to assess pain in paediatric patients of different ages
- Understand how to manage pain in children.

MODULE TWO

Introduction

To prescribe medicines safely, one needs to understand how the human body handles different medicines. In order to do this, one needs to have a basic understanding of clinical pharmacology. It is important to recognize that children handle medicines differently to adults, and therefore one needs to understand the interaction between age and clinical pharmacology; this is described below.

Pharmacokinetics

Pharmacokinetics is the relationship between the dose of a drug and its concentration in different parts of the body (usually plasma) in relation to time, and is defined numerically in a quantitative manner. Mathematical formulae are available that describe the interrelationship between clearance, volume of distribution and elimination half-life. These terms are described below.

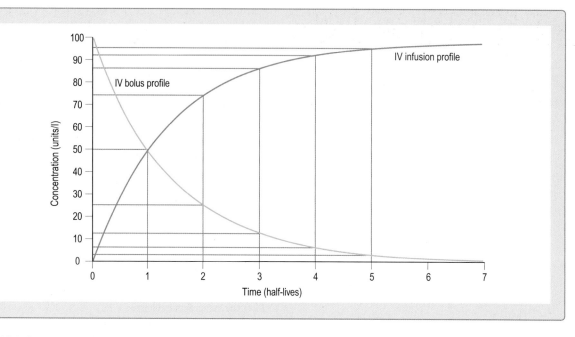

Fig. 10.1 Concentration–time profiles following a single intravenous bolus dose and during a constant rate infusion. Time is shown in half-lives. A total of 97% of the drug is eliminated and 97% of steady state is achieved in five half-lives.
(Reproduced from Thomson 2000, with permission.)

Absorption

If a drug is given intravenously, then 100% of the dose enters the blood stream. If a drug is given orally, then usually only a fraction is absorbed; the term 'bioavailability' is used to describe the percentage of the drug administered that reaches the systemic circulation. Absorption is often reduced following oral administration in the neonatal period.

Volume of distribution (V)

This is not a physiological volume, but rather an apparent volume into which the drug would have to distribute to achieve the measured concentration. Water-soluble drugs, such as gentamicin, have a V that is similar to the extracellular fluid volume. Drugs that are highly bound to plasma proteins have a low V. Differences between paediatric and adult patients stem mainly from the fact that neonates and young children have a higher proportion of body water and lower concentrations of plasma proteins.

Clearance

Clearance describes the removal of a drug from the body and is defined as the volume (usually of plasma) that is completely cleared of drug in a given time period. In adults, clearance is therefore described in relation to volume/time (ml/min). In paediatric

patients, clearance is also described in relation to body weight (ml/min/kg).

Elimination half-life

The elimination half-life is inversely related to the clearance. The elimination half-life is the time it takes for the concentration of a drug (usually in plasma) to fall to half its original value. By definition, therefore, 50% of the dose will be eliminated in one half-life. Five half-lives is the time required for 97% of the drug to be eliminated (Fig. 10.1). This is also the time required for steady state to be achieved following initial administration of the drug.

Therapeutic drug monitoring

Therapeutic drug monitoring (TDM) consists of measuring plasma concentrations of the drug in order to improve efficacy and reduce toxicity (Box 10.1). It is useful if there is a clear relationship between the plasma concentration and the clinical effect. A specific, precise and accurate analytical technique is required to measure plasma concentrations of a drug. TDM is recommended for aminoglycosides in order to reduce toxicity (p. 108). It may be beneficial in patients with poorly controlled epilepsy who are receiving carbamazepine, phenytoin or phenobarbital (Chs 24 and 28). It is also clinically useful with a variety of other medications. Interpretation of the plasma concentration of a drug requires details of the time of administration of the drug and time of collection of the blood sample, as well as an understanding of why TDM has been requested.

Key points

- Clearance is usually reduced in the neonatal period.
- The half-life is usually longer in the neonatal period.

Drug metabolism

The major pathways involved in drug metabolism are divided into phase 1 (oxidation, reduction, hydrolysis and hydration) and phase 2 (glucuronidation, sulphation, methylation and acetylation) reactions. As a general rule, the clearance of drugs in the neonatal period is reduced. For many drugs, adult clearance values are reached by the age of 2 years (Table 10.1).

The major pathway in phase 1 is oxidation, which involves the cytochrome P450 enzymes (CYP) that are present mainly in the liver. The major CYP enzymes are CYP3A4 and CYP1A2. CYP3A4 is responsible for the metabolism of many drugs such as midazolam, ciclosporin, fentanyl and nifedipine. CYP3A4 activity is reduced in the neonatal period and early infancy. There is considerable inter-individual variation in enzyme activity, and this results in considerable variation in plasma concentrations of drugs such as midazolam, despite usage

Table 10.1 Age and morphine clearance

Age group	Number of patients	Mean or median plasma clearance (ml/min/kg)	Range
Preterm neonates	72	3.5	0.5–9.6
Term neonates	44	6.3	0.6–39
Infants 1–24 months	11	13.9	8.3–24.1
Children 2–11 years	18	37.4	20.1–48.5
Adolescents 12–17 years	6	25.4	9–53.4

(Reproduced from de Wildt, Johnson & Choonara 2003, with permission.)

of similar doses. CYP1A2 accounts for 13% of total enzyme activity in the liver. Caffeine and theophylline are metabolized via the CYP1A2 pathway. Enzyme activity is reduced in the neonatal period but increases rapidly such that, by the age of 6 months, activity is approaching that of older children and adults.

Glucuronidation and sulphation are the two major phase 2 pathways. Glucuronidation is reduced in the neonatal period and there is compensatory sulphation. The development of glucuronidation varies, in that children who are 2 years old have rates of glucuronidation for morphine similar to that in adults (Table 10.1). In the case of paracetamol, however, adult rates of glucuronidation are not reached until puberty.

Drug toxicity

Almost 1 in 10 children in hospital will experience an adverse drug reaction (ADR), of which 1 in 8 will be severe. About 2% of children in hospital are admitted following an ADR. Children can experience a wide variety of ADRs.

Children are at risk of specific ADRs that do not affect adults, as growth and development are not an issue in adult patients. Differences in drug metabolism make certain ADRs a greater problem in children (e.g. valproate hepatotoxicity in young children, where toxic metabolites are more likely to be produced) or less of a problem (e.g. paracetamol hepatotoxicity following an overdose). There is a greater capacity for the sulphation of paracetamol in prepubertal children, which reduces the formation of toxic metabolites. The mechanisms of ADRs specifically affecting children are illustrated in Table 10.2.

Percutaneous absorption

The newborn infant has a higher surface area to weight ratio than both adults and children. Percutaneous toxicity can therefore be a significant problem in the neonatal period. Examples of this include the use of antiseptic agents such as hexachlorophene, which have been associated with neurotoxicity.

Protein-displacing effect on bilirubin

The sulphonamide, sulphisoxazole, was used as an antibiotic in neonates in the 1950s. It was associated with increased mortality due to the development of kernicterus. Sulphonamides have a higher binding affinity to albumin than bilirubin. Thus, the administration of sulphonamides results in an increase in the free fraction of bilirubin, which crosses the blood–brain barrier and causes kernicterus if the neonate is ill

Table 10.2 Major adverse drug reactions (ADRs) in paediatric patients

Year	Drug/compound	Age group	ADR	Mechanism
1886	Aniline dye	Neonates	Methaemoglobinaemia	Percutaneous absorption
1956	Sulphisoxazole	Neonates	Kernicterus	Protein-displacing effect on bilirubin
1959	Chloramphenicol	Neonates	Grey baby syndrome	Impaired metabolism
1979	Sodium valproate	Young children (< 3 years)	Hepatic failure	Abnormal metabolism?
1980	Salicylate	Children	Reye syndrome	Unknown
1990	Propofol	Children	Metabolic acidosis	Unknown Dose-related?
1996	Lamotrigine	Children	Skin reactions	Unknown Associated with co-medication with sodium valproate

(Reproduced from Choonara & Rieder 2002, with permission.)

and jaundiced. In most areas of paediatrics, protein binding is not a significant issue.

Impaired drug metabolism

Chloramphenicol was associated with the development of the grey baby syndrome in neonates. Infants developed vomiting, cyanosis and cardiovascular collapse, and in some cases died. The newborn infant metabolizes chloramphenicol more slowly than adults and therefore requires a lower dose. Reduction in the dosage prevents the development of the grey baby syndrome.

Altered drug metabolism

Paediatric patients may have reduced activity of the major enzymes associated with drug metabolism in the liver. To compensate for this, they may have increased pathways of other enzymes. This is thought to be one of the factors contributing to the increased risk of hepatotoxicity in children under the age of 3 years who receive sodium valproate. This increased risk is raised by the use of additional anticonvulsants alongside the sodium valproate, which may result in enzyme induction of certain metabolic pathways.

Drug interactions

Skin reactions to the anticonvulsant, lamotrigine, are more likely to occur in children than in infants. The incidence is significantly increased by co-medication with sodium valproate alongside the lamotrigine. The mechanism of this drug interaction is unknown.

Unknown

There are several examples of major ADRs that occur in children for which we do not understand the mechanism. Salicylate given during the presence of a viral illness will predispose children of all ages to develop Reye syndrome. By avoiding the use of salicylates in children with viral infections, the incidence of Reye syndrome has been dramatically reduced. Propofol is a parenteral anaesthetic agent with minimal toxicity when used to induce general anaesthesia. However, reports in the literature have indicated that when used as a sedative in critically ill infants and young children, it may be associated with a fatal outcome. The biological explanation for this is that children, in states of stress, are more dependent than adults on the use of fatty acids as fuel substrates. Propofol has been associated with failure of mitochondrial respiration and defects of fatty acid oxidation and its use in critically ill children can result in overall energy failure with clinical evidence of multiple organ and/or myocardial failure, resulting in death. Propofol infusion syndrome is defined as the sudden, or relatively sudden, onset of marked bradycardia during propofol infusion plus one or more of the following: (1) lipemic plasma; (2) a clinically enlarged liver secondary to fatty infiltration; (3) the presence of severe metabolic acidosis; and (4) the presence of muscle involvement with evidence of rhabdomyolysis or myoglobinuria. The syndrome is thought to be related to the total dose of propofol infused, i.e. high dose or prolonged duration is more likely to cause problems.

Fetal toxicity

The majority of medicines used during pregnancy do not result in harm to the fetus. Both health professionals and pregnant women usually over-estimate the risk of drug toxicity associated with the use of medicines during pregnancy. Thalidomide, however, is an example of how a drug that is relatively safe in adults can result in significant harm to the fetus (phocomelia) when it is given during a critical stage in pregnancy (24–27 days). The drug that is most likely to be associated with fetal toxicity at present is alcohol, which may result in the fetal alcohol syndrome. With the increasing use of recreational drugs by young women, it is highly likely that the major cause of fetal toxicity in the future will be associated with recreational drug use rather than prescribed medicines.

Key points

- Percutaneous toxicity can occur in newborn infants.
- The protein-displacing effect of medicines should be considered in sick preterm neonates.
- Paediatric patients, and neonates in particular, are more likely to have a reduced capacity to metabolize drugs than adults. Therefore lower doses are usually required.
- Sodium valproate should not be used as a first-line anticonvulsant in children under the age of 3 years.
- Drug interactions may increase the risk of an ADR.
- Propofol should not be used as a sedative in critically ill children.

One should always consider the possibility of an ADR being responsible for a child's symptoms. Recognizing which patients are at greater risk of ADRs can help reduce the overall incidence. Health professionals should try to follow guidelines. Suspected ADRs should be reported to the regulatory authorities.

Prescribing for children

Many medicines used in children are not licensed for such use. This is usually because the pharmaceutical company has not asked for a licence from the regulatory authorities. Additionally, many medicines given to children are off-label, i.e. used at a different dose or route than specified within the product licence or for a different age or different indication. The Medicines for Children Working Group of the European Academy of Paediatrics (EAP) recommends using the medicines for which there is the greatest amount of evidence to justify its usage. In certain circumstances, this may involve off-label use.

The metabolism of some drugs may be affected by one or a number of the following mechanisms:
- Certain illnesses, e.g. cystic fibrosis
- Clinical conditions, e.g. shock, which may affect the metabolism of drugs
- Liver and renal failure, which will delay the elimination of drugs and hence dictates reduced dosages.

One needs to recognize that not all medicines are prescribed, i.e. they can be obtained over the counter from a pharmacy either by a parent or, in the case of

Table 10.3 Types of medication error

Type of medication error	Number	Fatal
Incorrect dose	32	13
Incorrect drug	16	5
Incorrect strength	3	1
Omitted in error	4	1
Incorrect patient	4	–
Duplicate dose	3	–
Expired drugs	3	–
Incorrect route	3	3
Incorrect container	2	1
Incorrect label	2	–
Incorrect rate	2	2
Miscellaneous	6	3
TOTAL	80*	29

* Six children experienced more than one error each.
(Reproduced from Cousins et al 2002, with permission.)

adolescents, by children themselves. Parents may not always be aware of the active ingredient present in over-the-counter medicines and therefore a full history needs to be obtained before prescribing medicines such as paracetamol or ibuprofen. In adolescent girls, one also needs to be aware of the possibility of any possible teratogenic effects of medicines if they become pregnant.

Most medicines can be taken by a breastfeeding mother and will not cause a significant problem to the breastfed infant. One should not discourage mothers from breastfeeding because they are uncertain of possible toxic effects. Several formularies give detailed information regarding which medicines to avoid during breastfeeding.

Medication errors are a significant problem in paediatric patients. A review of press reports of medication errors described 29 deaths of paediatric patients in the UK only over a period of 8 years (Cousins et al 2002). The types of medication error are illustrated in Table 10.3. All health professionals will commit a medication error at some stage in their career. Systems need to be introduced to try to minimize the impact of these errors.

Incorrect dose is the most frequent type of medication error and is also the type of error most likely to be associated with a fatality. One therefore needs to have an accurate note of the child's weight, and dose calculations, especially on the neonatal unit and when using parenteral medicines, require careful checking. Tenfold errors are a particular problem in both neonates and children.

Incorrect drug is the second most common type of medication error and is also associated with significant fatalities. Incorrect route is a particular problem with intrathecal drugs and great care is required for medicines administered via this route (Box 10.2).

Key points

- Incorrect dose is the most frequent medication error.
- Tenfold errors are a significant problem in paediatric patients.
- Incorrect drug is a common type of medication error.

Use of antimicrobials

The choice of antimicrobial agent needs to be made in conjunction with the local microbiologist, who will be aware of local resistance patterns. A broad-spectrum antimicrobial is of value where the organism is unknown, but is not recommended if the organism is known and sensitive to more specific antibiotics. In general, one should aim to use the lowest effective dose of an antimicrobial agent, as drug toxicity is more likely to be associated with higher doses. This is especially the case with aminoglycosides. The preterm neonate handles drugs differently to the term neonate and therefore the frequency of administration of many antibiotics needs to be reduced in premature infants.

BOX 10.2 In the event of a medication error

- Inform the parents (and the child if old enough and if this is appropriate)
- Inform all relevant health professionals directly involved with the patient
- Discuss with the pharmacy/poison centre
- At a later stage, discuss with all relevant parties what lessons can be learnt from the medication error and whether a similar error can be prevented in the future
- Inform, if requested in your country, the legal advisors of your hospital and/or malpractice insurance company

---

The duration of antibiotic therapy needs to be carefully considered. Certain organisms, such as the meningococcus, are extremely sensitive and in the vast majority of cases 5 days' treatment is more than sufficient. Most hospitals have local antibiotic guidelines that should be followed.

The cost of medicines is usually an important factor in the choice of antibiotic. If there are two equally effective and safe drugs, then one would normally choose the cheaper medicine. In certain cases, however, the increased cost of the drug may be compensated by savings in nursing expenditure by allowing reduced frequency of administration of intravenous antibiotics.

Pain assessment and management (see also p. 288)

One always needs to consider the possibility of a child being in pain, as a result either of the disease process or of the interventions. The assessment of pain requires an age-appropriate, validated pain assessment scale. Self-reporting is the ideal, but the child needs to have the cognitive ability to do this and therefore needs to be at least 3 years old. It is also important that a pain scale that has been validated for an acute painful response is not used for children with chronic pain.

Self-report scales usually involve the child pointing to a photograph (the Oucher Scale) or a diagram of a child in pain (Bieri Faces Pain Scale, Fig. 10.2). The Oucher Scale has been validated in children as young as 3 years of age and the Bieri Faces Pain Scale for children aged 6 years and over. The Wong–Baker Faces Pain Scale is more reliable in children aged 8–12 years than in the 3–7-year age group. The Adolescent Paediatric Pain Tool is for children between the ages of 8 and 17 years.

Behavioural pain scales are used for preverbal children and include the Toddler–Preschooler Post-operative Pain Scale (TPPPS) and the Children's Hospital of Eastern Ontario Pain Scale (CHEOPS). These pain scales rely

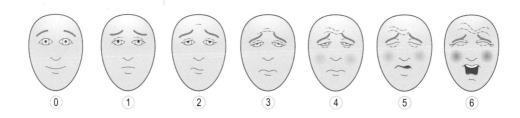

Fig. 10.2 Faces pain scale.
'These faces show how much something can hurt. This face [point to the left-most face] shows no pain. The faces show more and more pain [point to each one from left to right] up to this one [point to the right-most face]. It shows very much pain. Point to the pain that shows how much you hurt (right now).'
(Reproduced from Bieri et al 1990, with permission.)

on assessment of the child's behaviour and have been validated for children aged 1–5 years. The Faces, Legs, Activity, Cry and Consolability (FLACC) Scale has been validated for children aged 2 months–7 years.

There are numerous pain assessment tools for use in neonates (Bieri et al 1990). These rely on behavioural observation and, in some of the pain scales, measurements of pulse, blood pressure and oxygen saturation. For preterm neonates, it is important to use a scale that has been validated in preterm neonates (van Dijk et al, 2004).

Management involves the use of techniques such as distraction as well as analgesia. Paracetamol is the safest analgesic available and is the first-line drug to be used for paediatric patients of all ages with mild pain. Children who either do not respond to paracetamol or are unlikely to respond to paracetamol should receive a non-steroidal anti-inflammatory drug (NSAID) such as ibuprofen or diclofenac. Alternatively, codeine or dihydrocodeine can be administered orally. Patients with severe pain require opiates, and morphine remains the drug of choice. It can be administered intravenously, intranasally or orally. For certain painful conditions, e.g. change of dressings in burns patients, it may be more appropriate to use an inhaled equimolar mixture of nitric oxide and oxygen. This is an effective and safe analgesic with a short duration of action, which children can control themselves.

References

Bieri D et al 1990 The faces pain scale for the self-assessment of the severity of pain experienced by children: development, initial validation, and preliminary investigation for ratio scale properties. Pain 41:139–150

Choonara I, Rieder MJ 2002 Drug toxicity and adverse drug reactions in children — a brief historical review. Paediatric and Perinatal Drug Therapy 5:12–18

Cousins D et al 2002 Medication errors in children — an eight-year review using press reports. Paediatric and Perinatal Drug Therapy 5:52–58

De Wildt SN, Johnson TN, Choonara J 2003 The effect of age on drug metabolism. Paediatric and Perinatal Drug Therapy 5:101–106

Thomson AH 2000 Introduction to clinical pharmacokinetics. Paediatric and Perinatal Drug Therapy 4: 3–11

van Dijk M, Simons S, Tibboel D 2004 Pain assessment in neonates. Paediatric and Perinatal Drug Therapy 6:97–103

MODULE TWO

11

Julie-Clare Becher   Neil McIntosh   Pieter J. J. Sauer

Ethics and children's rights

LEARNING OUTCOMES

By the end of this chapter you should:
- Understand a parent's responsibility for his or her child
- Appreciate the rights of a child and how you can ensure them
- Understand confidentiality issues pertaining to children
- Know about the issues surrounding considerations of care reorientation
- Understand the importance of autopsy and the issues surrounding authorization
- Understand the importance of research for the future of children.

Introduction

The increasing availability of sophisticated medical technology has raised ethical and legal questions about the appropriateness of provision of care for children who may ultimately die or survive with severe disability. At the same time, society is demanding greater personal involvement in decision-making. The expertise of doctors and nurses in their field may not extend to the skills required to deal with problems of parental dissent, decisions about whether a severely damaged baby should be allowed to die or the extent to which parents should be involved in their child's management. Expertise in moral and legal argument is fundamental to such issues. This chapter aims to provide the reader with an understanding of how ethical and legal issues interact with clinical practice in paediatrics.

Children's rights and parental responsibilities

Rights may be defined as the entitlement for all individuals to have their worth and dignity respected.

MODULE TWO

The United Nations Convention on the Rights of the Child (UNCRC) declares that children are entitled to special consideration and care due to their immaturity and vulnerability. The European Union has endorsed this convention. The articles of this convention state that the primary consideration of actions affecting children should be the 'best interests of the child' (Article 3), and that it is every child's right to enjoy the highest attainable standard of health and to be able to access facilities for the treatment of illness and the rehabilitation of health (Article 24), subject to the resources available (Article 4). The Convention also recognizes the right of a child to 'freedom of expression, freedom to seek, receive and impart information and ideas of all kinds, regardless of frontiers' (Article 13), and states that the 'child who is capable of forming his or her own views has the right to express those views freely on all matters. The views of the child will be given due weight in accordance with the age and maturation' (Article 12). These rights, also pertaining to children, include the right to life, the right not to be subjected to degrading or inhuman treatment, and the right to private and family life.

The United Nations Convention on the Rights of the Child is endorsed in a number of EU regulations and proclamations. In 2000 the rights of the child were described in articles 24 and 25 of the Charter of Fundamental Rights in the EU. In 2007 the European Council accepted the 'EU Guidelines for the Promotion and Protection of the Rights of the Child'. These guidelines further describe the rights of a child.

http://www.childrenslawcentre.org/UNCRC_international.htm

European Convention on Human Rights

The Charter of Fundamental Rights in the EU

A child has autonomy and a separate identity to that of his or her parents, and respect for this is fundamental to trust and communication, even in the smallest child. Healthcare professionals have an important role in sharing information with children and listening to their needs, empowering them to make confident decisions with their parents about treatment. Support of parents, who may express different needs and desires to those of their child or those of staff, is also crucial in this process.

The principal role of parenthood is to provide care for a child and to raise him or her in emotional, moral and physical health. Parents can generally be expected to protect the interests of their child to a greater degree than anyone else, but parental rights do not equate to ownership and it is essential that these rights be

BOX 11.1 Unmarried fathers

Unmarried fathers can obtain parental responsibility by entering into a voluntary parental responsibility agreement with the mother or this can be granted by a court in most European countries. Legislation in countries like England and The Netherlands grants the father parental rights if he registers the child's birth jointly with the mother.

exercised for the benefit of the child and not for the benefit of the parent. Currently, biological parents are the legal parents unless the child has been adopted. The mother has parental responsibility, and so does the father if he is married to the mother at the time of birth or marries her thereafter (Box 11.1).

Adoptive parents have parental responsibility, as do others such as guardians or local authorities when granted these by the courts. Legal authorities may consent to treatment on behalf of a child or may limit parental responsibility in certain circumstances.

Consent, dissent and competency

The right to autonomy declares that each individual can decide what happens to his or her body. This applies to any act of touching, including medical treatment. Without consent, such violation of this right may constitute assault. Consent makes the act of touching for medical treatment lawful and such consent may be 'implied', as in the rolling up of a sleeve for a venepuncture, or 'expressed', as in verbal or written assent. Exceptions to the requirement for consent arise in the situation of an unconscious patient, where to delay until a patient is conscious would result in unreasonable treatment delays, and in the context of mental illness where non-consensual treatment may be instituted.

All healthcare decisions involve choices and, in the case of children, the question arises 'by whom?' Consent requires competence, a term which is difficult to define and assess (Box 11.2). In England and Wales a child of 16 or over is deemed legally able and competent to make decisions about his or her own medical treatment. However, case law has undermined the ability of such young people to refuse consent to a procedure or treatment where refusal might result in significant harm; this they can only do at 18. Under the age of 16, if competency is not present, consent is generally obtained on the child's behalf from a parent or other person exercising parental powers. However, if a child is deemed 'competent', that child is able to give consent or assent with the parental consent. Competency is difficult to define and assess (Box 11.2).

> **BOX 11.2 Competency**
>
> This involves a capacity to retain and comprehend information, and an ability to weigh up the risks and benefits to arrive at a choice and to understand the consequences of not consenting. It depends not only on the mental age of the child, but also on the complexity of the procedure or treatment and the experience of that child to date.

If the child is considered competent, encouragement should be given to that child to involve the parents in the decision-making. However, this is not mandatory and the consent of a competent child to treatment cannot be overruled by the dissent of a parent. Such competency of a 'mature minor' is often termed 'Gillick competence' and has been established legally in the case of a minor who won her right to be prescribed contraception without her parent's knowledge. Good practice takes account of children's views irrespective of their minimum legal age, and good standards of communication, such as informing, listening and respecting a child's views, are central to informed and ethical decision-making. Careful documentation would be necessary if one were to act against the young person's wishes.

🔄 http://www.gpnotebook.co.uk/simplepage.
cfm?ID=-1254817788

'Mature minor' (Gillick competency) and consent in children

Dissent or difference in opinion may arise between the healthcare team and parents, or between the members of the team, or between parents. When such disagreement arises, the reasons must be discussed. Parents may have a different understanding of the complex issues involved, and cultural and language barriers may compound the problem. Good-quality communication over time may result in consensus. It may be necessary to involve other specialists or to consider extended investigations to help resolve any uncertainty about prognosis. An opportunity should be allowed for parents to consult religious advisers or others of their choice. If they and the medical team continue to disagree about which management strategy is in the child's best interests and this cannot be resolved through local means (such as involving another colleague), it might be necessary to seek involvement from a legal authority. Legal support is always available for such matters and parents should be notified immediately about such a move so they can seek representation, and put forward their views and seek alternative opinions.

Dissent within the healthcare team may also occur and, although unanimity is not essential, consensus should be sought. If individuals express dissent, it is important to record such opinion in the notes and attribute to it weight in proportion with that member's experience or status. Such members may be given an opportunity to ask for a second opinion.

Clinical ethics committees have been encouraged by professional bodies in the United States and may be useful in developing policies or dealing with individual cases. In some countries where these committees exist, they mainly function to reflect what decisions are made by responsible physicians and how they are made. This is done as the physician remains legally and professionally responsible for any decision, not a committee.

Confidentiality

Doctors have a duty of confidentiality to all patients, including children. A child who is deemed legally competent has the right to expect that information about him or her will not be disclosed to a third party, including a parent, without the child's consent. However, such children should be encouraged to involve their parents wherever possible, if it is in their best interests to do so. It is only justified to disclose confidential information to a third party if it is thought a child may suffer or come to harm through non-disclosure. In such a case, the child should be informed of this decision prior to the third party being informed. Similarly, confidentiality with regard to a non-competent child should incur the same respect, and disclosure of any information pertaining to that child should first be discussed with the parent. Clinicians have a duty to safeguard children by sharing information with relevant agencies when there is manifest evidence of child abuse. In 2006 WHO published a booklet entitled 'Preventing Child Maltreatment: a guide to taking action and generating evidence'. This guide provides the necessary tools and information to governments, civil society and international organizations in their efforts to prevent and respond to violence against children. The organization of child abuse service centres is regulated differently in EU countries; nevertheless, action should be taken in all cases of suspected child abuse. All clinicians should be aware of recent data protection legislation that allows all individuals the right to access their medical records.

Sanctity of life and quality of life

Traditional Hippocratic medical ethics advocates respect for the sanctity of all human life, combined with a medical duty of care and a duty to act in the sole interest of the patient. However, some modern philosophy challenges this perspective as outdated and argues that 'personhood' with its attendant rights and obligations is dependent on the presence of consciousness and self-awareness, as well as an ability to reason and to have control over one's existence. In this view, newborn infants and those children with severe brain damage are not regarded as persons. However, the concept of the sanctity of life, although originating in religious tradition, is a central tenet in our society, where murder is perceived as wrong, vulnerability is protected and resources are provided to treat the sick and save lives where possible. Guidelines published by the World Health Organization emphasize that the care of the patient should be a doctor's primary responsibility and that doctors should strive to protect their patients from risk.

However, as neonatal and paediatric intensive care has advanced, it has become apparent that saving life may cause harm. Survival of an infant at all costs may lead to unbearable suffering or a bleak life of severe disability. Such individuals may be unable to have any meaningful interaction with the environment and lack ability to reason, both measures of quality of life. Despite the primary motivation of preservation of life in these situations, many clinicians find such 'therapeutic successes' at odds with the concept of 'the sanctity of life'. It is not always in a child's best interests to prolong life at all costs. Decisions not to provide or to withdraw life-sustaining treatment in the face of intolerable suffering are increasingly accepted as morally appropriate, and guidelines have been produced by the Ethical Committee of the European Academy of Paediatrics.

🌐 http://www.gmc-uk.org/guidance/good_medical_practice/index.asp

GMC, 'Good Medical Practice'

Withdrawal and withholding of life-prolonging treatment in children

The healthcare team has a duty of care, with the principal goal of sustaining life and restoring health. However, technological advances have led to an increasing ability to sustain life in infants and children who would otherwise have died. As a result, ethical dilemmas have arisen as to whether all attempts to prolong life are sensible or in the best interests of the child. In particular, concern has arisen as to the justification of continuing pointless treatment in patients who are not dying and to the prolongation of life in those who are dying or destined for severe disability.

BOX 11.3 Four situations where the withholding or withdrawal of curative medical treatment might be considered

- The persistent vegetative state
- The 'no-chance' situation
- The 'no-purpose' situation
- The 'unbearable' situation

In the consideration of the withholding or withdrawal of curative life-saving medical treatment four situations may be identified in which prolongation or initiation of active treatment may be considered unjustified (Box 11.3).

Despite potential differences in opinion between paediatricians in different EU countries, the following general statements can be made:

- In the event of futile treatment, the primary obligation of the paediatrician is to counsel the parents and let the patient die with minimal suffering. The decision lies primarily with the physician.
- Where a patient might survive with the help of neonatal intensive care but the outlook as to how the patient might survive is very poor, the paediatrician and parents should discuss the best interests of the infant. If parents and physicians believe that it is in the best interest of the infant to withhold further treatment, this should be done. If the parents ask for continuation of treatment, this should be done. Paediatricians should never stop treatment against parental wishes.
- In a situation where a patient is dependent on non-intensive medical treatment but the predicted life will be one full of suffering which cannot be relieved by any means, all possible interventions have to be used to alleviate the suffering. When suffering can be alleviated only by means which could, as a side-effect, shorten the life of the infant, these interventions are indicated.

These situations rely on a degree of certainty about death, cure or outcomes between the two, and if there is doubt about either of these extremes, the motivation should always be to protect life until a value judgment based on outcome can be ascertained. In such instances, advice from specialist colleagues or more detailed investigations may be warranted. It is essential that enough time be allowed to gather and disseminate information and to allow opinions to be expressed by all involved.

Historically, end-of-life decisions were taken by medical staff with or without involvement of the parents. Nowadays, parents increasingly want to share this responsibility. Doctors must help guide parents towards a decision that is medically appropriate and within the law and, in doing so, need to respect the fact that parents may have their own values, beliefs, priorities and resources. In addition, parents will have to live with the consequences of any decision made. Siblings must not be forgotten in the decision-making process; they may have important insights into the feelings of their brother or sister and may have differing views to those of their parents.

All members of the healthcare team should be involved in such decision-making and, although the final responsibility lies with the consultant in charge of the child, such decisions are virtually always taken by a multidisciplinary group involving nurses, social workers, family members and specialist medical staff who together form the 'moral community' within a paediatric unit.

It is important to remember that withholding or withdrawing life-prolonging treatment is not withdrawal of care. All dying children should receive warmth, loving human contact and feeds as tolerated, and should be assured of freedom from distress or pain by the use of sedation or analgesics. There should be a commitment to the family as a whole with the opportunity for parents to maintain close contact and participate in their child's care until death.

Omission, commission and the principle of double effect

Commission in this context refers to an act that has the certain result of death, and such deliberate killing of any individual is prohibited. However, the withdrawal of life-prolonging treatment in appropriate circumstances is accepted by the courts and is not regarded as a breach of the right to life. Omission refers to the withholding of treatment.

Ensuring that a dying child is free from distress is a sensitive matter that has attracted much debate. Legally, any treatment given to hasten death is murder but administration of medication to alleviate suffering is permissible, even if a side-effect may be to hasten death. This principle of 'double effect' is seen in the administration of opiates to prevent pain or distress where the drug may also have the effect of depressing respiration. Such a prescription is regarded as being for the benefit of the patient during life and not intended to cause or hasten death.

Refusal of blood products by Jehovah's Witnesses

The position of Jehovah's Witnesses in refusing donor blood transfusions in view of their personal deeply held religious beliefs is well known. This position includes the refusal of whole blood and red cells, white cells, platelets and plasma. Members who wilfully accept prohibited blood components have historically been disfellowshipped by their church and are considered outcasts. However, recent significant changes in policy mean that members can now remain silent about the medical treatment they receive and avoid punishment. Blood transfusions in the children of Jehovah's Witnesses have often raised medical dilemmas and ultimately involved the jurisdiction of the courts. Previously, decisions in favour of the clinician may have meant risking the subsequent ostracization of that child or family from the religious community. Although Jehovah's Witnesses are an increasingly diverse group, this recent policy change may mean that conflict in such cases will be less common. As this change may be interpreted differently by various members of the group, the clinician must explore the personal preference and conviction of parents before treatment and remember that breaches in patient confidentiality may result in significant punishment for the family. Withholding blood or blood products from a child when they are medically needed is considered unethical, as is refusal of permission by the parents for religious reasons. In these cases, a legal decision is sought in order to safeguard the wellbeing of the child.

Resource allocation

Decisions about funding experimental and expensive treatments raise ethical and practical dilemmas. A clinician has a duty of care to an individual patient. However, in a world where resources are scarce, clinicians and managers have an ethical duty to consider cost in rationing healthcare. Treatments or procedures must be justified in terms of cost-effectiveness, medical efficacy and maximum benefit to the community. A decision to offer one patient a particular treatment may deny treatment to another.

The principle of health gain maximization ranks procedures or treatments so that those that generate more gains to health for every unit of resource take priority over those that generate fewer. Gains to health may be measured by life expectancy, lives saved, 'quality-adjusted life years' (QALYs) or other outcomes. All individuals are regarded as equal in health gain maximization. Any departure from this ranking involves a loss of efficiency and a judgment that the value of one life is more important then the value of another. However, high-profile cases in the media have demonstrated the difficulties of weighing the needs of an individual and the interests of the community, and there may be situations where 'rescue' treatment may be justified for an individual, even when this may be at conflict with the priorities of the community as a whole (Ham 1999).

There are no current guidelines on how a paediatrician should act when facing such dilemmas. Therefore, the interest of the individual patient should prevail above financial constraints.

Post-mortem and organ retention

The usefulness of post-mortem in establishing cause of death, determining unrelated diagnoses and assisting grieving is well documented. In infants and children information may also be provided for genetic counselling. The post-mortem rate has been falling throughout the developed world over the last three decades, and this has been particularly so since well-publicized criticisms of post-mortem standards appeared in the media over the last decade. In particular, the practice of retention of organs from individuals without the knowledge or consent of relatives has led to a crisis in public confidence and a subsequent overhaul of the post-mortem consent and examination process.

Information, communication and knowledge are fundamental in rebuilding the public's trust in the post-mortem examination. As a result, the consent process is now unambiguous and explicit. Parents need to be assured that examination will only be carried out with their authorization and that any examination of their child will be with the utmost dignity and respect. The extent of the examination and retention of organs and the purposes for such retention must be fully explained to parents, and high-quality written information provided in order to aid their decision. The extent of examination and retention must correspond to the level of consent given. Any breach of such authorization now results in legal penalty. Historically it was common for doctors to withhold post-mortem results from parents in the belief that these details would result in distress. At present information from the examination should be freely available. This information is best provided and discussed at a meeting between the clinician, parents and involved support staff in the weeks following bereavement.

In specific instances, the coroner or procurator fiscal may ask for a post-mortem examination to ascertain cause of death, irrespective of parental consent. Such a requirement follows sudden, suspicious or accidental deaths or where death may have occurred due to medical mishap or the result of a medical treatment or surgical procedure. In this situation, tissue retention is not authorized unless specific consent has been obtained. The laws of each country will regulate if this information can and must be provided. Providing legal authorities with information obtained after a post-mortem that was performed with permission of the parents can be illegal in some countries. In these countries findings in the post-mortem can be used for prosecution only when the post-mortem was ordered by a legal institution.

Research in babies and children

Medical research is essential for advancing child health and wellbeing. Many disease processes in children have no close analogies in adults. Moreover, children have different physiology to adults and as a result drugs may have different pharmacokinetics (p. 105). Many disorders can only be understood in the context of a child's growth and development. Research in children can also advance our understanding of some adult diseases that are thought to have their origins in childhood.

Children require special protection in research, as they are less likely to be able to communicate their needs or protect their interests compared to adult subjects. The following are ethical considerations to keep in mind when children are involved in research:

- All proposed research should be approved by a research ethics committee.
- Entry into a study should be preceded by written informed consent from a parent following the provision of high-quality information and the opportunity to discuss the research with another member of staff. All language used should be appropriate to the intellectual level of the parent and supported with written information.
- Many parents will be under significant stress, particularly following labour and delivery or the diagnosis of significant morbidity. This may affect their ability to listen, comprehend and retain information.
- All risks involved in study participation should be shared with the parent.
- Parents should be assured that their child will receive the best possible medical care, irrespective of their participation in the study.
- Parents should understand that they are free to withdraw their child from the study at any time and that this will not affect the care their child will receive.
- Where parents give consent, agreement should also be sought from school-age children. A child's refusal to participate or continue in a study should always be respected.
- The researcher has an ongoing obligation to monitor the risks to each child and inform both the parents and the data monitoring committee of the progress of the study and any adverse effects.

BOX 11.4 Six principles about research with children

- Research involving children is important for the benefit of all children and should be supported, encouraged and conducted in an ethical manner
- Children are not small adults; they have an additional, unique set of interests
- Research should only be done on children if comparable research on adults could not answer the same question
- A research procedure that is not intended to benefit the child subject directly is not necessarily either unethical or illegal
- All proposals involving medical research on children should be submitted to the local research ethics committee
- Legally valid consent should be obtained from the child, parent or guardian as appropriate. When parental consent is obtained, the agreement of school-age children who take part in research should also be requested by researchers

- A data monitoring committee should be active in monitoring for significant side-effects and interim analysis.

Good quality research is essential for improving the efficacy and safety of clinical practice, and should be actively encouraged (Box 11.4).

Neonatal issues

Viability and outcome

For extremely preterm infants there is a close relationship between gestational age and mortality/morbidity, with significant decreases in mortality for each week of prolonged intrauterine survival. The decision to attempt to prolong a pregnancy may have to be balanced against considerable ongoing risk for both the mother and the fetus. Moderate to severe disability affects over a third of extreme preterm survivors, many of whom have needed prolonged intensive care. The emotional and financial burden of disability and handicap means that families require accurate information about the survival and prognosis for such infants. There are no randomized trials to advise clinicians facing such complex medical, emotional and social challenges about whether or not to resuscitate the extreme preterm infant. Recent statistics on short-term survival and long-term sequelae may already be outdated. The United Kingdom EPICURE study (Wood et al 2000) and a similar study of extremely preterm infants born in the United States in the mid-

1990s found a survival rate of 11–30% at 23 weeks' gestation, increasing to 34–76% by 25 weeks' gestation. Moderate to severe disability affected around 50% of survivors. In addition, pervasive behaviour problems at the age of 6½ years were seen in almost 20% of survivors compared to 3% in controls and hyperactivity in 30% of survivors compared to 9% in controls. In these infants born ≤25 weeks of gestation, cognitive ability was 20 points and mathematics 27 points lower than controls. There is also a relationship of mortality and morbidity with birth weight but outcome studies seldom explore the variable influences of growth restriction or gender. There is a well-described poorer outcome for multiple pregnancies.

In practice, accurate estimation of gestational age may be problematic in the absence of first trimester ultrasound, and fetal weight estimates are notoriously inaccurate. Obstetricians have more pessimistic views than paediatricians about survival in very early gestation deliveries, and all clinicians who are involved in counselling parents should be familiar with both national and local statistics for survival and long-term outcome. Counselling should be sensitive to ethnic and cultural diversity, and input from clergy, social workers or translators may be important.

The delivery of extremely premature infants and infants with severe congenital abnormalities raises issues about the initiation of resuscitation. Practices include the resuscitation of all infants, resuscitation according to previously defined parameters or application of an individualized risk assessment approach. Although absolute rules are inappropriate for such difficult issues, guidelines can provide a framework for acceptable practice but without prescriptive guidance. Current international guidelines advise that resuscitation is inappropriate where an infant has a condition or characteristic unlikely to result in survival or survival without extreme disability (Niermeyer et al 2000). The gestational age and birth weight used as cut off for initiation of resuscitation differ between EU countries. In some countries it is advised to start resuscitation at 23 weeks, whereas in other countries it is not advised below 25 weeks. In some countries a child with confirmed trisomy-13 or 18 will not be offered intensive care in contrast to other countries that might offer it. Approaches will depend on the ethical and moral opinion in each country. Sometimes it is difficult to obtain reliable or accurate information prior to delivery, and a trial of therapy may be instituted while full assessment of the infant is undertaken. Withdrawal of full support may follow ascertainment of status. Discussions with parents and obstetricians in the antenatal period are valuable and enable repeated communication with time for reflection and questions. It is important to develop a plan that has consensus for the family and clinician. Both parties should agree that in the face of uncertainty, evaluation and further investigations may be needed. Where the situation is complex or where there is irreconcilable disagreement, it is useful to involve other colleagues.

In all cases, the final decision not to initiate resuscitation should be made by a senior clinician; when one is not present, a junior doctor should initiate treatment until a more experienced doctor arrives. This approach allows time to gather information, counsel parents and allow parents some time to cherish their baby. The disadvantage is the danger that in some instances subsequent withdrawal of life-sustaining treatment may not result in death but in an infant with severe disability.

All treatment strategies have benefits and risks, and their availability does not necessarily justify their use. The provision of intensive care when there is evidence of severe neurological damage is ethically unjust. All centres offering intensive care should have a comprehensive and standardized method of follow-up ascertainment, and outcome data should be available for public consumption and for benchmarking with other centres.

References and further reading

British Medical Association Ethics Department 2003 Medical ethics today. BMJ Books, London

Ham C 1999 Tragic choices in health care: lessons from the child B case. British Medical Journal 319(7219):1258–1261

Niermeyer S, Kattwinkel J, Van Reempts P et al, International Consensus on Science and Contributors and Reviewers for the Neonatal Resuscitation Guidelines 2000 International guidelines for neonatal resuscitation: an excerpt from the guidelines 2000 for cardiopulmonary resuscitation and emergency cardiovascular care. Pediatrics 106(3):E29

Royal College of Paediatrics and Child Health Ethics Advisory Committee 2004 A framework for practice in relation to the withholding and withdrawing of life-saving treatment in children, 2nd edn. RCPCH, London

Wood NS, Marlow N, Costeloe K et al and EPICURE Study Group 2000 Neurologic and developmental disability after extremely preterm birth. New England Journal of Medicine 343(6):378–384

CHAPTER

12

Jonathan Darling   Eleanor J. Molloy

Practical procedures and investigations

LEARNING OUTCOMES

By the end of this chapter you should:

- Have reviewed your approach to learning and performing practical procedures
- Be able to perform specific common procedures
- Be able to discuss interpretation of investigations, particularly with regard to common X-rays.

Investigations in children

Procedures and investigations in children are often more difficult than those in adults. The smaller size of the child may make the technical aspects more challenging; the child may be less cooperative (or refuse outright!); and the distress caused may be greater — both to the child and the parents. Although investigations should not be done without good reason in any branch of medicine, this is particularly the case in paediatrics. Consider the test characteristics, the potential contribution to diagnosis and management, and the risks and costs of doing the test (p. 58).

Approach to practical procedures

You need to become competent in performing common practical procedures. The best way to achieve this is to be taught and supervised by an experienced practitioner. Many investigations will be explained in more detail in later chapters. The notes below are not meant to be a comprehensive manual, but practical tips to help you achieve success and avoid common problems.

Learning a new practical procedure

Only learn a procedure when you can practise it regularly with appropriate supervision and support near at hand. Make sure you know any relevant background physiology and anatomy, and any associated risks and how to minimize these. Watch experienced practitioners perform the procedure a number of times and take time to review it with them afterwards until you are sure you know what to do.

Perform the procedure (or part of the procedure) under close supervision by an experienced colleague. If you fail, do not make repeated attempts, as this is unfair to the child. Let the experienced colleague take over and complete the test, and then review afterwards with him or her how you can complete the procedure successfully next time.

You need to learn not only the technical aspects of performing the procedure but also how best to communicate to parents and children about what you are going to do before, during and after the procedure. This 'communication competence' is just as important as the technical competence that you need (Box 12.1).

In clinical postgraduate examinations, you could be asked to explain the need for a common or important investigation to proxy parents and/or their child. Such a task can be made appropriately challenging in various ways; for example, the parents may not be convinced that the test is necessary, or there may be some contraindications, and you may have to decide yourself if the test is appropriate. Make sure that you know what each investigation involves (watch as many as you can) and that you can clearly explain this to parents.

If at first you don't succeed …

Even the best operators have occasions where they fail to complete a procedure that they are usually good at. This is more likely when you are tired or relatively inexperienced. Do not keep repeating the procedure until you achieve success, since this is likely to be a fruitless exercise and may only lead to a fraught child and parents. Do not be embarrassed to ask somebody else to try.

Minimizing distress

For every procedure you perform, make it your goal to minimize any distress to the child and parents. Remember the golden rules of *p*reparation, *p*arents presence and *p*ain control. However, when blood sampling is performed on neonates it may be less distressing for parents to be absent.

Preparation

This includes having everything ready so that you look proficient and minimize anxious waiting. It also includes explanation to child and parent of what is involved, and arranging for other appropriate staff to be present to help you. For most procedures the presence of an experienced children's nurse can make a huge difference.

Parents present?

Decide together with the parents whether they will be present in the room for the procedure, and what part they will play. In general it is best to have at least one parent present, although often parents decline to watch a lumbar puncture in a younger child but wait nearby to cuddle and comfort the child afterwards.

Pain control

This is important (p. 108).

Distraction

Distraction can be a powerful tool in children. You will see many examples of it in use on paediatric wards and in clinics. Aim to build up your own repertoire of useful distractions, which may include funny toys, funny faces, flashing lights, projected images and blowing bubbles. For the younger infant, a feed may be all that is needed. Well-judged distractions like these can make an unpleasant procedure almost a happy occasion, and acquiring a good repertoire is an important part of your toolkit.

Local anaesthesia

Many procedures carried out without pain control in adults require local anaesthesia at the least in children. Make sure you are familiar with local anaesthetic creams and the procedures for their use in your hospital, and offer these in all but the most grown-up adolescents (and even these patients might appreciate them). For more painful procedures, or where a greater depth of anaesthesia is needed, infiltrate the area with up to 0.4 ml/kg of 1% lidocaine solution. Make sure that you allow time for it to take effect.

Analgesia

Prescribe at least paracetamol following any procedure where the child is likely to continue to experience pain afterwards.

Venepuncture and cannulation

Although many ask an experienced helper to squeeze the limb being cannulated to produce appropriate venous engorgement, it is worth buying a good-quality tourniquet and learning to adjust it to get exactly the right degree of compression each time. The problem with using a helper (particularly if it is a different person each time) is that the compression may vary considerably and you have little control over it. Learn a reliable method to secure any cannula you insert and try to ensure that it is easy to check for 'tissuing' of the cannula (e.g. by having a clear adhesive dressing over the tip), particularly if you are using irritant solutions containing calcium or high concentrations (> 10%) of glucose. Wherever possible, these should go through a central line; if they do have to go through a peripheral line, great care must be taken, with frequent monitoring (every 15 minutes or so) according to an agreed protocol with good documentation. Otherwise the child is at risk of unpleasant burn scars.

Capillary sampling

Capillary sampling is a useful technique and can be employed for nearly all samples, except those that

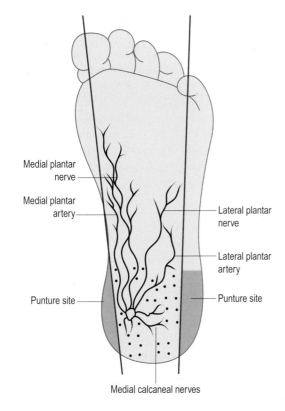

Fig. 12.1 Sites suitable for heelprick blood sampling

need to be sterile or require a large volume of blood. Use a capillary sampling safety device or an automated device wherever possible. If an automated lancet is chosen and the puncture depth is less than 2.2 mm, then this device can be used safely anywhere over the plantar surface of the heel, except the posterior heel in preterms < 33 weeks' gestation (Fig. 12.1). Make sure the heel (infants under 2 years) or finger (older children) is warm before you start. If a large sample is needed, wrap the target area in a warm wet towel for 5 minutes to induce hyperaemia.

Lumbar puncture

Positioning is key for this investigation, and having an experienced assistant hold the baby or child will greatly increase your chances of success. Lay the infant on his or her side, held by your assistant, such that the head and hips are flexed and the spine is curved with the convexity towards you. The plane of the spine should be horizontal (Figs 12.2 and 12.3). Full aseptic technique is essential including gloves, mask and gown.

An imaginary line joining the highest points of the iliac crests passes just above the fourth lumbar spine. You should insert the lumbar puncture needle in either the L3–L4 space or the space below (L4–L5).

In children over a year, use local anaesthesia, with a combination of topical anaesthetic cream, followed by local infiltration with lidocaine 1%, aspirating before each injection (to check you are not in the spinal canal or a blood vessel), and waiting a minute or so for each injection to take effect.

Aim towards the umbilicus through the flexed spine and make sure your needle entry point is in the plane of the spinous processes. Firmly advance the needle with the stylet in place. You may feel a faint 'popping' sensation as you pierce the dura, in which case stop and remove the stylet. The distance to advance in cm is 0.03 × height (in cm), which is about 1.5 cm in a baby and up to around 5 cm in an adult. In a baby, stop after 1.5 cm, remove the stylet and gently rotate the needle. If no cerebrospinal fluid (CSF) appears, then reinsert the stylet and advance the needle a little further. Repeat this until you are in the CSF space.

Take three sterile bottles (6 drops in each) labelled ready for microscopy, and then one for protein and a fluoride container for glucose. Do not forget to send blood for glucose measurement at the time of the lumbar puncture to allow comparison of blood and CSF glucose.

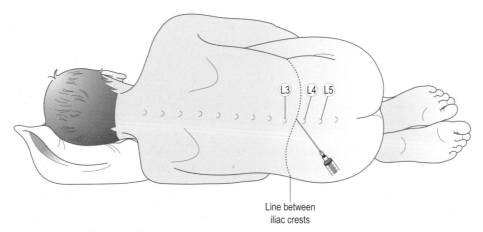

Fig. 12.2 Recumbent position for lumbar puncture showing correct site

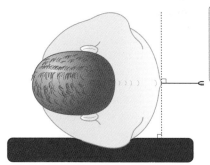

a) **Correct position.** The LP needle is at right angles to the plane of the back, which is perpendicular, at right angles to the plane of the couch, and near the edge of the couch. The LP needle is in line with the spinous processes.

Fig. 12.3 Lumbar puncture — achieving success.
Schematic representation of a view of the curled child, looking from the head (black oval) down the back.

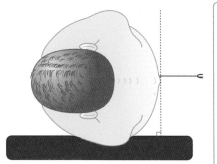

b) **Incorrect entry point.** The LP needle is not in line with the spinous processes. This can occur when
- the overlying skin is stretched while inserting the needle, so that skin recoil pulls the needle point out of line
- the spinous processes are difficult to feel due to overlying fat
- the child is moving at the time of insertion.

Remedy: *Take time to feel the processes, avoid skin stretch, and ensure your assistant can hold the child still.*

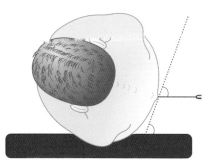

c) **Body roll.** The child's body has rolled so that the plane of the back is no longer perpendicular and at right angles to the couch. This is a common reason for a failed LP.

Remedy: *Have a second assistant view down the spine as shown in these pictures, or stop periodically and check yourself.*
Roll back to the correct position.
If this is difficult, adjust the plane of the needle to be at right angles to the plane of the back.

Contraindications to lumbar puncture

- Signs of raised intracranial pressure: altered pupillary responses, absent Doll's eye reflex, decerebrate or decorticate posturing, abnormal respiratory pattern, papilloedema, hypertension and bradycardia
- Recent (within 30 minutes) or prolonged (over 30 minutes) convulsive seizures
- Focal or tonic seizures
- Other focal neurological signs: hemiparesis/ monoparesis, extensor plantar responses, ocular palsies
- Glasgow Coma Score < 13 or deteriorating level of consciousness
- Strong suspicion of meningococcal infection (typical purpuric rash in an ill child) or state of shock (but perform lumbar puncture once the child is stable)
- Local superficial infection
- Coagulation disorder. In neonates, although raised intracranial pressure is a lesser concern because of the open fontanelle, if the fontanelle is bulging and tense, coagulopathy should be ruled out before LP.

Injection

Intramuscular injection is used for most immunizations, and is occasionally used for intramuscular antibiotics if access is difficult and only a short course is required. For immunization, check that the expiry date has not been reached, that it is the correct immunization for the child, and that appropriate consent and explana-

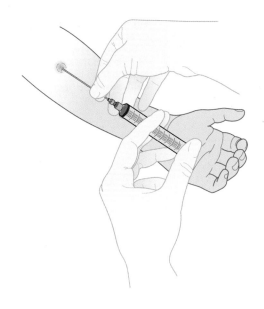

Fig. 12.4 Intradermal injection

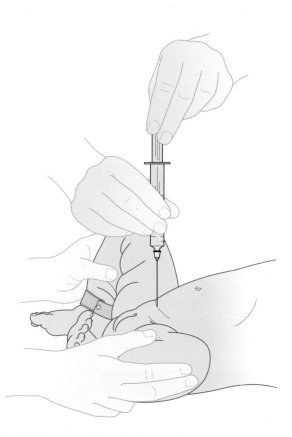

Fig. 12.5 Suprapubic aspiration of urine

tion have been given. Ensure that any powder is fully dissolved and then, using a sterile technique, draw up the full amount into the syringe. Use a 25G (green) needle and pinch a large fold of skin, either on the upper arm (around the insertion of the deltoid muscle) or in the anterolateral aspect of the thigh; in older children, skin in the upper outer quadrant of the buttocks may be chosen (to avoid the risk of sciatic nerve damage). Insert the needle into the muscle, exert some brief gentle suction to check you are not in a blood vessel, and then inject the contents. Remove the needle promptly and apply a dressing if needed.

Intradermal injections (Fig. 12.4)

Mantoux is given intradermally. Use a 26G needle (or smaller), stretch the skin between the thumb and forefinger of one hand, and with the other hand slowly insert the needle (bevel upwards) for about 2 mm into the superficial layer of dermis. Keep the tip of the needle almost parallel with the surface. Slowly inject the contents of the syringe. You should feel considerable resistance and see a blanched, raised bleb appear, showing the tips of hair follicles. If not, the needle is likely to be too deep. An amount of 0.1 ml should produce a bleb of about 7 mm in diameter.

Suprapubic aspiration of urine

(Fig. 12.5)

This procedure is useful in infants where there is doubt about the presence of a urine infection or a specimen is needed promptly before antibiotics are started (e.g.

in suspected sepsis). Portable ultrasound to check for a full bladder before proceeding increases the success rate from about 50% to 80%. There is no point performing this procedure if the child has just passed urine. Use a sterile technique, take a 5 ml syringe and attach a 25G (green) needle. Ask an assistant to hold the child's legs straight and hold the hands or arms with the other hand. Insert the needle downwards just above the pubic bone to a distance of about 2 cm. Gently aspirate urine into the syringe, then withdraw the needle and apply a small sticking plaster. Bacterial growth from a suprapubic aspirate is significant, even if less than 10^5 organisms per ml.

Pulse oximetry

This measures the percentage of haemoglobin that is saturated with oxygen. It is based on the fact that deoxyhaemoglobin and oxyhaemoglobin absorb red and infrared light differently. The change in the amount of light of both frequencies passing through a digit or earlobe with each pulse is measured. This allows calculation of the relative amounts of oxygenated and deoxygenated haemoglobin in arterial blood. Accuracy is affected by peripheral vasoconstriction, venous congestion, movement, bright or flickering ambient light, different forms

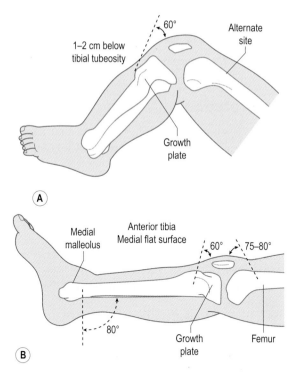

Fig. 12.6 Sites of intraosseous needle insertion showing the angles required to avoid the growth plate in the infant (A) and older child (B)

of haemoglobin and severe anaemia. Oxygen saturation has a non-linear correlation with partial pressure of oxygen (PaO_2). It is usually above 96% in children, and below 92% is considered to be hypoxia with a need for oxygen. However, during neonatal resuscitation a period of transition is allowed from in utero saturations of 70%, as recent evidence suggests that use of 100% oxygen is detrimental in this situation.

Intraosseus access

Learn this technique as soon as you start looking after sick children, since it gives you rapid vascular access even in a very shut-down child. It is taught on paediatric advanced resuscitation courses. Use the specially designed needle (Fig. 12.6) with the handle cupped in your palm. With a firm rotating action, insert it at 90° to the skin into the anteromedial aspect of the tibia about 2 cm below and medial to the tibial tuberosity. (This avoids the growth plate.) Alternative sites for intraosseous insertion in infants and children include the medial and lateral malleoli, distal femur and iliac crests. The distal femur location is approximately 1 cm above patella in the midline and malleoli sites are approximately 1 cm superior to the malleoli. The medial malleoli are generally easier to penetrate than the lateral malleoli. Once correctly inserted, the needle should feel solid in the bone. Remove the trochar and aspirate for blood samples, then push in fluid with a syringe.

Long lines

Fine, flexible central catheters inserted through a peripheral vein (usually antecubital or saphenous) are used especially in neonatal patients who will need total parenteral nutrition (TPN) for several days, to minimize the handling and trauma of repeated peripheral lines. Following full sterile technique including gown, gloves and mask, a butterfly needle is inserted into a peripheral vein, through which the line is passed until the length inserted matches that measured externally prior to the procedure. The needle is then slid out of the vein and either passed over the line or pulled into two parts to allow removal. Place the catheter tip in the superior or inferior vena cava well outside the heart to avoid the risk of tamponade, and use radio-opaque catheters or contrast injection to check the position regularly on X-ray (beware of migration).

Umbilical venous and arterial catheter insertion

Umbilical vascular catheterization is one of the commonest techniques used in the neonatal intensive care unit. Umbilical venous catheterization can be used for emergency resuscitation of the newborn and as a source of central venous access. Umbilical arterial catheterization allows arterial sampling and continuous blood pressure monitoring.

Interpretation of investigations

General principles

1. Check the basics (e.g. name, units, orientation of a film, normal ranges for the lab used).
2. Never assume that normal ranges in children are the same as for adults. Many are different and vary across age range (Box 12.2).
3. Consider repeating unexpectedly abnormal results. They may be due to artefact or sampling error.
4. List differentials and use a logical approach: for example, listing all categories of aetiology (sometimes called a 'surgical sieve') to ensure you consider all possibilities.
5. Take all the available information into account when interpreting results, including salient features from the history, examination and other investigations. Aim to find a diagnosis that will explain all if possible.

See page 59 for a discussion of interpretation of common investigations. Other investigations are discussed later in the text.

http://www.labtestsonline.org
http://www.labtestsonline.info

Information on investigations

Reference ranges

Most hospital laboratories make their own reference ranges available through an intranet system or in published form. It is best to use these whenever possible, since ranges (and the units used) can vary between laboratories.

BOX 12.2 Examples of differences in paediatric investigations

- Haemoglobin is high at birth (15–24 g/dl) and falls by 2 months
- White cell count is high at birth (10–26 × 10⁹) and falls slowly over first few years
- Alkaline phosphatase is higher than in adults throughout childhood due to bone growth, but especially so in preterm infants and during the adolescent growth spurt
- CSF protein and cell count are both higher in the neonatal period
  - Normal cells 0–4/mm³ (neonate up to 20/mm³)
  - Normal protein < 0.4 g/l (neonate up to 1.0 g/l)
- ECG: right axis deviation at birth which gradually becomes left axis deviation, reflecting the changes in the fetal circulation at birth and subsequent dominance of the left ventricle

---

Interpretation of X-rays

Develop a system for looking at X-rays that ensures you go through them logically without missing any important features. Always start with the basics: name and patient details, and orientation of both film and patient. Review films regularly with more experienced colleagues to help you improve your interpretation skills.

Chest X-rays (Fig. 12.7)

Basics (as above)
- Is the patient rotated (check symmetry of clavicles and ribs)?
- Was the film shot as postero-anterior (PA, usual) or antero-posterior (AP, may magnify the cardiac shadow)?

Lung fields
- Volume? (N.B. The number of posterior ribs above the diaphragm should be 8 or 9.)
  - Inadequate inspiration?
  - Hyperinflation: increased number of posterior ribs (10 in Fig. 12.7 — A), flattened diaphragm, ribs more horizontal.
- Collapse, consolidation, effusion:
  - Check for clarity of heart borders and both hemidiaphragms (including costophrenic

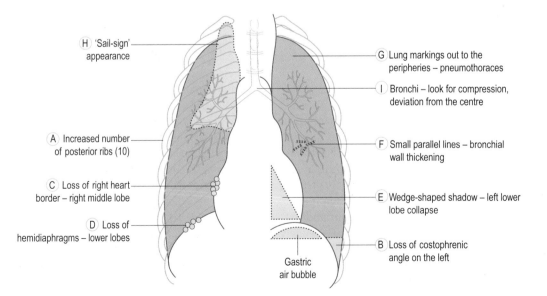

H 'Sail-sign' appearance

G Lung markings out to the peripheries – pneumothoraces

I Bronchi – look for compression, deviation from the centre

A Increased number of posterior ribs (10)

F Small parallel lines – bronchial wall thickening

C Loss of right heart border – right middle lobe

E Wedge-shaped shadow – left lower lobe collapse

D Loss of hemidiaphragms – lower lobes

B Loss of costophrenic angle on the left

Gastric air bubble

Fig. 12.7 Chest X-ray

Table 12.1 Guide to investigations you should have seen and/or performed

System/type	Investigation	Reference in European MasterCourse
Biochemistry	Urea and electrolytes (U&Es), creatinine	Ch. 39
	Glucose	Ch. 35
	Liver function tests (LFTs)	Ch. 38
	C-reactive protein (CRP)	Ch. 43
	Calcium and phosphate	Ch. 33
	Magnesium	Ch. 43
Microbiology and virology	Microscopy and culture	Ch. 43
	Viral culture	Ch. 43
	Polymerase chain reaction (PCR)	Ch. 43
	Respiratory syncytial virus (RSV) immunofluorescence	Ch. 43
	Bordetella pertussis culture	Ch. 43
	Viral titres	Ch. 43
	Hepatitis serology	Ch. 43
Haematology	Full blood count (FBC) and film	Ch. 42
	Erythrocyte sedimentation rate (ESR)	Ch. 42
	Plasma viscosity	Ch. 42
	Clotting screen	Ch. 42
	Sickle test	Ch. 42
	Advanced tests of clotting and platelet function	Ch. 42
	Platelet antibodies	Ch. 42
Immunology, infections, and allergy	Total and specific IgE	Ch. 43
	Functional antibodies	Ch. 43
	Coeliac screen	Ch. 43
	Immunoglobulins	Ch. 43
	IgG subclasses	Ch. 43
	Neutrophil function tests	Ch. 43
	Cell markers	Ch. 43
	Human immunodeficiency virus (HIV) testing	Ch. 43
	Autoantibodies	Ch. 43
	Immune complexes and complement	Ch. 43
	Human leucocyte antigen (HLA) typing	Ch. 43
Cardiology	Electrocardiography (ECG)	Ch. 40
	Echo	Ch. 40
Respiratory and ear, nose and throat	Peak flow	Chs 23 and 41
	Respiratory function tests	Chs 23 and 41
	Sweat test	Chs 23 and 41
Gastrointestinal and hepatobiliary	Test feed	Chs 25 and 38
	Endoscopy	Chs 25 and 38
	White cell scan	Chs 25 and 38
Renal, fluid and electrolyte balance	Plasma and urine osmolality	Ch. 39
	Urine electrolytes	Ch. 39
	Renal ultrasound	Ch. 39
	DMSA	Ch. 39
	MCUG	Ch. 39
	MAG3	Ch. 39
	Glomerular filtration rate (GFR)	Ch. 39
Neurology	Lumbar puncture	Chs 24 and 28
	Ultrasound head	Chs 24 and 28
	Computed tomography (CT) head	Chs 24 and 28
	Magnetic resonance imaging (MRI) head	Chs 24 and 28
	Electroencephalogram (EEG)	Chs 24 and 28
	Nerve conduction	Chs 24 and 28
	Creatine kinase	Chs 24 and 28
	Muscle biopsy	Chs 24 and 28
Oncology	Tumour markers	Ch. 50

Table 12.1 Guide to investigations you should have seen and/or performed (*cont'd*)

System/type	Investigation	Reference in European MasterCourse
Endocrine and metabolic	Thyroid function	Ch. 35
	HbA₁C	Ch. 35
	Glucose tolerance test	Ch. 35
	Metabolic screen	Ch. 35
	Tandem mass spectrometry	Ch. 35
	Follicle-stimulating hormone (FSH) and luteinizing hormone (LH)	Ch. 35
	Sex steroids	Ch. 35
	Cortisol	Ch. 35
	Growth hormone	Ch. 35
	Vitamin D	Ch. 35
Child protection	Skeletal survey	Chs 21 and 36
Rheumatology and orthopaedics	Tissue biopsy	Ch. 33
	Synovial fluid analysis	Ch. 33
	Athroscopy	Ch. 33
Genetic	Karyotype	Ch. 9
	Fluorescent in situ hybridization (FISH) testing for mutations	Ch. 9

angles — B on Fig. 12.7 shows loss of the angle on the left).
- Clues to site of consolidation: loss of right heart border — right middle lobe (C), loss of left heart border — lingula; loss of hemidiaphragms — lower lobes (D).
- Look carefully behind the cardiac shadow; e.g. left lower lobe collapse may show as a wedge-shaped shadow (E), often accompanied by increased lucency of the left lung field compared to the right.
- Bronchial wall thickening:
  - Common in viral infections, especially in the perihilar regions (look for small parallel lines, F).
- Pneumothoraces:
  - Use bright light if in doubt to check for lung markings out to the peripheries and include a lateral view (G).
- Lucency:
  - Is this symmetrical? Compare upper middle and lower zones. If uncertain, try covering the cardiac shadow with your hand.
  - Asymmetry if large collapse or foreign body.
- Other lung field changes:
  - Cystic (as in cystic fibrosis)
  - Ground glass (respiratory distress syndrome).

Heart and mediastinum
- Cardiac size and shape:
  - Cardiothoracic ratio (PA) < 0.55 under 2 years, < 0.50 above 2 years.

- Thymus:
  - May be quite large in small children, and have a flat lower border due to it resting on the horizontal fissure. This gives it the 'sail-sign' appearance (H).
- Trachea, carina (at the level of the 6th posterior rib) and bronchi (I):
  - Compression, deviation from centre, other signs of mediastinal shift?

Bones
- Check all carefully for fractures (especially ribs and clavicles) or other abnormality.

Other
- Look at other features visible on the film: upper abdomen, arms, neck, upper airway, soft tissues, and tubes and lines. Correct placement of endotracheal tube position (T4), UAC (T6-9), UVC (above the diaphragm) and longline position (central) needs to be verified.

Abdominal X-rays

These are useful for the acute abdomen, especially when obstruction or perforation is suspected. For the latter, combine with an erect chest X-ray to look for gas under the diaphragm (and also for pneumonia). Some units advise an erect abdominal film too. Check for pattern and amount of bowel gas, any fluid levels and bowel distension. A gasless abdomen is suggestive of obstruction, as are fluid levels on an erect film. Abdominal X-rays are generally not useful in constipation.

Skull X-rays

These are not now routinely done in children with head injuries since they do not reliably identify children who need a computed tomography (CT) head scan. They may be indicated in certain situations; for example, in suspected non-accidental head injury it is helpful to know whether a fracture is present. You need to be familiar with the appearance of normal vascular markings and sutures lines, so that you can distinguish these from fractures. Fractures tend to be blacker than vascular markings (because both tables of the skull are involved), and may have less-defined edges. If there are any branches, they do not taper uniformly as do vascular markings. Depressed fractures appear denser (whiter) on a radiograph.

http://www.rch.org.au/clinicalguide/index.cfm?doc_id=5033

The Royal Children's Hospital Melbourne has an excellent Clinical Practice Guidelines section with guidelines and further information (including videos) on most practical procedures

Table 12.1 indicates the procedures that you should have either performed or seen.

David Evans   Steven J. Novek   Alison Pike

13

Evidence-based paediatrics and audit

LEARNING OUTCOMES

By the end of this chapter you should:

- Be able to describe the structure used to formulate a clinical question
- Be able to identify the advantages of using the Cochrane Library as a starting point for searching evidence on the effectiveness of interventions
- Know how to compare and contrast bias and chance as sources of error
- Be able to critically appraise a randomized controlled trial
- Be able to interpret the commonly used measures of treatment efficacy
- Be familiar with secondary sources of evidence-based interventions
- Be able to briefly describe the purpose and process of clinical audit.

MODULE TWO

What is evidence-based medicine?

Evidence-based medicine (EBM) involves the 'integration of best available evidence with individual clinical expertise'. In other words, it means applying relevant, up-to-date research findings to the management of your patients.

There are many reasons why familiarity with the techniques of EBM has become increasingly necessary. Firstly, we now require evidence of efficacy from the results of randomized control trials (RCTs) reporting clinically relevant outcomes, whereas in the past, an understanding of pathophysiological processes was deemed sufficient. Secondly, evidence changes with the growth of our knowledge base through continued research, so that it is crucial that we develop techniques that search out the latest evidence. Thirdly, traditional medical education has evolved from the handing down of knowledge and skills from expert practitioners to apprentices. In the past, this may have placed too much reliance on believing the experts, thus inhibiting questioning behaviour.

What EBM is not!

EBM is not 'cookbook' medicine, threatening to take away an individual clinician's judgment (honed over years of experience). Clinical expertise and experience are very much required. It is still essential to make a correct diagnosis! Communication skills, enabling appreciation of your patient's values, are important in selecting whether a particular treatment choice would be in your patient's best interests.

It is not the primary function of EBM to ration or deny patient choice. Rather, it provides a framework by which healthcare interventions can be judged or compared, in terms of important patient outcomes. Some EBM interventions may save money (immunizations), and others may be very expensive (extra-corporeal membrane oxygenation [ECMO]). Whether achieving these outcomes is worth the financial expenditure is largely a political decision.

EBM is not restricted to RCTs and meta-analyses. The principles of EBM are also applicable to diagnosis (see Chapter 6, page 58), prognosis, and determination of harm.

The five steps of EBM

- Formulating an answerable clinical question
- Searching for the evidence
- Critical appraisal of the evidence
- Applying the evidence to help your patient
- Evaluation of your performance.

Step 1: Posing the question

Clinical questions fall into two broad categories: background and foreground. Background questions (What are the most common causes of neonatal sepsis? How does nephrosis cause oedema?) are usually asked by students, and focus on pathophysiology and other clinical sciences. Foreground questions focus on specific diagnostic or therapeutic decisions (should surfactant be given to a 30-week-gestation newborn prophylactically, or as rescue therapy?), and are usually posed by experienced clinicians. We must remember, however, that even the most astute specialist needs background information about some topics, and that novice clinical clerks can learn the evidence basis for the foreground of cutting-edge treatment decisions.

It is all too easy to practise without asking questions, as these have the annoying habit of exposing gaps in knowledge which then require time and effort to plug! When we do have questions about current practice, however, they often appear unstructured, too vague or too complex. Good questions should be focused on the medical problem and concentrated on outcomes of interest. The framework most commonly used to formulate clinical questions has four components:
- P: The patient with the pathology
- I: The intervention, diagnostic test or exposure of interest

- C: The comparison group (if relevant)
- O: The outcomes of interest.

Questions clearly focused using this mnemonic (PICO) have the greatest chance of being answerable (see example, Box 13.1).

Step 2: Searching for the evidence

What to search for?

We are looking for high-quality current studies that address our clinical question. Textbooks are unlikely to be sufficiently up to date and, despite their claims, expert colleagues may not be aware of all the relevant literature. When looking for evidence about the effectiveness of clinical interventions, we require data from RCTs. However, searching a bibliographical database, such as Medline or Embase, can be an unrewarding exercise unless a focused search strategy is employed.

How to search

Electronic searching of databases allows combinations of search keywords, most often combined with either 'AND' or 'OR' Boolean operators. For example, a search to address the surfactant question might have the following structure (PICO):
- P Infant, preterm OR Respiratory distress syndrome
  AND
- I Surfactant [C Rescue therapy]
  AND
- O Mortality OR Pneumothorax OR Chronic lung disease OR Intraventricular haemorrhage.

In this example, you do not need to specify the control group. The combination of terms 'Infant, preterm OR Respiratory distress syndrome' will result in the search returning articles containing either of the terms. The combination of 'Infant, preterm AND Surfactant' will return only articles containing both terms. There are many refinements to searching, such as using a combination of text word and medical subheadings, or using wildcard characters (useful for North American spelling, e.g. an?emia — for anaemia or anemia) and truncated words (e.g. neonat* — for neonate, neonates, neonatal, neonatology, etc).

We may begin our search with the largest database, housed at the US National Library of Medicine, accessible through various search engines, such as Medline or PubMed. Or, we may limit ourselves to a collection of articles that have already been critically evaluated for us to locate only the highest quality studies, such as the Cochrane Collaboration. Founded in 1993, the Cochrane Collaboration produces and disseminates systematic reviews of healthcare interventions, and promotes the search for evidence in the form of clinical trials. It was initially a British organization, but rapidly developed ties to other English-speaking countries, and has now spread to more than a dozen countries.

Medical librarians can offer expert tips and advice on how to make a search either more sensitive, which is useful when the initial strategy results in few articles, or more specific, which is useful when the initial strategy results in too many articles.

http://www.ncbi.nlm.nih.gov/sites/
entrez?db=pmc

PubMed search engine (free from US National Institutes of Health [NIH])

Here are the results for the above search using Medline:

		# of articles
Infant, preterm	OR RDS	42 872
Surfactant		73 762
AND		338
Mortality OR pneumothorax OR chronic lung disease OR intraventricular haemorrhage		226 285
AND		54

It would be great if every search found a definitive study that addressed our clinical question. More usually, search results fall into two categories. Either we fail to find a single relevant article or we find too many, as in the above example.

Let us consider the first situation. One reason for not finding a study is that, unfortunately, not all studies can be found by searching Medline. This is because they may be published elsewhere: in journals that are not listed on Medline (which favours English language journals) or in what is known as the 'grey literature' (abstracts, proceedings of meetings, university theses, etc.). Fortunately, the Cochrane Collaboration employs trained searchers to look through all the literature in its different types and languages.

http://www.cochrane.org
http://www.thecochranelibrary.com

Medline also has a database called 'All EBM Reviews' that allows you to search simultaneously seven EBM databases: ACP Journal Club, Cochrane Central Register of Controlled Trials (CCTR), Cochrane Database of Systematic Reviews (DSR), Cochrane Methodology Register (CMR), Database of Abstracts of Reviews of Effects (DARE), Health Technology Assessment (HTA), and National Health Service Economic Evaluation (NHSEED).

http://gateway.ovid.com

Ovid Medline search engine

If we repeat the above search in Medline, but change to the 'All EBM Reviews' database, we obtain a more reasonable total of 24 articles. If instead we run a similar search under the Cochrane website (using as our search terms: prophylactic surfactant for RDS), we obtain only 8 citations, and you may scan them easily and rapidly for results.

The Cochrane Library is restricted to information about healthcare interventions, but there are an increasing number of other secondary publications that address diagnosis, prognosis, harm, cost-effectiveness, etc. Later in this chapter we will review some of these EBM secondary sources.

Search strategies

The Centre for Evidence-Based Medicine in Oxford, UK gives very useful guidance on 'how to get the right stuff and avoid getting the wrong stuff'! This includes methods of altering the sensitivity and specificity of your searches, and also strategies to pick out the most relevant publication types (RCTs, cohort studies etc.) in order to answer different types of question (interventions, prognosis, harm, diagnosis, etc.). The site below also separates search methods into secondary sources, and primary sources with modifiers to make your search either more sensitive or more specific as needed.

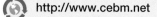

http://www.cebm.net

Step 3: Critical appraisal of the evidence

There are four main stages to appraising any evidence:

1. Relevance. This stage is largely intuitive (i.e. you are not going to waste time reading a paper if it is not relevant!), although using the PICO formulation helps you focus your attention and quickly decide whether the study is assessing the relevant intervention in the appropriate patients and reporting the important outcomes.
2. Validity. Can I believe the results? A dictionary definition of validity might include 'based upon or borne out by truth'. Why do we need to appraise validity? Surely, if evidence is published it must be correct? Although research fraud does exist, no one is suggesting that the majority of authors are trying to falsify claims, but there might be many reasons why the evidence you have just found will not be as valid as you hoped. Despite all the best intentions, a research study might not produce results that are 'based upon truth' as far as the researchers had anticipated (see Box 13.2).
3. Significance. Are the results likely to result in an important improvement? We will consider this in more detail in the section on assessing significance.
4. Applicability. Can I apply the results so that my patients receive similar benefits to the study participants?

The importance of validity

Box 13.2 describes a simple research experiment.

There are a number of reasons why the results obtained do not match those anticipated. These can be grouped into three categories:

BOX 13.2 Research study: an analogy

You are given a solid object and your task is to determine how many surfaces it has. You have been told that the object has a number of flat surfaces of equal area. Each surface has a number of dots but only one surface has one dot.

You suspect from your prior knowledge that the object is a die (hypothesis). Unfortunately, you cannot see or feel the object well enough to determine this by inspection (because of a visual impairment and peripheral neuropathy). Thus, you test your hypothesis by throwing the object and asking your friend to call out each time the surface with the single dot is uppermost. You throw the object 60 times, expecting your friend to call out on 10 occasions but, in fact, he calls out 15 times.

Think of the reasons why the result was not what you expected.

- Wrong hypothesis. Perhaps the object was a tetrahedron, not a die.
- Random error (chance). The confidence interval (CI) gives an indication of variation in results attributable by chance (see below, assessment of significance). In this example, the CI includes the possibilities that the object could have between three and seven sides. Performing a larger study (e.g. 600 throws) will reduce this variation and narrow the CI.
- Systematic error (bias). Was the die weighted? Was your friend lying? Is your friend also visually impaired? Is he innumerate? Do you also have a hearing impairment? In contrast to random error, statistics or CI are not helpful with these sources of bias; performing a larger study would just compound the error. The sources of bias need to be minimized by improving study design. In the vignette, one might want to test your friend's vision against a known standard beforehand (e.g. Snellen chart). Other ways of assessing the outcome might be to use two independent observers, who separately record their observations, or by filming the throws for validation purposes, etc.

How is this analogous to a research study? Well, in real life the truth is only ever inferred through observation. If we wish to study the effectiveness of surfactant therapy in the delivery suite, we cannot actually see the surfactant molecules benefiting the infant. We have to make observations on outcomes that we can measure, such as mortality or chronic lung disease. Unfortunately, these outcomes are not necessarily easy to define, and are subject to both random effects and systematic influences (gestation, presence of infection, etc.). Statistics help us assess random error, but good study design is essential and constitutes the only way of minimizing systematic error or bias.

The validity of a study is therefore determined by its design; good study design ensures validity by minimizing bias. Thus, the most appropriate place in an article to assess validity is in the description of methods. Unfortunately, this is often the least-read section of an article. Many of the teachings of EBM and critical appraisal courses are intended to equip readers with the skills to interpret the methods of the more commonly employed study designs in clinical medicine.

RCTs

One of the most important study designs used to assess the effectiveness of an intervention is the RCT. When assessing whether an RCT has reported valid claims, it is important to know what aspects of this design make it such a powerful methodology and hence which aspects of design must, where possible, be strictly adhered to in order to minimize bias.

> ## Problem-oriented topic:
>
> ### RCT ⚪⚪⚪⚪⚪
>
> Johnny is a 7-year-old boy with cystic fibrosis. He has good pulmonary function ($FEV_1 = 90\%$) and is growing along the 25% for height and weight, but he is colonized with *Pseudomonas*, and he has frequent pulmonary exacerbations that require hospital admission for intravenous (IV) antibiotics. His mother asks you if prophylactic oral antibiotics would improve his lung function and keep him from missing school.

Search Strategy:

Start with Medline, all EBM review database, using search terms: Cystic fibrosis and oral antibiotics. You find 18 articles listed. You select the article by A Clement et al from Paris, France, published in Thorax 61: 895–902 (2006), entitled, 'Long term effects of azithromycin in patients with cystic fibrosis: a double blind, placebo controlled trial'.

We will review the methods section, making reference to criteria published in the Users' Guide to the Medical Literature that explain how to tell whether the results of a therapy article are valid. Printing a copy of this article will help you to appraise it critically; excerpts from the article are reproduced in italics below. Furthermore, the Public Health Resource Unit of the UK National Health Service provides worksheets to help you in your appraisal of any RCT:

🌐 http://www.phru.nhs.uk/Pages/PHD/ resources.htm

Medline and Embase are large and unwieldy, but there are techniques to limit your searches. If you use PubMed, you can restrict your search to RCTs or meta-analyses by selecting limit to article type. Ovid Medline offers two options: you may limit a search by publication type (RCT or systematic reviews), or, even better, you may choose the 'all EBM reviews' database described above. This database includes only those studies that have already been critically appraised for validity (you still have to decide what's relevant!).

Secondary sources of evidence

We commented earlier that textbooks are next to useless for current treatment, years behind current evidence by the time they are published, and poorly referenced. But what if a textbook could be updated every 6 months, and if it focused on critically appraised evidence for treatments, and was extensively referenced? Three textbooks currently fit the bill for paediatrics: *Clinical Evidence* (in print and web-based); *Evidence-based Pediatrics and Child Health* (in print and web-based); and *UpToDate* (CD and web-based).

Clinical Evidence is published by BMJ Books, with a new edition published every 6 months, and a frequently updated website. It poses common questions from all areas of ambulatory paediatrics, reviews all available evidence, and then grades interventions based on the evidence. Treatments are listed as beneficial, likely to be beneficial, unknown effectiveness, unlikely to be beneficial, or trade-off between benefits and harm.

Evidence-based Pediatrics and Child Health is a traditional textbook published in 2004 by BMJ Books (2nd edition). It is divided into two halves: the first half reviews EBM principles in detail, and the second half addresses common ambulatory paediatric problems by critically appraising available evidence for key questions. The book's website is updated regularly as important new studies are published.

UpToDate is an electronic textbook that covers all medical specialties; it began as an internal medicine text, but paediatrics was completed in 2005. It may be searched for general disease-based information, but it focuses on evidence-based therapy, and it is extensively referenced, with automatic hyperlinks to Medline abstracts. Although not explicit in earlier editions, the *UpToDate* editors and authors have adopted standardized grading scales for the quality of evidence for treatment recommendations.

> ## BOX 13.3 Critical appraisal criteria for a paper on therapy
>
> ### Study design:
> Were patients randomized to therapy groups?
> Was therapy allocation adequately concealed?
> Were some eligible patients not enrolled?
> Were patients, caregivers, and investigators blinded to treatment groups?
>
> ### Data analysis:
> Were groups similar at the start of the trial?
> Were groups treated the same during the trial?
> Were all patients accounted for in follow-up?
> Were patients analysed in their assigned groups? (intention-to-treat)
>
> ### Results reporting:
> How large was the effect of therapy?
> How precise was the estimate of therapy effect?
> Were all important endpoints reported?

Finally, there is another website designed for secondary searches, called TRIP (Turning Research Into Practice), that allows you to search for a specific topic, and summarizes the available evidence based on quality and provenance:

http://www.tripdatabase.com/index.html

Study design

Inclusion criteria: cystic fibrosis (CF), age 6–21, ability to perform spirometry, forced expiratory volume in one second (FEV₁) > 40% predicted, ability to swallow pills.

Exclusion criteria: allergy to macrolides, chronic prior use of macrolides within 3 months, liver disease with transaminases > twice normal, kidney disease with GFR < half normal, or use of inhaled tobramycin, inhaled steroids, or recombinant human DNAase in the three months prior to the study.

All inclusion criteria are appropriate, although the FEV_1 > 40% limits possible benefits to mild-moderate CF. The final exclusion criterion is suspect, because it may have excluded many otherwise eligible patients using multimodal therapies, the norm in CF.

Randomization method

Randomization refers to the method of treatment allocation: how are patients assigned to either the treatment or control group? Did the investigators use some method analogous to tossing a coin to allocate each patient? In practice, nowadays we use computer-generated random numbers, but the idea is the same. We should insist on random allocation because this technique comes closer than any other design to dividing up the patients at the start of the trial into groups that are equally at risk for the outcome of interest. Randomization balances the groups for prognostic factors, which could accentuate or attenuate the effects of therapy if they were unevenly distributed when the trial began. These factors are called confounders, and there are other methods to avoid them, such as exclusion, stratified sampling, and matching. However, these other methods work only for confounders that are known before the study; randomization also works for unknown confounders that are detected only after the study is completed.

Randomization: double-blind, placebo-controlled, multicentre drug therapy trial of 12 months' duration. Stratification according to treatment centre and P. aeruginosa status. Allocation was assigned by a centralized randomized number generator at a non-participating centre, with enrolment of each patient locally, and then pharmacist calls to obtain assignment.

Allocation should be truly random (e.g. computer-generated random number lists). Other methods, such

as allocation by alternating assignment, hospital number, dates of birth, etc., are known as quasirandomization and are prone to selection bias.

Randomization is frequently stratified; although randomization should balance all the confounding variables, in trials with relatively small numbers, some variables may not be equally balanced. A common situation in which stratification is used is when an RCT evaluates the effectiveness of a treatment for a rare disorder, with many participating centres. Each centre will recruit only a modest number and stratifying randomization for each centre (i.e. its own random number list) will ensure that any centre-specific differences in treatment are balanced within the trial. It is also common to stratify for disease severity (if reliable markers of severity can be determined before trial entry), so that the groups contain patients of a similar prognostic profile.

Allocation concealment

This technique prevents prior knowledge of the treatment allocation before patient entry into a trial. It is particularly important in RCTs where the treatment is complex and resource-intensive and cannot be blinded. An example would be ECMO for severe respiratory failure in infants. This treatment requires the very sick infant to be transferred to a referral centre for the procedure, whereas the control might involve standard respiratory care at the original hospital. If the clinicians responsible for entering patients into the trial were to know what the allocated treatment would be before they enrolled the infant, this could bias selection for the study. For example, if the infant were extremely unstable and the clinicians were worried that the infant might not survive transfer, they would be more willing to enter the infant into the study if they knew that the allocated treatment was standard respiratory care at the original hospital. Selection bias in this way would result in the control group having a higher proportion of sicker infants than the intervention group.

The best method of concealing the allocation is to require the clinician entering a patient into an RCT to telephone and register the patient before randomization (and to report any markers of disease severity used for stratification). The patient is then entered into the trial before the clinician is told the allocated treatment. In our CF RCT above, the clinician was never told the assignment; only the pharmacist learned it! Less robust methods include using opaque-sealed envelopes, although eager clinicians have been known to attempt transillumination or steam treatment in an effort to find out the allocation!

Intention-to-treat analysis

Both treatment groups were evaluated at 0, 2, 4, 6, 8, 10, and 12 months. Any unused study drug was returned at each visit, and the pharmacist counted remaining pills to measure compliance. Patients who missed > 30% of pills were labelled noncompliant, but were analyzed with their originally assigned group.

There are many reasons why a patient's treatment deviates from what was allocated at randomization: misdiagnosis, being given the wrong treatment by mistake (it happens!), not complying with the treatment, withdrawal of consent, loss to follow-up. Despite all these mishaps, each patient's data should always be analysed according to the group allocated at randomization (intention-to-treat analysis). Randomization is the point in the study when patient characteristics (and confounding variables) are matched. There may be a systematic reason (i.e. connected to the treatment) why certain patients cannot comply with the protocol. Using the ECMO example, if infants do not survive transfer to the ECMO treatment centre, it would be misleading to disregard their data (the excuse being 'they did not receive ECMO') and, worse still, to analyse their data with the control group ('because they received standard care'). This is because the transfer is a necessary part of ECMO, and ignoring data from patients allocated ECMO but not surviving leads to an overestimation of any beneficial ECMO treatment effect.

The three techniques described above are mandatory for an RCT to be valid; there can be little excuse for not carrying out true randomization with allocation concealment and intention-to-treat analysis.

Follow-up: 82 patients were randomized: 40 to drug, 42 to placebo. Three patients dropped out of drug arm before study began, none from placebo arm. Two drug and four placebo patients were not compliant. All patients were analysed in their originally assigned groups (intention-to-treat).

35 patients completed the drug arm, and 37 the placebo arm.

So our study adhered to an intention-to-treat analysis of the patient data, and all enrolled patients were accounted for in the statistical analysis.

Blinding

The patients and all study investigators remained blinded to the treatment assigned until the study had been completed.

This is an important technique in RCT methodology but there may be pragmatic constraints on researchers' abilities to blind various aspects of a study. Blinding is useful when the outcome of interest is subjective (think about the 'placebo effect') or the definition is open to interpretation. The use of a placebo, indistinguishable

from the active treatment, controls the natural tendency in caregivers and parents to believe that new treatments confer benefit. However, it is not always possible or ethical to use a placebo or to blind caregivers (think of surgical procedures, or behavioural therapies). In these cases, it is important to try to blind the outcome assessment. For example, if the outcome is to be a severity score of lung disease on chest radiographs, the radiographs should be interpreted by someone who is unaware of the treatment allocation.

Systematic review and meta-analysis

A systematic review aims to summarize all the available evidence relating to studies addressing a defined clinical question. Systematic reviews that address questions about the effectiveness of interventions follow a rigorous methodology. They should comprise a comprehensive search for RCTs that address a focused question, evaluated with the use of explicit predetermined criteria, a critical appraisal of each study, and synthesis of the results. The review lists the characteristics of each RCT (which patients, which intervention compared to which control, and which outcomes are reported). A review will also draw the reader's attention to whether or not the trial employed sufficient methodology to protect against bias (allocation concealment, intention-to-treat analysis, etc.).

Strictly speaking, meta-analysis refers to the statistical technique of combining the results of a number of RCTs evaluated in the systematic review (although, confusingly, North Americans often use the term synonymously with the term systematic review). It is appropriate to combine results from RCTs only if: (a) the definitions of outcomes are sufficiently similar, and (b) the trials are of sufficient methodological quality. We will look at how to interpret the results of a meta-analysis in the section on assessment of significance.

Other study designs

Two other study designs deserve mention: cohort and case-control studies. These designs are frequently used in clinical epidemiological work to determine the answers to questions about prognosis, risks, harm, and diagnosis.

Cohort study

A cohort study is useful for examining what happens to a selected sample of patients exposed to a risk factor over time, compared with a non-exposed population — the comparison being in the form of relative risk.

Cohort studies are able to measure more than one outcome. For example, in children whose risk is prematurity, the outcomes might be death, cerebral palsy, or cognitive impairment. Cohort studies also allow temporal relationships to be observed. They are relatively expensive to run over a long timescale. The main sources of bias in cohort studies are:

- Selection bias. The population should be established at a common (early) point in their disease following exposure to the risk factor.
- Loss to follow-up. This needs to be minimized.
- Diagnostic (ascertainment, surveillance) bias. If the exposed group is being followed up more closely (e.g. with more frequent examinations) than controls, there is a greater chance of detecting an outcome (and at an earlier stage).
- Recall bias, if retrospective.

Case-control study

In this study design, cases are sought with the outcome of interest (e.g. autism) and controls are picked from the population who do not have this outcome. The prevalence of exposure to a number of risk factors is determined retrospectively and compared between the two groups (e.g. maternal infections, measles/mumps/rubella [MMR] vaccinations), in the form of odds ratios. The advantage of a case-control study is that it allows study of the impact of multiple risk factors on a rare outcome, in contrast to a cohort study, which examines the effect of a single risk factor on multiple outcomes. The disadvantage is that causal relationships between risk and outcome are not identified.

The main sources of bias are:

- Selection bias, particularly in the selection of controls. Ideally, this should be a random sample from the population, but often hospital-based controls are used because they are easily identified.
- Information (recall) bias. Exposure information is reported differently in cases and controls (e.g. parents with autistic children are more likely to recall a reaction to MMR vaccination, particularly if they are aware of the hypothesis).
- Information (observation) bias. The investigator, who may be aware of the hypothesis, interprets the information differently.

The major confounding variables (that are known) can be controlled for in the design of both cohort and case-control studies by matching. The results have to be adjusted for other known confounders by use of complex statistical techniques in the analysis, such as logistic regression. (In comparison, the statistical techniques for analysing the results of RCTs are relatively straightforward.) Unknown confounders remain unknown and cannot be controlled for in study design (unlike with randomization).

As noted earlier, the Public Health Resource Unit of the UK National Health Service also publishes appraisal checklists for systematic reviews, diagnostic test studies, cohort and case-control studies, as well as other study designs.

http://www.phru.nhs.uk/Pages/PHD/resources.htm

A note of caution

There is no such thing as a perfect clinical research study; this is because there are usually practical constraints upon clinicians (ethical, financial, time, wilful patients[!], etc.). The skill in appraising a study is not simply to 'pick holes' in someone else's endeavour, but rather to determine whether or not the problems you have noted compromise the study to the extent that the results are no longer reliable. Think to yourself, 'Do the problems with the study invalidate the results?' or 'Could I have improved the design?' and also 'Are these improvements actually feasible?'

Assessment of significance

Measurements of efficacy

Box 13.4 gives the definitions of some of the common measurements of efficacy derived from the results of RCTs. Conventionally, events are considered to be adverse outcomes (e.g. death, cerebral palsy, etc.) and therefore we are hoping for a reduction in the odds and risks of such events in the treatment group, compared with the control group. Thus, an odds ratio or a relative risk of less than 1 indicates that the treatment is associated with a lower risk of adverse outcome.

If the odds ratio or relative risk is greater than 1, the treatment is associated with increased risk. If the ratio is equal to 1, then the treatment is neither effective nor harmful.

p-values and 95% CIs

If any experiment or study were repeated, it would be unlikely to produce exactly the same results each time because of the random variation that occurs each time a different patient population is sampled. Therefore, there is a risk that the result yielded by a single study does not represent a true treatment effect in the population at large but, rather, a chance effect.

The p-value is the probability that the observed result has arisen purely by chance. It can be seen that if the p-value is small, then the result is unlikely to be a chance effect and, hence, more likely to be a treatment

Box 13.4 Measurements of efficacy commonly used in randomized controlled trials

	Event	No event	Totals
Intervention group	a	b	a+b
Control group	c	d	c+d

Odds ratio (OR)

Ratio of the odds of an event in the intervention group to the odds of an event in the control group

$$OR = \frac{a}{b} \Big/ \frac{c}{d} = \frac{a.d}{b.c}$$

OR < 1 Effective
OR = 1 Ineffective
OR > 1 Harmful

Relative risk (RR)

Ratio of the risk of an event in the intervention group to the risk of an event in the control group

$$RR = \frac{a/(a+b)}{c/(c+d)}$$

RR < 1 Effective
RR = 1 Ineffective
RR > 1 Harmful

Absolute risk reduction (ARR)

Difference in the risks of an event in the intervention group from that of the control group

$$ARR = c/(c+d) - a/(a+b)$$

ARR > 0 Effective
APP = 0 Ineffective
ARR < 0 Harmful

Number needed to treat for benefit (NNTB)

Number of patients needed to treat in order to prevent one adverse event

$$NNTB = \frac{1}{ARR}$$

NNT ≥ 1 Effective
NNT = infinity Ineffective
NNT ≤ −1 Harmful

effect. Conventionally, a p-value of <0.05 is taken as a low enough risk of a random effect (<5%) for the result to be 'statistically significant'.

While the p-value gives us a good idea of the risk of random error or chance effects, the CI provides more useful information. A CI is a range of values that is likely to include the true treatment effect in the population, the estimated range being calculated from the sample studied in the RCT. The confidence level (usually 95%) describes how confident we are that the true effect falls within that range. A 95% CI means that if the study were repeated 100 times, 95 of the studies would give a result within that range. Choosing a higher confidence level, such as 99%, would make us even more confident that the range included the true result.

The number of pulmonary exacerbations per patient was significantly reduced in the azithromycin group (1.5) compared with the placebo group (3.0), with the relative risk = 0.50 with 95% CI of 0.32 to 0.79, p < 0.005.

Time to remain free of exacerbations during the study was significantly longer in those receiving azithromycin (median 8.7 months) than in those given placebo (2.9 months), with a hazard ratio of azithromycin vs. placebo = 0.37 (95% CI 0.22 to 0.63)

Therefore, in our CF study, a decrease in the frequency of pulmonary exacerbations and a longer time before first exacerbation are both statistically significant results, unlikely to be explained by chance.

In the case of the odds ratio or relative risk, if the 95% CI includes the value 1, it means that we cannot confidently exclude the possibility that the treatment has no effect (and therefore the result is not statistically significant; that is to say, p > 0.05). An example of such a study is Egberts (1993) in Fig. 13.1. If the whole of the 95% CI for the relative risk or the odds ratio is

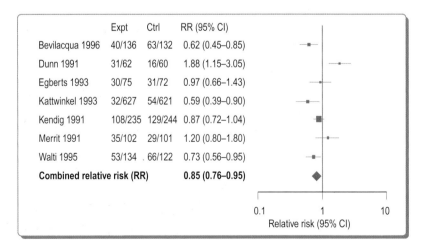

	Expt	Ctrl	RR (95% CI)
Bevilacqua 1996	40/136	63/132	0.62 (0.45–0.85)
Dunn 1991	31/62	16/60	1.88 (1.15–3.05)
Egberts 1993	30/75	31/72	0.97 (0.66–1.43)
Kattwinkel 1993	32/627	54/621	0.59 (0.39–0.90)
Kendig 1991	108/235	129/244	0.87 (0.72–1.04)
Merrit 1991	35/102	29/101	1.20 (0.80–1.80)
Walti 1995	53/134	66/122	0.73 (0.56–0.95)
Combined relative risk (RR)			**0.85 (0.76–0.95)**

Relative risk (95% CI)

Fig. 13.1 Forest plot: meta-analysis of randomized controlled trials comparing prophylactic surfactant therapy (Exp) with later surfactant treatment (Ctrl) for RDS. Outcome: death or chronic lung disease.

less than 1, the treatment effect is statistically significant (p < 0.05) (e.g. Bevilacqua [1996] in Fig. 13.1).

The width of the CI gives us some idea about how uncertain we are about the treatment effect. A very wide interval may indicate that more data should be collected before making a final decision on significance.

Sample size

A sample size calculation is performed before the study to provide an estimate of how many patients will be required to generate meaningful data. The sample size for an RCT is dependent upon four factors:

1. Event rates. If the outcome of interest is rare (e.g. death from acute asthma), the sample size will be greater than for studies with more common outcomes (e.g. death following leukaemia).
2. Treatment effect. Studies looking for small treatment effects will need to be larger than studies that are looking for larger, more obvious effects.
3. Significance (α). This is the level of probability below which you would accept that the results would not have occurred by chance (i.e. p-value $< \alpha$). The smaller the p-value with which you need to convince yourself the observed effect is real, the larger the study required.
4. Power (1-β). This is the ability of a study to detect a true treatment effect. RCTs are often powered to detect a true treatment effect 80% of the time; this means there is a 20% risk ($\beta = 0.2$) that the RCT will produce an equivocal result, despite the treatment being effective. Hence, one needs to be cautious about stating that a treatment is not effective, based upon the results of a small RCT of low power, since there is a fair chance that the RCT might have missed an unequivocal result. Studies that are designed to have more power require more patients.

We estimated that FEV$_1$ would decrease by 2% per year in patients not colonized by P. aeruginosa, and by 4% per year in patients who were colonized. We hypothesized that azithromycin treatment would slow the decrease in FEV1 by approximately 4% per year. Using this estimate, a planned sample size of 121 patients per group provided a power of 90% to detect the anticipated difference between treatments.

Only 82 patients were randomized during the study, instead of the planned for 240. Nevertheless, a treatment effect was discerned, as noted above in the results.

Meta-analysis

The results from a number of RCTs may be combined to give a more precise estimate of the treatment effect, as long as: (a) the definitions of outcomes are sufficiently similar, and (b) the trials are of sufficient methodological standard. The results can be displayed in the form of a forest plot. An example is given in Fig. 13.1, which comes from a Cochrane review of RCTs evaluating the effects of early prophylactic surfactant therapy versus delayed surfactant treatment for respiratory distress syndrome on death or chronic lung disease (Yost & Soll 1999). The studies that report a statistically significant beneficial treatment effect can be clearly seen because their point estimates and 95% CIs all fall to the left of the line on the graphical representation. Non-significant studies have 95% CIs that cross the line.

The results are combined in a meta-analysis, giving greatest weight to those studies that report results with higher precision (narrower 95% CIs). An advantage of a meta-analysis is that many small studies, each with equivocal results, may be combined to produce a more precise overall estimate of treatment effect. Also, if a treatment effect is seen to be consistent across all the studies (with varying, albeit similar, populations), one might be more confident that the treatment will be beneficial when applied outside the strict confines of a research study.

Clinical versus statistical significance

Although the results may be statistically significant, the treatment effect may not necessarily be clinically significant. For example, a bronchodilator is found to produce a 10% increase in peak expiratory flow rates in asthma (95% CIs 8–12%), but this statistically significant result might not result in a clinically significant improvement in symptoms.

In our CF study cited above, the results are statistically significant, but they are also clinically significant, because half the number of pulmonary exacerbations per year translates into time at home and in school instead of in hospital, as well as real cost savings; plus, there is the added benefit of a slowdown in the inexorable loss of pulmonary function so damaging in CF. We imagine that our patient and his parents will be happy to avoid one or two hospitalizations per year!

Determining whether the results from a study are clinically significant requires clinical judgment and depends on the values of your patient, which brings us to the penultimate step in EBM.

Step 4: Applying the evidence to help your patient

If we have determined that the results of a study are valid and significant, we then have to decide whether applying the evidence will benefit our patient. The following questions are useful when coming to such decisions:

1. Is your patient similar to those patients studied? Look at the eligibility or selection criteria. Was the frequency of outcome in the study what you would expect in your practice? For example, if the death rates were much higher than expected, perhaps the studied population might be more severely affected by the disease than your patient.

2. Do the potential side-effects of treatment outweigh the benefits? Did the study report all the side-effects that would be important to your patient? Does the benefit/risk ratio accord with your patient's expectations and values? Will your patient comply with the regimen?

3. Can you offer the treatment? Do you have the facilities to ensure the treatment is administered safely (e.g. technology, trained staff)? Do you have the required resources (e.g. time, money)?

Step 5: Evaluation of your performance

We need to learn from the process of practising EBM. Firstly, are we challenging our current practice and asking questions in an appropriately formulated manner? Can we find good evidence using searches with the right balance of sensitivity and specificity? Are we critically appraising papers relevant to our practice? Has the application of evidence led to an improvement in patient outcomes? This final step shares many of the concepts and techniques with clinical audit, or, as it is called in North America, 'performance improvement'.

Are you asking questions? Are your questions identifiable as either background or foreground, and do your foreground questions adhere to the PICO mnemonic? What is your working method to save your questions (personal digital assistant [PDA] entry, note cards)?

Once you are convinced that you are asking answerable clinical questions, how are your searches proceeding? Do you take advantage of the best secondary sources in paediatrics (see end of this chapter)? If you cannot find appropriate secondary sources, can you turn to primary sources rapidly and successfully? Do you have ready access to the necessary hardware and software to perform your search near the point of care, on the ward? After all, if you must leave the ward, cross a busy street, enter the medical school library, sign a waiting list for a computer terminal, and only then be able to search, we doubt that you will be enthusiastic about making evidence-based treatment decisions during rounds! Finally, are you finding high-quality evidence when you search? How do your searches compare with those of your professors, or the medical librarian?

When your search is successful, and you locate the evidence, how good are you at critically appraising it? Are you choosing the correct study designs for your clinical questions? Do you need a critical appraisal worksheet to help you analyse the article? We have found that critical appraisal skills improve rapidly when working as a group, such as in a modern evidence-based journal club. And finally, after you have critically appraised the evidence, how do you save the results for when you need them the next time? In a notebook of critically appraised topics (CATs), or in some more abbreviated form?

The ultimate step in evaluating your performance is to determine if your patients benefit from your efforts: does your application of high-quality evidence result in improved clinical outcomes? And this question leads to the clinical audit.

Clinical audit

Healthcare providers able to answer all of the above questions thoughtfully would be justifiably proud of their adoption of EBM principles, but we may go one step further, and ask if what we have learned translates into better health outcomes for our patients. A useful paradigm for quality improvement is the clinical audit cycle, illustrated in Fig. 13.2:

We may extend the CF RCT example above to an entire university-based CF specialty clinic. Once we have determined that our patient will benefit from long-term maintenance treatment with oral

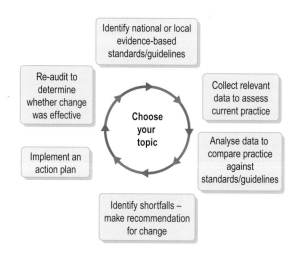

Fig. 13.2 The clinical audit cycle. As each cycle is successfully completed, the process spirals upwards towards a higher level of quality. The topic chosen should be a common clinical problem.

azithromycin, why should we not treat all our patients with azithromycin? How well are we already doing? And is there room for improvement?

We might want to confirm that higher-quality evidence exists than our single RCT before we reorganize our clinic, so we search the TRIP database with search terms 'oral azithromycin' AND 'cystic fibrosis'. A rapid review of the listed guidelines for North America and Europe shows that they are not CF-specific, but the single systematic review (Cochrane DSR, 2004) confirms that there is benefit, and since our French RCT above was published in 2006, it adds fuel to the evidence-based fire.

Next, we need to collect data to assess our current practice: how many patients do we follow? How many are already taking azithromycin? How many are not, and what are the reasons? If we find that most of our patients are already taking maintenance macrolides, and that the few who are not have allergies to macrolides, or unacceptable adverse effects, then we are finished. But if many of our patients are not taking azithromycin, then we are ready to make a plan to increase our numbers. It might be as simple as a note to start azithromycin at the next clinic visit, or perhaps a computerized reminder that pops up the next time the patient's parents call with a question.

Finally, we must analyse our results after a reasonable time frame. If we see all our CF patients in the clinic at least three times per year, then we could recheck our numbers in 6 months. And if we have prescribed azithromycin for all eligible patients, then we have succeeded; if not, it is back to step 4, and an attempt to make a more foolproof implementation plan.

Clinical audit may be applied to any problem, but it is most effective when used for high-volume problems, changes to which may make a difference in patient outcomes.

Further reading

EBM websites evolve rapidly, and aside from the two excellent textbooks listed below, there are many instructional tutorials, appraisal tools, EBM calculators, and CATs to be found on the internet, many with free access, but some restricted to subscribers.

References

Guyatt GH, Sackett DL, Cook DJ 1993 Users' guides to the medical literature. II. How to use an article about therapy or prevention. Are the results of the study valid? Evidence-Based Medicine Working Group. JAMA 270: 2598–2601

Moyer VA, Elliot EJ (eds) 2004 Evidence-based Paediatrics and Child Health, 2nd edition. BMJ Books, London.

Yost CC, Soll RF 1999 Early versus delayed selective surfactant treatment for neonatal respiratory distress syndrome. Cochrane Database of Systematic Reviews 4:CD001456; DOI 10.1002/14651858.CD001456

Strauss SE, Richardson WS, Glasziou P, Haynes RB 2005 Evidence Based Medicine: How to Practice and Teach EBM. 3rd edition. Elsevier/Churchill Livingstone, London

Useful websites

EBM lends itself particularly well to the internet. Early websites and electronic textbooks focused primarily on internal medicine, whereas paediatrics suffered a bit for lack of attention, but that early neglect is being rapidly corrected. Below you will find a compendium of valuable EBM websites with hyperlinks, as well as a brief description of what you will find at each site. Please remember that this discipline evolves at a brisk pace; if you have trouble finding a listed site, you can search for it using http://www.google.com.

Where to find evidence:
http://www.ncbi.nlm.nih.gov/pubmed/
US National Library of Medicine, PubMed search engine; free use; very sensitive, but you may limit a search to RCTs, meta-analyses, or guidelines

http://www.gateway.ovid.com
Ovid Medline search engine for NLM articles, only by subscription; very sensitive, but has same limits as PubMed; even better is the 'All EBM Reviews' database, which provides critically appraised evidence

http://www.thecochranelibrary.com
The Cochrane Collaboration; provided free by Wiley Interscience; may search by topic, MeSH terms, or alphabetically; all evidence has already been critically appraised

http://www.tripdatabase.com
Turning Research Into Practice (TRIP): this meta-search engine collates critically appraised evidence from all appropriate sources, and presents in an easy-to-interpret format; free use

http://www.clinicalevidence.com
Clinical Evidence, published by BMJ Books, UK, and updated every 6 months. Ambulatory paediatric topics, available by subscription. Click on 'Child Health' section for paediatrics

http://www.uptodate.com
UpToDate: electronic textbook, available only by subscription. Paediatrics section since 2005, updated every 4 months, explicit grading of evidence, and hyperlinks to Medline abstracts of references

http://www.guideline.gov
National Guideline Clearinghouse, USA. This is a compendium of EBM clinical guidelines from many sources; selection criteria are usually, but not always, specified.

Where to learn more about EBM:
http://www.hsl.unc.edu/Services/Tutorials/ebm/welcome.htm
EBM tutorial produced by the Health Sciences Library at the University of North Carolina, USA. The tutorial covers the first three steps in the five-step EBM process, and offers a practice exercise.

http://www.poems.msu.edu/EBM/
Michigan State University, USA. This web-based course focuses on reading and critical appraisal of articles about therapy, diagnosis, prognosis, and systematic reviews.

http://www.cebm.net

Centre for Evidence-Based Medicine, Oxford, UK. A treasure trove of EBM information, including courses, tutorials (click on EBM tools above), critical appraisal tools (EBM tools, then critical appraisal).

http://www.cche.net/usersguides/main.asp

Canadian Centre for Health Evidence; reprints of all User's Guides to the medical literature, as published in the *Journal of the American Medical Association* (JAMA) in 1994–95, by the EBM Working Group.

http://www.prhu.nhs.uk/Pages/PHD/resources.htm

Public Health Resource Unit of the National Health Service, UK. Appraisal tools developed for use in the Critical Appraisal Skills Program (CASP).

Where to find completed CATs:

http://www.med.umich.edu/pediatrics/ebm

University of Michigan, USA, website for evidence-based paediatrics. Compilation of CATs by subspecialty.

Paediatric journals with evidence-based sections:

http://www.evidence-basedchildhealth.com

Evidence-based Child Health: A Cochrane Review Journal. Founded in 2006, published quarterly, it reviews important paediatric Cochrane trials. It is available by subscription, but abstracts are free.

http://www.jpeds.com

Journal of Pediatrics. It has a relatively new section called 'Current Best Evidence', which summarizes relevant articles in a simplified CAT format.

http://www.adc.bmj.com/

Archives of Disease in Childhood, the journal of the Royal College of Paediatrics and Child Health, UK, and of the European Academy of Paediatrics. It has a section called 'Archimedes', which asks common clinical questions and then reviews the literature in a CAT format.

One cannot help but notice that all the above sites are located in the English-speaking world; EBM was first codified in the UK and then the USA, and Anglo-American universities have been at the forefront of the EBM movement. Nevertheless, continental Europe has been catching up with EBM, and below are some of the websites you may want to bookmark, especially any sites from your country of residence. The Cochrane Collaboration now has societies in more than a dozen countries, including France, Italy, Germany, the Netherlands, Norway, Denmark, Spain, Russia, Brazil, and China. So, although knowing English is still a great advantage when you need to search the medical literature, we are starting to provide high-quality evidence in many other languages, spoken cumulatively by more than half the world's population.

http://www.ecdc.europa.eu/en/Default.aspx

European Centre for Disease Prevention and Control

http://www.ceveas.it

Centre for the Evaluation of Health Care Efficacy, Modena, Italy

http://www.onderzoekinformatie.nl/en/oi/nod/clasgenees/

Dutch health information

http://www.medizin-forum.de/

German health information

http://www.inserm.fr/en/home.html

French National Health Institute

*Edited by Mitch Blair, Diego van Esso,
Adamos Hadjipanayis, Mary Rudolf*

Child public health

MODULE

THREE

Shimon Barak   Rachel Crowther   Francis B. Mimouni

CHAPTER

Epidemiology

14

LEARNING OUTCOMES

By the end of this chapter you should:

- Understand what child public health is and why it is important
- Be familiar with the broad characteristics of the child population in Europe — and the world
- Know about the key factors that affect the health of children, including wider determinants of health
- Recognize the main causes of mortality and morbidity in children
- Know about different types and structures of health, education and social care services for children
- Understand how to assess health and health needs in a population, including key data sources
- Know about different types of health inequality and how they affect children
- Understand the impact of poverty, stigma and social exclusion on child health
- Be familiar with key methods for measuring social deprivation
- Understand the particular health needs of certain vulnerable groups, including at-risk children, children from black and minority ethnic groups and children with disabilities.

MODULE THREE

Child public health

Doctors frequently see children out of their everyday context, and gain a sense of their family and social background largely at second hand. The children who pass through the doors of the hospital or primary-care setting are part of a wider population of children whose characteristics can be difficult to grasp from the perspective of a clinician. Child public health is concerned with this wider population — with children's daily

143

lives, and what goes on before and after encounters with healthcare professionals; with how to assess and measure the health and health needs of children; with how to improve their health and wellbeing, in the broadest sense, and tackle health inequality (Box 14.1). The size and nature of the 'population' varies enormously; child public health practitioners are involved in everything from large-scale international projects through the World Health Organization (WHO) to local community projects.

The child population

In 2005 the European population of children up to age 14 approached 125 million. Today, the major geographical areas find themselves at very different stages in the path to population ageing. Ageing is most advanced in Europe, where except for specific ethnic minorities like the Roma gypsies the number of persons aged 60 or over surpassed the number of children in 1995. By 2050, Europe will have twice as many older persons as children. In fact, in Europe only the older population is expected to increase in the future, whereas the population under age 60 is expected to decrease.

In 2001 there were 2.1 billion children worldwide aged under 18 and 613 million under 5. The world's child population is concentrated in the poorest countries, where child and infant mortality rates are highest. The life expectancy from birth in the world's poorest countries is only 51 years. The infant mortality rate for these countries is for instance 16 times higher than in the UK and the under-5 mortality rate is 22 times that of the UK.

Determinants of health in children

Children's health is affected by a wide range of factors that operate at many different 'levels', from within the child (e.g. genetic factors) to across the globe (e.g. international agreements such as the United Nations Convention on the Rights of the Child). Socioeconomic and environmental factors, especially poverty, play a very significant part and account for much of the variation between different children's experience of life and of health.

A commonly used framework for understanding the interaction of determinants and the various 'levels' is the Dahlgren and Whitehead model (Fig. 14.1). This places the individual in the centre and explores the influences on the child — see the boxes on the figure for details of each 'layer'.

Health inequalities

Introduction

Health inequalities can be defined as differences between the experience of health and wellbeing of different groups that result in an unfair distribution of morbidity and mortality in the population. The population in question might be that of the whole world or of a much smaller area or community. The extent of health inequality in the child population in Europe is considerable, even in the first year of life, and is continuing to increase. In the last quarter of the 20th century, as average levels of health improved, health inequalities grew wider. A large proportion of this inequality is socially determined: that is to say, it reflects differences in children's environments, circumstances, opportunities and resources. Children themselves have almost no control over these factors, but the remedies for this inequality lie within the power of society. We cannot avoid a collective responsibility for the experience of children who are less well off, in health terms, than others.

Types of health inequality

Differences in health, and in the distribution of determinants of health, can be identified between many different kinds of children. Factors include:

- *Gender*: e.g. the rise in smoking and binge drinking among young women in Europe
- *Geography*: e.g. differences in the prevalence of childhood obesity between European countries
- *Socioeconomic status*: e.g. differences in infant mortality between those born into families from manual and non-manual groups
- *Ethnicity*: e.g. greater rise in prevalence of and mortality from asthma among black children in the USA
- *Disability*: e.g. greater risk of child abuse among children with disabilities
- *Age*: e.g. differences in the type and overall risk of injury in children of different ages.

Causes of health inequalities

A complex web of factors contribute to the existence of health inequalities, and lead to differences in health

Age, sex and constitutional factors
- Some conditions have a clear **genetic** cause or predisposition — e.g. sickle cell disease, cystic fibrosis, Huntington chorea, Down syndrome.
- There is growing evidence of the impact of prenatal life on later health — e.g. Barker hypothesis (p. 6); specific insults such as rubella virus
- **Gestational age and birth weight** affect the incidence of cerebral palsy and other conditions. Preterm birth and low birth weight are significant causes of infant mortality
- There are gender differences in the pattern of mortality from many diseases in children.

Poverty and deprivation
Poverty is still the single most important factor affecting the health of children worldwide. It is discussed in more detail in the section on inequalities.

The media and commercial world
Aspects of the wider world have a growing impact on children as the reach of the media (including the worldwide web) push forward **globalization** and **consumerism. Marketing** (especially of unhealthy food) to children is an increasingly worrying trend. Politics, social policy and the legal world also have an impact on the circumstances in which children live.

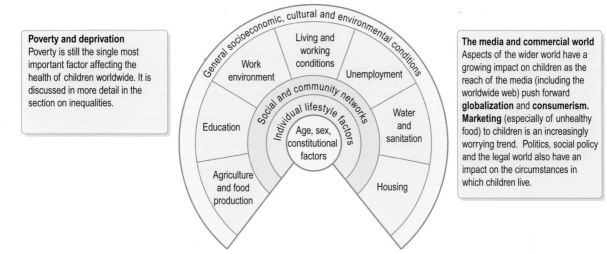

Individual lifestyle factors
Lifestyle and health-related behaviour are important determinants of health in older children and parental lifestyles can affect children directly (e.g. smoking in pregnancy and around young children; choices between breast- and formula feeding) and indirectly, by helping to shape habits (e.g. of diet and exercise) which children will carry into later childhood and adulthood. Such 'choices' are significantly affected by socioeconomic and environmental factors (e.g. the 'obesogenic' environment; social class gradients for smoking). Important aspects of lifestyle include:
- **Nutrition,** including breastfeeding and establishing a healthy diet at and after weaning. Many foods which are high in fat, calories, sugar and salt are cheap and readily available. The national School Fruit and Vegetable scheme aims to increase consumption of healthier foods.
- **Physical activity:** 40% of boys and 60% of girls get less than the recommended hour of physical activity a day. Fewer children walk to school, PE provision is poor in schools, many playing fields have been sold off and parents are often reluctant to allow children to play outside because of the lack of safe play areas.
- **Smoking:** Smoking in pregnancy increases the risk of low birth weight, stillbirth and infant death. Smoking in the same household as a young child increases the risk of sudden death and respiratory problems.
- **Risk behaviour** is on the rise among older children and adolescents, e.g. alcohol and drug misuse, sexual behaviour, physical risks and accidents, deliberate self-harm.

Social, family and community networks
- **Relationships between parents and children** affect the child's wellbeing and resilience in responding to stress and adverse events. Particularly important are:
  - **Early care and nurture** and the degree of **attachment** at 1 year of age.
  - **Parenting style,** boundary-setting and support, communication, shared family pursuits and culture.
  - **Abuse and neglect,** which are extreme examples of unhelpful parenting.
- **Family break-up and conflict:** Conflict and domestic violence can have a serious effect on children's health and wellbeing.
- **Family structure:** 23% of dependent children now live in single-parent households, and more than 10% live in reconstituted families. For children who receive continuous loving care this may be important, but for others living in a non-traditional family may have disadvantages. Other factors include birth order and number of siblings, and the proximity of extended family members.
- **Childcare and working patterns:** The government's plans for 'wraparound childcare' aim to support working parents and mean that more young children will spend more time in daycare. Benefits from extended contact with other children include a decreased risk of asthma and leukaemia, but extended separation at an early age may have less desirable implications for both mother and baby.
- **Maternal age, status and income:** Around 8% of babies are now born to a teenage mother, and 40% outside marriage (although most of these are jointly registered by both parents). Younger mothers tend to be on lower incomes and the health prospects for teenage mothers and their babies are poorer.

Fig. 14.1 The Dahlgren & Whitehead model of determinants of health

MODULE THREE

Physical environment

Several aspects of the physical environment affect children's health, including:

- **Housing,** e.g. quality (fitness for human habitation criteria), size, amenities. Damp housing increases the risk of childhood asthma; overcrowding increases the risk of infectious diseases, domestic violence and accidents.
- **Neighbourhood,** e.g. availability of parks and safe play areas; traffic (which causes pollution and road traffic accidents).
- **Poor air quality,** e.g. in inner city areas, can cause exacerbations of respiratory conditions.
- Exposure to **infectious agents,** e.g. food hygiene, handwashing practices, time spent in daycare and nurseries.

Wider social environment

- Qualities of local communities and networks such as **social inclusion** and **social capital** can have a significant impact on health, offering protection against some of the adverse effects of poverty and deprivation.
- Conversely, **social exclusion and stigma** may have a detrimental effect on the health and wellbeing of children from marginalized and minority groups who are less able to access services and participate in community life. These include the very poor, travelling families, asylum seekers, and ethnic and religious minorities, as well as children with disabilities or chronic illnesses.
- The **school environment** is very important for children: the healthy schools movement aims to promote positive ethos, pupil involvement and strong self-esteem, and to tackle bullying and unhealthy environments.
- Respect for **children's rights** is a fundamental responsibility for all. The United Nations Convention on the Rights of the Child is an international treaty which enshrines basic rights for all children, including the right to life, identity, protection and education.

Access to services

Many public services have an impact on children's health, either directly or indirectly. They include:

- **Health services,** including preventive, acute and community services, delivered by a range of health professionals.
- **Education services:** Educational attainment has a significant impact on self-esteem and wellbeing in children, and on later health.
- **Social services,** e.g. child protection and family support for children with disabilities.
- **Leisure services,** e.g. sporting facilities, youth clubs, after-school and holiday activities.
- **Transport services,** e.g. public transport, cycle lanes and safe routes to school.

Fig. 14.1 (*cont'd*)

status and outcome that can be clearly observed at a collective level. Some of the most important causes include:

- Socioeconomic factors
- Stigma and social exclusion
- Family circumstances and parenting
- The wider social and physical environment
- Lifestyle and behaviour (e.g. smoking, diet and physical activity, substance misuse, sexual behaviour)
- Access to services (e.g. the 'inverse care law', a term coined by Tudor Hart in 1971: those most in need are least likely to access and benefit from health services).

These factors are closely interrelated. Poverty and deprivation are more common among socially excluded groups, and social exclusion makes it harder to find a job (or to get a decent education) in order to climb out of poverty. Effective and empathetic parenting is much more of a challenge when living in poverty, and the impact of poor parenting can put children at a disadvantage in educational (and later employment) terms, as well as emotional and health terms. The quality of the built environment is very often poorer in areas where many of the residents are poor, and promotes crime and social fragmentation. Unhealthy lifestyles

are substantially affected by social and environmental constraints, such as the lack of availability of affordable fresh food in deprived areas. Most clinicians will have seen children whose lives tragically illustrate the clustering of disadvantageous circumstances, with inevitable consequences for their health and wellbeing both now and in later life, and often for the next generation too.

Key contributors to health inequality in children are described below.

Socioeconomic inequalities

A substantial proportion of health inequality is directly related to socioeconomic inequality. There is a clear social class gradient for most of the leading causes of morbidity and mortality in children, and poverty and social deprivation remain the most significant determinants of child health. The Joseph Rowntree Foundation has estimated that 1400 children's lives would be saved each year in the UK if child poverty were eradicated. Both *absolute poverty* and *relative poverty* are important, and the debate continues about the relative contribution of each.

Absolute poverty reflects the resources a family has available to pay for basic necessities such as accommodation, heating and lighting, food, clothing, transport etc. Various formulae (sometimes described as 'consensus' or 'subjective' measures of poverty) have been devised to calculate the minimum weekly or monthly requirement for a family of different sizes, and any whose income falls below this level is deemed to be living in absolute poverty. Absolute poverty can be tackled by boosting the resources of the very poor (e.g. by increasing state benefit levels, which are generally judged to be lower than the minimum needs of an average family), but most experts believe that is not enough to mitigate the health effects of poverty, because relative poverty also plays an important role.

Relative poverty reflects income inequality: how a family's resources compare to those of others. The European Union defines as poor those households whose income is 50% or less of the national average — sometimes known as the 'poverty line'. Relative poverty is important at every geographical level. In Scandinavian countries with a more even distribution of wealth, the health status of the whole population is better, not just that of people in lower-income brackets. At a local level, it is better in health terms to be poor in a poor neighbourhood than to be surrounded by better-off households. Relative poverty is believed to exert its effects partly through psychosocial factors such as a sense of marginalization and exclusion, low self-esteem and powerlessness, which can result in physiological changes such as hypertension and lowered immune response.

Poverty affects children's health in several different ways:

- *Effects of absolute poverty*: lack of money to pay for healthy food, suitable housing, clothing, heating, toys and outings.
- *Effects of relative poverty*: psychosocial stresses on parents increase the risk of conflict and domestic violence, depression and poor supervision of children (which may lead to accidents); children themselves can also experience psychosocial effects such as low self-esteem and hopelessness.
- *Effects of living in poor neighbourhoods*: lack of facilities (e.g. outdoor play areas) and services (e.g. poor schools); poor built environment, derelict spaces etc.; crime and violence.
- *Effects of social, cultural and environmental norms and constraints*: unhealthy lifestyle choices (e.g. smoking, binge drinking) may be encouraged by the limited alternative opportunities for pleasure or escape.

Stigma and social exclusion

Social exclusion is described as follows by the UK government's Social Exclusion Unit:

Social exclusion happens when people or places suffer from a series of problems such as unemployment, discrimination, poor skills, low incomes, poor housing, high crime, ill health and family breakdown. When such problems combine they can create a vicious cycle. Social exclusion can happen as a result of problems that face one person in their life. But it can also start from birth.

http://www.socialexclusionunit.gov.uk

Social exclusion is often closely related to poverty, but other factors affect an individual's, a family's or indeed a whole group's ability to benefit from the opportunities offered by their community and society. The sociological term 'stigma' refers to the negative interpretation placed by society on outward differences, including:

- Bodily characteristics (e.g. disability, obesity, significant birth marks)
- Skin colour
- Religious observance
- Language
- Clothes or other cultural appurtenances
- Illness (especially mental illness)
- Family and social background (e.g. children looked after by the local authority, asylum seekers and refugees)
- Age
- Gender
- Behaviour or lifestyle (e.g. travellers)
- Sexual orientation
- Evident poverty
- Poor hygiene
- Any other factors that set individuals apart.

Children have the capacity to be very accepting of others, but are also quick to pick up prevailing disapproval or mockery and, in circumstances that allow such behaviour, can rapidly learn that falling in with the disparaging of others reinforces their own position as part of the crowd. Thus children (as well as their parents and families) can feel the breath of intolerance directly and suffer the handicapping effects of social exclusion. These may include bullying, low self-esteem, anxiety and depression, a sense of worthlessness and lack of opportunities, difficulties in accessing services (including education and health services) and, in extreme cases, self-harm or physical violence at the hands of others. It is especially tragic when health and social inequalities are perpetuated through generations as a direct result of intolerance and inhumanity.

Vulnerable and at-risk children

Some children are at particular risk of poor health and/or social exclusion and may need help from one or more public agencies (health, social services, education etc.) to maintain their physical, mental and social wellbeing. These vulnerable children include those:

- With disabilities
- With emotional and behavioural problems
- With a history of abuse or who are at risk of abuse
- Whose families are homeless
- Who are looked after by the local authority ('in care')
- Who have a history of truancy or crime
- Who care for others (e.g. parents with health problems)
- Who have chronic illnesses, especially mental health problems
- Who misuse drugs or alcohol
- Who are teenage parents
- Who are children of asylum seekers, or have arrived in Europe as unaccompanied minors.

Some of these children are considered to be in need of more formal public support, and constitute a subgroup of vulnerable children deemed 'at-risk' and includes those:

- In need of protection
- In need of family support
- In public care.

Measuring poverty and social deprivation

Absolute and relative measures of poverty have been described above. Social deprivation is harder to measure than family income and outgoings, but various instruments have been developed to assess deprivation in a broader sense in local areas. The Townsend Index and Jarman Index have both been much used, and are often cited in studies that examine the correlation between deprivation and mortality, morbidity or hospital admission rates for certain conditions (e.g. childhood asthma or accidents), or which plot 'hot spots' of deprivation across a specific geographic or primary care area. These indices use four and eight items respectively, such as the percentage of the local population that is unemployed or does not own their home.

Such an index has been developed in the UK, and is called the Index of Multiple Deprivation 2007. It combines a number of indicators, chosen to cover a range of economic, social and housing issues, into a single deprivation score for each small area in England. It is available online (see below) and has a supplementary index on income deprivation affecting children. The IMD 2004 includes seven 'domains':

1. *Income deprivation* (e.g. number of households receiving benefits such as income support, working families' tax credit or asylum seekers' support)

2. *Employment deprivation* (e.g. number of claimants for unemployment or incapacity benefit)
3. *Health deprivation and disability* (e.g. comparative illness and disability ratio, emergency admissions to hospital)
4. *Education, skills and training deprivation* (e.g. children's average scores at Key Stages 2, 3 and 4; proportion leaving school at 16; secondary school absence rate)
5. *Barriers to housing and services* (e.g. overcrowding and homelessness; distance to nearest primary care physician, supermarket, primary school and post office)
6. *Living environment deprivation* (indoors, e.g. housing in poor condition or without central heating; outdoors, e.g. air quality, road traffic accidents with injury to pedestrians or cyclists)
7. *Crime* (e.g. recorded burglary, theft, criminal damage and violence).

Local scores are available for every 'Super Output Area' (SOA) in England — of which there are almost 32 500, with an average population of around 2000 — for each domain separately, together with an overall (weighted) score and rank. Summary scores are also available at district and county level. In the most deprived quintile (20%) of SOAs:

- A fifth of adults are 'employment-deprived'
- Almost half of children live in families which are 'income-deprived' (usually meaning on benefits).

Geographical inequality can be clearly illustrated by looking at the distribution of these most-deprived SOAs; most are in the North-East and North-West regions.

http://www.odpm.gov.uk

Preliminary report on Index of Multiple Deprivation 2004

The impact of health inequalities: childhood injuries

Childhood injuries offer a useful case study for examining the impact of health inequalities. Patterns of inequalities throughout European countries can be found in a European Report on child safety, which shows the 'report card' of 24 European countries that adhered to a strict reporting system:

http://www.eurosafe.eu.com/csi/eurosafe2006. nsf/wwwVwContent/l4downloads-111.htm

Even within a given country, significant regional disparities exist as well. For instance, in the UK, a recent report from the Health Development Agency *(http:// www.nice.org.uk)* reviews differences in the pattern

Table 14.1 Reasons for inequalities in childhood injuries*

Category	Examples of relevant factors
Age	• Physical development and motor coordination affect ability to avoid (or tendency to encounter) risk: e.g. ability to manage climbing frame/swings • Perceptual and intellectual development affect e.g. ability to judge traffic, awareness of danger • Changing attitudes, behaviour and nature of play/leisure activity with increasing age affect exposure to risk: e.g. deliberate risk-taking in adolescence, hazardous sport • Levels of supervision/independence affect degree of safeguards: e.g. cycling/walking alone to school or shops
Gender	• Differences in rates of development: motor, spatial, cognitive, intellectual • Differences in behaviour: gender-specific norms such as 'macho' risk-taking, nature of peer pressure and attitude to safety (e.g. cycle helmets) • Different choices of sport/leisure activity: e.g. contact sports such as football and rugby; greater overall physical activity levels in boys • Differences in levels of supervision/independence: perhaps greater tendency for parents to protect girls
Socioeconomic group	• Cost of safety equipment: e.g. stair gates, car seats, cycle helmets, reflective clothing, safety harnesses, cordless kettles, smoke alarms • Different levels of exposure to hazards, inside and outside: e.g. cigarette smoking (can lead to fires), unsafe electrical wiring, overcrowded housing, lack of garden/safe play areas, living on main road • Differences in parents'/carers' ability to supervise: e.g. single-parent families, very young mothers, stress/illness (especially mental health problems), parents' working patterns and childcare arrangements • Parents' attitudes to and awareness of risks, and access to information and services to help manage risk
Ethnicity	• Differences in environment and exposure to risk: e.g. different activities and patterns of behaviour, supervision/childcare arrangements • Access to information and services to help manage risk: e.g. language barriers, awareness of services (e.g. lower attendance at child health clinics where health promotion and safety advice is offered) • Especially for first-generation immigrants, lack of familiarity with hazards (e.g. road environment) and differences in expectation (e.g. children 'falling in with' peers)
Geography	• Factors relating to physical environment: e.g. safety of roads (including on-street parking, traffic volume, cycle lanes, pavements, underpasses) • Factors relating to social environment: e.g. community safety, level of collective responsibility for children, familiarity of neighbours

* Adapted from: Health Development Agency 2005 Injuries in children aged 0–14 years and inequalities.

of injuries to children for most of the categories of inequality listed above.

The explanations for these differences are complex and incompletely understood, but some relevant factors are listed in Table 14.1. It is helpful to bear in mind the different levels at which factors influencing injury risk can operate:

- The event itself and immediate circumstances surrounding the child's exposure to the hazard
- Intermediate factors affecting the child's exposure to risk
- Wider social, economic, cultural and environmental factors that shape the child's experience.

Approaches to preventing injuries in children are discussed in Chapter 17; you may like to consider whether targeted approaches might be needed for some of the different groups considered here.

Other examples of socioeconomic inequalities in child health include:

- *Infant mortality rate (age 0–1 year)*. Social class V has double the mortality rate of social class I, and the gap is still rising.

- *Child mortality rate (age 1–15 years)*. Social classes IV and V have almost double the rate of social classes I and II.
- *Mental health problems*. Prevalence in social class V is three times higher than in social class I.

Ethnicity and health

There is a dearth of child health data to illustrate differences in health outcome between ethnic groups, but infant mortality provides a good 'summary measure' that is routinely available and shows significant variation. For example, in 2003 the infant mortality rate (in England and Wales) for babies whose mothers were born in Pakistan was 10.5 per 1000 live births — more than double the national average — and for babies whose mothers were born in the Caribbean the rate was 8.5 per 1000. In the Netherlands the death rate of Turkish and Moroccan children is twice as high as that of native Dutch children and perinatal death rates are higher by a 2.2 ratio for Blacks, 1.4 for Hindustanis and 1.3 for Mediterraneans.

Several factors may affect the health and wellbeing of children from black and minority ethnic groups, including:

- *Socioeconomic factors*. Children from minority ethnic groups are on average more likely to live in poverty, and to suffer the effects of deprivation such as unsuitable, overcrowded accommodation.
- *Stigma and social exclusion*. Children from minority ethnic groups are more likely to suffer the effects of bullying and exclusion; lack of recognition of foreign qualifications may bar entry to employment for parents.
- *Cultural factors*. Differences in child-rearing and lifestyle may affect children's health. For example, family composition and relationship with the extended family affect the home environment; late weaning practices in Asian families can increase the risk of anaemia; peer pressure and cultural norms (especially in adolescence) may act in very different ways for children from different groups.
- *Barriers to access*. Language difficulties (and lack of interpreting services) and cultural barriers (e.g. women needing a chaperone to visit the doctor, lack of familiarity with appointments system, lack of awareness of entitlements) may impede access to health services (including antenatal and preventive child health services), social services, education and others (including transport, leisure, benefits).
- *Recent history*. Recent immigrants may be separated from extended family and friends and feel very isolated; poor healthcare (e.g. immunization programmes) and/or prevalence of infectious diseases (e.g. HIV, tuberculosis) in their home country may affect health directly; in addition, asylum seekers and refugees have often suffered traumatic experiences before and during their flight, may have lost relatives and friends to war or torture, and may have suffered the effects of infrastructure breakdown (including the loss of possessions or profession).
- *Genetic factors*. Some inherited conditions are more common in certain ethnic groups, e.g. sickle cell disease and thalassaemia; consanguineous marriage increases the risk of a range of rare congenital conditions.

It is clear that the picture is complicated, and that the experience of children from different backgrounds may be dramatically different — which is why simply comparing 'white' and 'non-white' children is over-simplistic and generally unhelpful in elucidating health inequalities and exploring their causes.

There is an accumulation of evidence pointing to an association between ethnic minority status and increased risk of child pedestrian injury in most countries. In the USA black children are involved two and three times more than the national average and a similar pattern has been reported in non Jewish children in Israel.

What can health professionals do to help?

- Adequate interpreting services are very important. They should always be provided by professionals, not members of the family, to avoid problems of incomplete communication or disclosure.
- Patience, persistence and sensitivity to cultural and other barriers are needed to ensure full and equitable access to services for children from all backgrounds. Failure to attend appointments is frustrating, but should not be accepted as a reason for giving up on a child.
- The school environment is crucially important to children's wellbeing, and much can be done at whole-school level to improve the experience of all pupils — and staff.
- Advocacy, partnership working and information sharing with other agencies are essential to ensure a coordinated and effective approach to addressing the needs of individual children and young people (e.g. ensuring that vulnerable children do not miss out on education — including Foundation Stage (nursery and reception year)).
- It is very important that all professionals working with children are sensitive to cultural issues but do not allow them to cloud their judgment about a child's wellbeing, as the Victoria Climbié case tragically illustrated.

Tackling health inequalities: policy, targets and progress

Eurothine is a European project which has made a major effort in furthering the description of health inequalities within the European Union. It is characterized by having the following specific objectives:

1. To develop health inequalities indicators, and to provide bench-marking data on inequalities in health and health determinants to participating countries.
2. To assess evidence on the effectiveness of policies and interventions to tackle the determinants of health inequalities, and to make recommendations on strategies for reducing health inequalities in participating countries.

3. To disseminate the results, and to develop a proposal for a permanent European clearing house on tackling health inequalities. Eurothine is fully described at the following web address:

 http://ec.europa.eu/health/ph_projects/2003/action1/action1_2003_16_en.htm#3

Through improving information and knowledge for the development of public health, this project aims to collect and analyse information on socioeconomic inequalities in health from different European countries in order to facilitate mutual learning that will help policy-makers at the European and national level to develop rational strategies for tackling inequalities in health.

The Eurothine project has led to the development of 'Health inequalities indicators', which are measures of 'health inequalities', defined as systematic variations between socioeconomic groups in the occurrence of a health indicator.

http://ec.europa.eu/health/ph_projects/2003/action1/docs/2003_1_16_rep3_en.pdf

It is indeed important to develop these proposals in each individual country in order to identify and tackle the determinants of health that sit behind health inequalities, including poverty, tax and benefits; education and employment; environment and housing; transport and pollution; and diet and nutrition.

In the UK, the government has included a commitment to reduce inequalities in a number of national public health targets, including two focused specifically on children (Box 14.2). Addressing health inequalities is also a key theme of the Children's National Service Framework.

The UK government's 2003 Programme for Action sets out wide-ranging plans for tackling health inequalities by improving the health of the worst-off in society, providing financial support for families (e.g. tax credits and benefits) and introducing public service changes to improve children's life chances.

Progress against national targets

Infant mortality

The Eurofound project, which monitors quality of life in European countries

http://www.eurofound.europa.eu/areas/qualityoflife/eurlife/index.php?template=3&radioindic=4&idDomain=1

reported universally improving figures of infant mortality (number of infants who die per 1000 live births) in all countries that provided data. Of note, in the UK, the latest Office for National Statistics (ONS) figures for infant mortality (quoted in a 2005 Department of Health update on the inequalities targets) show that the gap between manual groups and the population as a whole has *widened* since the target was set; infant mortality in manual groups was 19% higher than the total population in 2001–03, compared with 13% higher in the baseline period of 1997–99.

Child poverty

While no European country is immune to child poverty, it appears from a recent report published in 2000 by the European Children's Trust that as many as 50 million children may be living in poverty in Eastern Europe and the former Soviet Union. The study was based on figures gathered between 1993 and 1995. It showed that many families were having to leave their children in state orphanages as they were unable to feed them. This crisis has been building since the old communist system disappeared, with more than 160 million people living below the poverty line in recent years — twelve times more than at the collapse of communism. The report stated that Western countries should help expand services preventing family breakdown instead of providing direct aid. The report showed that 88% of the population in Kyrgyzstan live in poverty, while the figure is more than 60% in Ukraine, Uzbekistan and Kazakhstan. The United Nation Development Programme (UNDP) stated that: 'While the schooling of parents is strongly associated with that of their offspring, there is also evidence that investing in parental education can help remove many children from a situation of poverty and save their lives. Each additional year spent by mothers in primary school lowers the risk of premature child death by about

8%. Since attendance at a poor quality school may have little effect in reducing poverty outcomes, quality schooling is of great consequence too'

http://www.undp-povertycentre.org/newsletters/infocus2mar04eng.pdf

Key causes of morbidity and mortality in children

The health of children in Europe has improved significantly over the last century, and at the same time the pattern of morbidity and mortality has changed dramatically. Immunization and antibiotics have helped reduce the impact of infectious diseases, and 'high-tech' interventions have improved the chances of survival of premature babies and of children with conditions such as cancer or congenital heart disease. Social and environmental factors have played an even larger role, including the beneficial effects of increasing wealth, improved sanitation and housing quality, family planning and safer environments. Society faces new problems today — consumerism, the over-availability of processed and unhealthy food, the prominence of sedentary lifestyles, disaffection and the decline in traditional family structures, a growing gap between the income and health of the richest and poorest — and the pattern of child health reflects them all (Box 14.3).

The leading causes of death among children worldwide are shown below (Box 14.4).

BOX 14.3 Some key child health problems in the 21st century

Childhood obesity

Prevalence has risen by 0.8% per year over the last decade, due to changes in both caloric intake (diet) and output (physical activity). Almost all European governments have set a high-profile target to halt this trend. If it is not successful, life expectancy for current and future generations of children may be significantly reduced.

Emotional and behavioural/mental health problems

These are on the increase in children and young people. There are knock-on effects on the individual (jeopardizing educational achievement, employment prospects, success in establishing relationships), the family (increasing stress on parents and siblings; increasing the risk of violent behaviour towards future partners and children), teachers (who find it harder and harder to teach, and may be physically threatened by pupils) and society (increasing truancy and youth crime).

Teenage pregnancy and sexually transmitted infections

The impact on the health and wellbeing of teenage mothers and their children is substantial. The UK has the highest rates in Europe.

Accidents and injuries

These remain a significant cause of morbidity and mortality. The UK has the highest rates in Europe for injuries to child pedestrians.

Child abuse and neglect

These include fatal cases, estimated by the National Society for the Prevention of Cruelty to Children to number at least 100 per year.

Poor vaccine uptake

This is due to media scares and mistrust of official sources, leading to a significant risk of outbreaks of measles and increasing the exposure of pregnant women to rubella.

Increase in disabilities and chronic illness

Many disabilities are due to the improved survival of premature babies.

Substance misuse

This includes alcohol (binge drinking is an especially worrying trend), tobacco (smoking rates continue to rise, especially among teenage girls), drugs and glue-sniffing.

Suicide and self-harm

These are also on the rise; suicide now accounts for a third of deaths in 15–24-year-olds.

Social and health inequalities

These continue to increase as society becomes generally richer and healthier. The UK has the worst record in Europe on child poverty.

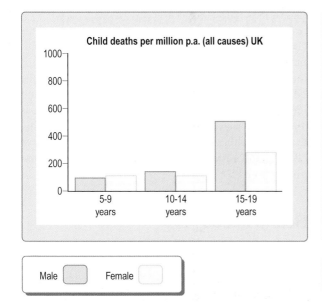

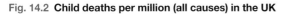

Male ☐ Female ☐

Fig. 14.2 **Child deaths per million (all causes) in the UK**

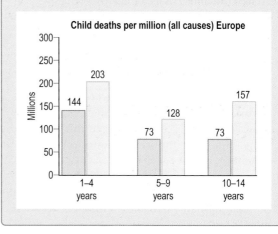

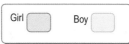

Girl ☐ Boy ☐

Fig. 14.3 **Causes of child death in Europe by age and sex.**

BOX 14.4 Main causes of death among children under 5

Worldwide

A total of 70% of the 10.6 million child deaths every year in children under 5 are due to six causes:

- Pneumonia (19%)
- Diarrhoea (18%)
- Neonatal infection (10%)
- Preterm delivery (10%)
- Malaria (8%)
- Birth asphyxia (8%).

Many of these are potentially preventable through simple interventions, such as providing clean water supplies, immunization and basic healthcare (especially antenatal and intrapartum care). Overall, 54% of child deaths are due to infections, and many occur as a direct or indirect result of absolute poverty.

Sources: Bryce et al 2005 Lancet.

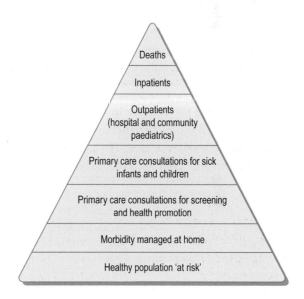

Fig. 14.4 **Pyramid of care**

The pyramid of care (Fig. 14.4)

By no means all children who become ill are cared for in hospital or even see a healthcare professional. Informal care by parents or others in the home is the norm, and advice may be sought from a variety of sources before a doctor is consulted: friends and relatives, the Internet or family health reference books, the community pharmacist etc. The percentage of infants cared for in the community, in primary care or in hospital varies widely from country to country, and largely depends upon the national medical system of the country.

Surveillance of health in the population

Many aspects of child health are monitored routinely. Child health surveillance is important for many reasons, for example:

- To find out about the child population in order to plan services (e.g. birth rate, mortality rate, proportion from minority ethnic groups, number with disabilities or particular diseases)

- To find out about usage of health services (e.g. children's admission rates to hospital)
- To pick up changes and trends that may require action (e.g. falling immunization coverage rates, which may leave the population susceptible to outbreaks of infectious disease)
- To assess progress against a target (e.g. prevalence of childhood obesity, infant mortality rates)
- To evaluate the success of public health programmes (e.g. the School Fruit and Vegetable scheme)
- To compare the health status of different groups and assess health inequalities (e.g. low birth weight or infant mortality in babies of mothers from different socioeconomic, ethnic or age groups, or childhood admissions to hospital in different areas of the country).

Some of these require the examination or assessment of every child in a particular age group or population; others rely on statistically valid sampling methods to draw conclusions about the population as a whole after studying a relatively small number of children. In general, public health surveillance does not require identifiable data about individual children, although it may need some demographic information about them to help interpret the results.

Collecting and interpreting health information relies on understanding a few basic measures:

- *Incidence* is the number of new events or cases in a population in a given period (e.g. number of babies born with congenital anomalies each year).
- *Prevalence* is the overall number (or proportion) of cases in a population at a particular moment in time (e.g. number of children with asthma in the population taken care of in a particular medical setting. Health Maintenance Organization (HMO) population).
- *Numerators* are the numbers of children, events or cases measured; they do not usually mean much without knowing how big the population is (e.g. 500 cases per year in a national population of 13 million children is a very rare condition; 500 cases a year in an HMO population of 30 000 children is a fairly common condition).
- *Denominators* provide the population size. They may include all children in a geographic area, a selected population group (e.g. children under 5, children looked after by the local authority) or another measure (e.g. infant mortality is expressed as a proportion of live births).
- *Rates* measure the frequency with which particular events occur in a defined population, taking the average population during a specified period (e.g. a year) as the denominator.

Health needs assessment

Health needs assessment is a key tool for public health practice. Although public health focuses on populations rather than individuals, the first step in most public health projects is still to make a 'diagnosis' and identify the problems to be addressed. Health needs assessment is also an important way of ensuring that the health service uses its resources in the most efficient and effective way to improve the health of the population.

Health needs

But what are 'health needs'? Clearly, this is partly a matter of opinion and perspective, so it is important to be clear about what kind of need is being considered:

- *Felt needs* involve a subjective perception of poor health — or of a risk to health — by an individual (e.g. abdominal pain) or a community (e.g. concern about a dangerous road).
- *Expressed needs* are felt needs that have been articulated, usually to gain the attention of those who might help address them (e.g. a doctor or the local council).
- *Normative needs* are needs defined — usually by a professional — in relation to an objective norm or standard, and may be perceived as requiring or justifying intervention (e.g. acute appendicitis, or a traffic 'black spot' where there has been a consistent pattern of fatal accidents).
- *Comparative needs* are identified by weighing up the health needs of one individual or community against another.

Public health may be concerned with all of these: with uncovering felt needs that have not been articulated; with balancing the expressed needs of communities and normative needs perceived by 'experts'; with comparing the health status and health needs of different communities to ensure that healthcare commissioning and service provision across a given area adequately reflect differences in need. Needs assessment also encompasses:

- *Health needs* — literally a 'need for health' — which include anything that affects children's (or communities') wellbeing, whether or not they can be 'treated' by health services. Some health needs require action outside the health sector to tackle determinants of health such as poverty, nutrition, housing, pollution, transport policy or employment opportunities.
- *Healthcare needs,* which are those for which effective healthcare interventions are available (e.g. infectious diseases, diabetes, congenital heart disease).

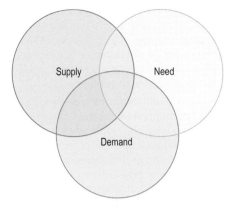

Fig. 14.5 Triad of need, supply and demand

Healthcare needs can be considered in more detail by looking at the triad of need, supply and demand (Fig. 14.5), which compares healthcare needs (usually normative needs), demand for healthcare (similar to expressed needs) and the supply of healthcare services for a particular condition.

The ideal is for need, supply and demand to coincide as far as possible, but where they do not, some action may be indicated. If healthcare is needed and demanded but not supplied (e.g. a local allergy clinic, or school-based sexual health advice for adolescents), then local authorities may want to consider introducing it. If it is demanded and supplied but not strictly needed (e.g. many instances of tonsillectomy, or antibiotic treatment for acute otitis media that will probably resolve spontaneously), then discontinuing or reducing provision may be appropriate. However, services that are needed and supplied but not demanded (e.g. child protection, some kinds of immunization) may be important.

Approaches to needs assessment

Health needs assessment can focus on a *condition* (e.g. childhood asthma), a *service* (e.g. the paediatric emergency department) or a *population group* (e.g. hearing-impaired children). Stevens and Raftery have identified three main approaches to needs assessment:

Epidemiological needs assessment: what data do we have?

- Essentially sets out to identify gaps in services for which there is both a need and an effective intervention.
- Brings together data from many sources to look at the characteristics and health status of the *population*, the *effectiveness* of interventions for the problem(s) under scrutiny, and the current *availability* of services locally.

- Offers a 'scientific' approach to health needs assessment, which considers the issues logically, and largely from the perspective of health professionals and policy makers.

A simple epidemiological needs assessment for childhood diabetes is outlined in Box 14.5.

Comparative needs assessment: what do other areas do?

- Compares services available locally with those provided for similar populations in other areas. For example, might look at models of care for children with diabetes in neighbouring districts to see whether any of them have services that seem more effective, more efficient or better suited to the needs of the local population.
- May seem an overly simple approach, but allows those commissioning healthcare to 'benchmark' their own local services against others, and looking at examples of good practice elsewhere is often very helpful.

Corporate needs assessment: what do stakeholders think?

- Involves a wide range of people and organizations who have views about health and healthcare, including children, parents, healthcare workers, support groups, policy makers, teachers and social workers.
- Brings together their different perspectives and experience to identify problems and make recommendations to address them.
- Major advantages are in allowing the views of professionals, parents, children and everyone who works with them to be considered together and in

avoiding an overly technical or professional focus — vital if services are to be child-centred and to properly reflect the wishes and needs of children and families.

These three approaches are complementary, and are often used in conjunction to build up a full picture of health needs. The balance between the three depends largely on the focus of the needs assessment. The example in Box 14.5 concerns a medical condition, but sometimes needs assessment is more exploratory, starting without any particular agenda or focus and aiming to find out about the problems and health needs of a particular community (e.g. children on a large deprived estate). In this case, the corporate element is likely to be the most important.

Specific techniques have been developed for conducting this type of needs assessment:

- *Participatory needs assessment* aims to involve members of the community fully, with 'experts' facilitating rather than leading the process.
- *Rapid appraisal needs assessment* allows a picture of health needs and problems to be built up very swiftly by gathering and sifting through a wide range of evidence and information from different sources.

Outcomes of needs assessment

The action taken as a result of needs assessment can be very varied and is certainly not limited to changes in health service provision. The outcomes depend very much on the problem and population studied. Before looking at the examples in Box 14.6, see how many different kinds of action, intervention or change you can list that might result from a health needs assessment for a particular condition or population group: for example, a sexual health needs assessment for young people in a local authority area with high rates of teenage pregnancy and sexually transmitted diseases.

Data sources

Child health surveillance and needs assessment both rely on information about the health of individuals and populations, but where does this come from? Much (though not all) is collected, directly or indirectly, by doctors and other health professionals. It is helpful to have some idea about what happens to information within the health service and how it is used — and to be aware of the wide range of information from other sources that can be useful in assessing or monitoring the health of the population.

> ### BOX 14.6 Examples of action taken as a result of needs assessment
>
> - Health promotion programmes (e.g. school-based projects to tackle smoking or provide sexual health advice to young people)
> - Changes to healthcare commissioning to reflect changed perception of priorities: developing new services (e.g. interpreting services for asylum seeker and refugee families) or reconfiguring others (increasing or decreasing availability, or changing the way they are delivered) to ensure that service provision reflects local need
> - Changes to other services (e.g. transport, leisure, community safety)
> - Community development projects (e.g. helping a community to start a new nursery or youth group)
> - Advocacy (e.g. championing children from traveller families or those caring for relatives, to help ensure their needs are met)
> - Developing new policies or strategies to tackle complex or long-term problems (e.g. promoting breastfeeding, reducing emotional and behavioural problems in a community)

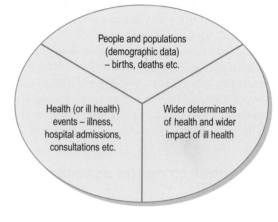

Fig. 14.6 **Different kinds of health information**

Different kinds of health information

Figure 14.6 illustrates some kinds of information which it is useful to collect; these are explored further below.

Different sources of health information

Box 14.7 illustrates the wide variety of sources of information about health.

Demographic data

Birth

Typical information recorded on birth certificates may include birth weight, the marital status of the mother, and whether the birth is registered jointly (i.e. by both parents) or singly. It also includes parents' occupations and places of birth. In most European countries hospitals pass basic information on each birth to the local Registrar of Births and Deaths, and parents are required to register the birth (and provide more information, including the child's name) within a few weeks of delivery. In many countries, birth registration is linked to the allocation of an HMO number, which entitles the child to use health services (e.g. register with a primary care physician).

Death

Typical information recorded on death certificates should include such data as the place and cause of death. Unexpected or unexplained deaths should be referred to a Coroner, whose records will contain more information, e.g. whether an inquest was held or a post-mortem conducted. Information on deaths in children can be used to generate neonatal, infant and child mortality rates, to examine causes of death (see above), and to compare rates in different areas, ethnic groups and sexes.

Census data

In the last part of the 20th century, population censuses became a global phenomenon. More than 90% of the present world population is counted and re-counted every few years. Despite remaining issues of statistical confidentiality, census samples of individuals and households are increasingly used as analytic tools by researchers within historical and present-day demography. They provide detailed information about the population, including age distribution, ethnic origin, occupation and long-standing illness and disability.

Health data

Information on morbidity and contacts with caretakers varies widely from one European country to the other, and depends upon the level of computer technology in an individual region and within an individual healthcare system is less comprehensive than demographic information.

Morbidity

Information on illness may be collected through various sources, including routine surveys, doctor-diagnosed illness and screening programmes (e.g. the neonatal blood spot programme). Incidence and prevalence can be calculated if the denominator population is known.

The use of a representative sample may provide a good estimate of health status and trends in a population as a whole. An example of such an approach may be found in the Health Survey for England based on a sample of households and which collects data on 4000 children (as well as adults) each year. It includes information on lifestyle (e.g. smoking, fruit and vegetable consumption), certain key conditions and long-standing illnesses, and nurse-measured height and weight. It is used to provide estimates about health status and trends in the population as a whole.

Contacts with a health maintenance organization (HMO)

In some countries, hospitalizations are recorded. For instance in the UK, the Hospital Episode Statistics (HES) include a range of information about patients attending outpatients or admitted to hospital, including discharge information recorded by junior doctors. They contain:

- Details about the hospital and consultant (e.g. specialty)
- Demographic information about the patient (e.g. NHS number, sex, birth date, postcode of usual address)
- Admission information (e.g. referring GP, admission/discharge dates, method/source of admission)
- Clinical information: diagnoses and procedures, coded using ICD–10 (International Classification of Diseases) and OPCS (Office of Population Censuses and Surveys) coding systems to allow analysis by type of disease and operation.

GP consultation data from the Royal College of General Practitioners are based on selected ('sentinel') practices. READ codes are used to classify health problems presenting in general practice. The fact that hospitalizations data are widely available in EU countries led to the development, for instance, of the APOLLO project, which has published an important report on injury-related hospitalizations in Europe. The aim of this project was to identify strategies and best practices for the prevention of injuries in Europe.

http://www.unav.es/ecip/memoria/2008/
Atlas_2004.pdf

Preventive health care

Local child health information systems should aim to provide a computerized database of all children living in the area. They are used to manage — and to record data about — preventive care services (e.g. immunization and routine health checks), and may also contain data on disability.

Chronic diseases

Information about the incidence and prevalence of some diseases — including congenital malformations, cancer, cerebral palsy, cystic fibrosis and diabetes — should be recorded in disease registers.

Household Surveys

The use of a representative sample here again may provide a good estimate of health and socio-economic variables. An example of such an approach may be found in the General Household Survey in the UK, which is an interview-based survey administered to a sample of around 12 000 households. There are questions about acute and chronic illness, healthcare contacts and health-related lifestyle. It also covers wider determinants of health such as housing, employment, pensions, leisure activities, education and the family.

Wider aspects of health

Wider determinants of health

At an international level, the WHO's survey of Health Behaviour of School Children allows comparisons to be made among European countries.

Wider impact of health issues

Information from many other sources also adds to what we know about children's health in the broader sense and about the impact of ill health on children's lives: for example, school attendance and educational achievement (both can be affected by health — and in turn have repercussions for later health); data from social services on children looked after by the local authority or on the child protection register; and police data on traffic accidents and incidents of domestic violence.

Structure of health and other related services

In 2002, the Union of National European Paediatric Societies and Associations published a report concerning the demography of delivery of care and training for the doctors who care for children in Europe. It also reported on specific factors that might explain the variation between countries regarding paediatric primary care (PPC) and community paediatrics (CP) as well as the extent of formal training provided for those who take care of children at the community level. An explanatory letter and a questionnaire with 12 questions regarding delivery of PPC and CP and training was mailed to the president of each of 41 national paediatric societies in Europe. Statistical data about population, country's income, and infant mortality rate (IMR) were also obtained from WHO data. It appears that in 1999, a total of 167 444 paediatricians served a population of 158 million children who were younger than 15 years and living in the 34 reporting European countries. The median number of children per paediatrician was 2094; this varied from 401 to 15 150. A paediatric system for PPC existed in 12 countries; 6 countries had a general practitioner system, and a combined system was reported from 16 countries. Paediatricians did not work at the primary care level at all in 3 countries. In 14 of 34 countries, paediatricians worked in various aspects of community medicine, such as developmental paediatrics, well-infant care, school physicians, and so forth. IMR was lower in countries with a higher income per capita. In addition, a paediatric system of primary care had a protective effect when looking at IMR as the outcome. Community-based teaching programs were offered to paediatricians and primary care physicians in a minority of countries only. Thus there is a considerable variation in both delivery of PPC and training for doctors who care for children. This study identified 3 different healthcare delivery systems for PPC, as well as 2 types of paediatricians who work in community-based settings. The study concluded that economic and sociopolitical issues, professional power, and geographical and historical factors may explain the differences in paediatric care among European countries.

Role of caretakers in the health of children

Parents

Parenting is arguably the most important factor contributing to the health and wellbeing of children, yet it is assumed that it comes naturally and does not need to be taught. The breakdown of the extended family compounds the situation, as parents are often isolated in bringing up children and responsibilities go unshared. Where parenting is good, children in quite adverse circumstances develop resilience to adversity. Where parenting is poor, particularly where it is neglectful or abusive, difficulties are passed from generation to generation.

It is now being recognized that parenting should be taught to young people while at school. The curriculum should address emotional wellbeing and discipline as much as the practicalities of caring for babies and young children. A further opportunity to impart good principles and practice comes at antenatal classes. Parenting groups too are helpful and are now becoming popular.

Childcare providers

Increasingly, mothers are working outside the home and have to find alternative care for their young children. Options include a nanny or minder in the home, or childcare outside the home. In many European countries child-minders who take other children into their own home have to be legally approved and registered with some type of social services authorities.

Alternative care varies considerably from country to country. In countries such as Denmark and France, childcare is primarily a matter for the public sector, and working couples are helped by well-established systems that seek to provide day care to families of all incomes. In contrast, in Britain, where the Government is committed to the free market, the private sector provides abundantly. Subsequently,

the costs of private child care put it out of reach for low-income working couples; these parents often make it with the help of relatives and friends. In France, nearly all children aged 3 to 5 attend free pre-primary school. Free after-school care is also widely available. Children under 3 can be placed in nurseries or in the homes of licensed baby sitters. Teams of doctors and nurses visit regularly to inspect centres and check on the health of the children. Parents pay according to income.

Education professionals

Compulsory education is education which children are required by law to receive and governments are required by law to provide. Compulsory education begins as early as 4 years of life (Northern Ireland), 5 years of life (UK, Malta), 6 years of life (Austria, Belgium, France), or even 7 (Bulgaria, Sweden, Poland).

> Euridyce report: http://www.nfer.ac.uk/ eurydice/briefingseurope/ school-starting-ages.cfm

Compulsory education usually includes:
- *Primary school* (5–11 years)
- *Secondary school* (until 16 years).

Educational provision for children with special needs is discussed on page 201.

Professionals involved in child health promotion and screening

Health visitors

Many EU countries customarily use health visitors. These are usually nurses who are specially trained in childcare and development. They work either in the framework of a baby clinic or with primary care physicians, and carry out duties of child health surveillance and health promotion programme for preschool children. This includes running child health clinics, visiting at home and providing support, particularly for those children and families identified as being in need or at risk.

School nurses

School nurses are specially trained nurses who work in a group of local schools. They are responsible for identifying children with medical needs, facilitating their care at school, providing liaison between professionals and supplying medical information to school staff. They may work together with school doctors or are responsible for reviewing all children and selecting those who need to be seen by the community paediatrician.

Practice nurses

These nurses are attached to primary care physicians' practices and provide immunization and other healthcare services to children, e.g. asthma review clinics.

Parents

Parents have a central role in enhancing the health of their children and they should be seen as partners in child health promotion.

Standards of Paediatric Care In Europe

There are, as mentioned earlier, 3 basic systems for paediatric care in European countries. The first one is a pure paediatric system (only paediatricians, in some cases up 18th/19th year, such as in the Czech Republic), a combined system (e.g. Germany), and a general practitioners' system only (e.g. United Kingdom, whereby paediatricians are secondary care physicians).

'Every Child Matters'

Integration of children's health in a healthy lifestyle has been the focus of multiple countries and multiple paediatric organizations. For instance we must describe briefly the 'Every child matters' program developed in the UK. Every Child Matters, or ECM for short, is a UK government initiative that was launched in 2003, at least partly in response to the death of Victoria Climbié. It is the title of the website http://www.everychildmatters.gov.uk, and led to the Children Act 2004. The word child applies to anyone under the age of 18. Its main aims are for every child, whatever their background or their circumstances, to have the support they need to be healthy, stay safe, enjoy and achieve, make a positive contribution, and achieve economic wellbeing. Each of these themes has a detailed outcomes framework attached to it which

requires multi-agency partnerships working together to achieve them. These include children's centres, early years, schools, children's social work services, primary and secondary health services, playwork, and Child and Adolescent Mental Health services (CAMHS). It is important that all professionals working with children are aware of the contribution that could be made by each service and plan their work accordingly. It is now in place in all schools throughout the United Kingdom and it is the central goal of 'Every Child Matters' to ensure every pupil is given the chance to be able to work towards the goals referenced within it. At the European level, some projects have been launched that attempt to tackle specific health issues such as the IDEFICS project. The IDEFICS study (Identification and prevention of Dietary- and lifestyle-induced health effects In Children and infants) is a 5-year multi-centre, pan European epidemiological study, funded by the European Commission. Focusing on 2- to 10-year-old children, it has the challenging objectives of both understanding the multi-factorial origin of childhood overweight and obesity and of preventing it and its related disorders.

http://www.eufic.org/article/en/health-and-lifestyle/food-for-all-ages/artid/Learn-healthy-living-european-intervention-strategy/

References

Acheson 1986. From Public Health in England: the report of the Committee of Inquiry into the Future Development of the Public Health Function (Cm 289) London: HMSO, 1988

Bryce J, Boschi-Pint C, Shibuya K, Black RE; WHO Child Health Epidemiology Reference Group 2005 WHO estimates of the causes of death in children. Lancet 365:1147–1152

Emigh RJ & Szelényi I: Poverty, ethnicity, and gender in Eastern Europe during the market transition. Greenwood Publishing Group, 2001: p.47

Katz M, Rubino A, Collier J et al 2002 Demography of pediatric primary care in Europe. Pediatrics 109:788–796

Rachel Crowther   Zsofia Meszner

CHAPTER

Screening

15

LEARNING OUTCOMES

By the end of this chapter you should:

- Understand the place of screening in preventive healthcare and why it is an important element of child health services
- Understand the theoretical background to screening and the parameters used to assess screening tests (sensitivity, specificity, positive and negative predictive value)
- Be familiar with the criteria used to evaluate new and existing screening programmes
- Appreciate the difference between screening and surveillance
- Appreciate the potential benefits and disadvantages of screening and the ethical issues involved for parents and professionals
- Understand the role of the national public health bodies in overseeing screening programmes and the policy context for child health screening
- Be familiar with current antenatal, neonatal and childhood screening programmes and those under development or consideration
- Appreciate the difficulties involved in ensuring universal coverage in screening programmes.

MODULE THREE

Introduction

Screening is an example of secondary prevention (Ch. 17), and which aims to prevent or mitigate the effects of a condition by identifying it early (usually before it is clinically apparent) so that treatment is more effective. Much attention has been focused on screening in early life, when there is considerable scope for identifying potentially serious conditions and reducing — or even eliminating — their impact. Consequently many of the routine screening programmes operate before birth and in childhood. Together they offer considerable benefits and form an important element of child health services.

In recent years, however, appreciation of the potential drawbacks of screening has grown. It is essential to have an appropriate means of testing before introducing a new screening programme, but that is not enough: careful thought must go into evaluating and designing screening programmes in order to maximize the balance of

Table 15.1 Screening and diagnostic tests

Condition	Screening test	Diagnostic test
Down syndrome	Serum markers (e.g. β-human chorionic gonadotrophin, β-hCG) and/or nuchal translucency	Amniocentesis or chorionic villus sampling (CVS)
Newborn hearing	Oto-acoustic emissions (OAE)	Auditory brainstem responses (ABR)

Table 15.2 False positives and false negatives

	Affected individuals (those with the condition — 'cases')	Unaffected individuals (those without the condition — 'non-cases')
Positive screening test	True positive	False positive
Negative screening test	False negative	True negative

benefit and harm (p. 164). The impact of screening, in economic, social and personal terms, needs to be considered alongside any beneficial health effects. It is also vital that the public understands that screening is not infallible, and that screening tests are offered with as clear an explanation as possible of what the results actually mean (p. 166). This chapter introduces the theory and practice of screening, considering the nature of screening tests, the policy context and the ethical and practical issues involved in delivering a screening programme.

Theoretical background: screening tests

A *screening test* is the first building block in a screening programme. Sometimes the screening test is a 'one-stop shop' that identifies affected or susceptible individuals immediately; examples include serological tests for rubella or HIV antibodies, or certain elements of the neonatal physical examination (e.g. checking for simple abnormalities such as extra digits). Often, however, the initial screening test merely identifies individuals who have a higher chance of having a particular condition, and a positive result leads to a second stage of testing involving a *diagnostic* test. Two examples are given in Table 15.1. Note that for Down syndrome the diagnostic test is invasive and carries a small but significant risk of abortion, while for newborn hearing screening the diagnostic test is simply a more accurate audiological test.

False positives and false negatives

Most screening tests are not 100% accurate either in detecting individuals who have the condition being tested for or in identifying those who do not. There are almost always 'false positives' and 'false negatives' (Table 15.2).

Individuals with both false positive and false negative are done a disservice by the screening test results. Although

false positives can usually be reassured after further testing (the diagnostic test), they (and/or their parents and families) may suffer considerable anxiety in the meantime, and there may be a more serious impact, such as lost time at work or school, or social stigma. In addition, the diagnostic test, which would have been unnecessary if the screening test had been more accurate or had not been offered at all, may be unpleasant or carry some health risk.

False negatives, on the other hand, are given false reassurance, which may have serious consequences later on: the birth of a child with a congenital condition the parents believed to have been excluded, for example, or the risk that individuals may ignore early symptoms of a condition they believe they do not have.

Sensitivity and specificity

It is clearly important to keep the number of false negative and false positive results from any screening test to a minimum. In technical terms, any test needs to be as *sensitive* and as *specific* as possible. Since the development of a test usually involves reaching agreement about where to set the cutoff for positive/negative results (e.g. at a particular level of a serum marker), there is generally a trade-off between sensitivity and specificity; set the cutoff too high and sensitivity will decline, although specificity will rise, and vice versa.

Sensitivity

- Is related to the number of false negatives: a test is less sensitive if it produces large numbers of false negatives (missed cases)
- Describes the proportion of affected individuals who are picked up by the test (i.e. who have positive test results)
- Is calculated by dividing the number of affected individuals with a positive test by the total number of affected individuals, i.e. (referring to Table 15.2)

BOX 15.1 Exercise: sensitivity and specificity

A new serum marker for Down syndrome has recently been piloted. The results are shown below. Calculate the sensitivity and specificity if this marker were to be used on its own as a screening test for Down syndrome.

- *Trial population*: 1000
- *Positive screening test results*: 82, of which all proceeded to amniocentesis or CVS and 17 were found to be carrying fetuses with Down syndrome
- *Missed cases*: 2 women with negative screening tests had an amniocentesis for other reasons, which detected Down fetuses, and another woman subsequently delivered a baby with Down syndrome

	Affected fetuses	**Unaffected fetuses**
Positive test	17 (true positives)	65 (false positives)
Negative test	3 (false negatives)	915 (true negatives)

Sensitivity = 17 ÷ (17 + 3) = 85%

Specificity = 915 ÷ (915 + 65) = 93.4%

In the second stage of the pilot, the cutoff for the new marker was lowered in an attempt to increase sensitivity. The results for this stage are shown below. Has the screening test improved? Which do you think is more important in this case: sensitivity or specificity? (Think about the implications of false negative and false positive test results.)

- *Trial population*: 2000
- *Positive screening test results*: 296, of which all proceeded to amniocentesis or CVS and 36 were found to be carrying fetuses with Down syndrome
- *Missed cases*: 4

	Affected fetuses	**Unaffected fetuses**
Positive test	36 (true positives)	260 (false positives)
Negative test	4 (false negatives)	1700 (true negatives)

Sensitivity = 36 ÷ (36 + 4) = 90%

Specificity = 1700 ÷ (1700 + 260) = 86.7%

by dividing true positives by (true positives + false negatives).

Specificity

- Is related to the number of false positives: a test is less specific if it produces large numbers of false positives
- Describes the proportion of unaffected individuals who are cleared by the test (i.e. who have negative test results)
- Is calculated by dividing the number of unaffected individuals with a negative test by the total number of unaffected individuals, i.e. (referring to Table 15.2) by dividing true negatives by (true negatives + false positives).

Both sensitivity and specificity are usually expressed as a percentage (Box 15.1).

Positive and negative predictive value

Other terms used to describe how well a screening test performs are *positive and negative predictive value*.

Positive predictive value (PPV)

- Asks the question: how helpful is a positive result in predicting whether an individual is affected by the condition being tested for?
- Describes the proportion of individuals with a positive test who actually have the condition
- Is calculated by dividing the number of affected individuals with a positive test by the total number of positive test results, i.e. (referring to Table 15.2) by dividing true positives by (true positives + false positives).

Negative predictive value (NPV)

- Asks the question: how helpful is a negative result in predicting whether an individual is unaffected by the condition being tested for?
- Describes the proportion of individuals with a negative test who are free of the condition
- Is calculated by dividing the number of unaffected individuals with a negative test by the total number of negative test results, i.e. (referring to Table 15.2) by dividing true negatives by (true negatives + false negatives).

Like specificity, PPV is lower when there are more false positives; and like sensitivity, NPV is lower when there are more false negatives. However, there is an important difference between the two sets of terms. Sensitivity and specificity are intrinsic properties of the screening test that remain the same whatever the characteristics of the population being tested. PPV and NPV, however, vary according to the prevalence of the condition in a particular population. Generally, where prevalence is low, PPV is lower too, but NPV is higher.

The development of new screening tests may raise important issues such as the acceptability of the test for families, the cost of the test and also the cost of care for a case *not* detected. It is clear that a framework for assessing a potential screening programme is required. Such a framework is shown in Box 15.2 facing.

Policy and practice: screening programmes

Screening programmes

Responsibility for managing screening programmes in each country and shaping screening policy in European countries (ECs) rests with the respective local public health committee which advises government ministers on screening issues, and states its purpose as follows:

Screening programmes are public health services that need to be managed at the level of a large population to monitor quality effectively, e.g. in the UK, this is carried out by the National Screening Committee (NSC). The first task of the NSC is to use research evidence to identify programmes that do more good than harm; the second is to make policy recommendations about those programmes that will do more good than harm at a reasonable cost. In policy-making, the evidence for screening is often limited, because of the rarity of the conditions being screened for.

It is clear from the previous section that evaluating any proposed screening programme involves considering many complex issues.

Although the general public has become more cautious in accepting medical opinion wholesale (witness falling immunization rates for the measles/mumps/rubella (MMR) vaccine following the 'autism scare'), faith in clinical tests tends to be high and lay people may find it hard to understand that a screening test may not necessarily give them the 'right answer'. There is a recognized danger of such situations and it is necessary to present and explain screening programmes so that the balance of benefit and harm is understood. Screening should be seen as a way of reducing the risk of suffering the ill-effects of a condition, rather than an infallible means of distinguishing those with and without it, and individuals should always be given fully informed choice about screening tests.

In order to fulfil this role, information should be drawn from a wide range of sources, and should be made available through the web, as in the UK through the Health Information Resources (formerly the National Library for Health).

http://www.libraries.nhs.uk/default.aspx

In addition, the 'Health for all Children' (4th edition) report set out carefully considered recommendations for screening and health promotion throughout childhood.

Criteria for screening programmes

In order to ensure that screening does more good than harm, and that all the relevant issues, difficulties and drawbacks are considered, a set of criteria should be developed for appraising the viability, effectiveness and appropriateness of existing and potential screening programmes as in the UK (Box 15.2). These build on the criteria first established by Wilson and Jungner, but set screening in the context of planned service provision for each condition, of meticulous quality control, and of informed choice for the public.

Benefit and harm: ethical issues in screening

Some ethical implications of screening programmes have been alluded to earlier (e.g. drawbacks for those with false positive and false negative results on screening tests). As well as ensuring that screening does more good than harm at population level, it is important to bear in mind the experience of individuals and to strive to maximize the balance of good over harm for each.

Screening in pregnancy and childhood is different from screening in adulthood. It requires parents to make decisions about and on behalf of their children, often before birth or very early in life. These are often emotionally charged times, and such decisions may be the first experience of the responsibilities of parenthood. Antenatal screening is usually directed at offering parents the choice of terminating an affected pregnancy, a life-or-death decision about a child who may be very much wanted, and neonatal screening involves facing up to the possibility that an apparently perfect baby may have something seriously wrong with him or her before the parents have even got used to

The condition

- The condition should be an important health problem
- The epidemiology and natural history of the condition, including development from latent to declared disease, should be adequately understood and there should be a detectable risk factor, disease marker, latent period or early symptomatic stage
- All the cost-effective primary prevention interventions should have been implemented as far as practicable
- If the carriers of a mutation are identified as a result of screening, the natural history of people with this status should be understood, including the psychological implications

The test

- There should be a simple, safe, precise and validated screening test
- The distribution of the test values in the target population should be known and a suitable cutoff level defined and agreed
- The test should be acceptable to the population
- There should be an agreed policy on the further diagnostic investigation of individuals with a positive test result and on the choices available to those individuals
- If the test is for mutations, the criteria used to select the subset of mutations to be covered by screening, if all possible mutations are not being tested, should be clearly set out

The treatment

- There should be an effective treatment or intervention for patients identified through early detection, with evidence of early treatment leading to better outcomes than late treatment
- There should be agreed evidence-based policies covering which individuals should be offered treatment and the appropriate treatment to be offered
- Clinical management of the condition and patient outcomes should be optimized by all healthcare providers prior to participation in a screening programme

The screening programme

- There should be evidence from high-quality RCTs that the screening programme is effective in reducing mortality or morbidity
- Where screening is aimed solely at providing information to allow the person being screened to make an 'informed choice' (e.g. Down syndrome, cystic fibrosis carrier screening), there must be evidence from high-quality trials that the test accurately measures risk. The information that is provided about the test and its outcome must be of value and readily understood by the individual being screened
- There should be evidence that the complete screening programme (test, diagnostic procedures, treatment/intervention) is clinically, socially and ethically acceptable to health professionals and the public
- The benefit from the screening programme should outweigh the physical and psychological harm (caused by the test, diagnostic procedures and treatment)
- The opportunity cost of the screening programme (including testing, diagnosis and treatment, administration, training and quality assurance) should be economically balanced in relation to expenditure on medical care as a whole (i.e. value for money)
- There should be a plan for managing and monitoring the screening programme and an agreed set of quality assurance standards
- Adequate staffing and facilities for testing, diagnosis, treatment and programme management should be available prior to the commencement of the screening programme
- All other options for managing the condition should have been considered (e.g. improving treatment, providing other services), to ensure that no more cost-effective intervention could be introduced or current interventions increased within the resources available
- Evidence-based information, explaining the consequences of testing, investigation and treatment, should be made available to potential participants to assist them in making an informed choice
- Public pressure for widening the eligibility criteria for reducing the screening interval, and for increasing the sensitivity of the testing process, should be anticipated. Decisions about these parameters should be scientifically justifiable to the public
- If screening is for a mutation, the programme should be acceptable to people identified as carriers and to other family members

MODULE THREE

this new presence in their lives. Cultural, religious and social factors may strongly influence parents' thinking, and the views and interests of others, including older children and perhaps the extended family, may need to be taken into account. Sometimes screening may be offered for a condition (e.g. sickle cell disease) that already affects one child in the family, and may therefore involve implicit judgments about the value of that child's life and stimulate reflection about what the parents might have done, had they known in advance that the first child was affected.

It is important not to underestimate the gravity of the burden these decisions place on parents. However, where testing will be, for the majority, no more than a brief incident soon forgotten, there is a balance to be struck between the obligation to provide full information and the risk of causing undue alarm by insisting that every single parent is briefed on the full range of consequences of every single test. Doctors and others involved in delivering screening programmes are often advised to test the water by asking parents whether they would like to know everything about every test in advance, or whether they would prefer the healthcare team to 'do what is usually done' and leave detailed discussion until there is an indication that something might be wrong. Does this seem a good approach to you? If you were a parent, how would you answer this question?

Some of the advantages and disadvantages of screening programmes are summarized in Box 15.3.

Screening and surveillance

It is important to be clear about the distinction between screening and surveillance: both useful public health activities, but with different purposes. Surveillance is concerned with the collection of data on health and disease from a variety of possible sources, with analysing and interpreting it, and with feedback to 'those who need to know' (e.g. those planning and delivering health services or responsible for healthcare policy). Surveillance is an epidemiological rather than a clinical tool, and does not generally involve patient-identifiable data (although sometimes individuals' records are identified in order to facilitate further investigation and follow-up).

The term 'surveillance' is sometimes used more loosely in paediatrics, to cover the broader elements of child health services that involve regular contact between health visitors, primary care physicians and others and the children and families they look after, and which aim to spot problems early, to offer reassurance and advice, and to 'keep an eye' on the child: a group of functions closer to the lay definition of surveillance as 'close observation'.

BOX 15.3 Advantages and disadvantages of screening

Advantages

- Better outcome for true positives if picked up early: may include lower morbidity and/or mortality, avoiding more unpleasant and severe treatment for later disease etc.
- Opportunity for parents to decide whether or not to proceed with affected pregnancy, and/or to prepare for birth of baby with health problems
- Reassurance for true negatives that they do not have the condition or are at very low risk
- Public health benefits: may include lower prevalence of condition, lower mortality, lower overall expenditure on the condition

Disadvantages

- Anxiety, further intervention and other possible risks for false positives
- False reassurance and possibly worse outcome for false negatives
- Cost of screening test for individuals: time, worry, discomfort or risk associated with procedure
- Those with positive screening test may face difficult decisions about how to proceed
- Cost of screening programme for NHS: N.B. opportunity cost (what else could this money be spent on?)
- Unless benefit of early intervention is absolutely clear, early diagnosis may mean longer period of 'illness' and/or unnecessary or excessive treatment

---

This use of the term is potentially unhelpful, however, for a variety of reasons, unless it involves collecting and collating data (rather than simply recording it in the parent-held record), it is *not* surveillance, and it may involve activities that are in effect screening but which do not meet the accepted criteria (often because there is insufficient evidence for the validity of the 'screening test' or the benefits of early intervention).

A topical example is childhood obesity. Although weighing and measuring all children in certain years of primary school is a useful public health surveillance exercise, until there is a remedy of proven effectiveness for those found to be obese (and everything possible has been done to prevent obesity in children), it is not acceptable to support the introduction of a screening programme for childhood obesity in which results are fed back to individual children and parents. It is better to divide child health 'surveillance' into screening and health promotion activities and to be clear about their precise purpose and justification.

Current antenatal, neonatal and child health screening programmes

A brief summary of antenatal, neonatal and childhood screening recommendations in ECs is set out in Boxes 15.4–15.7.

 http://www.euro.who.int/Document/ E88698.pdf

 http://www.euro.who.int/Document/Obs/ EuroObserver8_3.pdf

Contain more information on any screening programme or condition

Antenatal screening

Antenatal screening (Box 15.4) is included here because it inevitably involves the fetus as well as the mother. It falls into one of several categories, including programmes that aim to:

- Ensure optimal general health for mother and fetus, and identify complications of pregnancy and threats to the fetus early so that they can be mitigated through optimal antenatal care (e.g. screening for anaemia, atypical red cell antibodies and risk factors for pre-eclampsia)
- Identify specific conditions for which planned changes in management can benefit mother and fetus (e.g. screening for HIV and hepatitis B)
- Identify fetal abnormalities early so parents can be offered counselling and options for management, including termination of pregnancy (e.g. screening for Down syndrome, neural tube defects and other fetal anomalies).

Down syndrome (p. 94)

The Down syndrome screening programme, which is available in a number of European countries, aims to ensure that all pregnant women are offered screening in order to give parents informed choices about pregnancy outcome and reduce the number of babies born with *undiagnosed* Down syndrome.

Down syndrome tests

A variety of testing combinations have evolved, including up to four serum markers (various proteins and hormones assayed in a blood sample taken between 10 and 20 weeks' gestation) and ultrasound scanning for nuchal translucency (NT; the fluid area at the back of

---

BOX 15.4 Recommended policy on antenatal screening

Conditions for which all pregnant women should be offered screening (in most cases as part of routine antenatal care)

- Anaemia
- Bacteriuria
- Blood group, rhesus D status and atypical red cell alloantibodies
- Down syndrome
- Fetal anomalies
- Hepatitis B
- HIV
- Neural tube defects
- Risk factors for pre-eclampsia
- Rubella immunity
- Syphilis

Conditions for which screening should be offered in some cases

- Placenta praevia (given relevant history)
- Psychiatric illness (given relevant history)
- Sickle cell and thalassaemia (in high-prevalence areas — see below)
- Tay–Sachs disease (in at-risk populations)

Conditions for which screening should not be offered

- Bacterial vaginosis
- *Chlamydia*
- Cystic fibrosis
- Cytomegalovirus
- Diabetes
- Domestic violence
- Familial dysautonomia
- Fetomaternal alloimmune thrombocytopenia
- Fragile X syndrome
- Hepatitis C
- Herpes
- Human T-cell lymphotrophic virus (HTLV) 1
- Postnatal depression
- Predictors of preterm labour
- Streptococcus B
- Thrombophilia
- Toxoplasmosis

---

the fetal neck, the size of which is related to the risk of Down syndrome).

A combination of ultrasound and serum methods is ideal, but where NT measurement is not yet available, serum testing alone is acceptable. Markers used for second-trimester screening include alpha-fetoprotein (AFP), free β-human chorionic gonadotrophin (β-hCG), unconjugated oestriol (UE3) and inhibin A. First-trimester (10–14 weeks) screening generally uses β-hCG and placenta-associated plasma protein-A (PAPP-A).

Estimating the risk of Down syndrome from the results of any testing combination requires the use of specialist software that calculates the risk of an affected baby given the mother's age. (The background risk increases sharply with age, from 1:1500 at age 20 to 1:270 at age 35 and 1:100 at 40.) Women with an adjusted risk over 1:250 (about 5% of those tested) should be offered diagnostic cytogenetic testing, involving amniocentesis between 15 and 20 weeks, or chorionic villus sampling (CVS) between 11 and 13 weeks, together with appropriate counselling. Both carry a risk of miscarriage: around 2% for CVS and 1% for amniocentesis. Currently, around 90% of women choose to terminate confirmed Down syndrome fetuses. Testing should ideally take place early in pregnancy to avoid late decisions about termination.

As for any screening programme, maximizing sensitivity and specificity is important. The targets for the Down syndrome programme are:

- Detection rate of 60% or more and false positive rate of 5% or less by April 2005, progressing to
- Detection rate over 75% and false positive rate less than 3% by April 2007.

http://www.screening.nhs.uk/downs

Fetal anomalies

A recent Health Technology Assessment (HTA) review found that ultrasound screening before 24 weeks offered some benefits. In many hospitals all women are already offered a fetal anomaly scan at 18–20 weeks of pregnancy, and a national programme is now planned with working standards that aim to ensure a high-quality universal service. Anomaly scans cannot detect all abnormalities, but aim to identify those that:

- Are incompatible with life
- Are likely to be associated with high morbidity and long-term disability
- Might benefit from intrauterine therapy
- Will need investigation or treatment after birth.

HIV (Ch. 43)

Routine antenatal serological screening and treatment for HIV can substantially reduce the mother-to-child transmission of the infection. Most children infected with HIV acquire the infection from their mothers during pregnancy, birth or lactation ('vertical transmission'). If maternal infection is diagnosed during pregnancy, interventions are available that can reduce the risk of vertical transmission from 25% to around 2% (including antiretroviral drugs, delivery by caesarean section and advising against breastfeeding). Women found to be HIV-positive are also referred for specialist HIV treatment and advice, and virological follow-up is arranged for the baby.

Sickle cell disease and thalassaemia (Ch. 42)

Sickle cell and thalassaemia screening, as part of a national linked antenatal and neonatal screening programme, has three elements:

- Antenatal screening for thalassaemia
- Antenatal screening for sickle cell disease
- Neonatal screening for sickle cell disease.

Antenatal screening for sickle cell disease and thalassaemia aims to identify couples at risk of carrying an affected fetus early in pregnancy and to offer them the choice of prenatal diagnosis, potentially followed by termination. It should be offered in high-prevalence areas (where the estimated fetal prevalence of sickle cell disorder is 1.5 per 10 000 or more). Testing for relevant haemoglobin variants (e.g. HbS, HbC) should be offered to some women in low-prevalence areas on the basis of a question about ethnic origin (targeting high-risk groups, including those originating from Africa, the Caribbean, the Middle East, Asia and the Mediterranean).

Neonatal screening for sickle cell disease has been found to reduce morbidity and mortality in infancy. Identifying affected infants before the disease presents clinically (often with severe infections and splenic sequestration crises) enables babies to be given penicillin and vaccine prophylaxis and parents to be trained to recognize complications early and seek help. It is being introduced as part of the universal newborn blood spot programme, to complement antenatal screening.

http://apps.who.int/gb/ebwha/pdf_files/ WHA59/A59_9-en.pdf

Neonatal blood spot screening

The neonatal blood spot test is offered to babies at 3–8 days of age. It is usually delivered by midwives or paediatricians and involves the collection of capillary blood on to a card. Babies are usually tested for phenylketonuria (PKU), and congenital hypothyroidism (CHT), although other conditions may also be screened and this varies from country to country (for example in some European countries G-6-PD deficiency is tested as well). Both PKU, but more so, CHT, are conditions for which early intervention is highly effective, preventing irreversible neurological damage and consequent disability. Cystic fibrosis and sickle cell disease (both disorders for which testing is already established in some European countries) are being added to national programmes, using the same blood sample as for PKU and CHT screening.

The neonatal blood spot programme is one of the largest and most successful screening programmes in Europe. In the UK, for example, over 600 000 babies are screened each year, with uptake levels of over 99%, and about 250 babies with PKU or CHT are identified each year. As for most screening programmes, a positive screening result means that further diagnostic tests are indicated to confirm whether or not the child is affected. The UK Newborn Screening Programme Centre has been set up to monitor newborn blood spot screening (Box 15.5).

Several ECs have recently introduced neonatal screening for other inborn errors of metabolism made available by the development of tandem mass spectrometry. Rapid developments in biochemistry and genetics mean that screening for other conditions will continue to be regularly reviewed.

Duchenne muscular dystrophy (Ch. 28)

The condition was assessed against the WHO criteria in 2004 and newborn screening was not recommended. However, screening was introduced on a pilot basis in Wales (UK) and has not been discontinued.

Other neonatal screening

All newborn babies should be offered a routine physical examination that aims to detect a range of congenital conditions (Box 15.6). Universal newborn hearing screening is also in place in most countries now.

Universal newborn hearing screening

Approximately 0.1–0.3% of all babies with permanent hearing loss are born every year in ECs. Universal newborn hearing screening (UNHS) was first introduced in 2001 as a more accurate — and earlier — alternative to the infant distraction test (IDT). It offers benefits for:
- *Parents*. Parents would generally rather know earlier if their child has a hearing problem and can be helped to come to terms with and manage their child's condition.

BOX 15.5 Recommended policy on neonatal blood spot screening

Conditions included in the neonatal blood spot programme
- Congenital hypothyroidism
- Phenylketonuria
- Cystic fibrosis (soon to be added)
- Sickle cell disease (soon to be added)

Conditions for which screening is under review
- Medium chain acyl CoA dehydrogenase deficiency (MCADD)

Conditions for which screening should not be offered
- Biotinidase deficiency
- Cannavan disease (review against NSC criteria commissioned)
- Congenital adrenal hyperplasia
- Duchenne muscular dystrophy
- Galactosaemia
- Gaucher disease
- Organic acid metabolism disorder

BOX 15.6 Recommended policy on other neonatal screening

Conditions for which screening forms part of the routine physical examination of newborn babies
- Congenital cataract
- Congenital heart disease
- Congenital malformations
- Cryptorchidism
- Developmental dislocation of the hip

Conditions for which screening should also be offered
- Hearing

Conditions for which screening should not be offered
- Biliary atresia
- Neonatal alloimmune thrombocytopenia
- Neuroblastoma

- *Children*. There is increasing evidence of the benefits of appropriate intervention before 6 months of age in terms of language skills, speech, social and emotional development.
- UNHS is cheaper per child than the IDT and far more cost-effective, given its superior sensitivity and specificity.

Conditions for which screening is currently recommended*

- Growth
- Hearing
- Hyperlipidaemia
- Vision defects

Conditions for which screening is being reviewed

- Dental disease

Conditions for which screening should not be offered

- Autism
- Developmental and behavioural problems
- Hypertension
- Hypertrophic cardiomyopathy
- Iron deficiency anaemia
- Lead poisoning
- Obesity
- Scoliosis
- Speech and language delay

* See below for qualifications.

The UNHS is discussed in detail in Chapter 32.

http://www.nhsp.info/index.php

Screening in later childhood (Box 15.7)

Growth

Children should have their height and weight measured around the time of school entry and the 0.4th centile cutoff for height should be used to initiate referral.

Hearing

Screening for hearing loss in school-age children should continue while further research is undertaken.

Hyperlipidaemia

Screening should only be offered as part of a project on cascade screening of the relatives of patients with confirmed familial hypercholesterolaemia.

Vision defects

In line with the recommendation in the 4th edition of 'Health for All Children', screening for visual impairment in 7-year-old children should be discontinued, and screening should instead be offered between 4 and 5 years of age.

Obesity

Overweight and obesity in childhood are known to have significant impact on both physical and psychological health. However, further research into effective preventive measures is needed before screening for obesity should be supported.

Coverage in screening programmes

National screening programmes aim to offer testing to all individuals within the target population on the basis of informed consent. Among the parameters for quality control of screening programmes is the coverage rate achieved in practice (what percentage of eligible individuals have actually been offered screening, and/or have taken it up?). Several factors may affect coverage:

- Local difficulties within the programme — shortage of staff, problems with the call–recall system, laboratory issues etc. — which require the attention of the programme coordinator.
- Problems with access, which may — as for other aspects of healthcare — affect different groups differently, and often mean that deprived groups are less likely to benefit from services. It is important that screening programmes take account of 'hard to reach' groups (including, for example, women who book very late, or not at all, for antenatal care) and ensure that they promote equity and reduce health inequality, rather than increasing it by allowing those with the greatest health needs to miss out on screening.
- Individuals may make informed choices not to accept screening or not to proceed to diagnostic testing: for example, those who would not accept termination of an affected fetus.

The objective is to ensure that universal programmes offer universal access, and provide individuals with full information on which to base their decisions.

Reference

Hall DMB, Elliman D 2003 Health for all children, 4th edn. Oxford University Press, Oxford

Zsofia Meszner   Kathleen Skinner

CHAPTER

16

Immunization

LEARNING OUTCOMES

By the end of this chapter you should:

● Understand passive and active immunity
● Understand the principles and rationale behind the national immunization policies for children in European countries
● Understand the indications and contraindications of routine childhood immunizations, and know them
● Understand the reasons why some parents are resistant to immunization
● Understand the principles of disease outbreak control.

MODULE THREE

Introduction

Immunization is the process of protecting individuals from infection through passive or active immunity. Passive immunity is provided by administering antibodies, whilst active immunity is achieved through stimulating the individual's immune system by an inactive vaccine (toxoid such as tetanus, inactivated organism such as hepatitis A vaccine, or subunit vaccines such as acellular pertussis vaccine) or a modified, attenuated live organism such as measles/mumps/rubella (MMR).

Historical impact

After clean water, vaccination is the most effective public health measure for saving lives and promoting good health. Vaccination now refers to all procedures for immunization but first originated 200 years ago from the procedure to protect people from smallpox using the first vaccine derived from a cow infected with the vaccinia virus.

Diseases such as smallpox and polio used to cause widespread illness, disability and death but, because of vaccination, smallpox has been eradicated and polio is present in only a few countries in the world, with strong efforts ongoing to eradicate this as well. Most people in Europe will never have seen a child crippled by polio.

In the UK in the late 1990s, meningitis C was a major killer of children under 5 but since the introduction of the vaccine in 1999, the incidence rates and subsequent complications have plummeted.

Because immunization is so successful it may be easy to think that outbreaks cannot occur today; however, most childhood diseases have not disappeared. In Ireland, the Netherlands, Germany, Spain and Italy there have been outbreaks of measles in the last 5 years. Immunization is the safest way to protect children and the new diphtheria, tetanus, pertussis, polio and Hib (DTaP/IPV/Hib) immunization provides protection from five diseases in one vaccine.

Rationale

Infectious disease is different from other disease in many respects, including its non-linear nature. Herd immunity refers to the immunity of a group or community. The resistance to infection is the product of the number susceptible and the probability that those susceptible will come into contact with an infected person. The proportion of the population required to be immune varies with the agent, its transmission dynamics, the geographical distribution of susceptibles and immunes, and other environmental factors.

The herd immunity threshold is the proportion of immunes in a population above which the incidence of infection decreases. Therefore immunizing a greater proportion than this will ensure that infection will always decline and herd immunity is achieved.

For measles vaccination, coverage of 90% is required to prevent ongoing transmission, whilst for mumps this threshold is much lower.

The age at which vaccination is carried out is crucial; vaccination after the average age of infection cannot interrupt transmission.

Note that herd immunity is based on the following assumptions:

- Natural immunity is solid and lifelong.
- Vaccine immunity is solid and lifelong.
- Dynamic effects of antigenic diversity are negligible.

Since none of these is strictly true, eradication becomes more difficult.

Recommended routine schedules of vaccination in European countries

The current recommended routine schedules in European contries are outlined in Table 16.1. There have been several recent changes to the routine schedules in each country.

Inactivated polio vaccine (IPV)

IPV is used instead of the live oral polio vaccine (OPV) because the present risk of imported polio infection in Europe is low now that polio has been eliminated from large parts of the world through the global vaccination programme. OPV provided more effective community-wide protection but carried a small risk (about 1 case in more than 1.5 million doses used) of

Table 16.1 Recommended routine vaccination schedules in most European contries

When to immunize	What is given
2, 3 and 4, or 2,4 and 6, or 3,4 and 5, or 3 and 6 months old	Diphtheria, tetanus, pertussis (whooping cough), polio and Hib (DTaP/IPV/Hib) *and* meningitis C (MenC), and pneumococcus (PCV-7)
Around 12–15 months old	Measles, mumps and rubella (MMR, 2x)
12 or 18 months 3 to 5 or 6 years old	Diphtheria, tetanus, pertussis and polio (dTaP/IPV or DTaP/IPV) meningitis C (MenC) and pneumococcus (PCV-7) *and* MMR revaccination
11 or 13 to 18 years old	Diphtheria, tetanus, pertussis, polio (DTaP/IPV)

causing vaccine-associated paralytic polio (VAPP). IPV provides effective individual protection but carries no risk of VAPP.

Diphtheria, tetanus and acellular pertussis (DTaP)

A change has been made from using whole-cell pertussis vaccine to using acellular pertussis, which has been shown to be just as effective at protecting babies from whooping cough. The acellular vaccine causes fewer minor reactions of the type that was previously associated with the whole-cell vaccine. Due to the re-emergence of pertussis a booster dose in adolescence replaced Td in a number of countries.

Thiomersal

Thiomersal is a mercury-based preservative that has been used in some vaccines to prevent microbial contamination, or in the process of producing inactivated vaccines. Recently concern has been raised over the safety of thiomersal in vaccines, particularly regarding organo-mercury compounds linked to neurotoxicity.

All vaccines in the childhood immunization programme are now thiomersal-free in order to meet with World Health Organization (WHO) and internationally agreed aims of reducing the exposure of children to mercury where it can be avoided and where a safe effective alternative can be provided.

Additional vaccines available for children in selected European countries

Tuberculosis (TB, Ch. 43)

BCG (bacille Calmette-Guérin) targeting neonatal and other at-risk children is used in some European countries depending on local epidemiology.

The WHO recommendations to receive BCG are:

- All infants living in areas where the incidence of smear positive pulmonary TB is greater than 5/100 000, or an average risk of TB is <1%
- High risk neonates and infants in low TB burden countries
- Previously unvaccinated recent immigrants from high-prevalence countries
- Unvaccinated, tuberculin negative individuals exposed to *Mycobacterium tuberculosis* (Mtb).

The contact recommendations remain unchanged. The Mantoux test will be the standard method of tuberculin skin testing.

Pneumococcal vaccines

There are two types of pneumococcal vaccine: pneumococcal conjugate vaccine and pneumococcal polysaccharide vaccine.

Pneumococcal conjugate vaccine (PCV)

This contains polysaccharide from seven common capsular types, which are then conjugated to protein using similar technology to that for Hib and MenC vaccines. The seven capsular types cause about 66% of all pneumococcal disease and 82% of pneumococcal disease in children less than 5 years. The pneumococcal conjugate vaccine is recommended for all children aged between 2 months and 5 years. Newer pneumococcal conjugate vaccines (PCV-10, PCV-13) are already on the market or will soon be available in Europe.

Pneumococcal polysaccharide vaccine (PPV)

This can be used for adults and children over the age of 2 years. The antibodies it produces help protect against 23 types of pneumococcal bacteria, which cause about 96% of pneumococcal disease, though immunity declines with time and cannot be boosted. Its use in children is limited to those over the age of 2 years with high risk of pneumococcal invasive disease.

Hepatitis B

Some European countries recommend universal Hep B vaccine (HBV) for all babies, while others, depending on local epidemiology, recommend HBV for babies, whose mothers or close family have been infected with hepatitis B. The evidence so far suggests that people who develop immunity after vaccination stay immune for life.

Rotavirus (RV) gastroenteritis

Recently two different live, attenuated oral vaccines have been introduced for the prevention of rotavirus gastroenteritis for infants less than 6 months old.

Influenza

In the majority of European countries inactivated, trivalent seasonal viral vaccines are recommended against influenza for infants from 6 to 24–60 months and also for children at high risk for complications.

Chickenpox

A live attenuated varicella-zoster virus vaccine against chickenpox is available and incorporated into general recommendations in selected European countries.

Human papillomavirus (HPV) vaccines

There is convincing evidence for the role of HPVs in cervical cancer. The implementation of HPV vaccines into adolescent immunization programmes is a great challenge in European countries.

Tick borne encephalitis (TBE) vaccines

Inactivated viral vaccines are recommended for children over 12 months of age living in affected areas.

Hepatitis A (HAV)

Inactivated HAV viral vaccines against infectious hepatitis A is recommended for children living in high endemic areas and for those traveling to such places and/or having chronic liver disease of any etiology.

http://www.immunisation.org.uk
http://www.dh.gov.uk/en/Publichealth/
Healthprotection/Immunisation/Greenbook/
DH_145
http://www.who.int/immunization/documents/
positionpapers_intro/en

http://www.euvac.net

http://ecdc.europa.eu/en/activities/
diseaseprogrammes/Pages/Programme_on_
vaccine_preventable_diseases_and_invasive_
bacterial_infections.aspx

http://www.who.int/immunization_safety/
safety_quality/approved_vaccine_safety_
websites/en/index.html

http://www.euro.who.int/vaccine

Maintaining coverage in the face of complacency

Today it is clear that fear of the vaccine-preventable diseases has declined. Many parents will never see a case of measles. Whilst fear of the diseases themselves

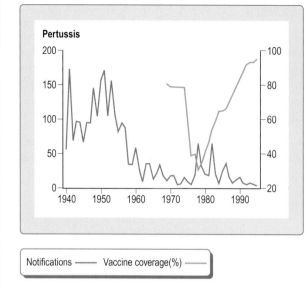

Fig. 16.1 Graph showing relationship between coverage and notifications of pertussis disease

has diminished, fear of the potential side-effects has increased, especially since it requires parents taking a proactive step to give their child vaccinations. In the 1970s, many parents were concerned about a possible link between pertussis immunization and 'brain damage', with major consequences for the uptake and consequent protection of the child population from pertussis disease (Fig. 16.1).

Overwhelming evidence shows the benefits and safety of childhood vaccination, and whilst it may seem that parental concern is misplaced, these are genuine anxieties that should be treated seriously and sympathetically whilst being countered with evidence from robust scientific trials.

MMR: the facts

Parents have been refusing MMR vaccine based on a belief that it is associated with autism. No vaccine has ever been studied in as much detail as MMR, and making a decision on whether to immunize with MMR should be easy for both doctors and parents, but it is the most frequently questioned and contested of all vaccines by parents from all walks of life.

The Wakefield et al study published in the Lancet in 1998 actually said, 'We did not prove an association between MMR vaccine and the syndrome described' and none of the studies since has found a link.

A review of the case histories of all autistic children born in the North Thames region between 1979 and 1994 (the time before and after the introduction of MMR in the UK in 1988) found:

- No increase in autism associated with the introduction of MMR in 1998

- No difference in age of diagnosis of autism between children who had been immunized with MMR and unimmunized children
- No difference in the MMR immunization rates between those children with autism and the general population in North Thames
- No link between the timing of MMR and the onset of autism.

It concluded there was no causal link between the MMR vaccine and autism.

Parents should be informed of all the ongoing trials and given the opportunity to study the evidence by themselves. They may worry that they cannot trust 'the government' but it should be remembered that vaccines are recommended for children on the advice of independent expert groups:

- The Royal College of Paediatrics and Child Health, the Health Protection Agency and the WHO all have a responsibility and mission to protect health and each recommends the MMR.
- MMR is the vaccine of choice in 90 countries.
- Single vaccines leave children vulnerable to diseases for longer periods of time.
- Past experience shows that uptake of single vaccines will be much lower.
- It is unfair and unkind to give children six injections when they can be better protected by just two.

http://www.immunisation.nhs.uk/Vaccines/MMR

Some frequent parental concerns

- *Vaccines cause long-term side-effects.* On the contrary, there is strong evidence to support the fact that allowing children to develop infections that were once considered part of growing up is much more dangerous.
- *Vaccines cause disease.* Vaccines have been linked to autism, bowel disease, brain damage, diabetes, multiple sclerosis and rheumatoid arthritis. No robust trials have ever proved this link. Many robust trials have indeed failed to find any link.
- *Vaccines do not work.* Evidence from notifiable disease statistics testifies to the dramatic drop in measles, mumps and rubella incidence, the almost complete eradication of Hib meningitis in European countries and the plummeting incidence of group C meningitis.
- *Clean water and healthy living are better than vaccines.* Undoubtedly these contribute to the decrease in spread of diseases but living standards increased in the 1960s and 1970s and whooping cough came back when vaccination coverage fell.

Table 16.2 Contraindications to immunization

General contraindications	What to do
Acute illness with fever or systemic upset	Immunization should be postponed until recovery has occurred in order to ensure symptoms are not wrongly attributed to an adverse vaccine reaction. Minor illness is not a reason to postpone immunization
Hypersensitivity or previous anaphylactic reaction to egg	Previous anaphylactic reaction to egg contraindicates influenza and yellow fever vaccines. MMR vaccine can be given safely

- *Multiple vaccines 'overload' the child's immune system.* From birth the immune system copes with many challenges every day. Highly purified, safety-tested vaccine is introduced into muscle tissue at the lowest effective dose, causing a natural immune response.

The bottom line is that having a vaccine is safer than having the disease.

Indications and contraindications

Withholding immunization may have consequences for both the individual concerned and the general public; therefore serious consideration should be given to all risks and benefits before taking this step. No opportunity for immunizing children should be missed, and so when in any doubt, advice should be sought from a consultant paediatrician, a consultant in communicable disease control or the immunization coordinator based in the local public health service. Hospitals may provide specialist immunization clinics for those children thought to be at high risk from severe adverse reactions. Contraindications to immunizations are shown in Table 16.2.

Siblings and close contacts of immunosuppressed children should be immunized against measles, mumps, rubella and chickenpox.

Conditions that are *not* contraindications

- Personal history of seizure not associated with fever (with no evidence of neurological deterioration)
- Personal history of seizure associated with fever with no evidence of neurological deterioration (but advice to be given on management of fever)
- Family history of seizures or any adverse reaction post-immunization

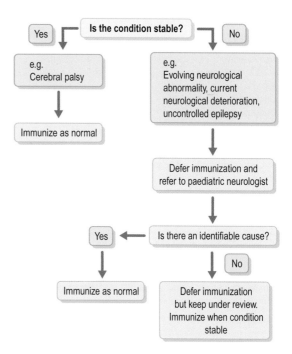

Fig. 16.2 Neurological conditions prior to immunization

- Previous history of natural pertussis, measles, rubella or mumps infection
- Contact with an infectious disease
- Asthma or hay fever
- Personal or family history of autistic spectrum disorders or inflammatory bowel disease
- Treatment with antibiotics or topical or inhaled steroids
- Breastfed child
- Pregnancy of child's mother
- History of neonatal jaundice
- Being under a certain weight
- Surgery (neither is recent immunization a contraindication to surgery or anaesthesia).

There are a number of 'special risk' groups where further consideration of the risks of the disease or vaccination need to be considered (Table 16.3). Figure 16.2 shows an algorithm for children with neurological disease.

http://www.ncbi.nlm.nih.gov/pubmed/19252428

Vaccination in the immunocompromised child: a probe of immune reconstitution.

Live vaccines — special risk groups

Certain individuals cannot mount a normal immune response to live vaccines and could suffer from severe complications, such as disseminated BCG infection. Do not offer live vaccines to the following:

Table 16.3 Special risk groups

Special risk groups	What to do

Certain conditions increase the risk of complications from infectious diseases, e.g.
    Asthma
    Chronic lung disease
    Congenital heart disease
    Down syndrome
    HIV (not all routine vaccines — see below)
    Small-for-dates babies
    Premature babies — the schedule should start from 2 months after their birth *not* from their expected due date
	Immunize as a matter of priority following routine schedule

Unimmunized children	Assume they are unimmunized and begin a full course of immunization following the standard schedule with some modifications for those 10 years and over
Uncertain immunization histories	Assume they are unimmunized and begin a full course of immunization following the standard schedule with some modification for those 10 years and over
Incomplete but known immunization history: for example, from coming to the UK part way through	Start on the routine schedule according to the child's age at presentation
Asplenia or functional hyposplenia increase the risk of bacterial infections, most commonly due to encapsulated organisms, particularly in the first 2 years after splenectomy	Follow the routine schedule and *also* give pneumococcal vaccine, Hib vaccine, influenza, meningococcal A and C
Haemodialysis increases the risk of hepatitis B and C	Screen patients for serological evidence of hepatitis B immunity; antibody-negative patients should receive three doses of hepatitis B vaccine
Renal transplant recipients and those with chronic renal disease	Consider annual influenza immunization, Hib and pneumococcal immunization

- All patients treated currently or within last 6 months with chemotherapy or radiotherapy for malignant disease
- All post-operative organ transplant patients currently on immunosuppressant drugs
- All patients receiving a bone marrow transplant within the last 6 months
- Children receiving prednisolone at a daily dose of 2 mg/kg for at least 1 week or 1 mg/kg/day for 1 month
- Patients with evidence of impaired cell-mediated immunity: for example, HIV-positive patients with current symptoms, those with severe combined immunodeficiency syndrome, those with DiGeorge syndrome.

Individuals from this list, who are exposed to measles or chickenpox and are susceptible on the grounds of history or antibody titres, should be given the appropriate immunoglobulin as soon as possible.

HIV-positive children

Whether or not they have symptoms, these children should receive the following:
- *Live vaccines*: MMR
- *Inactivated vaccines*: inactivated polio vaccine, pertussis; diphtheria; tetanus; polio; typhoid; cholera; hepatitis B and Hib

- *Contraindicated*: BCG vaccination
- *May also receive*: pneumococcal, rabies, hepatitis A and meningococcal A and C vaccines.

Safety of the yellow fever vaccine is not established; therefore it is contraindicated.

Consider measles, chickenpox or zoster normal immunoglobulin after exposure.

Principles of outbreak control — the UK example

It is not uncommon for the paediatric team to be asked for advice about control of an outbreak of an infectious disease in either a home, a nursery or a school setting. Meningococcal disease (Ch. 43) is a good example.

The peak ages for meningococcal disease are in children under 5 (especially infants) and in the late teens (15–19 years, including first-year college students). MenC vaccine is now given as part of the routine UK schedule to infants and is available to young people if they are under 24 years of age and unimmunized. During the first winter after its introduction in 1999 there was a 75% reduction in incidence of group C disease in children under 1 and in young people between 15 and 17 years (Fig. 16.3). The previous year had seen 1500 cases of group C disease, with 150 deaths.

Meningococcal disease is communicable and close, i.e. household or mouth-kissing, contacts are at

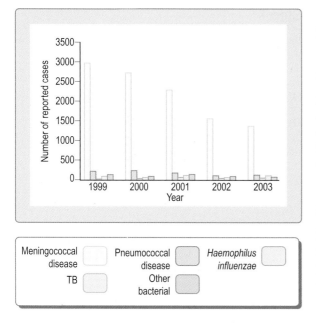

Meningococcal disease | Pneumococcal disease | *Haemophilus influenzae*

TB | Other bacterial

Fig. 16.3 Reported cases of meningococcal disease and other bacterial meningitis, England and Wales, 1999–2003

increased risk; however, the risk of a secondary case is only about 1 in 200.

Between 5 and 10% of adults carry meningococcus in the nasopharynx, whilst 25% of young adults, especially those living in close proximity in boarding schools or residential establishments, may be carriers. Smoking and concurrent upper respiratory tract infections (URTIs) increase the risk of invasive disease.

Public health responsibilities

Below are given some of the steps you need to consider.

Step 1

Decide whether the case is confirmed, probable or possible:
- *Confirmed case*: invasive disease (meningitis, septicaemia, or infection of otherwise normally sterile tissue) in which *Neisseria meningitidis* has been isolated or identified
- *Probable case*: clinical diagnosis in which the Health Protection Team, in consultation with the clinician managing the case, considers that meningococcal disease is the likeliest diagnosis
- *Possible case*: as for probable, but it is considered that diagnoses other than meningococcal disease are at least as likely (including cases treated with antibiotics whose probable diagnosis is viral meningitis).

Public health action is required for confirmed and probable cases only.

Step 2

Ensure specimens are taken to maximize the possibility of identification of the organism; throat swab, blood culture and polymerase chain reaction (PCR) on EDTA blood, and acute serum should always be carried out. Consider a cerebrospinal fluid/rash aspirate.

Step 3

Identify the group of close contacts and ensure they receive appropriate prophylaxis within 24 hours when possible:
- Rifampicin, ciprofloxacin and ceftriaxone are all recommended for use in preventing secondary cases of meningococcal disease, but rifampicin is the only antibacterial licensed for this purpose. Rifampicin is recommended for all age groups. Ciprofloxacin is recommended as an alternative agent to rifampicin in adults and children aged 5 years and above.
- Close contacts of confirmed cases due to vaccine-preventable strains of *N. meningitidis* (A, C, W135 and Y) should be offered vaccination up to 4 weeks after onset of symptoms in the index case.
- MenC vaccine should be offered to all unimmunized index cases under 25 years, irrespective of serogroup found.

Chemoprophylaxis acts in two ways: by eradicating carriage in established carriers who pose a risk of infection to others, and by eradicating carriage in those who have newly acquired the invasive strain and who may themselves be at risk. There is a small risk of meningitis developing in contacts, even if they are given prophylaxis; therefore, close contacts should be made aware of key meningitis symptoms and advised to seek urgent medical treatment if they occur.

Chemoprophylaxis is rarely required for cases now that first-line treatment is with ceftriaxone, which efficiently eradicates carriage.

Step 4

Give advice and information about the risks of secondary cases.

Risks of second cases within 4 weeks are as follows:
- *Background risk*: 2–6 in 100 000
- *Household members*: 1 in 300 if prophylaxis not given
- *Pre-school group*: 1 in 1500
- *Primary school child*: 1 in 18 000
- *Secondary school student*: 1 in 33 000.

Step 5

Investigate whether there are linked cases. If there is a second related case, e.g. in the same school, this constitutes an outbreak and would require a multidisciplinary Outbreak Control Team to manage it.

Step 6

Liaise with and inform primary care physicians, employers and head teachers, where appropriate.

Step 7

Be available to reassure the public when the case reaches the media.

Step 8

Decide who else needs to be informed.

Rachel Crowther   Giorgio Tamburlini

Health promotion and disease prevention

LEARNING OUTCOMES

By the end of this chapter you should:

- Understand the terms health promotion, disease prevention and health protection, and how these relate to child and adolescent health
- Understand the importance of thinking 'upstream' about the determinants of health
- Understand why improving the health of the population is everyone's concern and the importance of partnership working to improve health
- Know about different approaches to improving health
- Appreciate the different levels at which health promotion and disease prevention can operate
- Be able to suggest examples of health promotion and disease prevention at various levels for different conditions relevant to child and adolescent health
- Understand the difference between universal and targeted approaches to health promotion and disease prevention and the 'population paradox'
- Be aware of opportunities for health promotion in everyday practice, and the skills required to be a health-promoting doctor.

MODULE THREE

Health and health improvement

Definitions and meanings are important in the area of health promotion and preventive health care because they help to identify what we are trying to achieve. Before reading further, think for a moment about what you understand by the following terms, which will be explored in this chapter. How easy is it to come up with succinct definitions?

- Health
- Health improvement
- Health promotion
- Health protection
- Disease prevention.

- The absence of disease (medical or deficit model)
- A state of complete physical, mental and social wellbeing and not merely the absence of disease or infirmity (WHO)
- A function of individual lifestyle, the environment, human biology and healthcare provision (Lalonde)
- The ability to realize aspirations, satisfy needs and change or learn to cope with the environment
- A resource for living, not the object of living … a positive concept emphasizing social and personal resources as well as physical capabilities (Ottawa Charter for Health Promotion 1986)

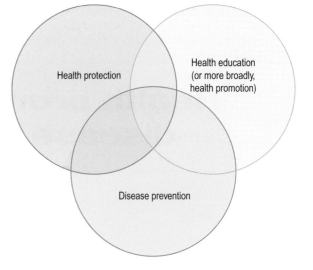

Fig. 17.1 **Summary of different means of improving health**

What is health?

Although it may seem a straightforward concept, the question of what health is, and how to define it, has generated considerable debate. Doctors have tended to see it simply as an absence of disease — sometimes called the 'deficit model', since it does not recognize the positive aspects of good health. The World Health Organization (WHO) has addressed this shortcoming in its much-used (though arguably rather idealistic) definition, which conceives of health as a state of complete wellbeing. Others have seen it in terms of its determinants — what affects health — or in terms of function: not what health is, but what it enables us to do.

Some commonly used definitions of health are listed in Box 17.1. The most appropriate choice depends partly on the circumstances, but in the field of health promotion, when we are seeking to foster optimum health across a population, a wider interpretation is needed that embraces the notion of wellbeing and includes different dimensions of health.

Health improvement

'Health improvement' is often used in a very general way to encompass all activities that aim to enhance health — including both preventive and curative medical services, and other functions undertaken by a wide range of organizations and individuals. Health improvement plans have been used, for example, as a means of setting out clearly the means by which national and local health authorities and other partners aim to maximize the health of their population.

In this chapter, health improvement is defined more narrowly, as a broad term for 'upstream' interventions that tackle the determinants of health, as opposed to 'downstream' therapeutic interventions. Acting upstream to prevent ill health and to promote health in its broadest sense is one of the key features of public health and, as will become clear in this chapter, improving health is an important responsibility for everyone involved in health care, as well as many other fields of public and private life. Different means of improving health have been summarized by Tannahill (Fig. 17.1).

Health protection involves a wide range of activities that aim to protect the population from hazards, including infectious diseases, environmental threats and child abuse and neglect. These activities are usually provided by a variety of agencies and functions. The term has also been used to describe other measures such as seatbelt legislation, usually introduced (and often enforced) by the government or government agencies.

Whose responsibility is health improvement?

Improving health is an essential component of any health system's agenda; indeed, if the health of the population is not improved by the combined activities of the health authorities, then it might be seen to have failed in its main purpose. International agencies such as the World Health Organization, the European Commission and national governments have recently placed increasing emphasis on prevention, and on making health improvement the responsibility of all health professionals. Health professionals' commitment to improving health as well as tackling disease is vital. This is especially so in the case of children: all professionals share a responsibility to protect and care for children and to promote their best interests, and this includes action along the life cycle from the periconceptional period to adolescence, to ensure the best possible health for them, now and in the future.

It is also very important to recognize that improving health is not just the business of the health authorities. A very wide variety of factors affect health, many of which are beyond the scope of health professionals; consider, for example, poverty, traffic, pollution, parenting and school attendance, to name just a few key influences on child health. Partnership working is therefore crucial, and our achievements would be severely limited if we were to ignore the potential contribution of others.

Evidence-based health improvement

The value of evidence-based medicine is well established in medical practice and education. It is just as important in public health practice as in clinical practice to ensure that what we do is effective and makes the best use of scarce resources, but it is less easy to establish an evidence base for health improvement than it is for many therapeutic interventions. Evidence-based medicine relevant to this course is discussed in Chapter 13.

Disease prevention

Disease prevention can be seen as the 'medical' end of the health improvement spectrum, related to the deficit model (health as absence of disease) rather than the positive WHO model. It tends to focus on the prevention of specific diseases or conditions, but quite often involves reducing risk factors that have a more general benefit for health; for example, tackling obesity to prevent type 2 diabetes in children confers many other advantages too. Three different levels of prevention are usually described.

Primary prevention

This involves stopping a disease, condition or insult from occurring in the first place.

Examples include the prevention of:
- Infectious diseases, by immunization and breastfeeding
- Sudden unexplained death in infancy (SUDI, SIDS), through the 'Back to Sleep' campaign
- Child abuse, through interventions to support vulnerable children and families
- Teenage pregnancy through the provision of appropriate contraceptive advice

- Neural tube defects, by encouraging folic acid consumption before conception and in early pregnancy.

Secondary prevention

This involves preventing or mitigating the *effects* of a disease, condition or insult, often by identifying it early so treatment is more effective. Examples include child health screening programmes.

N.B. Sometimes 'secondary prevention' is used in a different way, to mean preventing recurrence after a first episode: for example, of child abuse.

Tertiary prevention

This involves slowing the progress and/or managing the consequences of an established disease, condition or insult.

Examples include:
- Optimum management of children with chronic diseases, such as diabetes mellitus, asthma or cystic fibrosis, to maximize their health (now and in the longer term) and minimize the impact of the disease on the child's everyday life
- Appropriate education, therapy (physiotherapy, occupational therapy, speech and language therapy), medical treatment and family support for a child with complex disabilities (pp. 202–203).

Example: dental caries

The prevention of dental caries offers a good illustration of preventive action at all three levels.

Primary prevention

- Fluoridation of the water supply
- Regular tooth-brushing and good oral hygiene (involves providing advice to parents and children through a range of channels — dental health promotion)
- Avoiding sweets and fizzy drinks, or limiting them to specific times after meals (involves providing advice — link to nutrition and healthy eating, and the prevention of obesity)
- Fissure sealants (preventive dental care).

Secondary prevention

- Regular dental checkups to ensure decay is spotted and treated early (involves ensuring that

all children in the local area have access to NHS dentistry)
- Identifying gingivitis and advising on treatment
- Removal of plaque by hygienist.

Tertiary prevention

- Filling of cavities — or in extreme cases, removal of teeth.

Example: childhood injuries

Key facts

- Childhood injury prevention has been very successful; the number of deaths in many European countries has dropped significantly in recent years.
- However, injuries and accidents remain very common; on average, 1 in 5 children attend the accident and emergency department each year, having sustained an injury. 'Injury and poisoning' is a leading cause of death in children (p. 152) and also causes significant morbidity.
- There is a strong social class gradient in childhood injuries, with those in lower socioeconomic groups being most at risk.
- Non-accidental injury is an important cause that must always be borne in mind.
- Childhood injuries occur in many different settings — at home, on the roads, in other public places — as the clinical histories below illustrate. Head injuries, and other types of injury, can occur at any age, but the patterns vary at different ages. Common types of injury include:
  - *Toddlers*: falls, scalds, poisoning, drowning
  - *Older children*: road traffic accidents (usually as pedestrian or cyclist), and injuries sustained while playing sport
  - *Adolescents*: often related to risk behaviour— joy riding, extreme sports, experimenting with substance use etc.

Problem-orientated topic:

head injury ● ● ● ● ●

Three children have been admitted to the local hospital via the accident and emergency department in the last fortnight with moderate to severe head injuries.

Jonas is 18 months old and was brought to hospital by ambulance after falling at home. His mother was out at the time, running an errand for her mother-in-law, and Jonas was being looked after by his 6-year-old brother and an uncle with learning difficulties. The history is confused but the brother reports that Jonas wanted to come downstairs, and when they tried to stop him the toddler screamed and struggled and eventually fell down the stairs, landing on the uncarpeted floor in the hall.

Janina is 2¹/₂ years old and sustained her injury in the local supermarket while out shopping with her mother. She had refused to be strapped into the trolley and insisted on climbing to and fro between the main part of the trolley and the seat at the back, helping herself to chocolate biscuits, while her mother made her way round the shop. A member of the public was worried by her behaviour and tried to intervene, whereupon Janina became angry and frightened and lost her balance, falling head-first on to the tiled floor. She was unconscious on arrival.

Andrius is 10 and was out with friends riding his bike around their housing estate at dusk. When a car came round the corner he tried to swerve to the side of the road but lost control of the bike, colliding with the car's bumper, and was thrown across the road and on to the pavement. He was not wearing a cycle helmet or any reflective clothing. The other children reported that the car was going 'very fast', but it may not have been travelling over the 50 kilometres an hour speed limit. The council has recently put up signs on the roads in the estate warning motorists of children playing nearby, and has been deliberating about imposing a 35 kilometres an hour limit and installing speed bumps and other traffic calming measures to help enforce it. Andrius had multiple injuries including a skull fracture.

Q1. What could be done to prevent these injuries?

Q2. Can you give examples of primary, secondary and tertiary preventive measures?

Q1. What could be done to prevent these injuries?

It can be helpful to think about the kinds of action that can be taken at different organizational levels — individual, community/environment and policy (p. 184) — and by different agencies. For example:

Individual level
- Advice to parents and children from health visitors, primary care paediatricians, family doctors, school nurses and others
- Providing access to safety equipment for those who cannot afford it.

Community/environmental level
- Action by supermarkets to encourage the use of safety straps in trolleys
- Action by local authorities to improve road safety (traffic calming, safe areas for playing, cycle lanes)
- Installing soft flooring in community playgrounds and other improvements to the environment to protect or separate children from hazards.

National/policy level
- Legislation on seatbelts
- Reduction of speed limits in built-up areas.

Q2. Can you give examples of primary, secondary and tertiary preventive measures?

Primary prevention — preventing accidents from occurring
Examples include:
- Promoting the use of safety equipment such as stair gates, safety harnesses and fluorescent clothing for cyclists. Approaches include individual advice to parents from health visitors, primary care paediatricians, family doctors and others; health education in schools; programmes linked to hospital accident and emergency departments (e.g. injury minimization and prevention — IMPS) and media campaigns to raise awareness of hazards.
- Promoting road safety to reduce the likelihood of road traffic accidents. Approaches include cycle proficiency training, traffic calming and the provision of cycle lanes and safe areas to play and cycle (e.g. parks with cycle tracks).

Secondary prevention — mitigating the impact of accidents and reducing the likelihood of them resulting in serious injury
Examples include:
- Promoting the use of seatbelts in cars, cycle helmets etc. Approaches may be similar to those

---

BOX 17.2 Exercise

Can you apply the same approach to identify examples of primary, secondary and tertiary prevention for congenital malformations and meningococcal disease?

Prevention of congenital malformations: some examples
- *Primary*: folic acid before conception and in early pregnancy; advice on nutrition and other activities in pregnancy to avoid listeria and toxoplasmosis
- *Secondary*: antenatal screening to pick up malformations early and offer information/termination
- *Tertiary*: information/support/discussion of treatment options after delivery

Prevention of meningococcal disease: some examples
- *Primary*: immunization (especially group C)
- *Secondary*: prophylaxis for contacts after a single case
- *Tertiary*: rehabilitation for children damaged by meningitis, e.g. providing hearing aids for those with deafness resulting from the disease

---

listed above, but also include legislation (e.g. for seatbelts, motorcycle helmets).

Secondary prevention — preventing a second episode
Examples include:
- Offering support to families where children are at risk of injury through poverty, poor supervision or neglect (in extreme cases) through the child protection system.

Tertiary prevention — managing the consequences of injury
Examples include:
- Provision of effective emergency services, neurosurgical units and rehabilitation facilities to optimize the long-term outcome for children with head injuries.

More examples are given in Box 17.2.

Health promotion

Health promotion is a broader endeavour than disease prevention. The definitions in Box 17.3 capture the key features of health promotion.

The aims of health promotion

Health promotion seeks to benefit both individuals and whole populations. At the individual level, it is most

Health promotion is:

- 'The process of enabling people to increase control over the determinants of health and thereby improve their health' (Nutbeam 1985)
- 'Any activity or program designed to improve social and environmental living conditions such that people's experience of well-being is increased' (Labonte & Little 1992)
- 'A combination of health education and related organizational, political and economic programs designed to support changes in behavior and in the environment that will improve health' (US Department of Health, Education and Welfare 1979)

simply seen as aiming to improve physical, mental and social wellbeing. At population level, the WHO (Health for All in Europe) sets out the aspirations of health promotion as follows:

- *To ensure equity in health* by reducing gaps in health status between and within countries
- *To add life to years* by ensuring the full development and use of people's physical and mental capacity to derive full benefit from life
- *To add health to life* by reducing disease and disability
- *To add years to life* by reducing premature deaths and thereby increasing life expectancy.

Different types of health promotion activity

The Ottawa Charter for Health Promotion (1986) defined five aspects of health promotion, which provide a useful overview of activities in this field:

1. **Building healthy public policy,** e.g.:
   - Taking account of the health impact of all policy decisions — such as the design of new buildings and roads
   - Legislation — including regulations to protect, promote and support breastfeeding, laws on seatbelts, drink-driving, and restrictions on the sale of tobacco, solvents and alcohol
   - Fiscal policy — including taxes on fuel, cigarettes and alcohol
2. **Creating supportive environments,** e.g.:
   - Local and national policies on transport and smoking
   - Encouraging active transport — walking and cycling
   - Increasing the availability and accessibility of healthy food
   - Making healthy choices easier in every aspect of life

3. **Strengthening communities,** e.g.:
   - Encouraging genuine participation and involvement in local democracy
   - Promoting ownership and control by communities, and enabling them to make decisions about issues affecting their health and to set priorities for action
4. **Reorienting health services,** e.g.:
   - Improving access and reducing inequalities in health service provision
   - Focusing on the health needs of the individual as a whole person rather than on the illness, and sharing power in decision-making
5. **Developing personal knowledge and skills,** e.g.:
   - Providing information and health education
   - Promoting problem-solving and coping skills to help individuals increase control over their health.

Health promotion can thus operate in many different ways and at many different levels. A simpler framework considers action at:

- *Individual level* (e.g. health education and empowerment)
- *Community level* (e.g. social action and community development)
- *Policy level* (e.g. lobbying and advocacy directed at healthy public policy).

It is always more effective to combine action at two or three different levels than to focus only on one, and to involve as wide a range of stakeholders as possible. Health promotion is very much about partnership: with individuals and communities, with other statutory and voluntary agencies, and with the worlds of commerce and the media.

Health promotion at individual level

In the past, there was a tendency to perceive individual-level health promotion as a matter of simply instructing people as to how to live and act in order to be healthy, and seeing it as their own responsibility to make the necessary changes (giving up smoking, losing weight, taking more exercise etc.) to achieve better health. Although individual responsibility and control is an important concept, there is much greater understanding now of the impact of societal and environmental constraints on choices and behaviour; hence the emphasis on structural and social changes to make healthy choices easier (e.g. walking or cycling to school rather than driving children there; eating five pieces of fresh fruit and vegetables a day). This is particularly the case for children. Box 17.4 below summarizes some of the key influences on 'lifestyle choices' for children of different ages.

Infancy and early childhood

- Choices are largely made by parents or other adults, e.g. breast- vs formula feeding; weaning and later diet; second-hand smoking; sleeping position; leisure pursuits (television, playing outside); parenting style, affection and control
- Parental choices are heavily constrained by factors such as cost, convenience, knowledge and perceptions, habit and cultural norms

Later childhood

- Children have increasing scope to make decisions for themselves (e.g. meals at school, physical activity, experimenting with tobacco, alcohol and other substances) and also have an influence over their parents and carers through 'pester power'
- Children's habits and decisions are strongly shaped by parental and family norms, by peer pressure, by media campaigns aimed at children, and, as for adults, by cost and convenience

Health education

There is still, nevertheless, an important role for health education, which was defined by Ewles and Simnett as 'planned interventions or programmes for people to learn about health, and to undertake voluntary changes in their behaviour'. In terms of the Ottawa Charter categories set out above, this involves developing personal knowledge and skills.

Health education is often delivered to individuals in groups (e.g. children in schools) and includes not simply providing information, but also building skills and self-esteem. The key outcome is often seen as improved *health literacy*, defined by Nutbeam as 'cognitive and social skills which determine the motivation and ability of individuals to gain access to, and understand and use information in ways that promote health'. Health education is an active, rather than a passive, activity, recognizing that interventions to change behaviour and lifestyle can only succeed through individuals' conscious participation.

Empowerment

Another important concept in the field of individual health promotion is that of empowerment, defined as the process of helping people to develop a sense of:

- *Agency* (the ability to have an influence on the world)
- *Self-efficacy* (belief in the capacity to have an influence)
- *Personal autonomy* (the ability to speak and act independently of others).

Together, these enable individuals to take charge of their own destinies and their health.

Health promotion at community level

Community level health promotion is important for a number of reasons:

- The physical and social environment has a powerful influence on health, both directly (e.g. pollution, bullying) and indirectly, by affecting individual behaviour (e.g. choices about food), and the local environment is best tackled through a local approach.
- There are important group effects when programmes operate at the level of settings (e.g. schools, young offenders' institutions), involving all members of these communities and seeking to improve policies, ethos and culture (p. 190).
- The participation of users in the planning and running of services makes them more appropriate to the local population.
- Communities have untapped resources that may be directed towards promoting health concerns.
- People have the right and responsibility to be involved in improving their collective life.

In terms of the Ottawa Charter categories set out above, action at this level includes creating supportive environments and strengthening communities.

Community development

Community development involves working with a community (which may be a village, a housing estate, a school, or an interest group such as a parents' collective) to identify areas of concern and to improve health and wellbeing. It is 'done with' the community rather than 'done to' them and indeed, in an ideal world, involves only minimal support and advice from 'experts' to encourage and enable local action.

Healthy Schools

The European Network of Health Promoting Schools emphasizes the entire organization of the school as well as focusing upon the individual. At the heart of the model is the young person, who is viewed as a whole individual within a dynamic environment. Such an approach creates a highly supportive social setting which influences the visions, perceptions and actions of all who live, work, play and learn in the school.

http://www.euro.who.int/document/e74993.pdf

For example, the UK National Health School Programme focuses on a whole-school approach to the five national outcomes for children:

- Being healthy
- Staying safe
- Enjoying and achieving
- Making a positive contribution
- Achieving economic wellbeing.

There are four core themes for healthy schools:

- *Personal, social and health education,* including sex and relationship education and drug education (alcohol, tobacco and volatile substance abuse)
- *Healthy eating*
- *Physical activity*
- *Emotional health and wellbeing* (including bullying).

The government of the UK aims to involve every school in the programme. The aims include supporting children and young people in developing healthy behaviours, helping to reduce health inequalities and promoting social inclusion. The intended benefits for schools as a whole include:

- Improving behaviour and attendance (schools with Healthy School status have less fear of bullying)
- Improving educational achievement (schools with Healthy School status have better results for government assessments at Key Stages 1 and 2)
- Reducing and halting the increase in childhood obesity
- Promoting positive sexual health and reducing teenage pregnancy
- Reducing young people's drug, alcohol and tobacco use (schools with Healthy School status have less use of illegal drugs).

The programme emphasizes pupil involvement as well as the commitment of staff, parents, governors and others associated with the school. Examples of projects that might contribute to a school achieving National Healthy Schools status include:

- Introducing a breakfast club or break-time stalls selling healthy drinks and snacks
- Introducing a school council with pupil representation to feed into policy decisions and ensure pupils' voices are heard
- Introducing a peer listening and counselling service run by pupils, for pupils
- Improving playground facilities or introducing lunch-time activity clubs.

Health promotion at policy level

The third level for health promotion involves policy: often at national level, though international (and more local) policy is important too. In terms of the Ottawa Charter categories set out above, action at this level includes building healthy public policy and reorienting health services (although the latter can also be seen as operating at local and individual level). Healthy public policy includes areas outside health, e.g. transport, education, and social and fiscal policy.

Clearly, 'high-level' decisions can have a significant impact on individuals' health — affecting, for example, their disposable income (including benefits), the cost and availability of goods, public sector service provision, their exposure to advertising and other media influences, the safety of their environment, and opportunities for employment and training. Although such decisions are largely the responsibility of local and national government, individuals can influence them not merely by participating in elections, but through advocacy and lobbying. *Advocacy* means speaking out publicly in support of an individual, group or cause, and *lobbying* means putting pressure on government: for example, to encourage healthy public policy.

Examples of health promotion and disease prevention in key areas of child health

Childhood obesity (Box 17.5 and p. 259)

The importance of the childhood obesity 'epidemic' has been recognized by International Agencies such as WHO, by the European Commission and by national governments.

The impact of childhood obesity is far-reaching, and obese children are more likely to suffer from:

- Early signs of risk factors for heart disease (e.g. high blood pressure or arterial intimal changes)
- Type 2 diabetes, traditionally 'maturity onset', which is being seen increasingly in obese children and has been dubbed 'diabesity'
- Other medical problems, including sleep apnoea, orthopaedic problems and benign intracranial hypertension
- Social isolation and bullying, poor self-esteem and depression
- Reduced mobility and lower levels of participation in sport and physical activity, which in turn perpetuate obesity
- Lower levels of educational achievement
- A higher risk of becoming obese adults (up to 25%), with all the associated long-term health

- Childhood obesity is a growing problem. Surveys have shown the prevalence of overweight among school age children to be as high as 35% in many European countries and some of them have reported prevalence rates increasing year by year
- Annual increases in prevalence of overweight children (including obesity) rose from typically below 0.5 percentage points in the 1980s, to over 1.0 percentage points in the late 1990s. Obesity rates have doubled in 6-year-olds and trebled in 15-year-olds in the last 10 years
- Rates are higher for girls than boys: up to 30% of girls aged 2–15 are overweight or obese in some areas of England
- If the increase continues, parents' life expectancy may exceed their children's, with obesity becoming the chief cause of premature death
- Both energy input (diet) and output (physical activity) play a part
- Children eat on average double the necessary amounts of saturated fat, salt and sugar per day
- 40% of boys and 60% of girls get less than the recommended hour of physical activity a day

risks. The risks are even higher if both parents are overweight or obesity persists into adolescence.

Action to tackle obesity

Childhood obesity is a key public health problem that needs a collaborative, multisectoral approach. Since treatment is difficult and of limited effectiveness, the emphasis must be on prevention. Concerted action is needed, which tackles both the input and output sides of the equation, operates at different levels and involves a wide range of stakeholders and agencies.

Examples of action at different levels might include:
- Physical activity:
  - *At individual level*: exercise prescriptions, cycle proficiency training
  - *At community level*: better and more equitable access to local leisure facilities and sports clubs
  - *At policy level*: transport policy designed to promote walking and cycling and reduce traffic danger to child pedestrians and cyclists
- Food:
  - *At individual level*: classroom activities to teach children about healthy eating and food preparation
  - *At community level*: farmers' markets and local food cooperatives to increase availability of cheap, fresh, local produce
  - *At policy level*: agreement on labelling to help consumers choose healthy food.

Examples of action by different agencies might include:
- Schools (e.g. as part of the National Healthy Schools Programme):
  - 'Safe Routes to School' schemes and 'walking buses' (organized and supervised walking routes for groups of children)
  - Changing to healthy vending machines (e.g. selling fruit and other healthy snacks)
- Local authorities:
  - Allotment schemes to encourage growing fruit and vegetables
  - Improving street safety and outdoor play spaces
- Media and commercial worlds:
  - Schemes to market sport and exercise as 'cool' by celebrities
- Food manufacturers:
  - Reducing sugar, salt and fat content of food
- Supermarkets:
  - Offering ranges of fruit and vegetables to appeal to children
  - Promoting the '5 a Day' message
- Agriculture:
  - Research into production of lower-fat foods
- National government:
  - Food pricing policies to shift balance away from junk foods
  - Setting nutritional standards for school catering.

The UK Health Development Agency's evidence briefing, 'Management of obesity and overweight' (Oct 2003), summarizes evidence of effectiveness of strategies to tackle obesity, including those that aim to:
- Prevent obesity and overweight in children (e.g. multifaceted school-based interventions)
- Treat obesity and overweight in children (e.g. interventions that involve parents, including exercise and behaviour modification programmes).

The available evidence for effective interventions in pre-school children indicates the need for multi-faceted interventions on micro (family) and macro (social) determinants focussed on:
- Reducing low birth weight
- Increasing breastfeeding
- Improving physical activity and nutrition
- Controlling marketing of breast milk substitutes, unhealthy foods and beverages

For school children and adolescents, the evidence indicates the need to implement multi-component interventions including providing new opportunities for physical activity, reduce TV viewing, reduce the consumption of sugar sweetened beverages. Educational interventions should not be implemented only at school or at family level, but require combined action.

MODULE THREE

187

- Attachment is determined by the quality of the early interaction between the primary caregiver and the baby
- Poor attachment leads to lower self-confidence, higher anxiety, aggression and stress, and less success in forming relationships in later childhood and adulthood
- Secure attachment leads to greater resilience to stress and adversity and seems to mitigate some of the detrimental health effects of poverty and deprivation

BOX 17.7 Parenting in later childhood

- Different styles of parenting may be 'helpful' or 'unhelpful' in nurturing the child's emotional health and self-esteem, and his or her later predisposition to conduct disorder and antisocial behaviour
- The parents' approach to discipline is particularly important; a balance is needed between clear, consistent and appropriate boundary-setting, and warmth, empathy and encouragement
- Less helpful parenting styles may be cold and punitive, overly permissive or neglectful of the child and his or her needs

Parenting

For most children, parents and families make up the closest 'layer' of their environment and constitute the most immediate influence on their health and wellbeing. Particular aspects of family life that affect children's health (apart from lifestyle factors such as eating and smoking habits, and economic factors such as employment and family income) include:

- Family size and composition, including the extended family
- Family relationships, culture and communication
- Early relationships and attachment
- Parenting skills and style
- Domestic violence, conflict and family breakup.

Parenting is an important determinant of mental health in children, and is an often-undervalued skill. Parenting is important both in very early life (e.g. establishing secure attachment to the mother in the first year) and throughout childhood (Boxes 17.6 and 17.7).

Abuse and neglect (Chs 21 and 36)

Child abuse is the most extreme example of unhelpful parenting and can have a serious and long-lasting effect on children's physical and mental health. Abuse may be physical, emotional or sexual, and severe neglect is also recognized as a form of abuse. Children who have been abused are more likely to abuse their own children and partners when they grow up, perpetuating a vicious cycle. Identifying and tackling child abuse is the responsibility of all who work with children.

Action to tackle unhelpful parenting

Individual level

- Several programmes have been shown to help promote attachment, especially for 'high-risk' mother–baby relationships (e.g. teenage mothers, mothers with mental health problems or families experiencing severe social stress).
- Interventions can also help parents of older children to alter their parenting style and improve the health and wellbeing of their children — and often themselves.
- Family support (often involving several agencies) can help prevent abuse in families where a risk has been identified.

Community level

- Some parenting programmes are offered to parents through home visiting, day-care centres and schools, and may have a component delivered directly to children in the classroom too.
- Linking to a Healthy Schools project can be helpful in achieving a consistent change throughout the child's environment.

Policy level

- Legislation and information, education and communication campaigns on physical punishment of children by parents aim to reduce violence against children, which is an inappropriate element of parenting.
- Criminal Records Bureaus' checks on all staff working with children can help prevent known abusers from coming into contact with children.
- In the case of abuse or an identified risk of abuse, all agencies working with children should have identified child protection procedures, overseen by local Area Child Protection Committees.

Sudden unexplained death in infancy (SUDI, SIDS, Ch. 49)

Risk factors for SUDI include:

- Sleeping prone
- Parental smoking
- Co-sleeping (bed-sharing) with parents, especially on a sofa or when parents have taken alcohol or drugs

- Premature and low-birth weight babies
- Children of very young mothers
- Poverty and deprivation
- Postnatal depression
- Male gender (male babies being at slightly increased risk).

Inappropriate medical advice that babies should sleep on their fronts has been blamed for a rise in SUDI deaths in the 1960s and 1970s. The rate of SUDI remained around 2 per 1000 live births in the 1970s and 1980s. Following clear evidence that prone sleeping increased the risk of SUDI, the 'Back to Sleep' (or 'Reduce the Risk') campaigns were introduced in most European countries in the 1990s, since when the rate of SUDI has fallen dramatically. This is a powerful example of a successful prevention campaign and also illustrates the importance of ensuring that the health promotion messages conveyed to parents and the population at large are the right ones.

Action to tackle SUDI

The most important aspect of prevention is consistent and appropriate advice to parents, delivered through as many routes as possible and including action at individual level (e.g. contact with health professionals), at community level (e.g. communication through antenatal and postnatal groups) and at policy level (e.g. clear policies and guidance for health professionals, supported by leaflets, media campaigns etc.).

Advice should include:

- Putting babies to sleep on their backs, with the head uncovered and feet placed to the foot of the cot to prevent wriggling down under the covers — ideally in a cot in the parents' room for the first 6 months
- Preventing the baby getting too hot
- Stopping (or reducing) smoking in pregnancy — mothers and partners
- Keeping babies away from cigarette smoke
- Avoiding co-sleeping on a sofa or armchair, or if either parent smokes, has been drinking or taking drugs, or is very tired.

Smoking

Cigarette smoking affects children's health in a variety of different ways. Smoking by parents and other adults is an important starting point, since it significantly affects a child's intrauterine and early postnatal environment and subsequent health:

- *Smoking in pregnancy* increases the risk of stillbirth, preterm delivery and low birth weight.

BOX 17.8 Smoking in children and young people

- In Europe, at the age of 15, 7–37% of boys and 7–48% of girls are weekly smokers, most of them smoking daily. The most striking feature of weekly smoking behaviour is the increase between ages 13 and 15 and the emerging variation in rates across countries.
- In the UK, 10% of 11–15-year-olds smoked regularly in 2002; rates are higher in 16–19-year-olds and are falling more slowly
- In the UK, more children from manual social classes smoke
- In the UK, girls are a particular worry: 29% of 15-year-old girls are regular smokers
- In the UK, rates are lower in young people from several ethnic minority groups: Indian, Pakistani, Bangladeshi and Chinese

Source: Health Behaviour in School-aged Children (HBSC) 2005/2006 survey and Office for National Statistics 2004 The health of children and young people

---

- *Smoking by parents or others in the household during a child's early life* increases the risk of asthma and other respiratory problems, pneumonia, meningitis, glue ear and SUDI.
- *Exposure to smoke during childhood and modelling of smoking behaviour by parents and others* increase the chances of the child taking up smoking, which confers a long and familiar list of long-term risks.

Smoking is more common in low-income families, so that children in lower social classes are more likely to be exposed to all these risks. Although young people from all social classes experiment with smoking in their teens, those from higher social classes are more likely to quit as they enter adulthood. Marketing campaigns aimed at adolescents, peer pressure and low self-esteem (e.g. related to lack of educational attainment and poor opportunities for employment) also encourage unhealthy choices in young people (Box 17.8).

Action to tackle smoking

Action can be taken at different levels:

- *Individual level*: e.g. offering information, advice, access to expert help. The availability of specialist smoking cessation services is important.
- *Community level*: e.g. interventions in schools and with community groups, enforcing ban on under-age cigarette sales.
- *Policy level*: no smoking in public places, taxation — but raising taxes on cigarettes deters rich smokers more than poor.

The UK Health Development Agency's evidence briefing, 'Smoking and Public Health' (April 2004), summarizes evidence of effectiveness of smoking cessation strategies, including:

- Deterring young people from starting smoking (e.g. school- and community-level interventions, media campaigns, interventions with tobacco retailers)
- Helping all smokers stop (e.g. role of health professionals, counselling, pricing of cigarettes, media campaigns)
- Helping pregnant women stop (e.g. giving stop smoking leaflets during routine antenatal care)
- Tackling inequalities (little evidence available).

Problem-orientated topic:

health promotion ● ● ● ● ●

You are charged with planning a health promotion programme to promote sexual health in teenage girls.

Q1. What would you aim to achieve?

Q2. Can you come up with examples of action at individual, community and policy level to illustrate how you might approach the problem?

Q1. What would you aim to achieve?

The major aim would be to reduce sexually transmitted diseases and prevent teenage pregnancy by:
- Improving access to contraceptive advice
- Improving knowledge of sex and sexual health
- Empowering young women to take charge of their bodies and control their sexual activity
- Building self-esteem (the best way to reduce under-age conceptions).

Q2. Can you come up with examples of action at individual, community and policy level to illustrate how you might approach the problem?

- *Individual level*: peer-led sessions to discuss sexual health issues and build confidence and self-esteem; Teenage Health Freak website
- *Community level*: Interventions in schools and other places attended by teenagers to offer confidential accessible information, advice and contraceptive services

BOX 17.9 Advantages of a universal approach

- Often everyone stands to benefit: e.g. from adding fluoride to drinking water to prevent caries
- No stigma attached: e.g. difference between health visiting and social services involvement
- Often hard to define who is 'at risk'; therefore treat all
- May have 'knock-on' benefits for others: e.g. herd immunity, altered attitude or behaviour in peer group
- May be easier and/or cheaper to deliver to all than to select out target group: e.g. School Fruit and Vegetable Programme

BOX 17.10 Advantages of targeted approach

- May be a better use of limited resources
- Those who perceive themselves as low-risk may ignore advice or opt out of programme, thus wasting resources
- Sometimes very clear who is at risk and who is not: e.g. by family history, sex, ethnic group
- Even if everyone would benefit a little, may be better to focus on those who could benefit a lot
- More effective for reducing inequalities (direct resources at worst off or those with poorest health, to reduce gap)

- *Policy level*: improve facilities for teenage mothers to continue their education, to try to break the cycle of deprivation and recurrence.

Universal and targeted approaches

Sometimes there is a choice between a universal approach to health promotion or disease prevention, which encompasses a whole population or community, and a targeted approach, which focuses on an identified high-risk group (e.g. defined by age, race, gender, occupation or geography) (Boxes 17.9 and 17.10).

Think about the following examples while you consider the advantages and disadvantages of each approach:
- Immunization
- Screening for thalassaemia
- Screening for Down syndrome.

Clearly much depends on the particular condition, intervention and situation. Factors to consider when choosing between universal and targeted approaches include:

- How common is the condition?
- How well defined are the risk factors (and the cutoff for the at-risk group)?
- How will the programme be delivered (e.g. media campaigns vs individual screening)?
- How will the intervention be perceived?
- How expensive is the intervention (and how expensive to select out an at-risk group)?
- Is there likely to be a 'group effect'?

The population paradox

The population paradox was described by the famous epidemiologist, Geoffrey Rose, and provides a powerful argument for the universal approach to health promotion and disease prevention. Rose noted that even when a risk factor can be clearly linked to a disease, most cases may occur in low-risk groups simply because these contain far more people. To take a simple numerical illustration, a 1 in 10 risk applied to 10 000 people will lead to 1000 cases — ten times fewer than the number of cases produced by a 1 in 100 risk applied to a million people. The classic example in adult health is serum cholesterol or blood pressure and the risk of myocardial infarction; in child health an obvious example is Down syndrome and maternal age.

The paradox can be represented as in Figure 17.2, where a universal approach would seek to shift the entire risk distribution to the left, while a targeted approach would aim to 'cut off the tail' at the top end of the distribution. It is clear which would have a more significant effect at the population level. However, the 'number needed to treat for benefit' is much higher for the universal approach, so much still depends on the cost of the intervention.

Improving health in everyday practice

International Agencies, national and local health authorities are committed to improving health across the population and to making health improvement the responsibility of all its staff. But what can individuals do in their everyday clinical practice to promote health and prevent disease? What is the role of doctors, in a field that relies on partnership working across such a wide range of individuals and agencies? What opportunities are there and what skills are required?

The most important answer is to be aware of the importance of this aspect of practice, and to ask yourself regularly, 'How could I, as a doctor working with other professionals and agencies, make a difference to the way this patient, condition or service is managed?' The list

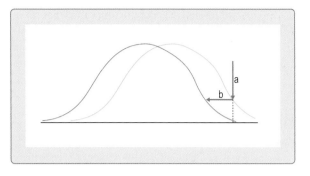

Fig. 17.2 Is it better to 'cut off the tail' (a) through a targeted approach, or to shift the whole population's risk profile downwards (b) through a universal approach?

below is not exhaustive, but contains some examples of action that individual doctors can take to promote child health:

- Advising parents about avoiding risks:
  - Sleeping position and SUDI
  - Safety in the home (cordless kettles, stair gates, smoke alarms) and in the outdoor environment (road traffic, waste sites, water ponds)
  - Cycle helmets and cycle proficiency training
  - Child car seats and restraints
  - Pets, smoking and asthma
- Being alert to the presence of conditions or risks that might threaten health and offering appropriate advice and/or referral:
  - Obesity and overweight
  - Smoking (children or adults)
  - Exposure to environmental pollutants
  - Short stature, failure to thrive etc.
- Knowing about and offering advice on preventive and health promotion services:
  - Breastfeeding and complementary feeding
  - Immunization
  - Smoking cessation
  - Parenting classes and support for vulnerable families
  - Dental health care
- Recognizing and acting on signs of abuse and neglect
- Knowing about services provided by other agencies and liaising effectively with them:
  - *Social services*: asylum seekers; children at risk of abuse or neglect; children with disabilities
  - *Education*: children with complex health needs; using school staff and services to best effect
  - *'Connections'* careers and employment services
  - *Drug action teams* and facilities
  - In some cases, the *police* and *the judiciary services*
- Advocacy and lobbying:
  - *Individual level*: e.g. supporting request for rehousing for child with severe asthma

- *Community level*: e.g. supporting campaign for a new NHS dental centre in the middle of a local housing estate
- *Policy level*: e.g. lobbying for more resources for children within the NHS.

References

Labonte & Little 1992. From Rootman I et al (eds) 2001. Evaluation in health promotion. Principles and perspectives. WHO Regional Publications, European Series, N° 92, p. 10. WHO Office for Europe, Copenhagen

Nutbeam 1985. From Rootman I et al (eds) 2001. Evaluation in health promotion. Principles and perspectives. WHO Regional Publications, European Series, N° 92, p. 10. WHO Office for Europe, Copenhagen

Ottawa Charter for Health Promotion Downloadable from http://www.who.int/hpr/NPH/docs/ottawa_charter_hp.pdf

US Department of Health, Education and Welfare 1979. From Rootman I et al (eds) 2001. Evaluation in health promotion. Principles and perspectives. WHO Regional Publications, European Series, N° 92, p. 10. WHO Office for Europe, Copenhagen

Jackson-Leach R, Lobstein T. Estimated burden of paediatric obesity and co-morbidities in Europe. Part 1. The increase in the prevalence of child obesity in Europe is itself increasing. International Journal of Pediatric Obesity. 2006; 1: 26–32

European Strategy for Child and Adolescent Health. WHO European Office for Europe, 2008 (http://www.euro.who.int/document/e91655.pdf).

Currie C et al, eds. Inequalities in young people's health. Health Behaviour in School-aged Children international report from the 2005/2006 survey. Copenhagen, WHO Regional Office for Europe, 2008

Edited by Mitch Blair, Diego van Esso,
Adamos Hadjipanayis, Mary Rudolf

Community Child Health

MODULE FOUR

Susan M. Gentle   Valerie Harpin   Fernand M. Pauly

CHAPTER

18

Childhood disability

MODULE FOUR

LEARNING OUTCOMES

By the end of this chapter you should:

- Understand concepts of disability and be familiar with the terminology in use
- Be aware of cultural attitudes to disability
- Know the causes of disability in childhood
- Be able to identify abnormal patterns of development
- Know when further assessment and investigation is required
- Understand the need for a multidisciplinary approach to management
- Appreciate the impact that disability has on the family
- Know about the role that various agencies have in providing services for the child with a disability
- Recognize the most common complications in specific disabilities
- Acquire basic knowledge about monitoring children with disabilities.

Concepts of disability and terminology

Before considering clinical aspects of disability we need to think about what the terminology used in relation to disability means and why this might be important. There are three groups of people who must be considered: (a) our fellow professionals with whom we need to be able to communicate clearly, (b) the affected children or young people who have to bear the weight of these words and (c) their parents who need to understand the terms we use. We need to avoid terms to which stigma is attached. Sadly many words previously used by professionals may now be terms of abuse in the playground, e.g. 'spastic', 'cretin' or 'retarded'. Use of the term 'mongoloid child' cannot be accepted because of the ethnic allusion. Even some medical expressions like 'deafness', 'dribbling', 'multiply disabled' may profoundly distress the families concerned. We must always look for gentler terms while understanding that whatever the terminology used, it is never easy for the parents to accept a situation that they always feel is deeply unfair.

Four common terms used in association with children with disability are disorder, impairment, disability and handicap (Box 18.1). In Table 18.1 you will see accepted definitions of these terms based on the World Health Organization (WHO) International Classification of Impairments, Disabilities and Handicaps (ICIDH). How do these definitions compare with yours?

BOX 18.1 Exercise

What do you understand by these terms? Spend a few moments trying to define them:

- Disorder
- Impairment
- Disability
- Handicap

Table 18.1 Feedback: defining the terminology

Term	Definition
Disorder	Medically definable condition or disease
Impairment	Loss or abnormality of psychological, physiological or anatomical structure or function
Disability	Any restriction or lack (resulting from an impairment) of ability to perform an activity in the manner or within the range considered normal for a child of that age
Handicap	The impact of the disability on the person's pursuits or achievement of goals that are desired by him/her or expected of him/her by society

BOX 18.2 Exercise

One way to find out whether a definition of a term is a working definition is to try to apply it to some clinical situations. Have a go at identifying the disorder, impairment, disability and handicap in the conditions below:

- Spastic diplegia
- Sensorineural hearing loss
- Epilepsy

The distinction between disability and handicap is particularly important. One of our aims when looking after children with disabilities should be to minimize the handicap i.e. the negative social consequences that results from that disability. Some disabled people say that the handicap lies in society, not with them: this is the case, for example, with paraplegic children who are autonomous, who can get to their friends' houses alone with their wheelchair as long as they do not encounter any insurmountable obstacles in their path. We can help by teaching the child to overcome or compensate for the disability and by advocating for changes in attitudes to disability in society.

Some parents prefer to describe their child as a child with 'special needs' rather than as either disabled or handicapped. This terminology is also widely used by professionals, not only in discussions with families, but also in a more formal context, such as the educational setting when a child may have a 'statement of special educational needs' (see below).

An exercise for you to complete is given in Box 18.2 (see Table 18.1 for definitions and Table 18.2 for feedback after doing the exercise). For the sake of clarity, keep in mind that the disorder (disease, trauma) is the cause of a dysfunction (impairment) resulting in a functional deficit (disability) which is the cause of a social disadvantage (handicap).

In response to a move away from the entirely medical model of disability, the ICIDH has developed the International Classification of Functioning, Disability and Health (ICF). The stated aims are as follows:

- To provide a scientific basis for consequences of health conditions and to standardize help and treatment services
- To establish a common language to improve communications
- To permit comparison of data across countries, healthcare disciplines, services and time

Table 18.2 Applying the terminology

Disorder	Impairment	Disability	Handicap
Spastic diplegia	Increased muscle tone most marked in lower limbs, (for example in the context of severe prematurity)	Delayed gross motor milestones and abnormal gait. May not walk independently or only with walking aids	Inability to join in with all playground games/physical education or walk to school
Profound sensorineural hearing loss (e.g. following meningitis)	Hearing loss secondary to a lesion in the cochlea and/or neural pathways to auditory cortex	Impaired hearing and delay in speech and language development	Inability to communicate with most strangers. Difficulty understanding spoken conversation
Epilepsy (for example due to a genetic disease)	Tendency to recurrent seizures + Possible dysfunction of certain brain areas even without fits	– Risk of injury during seizures – Learning difficulties – Frequent attention disorders Recurrent seizures may prevent a child from functioning normally at school	– Impossibility of undertaking some risky activities if fits are not well-controlled (e.g. swimming, riding) – May cause poor school performance justifying a special school programme – Look for adapted and supervised sporting activities.

- To provide a systematic coding scheme for health information systems.

The stress is on functioning rather than disability, so the ICF has sections on:
- Body functions and structures rather than impairments
- Activities rather than disability
- Participation rather than handicap.

http://www.who.int/icf/icftemplate.cfm

Further details of definitions

Cultural attitudes to disability

Cultural issues should be in the back of your mind all the time. These are some key points relating to disability:
- Attitudes to disability differ in different cultures, e.g. acceptance of disability as the will of God; however, in recent years more and more people systematically think that a handicap is either due to a medical error or to something which should at least have been prevented by the doctor.
- Communication: we use a lot of terms that are hard for people to understand, even more so if the local language is their second language
- Consanguineous marriages are common in some ethnic groups, with a higher risk of recessive genetic disorders. It is important to offer genetic counselling but you need to take cultural differences into account when doing this.
- Attitudes to abortion as a method of preventing the birth of a disabled child have a strong cultural base.
- Expectations of children's development depends in part on the 'sociocultural group'.
- Within the deaf culture, some people choose to have a deaf child rather than a hearing child.
- The cultural background is relevant in all health settings, such as dietary needs, recognition of fasts and festivals, issues around death, attitudes to medicines, surgery and blood transfusions and concerns about the gender of the professional treating an adolescent girl.

The epidemiology of disability

Disability in childhood is relatively common. The prevalence of physical and multiple disabilities in children is estimated to be approximately 10–20 per 1000. The more common causes of disability are shown in Table 18.3.

Table 18.3 The more common causes of childhood disability

Type of disability	Incidence
Physical and multiple disabilities	
Cerebral palsy	2.5 per 1000
Spina bifida	0.3 per 1000
Muscular dystrophy	0.2 per 1000
Severe learning difficulty	4.0 per 1000
Chromosomal abnormalities	4.0 per 1000
Central nervous system abnormality	1–2 per 1000
Special senses	
Severe visual handicap	0.4 per 1000
Severe hearing loss	1.0 per 1000

Presentation of disability

Children with disabilities may be identified as a result of parental suspicion or concern on the part of health or other professionals. Their presentation occurs at different times, depending on the problem. A syndrome or central nervous system abnormality may be identified in the antenatal period or at birth. Deafness, motor handicaps and severe learning disabilities often become apparent during the first year. Moderate or even severe learning disabilities, language disorder and autism may not be recognized until the child is 2 or 3 years old, when the family or health visitor questions the child's developmental progress. Finally, children may present after life-threatening events such as head injury or encephalopathy. An important point to keep in mind is that usually the parents are the first people alerted by their child's abnormal development (for example movement deficit in cerebral palsy, speech delay in autistic syndrome) and doctors are often criticized for not adequately taking their anxieties or questions into account.

Developmental problems and disability in primary care

Problem-orientated topic:

developmental delay

Janka is 3 years old. Her parents have been concerned about her development, and have consulted their health visitor. She asks you to assess her.

You find that she falls over frequently; she shows no interest in toys and does not seem to know what they are for; she can only say a few single words; she has difficult outbursts when she seems in a world of her own; and she has major problems with sleeping and is not yet toilet-trained.

Continued overleaf

197

Q1. What are the important aspects to focus on in your history and physical examination?

Q2. When should you become concerned that a child's development is delayed and referral is required?

Q3. What is the role of a child development team?

Q4. What impact does a disabled child have on the family?

Q5. What educational options are there likely to be for Janka?

Q6. When a child is disabled, what agencies need to be involved and what support is available?

Q1. What are the important aspects to focus on in your history and physical examination?

The history is of paramount importance. Children are quite likely to be uncooperative when relating to an unfamiliar person and in unfamiliar surroundings, and a reliable parent's report can provide much information.

The history should include an assessment of the following:

- Parental anxieties
- Family history
- Pregnancy and birth history
- Past medical history
- History of developmental milestones
- Current developmental skills.

Allowances for prematurity (i.e. use of the adjusted age) must be made during the first 2 years, but beyond that period catch-up in development rarely occurs. Parents often find it difficult to recall their child's developmental milestones, although, often in the event of delay they are likely to be more accurate. Often, information obtained from the history will be linked to their anxieties or guilt. Try to use photos and films of the family to obtain a reliable medical history. Try to specify the developmental milestones by connecting them to social stages: Was he/she already walking at Christmas? Was he/she talking when he entered nursery? Of particular importance in taking a history is the identification of any regression in skills.

Your physical examination should include the following; however, you can often save time and improve your analysis by getting the parents to complete a questionnaire on their child's development and asking them about their expectations (i.e. the 'Ages & Stages Questionnaires' at **http://www. agesandstages.com**).

Developmental skills

You should attempt to evaluate Janka's development before carrying out any other part of the physical examination, as undressing her is likely to arouse some antagonism. When you meet a child who may have a neurodisability, you will find it helpful to think through the following areas systematically:

- Gross motor
- Fine motor
- Spontaneous behaviour (and organization of play)
- Hearing and Vision
- Communication (verbal and non-verbal)
- Self-care and independence
- Interactions with other people
- Chronic illness, e.g. chest or heart problems.

In addition, you must assess factors such as alertness, responsiveness, interest in surroundings, determination and concentration, which all can positively influence a child's attainments.

Janka may well not cooperate with particular tasks, particularly if she is tired, shy or at the stage of stranger anxiety. You can gain a great deal of information from simply observing her at play while taking the history.

General examination

You need to carry out a complete physical examination in order to identify medical problems. Particularly relevant are dysmorphic signs, microcephaly, poor growth, signs of neglect, abnormalities of the eyes and ears, skin or hair pigmentation disorders, organomegaly (spleen, liver, thyroid etc) hollow feet (*pes cavus*) or scoliosis.

Neurological examination

This needs to be thorough, looking for abnormalities in tone, strength and coordination, deep tendon reflexes, clonus, cranial nerves, primitive reflexes, movements and problems with balance. It will always be necessary to check for evidence compatible with convulsions/ absences by asking specific questions about such things as atypical daydreaming, unexplained falls, brief head nods, clusters of trembling, unusual jerks of the legs, excessive starts or jumps.

Q2. When should you become concerned that a child's development is delayed and referral is required?

Normal developmental milestones are covered in Module 1. It is important not only to know the normal range of development but also to appreciate when development is so delayed or disordered that an expert opinion should be obtained. Box 18.3 provides you with some developmental warning signs that can guide you in your decision whether to refer.

Table 18.4 The child development team

Professional	Role
Developmental paediatrician	Diagnosis of medical problems Advice on medical issues and coordinaton with other doctors
Physiotherapist (also called kinesitherapist)	Assessment and management of gross motor difficulties, abnormal tone and prevention of deformities for example in cerebral palsy or muscular diseases Provision of special equipment including training with braces or walking aids
Occupational therapist (also called ergotherapist)	Assessment and management of fine motor difficulties Advice on toys, play and appliances to aid daily living
Speech and language therapist (also called orthophonist or logopedist)	Advice on feeding Assessment and management of speech, language and all aspects of communication also assisted with pictures, signs and a PC
Psychologist	Support and counselling of family and team Cognitive assessment (developmental and/or neuropsychological evaluation) Psychotherapy if necessary
Special needs teacher	Advice on special educational needs
Social worker and/or health visitor	Support for the family Advice on social service benefits, respite care etc. and liaison with the local health visitor

BOX 18.3 Developmental warning signs

At any age
- Parental concern
- Regression in previously acquired skills

At 10 weeks
- Not smiling

At 6 months
- Persistent primitive reflexes
- Persistent squint
- Hand preference
- Little interest in people, toys, noises

At 10–12 months
- No sitting
- No double-syllable babble
- No pincer grasp

At 18 months
- Not walking independently
- Fewer than six words
- Persistent mouthing and drooling

At 2¹/₂ years
- No 2–3-word sentences

At 4 years
- Unintelligible speech

Janka's development is severely delayed in all areas, notably gross motor, communication and language as well as social skills. Such global developmental delay at the age of 3 is indicative of severe or at best moderate learning disability and she should be referred to your local Child Development Centre.

Q3. What is the role of a child development team?

The child development team is a multidisciplinary team of professionals who are involved in assessing and managing children with complex difficulties. The members of the team (Table 18.4) and the manner in which they work may vary from centre to centre, and their roles may overlap considerably in practice.

Janka's management will go beyond diagnosis, explanation of the problem and providing therapeutic input. It will involve supporting the family while they come to terms with the child's difficulties and learn how to cope. It also involves a great deal of liaison work with other professionals, both medical and non-medical.

One of the major benefits of the team approach lies in the coordination of care, so ensuring that the various professionals communicate with each other well and that the family does not receive a mixture of contradictory advice. The work of the team involves the following aspects.

Giving a diagnosis

The diagnosis of a disability is usually devastating and the way that the news is initially broken is of long-lasting importance to the family. The session has to be conducted by a senior doctor in the presence of both parents. The doctor must provide necessary and practical information so that the parents feel competent to better meet their child's needs.

Discussions should focus on foreseeable developments in the up-coming six-month period avoiding uncertain (and often imprecise) speculations about the child's long-term future. Notifying parents of a serious condition in their child must always leave a glimmer of hope for parents who expect practical advice from the doctor as to how they can parent a child who is different. The doctor must offer psychological support and if possible give the parents the address of a mutual help and support group. The doctor must check that his/her message has been understood by getting the parents to talk about what they have been told. The doctor must suggest a second meeting shortly afterwards to answer any questions unasked during the shock of the first declaration of disability. The empathy that the doctor must express for the parents must not be perceived as inconsideration on his/her part of the intrinsic and untouchable value of the handicapped child (i.e. One must never say: 'I'm sorry for you having a child like this').

On leaving the doctor's office, the family should have the addresses, meeting dates and telephone numbers for help and support to be provided in the weeks to come. It should be noted that often the medical diagnosis is very incomplete at the start and it is the child's development which will better define it (e.g. in the case of learning difficulties). If a baby is born with congenital anomalies, the session should take place directly after birth, when possible with the baby present.

Medical management

Parents' attendance at development meetings about their child (with the psychologist, speech therapist, etc.) will be very useful for them to better understand their child's specific difficulties and strong points. The child's disability will therefore be apparent to his/her parents and so they will be more able to come to terms with the official statement of the medical diagnosis. Once the child's difficulties have been fully assessed, appropriate therapeutic input is required. This may be delivered in the child development centre, at home or at nursery. Once the child is in full-time school, the services are delivered there by community therapists, whose task is not only to work with the child but also to advise school staff. The doctor will often have to divulge medical confidentiality with the different parties involved, in the immediate interests of the child and following consent from the parents. This openness of medical confidentiality covers the functional aspects of the child's disability but medical confidentiality is to be protected as regards genetic data and other aspects with guilt-inducing connotations for the parents (e.g. smoking or infectious diseases during pregnancy).

Genetic counselling

A genetic cause may be suspected in a number of child disability situations. A genetic assessment can only be done if both parents give their consent and if they have been informed about the potential consequences of the genetic diagnosis (e.g. feelings of guilt in cases of X-linked transmission or even situations of genetic

diseases which could affect several generations of one family but with variable expression; e.g. Steinert disease). When a child has been diagnosed as having a disability, the family will want to know the genetic implications for themselves and their relatives. Many disabilities have a genetic basis, in which case informed advice must be provided. In general genetic testing is not undertaken in the siblings of the 'target' child if these are minors and if the genetic diagnosis does not provide any therapeutic benefit.

The genetic evaluation is only rarely urgent but may be so at the request of the parents if they are planning another pregnancy.

http://www.orpha.net

An excellent internet portal for rare diseases and orphan drugs that can be consulted in different languages.

Q4. What impact does a disabled child have on the family?

Families differ greatly in their reaction to having a child with a disability. However, on first receiving the news, they all tend to pass through similar emotional stages to those experienced in coping with bereavement. The first reaction is one of shock, when often only a small proportion of what is said is taken in. Negative feelings of fear and loss, anger and guilt then follow. Gradually adaptation follows and leads to the final stage of acceptance. Some parents have difficulty in reaching this last stage, in which case supportive counselling by a psychologist may be necessary.

The family needs to adapt again at each stage of the child's development. Independence becomes an issue at each step and an important part of the child's education is to foster this, so it must be addressed as part of his or her special educational needs.

Good liaison is needed with school, and the school needs to be prepared and informed about any anticipated difficulties. If the child needs occupational therapy, physiotherapy or speech and language therapy, the staff will need to work with the therapists in order to implement their recommendations. In some circumstances the school may need to make alterations to accommodate physical disabilities. Special guidance or counselling may be required, and help may be needed to integrate the child into the classroom.

Having a child with a disability places extra pressure and stresses on any family. It is important therefore to determine how much support is available. Informal support in terms of family and friends can be variable, and additional support is often appreciated.

Q5. What educational options are there likely to be for Janka?

There are a number of possible educational options for children with special needs but these vary greatly from one country to another and may even vary from one region to the other within the same country. The majority of European countries make a great effort to promote the integration of 'disabled' children in mainstream schools, particularly in preschools.

Preschool

- *Preschool teachers* are often the first contact from the Education Department. They will usually get to know the family well and provide key support in the preschool years. There may be specialist preschool teachers for deaf and visually impaired children. They usually visit the home to work with the child and advise the parents on the best ways to help the child. This should be in the first year of life if it can be confidently assumed that there will be special needs at school age, e.g. Down syndrome, severe deafness.
- *Portage workers* have a similar role. Portage is a particular method of helping young children, which follows a specific programme of developmental steps.
- *Mainstream nursery school* with or without support.
- *Day nurseries, family centres and preschool playgroups* with or without support.
- *Special nursery school, unit or other group* for children with disabilities.

School age

- *Mainstream school.* The inclusion of children with special educational needs in mainstream school has been a core principle of Education Acts since 1981. The extent still varies across the country but there is a presumption of inclusive education where that meets the parents' wishes, meets the child's needs and is not incompatible with the efficient education of other children.

  The amount and type of support needed will vary according to the disability and severity. Physical disability may best be helped by structural changes in the school (lifts, ramps, toilets adapted for disabled people, premises for nursing care etc.); visual impairment by modifications for the child (enlargement of written material, better lighting etc.); severe hearing impairment may need the support of a signing assistant. Classroom support can range from occasional advice to one-to-one help full-time, including help during break times, nurses for vesical-sphincter care.

Local authorities may have specialist teams of teachers (e.g. sensory impairment, autism, behaviour difficulties), whose expertise can be called upon by schools to advise on management. Physiotherapy, psychomotricity and speech therapy sessions should be arranged within the school setting if possible, and during school hours so that families do not have to attend these sessions after school (refer to the risks of family burnout).

- *Special schools.* These are schools where all the children have special needs and the staff has special expertise in those needs. They may cater for a particular special need (e.g. deafness, visual impairment, autism) or be available for children with various or multiple special needs. Class sizes are small and children get a lot of individual attention. There have been major changes in the needs of children attending special schools, with the children generally having the most specialized needs. We are observing a growing number of multi-disabled children due to their increased life expectancy as a result of medical advances (with more frequent recourse to gastrostomy and non-invasive ventilation). It is still very difficult to educate these children in mainstream schools. Special schools may have links with a mainstream school to provide the children with some opportunity to interact with their mainstream peers and to give them access to a wider range of facilities. Some special schools are run by voluntary organizations. There may be boarding facilities at these schools because of the wide geographical area they cover.
- *Special units in mainstream schools.* These are a compromise between special school and full inclusion. The unit may be for a particular type of disability or for a range of disabilities.

The debate continues around the merits of mainstream and special schools for children with disabilities. It is vital to listen to the child/young person and family and consider their needs flexibly.

BOX 18.4 Services available for children with a disability

- Health services:
  - Primary care team
  - Disability team (Table 18.4)
- Education (see above)
- Social services
- Voluntary sector

Identification of special educational needs (SEN)

There have been many legislative measures around education. In the UK, all the Education Acts since 1944 have now been consolidated into the 1996 Education Act.

In response to the 1996 Education Act and the SEN and Disability Act 2001, a new Code of Practice came into being in 2002. This document is available from the Department for Education and Skills (DFES) website.

🌐 http://www.dfes.gov.uk/publications

The assessment process

When a school and family first recognize that a child has special educational needs, they first consider what can be done by the school to support the child. If these measures cannot meet the child's needs, an assessment of special educational needs is initiated and a statement of educational needs may be issued.

In the UK, the special educational needs coordinator (SENCO) is a teacher with special expertise in this area.

Medical advice for education

There are different levels and different degrees of formality for giving advice to schools about individual children with special needs. This may involve discussion of the child's difficulties with teachers or writing a letter to the school. The child's and parent's consent should always be sought and it is useful to include this request routinely in your outpatient sessions. You must always consider that the teacher is often concerned about not being able to meet the disabled child's medical needs. These must be at best played down, with clear instructions on dealing with complications (e.g. what to do in the case of epileptic fits), explain the principles of the technical aids and make sure you are available by telephone or e-mail. Educational integration has little chance of success if the teacher feels overwhelmed and alone when faced with the specific needs of the child and sometimes with unrealistic parental demands as well.

Medical reports for statutory assessment

During an assessment of special educational needs, input is sought from the school or nursery, parents/carers and the health services and social services involved.

🌐 http://www.dfes.gov.uk/publications

'The Role of Health Professionals', with helpful information about the health professional's role and guidance on writing medical advice

Q6. When a child is disabled, what agencies need to be involved and what support is available?

See Box 18.4. These services are described in detail below. However there are considerable differences between different countries as regards allowances, school systems and medical centres. You must obtain information from the Health Ministry in your own country in order to better advise families.

Agencies with a responsibility for childhood disability

Statutory services

Statutory services try to meet the needs of children and young people with disabilities and their families. It is particularly important to see how these services are coordinated. Much is said about multidisciplinary, interdisciplinary, interagency and multi-agency working. Putting it into practice so that an individual family can see it working is not so easy. Indeed we know that parents often feel that it is not working for them. Families' views must be taken into account when services are offered to them and in ongoing service review.

Health services

There are two important health teams with overlapping but distinct functions:
- The primary healthcare team (PHCT)
- The disability team.

The PHCT, particularly the primary care physician and health visitor, have usually been involved from the start and it is important that they remain fully informed in order to give continuing support to the family. Once a child gets into school, the school nurse becomes a key health professional in the PHCT.

The disability team varies from place to place. There is usually a core team of at least a paediatrician, physiotherapist, occupational therapist, speech and language therapist, psychologist and nurse. They usually work from a central base and are involved in the initial assessment of a child referred with a disability.

Communication between all involved professionals is vital. Parent-held Child Health Records can help with this, as long as they are used and kept up to date. In some European countries, properly completed health records constitute an excellent tool of communication between the professionals involved. Specialized health records (e.g. for trisomic children, epileptic children, and children with cystic fibrosis) are of great value to ensure good continuity of care.

Disability services and teams

In the UK, the Court Report, 'Fit for the Future' (HMSO 1976), recommended that each health district established a district handicap team, with two types of function:
- Clinical:
  - To provide investigation, assessment and coordinate management of children with complex disorders
  - To provide parents, teachers and others with advice and support on management of the child
  - To provide primary and supporting specialist services to special schools
- Operational:
  - To be involved in epidemiological surveys, monitoring effectiveness of services and maintaining quality
  - To organize training for professional staff.

More or less comparable models exist in the majority of European countries: this is a case of undertaking a 'neutral' multidisciplinary evaluation to determine the objectives and retain the methods indispensable to the project's success.

Organization of services (pathways of care)

For a given child, there are generally a number of parties involved and this can lead to confusion for families as well as for professionals.

One of the key things parents ask for is a 'joined-up service'. This is not only geographical (services on the same site) but also involves professionals who communicate with each other so that the parents do not have to keep repeating the story. Families also highlight their need for general and disorder-specific information. Some families, especially if their children are not making the progress hoped for, will not be satisfied with the school and re-education provision which you nevertheless deem to be adequate. You must do everything to maintain close contact with these families who sometimes express their despair blatantly. Other families do not want an 'all-in-one' programme and prefer to find personal solutions for their children sometimes with recourse to non-validated or barely validated methods.

Social services

Social work input can be invaluable for many families. Input may be diverse, ranging from practical tasks to emotional support, e.g. around the time of diagnosis of severe or complex difficulty. Social services have certain statutory responsibilities:
- To provide services for children in need
- To ensure services are coordinated
- To include families in decision-making
- To collaborate with the education authority to assess the needs of school-leavers with disabilities.

Social work services may advise on:
- Grants and allowances
- Respite care facilities
- Leisure activities
- Day care facilities.

Financial help

Caring for a child with a disability is expensive. Consider the following:
- Reduced income:
  - A parent giving up work or not starting work in order to care for the child
  - A parent choosing to turn down a promotion that means moving away
  - Loss of earnings when time is taken off for hospital visits
- Increased expenditure:
  - Transport: for hospital and therapy visits; general increased transport costs, e.g. taxis (imagine taking a child with severe behavioural problems on a bus or taking the underground with a wheelchair); a wheelchair-adapted car
  - Food: parents may want to 'feed the child up'; food wasted through feeding difficulties
  - Household goods: telephone needed; washing machine and drier for extra washing; freezer — difficulty getting to the shops frequently
  - Housing: adaptations (adapted bathroom, access ramp); moving to a larger house
  - Equipment (e.g. a specialized therapeutic bike) and special toys
  - Hospital admissions: transport to visit daily; child-minding for other children.

This is an endless list!

Anyone involved in caring for the child should be able to advise parents on how to access help and should have a knowledge of what is available.

Disability Living Allowance (DLA)

In the United Kingdom families can obtain an allowance for any child who has 'substantially' higher needs than those of a non-disabled child of the same age. There are two components: care and mobility.

Invalid Care Allowance

This is an additional allowance, which is available for the person caring for the child.

Income Support

This is a means-tested benefit for all low-income families and has a disabled child's premium.

Fares to hospital

These are available for those on income support.

The Family Fund Trust

This is an independent organization, registered as a charity. It provides information (such as the benefits checklist) and grants for special requests related to the care of children with disabilities.

 http://www.familyfundtrust.org.uk

Contact a Family

Contact a Family also produces guidance for parents on benefits.

 http://www.cafamily.org.uk

Other possible sources for help for families are:

- Toy libraries
- Equipment loan facilities
- Disabled person's railcard
- Local charities
- Local transport schemes
- Holiday organizations
- The local Citizens' Advice Bureau
- Families and professionals can obtain a great deal of information from the European Academy of Childhood Disability at:

 http://www.eacd.org

An excellent source of information about specific conditions and syndromes, primarily for families but also for professionals. It also provides information about parent support groups

The voluntary sector

Parents can be helped by local and national support groups with many of the issues so far covered in this chapter. Parents should be informed of any voluntary organizations that might be of help to the family. Many parents wish to make contact with other families experiencing similar problems. These mutual aid and support groups often provide fundamental support with exemplary solidarity. Some of these facilities have become very large non-governmental organizations

undertaking major lobbying (e.g. Association Française contre les Myopathies — French Myopathy Association).

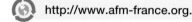 http://www.afm-france.org.

Specific conditions causing disabiliity

There are many possible causes of childhood disability. The most common ones are summarized here and are described in more detail in Chapter 29.

Severe learning disability (Ch. 29)

The incidence of mild/moderate learning disability (IQ 50–70) is 5 per 1000 and that of severe learning disability (IQ < 50) is 3.8 per 1000. In almost all cases of severe learning disability a cause is found. (Around 25% have a chromosome abnormality, and 80% of these have Down syndrome.) Other important causes include congenital brain malformations, acquired brain injury (e.g. intraventricular haemorrhage in a preterm infant or encephalitis) and metabolic defects (especially if unexplained illness or seizures occur).

Cerebral palsy (Ch. 29)

Incidence is approximately 1:400 births. Although the initial brain lesion is non-progressive, the effect on the child changes with time. Cerebral palsy is mostly due to factors before birth but may also follow infection, difficult or preterm birth or an accident in early life.

In monitoring children suffering from cerebral palsy you must:

- recognize dysplasia of the hips by asymmetry or limitation of the abduction of the hips early on because the risk of secondary hip dislocations is high
- check during each medical examination the appropriateness of the braces according to the child's growth
- discuss focal treatment for spasticity (particularly botulin), regional treatment (implantable baclofen pump) and general treatment (muscle-relaxant drugs p.o.).

Children with this condition frequently have additional difficulties (learning problems, epilepsy, sensory impairment). A multidisciplinary approach to care is essential.

Epilepsy (Chs 24 and 28)

This has been defined as epileptic seizures or attacks, which are transient clinical events resulting from abnormal or excessive activity of a more or less extensive collection of cerebral neurons. Epilepsy is classified as partial (simple or complex) or generalized. Several studies have highlighted the false diagnosis rate in epilepsy, with both under- and over-diagnosis, and this may be as high as 25% of cases. The most important step in making the diagnosis is to take a thorough and accurate history. With a team of professionals caring for disabled children, each team member must have training enabling him/her to recognize and describe an epileptic fit and how to react in an emergency (standardized protocol). Communication between the parties involved can be improved by keeping a diary of seizures.

Visual and hearing impairment

(Chs 31 and 32)

It is vital to assess vision and hearing in all children with a disability because it may further affect development, often avoidably, and also because vision and hearing problems are more common in this group of children. Sometimes disabled children cannot be accurately assessed by normal testing and specialist referral is required. Hearing deficiencies should be looked for systematically using the auditory brainstem response test (not only by oto-acoustic emissions) in cases of severe prematurity, bacterial meningitis or following neonatal resuscitation.

Specific learning disabilities (Ch. 29)

Children are defined as having specific learning difficulties if they have more difficulty than expected in an area of learning, which is not accounted for by general learning disability. This is a complex topic covering developmental coordination disorder, attention deficit disorder, dyslexia, dyscalculia, language disorder and social skills difficulties.

Medullary (spinal cord) paralysis

(Ch. 28)

Medullary paralysis may be in connection with myelomeningocoele, a medullary tumour or trauma.

Neuropathic bladder sometimes goes unnoticed on the clinical level especially in unweaned infants. It is detected systematically by vesico-renal ultrasound scans.

These children often present cutaneous anaesthesia in the feet predisposing them to ulcers which must be protected by good care of the toenails and by selecting appropriate footwear.

The paediatrician must undertake a full neurological examination at least once a year to detect secondary neurological aggravations in time in keeping with thetered cord syndrome or syringomyelia (also check for Arnold Chiari malformation).

Muscular dystrophies (see p. 381)

(see p. 381)

A large number of different situations and diseases fall under this term. For follow-up purposes we will recall the following:
- Nocturnal hypoventilation with or without apnoea must be carefully looked for especially in cases of morning asthenia.
- In Duchenne dystrophy the use of steroids and angiotensin inhibitors should be considered.
- In cases of progressive muscle diseases; long-term adaptation of the family home, family car and at school must be planned in advance, so that the child can use an electric wheelchair autonomously.
- In certain neuromuscular diseases, learning difficulties and/or communication problems may be severe (Duchenne MD, myotonic dystrophy, Fukuyama disease).

Treatment protocols and theoretical information can be consulted at the website of the Neuromuscular Disease Center, Washington University.

http://neuromuscular.wustl.edu/

Head trauma and other acquired brain lesions

The after-effects of cranial traumas, as well as lesions in connection with meningo-encephalitis or brain tumours are especially hard for families to live with who remember the 'normal' child they knew before. Psychological support is often required and even more so for these children who often have behavioural problems which clearly worsen the social consequences of their mental impairment. Convulsive fits may appear after the trauma and they should be identified by means of a targeted history.

Children with multiple disabilities

This in an umbrella term for children in a very high dependency situation due to their major mental deficiency combined with somewhat severe motor deficits, who have no effective verbal communication and often have sensory disorders as well. The children may have congenital malformations, affect-effects as a result of their prematurity or neonatal resuscitation and even children with acquired brain injury (head trauma, progressive neurodegenerative or metabolic diseases, infectious diseases) may fall into this category. Concentrate in particular on the following aspects:

- Is the dietary intake comfortable for the child and acceptable for the family (undertake an assessment with the speech therapist or paediatric nurse).
- Is the child's nutritional state satisfactory? If required arrange for food supplements, space out the gastro-oesophageal reflux very often present (consider resorting to a gastrostomy +/- Nissen procedure).
- Is the child receiving prevention from osteopenia which is generalized in tetraplegics (vitamin D and calcium supplements, adapted physiotherapy programmes, blood checks and regular osteodensitometries).
- Is the child presenting chronic or acute pain? This should be assessed by questionnaires specific to this group and enable adaptation of pain management.
- Can the family (parents and siblings) cope with the constraints associated with the disabled child: you must be able to detect family burnout early on; talk to the parents and siblings about their daily life; propose periods of time-out (specialized day-care centres, weekend short-term care, adapted holidays).
- Is everything possible being done by the physiotherapist and occupational therapist for the child to maintain a comfortable sitting position, indispensable for the child's social life? The opinion of a team specialized in cases of dysplasia of the hips and cases of progressive scoliosis will be required regularly.

The medical problems experienced by these children often necessitate ethical discussions with the families concerned as regards the best choice of treatment.

A great deal of information on rare and progressive diseases can be found at the Rare Diseases Task Force website:

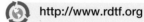 http://www.rdtf.org

Acknowledgments

We would like to thank the contributors to the Sheffield Distance Learning Course in Paediatric Neurodisability, and in particular Dr Helena Davies, Professor David Hall and Dr Connie Pullan.

Wolf-Rüdiger Horn   Elke Jaeger-Roman   Aidan MacFarlane

CHAPTER

19

Adolescent health and health problems

LEARNING OUTCOMES

By the end of this chapter you should:

- Understand and be able to apply the concepts of 'confidentiality' and 'informed consent' when dealing with adolescents
- Understand why the needs of adolescents may be different from those of children/ adults
- Know broadly what health problems are more specific to adolescents
- Have the skills and sensitivity to deal with the emotional and information needs of young people when they consult you
- Have the skills to diagnose and treat specific disorders relating to adolescence.

What is adolescence?

A definition of adolescence

Adolescence begins with the onset of physiologically normal puberty, and ends when an adult identity and behaviour are accepted. This period of development corresponds roughly to the period between the ages of 10 (from the beginning of the 10th year) and runs till 19 years (the end of the 19th year), which is consistent with the World Health Organization's definition of adolescence.

Note that adolescence contains biological, psychological and social elements (Fig. 19.1).

The key health problems of adolescence include the following, which are not all considered in detail in this chapter, but elsewhere in these books:

- Growth and puberty (Chs 22 and 25)
- Nutrition, exercise and obesity (Chs 4 and 22)
- Sexual and reproductive health
- Common medical conditions of adolescence (including acne, common orthopaedic diseases, functional/psychosomatic disorders, sleep disorders, fatigue and chronic fatigue syndrome)
- Chronic conditions/disabilities (Chs 29 and 32)
- Mental health problems (Ch. 29)
- Eating disorders
- Substance use and misuse, including smoking
- Injuries and violence, including accidents, self-harm, abuse etc. (Chs 36 and 49).

Sex and sexually transmitted infections

Teenagers and sex: some facts

- 30% of boys and 24% of girls have had sex by the age of 15 (with considerable variations across European countries)

MODULE FOUR

207

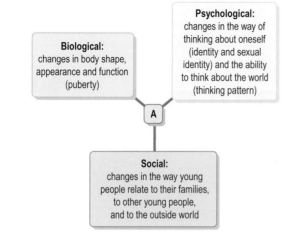

Fig. 19.1 **Adolescence (A) contains biological, psychological and social elements**

- 30 to 40% of teenagers reported not to know exactly how the first sexual intercourse came about
- 72% of 15-year-old girls and 81% of 15-year-old boys used a condom at last intercourse
- 26% of 15-year-old girls were on a contraceptive pill at last intercourse
- 10% of sexually active teenagers are infected with *Chlamydia*; in some countries teen infections almost doubled during the 1990s
- 25% of all new HIV infections are identified in young people under 21 years
- 1% (Netherlands) to 6% (Great Britain) of all newborn babies are born to 15- to 19-year-old teenagers

Teenage sexual behaviour is largely dependent on personal living conditions. Boundaries between normal, experimental and risky sexual behaviour are often difficult to define because adolescents and adults have different views of life. Unintended pregnancy and STIs are the most important negative consequences of teenage risk behaviour. Sexual education improves sexual behaviour but does not increase early sexual activity.

Risk factors for STIs and/or teenage pregnancy

- early puberty; early sexual activity
- narrow vaginal introitus which can lead to injuries
- unprotected sex
- a great many sexual partners
- anal or oral sex; homosexuality
- poverty; social exclusion; unemployment; school disconnectedness and failure
- alcohol and drug consumption; delinquency
- history of sexual and physical abuse
- limited access to emergency contraception
- mental handicap and mental health problems

The evidence base for reducing teenage pregnancy and STIs: the means and motivation

A key aspect in prevention is the availability of accurate information to young people in their own media, and sex education in schools and in out-of-school settings; this should focus on providing knowledge and skills, on delaying first sex, on the risks of unprotected sex, and on effective contraceptive/condom use. Open discussion with parents and carers has been shown to facilitate healthy sexual practices. Easy access to confidential youth-friendly contraceptive/sexual health services is important. Teenage pregnancy prevention aims at a multifaceted approach, with *all* factors in place and intensive delivery to at-risk groups, combined with additional motivation to delay early pregnancy.

Problem-orientated topic:

itchy and sore penis in a sexually active boy ⬤⬤⬤⬤⬤

Ambrius is a 16-year-old boy who asks you for an HIV test. On questioning, he reports that 2 days ago he first felt some tingling at the tip of his penis. He then noticed small red bumps which became sore. Urination was painful and he could feel swollen lumps in his groin. Now he is extremely worried and fears the worst, i.e. that he has contracted HIV.

Two weeks ago Ambrius went to a 'really good party', where everybody had lots of beer and other drinks. He had sex with a nice girl who he met for the first time. He did not use a condom because the girl said she was on contraceptive pills.

vaginal discharge in a sexually active girl ⬤⬤⬤⬤⬤

Kada is a 15-year-old girl who presents with a vaginal discharge. She has had very little information about sex because her parents refused to allow her to attend sex education classes at her school. She recently began having sex without using any form of contraception, out of fear that she would otherwise lose her boyfriend who is at the

Continued overleaf

same school. She knows this discharge could mean that she has an STI, but she refuses to discuss using contraceptive methods because she now intends to break up with her boyfriend, who she thinks has infected her, and says that she will never have sex again.

Q1. What are the issues here of confidentiality and consent? Do the parents need to know?

Q2. How do you investigate the STIs in these two patients?

Q3. How do you ensure that they do get information about healthy sexual behaviour, prevention of STIs and about contraception in the future?

Q1. What are the issues here of confidentiality and consent? Do the parents need to know?

Involvement
Article 12 of the United Nations Convention on the Rights of the Child states that:

Parties shall assure to the child who is capable of forming his or her own views, the right to express those views freely in all matters affecting the child, the views of the child being given due weight in accordance with the age and maturity of the child.

Confidentiality
(This is also discussed in detail in Chapter 11.)

The basic philosophy is that 'the professional should not disclose anything learned from a person who has consulted them, or whom he or she has examined or treated — without that person's agreement.' Children and young people are entitled to the same standards of confidentiality as other patients. This means that their rights are not absolute but can only generally be overridden when there is clear justification, such as the risk of significant harm. Where an exceptional reason justifies disclosure without consent, children should be told that their secrets cannot be kept. In the absence of any such reason justifying disclosure, they should be encouraged but not forced to share their health information with their parents.

Consent
Adolescents under 16 years of age can consent to examination and treatment, provided they have sufficient understanding and intelligence to enable them to understand fully what is being proposed. Consent for treatment of a person under 18 can therefore come from any one of the following:

- A competent child
- A person or local authority with parental responsibility
- A court
- A person caring for a child, but only if it is reasonable in the circumstances to safeguard or promote the child's welfare.

Q2. How do you investigate the STIs in these two patients?

Genital herpes (HSV type 1 and 2) is a very common genital infection which can occur after oral, anal or sexual intercourse. Generally, a person can only get HSV-2 infection during sexual contact with someone who has a genital HSV-2 infection. Transmission can occur from an infected partner who does not have a visible sore and may not know that he or she is infected. HSV-1 can cause genital herpes, but it more commonly causes infections of the mouth and lips, so-called 'fever blisters'. Genital HSV-1 outbreaks recur less regularly than genital HSV-2 outbreaks. Most individuals with HSV-2 infection never have sores, or they have very mild signs that they do not notice or that they mistake for insect bites or another skin condition, therefore they frequently are not aware of their infection. However, if signs and symptoms occur during the first outbreak, they can be quite pronounced, usually occurring within two weeks after the virus is transmitted, and the sores typically heal within two to four weeks. Other signs and symptoms during the primary episode may include a second crop of sores, and flu-like symptoms, including fever and swollen glands.

In 2003, women aged 16–24 accounted for 73% of all *Chlamydia* diagnoses in women, 69% of gonorrhoea, 35% of syphilis and 62% of genital warts diagnosed in genitourinary medicine (GUM) clinics in England, Wales and Northern Ireland.

In 2003, young men aged 16–24 accounted for 55% of all *Chlamydia* diagnoses in men, 41% of gonorrhoea and 44% of genital warts diagnosed in GUM clinics in England, Wales and Northern Ireland.

As adolescents have the highest rate of STIs and the highest rate of complications after STIs (ascending infections, adnexitis, transmission of some infectious agents during pregnancy or at birth, sterility), a screening programme for *Chlamydia* infection should also follow after the diagnosis of a specific STI. Procedures which allow a diagnosis in urine specimen like PCR (polymerase chain reaction) or LCR (ligase chain reaction), or blood tests or swabs for cultures (when taken by the adolescents themselves) are well

Table 19.1 HIV-infected individuals and AIDS cases in the UK by age group at diagnosis and sex (% of total cases)

	Male				Female				Total			
	HIV		AIDS		HIV		AIDS		HIV*		AIDS	
Age group (years)	No	%	No	%	No	%	No	%	No	%	No	%
0–4	471	1	224	1	432	2	223	6	905	1	447	2
5–9	262	1	73	0	157	1	52	1	421	1	125	1
10–14	232	0	49	0	76	0	26	1	309	0	75	0
15–19	949	2	71	0	647	3	34	1	1598	2	105	0

* In some cases sex not given.

accepted. A proper diagnosis should be made and the infection treated accordingly.

The common STIs of adolescence

- *Gonorrhoea* has an incubation period of only a few days. Males and females may experience a urethral discharge. Women are at risk of long-term serious complications such as infertility and ectopic pregnancy. It is possible to have long-term infection without obvious symptoms. Treatment is with antibiotics.
- *Chlamydia* causes an often symptomless infection but may be associated with vaginal bleeding, discharge, abdominal pain, fever, and inflammation of the cervix in women and watery discharge from the penis in men. Long-term complications may be severe, particularly in women, as it can lead to pelvic inflammatory diseases, ectopic pregnancy and infertility. It is easy to treat with antibiotics.
- *Genital warts* are caused by human papillomavirus (HPV) and are found around the penis, anus and vagina. Certain types of HPV are associated with cervical cancer. Warts often disappear without treatment but can also be removed by freezing, burning and laser treatment. Immunization against HPV types 16 and 18, which are responsible for 70% of cervical cancers, is now advised for girls before first sexual contacts in many European countries.
- *Syphilis* has an incubation period ranging from a few days to 3 months. Symptoms are non-specific, though illness usually begins with painless, highly infectious sores anywhere around the body but usually at the site of infection. Syphilis can cause miscarriage and stillbirth, but can be cured with antibiotics.
- *Genital herpes* is a common infection caused by herpes simplex virus type 2 or type 1. Symptoms include small blisters in the genital area, which break down to give painful ulcers. Herpes may cause pain on urination. Genital herpes can be treated with Aciclovir or Famciclovir.
- *HIV infection* — see Table 19.1 and Chapter 43.

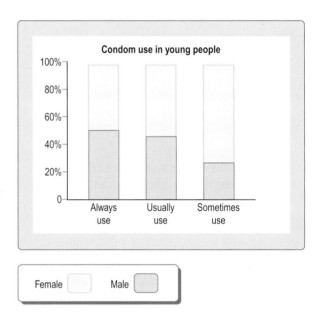

Fig. 19.2 Regular condom use amongst 16–19-year-olds by gender.
   The graph shows the clear gender difference for the 'sometimes use' group.

Q3. How do you ensure that they do get information about contraception in the future?

There has been a sustained increase in condom use and a decline of men and women reporting no contraceptive use at first intercourse (Fig. 19.2). Contraceptive use generally increases with age, and 'the pill' followed by the 'male condom' are by far the most common methods used by adolescents.

Legal issues relating to contraceptive advice to adolescents

A young person can be given contraceptive advice, even under the age of 16, if:

- The young person understands the doctor's advice
- The doctor cannot persuade the young person to inform his or her parents, or to allow the doctor to inform the parents

Table 19.2 Psychopathology of eating disorders

	Anorexia nervosa	Bulimia nervosa
Strict dieting	+++	+++
Self-induced vomiting	+	++
Laxative misuse	+	++
Over-exercising	++	+
Bulimic episodes ('binges')	+	+++
Ritualistic eating habits	++	–
Anxiety when eating with others	+++	+++
Over-evaluation of shape and weight	+++	+++
Depressive symptoms	+	+++
Anxiety symptoms	+	++
Obsessional symptoms	++	+
Impaired concentration	+++	+++
Social withdrawal	+++	+
Substance abuse	–	+

- The young person is likely to begin or continue having sexual intercourse with or without contraception
- The young person's physical and/or mental health are likely to suffer unless he or she receives contraception
- The young person's best interests require the doctor to give contraceptive advice, treatment or both, without parental consent.

Eating disorders (Table 19.2)

Problem-orientated topic:

eating disorder ● ● ● ● ●

Mirriam is a 15-year-old girl who comes to the clinic with her mother. Her mother is concerned because Mirriam has been losing weight for the past 3 months and the school has reported a falling off in her academic work, despite her previously being a high achiever. The mother says that Mirriam has been eating alone in her room and refusing to have dinner with her family. The father is a lawyer and the mother is a retired dancer. Mirriam started having regular periods at 11, but she has had no menstrual bleeding for the last 2 months. She avoids fat and sweets, never eats breakfast and exercises 5 days a week. Her oldest brother teased her about being fat when she was younger, around the time her periods started. She has few friends. From the school letter, you calculate a body mass index (BMI) of 16, which is under the 5th percentile for age and gender. Mirriam refuses to be either weighed or examined.

Q1. What initial assessment should you make?
Q2. What tests do you want to arrange?
Q3. Who can you treat yourself and who do you refer?

Q1. What initial assessment should you make?

Recommended screening questions for eating problems
- Do you worry about your weight?
- How much would you like to weigh?
- What do you eat and what do you do for exercise?

Note: early detection normally improves outcome.

Risk factors for developing eating disorders in adolescence
- Female sex
- Repeated dieting
- Being teased about weight and dieting
- Perfectionism
- Depressed mood

Engagement can be difficult but developing a good relationship and getting a clear history are paramount. Clinical (with weight and height), psychological and behavioural assessment of the young person is necessary to identify the type of eating disorder and its acute and long-term risk.

Diagnostic criteria for anorexia nervosa and bulimia nervosa (based on ICD-10)
Anorexia nervosa (AN)
- Body weight is maintained at least 15% below that expected or BMI is 17.5 or lower
- Self-induced weight loss by avoiding 'fattening foods' plus self-induced vomiting; purging; excessive exercise; use of appetite suppressants or use of diuretics
- Body image distortion in which dread of fatness persists as an intrusive, overwhelming idea

- Endocrine disorder of the hypothalamic-pituitary-gonadal axis, manifesting as amenorrhoea in women and loss of sexual interest and potency in men.
- If onset is pre-pubertal, puberty is delayed or arrested; with recovery, puberty is often normal, but the menarche is late.

Bulimia nervosa (BN)
- Persistent preoccupation with eating; overeating episodes in which large amounts of food are eaten in short periods of time
- Patient tries to counteract the 'fattening' effects of the overeating episodes by self-induced vomiting, purgative abuse; alternating starvation and eating; use of appetite suppressants, diuretics
- Morbid dread of fatness; patient sets her- or himself a precise weight threshold well below the healthy weight considered for this age.
- Often a history of previous anorexia nervosa, with the interval ranging from a few months to several years.

Presentations
- *Anorexia nervosa.* It is often not the patient herself/himself who makes contact, but rather someone else (e.g. parent, school etc.). The presentation features normally include weight loss, undereating and over-exercise, though patients may also present with non-specific physical symptoms. It is also normal for the patients themselves to deny that there is a problem.
- *Bulimia nervosa.* Usually patients consult alone (after a considerable delay), with the complaint that they are unable to control their eating. They may also present with non-specific physical or psychiatric symptoms (e.g. menstrual disturbance, depression).

Q2. What tests do you want to arrange?

Laboratory investigations should be limited to routine blood tests, which can be normal even with extreme weight loss. Complications may show up as:
- Decreased levels of sodium, potassium, organic phosphate and calcium (leading to osteoporosis; increased risk of bone fractures)
- Anaemia (iron deficiency); leucopenia and thrombocytopenia
- Euthyroid sick syndrome with normal TSH but low T3 and reduced T4 levels
- Raised urea nitrogen concentration with increased risk of renal stones
- Hypotension; sinus bradycardia; electrocardiography (ECG) may show prolongation

of the Q-T interval and other cardiac dysrhythmias; echocardiogram may show mitral valve prolapse and pericardial effusion.

Q3. Who can you treat yourself and who do you refer?

The management of a young person with an eating disorder has to tackle medical, nutritional, psychological and psychiatric aspects and should best be delivered by healthcare providers who are trained in this field. A shared management plan needs clear agreement about who is responsible for which part of the treatment. This should be communicated to the patient and the family.
- Weight monitoring should be established with a clear goal concerning an agreed weekly or monthly weight gain plus a plan to follow if weight falls. (Calculation of necessary caloric intake for adequate weight gain should take into account the level of activity of the young person.)
- Psychotherapy, mainly by means of cognitive behaviour therapy, is the method of choice for eating disorders. Parents, siblings and other carers should be included in the therapeutic involvement.
- Admission to hospital is generally avoided unless there is need for urgent weight restoration (very rapid weight loss or BMI substantially below the second percentile) and/or signs of physical compromise or a high risk of suicide.

There is no clear evidence that drugs have a role in the management of AN. In older adolescents with BN, antidepressants (especially selective serotonin-reuptake inhibitors) seem to be effective.

Substance abuse

Problem-orientated topic:

substance abuse   ● ● ● ● ●

The mother of a 16-year-old boy attends with her son and asks for him to have a urine test for drugs because of a marked change for the worse in his behaviour at home and at school. On questioning, the son says that, although he smokes a packet of cigarettes a day and binge-drinks at weekends, he is not otherwise 'into' taking illegal drugs but would like some information from you about the good and bad aspects of smoking cannabis.

Continued overleaf

Q1. What advice would you give him about smoking and excessive drinking?

Q2. How would you assess the risk of substance abuse in him?

Q3. What is the evidence of the effectiveness of drug intervention programmes?

Q1. What advice would you give him about smoking and excessive drinking?

According to a WHO survey in 2008, the weekly smoking rate among 15-year-olds in European countries is 19% (males 18%, females 19%). In the same age group the rate of adolescents who have been drunk at least twice in their life time is 33% (males 37%, females 30%) with relatively high rates of drunkenness in northern European countries. Recent (last 30 days) cannabis use was reported by 6% of the 15-year-olds (males 8%, females 6%). Smoking and excessive drinking are associated with a number of other risky behaviours, such as fighting and engaging in unprotected sex.

Effective methods for the prevention of starting smoking and drinking at an early age include banning advertising plus banning 'hidden advertising' on TV or in films, as well as increasing the price of cigarettes and alcohol.

Effective methods for giving up smoking and reducing alcohol and cannabis use include brief medical interventions. Motivational interviewing techniques have shown good results, especially when using 'decisional balance', i.e. before talking about the possible risks of substance use ('bad aspects') the health professional should question which benefits the young person expects from the use of the respective drug ('good aspects'). They can then try together to develop harm-reducing steps. The adolescent can also be encouraged to take advantage of helpful websites or in case of severe problems should be advised to see a drug councelling agency or a mental health service.

Q2. How would you assess the risk of substance abuse in him?

When you are taking a history, it is important for you to be aware of factors that are associated with an increased risk of substance abuse (Box 19.1).

General signs of drug abuse include:

- Physical:
  - Fatigue
  - Repeated health complaints
  - Red and glazed eyes

BOX 19.1 Risk factors for the problem use of substances in adolescence

- Genetic predisposition
- High experience-seeking
- High psychological distress
- Poor life skills
- Conduct disorder, impulsivity
- Mental disorders
- High level of use among friends
- High level of use among family members
- Physical or sexual abuse
- Childhood neglect
- Delinquency
- Poor academic achievement, school disconnectedness
- Unemployment, homelessness
- Separation or divorce of parents during childhood

- Emotional:
  - Personality change
  - Sudden mood changes
  - Irritability
  - Irresponsible behaviour
  - Low self-esteem
  - Poor judgment
  - Depression
  - General lack of interest
- Family:
  - Starting arguments
  - Negative attitude
  - Breaking rules
  - Withdrawing from family
  - Secretiveness
- School:
  - Decreased interest
  - Negative attitude
  - Drop in grades
  - Many absences
  - Truancy
  - Discipline problems
- Social problems:
  - New friends who make poor decisions and are not interested in school or family activities
  - Problems with the law

Be aware that many behaviours that parents tend to complain about are part of normal adolescent development: changes in mood, breaking rules, withdrawing from the family and/or showing no interest in learning.

Q3. What is the evidence of the effectiveness of drug intervention programmes?

School-based programmes aimed at adolescents can delay the start of substance misuse by non-users for a short time. Life skills training is one of the only programmes that has been extensively evaluated and for which there is some research evidence of a small but positive impact on drug use.

Acne

Acne vulgaris is the most common skin problem for which adolescents seek advice. 85% of all young people are affected to varying degrees at some stage of puberty. The severity of acne reaches its peak in late adolescence around the ages of 16 to 18. For most, acne reduces by the mid-20s; however, very sensitive people may continue to have the disorder until they reach their 40s. Affected are mainly the face (forehead, cheeks and area around the mouth), breast and back.

Acne is caused by a number of factors that can be attributed to the increased production of androgens during puberty

- Formation of comedones: the epithelium of the sebaceous glands proliferates; lipids and keratin are retained in the glands
- Seborrhoea: production of lipids in the sebaceous glands increases
- Inflammation and papules, pustules and nodules: though *Propionibacterium acnes* is a physiological bacterium of the skin and pores, its bacterial count increases during puberty and can lead to bacterial superinfection

Factors that may exacerbate acne include:
- Working in a damp environment with oil, grease and other chemicals
- Stress or emotional tension
- Squeezing or picking at the pimples
- In adolescent girls, menstrual periods
- Certain medicines and chemicals
- Hair gel and -spray may plug up the pores
- Some feel that certain foods (like chocolates, nuts, pork meat, fat, etc.) worsen their acne (although research has not yet proven that nutrients with high glycemic index or milk products influence acne)

Problem-orientated topic:

facial spots ● ● ● ● ●

Attila is a 14-year-old boy who consults you and is accompanied by his father. They explain how Attila is being teased because of his many spots and that it has started to affect his mood and confidence. His father is particularly worried about Attila not wishing to continue on the school swimming team because of acne on his torso.

Q1. How would you advise Attila to manage his acne?

Q1. How would you advise Attila to manage his acne?

General management includes:
- Washing the face twice a day with a mild cleanser (no soap)
- Using water-based moisturizers (no greasy or oily creams which block the pores)
- Keeping hair clean (no gel or spray) and out of the face
- Not squeezing or picking at the pimples. This makes them worse and may cause scarring.

Specific treatment depends on the severity of acne and whether the acne is predominantly comedonal or inflammatory:
- Comedolytic therapy ('peeling'): with benzoylperoxide (BPO), topical retinoids, azelaic acid or adapalene
- Topical anti-inflammatory therapy: with erythromycin or clindamycin preferably in combination with BPO
- Oral antibiotics for moderate to severe inflammatory acne, when topical treatment is not adequately effective: doxycycline and minocycline

Girls may profit from a combination contraceptive pill, e.g. cyproterone acetate and ethinyl estradiol.

In severe cases treatment with systemic isotretinoid can be used, preferably by specialists (contraception is necessary).

Julia Colomer Revuelta   Melanie Epstein

Emotional and behavioural problems: primary care aspects

MODULE FOUR

LEARNING OUTCOMES

By the end of this chapter you should:

- Know the common problems presenting in primary care
- Understand the common predisposing and protective factors related to mental health problems
- Know how to manage common problems presenting in preschool and school-age children.
- Have developed an approach to diagnostic formulation
- Be able to approach a consultation with a family presenting with an emotional or behavioural problem.

    Take the opportunity where possible of sitting in with an experienced community paediatrician or mental health professional for some observational experience.

Introduction

This chapter covers clinical aspects of child mental health, and how they present and need to be managed in primary care.

Children may have mental health needs if their abilities in any one of the following areas are impaired (Spender et al 2001):

- The ability to develop psychologically, emotionally, intellectually and spiritually

- The ability to initiate, develop and sustain mutually satisfying personal relationships
- The ability to become aware of others and to empathize with them
- The ability to use psychological distress as a developmental process, so that it does not hinder or impair further development.

In children, it is vital to consider their developmental stage. Child mental health problems arise when the degree of psychological distress and/or maladaptive behaviour is outside the normal limits for the child's age, developmental stage and context. This may depend on the values, thresholds for concern and culture of the family. Children are therefore presented as having emotional and behavioural problems according to the perceptions of the adults around them. Sometimes the behaviour is appropriate developmentally, but is not understood. Sometimes, a mild problem in some families may be seen as a major difficulty by others. Alternatively, serious problems may be overlooked. It is also important to remember that children may be presented as a symptom of another problem in a parent or the family.

Significant problems can be defined not by symptoms alone, but by interference with a child's functioning. Children present mental health problems in many different ways. Thus a child who is not doing well at school, who stops going to school, who does not make friends and who is very disruptive at home is likely to have mental health needs.

Mental health problems in children are associated with educational failure, family disruption, disability, offending and antisocial behaviour, placing demands on social services, schools and the youth justice system. Untreated mental health problems create distress not only in the children and young people, but also for their families and carers, continuing into adult life and affecting the next generation.

Prevalence of emotional and behavioural problems

Emotional and behavioural problems are relatively common in children and young people. It is estimated that between 10 and 25% of 0–18-year-olds are suffering from emotional and behavioural problems. Up to 15% of children and young people have mild emotional and behavioural problems. A further 7–10% have moderate or severe problems requiring specialist psychiatric assessment. Only 2% of children up to 16 years old have mental health disorders that are severe enough to be disabling.

About 2–5% of children seen in primary care settings are presented by their parents, with emotional and behavioural problems as the main complaint. The most frequent problems according to age are the following:

In preschool children (under 5 years of age)

- Waking and crying at night
- Over-activity
- Difficulty settling at night
- Refusing food.

In middle childhood (age 6–12 years)

- Persistent tearful, unhappy mood
- Bedtime behavioural rituals
- Night terrors/other disturbances of sleep
- Bedwetting
- Inattentive over-activity
- Faecal soiling.

In adolescence (age 13–18)

- Appreciable misery
- Social sensitivity
- Evident anxiety
- Suicidal ideas.

About 10% of adolescents suffer from more complex depressive moods. This is in addition to those diagnosed as having a psychiatric disorder, such as major depression.

Will the problem go away by itself?

Mild or moderate psychological problems are relatively persistent, particularly when linked with continuing problematic family relationships and attachment difficulties. Two large studies have shown that at least half of 3-year-olds rated as having behaviour problems were still displaying problems several years later.

Factors influencing the development of mental health problems

The presenting features of mental health problems in children can be associated with one or more biological, psychological or social factors. The sorts of factor that can impact on a child's mental health are shown in Box 20.1.

Some children who live with adverse circumstances or a combination of risk factors develop fewer or no more long-term problems than others. This is known as resilience.

The overarching factor contributing to resilience is mediated through attachment, and consists of having at least one adult who believes in and cares about the child. Three key groups of factors appear to protect children

BOX 20.1 Predisposing factors

The child
- Genetics and temperament (the child's inbuilt personality style)
- Acute or chronic illness
- Specific or general learning difficulties
- Language and other developmental disorder
- Sexual, physical or emotional abuse
- Lack of a secure attachment figure in the first few years of life

The family
- Parental discord
- Parental coldness or irritability towards the child
- Parental mental health problems or substance abuse
- Neglect
- Criminality
- Economic circumstances

The environment
- Overcrowding
- Homelessness
- Discrimination
- Refugee status

Life events
- Parental separation
- Acute illness
- Bereavement
- Experiencing or witnessing sudden and extreme trauma

School
- Bullying, victimization
- Inappropriate curriculum

BOX 20.2 Protective factors

The child
- Easy temperament
- At least average intelligence
- The capacity to process experiences in a positive way
- A sense of humour
- A sense of self-mastery

The family
- High warmth/low criticism
- Appropriate boundaries and discipline
- Absence of parental discord
- A secure attachment relationship with at least one parent

The social environment
- Affectionate ties with parent substitutes
- External support system
- Positive school experiences
- Opportunities for meaningful social roles and experiences

and adolescents (Spender et al 2001). Factors that are recognized to protect a child from the development of mental health problems are shown in Box 20.2.

Consultation skills

Parents often turn to their doctor for help with their child's emotional and behavioural problems. If conducted well, the consultation in itself can be therapeutic. To achieve this it is essential that you are skilled at listening and communicating, and convey empathy to the family.

It is useful to start from the premise that all parents want to do the best they can for their children and your role is to build on strengths in order to remove obstacles to a natural state of affairs. In doing this you are modelling the relationship you would like the parents to provide. In prevention, an approach focused on relationship building and treating the mother as the person with responsibility to promote the development of her child has been demonstrated to be more successful than one that is didactic.

Listening

Allow adequate time for the appointment and listen well. Hear a full account of the problem. This in itself can be therapeutic, and can lead the family to find solutions themselves.

Personal skills and attitudes

Know yourself

What are the cultural values, life experiences and personal attributes you bring to the consultation?

Maintain a respectful and non-judgmental attitude

This is best done by drawing on your skills of scientific enquiry and your natural curiosity and empathy. How-

217

ever, being human, we all experience other responses such as feeling critical, hopeless or frustrated, or an identification with the parents at times. It is useful to notice and be aware of the responses that you have. These can all give you more information.

Self-maintenance

Like a well-tuned car, your consultation is more likely to run smoothly if your physical and emotional needs are taken care of. In a busy job, considering work–life balance is sometimes a tall order. However, if you put yourself on hold for too long, your ability to be compassionate and curious is likely to feel harder to access.

Reflections

Sometimes, even with the best of intentions, consultations do not go as planned. If so, ask yourself:
- Does this give me any more information about the presenting problem or the process that is happening with the family?
- Do I need consultation with a colleague or another professional to help make sense of that?
- Does this tell me anything about myself?
- What did I like about how I was with this family?
- Would I do anything differently next time?

The consultation (Box 20.3)

You need to obtain as full a picture as possible of the problem, the child, the family and the environment, and it is important that the focus does not rest on the child alone. You need to understand the broader picture and see the difficulties in the context of the family and the child's environment. It is important to obtain the perceptions of each parent, where possible, as well as those of the child. It is helpful to bear in mind the predisposing and protective factors outlined in Boxes 20.1 and 20.2, and to think how these may be an influence on the child's behaviour.

As in any paediatric consultation, you need to take a structured approach. The following is the relevant background information you should obtain:
- History of the pregnancy and birth. It is usual when dealing with children to ask about the medical aspects of these. Remember also that pregnancy involves psychological preparation for a child, as well for the mother's changing identity.
- Prematurity and admission to a neonatal unit.

> **BOX 20.3 Key points: approach to the child with emotional and behavioural problems**
>
> - Allow adequate time to make a full assessment
> - Obtain as full a picture as possible of the problem, the child, the family and the environment. Involve the child in a developmentally appropriate way
> - Think about behaviour as a form of communication. Use observation of the family and child, as well as history-taking
> - Address family and school issues, as well as the child's problems. Where relevant, confer with others involved, such as grandparents, teachers or child-minders
> - Support parents in providing developmentally appropriate and consistent boundaries with love and affection. Focus on strengths and encourage parents to praise and reward good behaviour, rather than focusing on negatives
> - Do not wait for a child to grow out of a problem. Problems tend to persist or re-emerge at the next developmental stage
> - Medication has a very limited role and should only be prescribed by specialists

- Developmental milestones.
- Any medical problems.
- Establishment of routines around feeding and sleeping.
- History suggestive of maternal depression.
- Any history of separations.
- Any major losses, e.g. loss of parent, death of family member, moving house.
- The child's temperament and personality.
- Who else looks after the child and, if the child attends playgroup or nursery, how he or she has integrated.
- Sources of support to mother. It is usual to consider that a young single mother may be isolated. Older women or professional women who do not have a peer group with children, or people with no extended families, may also be isolated.
- Where possible, some assessment of the parental relationship.
- Any other professional involvement with the child, e.g. social worker — which may lead you to ask about any child protection issues.
- Family and social history. It is useful to draw a family tree, and also ask if the child reminds the parent of anyone.

Diagnostic formulation

In medicine, we generally learn that it is best to make one diagnosis that will explain all symptoms, rather than diagnosing more than one problem. This is not always the case when considering emotional and behavioural problems, and it is appropriate to formulate a broader picture. The 'four Ps' (Box 20.4) can help you to draw up your diagnostic formulation.

It is also useful to consider factors that promote change. This is linked to the protective factors, but will also include motivation to change and insight into the problem. The more you can harness that motivation, particularly if the family can find their own solutions, the more likely change will occur.

Management of emotional and behavioural problems

Many parental concerns relate to normal behaviour: for example, food fads in toddlers or night-waking in infants, and it may be adequate simply to provide reassurance. Other concerns relate to difficult behaviour, and you should be able to provide guidance on parenting. Helpful principles are shown in Box 20.5.

Star charts

A useful strategy in overcoming difficult behaviour is using a star chart, which can be adapted to improve and motivate a variety of behaviours, from enuresis to temper tantrums and disruptive behaviour at school. A calendar is drawn up and each day the child has behaved well, a star or smiley face is awarded. A prize can be given when an agreed number of stars have been earned. This can be very effective in reinforcing desirable behaviour, while alleviating focus on the negative.

Table 20.1 Behaviour indicative of serious disturbance

Behaviour	Disturbance
Deliberately destructive	Low self-esteem Hostile relationships Possible conduct disorder
Deliberate self-harm	Severe distress Loss of attachment Low self-esteem
Running away	Lack of affection Severe distress
Encopresis	Lack of self-worth Inadequate care
Age-inappropriate sexual behaviour	Sexual abuse

Time out

Time out is a strategy that is useful during an episode of difficult behaviour. The child has to stay in a quiet spot for a fixed short period of time. One minute per year of age is a good guide, and a kitchen timer is a useful way of enforcing the time. This method allows the child (and the parent) time to cool off, and also gives the parent a clear but limited non-violent means of discipline.

Involving other professionals

An important aspect of good management involves arranging a follow-up appointment. Other professionals may also be available to provide support and help for the child. The health visitor is a particular asset for preschool children, as is the teacher for the child at school. More intransigent cases may require referral to Child and Adolescent Mental Health Services. The sort of behaviour that is indicative of serious abuse is shown in Table 20.1. Any of these behaviours may be associated with abuse, and it is also important to consider the presence of child protection issues.

Emotional and behavioural problems presenting in the preschool child

Problems presenting in the preschool child are generally those of self-regulation and routines, and depend on the age and stage of development. They include problems with crying, sleep, feeding, toileting and behaviour. Babies may be communicating to their parents, through, for example, poor sleep patterns, excessive crying, difficulties with feeding, restlessness and gastric disturbance, that they are anxious and tense, distressed or fearful. Parents may not know how to respond to these communications with support and empathy, or may misread a baby's cues because of their own history or previous events in the baby's life, or simply a lack of knowledge of what is normal. Supporting families to provide an appropriate response is essential, in order to reduce the incidence of emotional and behavioural problems and their consequences in later life. Parents may be concerned that there is something wrong with the child, and in some cases there may be a medical problem. Differentiating between normal or abnormal behaviour, as well as knowing when further treatment is necessary, is important.

Crying

This is a common paediatric problem. A normal healthy baby cries for between 1 and 3 hours a day. Parents normally start to notice and pick out different types of crying, such as hunger, pain and boredom, by the time the baby is 1–14 days old.

About 10% of babies may cry excessively, more than 3 hours in 24. Reasons why babies may cry excessively include:

- Temperament and sensitivity to environmental change.
- Prematurity or difficult birth/special care admission.
- Environmental change. Some babies can be more sensitive to changes in their surroundings or care routine.
- New developmental stage in learning or growth.
- Tension. Babies sense when their parents are tense and it can affect their behaviour. This can be a bit confusing, and can become a circular situation.
- Colic. This can cause excessive crying in the first 3 months (Ch. 24).

http://www.cry-sis.org.uk

General advice to parents with babies who cry excessively, or are sleepless or demanding

Poor sleep patterns

> **Problem-orientated topic:**
>
> **a baby who will not sleep**
>
> Maria S. brings her 2-year-old daughter, Sofia, to see you. Maria says she is exhausted because Sofia will not sleep through the night. She does not settle down to sleep, and when she does eventually go to sleep, she wakes up at some point in the middle of the night. Often mum resorts to bringing Sofia into her bed because she is so tired. She would like some help in establishing a sleep routine.
>
> Q1. What should you ask about in the history?
> Q2. Can you give a brief diagnostic formulation?
> Q3. What will help you with your assessment?
> Q4. What advice can you give?

Q1. What should you ask about in the history?

It is important to obtain a full assessment of the problem, including parental views.

Sleep routines

Ask about daytime sleeps and bedtime routines. Ask about any other children and their routines. Sometimes the advent of a new baby, another significant change at home or conflicting needs of different children will impact on sleep routines.

Parental concerns

What does the mother feel is the main problem? There is a suggestion here that her tiredness is significant. Ask more about this and how it is affecting her. It takes a fair amount of will and energy to address a sleep problem. Are there concerns about the effects of sleeplessness on the child? Ask about sources of support. Is there a partner/grandparents/other support? What are they doing? Are mum and partner in accord about family rules, or is one somehow undermining the other?

Birth and early history/family history

A general paediatric history will help your assessment of whether this is an isolated problem, or whether there are other issues with routines such as feeding or with the child's behaviour. Children with neurodevelopmental problems may be more likely to have sleep difficulties and may need specialist help. Problems with the birth, illness in the child, or unresolved grief in relation to the death or significant illness of another child or family member may lead to parental anxiety, contributing to difficulty enforcing boundaries or leaving the child to go to sleep.

Medical problems

Are there any factors suggestive of medical problems in the history? In particular, ask about any night-time cough suggestive of asthma, snoring and early morning grogginess suggestive of obstructive sleep apnoea, or itch associated with eczema or scabies. Your examination will then be guided by your assessment of the presence of medical problems.

The child

A healthy child depends on stimulation and attention (whether negative or positive) for survival and development, and therefore it can be viewed as normal for a child to learn when it is possible to control a parent at bedtime to provide this.

You may have an idea from the general history as to whether the child may have a difficult temperament (p. 217), with poorly established circadian rhythms. In some cases the problem may be more that the child is afraid to go to sleep. This may occur in the presence of insecure attachment and separation anxiety, domestic violence or sexual abuse.

On further questioning you find out that Sofia was born by emergency section for fetal distress, and was in Special Care overnight. Maria admits she was terrified at the time. She says she is still a bit anxious about Sofia. When you ask about the sleep routine, Maria says she tends not to leave Sofia to go to sleep on her own, and does not like to leave her to cry. Sofia never seemed to settle into routines easily as a baby, but has had no other health problems. Mum says she has come to clinic now because she has become short-tempered with Sofia, and she does not want this to continue. She has given up her job in the media, which involved travelling away from home, to look after Sofia. She says she realizes she has lost touch with her friends and has made an arrangement to meet one of them for lunch. Her husband works a lot of late nights, but he helps with childcare when he is there.

BOX 20.6 Sleep problem: failure to settle as well as night-waking

Predisposing
- Difficult birth history
- Mother–baby separation
- Maternal anxiety for child's health/survival at birth — ?unresolved
- Difficult temperament

Precipitating
- Mother exhausted, has become short-tempered, ?depressed

Perpetuating
- Entrenched pattern between mother and child
- Father not home most bedtimes
- Lack of social support

Protective
- Father supportive when around
- Mother reconnecting with social support
- Mother has insight and is taking responsibility for the problem

---

Q2. Can you give a brief diagnostic formulation?

See Box 20.6.

Promoting change

Maria has recognized that there is a problem, has thought of some solutions herself, and is also asking for help and advice.

Q3. What will help you with your assessment?

A sleep diary may be helpful to obtain a more detailed picture of Sofia's sleep pattern, and to see what specific factors may be perpetuating the problem, as well as where change can most easily be instituted. Information obtained from the diary will include the child's wake time and mood on waking, any naps during the day, bedtime routines and going to sleep time, as well as times and duration of night-waking. In each case the parent's actions or responses are recorded as well. In some cases filling in the sleep diary may be therapeutic in itself, as parents may gain more insight into the problem.

Depression

It is worth asking more about how the mother feels to see whether she might be depressed. Further physician and/or nurse, social worker or other health care professional involvement may be useful. Depressed mothers are a high risk, as depression may interfere with their ability to tune into their baby's signals and provide a sensitive, emotionally nurturing and care-giving environment. Postnatal depression is linked to an increase in insecure attachment in toddlers, behavioural disturbance at home, less creative play and greater levels of disturbed or disruptive behaviour at primary school, poor peer relationships, and a decrease in self-control with an increase in aggression.

Q4. What advice can you give?

First give an explanation. Parents may find it helpful to know how common sleep problems are and that they can be solved, but that this takes some energy and persistence. Explain that the fact that the problem is getting worse may imply that the treatment is actually working. It may be useful to explain that all children wake up at night, but that some children have not yet learned how to settle themselves back to sleep. Give this advice in the context of support and reassurance. Around 50% of night-wakers like Sofia have a problem settling to sleep. In these cases, the first problem to tackle is the settling to sleep.

Helpful advice for parents

- Learn to read your child's cues of tiredness.
- Choose an appropriate time to enforce the sleep routine.
- Ensure all carers are involved and will agree to be consistent.
- Have a relaxing routine leading up to bedtime, e.g. warm bath, snack, story.
- Set a bedtime, enforce firmly and calmly say goodnight.
- If the child cries, ignore; if that is too much, at least give no positive attention.
- If the child gets out of bed, return him or her promptly and firmly.
- Give positive reinforcement (e.g. star or sticker chart) following good nights.
- Be consistent. Giving in now and again will reinforce the unwanted behaviour.
- Sleep problems can be solved. Get support when problems arise.

http://www.cry-sis.org.uk/

For more detailed advice to parents, follow the link to sleep problems

Who else can help?

If you are limited by time constraints, basic advice has not worked or the problem seems more complex, it may be appropriate to involve other health care professionals. If the problem still fails to respond or

you identify more complex underlying issues, consider referral to a Child and Adolescent Mental Health service.

Tantrums and difficult behaviour

Tantrums are a normal part of childhood development and peak between the ages of 18 months and 3 years. Frustration, anger and tantrums are typical for toddlers, and may involve hitting, biting and other potentially harmful behaviour. Some babies and toddlers may resort to breath-holding (p. 296) as part of the tantrum, and this is often a frightening event to witness. Parents often talk about these episodes in the context of the 'terrible twos'. In some cases, parents feel they are wilful on the part of their children. This is not the case. Children are merely 'testing' how to express and contain their feelings safely and how to assert their developing will and individual personality.

> **Problem-orientated topic:**
>
> **tantrums** ● ● ● ● ●
>
> Adriana, a 37-year-old mother, brings her 2¹/₂-year-old child, Natalia, to see you. She is complaining about Natalia's behaviour. The child seems to shout and get cross very often, for no apparent reason. This may then be followed by a full-blown tantrum. Mum says she has tried everything to stop this, but with no success. She is worried the neighbours will think she is hurting her child. Sometimes Natalia nips or hits her little sister. This has been happening for the last few months. Mum is worried that Natalia's younger sister is starting to copy her.
>
> Q1. What further information will help you with your assessment?
> Q2. What advice can you give parents about tantrums?

Q1. What further information will help you with your assessment?

Parental concerns

You have obtained some information about these already. Adriana has already told you she is concerned about the impact on her younger child and about the reaction of the neighbours.

Developmental history

It is important to take a full developmental history. Natalia was found to have been slow to talk, and to have only just started to say two words together. Delayed speech development may be associated with frustration. Other language or comprehension problems may mean the child does not understand what is expected of him or her. Wider developmental or cognitive difficulties may mean that tantrums may be more severe or persistent. Any family history of deafness or developmental delay may be significant.

General health

Check whether there has been a hearing test, and whether there have been any episodes of otitis media or upper respiratory tract infections. Ongoing or fluctuating hearing loss may be associated with behaviour problems.

Does the child have any symptoms of pain, discomfort or tiredness that may be affecting behaviour? Has the child had a significant head injury?

Ask about any medications. Anticonvulsants or night-time sedatives, for example, may affect behaviour.

Parental factors

Try to assess whether there is consistency of parental discipline from day to day and also between parents.

It is useful to know how other members of the family deal with anger, but this information is difficult to ascertain. A child whose sibling or parent is modelling tantrum behaviour is less likely to learn to deal with frustration or conflict. A child who is experiencing severe anger or witnessing domestic violence is unlikely to respond to simple behavioural measures.

Are there any particular parental stresses or issues of lack of support that make it more difficult to manage the child?

ABC diary

This can be used for almost any type of behavioural problem. Ask the parent to record relevant details of the most recent tantrums according to the following format. It is important that parents understand what the headings mean and the purpose of keeping the diary:

- A — antecedents
- B — behaviour
- C — consequences.

This can also be used to help you with history-taking and in formulating specific management strategies.

Q2. What advice can you give to parents?

The Royal College of Psychiatrists (UK) has some useful information designed for parents (also useful for professionals) that is easy to read and evidence-based. There are 36 fact sheets on a variety of emotional and

behavioural topics, many of them translated into 14 languages. These can be downloaded or bought as a collected volume.

 http://www.rcpsych.ac.uk/info

For advice on dealing with tantrums, follow the links to 'Leaflets for Young People' and then to 'Mental Health and Growing Up', 3rd edn, leaflet 3

The over-active child

> **Problem-orientated topic:**
>
> **an over-active child**
>
> Diego, a 3-year-old boy, is referred by his paediatrician or family doctor because his parents are concerned that he is hyperactive. They complain that Diego will not do as he is told. He talks continually but rarely listens. His mother says he is restless, does not sit still and moves from one thing to another. He does not like to go to sleep, and does not usually to go to bed before 9.00 pm. The only time he does sit still is when watching his favourite television programme. Mum would like him to be more like his sister, who she describes as her 'little helper', and who loves to sit and draw. Dad is not too worried because he says he has been told he was like that as a child. The family have a very small garden, and Diego does not have any friends who live nearby. He attends nursery part-time, where he is described as having no problems. During the interview, Diego explores the workings of your examination light and stethoscope, and opens all the boxes of toys. He is told off eight times. He takes the blocks out and sits absorbed making an elaborate castle, and playing a game that you can hear involves Spiderman. His parents are absorbed talking to you about him and do not appear to notice.
>
> Q1. Is Diego hyperactive?
> Q2. What advice can you give to his parents?

Q1. Is Diego hyperactive?

He is not. Many parents worry that their children have attention deficit hyperactivity disorder (ADHD),

223

when in fact their behaviour is in the range of normal. ADHD is a syndrome complex that requires the child to have specific symptoms of inattention, hyperactivity and impulsivity at home and at school (Ch. 29). When interpreting the criteria, it is essential to take the child's age and developmental stage into account. Many 2–3-year-olds are normally over-active and have a short attention span. If these behaviours are present in a child older than 4 at home and at school, then ADHD may be in your differential diagnosis.

Q2. What advice can you give to his parents?

- Reassure the parents.
- Encourage parental consistency.
- Advise them to 'catch the child being good' and praise him specifically for desired behaviour.
- Talk about how Diego can be given more opportunities for energetic play and for play with friends.

If parents want to change the sleep pattern, talk about sleep routines or think about involving other healthcare professionals. Most of the advice is the usual advice about good parenting. Many parents find it useful to have some written information.

http://www.rcpsych.ac.uk/info

'Mental Health and Growing Up' series, leaflet 2: 'Good Parenting'. Mental Health and Growing Up series is translated into different languages.

Emotional and behavioural problems presenting in the school-age child

Obtaining a history

School life brings its own problems and also affects how the child adjusts to difficulties at home. It is important to find out how the child has made the adjustment to school, and about relationships with teachers and peers, as well as about academic achievement in different areas. It is vital to involve children directly and this starts with taking a history from the children themselves. Having started school, they have their own life.

When speaking to the child, think how you can support his or her attempts to communicate.

Either sit down or position yourself at the same level as the child. Try to talk with the child, rather than at the child. Use simple words and ideas, and check that the child understands you. Start off with a (hopefully) neutral subject. It is sometimes helpful to use drawings and play as a way of getting alongside the child. This also

gives you the opportunity to make an observation about the child's fine motor skills. Let children tell you about their drawing, rather than interpreting this for them.

It is worth remembering that further information can be obtained from school, although of course you should only contact school with the parent's permission.

> **Problem-orientated topic:**
>
> **the child who is struggling at school** ●●●●
>
> Miguel, age 6, is brought to see you, by his mother. She says his teacher told her on parents' evening that Miguel is having a lot of difficulties at school. He has problems with his writing and is a bit clumsy. He does not pay attention in class. She is concerned and would like some help for him. Miguel has been otherwise healthy and his developmental milestones have been within normal limits. He was happy and had friends in nursery.
>
> Mum says their relationship is quite intense, as there are just the two of them at home. You ask about Miguel's father. Mum says that after dad kept breaking promises to come and see Miguel, she has stopped him seeing his father as he gets too upset. You ask Miguel what he thinks the problem is and he says that there are a group of boys who pick on him at school. He does not want to talk any more. You ask him to draw you a picture. He draws a picture of a boy with spiky hair, that you notice looks a bit like him. You ask him to tell you about his picture. He tells you that this is a picture of the boy they call stupid. You notice his mother looks upset as he says that.
>
> Q1. Can you give a brief diagnostic formulation?
> Q2. What is your management plan?

Q1. Can you give a brief diagnostic formulation?

See Box 20.7.

Q2. What is your management plan?

1. Ask mother and Miguel what specific help they would like.

2. If examination confirms evidence of difficulties with fine motor skills and incoordination, consider referral for occupational therapy assessment.
3. Refer for hearing test.
4. Find out from the teacher more about Miguel's abilities and how he is at school. It may be useful to talk to the school special needs coordinator.
5. Talk about the possibility of Miguel being bullied and how you can support mother, if necessary by talking to the school and making an appropriate plan.
6. Discuss Miguel's referral to Child and Adolescent Mental Health Services for work on his self-esteem and relationship with his father. It is important when making such a referral to check that the family want to engage in this process. Further discussion may shed some light on the 'intense relationship' between Miguel and his mother, and whether they need some help with this.
7. Talk to the mother about what support she has, and whether she has work or interests outside the home.
8. Arrange a follow-up appointment.

Recurrent and unexplained symptoms

Children who have recurrent symptoms, such as abdominal pain (Ch. 25) or headaches (Ch. 24) that do not respond to treatment, may have mental health problems. These may occur if the symptoms are primarily functional, or if the child has first had a primary illness. An underlying emotional component is also likely if a child has unexplained symptoms such as complaining of inability to walk in the absence of any abnormal physical signs or demonstrable pathology. In all these cases, help from Child and Adolescent Mental Health Services can be sought. Rarely, recurrent or unexplained symptoms can be a presentation of fabricated or induced illness (Ch. 21), and additional consultation with an appropriate consultant paediatrician and social services will be necessary.

Unwanted habits and behaviour

Parents may complain about a range of behaviours that occur normally. These include thumb-sucking, head-banging, body-rocking, nail-biting, hair-pulling, teeth-grinding, simple tics and masturbation. It is useful to know some simple facts, and to know when reassurance and some simple behavioural tips are appropriate. As is usual when dealing with children's behaviour, it is more helpful for the parent to 'catch the child being good', rather than chastising the child or trying to stop the undesired behaviour, as this may lead to reinforcement. In many cases, children may not be able to control these habits until they grow older.

Masturbation

This is common in both sexes in preschool children. The usual problem is the issue of its social acceptability. If parents wish to limit masturbation, it usually responds to common-sense techniques like ignoring the behaviour or distraction. Alternatively, children can be encouraged to masturbate in private.

Nail-biting and thumb-sucking

About 25% of children between 3 and 6 years of age suck their thumbs or bite their nails. Thumb-sucking is normal in early infancy. However, beyond a certain age, it makes the older child appear immature and may interfere with normal alignment of the teeth. It is a difficult habit to influence, and it is best to ignore it as it resolves over time. The child who actively tries to stop thumb-sucking should be given praise and encouragement.

Nail-biting is a difficult habit to break, unless the child has some motivation to do so. Application of bitter-tasting nail varnish can be helpful. In some children nail-biting is a sign of tension.

Food refusal

Feeding problems are very common in young children. About 10% of young children demonstrate some problem with food refusal between 9 and 15 months of age, and start to refuse food offered to them. It is common for this to be associated with food faddiness. This occurs in association with children's developing sense of self as they assert their autonomy by closing their mouth and turning away. Sometimes it may be associated with coercive or rushed feeding. At later stages, about one-third of 5-year-olds have a mild to moderate eating problem. In all these cases, as long as a child is thriving, some common-sense advice about nutrition and behaviour is probably all that is needed. (See also page 31.)

Enuresis

Urinary continence is generally achieved by the age of 3 or 4. Around 10% of 5-year-olds, 5% of 10-year-olds and 2% of teenagers still have enuresis. There is often a family history in children with enuresis. Failure to achieve toilet training or regression to wetting may be a sign of stress. Common precipitating events include the birth of a sibling, a death in the family, a move to a new home and marital conflict. Enuresis may also result from inadequate or inappropriate toilet training. It is fully discussed on page 331.

Encopresis

Encopresis, or the passage of faeces in inappropriate places, usually indicates a serious emotional disturbance. It needs to be distinguished from soiling, which results from leakage of liquid faeces around hard stool when a child is constipated. However, secondary psychological problems can still result when the problem is not recognized or understood. Constipation and soiling are discussed on page 308.

Reference

Spender Q, Salt S, Dawkins J et al 2001 Child mental health in primary care. Routledge, London. This is a comprehensive easy-to-read book for non-mental health practitioners. It contains a useful chapter on behavioural techniques for use by enthusiastic professionals in primary care

Malcolm Levene   Raisa H. K. Lounamaa   Neela Shabde
Amanda J. Thomas

Child protection in the community

LEARNING OUTCOMES

By the end of this chapter you should:

- Know and understand which children are most susceptible to child abuse
- Know and understand the legal framework protecting children
- Know and understand the roles and responsibilities of the primary care doctor in protecting children
- Know and understand the framework for interagency working
- Know how child abuse and neglect may present in primary care
- Understand the importance of being familiar with the reporting mechanisms for suspected abuse
- Be familiar with the Child Protection Case Conference and if the child is the subject of a child protection plan
- Understand the emotional and developmental impact of abuse
- Understand the needs of looked-after children
- Understand how children with emotional abuse and neglect present and are managed.

Introduction

Protecting children from intentional or indeed unintentional harm is the role of all doctors, whether they work in primary care or as a paediatrician, although their role in protecting children will differ. There is a basic level of knowledge that all such doctors must possess in order to be able to fulfil this function. This chapter describes the basis of child protection from the point of view of a primary care doctor and Chapter 36 describes this from a paediatric trainee's perspective.

These two chapters give an overview of child protection, but in Britain it is a requirement that all paediatric trainees undergo a formal educational programme for doctors, including a training day organized by the Royal College of Paediatrics and Child Health (RCPCH), the National Society for Prevention of Cruelty to Children (NSPCC) and the Advanced Life Support Group (ALSG). These chapters are not intended as a substitute for this formal training but rather as an overview and summary of material that is available through the College.

The responsibility for child protection is not primarily a medical one and the underlying principle of child protection is sharing concerns on a multi-agency basis, developing solutions and maintaining safety networks for children and their families.

What is child abuse?

Child abuse is the description given to a varied set of actions or omissions considered to be harmful to children. These can be defined under a number of categories, which are described in more detail both in this chapter and Chapter 36:

- Neglect
- Emotional abuse
- Physical abuse
- Sexual abuse
- Factitious or induced illness (child medical abuse).

Child abuse occurs in all social classes and is most frequent in vulnerable families. Risk factors for abuse include:

- Prematurity, separation and impaired bonding in the neonatal period
- Children with a difficult temperament (behaviour more a consequence than a risk factor)
- Chronic illness/disability in the child
- Poverty/single-parent status/step-parent or cohabitee present
- Male unemployment
- Domestic violence
- Absence of social support
- The carer who was abused in childhood

- History of parental mental health problems/illnesses
- Alcohol and substance abuse
- Large family size.

The legal framework

Child protection in most countries is guided by a legal framework which often incorporates principles within the United Nations Convention on the Rights of the Child and the European Convention on Human Rights. Children are protected by multi-agency working, promoting children's welfare and protecting them from abuse and neglect. The UK Department of Health (2006) document, 'Working Together to Safeguard Children', summarizes the UK legislation and is a good example of principles for professionals working with children. The emphasis is on:

- Focusing on the child and family rather than the injury
- Identifying roles and responsibilities of different agencies and practitioners
- Placing child protection procedures within the remit of a local organization with responsibility for coordinating interagency working (in the UK, the Local Safeguarding Children Board — LSCB)
- Describing processes to be followed when there are concerns about a child and actions to be taken to safeguard and promote the welfare of children suffering, or at risk of suffering, significant harm.
- Providing guidance on child protection for children in specific circumstances, such as children living away from home or children with disabilities.

The role of primary care professionals in child protection

The doctor represents an important partner in the network of child protection. The primary care doctor, together with the practice-based health visitor, is in an excellent position to provide a pivotal overview of the child within the family. The first concern about child abuse may arise from the doctor's concerns about injuries, failure to thrive, abnormal behaviour or disclosure by the child. Alternatively his or her concerns for the child may be aroused by evidence of domestic violence, parasuicide attempts, mental illness in the family or the parent's inappropriate emotional response to the child. Doctors must recognize their own role as a cog in the multi-agency wheel that must turn efficiently to protect children (p. 229).

The responsibilities of doctors with regard to child protection are summarized in Box 21.1.

The basic principles for doctors involved in child protection are:

- Recognition of the problem
- Reporting of suspicions
- Contributing to the investigation of the problem.

Table 21.1 summarizes knowledge, skills and attitudes that all doctors must develop in order to discharge their responsibilities in protecting children adequately.

The doctor must be able to balance the needs of the adults against those of the child. Struggling families should be given support to raise their children in a safe environment, but children may need to be protected if their parents are harming them. The needs of the child must be paramount. Parents who themselves have been abused and neglected may find it difficult to love and care for their children in an acceptable way. It should be recognized that they may potentially require a range of support. Health visitors are particularly well placed to identify early markers of potential abuse and neglect and to introduce services to support the family.

Interagency working — working together

This describes working together and sharing responsibility, which require that agencies and professionals, including paediatricians:

- Share information
- Collaborate and understand each other's roles and responsibilities
- Work in partnership with one another and with children and their families to plan comprehensive and coordinated services
- Recognize vulnerable children and coordinate services from various appropriate agencies, including the voluntary sector
- Work with adult services, particularly mental health
- Work to protect children and cooperate with the criminal justice system in the prosecution of the perpetrator in accordance with the national legal framework and national guidelines.

The Framework for the Assessment of Children in Need and Their Families provides the foundation for a systematic assessment of children and families. The framework triangle embraces three key areas:

- The child's developmental needs
- The parental capacity
- The wider family and environmental factors.

The process ideally draws on the contribution of a range of agencies in the comprehensive assessment of the child and family. The framework emphasizes that the assessment is a process, not a single event, and that the resulting interventions arise from the conclusions of this.

Table 21.1 **Summary of the doctor's role in protecting children***

Stage	Knowledge	Skills	Attitudes
Recognition	Predisposing factors Clinical indicators	Clinical acumen Developmental examination	Acceptance that abuse is prevalent
Reporting	Local reporting arrangements Role appreciation When to intervene	Communication skills Documentation	Principle that protecting the child is paramount Acknowledgment of adverse effects of abuse and neglect
Investigation	Role appreciation Role of others	Communication skills Report writing	Willingness to share information Cooperation with other agencies Coping skills

* Adapted from Bannon MJ, Carter YH 2003 Protecting Children from Abuse and Neglect in Primary Care. Oxford University Press, Oxford.

In the UK, all NHS trusts, be they primary, secondary or tertiary care providers, should have a named doctor and named nurse for child protection who take a professional lead within the Trust on child protection matters. Their responsibility includes education, support and supervision. Each local area must have a designated doctor and nurse for child protection at primary care level who work closely with the named professionals in supporting activities within Trusts.

Presentation in primary care

The basic principles involved in child protection are:
- Recognition and reporting
- Contributing information to the multi-agency investigation and risk assessment
- Providing support for the child and family.

The doctor in primary care has a responsibility to recognize the possibility of child abuse, and if uncertain, to report his or her concerns to others with responsibilities and greater experience in investigating the problem.

Recognition of the problem

'If you don't think, you won't diagnose.'

Presentation of abuse

The child may disclose an incident of abuse in confidence to a doctor. Disclosure to a relative, friend or professional is probably the most common way in which child sexual abuse comes to light. Doctors should be aware of the pitfall of promising confidentiality before being told the child's secret. There is no place for confidentiality where there is suspected abuse or neglect. The child should be informed that the information will be passed on to the agency and to professionals (the social services in most countries) with responsibility and powers to help and protect the child and other children. A doctor should never interrogate a child if she or he has disclosed abuse, as this may compromise the subsequent legal process, but gentle and non-leading questioning may be appropriate. The doctor should have no ethical dilemma as to whether this information should be reported to the statutory agencies for child protection. In most countries the reporting is supported by legislation which incorporates principles that protection of children and young people as patients overrides the duty of confidentiality to the patient.

Good communication skills with children and young people are very important.

There is no simple diagnostic test for child abuse and often the symptoms are subtle or non-specific. In some cases the diagnosis is straightforward, but in others — for example, where the parent vigorously denies any abuse — the situation is more difficult. The doctor does not need to be certain of the diagnosis to raise concern. The doctor's responsibility is first and foremost to report his or her suspicions and share those concerns with others.

The main presenting features of the different forms of child abuse are discussed below and in Chapter 36. A summary of the major presenting features are:
- Presentation with injury that is inconsistent or unexplained
- Allegations or disclosure of abuse from a child, carer or neighbour
- Pattern of poor and inadequate care of the child, failure to thrive
- Presence of individuals in the household who are suspected or known to be a risk to children
- Repeated visits or contacts for minor trivial or unexplained complaints with primary care providers, e.g. paediatrician, primary care physician, emergency department
- Failure to turn up for review of complaints, missed appointments
- Accumulated concerns about the child or family from various members of the primary care team.

Reporting

'Doing nothing in suspected cases is not an option.'

It is the doctor's responsibility to report concerns about an individual child to the appropriate authorities. This usually means a discussion between the doctor and either a local paediatrician or the local social services department, which will provide an out-of-hours service if you feel that there is an urgent risk to the child. The referral should be followed up with written notification. The primary care doctor does not need to be an expert in child protection. Further investigations will be taken forward by an experienced paediatrician. The notifying doctor's responsibility is for vigilance and reporting. Accurate notes written at the time of referral are essential.

Intervention and investigation

'If in doubt, ask for help or advice.'

In most countries, intervention is coordinated through social services, who have a statutory responsibility to respond when notified of a child suspected to be suffering, or likely to suffer, from significant harm.

Emotional impact of abuse

Many children who have been abused may show little evidence of psychological problems in childhood, but this represents a 'latent' phase that may manifest later in life as emotional disorder. In adolescence this may take the form of truancy, violence, substance abuse or mental health problems. Those children who are most damaged may themselves show self-damaging behaviour, become drug and alcohol abusers, or turn to prostitution or violence.

Emotional abuse has the most damaging effect in later life, with the inability to form normal relationships and hence the perpetuation of the risk of abuse to the next generation of children. Its long-term effects are greater than in children who have suffered physical abuse alone.

Persistent neglect has a pervasive effect on the child's self-esteem, with consequent effects on intellectual, physical, social and emotional development that are correlated with school failure. These effects may also result in later failure to develop normal relationships. It is suggested that this may result later in life in maternal depression, drug abuse and antisocial or criminal activities.

Looked-after children

A child is looked after when he or she is in local authority care or is being provided with accommodation by the local authority for more than 24 hours. A looked-after child can be accommodated voluntarily with his or her parent's/guardian's agreement or following a court order. Children can be cared for by extended family members, foster carers or another responsible adult or in a residential home/school. At any one time approximately 60 000 are in care and approximately 80% are in care due to abuse and neglect. Looked-after children are particularly vulnerable to further abuse and neglect, are the most socially excluded of all children, and as a group have poor experiences of education and very low educational attainment. Around 67% of looked-after children have mental health problems in later life. About half of the prison population and young people living rough report having been in care.

Children who are looked after should have a health needs assessment (which may include a physical examination), either before their placement or as soon as is reasonably practical after a placement is made. The health needs assessment should be carried out by a registered medical practitioner (ideally, one who is paediatrically trained), who should prepare a report and a future healthcare plan. A review health assessment should be carried out twice yearly if the child is under 5 years and annually for children over 5 years. Health assessments should cover a range of issues beyond those of physical health, which include developmental health and emotional wellbeing. Primary care teams and paediatricians have an important role to play in the identification, recording and coordination of the healthcare needs of looked-after children.

Adoption

Adoption of a child, through an adoption order, transfers all parental responsibility to the adopters. All children require a health assessment prior to adoption, with provision of a report regarding the child. Primary care teams and paediatricians have an important role in provision of health assessments for the adoption panel.

Child neglect

Problem-orientated topic:

neglect

Emil, aged 15 months, is referred because of pallor and delayed development. He is the youngest of four children, and on examination he is dirty and his clothes are unkempt. The mother is an alcoholic and the father is in prison. The three older children attend school sporadically, none is fully immunized and all have speech and language delay.

Q1. What is the most likely cause of Emil's problems?

Q2. How would you define child neglect?

Q3. How would you assess this case?

Q4. How would you manage this child and family?

Q1. What is the most likely cause of Emil's problems?

Emil is most likely to be suffering from a form of abuse referred to as neglect. Neglect may take several forms:

- Neglect of the child's physical needs, e.g. nutrition (Emil's anaemia arising as a result of a diet low in iron, resulting in pallor)

- Failure to pay attention to the child's personal hygiene, clothing etc. (Emil is dirty and unkempt)
- Failure to provide stimulation and education (developmental delay in Emil and frequent school absences in the older siblings)
- Neglect of the child's medical needs (neither Emil nor his siblings are fully immunized)
- Neglect of supervision and lack of awareness of safety issues
- Neglect of interaction with adults and with other children of the same age
- Failure to provide affection and appropriate nurturing.

Q2. How would you define child neglect?

The UK Department of Health defines neglect as:

persistent failure to meet a child's basic physical and/or psychological needs, likely to result in the serious impairment of the child's health or development. It may involve a parent or carer failing to provide adequate food, shelter or clothing, failing to protect a child from physical harm or danger, or the failure to ensure access to appropriate medical care or treatment. It may also include neglect of, or unresponsiveness to, a child's basic emotional needs.

Families in whom a child is subject to neglect have been described as those that 'are low on warmth and high on criticism'. Repeated criticism reminds the child that he or she is unloved (emotional abuse), with a consequent risk of neglect or other forms of abuse including either physical or sexual. Another common family trait is a lack of consistency in disciplining the child.

In the UK, neglect is the most common reason for the need of child protection procedures. Persistent neglect has a pervasive effect on the child's self-esteem, with consequent effects on intellectual, physical, social and emotional development that are correlated with school failure. These effects may also result in later failure to develop normal relationships and to parent one's own child. This may result later in life in maternal depression, drug abuse and antisocial or criminal activities.

Q3. How would you assess this case?

History
- Assess the parent's knowledge and understanding of the child's health and developmental needs.
- Document the family's social history, financial resources and support networks.
- Assess the parent's relationship with the presenting child.
- Is there a history of substance abuse in the family?

Examination
- Is Emil smelly, dirty or unkempt, and does he have untreated medical conditions, e.g. squint, and infections or infestations? What is his dental care like?
- Observe parent/child interactions (or the lack of them) during the consultation.
- Assess the child's growth and development. Speech and language are particularly affected. The child may be stunted, underweight or overweight.
- Does the child look pale — anaemia or prison pallor?

Q4. How would you manage this child and family?

- Involve other agencies (primary health care, social services, education) and obtain further information on the family. The health visitor or teacher may be particularly well placed to provide this.
- Participate with other agencies in the assessment and treatment plan, including follow-up of the child.
- Identify the child's unmet needs (health, social, developmental, educational).
- Refer for speech and language therapy, if appropriate.
- Request a multi-agency assessment using the Framework for Assessment of Children in Need and Their Families.

Emotional abuse and emotional neglect

Problem-orientated topic:

soiling

Aleksi is 8 years old and is referred to you with soiling. His attendance at school is erratic, and when he does attend, he is described as aggressive to teachers and pupils and verbally abusive. He has been suspended from school for violence on two occasions. He is reported to have no friends. His mother describes him as 'evil'.

Q1. What do you think is the cause of his problems?

Q2. How would you assess this child and family?

Q3. What management options are available for him?

Q1. What do you think is the cause of his problems?

All children need to be loved and respected within a secure, consistent and emotionally warm environment. Failure to provide this emotional support may cause severe long-term problems and children may be unable to form long-term relationships and achieve successful parenting themselves. This perpetuates the abuse when the child becomes a parent. The long-term adverse effects of emotional abuse are thought to be greater than the effects of physical abuse. Physical and sexual abuse almost invariably involves some component of emotional abuse.

The UK Department of Health has defined emotional abuse as:

persistent emotional ill-treatment of a child such as to cause severe and persistent adverse effects on the child's emotional development. It may involve conveying to children that they are worthless or unloved, inadequate, or valued only insofar as they meet the needs of another person. It may feature age or developmentally inappropriate expectations being imposed on children. It may involve causing children to feel frightened or in danger, or the exploitation or corruption of children. Some level of emotional abuse is involved in all types of ill-treatment of a child, though it may occur alone.

Harmful behaviour leading to emotional abuse and emotional neglect includes:
- Inconsistent parenting
- Exposure to violence between the parents
- Excessive anxiety about a child's health
- Scapegoating
- Induction of fear or insecurity
- Developmentally inappropriate roles and expectations of the child, such as caring for disabled parents
- Rejection
- Isolation of the child in a room alone with little social contact
- Exposure to degrading or humiliating practices
- Ignoring
- Corrupting or encouraging criminality.

Unlike physical or sexual abuse, emotional abuse is readily observable in the consulting room or family home. The primary care doctor and health visitor are well placed to detect emotional abuse through their observations and knowledge of the family situation. Domestic violence and frequent attendance at GP surgeries for stress-related complaints are features suggestive of the fact that a child in the family may be suffering from emotional abuse or neglect.

At-risk children and those families where there is heightened risk include:

- Children who are unwanted, e.g. of the 'wrong' sex
- Disabled/chronically ill children
- Children of vulnerable parents (alcohol or drug abusers, mentally ill, domestic violence).

Q2. How would you assess this child and family?

The presentation may vary, depending on the age of the child.

Babies
- Feeding difficulties, excessive crying, poor sleep patterns
- Failure to relate to care-givers (who may describe them as 'a difficult baby, doesn't feel like he belongs to me' or 'he doesn't love me').

Toddlers and preschool children
- Head banging or excessive rocking
- Aggressive behaviour
- Developmental delay
- Poor growth — failure to thrive.

School-age children
- Wetting and soiling
- Relationship difficulties
- Poor school performance
- ADHD type symptoms
- Truancy and antisocial behaviour
- Feeling worthless and unloved.

Adolescents
- Depression
- Self-harming
- Substance abuse
- Eating disorder
- Oppositional, aggressive and delinquent behaviour.

Q3. What management options are available for him?

Increasing social support for the family may ease family stress, and recognizing and treating specific problems such as developmental disorders in the child are important. 'Sure Start', where available, may also provide satisfactory intervention for problem families. Interventions to protect mothers from domestic violence are also important. More difficult cases may benefit from referral to Child and Adolescent Mental Health Services.

- The 'fat clinical note' sign, indicating persistent or recurrent illness, often with multiple investigations
- 'Doctor shopping': frequent referrals to different doctors, and regularly falling out with doctors because they do not take the child's symptoms seriously
- No firm diagnosis made and, when one condition gets better, another starts
- Discrepancy between severe symptoms and a well-looking child
- The over-attentive or over-anxious mother
- Symptoms that resolve when the child is separated from the carer (perpetrator)

Factitious or induced illness

This condition, previously known as Munchausen syndrome by proxy, also referred to as 'Child Medical Abuse', is relatively uncommoly recognized in paediatric practice. In this condition, a parent (usually the mother) invents, induces or exaggerates symptoms of an illness in her child to obtain some form of gratification. This may be sympathy, attention, publicity or money.

Features of this condition are shown in Box 21.2.

Presenting features

Clinical features suggestive of factitious or induced illness (FII) include:

- Poisoning with drugs or household items such as salt, in order to induce symptoms.
- Unexplained blood in the urine, vomitus or stool (blood added).
- An acute unexplained life-threatening event that only occurs when the parent is present. Covert video surveillance in hospital has revealed that the cause is most likely to be deliberate suffocation by the parent.
- Repeated apnoeic attacks or fits never witnessed by others.
- Fever (reported; not necessarily documented on examination).
- Failure to thrive (milk poured down the sink).

Management

Primary care physicians are in a good position to notice if parents are consulting numerous health providers, as they should have appropriate letters etc. The doctor's priority is to ensure that the child avoids

ongoing harm. FII may be fatal. Share information with other clinical carers, such as nurses and other specialists. Refer to the social services or police if you have continuing concerns rather than proof of FII.

It is not necessary to share your concerns with the parents if, by doing so, you may put the child at risk. It is important to consider carefully the risk of disclosure of concern to the family before adequate discussions have taken place and protection has been achieved for the child.

Physical and sexual abuse

As well as emotional abuse and neglect, physical and sexual abuses are also common and important conditions. Serious injury and child sexual abuse may present either to primary care or in hospital. They may require specialized forensic skills to diagnose and document for court. These two conditions are discussed in more detail in Chapter 36 and the section below represents a summary of features that are important for doctors in primary care. It should be read in conjunction with Chapter 36.

Physical abuse

The doctor must be alert to the varied ways in which physical abuse may present. The common types of injury that may result from physical abuse include:

- Bruising from blows, kicks or beating with objects
- Fractures: for example, from grabbing limbs, direct blows or shaking
- Bites (distinguish between animal and human dental patterns)
- Burns from being held in direct contact with hot objects or scalds from forced immersion
- Intra-oral injuries suggesting forcible insertion of bottles or spoons.

Important features that should arouse suspicion of physical abuse are:

- Multiple superficial injuries of varying type, size and age
- Delay in presentation
- Bruises or marks with characteristic features of inflicting instruments
- Injuries not consistent with the history
- Injuries not consistent with the child's developmental age, for example fracture in a child not yet cruising or in a child less than 1 year of age
- Injuries to an infant's central nervous system.

Important sites for inflicted bruises include the face, lower jaw, ears, neck, buttocks, trunk and proximal parts of limbs. Accidental injury is most commonly found on the bony prominences, e.g. shins, elbows or forehead. Common patterns include fingertip or handslap marks, pinch marks, localized petechiae, e.g. around the neck, and marks of implements, e.g. belt, strap, stick or shoe.

A thorough medical examination, including assessment of growth, development and behaviour, is essential in all cases of suspected child abuse. It is essential to document carefully the number, distribution and pattern of all bruises and injuries. Up to a half of all mobile children have at least one bruise and many have more than one, although more than ten are suspicious.

Burns and other thermal injuries occur commonly in childhood and often present to primary care doctors. A relatively small number are due to child abuse, but are known to be under-recognized. Thermal injury includes burns and scalds that may be caused by hot water, food or steam, cigarettes, lighters or matches, friction from being dragged across a carpet, electrical shocks, hot metal objects such as an iron or radiator, or chemical burns. Cigarette burns cause deep circular craters 0.5–1 cm in diameter, which scar. Accidental brushed contact causes superficial injury roughly circular but with a tail.

Child sexual abuse

Sexual abuse in children will not be recognized if it is not considered by the clinician. A high index of suspicion must exist and healthcare professionals must acknowledge that child sexual abuse may occur in any family. The abuser is most commonly a member of the household, an extended family member or a family friend. In the vast majority of cases the child knows the abuser, who may be either male or female. Sexual abuse of children by strangers is uncommon. Professionals dealing with children need to be aware of the variety of forms that sexual abuse can take and that in the majority of cases there will be no physical signs of the abuse. Exposing the child to inappropriate touching or sexual acts between adults constitutes child sexual abuse. There is also an increasing awareness that adolescents but also younger children are at risk of sexual abuse through the internet.

Child sexual abuse has both short- and long-term effects.
- Short-term:
  - Behavioural problems
  - Difficulties forming friendships
  - School failure and truancy
  - Difficulty in forming trusting relationships
  - Sexually transmitted diseases, pregnancy

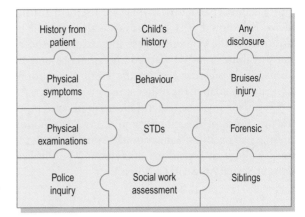

Fig. 21.1 **The jigsaw of sexual abuse**

- Long-term:
  - Sexual relationship difficulties
  - Mental health problems
  - Social dysfunction
  - Greater likelihood of patients abusing their own children.

There are very few pathognomonic signs of sexual abuse and the diagnosis is usually made by piecing together a jigsaw of information from many sources (Fig. 21.1).

Diagnosis may be suspected from the following features:
- *Disclosure*. This is the most common way in which the condition is diagnosed and children rarely fabricate disclosure of sexual abuse. If a child discloses in confidence, he or she must be told that the information will be passed on for his or her protection, as well as for the protection of other children. The doctor should have no ethical dilemma as to whether this information should be disclosed, as the protection of the patient overrides the duty of confidentiality to the patient.
- *Vaginal discharge or urinary symptoms*. A vulval swab and urine culture (and PCR) should be taken. Do not insert the swab into the vagina but take the specimen from the labia in a prepubertal child. If a vulval swab identifies a sexually transmitted disease, immediate referral to a child protection team should be made.
- *Rectal or vaginal bleeding* with no obvious explanation
- *Behavioural disturbances*. These are a common result of child sexual abuse and may include self-harm, mutilation, aggression and sexualized behaviours.
- *Pregnancy*.

If a doctor suspects child sexual abuse, this information must be passed on to social services. Discussion

235

with a named paediatrician may be useful if further advice is required. The primary care-giver should be informed of the referral, unless there is any concern that the abuser may be warned and evidence may be destroyed or pressure put on the child to withdraw disclosure or change his or her story.

The doctor must keep careful and accurate contemporaneous notes of the interview and any examination findings. All paediatricians should be familiar with the Royal College of Physicians document, 'The Physical Signs of Sexual Abuse in Children'.

Acknowledgments

We are very grateful to Dr Chris Hobbs for helpful advice.

Reference and further reading

Bannon MJ, Carter YH (eds) 2003 Protecting children from abuse and neglect in primary care. Oxford University Press, Oxford

Reece RM, Christian CW (eds) 2009 Child Abuse. Medical Diagnosis & Management. American Academy of Pediatrics

Roesler TA, Jenny C 2009 Medical Child Abuse. Beyond Munchausen Syndrome by Proxy. American Academy of Pediatrics

Edited by Diego van Esso,
Adamos Hadjipanayis, Malcolm Levene

Common Problems in Primary Care

MODULE FIVE

Stefan Riedl   Mary Rudolf

Growth: normal and abnormal

LEARNING OUTCOMES

By the end of this chapter you should:

● Know when a child's growth is of concern
● Know how to diagnose the common and important conditions responsible for poor growth
● Know the causes of poor weight gain in young children and babies
● Appreciate the stresses of having a child with weight faltering (failure to thrive), especially if there are eating difficulties, and be able to advise carers on management
● Know how to advise a child who is suffering from obesity
● Be able to weigh and measure a baby and child accurately
● Be able to plot measures on a growth chart, correcting for prematurity when appropriate
● Be able to calculate body mass index (BMI).

The basic science of growth

Normal growth occurs as a complex interplay between:
• Genetic influences
• Hormonal factors
• Nutritional availability
• Environmental exposure.

Poor growth may result from endocrine abnormalities, disease or poor environment.

Factors influencing growth

There are important differences between the factors influencing normal prenatal and postnatal growth.

Fetal growth

http://www.sciencedirect.com

Follow links to Gluckman PD, Hanson MA 2004 Maternal constraint of fetal growth and its consequences. Seminars in Fetal and Neonatal Medicine; 9:419–425

Growth before birth occurs as an interaction between genetic and environmental influences. A landmark study of mating large male Shire horses with small female Shetland ponies showed that maternal size was a major constraining factor in the prenatal growth of the foal. This has obvious evolutionary advantages in ensuring that the fetus does not grow too large

MODULE FIVE

to obstruct labour, predisposing to the death of the mother.

The factors affecting normal fetal growth are as follows.

Environmental factors

In normal pregnancies environmental factors have the major influence on fetal growth. 'Maternal constraint' limits fetal growth, which is a complicated relationship between uterine capacity and the ability of the placenta to provide sufficient nutrients. In multiple pregnancy the total weight of the babies is more than that of a singleton, although the individual weight of the babies is less than that of a singleton. This suggests that the availability of transplacental nutrients is a greater factor than uterine capacity.

Hormonal factors

Assuming sufficient supply of nutrients from the placenta, the hormonal milieu is important in determining embryonic and fetal growth. Insulin and insulin-like growth factors (IGFs) are the major prenatal trophic hormones. It appears that IGF-2 is particularly important in embryonic growth, and IGF-1 in later fetal and early infant linear growth. Insulin stimulates fat deposition (Ch. 47). Growth hormone has no effect on early human growth.

Placental factors

Normal placental function is essential for prenatal growth (Ch. 45) and the most common cause for intrauterine growth restriction is placental insufficiency. The placenta not only provides all the fetal nutritional needs, but also contributes to the fetal hormonal milieu necessary for normal growth. Maternal diet can influence nutritional availability to the fetus, which has major implications for pregnancy in developing countries where the maternal diet may be poor (Ch. 37).

Genetic factors

Genetic factors have a minor effect on fetal growth and the paternal genomic contribution has virtually no effect in determining birth size. Maternal environmental effects override fetal genetic contribution to prenatal growth.

Childhood growth

Genetic factors

Genetic factors largely account for final adult height, which generally can be anticipated to lie between the midparental centiles (average of parents' height (cm) + 6.5 (if boy), – 6.5 (if girl) = mid parent corrected height). The genotype is also a major determinant of final height. The Y chromosome controls the major genetic effects, as evident by males (XY) being taller than females (XX). Turner syndrome (XO) females are shorter than XX

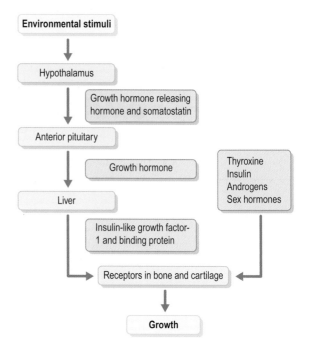

Fig. 22.1 Hormonal factors influencing growth

females, and males with the XYY pattern tend to be taller than average XY males. Males with Klinefelter's syndrome (XXY) are no shorter on average than normal XY males.

Hormonal influences (Fig. 22.1)

Human growth hormone (hGH) is secreted by the anterior pituitary and is expressed in two main forms by at least five genes on chromosome 17. hGH regulates protein synthesis and fat breakdown for energy use. It is particularly important for cartilaginous development within the epiphyses and consequently influences height. The production of hGH is stimulated by growth hormone releasing factor (GRF) from the hypothalamus. A growth hormone release-inhibiting factor (somatostatin) is also produced by the hypothalamus as well as other tissues and inhibits hGH release as well as acting on its remote receptor sites. The influence of higher brain centres on hypothalamic function may explain why adverse emotional factors may affect growth.

Insulin and IGFs, also termed somatomedins, are produced in liver and other organs and circulate in the blood. They have the effect, like insulin, of stimulating protein synthesis and depressing catabolism.

Other pituitary-derived hormones, such as thyroid and parathyroid hormone, have an important effect on maturation and growth, and hypothyroid children grow poorly. Sex hormones regulate the onset of puberty and are responsible for the adolescent growth spurt (see below). They also ultimately cause fusion of the epiphyseal centres and so cause linear growth to cease. Adrenal hormones have an influence on growth and excess corticosteroids have a profound suppressant effect (Ch. 35).

Nutrition

The availability of adequate nutritional substrate is essential for normal growth, and starvation inhibits growth in children. Malnutrition also delays the onset of puberty, which can have an important effect on final height.

Environmental factors

Factors known to affect growth include:
- *Socioeconomic status.* Adult height is on average 4.5 cm greater in socioeconomic class I, compared with class V.
- *Disease.* Any chronic disease can cause stunting of growth.
- *Emotional environment.* An adverse emotional environment can slow growth. This is probably mediated through hypothalamic factors.
- *Altitude.* This is probably mediated through lower oxygen saturation levels.

Periods of growth

Growth in infancy

At birth, a baby's weight and length are influenced mainly by intrauterine factors. The rate of growth in the first year of life is more rapid than at any other age. Between birth and 1 year of age, children on average increase their length by 50% and triple their birth weight. Head circumference increases by one-third. Crossing centiles is initially common, but by the age of 2 most children have attained their genetically destined centile, and the baby has changed in shape to take on the appearance of the lean and more muscular child.

Growth in the preschool and school years

In the preschool years a child continues to gain weight and height steadily. Beyond the age of 2 or 3 years until puberty, the growth rate is steady at about 3–3.5 kg and 6 cm per year, and centile crossing is not usually seen.

http://www.who.int/childgrowth/standards/en/

A number of different WHO growth charts can be downloaded from this site

http://www.rcpch.ac.uk/Research/
UK-WHO-Growth-Charts

New UK-WHO growth charts for boys and girls from birth to 4 years of age

Growth in adolescence

Adolescence is characterized by a growth spurt, which occurs under the influence of rising sex hormone levels. During the 3 or 4 years of puberty boys grow about 25 cm and girls 20 cm, and it is normal for centiles to be crossed until final height is achieved, which usually is located midway between the parental centiles.

Growth in adverse circumstances and catch-up growth

During a period of illness or starvation the rate of growth is slowed. After the incident the child usually grows more rapidly so that catch-up towards, or actually to, the original growth curve occurs. The degree to which catch-up is successful depends on the timing of the onset and the duration of slow growth. This is particularly important in infants who have suffered intrauterine growth retardation and who may have reduced growth potential.

In nutritionally compromised children, weight falls before height is impaired and head growth is the last to be affected. If growth has been slowed for too long or into puberty, complete catch-up is not achieved. There are important therapeutic implications in the early detection of children with abnormal growth velocity patterns, as early treatment is more likely to ensure that acceptable adult height is achieved.

Head growth

Although there is a tendency for large babies to have large heads and small babies smaller heads, head size is largely independent of body size. Head growth is driven by the growth of the brain, and if for any reason the brain fails to grow normally, the head will be small, so that it is common to find that children with developmental problems have microcephaly. Rapid head growth is a cause for concern and may result from raised intracranial pressure, when the sutures become pushed apart. So saying, pathological causes of unusual head size are uncommon and the most common explanation for both small and large heads in otherwise normal individuals is familial.

Short stature

http://www.sciencedirect.com

Follow links to Grote FK, van Dommelen P, Oostdijk W, de Muinck Keizer-Schrama SM, Verkerk PH, Wit JM, van Buuren S 2008 Developing evidence-based guidelines for referral for short stature. Archives of Diseases in Childhood; 93:212–217

See also Chapter 35.

Problem-orientated topic:

a short child

Abellona is 12 years old. She attends her doctor's office because she is short.
She is in general good health, but has recently become rather withdrawn and is having a difficult time at high school, where she has been recurrently teased about her height. Her father is 168 cm. Her mother is 160 cm and had menarche at the age of 15 years.

Abellona's height is 127 cm (below 0.4th centile) and her weight is 26 kg (0.4th centile) (Fig. 22.2).

Q1. When should one become concerned about short stature?

Q2. What is the likely cause of Abellona's short stature?

Q3. What other conditions should be considered?

Q4. What should you look for in your clinical evaluation?

Q5. What investigations might be appropriate?

Q6. When is referral indicated?

BOX 22.1 Guidelines for concern beyond the age of 2 years

According to ethnicity, different growth charts with different normal ranges are used across Europe.

The short or tall child

Height or weight beyond the dotted lines on the growth chart (> 99.6th or < 0.4th centile) is outside the normal range and pathology is more likely to be found. Many children whose height or weight lies in the shaded areas are normal but an evaluation needs to be considered.

Crossing of centiles

As a rule of thumb, one should be concerned if two centile lines are crossed.

Discrepancy between height and weight

There is a great deal of variation as regards leanness and obesity. The child who is very thin or overweight may have a problem.

Discrepancy with parental heights

A child should be evaluated if there is a large discrepancy between the child's height centile and the midparental centile. The child of tall parents who has a growth problem should not wait until he or she falls below the second centile to be evaluated.

Parental or professional concern

A good clinical evaluation should be carried out in any child when the parents or other professionals are concerned about growth.

Q1. When should one become concerned about short stature?

Given the social disadvantage of being short, especially for a man, it is not surprising that short stature commonly causes concern. Box 22.1 provides some guidance as to when growth in childhood may be of concern.

Q2. What is the likely cause of Abellona's short stature?

Abellona's parents are both relatively short and her mother had menarche late, so familial short stature and maturational delay are likely explanations. However, it is important to exclude organic problems. A good clinical evaluation and a growth chart should help you decide if the cause is pathological rather than physiological.

Q3. What other conditions should be considered?

It is important to exclude organic problems, particularly if there is a falloff in growth over time (p. 246). The causes of short stature are shown in Box 22.2.

Q4. What should you look for in your clinical evaluation?

Key points

- A good history and physical examination will identify most pathological causes of short stature.
- The child's height must be related to the parents' heights.
- Emotional and social *consequences* of the short stature should be identified.

History

Your history needs to focus on symptoms suggestive of underlying conditions, such as intracranial pathology, hormone deficiency, chronic illness and gastrointestinal symptoms.

- *Medical history.* Headache, diarrhoea and abdominal pain, constipation, cough, wheeze and fatigue are particularly relevant. Chronic conditions such as asthma, arthritis or diabetes may be significant, as is any chronic medication.
- *Family history.* A child's growth cannot be interpreted without reference to parental and siblings' heights. Ask about parental onset of

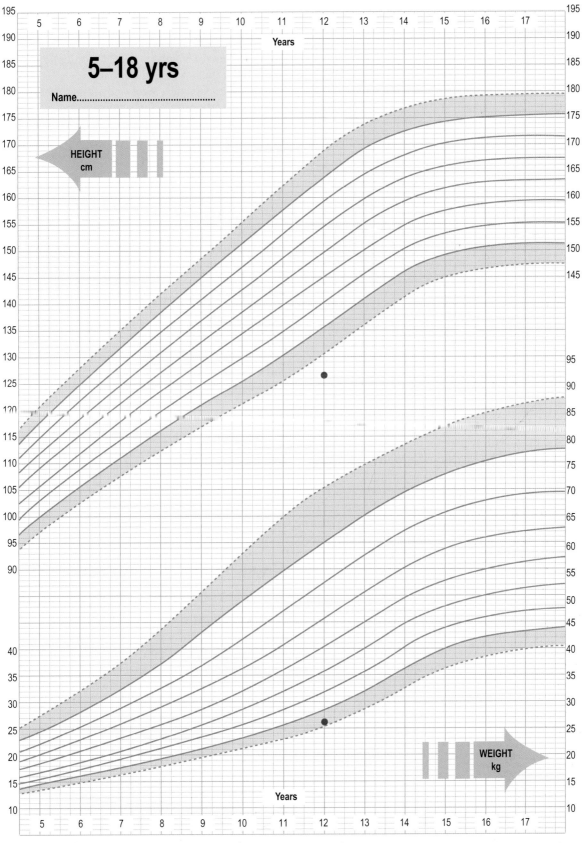

Fig. 22.2 Abellona's growth chart

BOX 22.2 Causes of short stature

Physiological causes

- Normal variant (often familial, also known as 'constitutional short stature')
- Maturational delay (often familial)

Pathological causes

- Endocrine:
  - Hypothyroidism
  - Corticosteroid excess
  - Growth hormone deficiency
- Chronic illness:
  - Inflammatory bowel and coeliac disease; chronic renal failure may be occult
- Genetic:
  - Turner syndrome
  - Other genetic syndromes
  - Skeletal dysplasias
- Intrauterine growth retardation
- Psychosocial

puberty, as maturational delay is common and often familial. Maternal menarche after the age of 14 years is suggestive. Onset of paternal puberty is harder to identify.

- *Birth history*. Low birth weight is significant. A child born severely preterm or small for gestational age (SGA) may have reduced growth potential, particularly if height as well as weight is affected.
- *Psychosocial history*. Psychosocial factors can severely stunt a child's growth, and you must be alert to the possibility of emotional neglect and abuse. When assessing any short child you should also find out about any social or emotional difficulties *resulting* from his or her stature.

Examination

A very thorough examination is required, focusing particularly on the following:

- *Pattern of growth*. Where possible, you should review previous growth measurements, as they provide important clues to the aetiology of the

condition. Falloff in growth usually indicates a medical condition requiring treatment.

- *Anthropometric measures*. Take careful measures of weight and of length (to age 24 months) or height and plot them on a growth chart.
- *General examination*. Signs of hypothyroidism, body disproportion, and signs of Turner syndrome (Ch. 35) and dysmorphism are particularly important to identify. Examine each organ system in turn, looking for evidence of occult disease.

Q5. What investigations might be appropriate?

Your clinical evaluation should guide any investigations. If you find a decrease in growth velocity, investigations are always required (Table 22.1).

Q6. When is referral indicated?

If a physiological cause — namely, constitutional short stature or maturational delay — is likely, the child can be followed in primary care. The growth rate needs to be periodically checked, and the family should be reassured that there is no underlying pathological problem. In addition it is important to address any psychosocial difficulties the child is having, and occasionally psychological counselling is required.

Reduction in growth rate is a definite indication for paediatric assessment (p. 246). Boys with maturational delay may benefit from testosterone. The use of growth hormone in children with physiological short stature is controversial and probably confers little benefit on final adult height.

Causes of short stature (Box 22.2)

Physiological causes of short stature

Normal variant short stature

Stature is largely genetically determined, and short parents tend to have short children. In normal variant short stature, the history and physical examination are normal, and the bone age is appropriate for age. Often reassurance

Table 22.1 Investigations in a child with short stature

Investigation	Relevance
Blood count, plasma viscosity or erythrocyte sedimentation rate	Inflammatory bowel disease
Urea and electrolytes	Chronic renal failure
Coeliac antibodies	Screening test for coeliac disease
Thyroxine and thyroid-stimulating hormone	Hypothyroidism
Karyotype (in girls)	Turner syndrome
Growth hormone tests	Hypopituitarism, growth hormone deficiency
X-ray of the wrist for bone age (Fig. 22.3)	Delayed bone age suggests maturational delay, hypothyroidism, growth hormone deficiency or corticosteroid excess. A prediction of adult height can be made from it

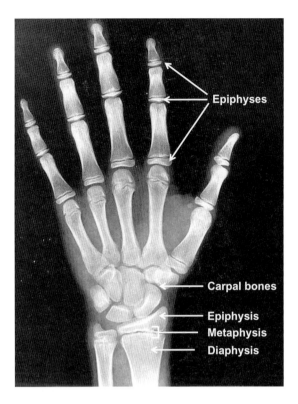

Fig. 22.3 X-ray of the left wrist taken for bone age. The development of the various bones is assessed to give an estimate of the child's skeletal maturity.

Labels on image: Epiphyses, Carpal bones, Epiphysis, Metaphysis, Diaphysis

which occurs particularly in girls. Thyroid deficiency has a profound effect on growth, and may present as short stature. Other features include a falloff in school performance, constipation, dry skin and delayed puberty. Investigations include a low T4, high thyroid-stimulating hormone (TSH) and antithyroid antibodies. Treatment is usually lifelong replacement of thyroid hormone.

Corticosteroid excess

Cushing syndrome and disease are extremely rare in childhood, growth suppression from exogenous steroids being much more common. In children requiring long-term high-steroid therapy, the deleterious effects on growth can often be minimized by giving the steroids on alternate days.

Growth hormone deficiency

Growth hormone deficiency is a rare cause of short stature. It may occur secondary to lesions of the pituitary such as tumours or cranial irradiation, or can be isolated, when it may or may not be accompanied by deficiency of other pituitary hormones.

The diagnosis is made by growth hormone testing. Brain imaging is needed to identify any underlying pathology. Deficiency is treated with daily subcutaneous injections of synthetic growth hormone until the child stops growing.

Other causes of short stature

Chronic illness

Any chronic illness can lead to stunting of growth. However, chronic illnesses rarely present as short stature because the features of the illness are usually all too evident. Chronic conditions that may present with poor growth, in advance of other clinical features, include inflammatory bowel disease, coeliac disease and chronic renal failure.

Turner syndrome (Ch. 35)

Turner syndrome (gonadal dysgenesis) is an important cause of short stature and delayed puberty in girls. It is a genetic disorder caused by the absence of one X chromosome. The resulting phenotype is female, with gonads that are merely streaks of fibrous tissue. Intelligence is usually normal, and characteristic features include webbing of the neck, shield-shaped chest, wide-spaced nipples and a wide carrying angle. Some girls are only diagnosed in adolescence when puberty fails to occur.

Girls with Turner syndrome should be followed in an endocrinology clinic, where they are generally given hormonal treatment to promote growth. Puberty must be initiated and maintained by oestrogen therapy.

is all that is required. Social difficulties are common in the adolescent years, particularly for boys, and occasionally children need psychological support at this time.

Maturational delay

Children with maturational delay are often called 'late developers' or 'late bloomers'. The biological clock operates more slowly than usual. Children in this circumstance are short and reach puberty late, their final height depending on their genetic constitution, which may be normal. A family history of delayed puberty and menarche is often obtained, and the bone age is delayed.

Most families simply require reassurance that final height will not be affected, but occasionally teenage boys find the social pressures to be so great that it is helpful to trigger puberty artificially with testosterone, thus causing an early growth spurt. This treatment does not have an effect on final height.

Endocrine causes of short stature

(See also Chapter 35.)

Hypothyroidism

Hypothyroidism may be congenital or acquired as autoimmune thyroiditis (Hashimoto syndrome),

Table 22.2 The differential diagnosis of short stature

Diagnosis	Growth pattern	History	Physical examination	Bone age
Constitutional short stature	Steady growth below the centile lines	Short parents	Normal	Normal
Maturational delay	Usually short, with falloff of growth in early teens	Family history of delayed puberty/menarche	Delay in developing secondary sex characteristics	Delayed
Endocrine disorders (hypothyroidism, Cushing, growth hormone deficiency)	Falloff of growth	Symptoms of hypothyroidism, on inhaled or oral steroids, symptoms of brain tumour	Signs of hypothyroidism or Cushing, rarely signs of brain tumour	Very delayed
Chronic illness	Falloff of growth	Symptoms of inflammatory bowel disease, malabsorption, fatigue	Ill-looking, symptoms of underlying illness, although inflammatory bowel disease, coeliac disease and chronic renal failure may be occult	Delayed ±
Genetic syndromes	Slow growth below centiles	–	Signs of Turner or other dysmorphism	Variable
Intrauterine growth retardation	Short from birth	Small for gestational age	Normal but small	Normal
Psychosocial	Variable depending on social circumstances	Adverse circumstances	Unhappy, signs of neglect or abuse	Usually normal

Other genetic syndromes

Short stature is a common feature in many genetic syndromes. Dysmorphic features are usual and learning disability is common.

Skeletal dysplasias

The skeletal dysplasias are a group of disorders where body disproportion occurs, resulting in shortened limbs. The most common of these is achondroplasia, which is inherited as an autosomal dominant trait.

Intrauterine growth retardation

Intrauterine growth retardation can result from a variety of causes (Ch. 45). The impact on postnatal growth depends on which stage of the pregnancy the growth retardation occurred. If the insult occurred early in gestation, the baby is born not only underweight but also short and often with a small head. If length is short, newborns may have reduced growth potential and remain short throughout life. If catch-up growth occurs, it does so in the first 2 or 3 years.

Psychosocial causes of short stature

Adverse psychosocial factors can severely affect a child's growth. In the young child it is referred to as failure to thrive (p. 248). The true incidence of psychosocial poor growth is unknown, but it is likely that it is quite common. On being placed in foster care, children often have a growth spurt, even when growth has previously been apparently normal.

The differential diagnosis of short stature is given in Table 22.2.

Plateauing in growth

Problem-orientated topic:

a child with plateauing growth

Kaatje is 8 years old. Her mother is concerned, as she does not seem to be following the same growth pattern as her brother and sister did. She brings you the height measures she has taken each year on Kaatje's birthday (Fig. 22.4). Kaatje is not short, but she seems to have crossed centiles.

Q1. Should you be worried?

Q2. What conditions might cause a falloff in growth?

Q3. What should you do?

Q1. Should you be worried?

Measurements made at home are likely to be very inaccurate; however, Kaatje's growth since she was measured by the school nurse at school entry suggests that there has indeed been reduced growth velocity.

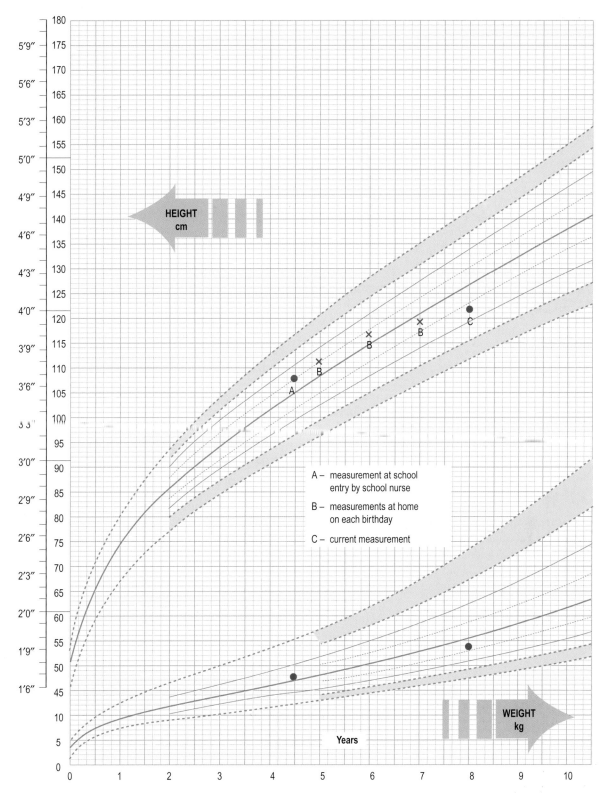

A – measurement at school
entry by school nurse

B – measurements at home
on each birthday

C – current measurement

HEIGHT cm

WEIGHT kg

Years

Fig. 22.4 Kaatje's growth chart

- Endocrine:
  - Hypothyroidism
  - Corticosteroid excess
  - Growth hormone deficiency
- Chronic illness:
  - Inflammatory bowel and coeliac disease; chronic renal failure may be occult
- Psychosocial

You should therefore be concerned. Falloff in growth is always worrying and merits investigation. If initially tall, the child may not be short in relation to peers.

Q2. What conditions might cause a falloff in growth?

The causes of falloff in growth are shown in Box 22.3.

Q3. What should you do?

The clinical approach and management of falloff in growth are the same as those described in the previous section, but the chance of finding pathology is higher. Any child with plateauing of growth needs a referral to a paediatrician or paediatric endocrinologist.

Tall stature

Tall stature is only rarely pathological and is usually simply a variant of normal. Tall women often encounter social difficulties and tall girls may present for help. Obese children tend to be tall for their age but on the whole reach puberty early, and so their final height is usually in the normal range.

Rapid growth can very rarely be a sign of hormonal disturbance such as giantism (growth hormone excess) or precocious puberty. These are discussed in Chapter 35.

Faltering growth and failure to thrive

Problem-orientated topic:

a child with faltering growth

Galyn is 15 months old. He started life on the 50th centile but at 12 weeks his weight started dropping off (Fig. 22.5). He has had a series of ear infections but no serious illnesses. He is developing normally but has become difficult to feed. His mother is desperately anxious, and meals are now taking up to 1 hour in length.

Q1. Does Galyn have a growth problem?

Q2. How should one define failure to thrive and growth faltering?

Q3. What are the possible causes for Galyn's growth pattern?

Q4. What clinical pointers should you look for in your clinical evaluation?

Q5. What investigations are indicated?

Q6. What strategies and advice might be useful in Galyn's situation?

Q1. Does Galyn have a growth problem?

Infants commonly cross centiles during the first 2 years of life. When they cross down this often causes concern, although it is usually physiological and due to the baby moving to its genetically intended centile. However, poor weight gain can also be an indication of psychosocial or (more rarely) medical problems. Expertise is required to differentiate the normal infant from the one who is failing to thrive.

Q2. How should one define failure to thrive and growth faltering?

Failure to thrive implies both a failure to grow and a failure of emotional and developmental progress. The term is sometimes considered pejorative and is being replaced by growth or weight 'faltering'. Both terms usually relate to poor weight gain in a toddler or baby, although they may also be used in reference to an older child, and may also refer to height.

There are no established criteria for defining failure to thrive. However, the following can act as guidelines as to when a clinical evaluation is advisable:
- Weight below the 2nd centile
- Height below the 2nd centile
- Crossing down two centile channels for height or weight.

Q3. What are the possible causes for Galyn's growth pattern?

The causes of weight faltering are listed in Box 22.4.

In the past children were classified as having organic (OFTT) or non-organic failure to thrive (NOFTT). Children more often than not do not fall simply into one category or the other, but fail to gain weight well for a combination of reasons. It is important to identify all the factors involved.

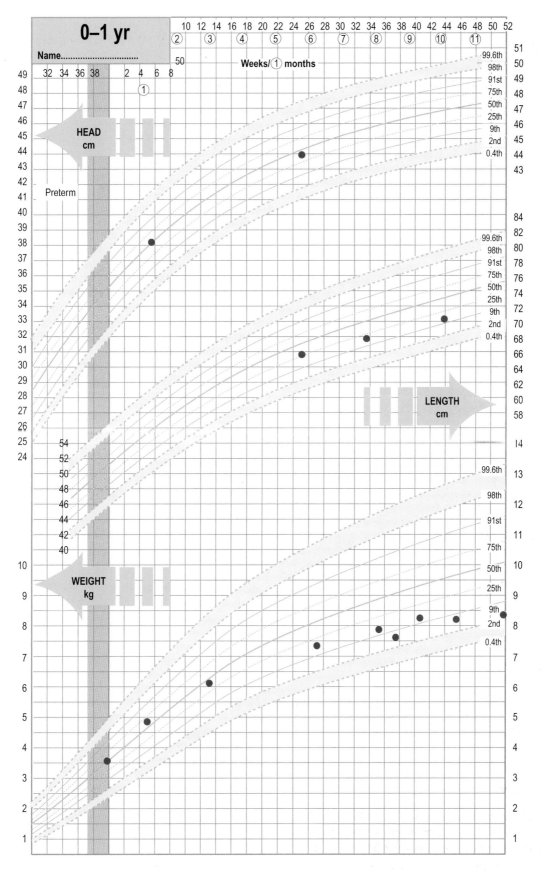

Fig. 22.5 **Galyn's growth charts.**
(a) 0–1 years

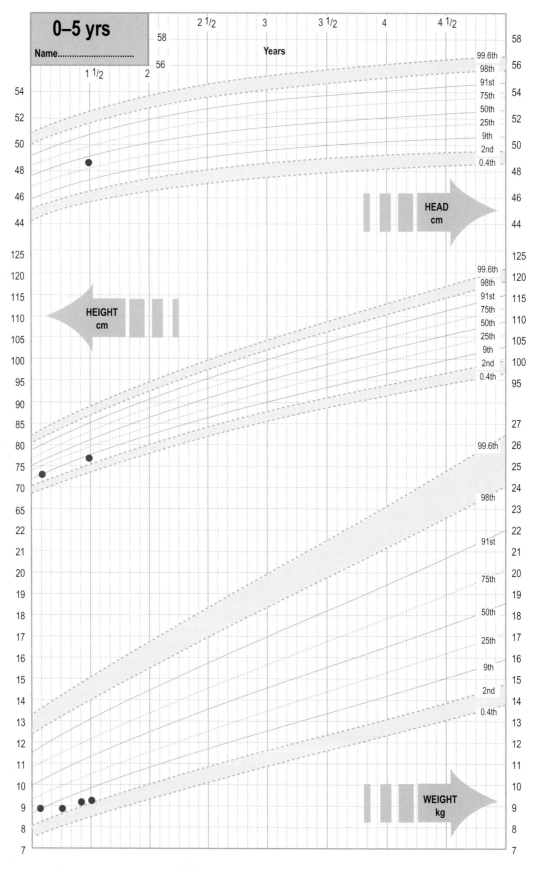

Fig. 22.5 (cont'd)
(b) 0–5 years.

BOX 22.4 Causes of weight faltering (failure to thrive)

Environmental/psychosocial (non-organic)
- Maternal depression/psychiatric disorder
- Disturbed maternal–infant attachment
- Eating difficulties
- Neglect

Medical
- Gastro-oesophageal reflux
- Malabsorption
- Chronic illness
- Endocrine dysfunction

Genetic
- Genetic constitution
- Intrauterine growth retardation
- Genetic syndromes

Q4. What clinical pointers should you look for in your clinical evaluation?

Key points
- You must differentiate the normal baby who is crossing centiles from the baby who is failing to thrive.
- Identify any symptoms and signs that suggest an organic condition.
- Only perform laboratory investigations if there are clinical leads in the history and physical examination.
- Identify psychosocial problems that might be affecting the baby's growth.

It is very distressing for the family when a young child fails to thrive, so your evaluation needs to be carried out sensitively. The purpose of the evaluation is first to differentiate the child demonstrating normal growth faltering from the child with a problem, and then to identify the contributing factors, whether organic or non-organic.

History
- *Nutritional history.* Obtain a good dietary history. Include questions about any feeding difficulties, which may have been present from birth but often develop at weaning and in the toddler years. Eating difficulties may be the *cause* of the failure to thrive, or may be generated from the anxiety that naturally occurs when a baby grows poorly because of other causes. It is helpful to ask the mother to keep a food diary for a few days, recording all that the baby has eaten.
- *Review of symptoms.* Most organic conditions are identifiable by history. Diarrhoea, colic, vomiting, irritability, fatigue and chronic cough are the most important features to elicit.
- *Past medical history.* The birth history is important. A low birth weight may indicate adverse prenatal conditions that affect growth potential. Recurrent illness of any nature may affect growth.
- *Developmental history.* This is needed for two reasons. Firstly, failure to thrive may affect a baby's developmental progress and, secondly, the child who has neurodevelopmental problems from any cause often has associated eating difficulties that may be limiting nutritional intake.
- *Family history.* Relate the child's growth to that of other family members. Medical problems affecting other children in the family may suggest a diagnosis. A good social history should identify psychosocial problems that may be causing or at least contributing to the problem.

Examination
You need to carry out a full physical examination to complement the history. Occasionally clinical signs alone can indicate a cause for the poor growth.
- *General observations.* The baby's appearance is important. The healthy small baby will look very different from the neglected or ill child. The child who is malnourished for whatever reason will appear thin, with wasted buttocks, a protuberant abdomen and sparse hair. A neglected child may look unclean and uncared for. Observations must also extend to the mother and how she relates to the baby, which can provide valuable clues to maternal–infant attachment difficulties.
- *Growth.* Plot growth on a growth chart and compare current measurements with previous. The pattern of growth can be very helpful in the diagnostic process. Figure 22.6 shows growth charts that are illustrative of common conditions.

Q5. What investigations are indicated?

There is good evidence that 'fishing' for a diagnosis by carrying out multiple investigations is a futile exercise. Investigations should only be carried out if clues to a problem are obtained from the history and physical examination. The only exception is a blood count and ferritin level, as iron deficiency is extremely common in this group of children, and can affect both development and appetite. Other investigations that may be helpful, if clinically justified, are shown in Table 22.3.

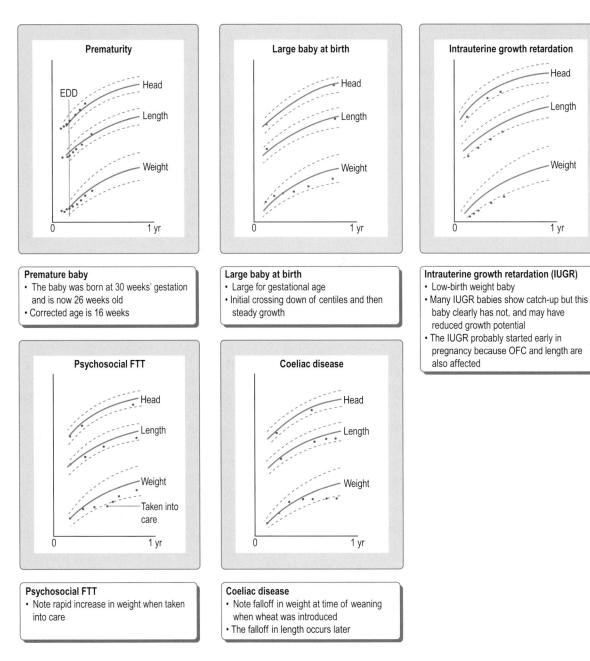

Fig. 22.6 **Growth charts illustrating five common conditions in infancy.**
(EDD = expected delivery for dates; OFC = occipito-frontal circumference.)

Q6. What strategies and advice might be useful in Galyn's situation?

The ability to nurture a baby is perhaps the most basic attribute of parenting. When a child fails to thrive it usually causes extreme distress, anxiety and feelings of inadequacy. It is important therefore that a normal, healthy but small baby is not wrongly labelled as having a problem. On the other hand, it is important that both organic and psychosocial problems are identified and addressed, as failure to thrive has important consequences on the child's developmental progress as well

as growth. A thorough clinical evaluation, together with information from the health visitor, can usually sort out the problem. Helpful advice regarding the young child with eating difficulties is shown in Box 22.5. Occasionally admission to hospital for observation may be required.

Causes of failure to thrive (Box 22.4)

Non-organic weight faltering

The most common causes for weight faltering are psychosocial. The problems include difficulties in the

Table 22.3 Investigations to consider in the evaluation of failure to thrive

Investigation	What you are looking for
Full blood count, ferritin	Iron deficiency is common in failure to thrive and can cause anorexia
Urea and electrolytes	Unsuspected renal failure
Stool for elastase and fat globules	Pancreatic insufficiency and malabsorption
Coeliac antibodies, jejunal biopsy, sweat test	Coeliac disease and cystic fibrosis are causes of malabsorption
Thyroid hormone and thyroid-stimulating hormone	Congenital hypothyroidism causes poor growth and developmental delay
Karyotype	Chromosomal abnormalities are often associated with short stature and dysmorphism
Hospitalization	Hospitalization can be a form of investigation. Observation of baby and mother over time can provide clues to the aetiology

---

BOX 22.5 Helpful advice for a child with eating difficulties

Dietary advice

- Offer meals and snacks frequently to stimulate the appetite
- Start with food that the child likes
- Give only small amounts to start with and offer more if food is eaten
- Increase caloric intake naturally rather then by supplements, e.g. full-fat milk, cheese, yoghurt and butter added to mashed potato, pasta etc.
- Reduce fluid intake if > 500 ml per day, as this can reduce appetite
- Limit use of a dummy to encourage food intake and language development
- Never force-feed

Mealtimes

- Make mealtimes relaxed social events
- Let the child touch and play with food and encourage independent eating
- Limit mealtimes to 30 minutes, as little extra is gained by longer meals
- Praise the child for eating but pay little attention to aversive behaviour

---

home, limitations in the parents, disturbed attachment between the mother and child, maternal depression/psychiatric disorder and eating difficulties. Neglect is the underlying factor in only a few children.

Clinical features

Weight gain is usually first affected, but a reduction in linear growth and head circumference may follow and the child's developmental progress may be delayed. The family circumstances may range from the child from a caring home who is well looked after, with parents who are anxious and concerned and interact well with the child, to the neglected child. Eating difficulties, where the child has a minimal appetite or refuses to eat, are common. Meals are very stressful

and the parents may be drawn into excessive measures (sometimes force-feeding) to persuade the child to eat. At the other end of the spectrum is the neglected child who shows physical signs of poor care and emotional attachment. In this case the problem is often denied and compliance with intervention is poor.

Management

Management must be tailored to fit the problem. Most families can be helped by appropriate intervention, usually consisting of dietary advice and psychological support. Practical support can ease the stress, and nursery placement can be very helpful in this regard, as well as helping to resolve eating difficulties. In those cases where neglect is the cause and the family are not amenable to help, social services must be involved.

Prognosis

With appropriate intervention, the problem usually resolves or at least stabilizes. A few children need to be removed from their homes.

Genetic and organic causes

Gastro-oesophageal reflux

Vomiting and possetting are common complaints in a baby, and usually do not deleteriously affect growth. However, occasionally reflux can cause failure to thrive, particularly if associated with oesophagitis, which causes pain and anorexia.

Malabsorption

Malabsorption is an important cause of failure to thrive. Symptoms of diarrhoea and colic are usually present as diagnostic clues. The most common causes of malabsorption in childhood are coeliac disease and cystic fibrosis. In the former, the growth curve characteristically shows a falloff in weight coincident with the introduction of gluten to the diet.

Chronic illness

Children and babies with any chronic illness can fail to thrive. They rarely present as a diagnostic dilemma,

Table 22.4 The differential diagnosis of weight faltering/failure to thrive

Diagnosis	Growth pattern*	History	Physical examination
Constitutional	Steady growth below centiles, or 'catch-down' for larger baby	Short parent(s)	Normal
Psychosocial	Crossing down of centiles at any age	Eating difficulties common, maternal depression may be present	Usually normal but poor or disturbed maternal–infant attachment may be evident
Coeliac disease	Crossing down of centiles classically occurring at introduction of wheat solids	Frequent stools or diarrhoea, irritability	Distended abdomen, wasted buttocks
Cystic fibrosis	Crossing down of centiles	Appetite often fine, chest infections, diarrhoea	Poorly child Protuberant abdomen, decreased muscle mass, chest signs possible
Gastro-oesophageal reflux	Crossing down of centiles early in life	Vomiting, irritability, occasionally apnoea	Normal
Intrauterine growth retardation	Low birth weight with subsequent poor weight gain, length and head circumference may be reduced	Possible placental insufficiency, difficult pregnancy, smoking, alcohol	Small normal, look for signs of intrauterine infection (TORCH — *to*xoplasmosis, *rubella* cytomegalovirus, *herpes* simplex virus)
Neglect	Crossing down of centiles, catch-up if removed from home	Difficult or troubled family circumstances	Poorly cared for, nappy rash, developmental delay common

* Refers to weight in the first instance.

as the manifestations of the disease are usually evident. However, organic failure to thrive may be compounded by psychosocial difficulties and these need to be addressed. Very rarely, chronic disease can be occult and present as failure to thrive.

Genetic constitution
Small parents tend to have small children and the small healthy normal child of short parents should not arouse concern. Usually in this case growth is steady along the lower centiles, but the large baby born to small parents may cross down centile lines before settling on the destined line.

Intrauterine growth retardation
If a fetus experiences adverse uterine conditions its growth may be retarded. When this occurs early in gestation, length and head circumference in addition to weight can be affected. In this circumstance the potential for postnatal growth may be jeopardized. The cause of the intrauterine growth retardation should, where possible, be identified.

Genetic syndromes
Dysmorphic syndromes are not uncommonly associated with short stature. If dysmorphic features are present, the diagnosis can be suspected. An important syndrome causing shortness is Turner syndrome (Ch. 35).

Endocrine dysfunction
Congenital hypothyroidism causes failure to thrive and developmental delay. Most cases are detected through neonatal screening.

The differential diagnosis of weight faltering/failure to thrive is given in Table 22.4.

Unusual head growth

The head grows rapidly in the first 2 years of life and then slows down, but continues to grow throughout childhood. In the early years the sutures are open, and then fuse around the age of 6 years. Prior to fusion they can separate in response to raised intracranial pressure. The posterior fontanelle usually closes by 8 weeks of age, and the anterior by 12–18 months.

Head size is not directly proportional to body size, but large children are more likely to have large heads, and vice versa. As in body growth, it is not unusual for head circumference measurements to cross centiles in the first year. However, when this occurs, clinical assessment is needed to exclude pathological causes.

The large head

(See also p. 294–5.)

Problem-orientated topic:

a child with a large head

The health visitor measures Jason's head at the 8-week check. She notes that the head circumference has crossed centiles since the

Continued overleaf

newborn examination (Fig. 22.7). Jason has been developing normally and is smiling and able to lift his head in the prone position. His parents describe him as easygoing and have no concerns.

Q1. Is this a worrying pattern of head growth?

Q2. What symptoms and signs should you look for in your clinical evaluation that might suggest hydrocephalus?

Q3. How do you advise the parents and health visitor?

Q1. Is this a worrying pattern of growth?

A large head is usually a normal variant, and often is a familial feature. An unusually large head may indicate hydrocephalus, in which case evidence of raised intracranial pressure may be present. Large heads may also be a feature of certain genetic syndromes. The causes of a large or enlarging head are shown in Box 22.6.

Q2. What symptoms and signs should you look for in your clinical evaluation that might suggest hydrocephalus?

Key points
- An enlarging head is a greater cause of concern than a steadily growing large head.
- Parental head size is helpful in deciding if this is a normal variant.
- Assess the baby's developmental skills.
- Evidence of raised intracranial pressure indicates hydrocephalus or subdural collection of fluid.

History
- *Is the baby developing normally?* Abnormal developmental progress in a child with a large head is strongly indicative of pathology.
- *Are there symptoms of raised intracranial pressure?* The baby with hydrocephalus or subdural effusion is likely to be irritable and lethargic, have a poor appetite and vomit.

Examination
- *Growth measures.* The pattern of head growth is important. Crossing of centile lines is a greater cause of concern than steady growth of a large head. Length and weight indicate whether the head is disproportionately large (Fig. 22.7).

BOX 22.6 Causes of a large or enlarging head

- Normal variation (often familial)
- Hydrocephalus
- Subdural effusion or haematomas
- Feature of certain dysmorphic syndromes

- *Signs of hydrocephalus.* The child with hydrocephalus has characteristic features (see below).
- *Development.* A developmental examination should accompany the developmental history.

Q3. How do you advise the parents and health visitor?

Frequent measurements of head circumference can generate anxiety, and should not be performed if the head size is considered to be a variant of normal. When raised intracranial pressure is suspected, immediate investigation is required, along with referral to neurosurgery. If the anterior fontanelle is still open, a cranial ultrasound can be performed to detect hydrocephalus, effusions or haemorrhage. If the fontanelles are closed, computed tomography (CT) or magnetic resonance imaging (MRI) scans are required to delineate underlying pathology.

Pathological causes of a large head

Hydrocephalus

Hydrocephalus may result from a congenital abnormality of the brain such as aqueductal stenosis, or be acquired as a result of intracranial haemorrhage, infection or tumour. Premature babies with severe intracranial haemorrhage are particularly at risk. Hydrocephalus is commonly associated with neural tube anomalies and occurs in 80% of babies with spina bifida (Ch. 28).

Clinical features
Clinical features include irritability, lethargy, poor appetite and vomiting. In infants, the anterior fontanelle is wide open and bulging, the sutures are separated and the scalp veins are dilated. The forehead is broad and the eyes deviated down, giving the 'setting sun' sign. Spasticity, clonus and brisk deep tendon reflexes are often demonstrable. In older children the signs are more subtle, with headache and a deterioration in school performance.

Management
Cranial ultrasound, CT and MRI scans provide information that determines the appropriate neurosurgical procedure.

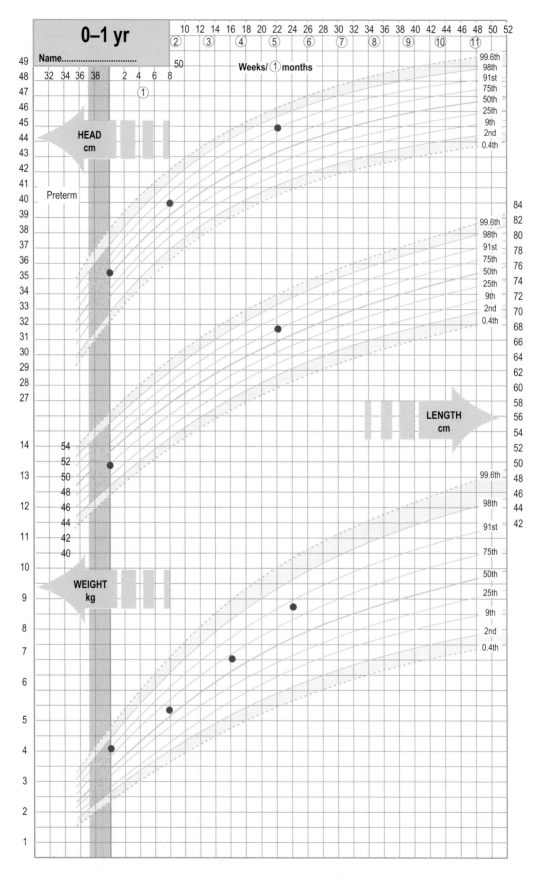

0–1 yr

Weeks/① months

Preterm

HEAD
cm

LENGTH
cm

WEIGHT
kg

99.6th
98th
91st
75th
50th
25th
9th
2nd
0.4th

Fig. 22.7 Jason's growth chart

Prognosis

Children with hydrocephalus are at increased risk for a variety of developmental disabilities and learning difficulties, particularly related to performance tasks and memory. Visual problems are also common. For these reasons it is important that they receive long-term follow-up.

Subdural effusions and haematomas

A subdural haematoma is a collection of bloody fluid under the dura. It results from rupture of the bridging veins that drain the cerebral cortex. Although any form of head trauma may produce subdural bleeding, a physically abused infant who is forcibly shaken is particularly susceptible to this injury (Ch. 36). Subdural haematomas may be acute or chronic, in which case they may eventually be replaced by a subdural collection of fluid. Subdural haematomas can lead to blockage of cerebrospinal fluid flow and hydrocephalus.

Clinical features

Although an enlarging head is a feature, the infant is more likely to present with fits, irritability, lethargy, vomiting and failure to thrive. Signs of raised intracranial pressure and retinal haemorrhages are common. Diagnosis is made by radiological imaging.

Management

Management is neurosurgical. All cases of subdural haematoma should be evaluated thoroughly for the possibility of abuse.

Prognosis

The prognosis for recovery is variable and depends on the associated cerebral insult.

The small head (microcephaly)

Problem-orientated topic:

a child with a small head

Dimitra is a 9-month-old baby. She was born small for gestational age and her growth has always been borderline, with her weight, length and head circumference now all between the 0.4th and 2nd centiles (Fig. 22.8). There are no dysmorphic features. Dimitra has just now achieved sitting with support and she has reasonable head control. She began to reach out for objects at 7 months and has just started transferring from hand to hand. She vocalizes with vowel but not consonant sounds.

Q1. Does Dimitra have microcephaly?

Q2. What do you need to focus on in your clinical evaluation?

Q3. Does Dimitra need to be investigated?

Q1. Does Dimitra have microcephaly?

By definition microcephaly is a head circumference below 2 standard deviations (below the 2nd centile). Dimitra therefore does have microcephaly; the question is whether this is of concern. A small head can be familial, in which case it can be quite normal. However, a small head may indicate limited brain growth, which can result from a number of perinatal insults. Very rarely poor head growth occurs as a result of premature fusion of cranial sutures (craniosynostosis). The causes of microcephaly are shown in Box 22.7.

Q2. What do you need to focus on in your clinical evaluation?

Key points
- Determine whether the child is developing normally.
- Check parental head size.

History
- *Is the baby developing normally?* If a baby is developing normally, it is unlikely that the head size is a cause for concern. If developmental delay is present, the baby needs to be evaluated for perinatal insults or genetic syndromes.
- *Past medical history.* The perinatal history may throw light on factors such as infection, alcohol or hypoxic–ischaemic events that may have affected brain growth.

Examination
- *Growth measures.* Length and weight of the baby indicate whether the head size is disproportionately small. The pattern of head growth is important. Crossing of centile lines is a greater cause of concern than steady growth of a small head.

BOX 22.7 Causes of microcephaly or poor head growth

- Normal variant (often familial)
- Limited brain growth:
  - Perinatal insult to the brain, e.g. hypoxic–ischaemic insult
  - Genetic syndromes usually associated with learning disability
  - Neurodegenerative conditions
  - Craniosynostosis (p. 259)

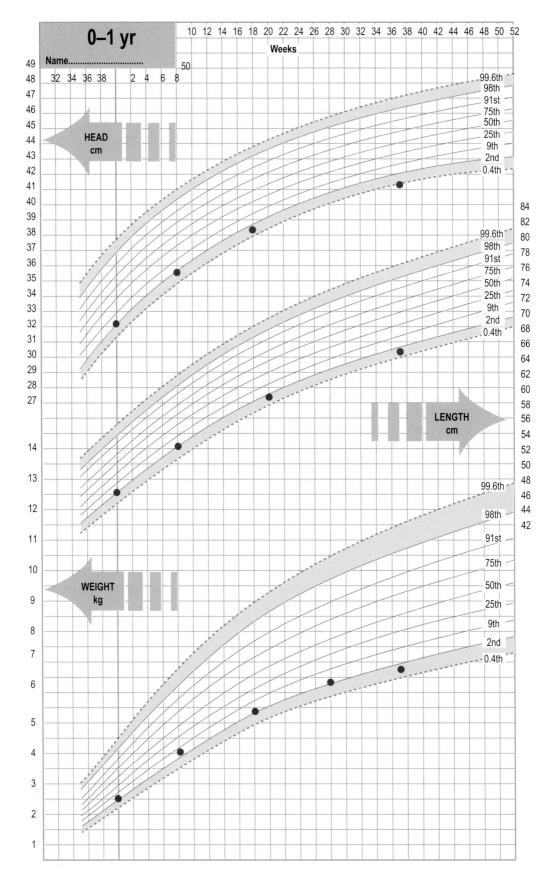

0–1 yr

Weeks

HEAD cm

LENGTH cm

WEIGHT kg

99.6th
98th
91st
75th
50th
25th
9th
2nd
0.4th

Fig. 22.8 Dimitra's growth chart

- *Parental head size.* Microcephaly in normal individuals is often familial.
- *Developmental skills.* Confirm the developmental history by carrying out a good developmental assessment.
- *Dysmorphic features.* Dysmorphic features suggest the diagnosis of a genetic syndrome.

Q3. Does Dimitra need to be investigated?

Dimitra has microcephaly and developmental delay, so she does merit investigation. If she did not have delay, there would be less concern. The level of developmental delay merits a good developmental evaluation and she should be referred to a developmental paediatrician. A karyotype and neurometabolic screen are indicated if a neurodegenerative or dysmorphic syndrome is suspected. An MRI might be helpful to determine underlying pathology. A skull X-ray is unlikely to be helpful unless craniosynostosis is suspected, in which case premature fusion of the sutures is seen.

Pathological causes of microcephaly

Cranial insults

A variety of insults to the developing brain can affect brain growth detrimentally and lead to microcephaly. These include:
- Hypoxic–ischaemic encephalopathy (Ch. 47)
- Congenital infections (Ch. 47)
- Genetic disorder or syndrome
- Toxins, such as alcohol
- Malnutrition
- Meningitis.

Developmental disorders

Many dysmorphic syndromes are accompanied by microcephaly. The most common of these is Down syndrome.

Craniosynostosis (craniostenosis)

In this rare condition premature fusion of the sutures occurs. Very rarely all the sutures are involved, so restricting growth of the skull and, as a consequence, growth of the brain. This results in a rise in intracranial pressure. The diagnosis is made on plain skull X-ray and urgent neurosurgical intervention is required.

Obesity

Obesity is increasing as a problem in childhood. The vast majority of overweight children have nutritional obesity, and this diagnosis can be simply made on the basis of the clinical evaluation. The importance of identifying the obese child is principally in order to provide support and advice and to attempt to prevent the complications of obesity later in life. Although there is a folk belief that obesity is caused by a child's 'glands', this is very rarely the case.

Basic science of weight control

Body weight depends on the interaction of many genes, and twin studies have shown that 50–90% of BMI variability is genetically determined. The individual's response to high caloric intake is subject to strong genetic influence. Weight gain in children is a normal process, but its control is complicated and not yet fully understood.

There are four important factors:
- Food intake
- Signals from adipose tissue
- Central control
- Satiety signals.

Signals from adipose tissue

Under normal circumstances the amount of body fat influences food intake, requiring hormonal signals to be sent from fatty tissue to the brain to modify appetite. The most important appetite control hormone is leptin, although insulin also has a role. Increased adipose tissue causes increased blood leptin levels. One important function of leptin is to inform hypothalamic neurons about levels of energy stored in the body. High leptin levels stimulate receptors within the hypothalamus to inhibit the release of neuropeptide Y(NPY), a potent orexigenic agent, and increase the secretion of hypothalamic melanocyte-stimulating hormone (aMSH), an important mediator of satiety: the overall effect is to reduce appetite.

Conversely, food deprivation reduces plasma leptin levels, stimulating appetite (Fig. 22.9).

Satiety

A meal causes upper bowel distension and stimulates the brain to stop eating; this is mediated through hormones such as cholecystokinin (CCK), released by the bowel. The neurotransmitter serotonin is a primary satiety factor within the brain, and when released, reduces food intake.

 http://www.sciencedirect.com

Follow the links to English PJ, Wilding PH 2002 Applied physiology: the control of weight. Current Paediatrics 12:130–137

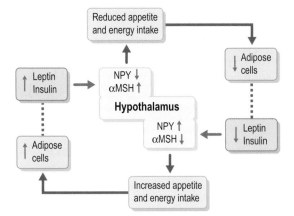

Fig. 22.9 Physiological mechanisms involved in appetite control; see text for details of hypothalamic control

Problem-orientated topic:

obesity ● ● ● ● ●

Kostantina is 10 years old. She comes to see you with her mother as she is troubled by her weight. As you can see from her growth chart (Fig. 22.10), she was always a big girl, and started to put on weight significantly when she was 3 years old. The family are concerned that she has a glandular problem causing her obesity.

Q1. Might there be a hormonal cause for Kostantina's obesity?

Q2. What should be included in your clinical assessment?

Q3. Should Kostantina have any investigations?

Q4. What treatment options are there?

Q5. What are the major complications of obesity?

Q1. Might there be a hormonal cause for Kostantina's obesity?

The best guide to whether there might be a medical cause for Kostantina's obesity is her growth chart. Children with nutritional obesity tend to be tall for their age, whereas those with a hormonal or syndromic cause are short or grow poorly (Fig. 22.11). The causes of obesity are shown in Box 22.8.

Q2. What should be included in your clinical assessment?

Key points

- Exclude rare causes of obesity, remembering that most of these children will be growing poorly.

BOX 22.8 Causes of obesity in childhood

Common
- Nutritional

Rare
- Hypothyroidism
- Cushing syndrome or disease
- Hypothalamic damage (tumours)
- Syndromes: Prader–Willi, Down

- Calculate the BMI and plot it on a BMI growth chart.
- Assess the child for early complications resulting from obesity.
- Obtain a clear picture of the child's lifestyle, focusing on physical activity and diet.
- Find out about emotional and behavioural problems.

Weight alone is not a measure of obesity in childhood, but must be related to the child's height. Your clinical evaluation should firstly focus on excluding the rare endocrine and genetic causes of obesity. As all of these are accompanied by poor growth, they can be excluded on clinical grounds fairly easily. You then need to assess those aspects of the child's lifestyle that predispose to obesity and any emotional and behavioural difficulties the child is having.

History

- *Diet.* Ask what the child and family eat on a normal day, bearing in mind that this may be a sensitive issue. Nevertheless it can form a basis for advice.
- *Lifestyle.* Ask about physical activity during the day and also about sedentary activities.
- *Sleep problems.* Sleep apnoea is a common complication of obesity, so ask about snoring and about lethargy or tiredness during the day
- *Complications.* Musculoskeletal symptoms are common due to the increased load on the joints. It is rare for diabetes or cardiovascular disease to develop in childhood, although there may be biochemical indicators present.
- *Emotional and behavioural problems.* Social and school problems are very common. Children may be bullied or be bullies, or may suffer from significant depression.
- *Learning difficulties.* Children with a genetic syndrome associated with obesity are likely to have special educational needs.
- *Physical symptoms.* Ask about any physical symptoms that might suggest hypothyroidism or Cushing disease (Ch. 35) as a cause.

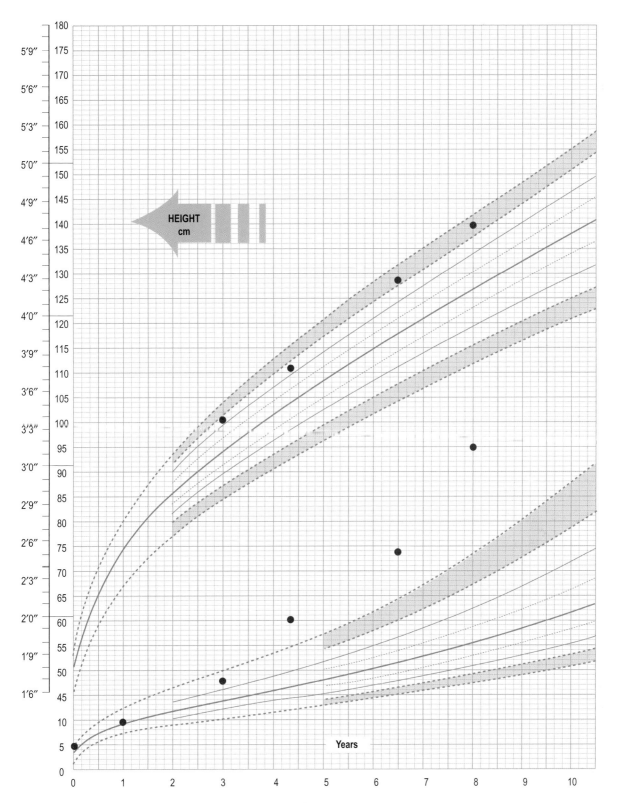

Fig. 22.10 **Kostantina's growth chart**

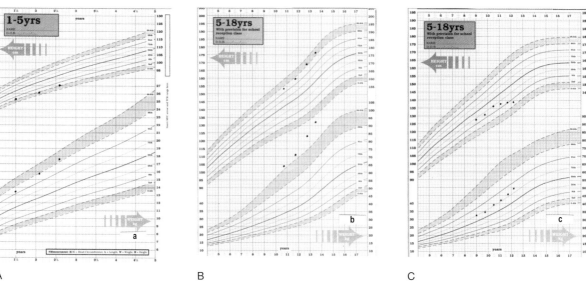

Fig. 22.11 Growth charts illustrating different causes of obesity.
(A) Obesity with short stature suggests a syndromic or hypothalamic cause; (B) obesity with tall stature suggests nutritional obesity; (C) obesity with falloff in growth suggests a hormonal cause.

Table 22.5 Investigations that may be indicated in the obese child

Aim	Investigation	Relevance
Looking for a cause	T4, TSH	Low T4 and high TSH are found in hypothyroidism
	Urinary free cortisol	High in Cushing disease
	Karyotype and DNA analysis	Genetic syndrome
	MRI of the brain	Hypothalamic cause
Looking for consequences of obesity	Urinary glucose, fasting glucose and insulin or an oral glucose tolerance test	Diabetes
	Fasting lipid screen	Hyperlipidaemia
	Liver function tests	Fatty liver

- *Family history.* As obesity is a familial condition (genetically and environmentally), a family history is important. It is important to ask about any family members who have developed, or died from, diabetes or early heart disease.

Examination

- *Growth.* This is the most important indicator of a non-nutritional cause. In nutritional obesity, the child is relatively tall. With pathological causes, the child either is short or demonstrates a falloff in height as the weight increases (Fig. 22.11). You should also calculate the BMI and plot this and waist circumference on the appropriate charts (Fig. 22.12).
- *Signs of an endocrinological cause.* In the child with poor growth, look for signs of hypothyroidism (goitre, developmental delay, slow return of deep tendon reflexes, bradycardia) and steroid excess (moon face, buffalo hump, striae, hypertension, bruising).

- *Signs of dysmorphic syndromes.* Certain dysmorphic syndromes are characterized by obesity. These children are invariably short. Look in particular for microcephaly, hypogonadism, hypotonia and congenital anomalies.
- *Signs of complications.* Check the blood pressure and look for acanthosis nigricans (a dark velvety appearance at the neck and axillae), as this is a sign of insulin resistance.

Q3. Should Kostantina have any investigations?

Investigations (Table 22.5) are required if you are concerned that there is a non-nutritional cause for the obesity, particularly if the child is short, is dysmorphic, is demonstrating a falloff in height or has learning difficulties. In this case thyroid function tests, diurnal cortisol levels and genetic studies are indicated. If the child is very obese, investigation for heart disease, diabetes and steatohepatitis may be needed.

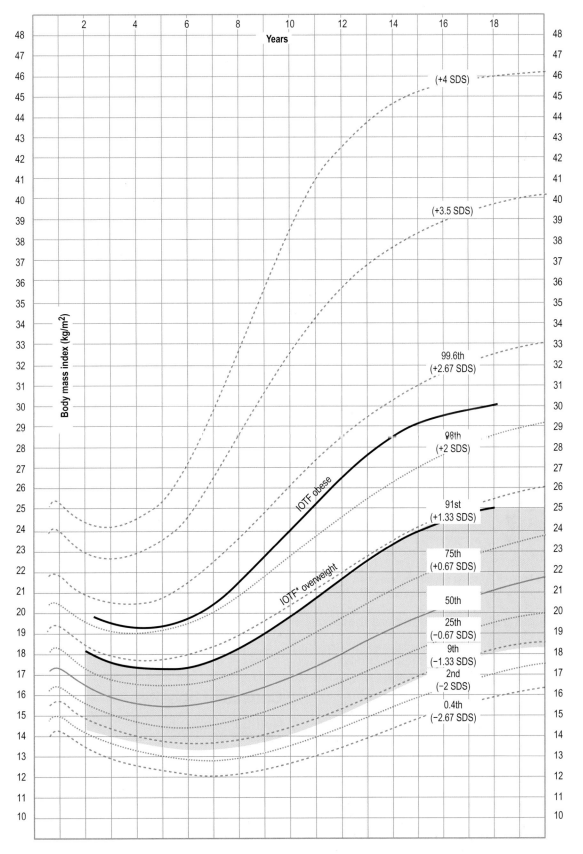

Fig. 22.12 (a) BMI chart (* IOTF — International Obesity Task Force; http://www.iotf.org)

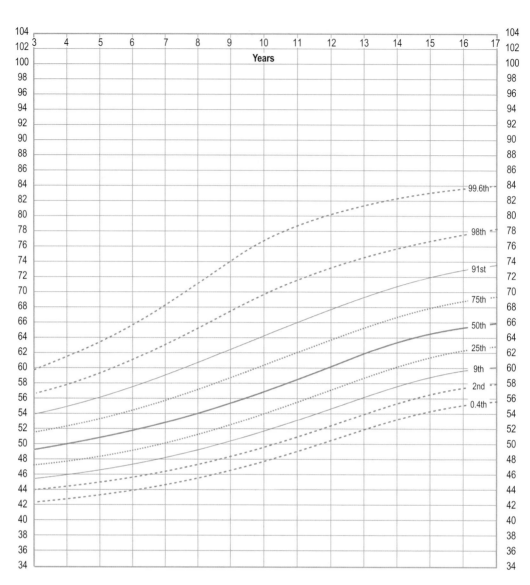

Fig. 22.12 (cont'd) **(b) waist circumference chart**

Q4. What treatment options are there?

Lifestyle management is the mainstay of treating obesity (as discussed below). At present there are no medications licensed for use in children.

Q5. What are the major complications of obesity?

Complications of obesity include:
- Psychological problems
- The metabolic syndrome: hyperinsulinism, hyperlipidaemia and hypertension
- Diabetes mellitus
- Cardiovascular disease
- Respiratory disorders, including obstructive sleep apnoea

- Musculoskeletal problems
- A predisposition to polycystic ovary syndrome.

Causes of obesity

Nutritional obesity

The metabolic factors that predispose some individuals to becoming obese have yet to be determined. The correlation between nutrient intake and development of obesity is not simple.

Clinical features

Nutritionally obese children tend to be tall for their age but develop puberty early, so that final height is not usually excessive. Boys' genitalia may appear deceptively small if buried in fat. Knock-knees are common. Obese children have a high incidence of emotional and behavioural difficulties.

Management

Obese children are often the victims of teasing by peers and psychological disturbance is common. If this is not addressed, it is unlikely that lifestyle change will be achieved. Even if weight control is not successful, continuous support is necessary to help these children cope with their condition. In advising on lifestyle it is essential that the family as a whole is engaged rather than targeting the child. Increasing physical activity is key. Reducing sedentary activity is especially important, and walking to school or swimming may be more acceptable than organized sports. In planning a diet, basic nutritional needs must be met. Rapid decreases in weight should not be attempted and during the growing years maintenance of weight, while the child increases in height, is a reasonable goal.

Prognosis

Despite medical intervention, reduction of obesity once it is well established is difficult. Psychological difficulties may well persist into the adult years. Society deals harshly with the obese and studies show that obesity is a handicap later in life. In childhood overt medical complications are few, although metabolic markers for cardiovascular disease, diabetes and fatty liver are common. Obese children are more susceptible to musculoskeletal strain and slipped capital femoral epiphyses. Rarely, insulin-resistant diabetes mellitus develops in childhood. For obese adults, morbidity is significant, with diabetes and hypertension common, leading to early mortality from ischaemic heart disease and strokes. Gallstones and certain cancers are also more prevalent.

Prevention

As in most conditions, prevention is better than cure. There is some evidence that breastfeeding in infancy is protective and promotion of good nutrition in the early years, when food habits are developing, is important. Physical activity needs to be encouraged in all children, not simply the obese. There is a need for these health issues to be addressed in school, particularly during adolescence, when high intake of high-fat foods and decrease in exercise are common. If intervention is provided early in the course of obesity, weight control is likely to be more successful.

Inês Azevedo   Simon Frazer

Heart and lung disorders

LEARNING OUTCOMES

It is important for primary care clinicians to have a structured approach to common respiratory and cardiac problems. By the end of this chapter you should be able to:

● Formulate a differential diagnosis for the common cardiac and respiratory problems that present to primary care

● Undertake an initial assessment and instigate the appropriate treatment for these illnesses

● Decide on when it is appropriate to refer to secondary/tertiary care services for further assessment of common respiratory and cardiac disorders.

Introduction

In Europe, respiratory illness remains one of the most common reasons for parents to take their child to their physician and for attendance at the accident and emergency department with a medical problem. Although the mortality from respiratory illness in developed countries is low, acute respiratory illness remains one of the leading causes of childhood death world-wide.

Unlike in adults, acquired cardiovascular disease in children is very rare in Europe. Congenital cardiac malformations are much more common, affecting up to 6 per 1000 live births.

Murmurs

(See also Ch. 40.)

Problem-orientated topic:

a child with a heart murmur ● ● ● ●

Milan is a 7-year-old boy who has come to the surgery with sore throat and fever. During the examination you detect a soft ejection systolic murmur in the pulmonary area. He has a red throat and otherwise looks relatively well.

Q1. What further features on history and examination would be important?

Q2. Would you refer this boy for further assessment?

BOX 23.1 Features of innocent ejection murmurs

- Systolic
- Soft blowing (pulmonary area) *or*
- Short buzzing (aortic area)
- Symptom-free
- Sign free: normal pulses (palpable femoral pulses), no palpable thrills or heaves, heart sounds normal, no radiation of murmur and no signs of cardiac failure or cyanosis

---

Q1. What further features on history and examination would be important?

Although children with structural cardiac defects often have murmurs on clinical examination, the majority of murmurs heard in childhood are innocent. It is common for primary care physicians to detect murmurs in children, particularly in those presenting with a febrile illness, when the cardiac output is increased. It is therefore important to identify features that would discriminate between innocent and pathological murmurs.

There are two main types of innocent murmur:

- *Ejection murmurs.* These are caused by turbulent blood flow through the main outflow vessels of the heart. They are heard loudest in the aortic and pulmonary areas (Box 23.1).
- *Venous hum.* A continuous, low-pitched rumbling murmur is heard below the clavicles. It is caused by turbulent blood flow through the major head and neck vessels. The murmur will disappear when the child lies supine.

Q2. Would you refer this boy for further assessment?

Children with abnormal features on history or examination should be referred for further assessment. Murmurs detected in infancy need particular attention. It is now common practice in many centres for murmurs detected in the neonatal period to be referred for cardiology assessment, as the proportion of pathological murmurs is much higher within this group.

Chest pain

(See also Ch. 40.)

Problem-orientated topic:

a child with chest pain ● ● ● ●

Daan is a 12-year-old boy who has been brought to see you by his parents. They are concerned that he has developed chest pain after playing sport yesterday. He has some left-sided chest wall tenderness on examination.

Q1. What further features of the history and examination would be important?

Q2. What causes of chest pain should you consider in your assessment?

Q3. When would you refer a patient for further assessment?

Q1. What further features of the history and examination would be important?

Chest pain is a common problem, particularly in the older child. Parents are often anxious and concerned that chest pain is caused by cardiac disease. However, it is unusual for cardiac conditions to present with chest pain in children and studies have estimated the incidence of cardiac-related disorders in children presenting with chest pain at around 1%. It is therefore important to distinguish features from both history and examination that will discriminate between benign chest pain and more significant pathology.

Q2. What causes of chest pain should you consider in your assessment?

See Table 23.1.

Table 23.1 Causes of chest pain in children

Type of pain	Associated features
Musculoskeletal	Local tenderness, pain exacerbated by inspiration or exercise Possible history of trauma
Respiratory	Acute onset of pleuritic pain, often unilateral with symptoms and signs of respiratory disease ± scoliosis Exercise-induced pain with wheeze or dyspnoea
Gastrointestinal	Burning retrosternal pain, epigastric tenderness

Cardiac
  Ischaemic pain
 	
  Pericardial
	
	Gripping, crushing ± radiation to neck, jaw and arms
	Dyspnoea and pallor ± palpitations
	Central sharp pleuritic pain, worse when supine

Psychogenic	History of stress factors, hyperventilation or panic attacks
Others	Shingles, nerve compression, mediastinal tumours, fibrocystic breast disease Gynaecomastia

Musculoskeletal causes

This is by far the most common cause of chest pain in children. Most children will experience short-lived lateral chest wall discomfort in relation to exertion that disappears on resting. This is what is commonly referred to as a 'stitch'. Trauma and muscular strains are also frequent innocent causes of chest pain. The presence of localized tenderness is almost always secondary to a musculoskeletal cause.

Central chest pain with associated tenderness along the costochondral margin is common with costochondritis. This is often a short benign self-limiting illness that responds to simple analgesia and avoidance of strenuous activity.

Precordial catch syndrome is a common childhood condition associated with stabbing left-sided anterior chest wall pain in the absence of respiratory and cardiac disease.

Coxsackie B viral infection (Bornholm disease) causes pleuritic chest pain (pain exacerbated by normal respiration) and chest wall tenderness in association with an upper respiratory tract infection and fever. Resolution often occurs within 1 week.

Respiratory causes

Asthma is a common condition that can cause mild chest discomfort and tightness on exertion. A history of wheeze and atopy supports the diagnosis. Symptoms should improve with inhaled bronchodilators.

Children who have pneumonia will frequently experience chest pain and discomfort secondary to muscular strain caused by excessive coughing.

Involvement of the pleura, as seen with a pleural effusion or empyema, will result in localized pain that is often worse on inspiration. There should be signs of acute illness and respiration is often shallow in an attempt to reduce pain. Air entry will be reduced on auscultation and resonance is dull on percussion. There may also be associated scoliosis in an attempt to reduce movement on the affected side.

Spontaneous pneumothoraces are occasionally seen in children with asthma or Marfan syndrome and occasionally in healthy normal children. On auscultation air entry is reduced on the affected side, but the percussion note is increased.

Children with sickle cell disease (Ch. 42) can develop an 'acute chest syndrome' as a complication of their condition. Pneumonia and vaso-occlusion of the pulmonary arterioles result in chest pain associated with tachypnoea and signs of consolidation. This is a serious and potentially dangerous complication that needs urgent inpatient assessment.

Deep venous thrombosis and pulmonary embolism are extremely rare during childhood.

Gastrointestinal causes

Gastro-oesophageal reflux can cause oesophageal irritation and burning retrosternal pain, often with food contents or acid being regurgitated into the mouth. Symptoms are often exacerbated when the child lies supine.

Epigastric tenderness in association with chest pain is suggestive of peptic ulcer disease. However, this is an unusual cause of chest pain in children.

Diaphragmatic irritation in association with a number of gastrointestinal disorders (e.g. pancreatitis) can cause chest pain in children. Other features on history and examination that suggest a gastrointestinal cause will almost always be present.

Cardiac causes

Cardiac chest pain is the result of either myocardial ischaemia or pericardial disease.

Ischaemic chest pain is often described as gripping or tight. There may be radiation to the neck, jaw or arm. Pallor, shortness of breath and palpitations are common. Ischaemic pain may occur in children with coronary artery disease (Kawasaki disease, anomalous coronary arteries, familial hypercholesterolaemia) or in association with tachyarrhythmias (supraventricular tachycardia, ventricular tachycardia).

Pericardial pain is often a central sharp stabbing pain that is exacerbated particularly in the supine position and by normal respiration. Pain may radiate to the shoulder or back. A pericardial rub may be detected (pericarditis) or the heart sounds may be decreased (pericardial effusion).

Aortic dissection should always be considered in children with chest pain and Marfan syndrome.

Psychogenic causes

Around 30% of all chest pain in children, particularly the older child, is secondary to stress and anxiety. Episodes of pain are commonly associated with hyperventilation and panic attacks. It is important to identify possible triggers and situations in which symptoms arise (e.g. bullying).

Q3. When would you refer a patient for further assessment? (Box 23.2)

In the majority of cases, chest pain will be benign in nature. A detailed history and examination should help distinguish those who need further assessment. For the majority of children, simple analgesia and reassurance are all that is required.

Palpitations

Problem-orientated topic:

a child having palpitations

Lieke is a 14-year-old girl who is concerned about episodes where she becomes aware that her heart is thumping and fast. She is extremely worried by these episodes and often hyperventilates.

Q1. What further features on history and examination would be important?

Q2. What are the common causes to consider?

Q3. What investigations would you perform?

Q4. How would you manage this patient's care?

Q1. What further features on history and examination would be important?

It is not unusual for children to become aware of their heart beat, particularly during periods of excitement or anxiety. In the majority of cases this is a normal phenomenon.

It is important to note the general health and emotional state of the child during the episode. Anxious children may experience palpitations associated with hyperventilation and discomfort within stressful situations.

Children who present with episodes of recurrent palpitations need careful assessment. It is important to highlight any family history of arrhythmias or sudden death. Palpitations that start and stop suddenly are more suggestive of a cardiac arrhythmia. Episodes associated with pallor, chest pain, dyspnoea or syncope will need further investigation for a possible cardiac cause.

Q2. What are the common causes to consider?

These include:
- Fever
- Anxiety/exercise
- Anaemia
- Hyperthyroidism
- Cardiac arrhythmia (Ch. 40).

Q3. What investigations would you perform?

When a cardiac arrhythmia is suspected, it is important to arrange a paediatric assessment and a 12-lead ECG. It is particularly important to assess the PR and QT corrected (QT_c) interval of the ECG.

The PR interval may be short in children with accessory electrical pathways between the atria and ventricles. This is often associated with episodes of supraventricular tachycardia (SVT). SVTs are the most common arrhythmias seen during childhood and are associated with very fast (> 210 beats per minute) regular tachycardias.

The QT interval is variable and dependent on the child's heart rate. This can be corrected for and most ECG machines will report the QT_c. Children with

MODULE FIVE

269

prolonged QT syndrome have QT_c intervals > 440 ms and are prone to episodes of ventricular tachycardia (VT) and sudden death. There is often a significant family history.

A normal PR and QT_c will not exclude paroxysmal arrhythmias. It is often difficult to detect arrhythmias when episodes are infrequent. A prolonged ambulant ECG recording is useful, but is dependent on episodes occurring during the period of monitoring.

Q4. How would you manage this patient's care?

The management is dependent on the likely cause. The case should be discussed with a paediatrician or paediatric cardiologist if there are concerns that the episode may be a possible arrhythmia (Ch. 40). Children experiencing anxiety-related palpitations should be reassured and offered support with any major stressors (e.g. bullying).

Syncope

(See also p. 295.)

Problem-orientated topic:

a child with syncope ● ● ● ● ●

Sanne is a 12-year-old girl who has presented to the surgery after collapsing in assembly. She remembers feeling dizzy initially before falling to the floor and blacking out.

Q1. What further features on history and examination would be important?

Q2. What differentials should be considered?

Q3. How would you manage this symptom?

Q1. What further features on history and examination would be important?

Syncope or 'fainting' is a frequent occurrence during childhood. It is commonly benign and often neurally mediated. Serious and life-threatening causes are rare. Investigations are often normal and are not routinely required.

A careful history, examination including blood pressure (standing and supine) and an optional ECG are useful if there is any worry that this is not a simple faint.

Episodes that occur when the child lies supine or in relation to exercise should raise alarm bells. Likewise,

---

BOX 23.3 Differential diagnosis of syncope

Vasovagal syncope 'faint' (p. 295)

- Neurally induced bradycardia and hypotension
- Common particularly in older children (9–14 years)
- Occurs when upright; may be triggered by pain, emotional stimuli, heat exposure or prolonged standing
- Associated dizziness, nausea, blurred vision or pallor
- Secondary anoxic seizures can cause stiffening or fine twitching
- Recovery often rapid after lying down

Reflex anoxic seizures — 'pallid breath-holding spells' (p. 295)

- Young children (6 months to 3 years)
- Neurally induced transient asystole that occurs in response to pain or emotional stimuli
- Marked pallor, secondary anoxic seizures common

Cardiac

- Rare
- May be associated with palpitations, dyspnoea or chest pain
- Family history of sudden death

Epilepsy

- Uncommon to have isolated collapse without tonic or tonic–clonic phases
- Recovery is often slow — 'post-ictal phase'

Factitious

- Unwitnessed episodes
- Inconsistent story and inappropriate parental or child response

---

a family history of sudden unexpected death would cause concern.

Q2. What differentials should be considered?

See Box 23.3.

Q3. How would you manage this symptom?

Parents are often worried that there is a serious and life-threatening cause. It is important to reassure the child and family. Vasovagal syncope tends to improve with age. Increased water and salt intake may help those with frequent episodes.

BOX 23.4 Common causes of acute febrile illness in children

Systemic
- Viral: influenza, viral exanthems (chickenpox, rubella, measles)
- Bacterial: meningococcal septicaemia, staphylococcal toxic shock
- Inflammatory: Kawasaki disease

Upper respiratory tract
- Common cold, pharyngitis, tonsillitis, otitis media

Lower respiratory tract
- Pneumonia, bronchiolitis

Renal
- Urinary tract infection, pyelonephritis

Gastrointestinal
- Gastroenteritis, appendicitis

Neurological
- Meningitis

Musculoskeletal
- Septic arthritis, osteomyelitis

Persistent fever
- See Chapter 40

Respiratory tract infections

Problem-orientated topic:

febrile respiratory illness

Rupert is a 4-year-old boy who has been unwell with fever and cough for 3 days. He looks unwell and has a temperature of 39.5°C. He is tachypnoeic and grunting.

Q1. What are the main differential diagnoses to be considered?

Q2. What investigations should you consider?

Q1. What are the main differential diagnoses to be considered?

Infective or inflammatory disorders are most likely and these are listed in Box 23.4.

Q2. What investigations should you consider?

Screen for infection is important, which as a minimum in primary care includes urine for culture

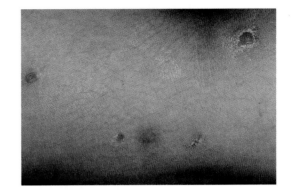

Fig. 23.1 **Chickenpox**

and sensitivity if there is no focus. A toxic febrile child should be referred to a hospital. A chest X-ray should be considered in Rupert's case. If there are concerns about meningococcal septicaemia, then immediate antibiotic treatment should be given (Ch. 43). In hospital, blood cultures and lumbar puncture are necessary if Rupert shows signs of altered consciousness or a stiff neck, or has a purpuric rash.

Non-specific viral illness

Febrile illnesses, with non-specific features of malaise, headache, nausea, cough and myalgia, are often caused by viral infections such as influenza. There are no specific clinical findings on examination and it is important to exclude clinically other causes of these symptoms. Management should be aimed at symptomatic relief with analgesia and antipyretics.

Viral exanthems

Chickenpox (see Ch. 43) and other viral exanthems (measles, rubella etc.) present with features similar to influenza early on in the illness, before the onset of their characteristic rashes.

Chickenpox

Chickenpox is a common infection that is spread by droplet inhalation of the varicella zoster virus from contacts with either chickenpox or shingles (Fig. 23.1). The majority of children have a relatively mild illness when they contract it at an early age. Those who escape childhood infection are at a greater risk of developing the associated complications of chickenpox. Children who have impaired immunity (long-term corticosteroids, immunosuppressant therapy and treatment for malignancy) are at a significant risk of severe and fatal disease. Babies born to mothers who have developed chickenpox between 5 days before and 2 days after delivery are also at increased risk of severe neonatal varicella.

Clinical features

The incubation period between contact and disease is 14–21 days. Spots appear in crops initially on the face and trunk. What initially begins as a macule quickly progresses into a papule, followed by vesicle formation. New crops continue to develop, whilst the earlier crops form pustules before finally crusting over. The rash often causes intense itching. Constitutional symptoms are variable, ranging from mild fever and upset to signs of toxicity in those with more severe disease. The child remains infectious from 48 hours before the onset of the rash until all the crops have crusted over.

Complications

- Secondary bacterial infection
- Encephalitis (typically post-infectious with cerebellar involvement and ataxia)
- Pneumonia
- Disseminated haemorrhagic chickenpox
- Arthritis, hepatitis, pancreatitis, nephritis and thrombocytopenia.

Scarring and secondary bacterial (*Staphylococcus aureus* and *Streptococcus*) infection of the lesions are common complications. Other complications are less common in children.

Management

Immunocompetent children with chickenpox require symptomatic treatment only. Calamine lotion and cool baths are soothing. Oral antihistamines may help ease the itching. Immunocompromised children and babies with peripartum exposure should receive zoster immunoglobulin (ZIG) within 96 hours of contact. Those who develop features of chickenpox despite ZIG should receive intravenous aciclovir.

Vaccination against varicella is common in the US but at present this has not been routinely adopted in European countries.

Upper respiratory tract infection (URTI)

In children, the majority of respiratory infections affect the upper respiratory tract (ears, nose and throat). Viruses are by far the most common pathogen.

The most common URTIs include:

- Common cold
- Pharyngitis
- Tonsillitis
- Otitis media.

Pharyngitis

Children often present with sore throat and fever. The oropharynx is inflamed and erythematous. Pharyngitis is most commonly due to viral infection.

> **BOX 23.5 Indications for adenotonsillectomy**
>
> - Recurrent severe tonsillitis
> - Glue ear (with grommets)
> - Obstructive sleep apnoea

Tonsillitis

Tonsillitis can cause children to present with sore throat, fever, malaise, abdominal pain, vomiting or meningism. On inspection the throat and tonsils are inflamed, often with pus on the surface of the tonsils. Cervical lymphadenopathy is a common feature.

Group A β-haemolytic streptococci and Epstein–Barr virus (EBV, glandular fever) are common causes. Clinically it is difficult to distinguish between bacterial and viral infections of the pharynx and tonsils. For most children treatment should be symptomatic, with prescriptions of analgesia, an antipyretic (paracetamol) and regular oral fluids. It would not be unreasonable to prescribe antibiotics to children with marked constitutional disturbance and high fever or those with pus on the tonsils. Oral penicillin V would be the treatment of choice in this situation. Amoxicillin should be avoided in children with tonsillitis, as it can precipitate a generalized erythematous rash in those with EBV infection. Nevertheless, it is a reasonable option in countries where oral penicillin V is not available or when children reject penicillin V because of its bitter taste.

Recurrent viral pharyngitis is common and often prompts parents to request adenotonsillectomy inappropriately (Box 23.5). Recurrent URTI and large tonsils are not an indication for routine tonsillectomy. Children often have large normal tonsils which later regress in size.

> **BOX 23.6 Common conditions predisposing to acute otitis media**
>
> - Down syndrome
> - Cleft lip and palate
> - Other craniofacial abnormalities
> - Immunodeficiency

Acute otitis media (AOM) (see also Ch. 32)

AOM is very common, with approximately 1 in 4 children having had at least one episode in the first decade of life. Otitis media occurs more frequently in children with associated structural abnormalities of the upper airway that affect the drainage of the Eustachian tube and aeration of the middle ear (Box 23.6). Common pathogens include viruses, *Pneumococcus, Haemophilus, Moraxella catarrhalis*, β-haemolytic streptococci and *Strep. pyogenes*.

Clinical features

Young children with acute otitis media often present with non-specific features of fever, irritability and vomiting. All children who present with fever should have their ears examined, particularly children who are noted to be pulling at their ears.

The eardrum in AOM may appear injected or bulging, often with loss of normal light reflection. If perforation has occurred, the view may be obscured by purulent discharge.

Complications of AOM (mastoiditis and meningitis) are uncommon. Recurrent otitis media predisposes to glue ear and conductive hearing loss.

Management

The use of antibiotics in AOM has been subject to large reviews by both the American Academy of Paediatrics (AAP) and the Scottish Intercollegiate Guideline Network (SIGN). Both agree that the majority of children (older than 2 years) with AOM will improve spontaneously, without the need for oral antibiotics. Instead of being prescribed antibiotics initially, children should be given paracetamol analgesia and a policy of delayed antibiotic prescription should be adopted (antibiotics to be collected at the parent's discretion after 72 hours, if the child has not improved). Children older than 2 years with severe AOM (moderate to severe otalgia and fever > 39°C) should be prescribed early antibiotics. Broad-spectrum antibiotics such as amoxicillin (± clavulanic acid) should be prescribed for 5 to 10 days in severe cases.

At present there is little evidence for the correct management of children under the age of 2 years presenting with AOM; the AAP recommends antibiotics for all cases of AOM in this age group.

🌐 **http://adc.bmjjournals.com/**

Archives of Disease in Children: Education and Practice. Follow links to 'Comparison of Two Otitis Media Guidelines', and to 'Community-acquired Pneumonia in Children: a Clinical Update'

🌐 **http://www.sign.ac.uk**

SIGN. Follow links to guidelines on 'Diagnosis and Management of Childhood Otitis Media in Primary Care'

Glue ear (see also Ch. 32)

Glue ear is defined as the persistence of fluid in the middle ear in the absence of signs of active inflammation. It is the most common cause of conductive hearing loss in children. It is associated with an increased risk of speech and learning difficulties in affected children. It occurs commonly following AOM, although the majority of children with AOM and middle ear effusion will resolve spontaneously within 3 months. Like AOM, it is more common in children with structural ear, nose and throat (ENT) abnormalities.

Assessment

- Inspection of tympanic membrane (retracted drum and loss of light reflection)
- Hearing assessment appropriate to child's age
- Tympanometry.

Management

Glue ear will spontaneously resolve after 3 months in most children. Those cases persisting beyond 3 months need further assessment. There is little evidence of significant short-term and long-term effects of medical therapy for glue ear (decongestants, mucolytics, anti-histamines, antibiotics and systemic steroids). Children with glue ear and significant hearing loss will require insertion of aeration tubes (grommets). This is often combined with adenoidectomy for better resolution of symptoms.

Chronic suppurative otitis media (CSOM)

CSOM is a condition of chronic middle ear infection associated with perforation of the eardrum and intermittent or persistent ear discharge. Children with CSOM should be referred for ENT assessment.

There are two broad groups:

- 'Safe' CSOM. Perforation occurs in the central aspect of the eardrum.
- 'Unsafe' CSOM. Perforation occurs in the margins of the eardrum or severe retraction of the drum. This is associated with increased risk of VII cranial nerve palsy, abscess formation and intracranial complications.

Lower respiratory tract infection (LRTI)

Infections of the lower respiratory tract are commonly caused by viruses. *Pneumococcus*, *Haemophilus* and *Mycoplasma* are important pathogens in bacterial pneumonia.

The common LRTIs are:

- Pneumonia
- Bronchiolitis.

Community-acquired pneumonia (CAP)

Pneumonia (Box 23.7) occurs more frequently in children under 5 years of age. Viruses alone account for up to one-third (14–35%) of all childhood CAP. A good proportion (8–40%) of CAP represents mixed infection.

BOX 23.7 Common pathogens in community-acquired pneumonia

Respiratory viruses
- Respiratory syncytial virus (RSV)
- Adenovirus
- Influenza
- Parainfluenza
- Metapneumovirus

Mixed
- Common viruses plus bacteria

Bacteria
- Common: *Streptococcus pneumoniae, Mycoplasma, Haemophilus influenzae*
- Others: *Chlamydia trachomatis, Bordetella pertussis, Staphylococcus aureus, Mycobacterium tuberculosis* (TB)

Age is a reasonable predictor of likely pathogen; children under the age of 5 are more likely to have a viral cause, although *Strep. pneumoniae* is important.

Viruses are less common in children over the age of 5, and when a bacterial cause is found, it is most commonly *Strep. pneumoniae* or *Mycoplasma* infection.

Clinical features

Fever, dyspnoea and cough are common symptoms reported in children presenting with pneumonia. Feeding difficulties associated with respiratory distress are particularly common in small children. Older children with pneumonia occasionally present to surgeons with abdominal pain secondary to diaphragmatic irritation.

Signs of pneumonia include:
- Fever
- Tachypnoea
- Recession and nasal flaring
- Grunting
- Cyanosis
- Decreased chest expansion
- Dullness to percussion
- Decreased air entry
- Crepitations
- Bronchial breathing (consolidation).

Tachypnoea and fever are good indicators of pneumonia, although both can be present in other conditions such as asthma. Chest signs may be unilateral (lobar pneumonia) or bilateral (bronchopneumonia).

Mycoplasma infection can often cause wheeze, cough and bilateral chest signs, making the distinction between *Mycoplasma* infection and asthma difficult. It is therefore important to consider *Mycoplasma* infection

in older children with wheeze that fails to respond to conventional asthma therapy.

No one sign on its own is diagnostic of pneumonia. It is the combination of signs that will aid the clinician in the consideration of a possible diagnosis of pneumonia. The absence of all signs is probably of more use in excluding pneumonia. However, pneumonia should still be considered in all acutely ill children under 5 years of age who present with fever of > 39°C with no alternative cause, even in the absence of respiratory symptoms or chest signs.

Complications

Complications of CAP affect only a small proportion of children. They include:
- Pleural effusion and empyema
- Septicaemia
- Lung abscess
- Secondary sepsis: osteomyelitis, septic arthritis.

Investigations

The ideal investigation will confirm the diagnosis of pneumonia and distinguish between bacterial and viral causes. Unfortunately there is no rapid and reliable test that can fit both of these criteria.

- *Blood tests.* Acute phase reactants (erythrocyte sedimentation rate, white cell count and C-reactive protein) are unreliable in distinguishing between bacterial and viral pneumonia. The yield from blood cultures in children with pneumonia is low and results can take up to 48 hours before they are available. Thus they have little impact on the initial decision to treat or not to treat with antibiotics. Routine collection of blood cultures should be reserved for children who require admission to hospital for suspected pneumonia.

  Paired serology for *Mycoplasma* infection is useful in cases of pneumonia that are not responding to treatment. Again it has no impact on the initial decision to treat or not to treat because of the delay in receiving results.
- *Nasopharyngeal aspirate (NPA).* This is recommended to identify respiratory viruses in children < 18 months of age.
- *Chest X-ray (CXR).* Consolidation on the CXR is the most consistent sign of infection and is considered the most reliable method of confirming the diagnosis of pneumonia (Figs 23.2 and 23.3). More subtle changes are subject to large differences in interpretation, reflecting the differences in opinion amongst clinicians and radiologists. Radiological findings may lag behind clinical signs, so a negative CXR does not always exclude pneumonia when there are clear clinical signs. Secondly, studies suggest that radiological

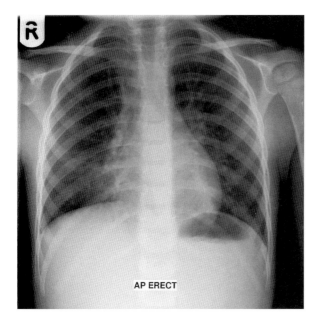

Fig. 23.2 **Chest X-ray in right middle lobe pneumonia**

BOX 23.8 Indications for chest X-ray: British Thoracic Society guidelines

- For diagnosis of children < 5 years with pyrexia of unknown origin
- If complications are suspected
- If there are atypical symptoms or no response to treatment
- Only for follow-up of children with lobar collapse, apparent round pneumonia or ongoing symptoms

consolidation alone cannot be used to assume bacterial infection.

Routine CXR is not required to confirm the diagnosis of pneumonia in children who are well enough to be managed at home. The CXR is useful for confirming the diagnosis and identifying any complications (pleural effusions) in those

admitted for hospital treatment. Interpretation of radiological signs should always be taken in context of the child's age and clinical status (Box 23.8 and Fig. 23.4).

Management

Young children with mild features of infection do not require investigation or treatment with antibiotics. For all other children, antibiotic treatment is recommended.

The majority of children in the community will respond to oral antibiotics prescribed for 5–7 days. Amoxicillin is a good first choice of antibiotic for children with CAP. In the under-5s it is effective against

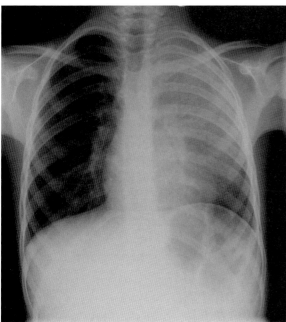

A

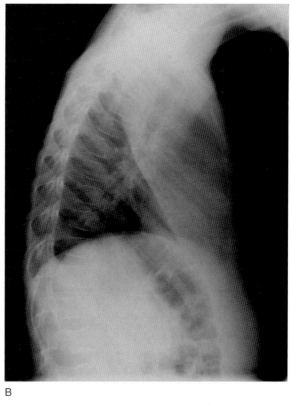

B

Fig. 23.3 **Chest X-ray in left upper lobe pneumonia.**
(A) PA sitting; (B) lateral.

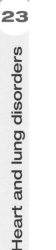

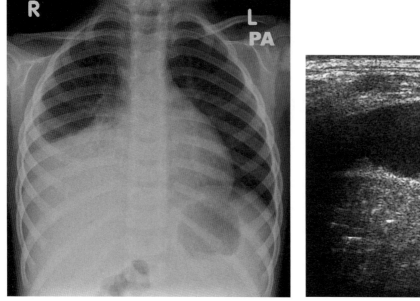

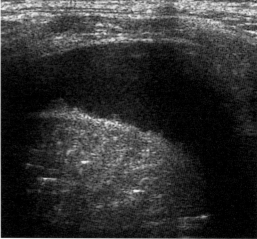

A   B

Fig. 23.4 Right-sided pleural effusion secondary to chest infection.
(A) PA X-ray; (B) ultrasound showing fluid collection above the right diaphragm.

most bacterial pathogens. Macrolide antibiotics (erythromycin, clarithromycin) are good first-line treatments in older children when *Mycoplasma* or *Chlamydia* infection is suspected. If *Staph. aureus* is suspected, then a combination of flucloxacillin and amoxicillin should be prescribed.

The child well enough to be cared for at home on oral antibiotics should be reviewed by a primary care physician if there are any signs of deterioration or if there is no improvement after 48 hours of treatment.

Intravenous antibiotics should be used in the treatment of pneumonia in children who are unable to absorb oral antibiotics or those with features of severe disease. In such circumstances the total (intravenous and oral) course of treatment should be extended to 10 days.

Criteria for admission are as follows:
- The child is vomiting and unable to tolerate oral medication.
- There are signs of severe disease (Box 23.9).
- There are social concerns about the parents' ability to monitor the child effectively.

Wheeze

Problem-orientated topic:

a wheezing child

Emma is a 3-year-old girl who attends the primary care clinic with a 1-day history of

---

BOX 23.9 Signs of severe disease

- Oxygen saturations < 92% on air
- Respiratory rate > 70/min in infants
- Respiratory rate > 50/min in older children
- Chest recessions, nasal flaring, grunting and apnoea
- Feeding < 50% normal fluids
- Signs of dehydration

---

noisy breathing. On examination she is coryzal, her temperature is 36.8°C and the respiratory rate is 32, and on inspection she has mild respiratory distress. On auscultation of the chest she has good air entry but has widespread bilateral wheeze.

Q1. What differential diagnoses should be considered with a child who presents with wheeze?

Q2. What further history and examination would be useful?

Q1. **What differential diagnoses should be considered with a child who presents with wheeze?**

See Box 23.10.

Asthma

- Recurrent episodes of cough and wheeze, responsive to inhaled bronchodilators
- Cough, often worse at night
- History of atopy in child or other family members
- Triggers: viral infections, exercise, smoke, pollution, animal dander, house dust mite, cold weather and stress

Bronchiolitis

- Majority of cases < 9 months
- Occurs in winter epidemics
- Coryza, cough, dyspnoea and difficulty in feeding; apnoeas in small babies; poor response to bronchodilators
- Crackles and wheeze on auscultation
- CXR: hyperinflation, patchy perihilar changes ± collapse
- 80% RSV-positive on NPA

Viral-induced wheeze

- Wheeze with infection
- Often past history of bronchiolitis
- Variable response to treatment; may progress to asthma

Mycoplasma pneumoniae

- Older children with wheeze and cough that fail to respond to conventional asthma therapy

Inhaled foreign body

- Toddler with history of choking
- Rapid onset of wheeze and cough
- CXR shows hyperinflation or segmental collapse
- Poor response to inhaled bronchodilators

Heart failure

- Crackles and wheeze on auscultation
- Murmur and hepatomegaly are common
- Enlarged heart on CXR

Q2. What further history and examination would be useful?

At 3 years of age Emma is too old for bronchiolitis, and an inhaled foreign body would also be unlikely at this age. She had mild bronchiolitis as a baby but was never troubled by her breathing until 3 months ago. Her father had asthma as a child. On examination she has eczema. There were no murmurs or hepatomegaly detected. This makes asthma the most likely diagnosis.

Asthma

Children who are genetically predisposed to asthma develop inflammation and hyper-reactivity of the small airways in response to infection, environmental triggers or exercise. Symptoms are the consequence of small airway obstruction secondary to mucosal oedema, excess mucus production and bronchoconstriction.

The diagnosis of asthma is based on history and response to conventional treatment in the absence of features suggesting alternative diagnoses. Children with asthma have recurrent episodes of cough, wheeze and dyspnoea. Exercise-induced symptoms are common. The reversibility of airway obstruction with inhaled bronchodilators and steroids is an essential feature of asthma. Atopy, the tendency to have eczema, hay fever, allergy and allergic rhinitis, is common amongst asthmatics and their family. One-third of asthmatic children suffer from eczema and almost a half have allergic rhinitis.

Management

The treatment of asthma can be divided into two areas:
- Acute treatment
- Preventing exacerbations/minimizing impact of disease on lifestyle.

Management of acute exacerbation in primary care

The immediate treatment of asthma in primary care depends on the presence or absence of severe or life-threatening features (Box 23.11).

Mild to moderate attacks that show no features of severe or life-threatening asthma can be managed with inhaled β_2-agonists (salbutamol or terbutaline) delivered via a large-volume spacer device. Children aged < 3 years will require a spacer with a face mask rather than a mouthpiece. Children > 3 years should be assessed on an individual basis.

Two to four puffs of salbutamol regularly according to clinical response might be sufficient for mild attacks. Up to ten puffs may be needed initially for more significant exacerbations. Children with acute asthma in primary care who have not improved after receiving an initial dose of ten puffs of inhaled β_2-agonist should be referred to hospital for further assessment. Further doses of inhaled bronchodilator should be given if a nebulizer is unavailable whilst awaiting transfer.

The early use of oral steroids for acute asthma can reduce the need for hospital admission and prevent relapse of symptoms (Table 23.2). There is no evidence to support the use of inhaled steroids as alternative or additional treatment to oral steroids for the treatment

BOX 23.11 Clinical features of severe and life-threatening asthma

Acute severe

- Cannot complete sentences in one breath or too breathless to talk or feed
- Pulse > 120 bpm in children aged > 5 years
- Pulse > 130 bpm in children aged 2–5 years
- Respiration > 30 breaths/min in children aged > 5 years
- Respiration > 50 breaths/min in children aged 2–5 years

Life-threatening

- Silent chest
- Cyanosis
- Poor respiratory effort
- Hypotension
- Exhaustion
- Confusion
- Coma

Table 23.2 Prednisolone dose

Age	Dose
< 2 years	10 mg
2–5 years	20 mg
> 5 years	30–40 mg

of an acute exacerbation. The effects of oral steroids start to become apparent within 3–4 hours of commencing treatment.

Severe or life-threatening asthma requires urgent referral for inpatient care. Nebulized bronchodilator therapy with salbutamol or terbutaline should be commenced prior to arrival of the paramedic team. If no nebulized therapy is available, then inhaled bronchodilators should be administered through a large-volume spacer.

Preventing exacerbations/minimizing impact of asthma on lifestyle

The aim of asthma therapy is to:

- Achieve good symptom control
- Minimize restriction of activities and exercise
- Have a minimal need for reliever therapy
- Reduce exacerbations
- Improve lung function (peak flow > 80% of predicted)
- Avoid side-effects of therapy.

In order to monitor the success of asthma therapies, it is important to assess regularly:

- Frequency and severity of cough, breathlessness and wheeze
- Any sleep disturbance
- Usual exercise tolerance

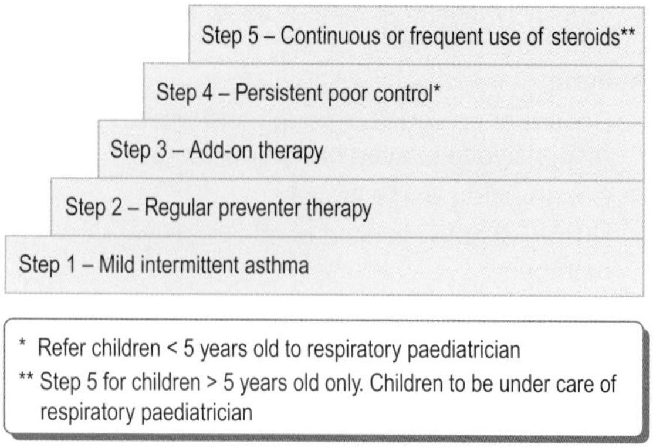

Step 5 – Continuous or frequent use of steroids**

Step 4 – Persistent poor control*

Step 3 – Add-on therapy

Step 2 – Regular preventer therapy

Step 1 – Mild intermittent asthma

* Refer children < 5 years old to respiratory paediatrician

** Step 5 for children > 5 years old only. Children to be under care of respiratory paediatrician

Fig. 23.5 Stepwise management of asthma in children

- Avoidance of activities/exercise because of symptoms
- Number and severity of exacerbations over past 6–12 months
- Number of days missed from school because of asthma
- Any chest deformity/Harrison sulci (poor control)
- Growth.

The stepwise management of asthma is illustrated in Figure 23.5. Patients should commence therapy at the step most appropriate to the severity of their asthma. In order to achieve control, stepping up the treatment may be required, in the same way as treatment should be stepped down when asthma has been well controlled and stable. This model stresses the importance of regular monitoring and review of medication.

Step 1: Mild intermittent asthma

Children with mild symptoms should be prescribed inhaled bronchodilators with β_2-agonists (salbutamol/terbutaline) as required.

Step 2: Regular preventer therapy

Regular inhaled corticosteroids should be considered in children who are symptomatic or using β_2-agonists more than three times per week, waking one or more night per week with asthma or having significant exacerbations. In children a reasonable starting dose would be 200 µg/day of budesonide equivalent split over two doses. (*N.B. 100 µg of inhaled budesonide is equivalent to 100 µg of beclomethasone or 50 µg of inhaled fluticasone.*) Children older than 12 would start at 400 µg/day. If steroids are not acceptable to the family, then a leukotriene receptor antagonist would be an acceptable alternative if symptoms are not too worrisome.

Step 3: Add-on therapy

Children who are still symptomatic after step 2 should receive additional therapy and referral to a paediatrician with respiratory training should be considered. This is very dependent on the child's age:

- *< 2 years.* Go to step 4 and refer to a paediatrician with a respiratory interest.
- *2–5 years.* Give a trial of an oral leukotriene receptor antagonist (e.g. Singulair).
- *> 5 years.* Use a long-acting bronchodilator (LABA) with β_2-agonist (e.g. salmeterol):
  - If there is a good response, then continue LABA.
  - If there is a partial response but control is still poor, continue LABA and increase the dose of inhaled corticosteroids to 400 µg/day (if 5–12 years) or 800 µg/day (if >12 years) of budesonide equivalent.
  - If there is no response, stop LABA. Increase the daily dose of inhaled corticosteroids to 400 µg/day (if < 12 years) or 800 µg/day (if > 12 years) of budesonide equivalent and consider an oral leukotriene receptor antagonist or oral theophylline.

Step 4: Persistent poor control

It is important to question the diagnosis of asthma in those children with persistent poor control. Children younger than 5 years should be referred to a paediatrician with a respiratory interest for further assessment. Children older than 5 years should have their inhaled corticosteroids increased to 800 µg/day of budesonide equivalent and referral should be considered.

Step 5: Oral steroids

Children older than 5 years may be considered for regular or intermittent oral prednisolone. This should be under the direct supervision of a paediatrician with a respiratory interest.

Key point

- Before stepping therapy up and down, always check inhaler technique, compliance and possible elimination of trigger factors.

Inhaler devices

- *Metered-dose inhalers (MDI).* See Figures 23.6–23.9.
- *Breath-actuated MDIs.* See Figures 23.10 and 23.11.
- *Dry powder inhalers.* See Figures 23.12 and 23.13.

The choice of drug delivery for stable asthma should be based on patient preference and an assessment of correct usage. Many patients may struggle to use an MDI without spacer correctly and it is better to suggest a dry powder device, MDI with spacer (± mask) or breath-actuated MDI inhaler. It is important to consider prescribing more than one device. An MDI with spacer is as effective as a nebulizer for treating mild to moderate exacerbations of asthma, but many children will not

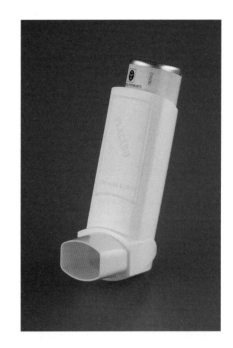

Fig. 23.6 Pressurized aerosol metered-dose inhaler (MDI)

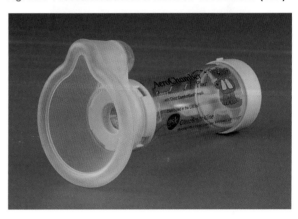

Fig. 23.7 AeroChamber spacer device

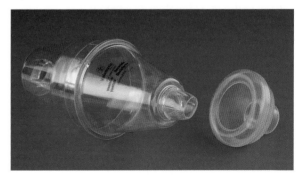

Fig. 23.8 Volumatic spacer inhaler

carry a spacer on their person and will need a smaller device for ease of access to treatment. It would be good practice to give every child a spacer and MDI for acute exacerbations as well as their preferred choice of inhaler.

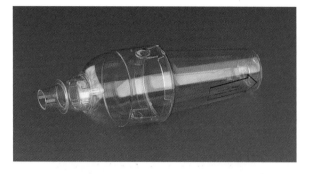

Fig. 23.9 **Nebuhaler spacer inhaler**

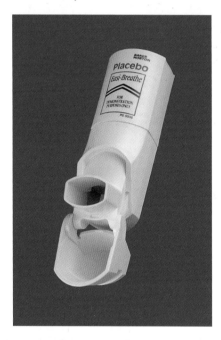

Fig. 23.10 **Easi-Breathe aerosol inhaler**

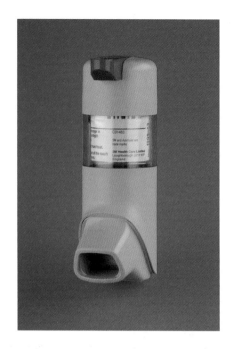

Fig. 23.11 **Autohaler aerosol inhaler**

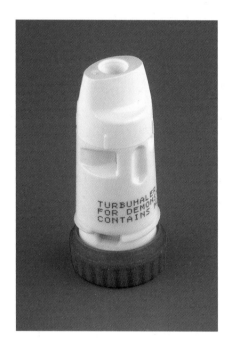

Fig. 23.12 **Turbohaler powder inhaler**

Generally, breath-actuated and dry powder devices are for children older than 5 years of age. Children under 5 years should have a spacer device. The aerochamber with mask is better for small children. Often from about 3 years children will be able to start using a large-volume spacer or blue aerochamber with mouthpiece, which improves drug delivery.

When to refer
See Box 23.12.

 http://www.brit-thoracic.org.uk/

British Thoracic Society (BTS). Follow links to guidelines on BTS/SIGN 'British Guideline on the Management of Asthma' and 'Guidelines for the Management of Community-acquired Pneumonia in Children'

http://www.ginasthma.com/

Follow links to Global Strategy for the Diagnosis and Management of Asthma in Children 5 Years and Younger

Bronchiolitis

Bronchiolitis (Box 23.13) is a common viral respiratory tract infection occurring in annual winter epidemics. It affects children under the age of 18 months, although the majority of cases occur in those who are less than 9 months of age.

RSV accounts for 75–80% of hospitalized cases, the remainder being caused by adenovirus, influenza and parainfluenza viruses, metapneumovirus, bocavirus

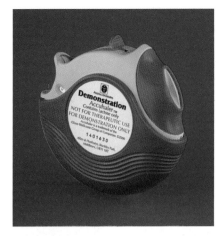

Fig. 23.13 **Accuhaler (dry powder for inhalation)**

or other respiratory viruses. It is one of the most common reasons for acute presentation to primary and secondary care during the winter period.

There is currently no vaccine against RSV infection. High-risk infants (those with congenital heart disease and ex-premature infants with chronic lung disease) are offered passive immunity with monoclonal antibodies to RSV. This is given as monthly intramuscular injections during the winter months.

Investigations

Pulse oximetry is essential in all bronchiolitic children with signs of respiratory distress. NPAs are sent for immunofluorescence to RSV and other common respiratory viruses. In most children bronchiolitis is a clinical diagnosis and routine CXR adds little benefit. Where the clinical features are atypical (high fever, unilateral signs, prolonged illness) or when the child shows signs of severe respiratory distress, a CXR and basic blood parameters (full blood

count, urea and electrolytes and blood cultures) may be useful.

Management

The majority of children with bronchiolitis will be managed safely in their own home, with reassurance and advice to parents on when to return. Indications for admission include low oxygen saturations, signs of severe respiratory distress, apnoeas, poor feeding, parental anxiety and infants who have risk factors for more severe disease.

Children admitted with bronchiolitis and poor feeding will often require either nasogastric or intravenous fluids. Humidified oxygen is delivered by nasal cannula. Handling of the infant should be kept to a minimum. Routine antibiotics are not prescribed unless there is evidence of secondary infection. Ribavirin is rarely used in most centres. Inhaled and oral steroids are of no benefit in the treatment of bronchiolitis.

Complications

Most children will recover from bronchiolitis within 1–2 weeks. A high proportion of children will develop wheeze with subsequent viral infections in the first few years following bronchiolitis.

Bronchiolitis obliterans is a rare complication of bronchiolitis infection. Most cases occur with severe viral infection, most commonly adenovirus. Chronic inflammation of the airway is associated with more permanent damage to the small airways.

Inhaled foreign body

Foreign body inhalation must always be considered in children presenting with acute respiratory difficulties or pneumonia that is failing to respond to treatment.

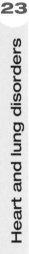

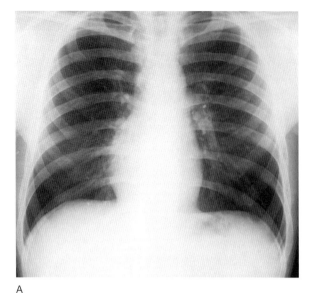

A

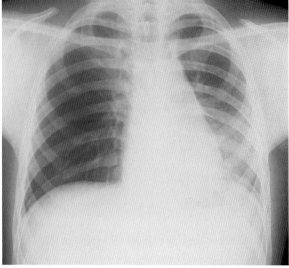

B

Fig. 23.14 Inhaled foreign body.
(A) Inspiratory X-ray film; (B) expiratory X-ray film.

Mobile toddlers who place everything into their mouth are at the greatest risk of inhaling small objects such as peanuts or beads. Thankfully the death rate from inhaled foreign body in childhood has fallen in recent years, partly related to increased public awareness.

Clinical features

The clinical features following inhaled foreign body are related to the position of lodgment. The most common place for lodgment of a foreign body in children has been shown to be the right main bronchus, accounting for 42%, whereas 17% will become lodged in the larynx or trachea.

Wheeze is a common feature if the main stem bronchus is involved, stridor can occur with high obstruction and chronic cough occurs with segmental collapse. The wheeze associated with foreign body inhalation is often fixed and sometimes unilateral, and the response to bronchodilator therapy is poor. Children with recurrent pneumonia, where there is failure of a collapsed lobe to re-expand, may have a distally lodged foreign body. Children with undiagnosed foreign body aspiration are at long-term risk of bronchiectasis in the affected lobe.

Often, but not always, there will be a history of choking associated with rapid onset of breathing difficulties, but there is often a delay between the choking episode and presentation. A careful history is essential to avoid overlooking this important diagnosis.

Diagnosis

The diagnosis of inhaled foreign body is supported by radiological changes on CXR; however, a normal CXR does not exclude the diagnosis (Fig. 23.14).

Management

If foreign body aspiration is strongly suspected, rigid bronchoscopy should be performed under general anaesthesia.

Cough

Problem-orientated topic:

a child with recurrent disturbing cough ●●●●●

Jayden is a 6-year-old boy who presents to his local surgery for the second time with a history of disturbing cough over the past 3 weeks. When he first presented to the surgery he was prescribed oral amoxicillin for a presumed lower respiratory tract infection.

The cough is not associated with any fever or productive sputum. He has not travelled recently and there has been no infectious contact. The family did not notice any choking before the onset of symptoms. Although his cough is worse at night, he has never been particularly troubled in the past and there is no associated wheeze.

Jayden has been previously fit and well. There is no history of atopy. Both parents are smokers.

Continued overleaf

Clinical examination is unremarkable. His height and weight are on the 50th centile. His peak flow is 98% predicted for his height.

Jayden and his mother are increasingly concerned about the duration of his symptoms.

Q1. What differential diagnoses should be considered in a child with recurrent cough?

Q2. What do you think is the most likely diagnosis?

Q1. What differential diagnoses should be considered in a child with recurrent cough?

See Box 23.14.

Asthma is a common cause of chronic cough in children. Although Jayden has a cough that is worse at night, the fact that he has never been troubled previously, the absence of wheeze, the lack of family history of atopy, and the normal peak flow readings would go against asthma as a likely cause of his symptoms. It would be unusual for cystic fibrosis or primary ciliary dyskinesia to present at this age in a child who is otherwise well and thriving. Likewise, there is nothing in the history to suggest recurrent infections and immune deficiency. It would be unusual for a 6-year-old to inhale a foreign body and without a significant history this would be extremely unlikely. The lack of fever, foreign travel or contact with TB would rule out TB as a likely cause in European countries with a low TB rate.

BOX 23.14 Causes of recurrent or persistent cough in children

- Prolonged infection (viral, *Mycoplasma*, pertussis, TB)
- Postnasal drip (rhinitis)
- Gastro-oesophageal reflux
- Asthma
- Inhaled foreign body
- Cystic fibrosis
- Primary ciliary dyskinesia
- Immune deficiency
- Habit
- Smoking (including passive)

Q2. What do you think is the most likely diagnosis?

In Jayden's case, the most likely cause of cough is prolonged infection with *Mycoplasma*, pertussis or viral pathogens. It would be appropriate to reassure Jayden and his parents that it is not unusual for a cough to last several weeks before disappearing. A 7–10-day course with a macrolide antibiotic (erythromycin or clarithromycin) would be appropriate if *Mycoplasma* or pertussis infection were suspected.

It is well recognized that parental smoking is a significant risk factor for recurrent episodes of cough and wheeze during childhood. It may be appropriate to highlight the risks and offer smoking cessation support.

Pertussis (whooping cough)

Whooping cough is an infection characterized by paroxysms or spasms of cough associated with vomiting and inspiratory whoop. The majority of children affected by the disease are under the age of 5 years, with those under 12 months being more severely affected. In small children the typical whoop is often absent. However, apnoeas and cyanotic episodes are more frequent. The paroxysmal stage is often preceded by an early catarrhal stage associated with rhinorrhoea, malaise, conjunctivitis and fever. The paroxysmal stage can typically last up to 10–12 weeks.

Complications
- Pneumonia
- Encephalopathy
- Bronchiectasis (late).

Before vaccination, mortality and morbidity were high, especially among infants. Although rare, complications remain a cause for concern, particularly in small infants in whom cyanotic or apnoeic episodes require hospitalization.

Diagnosis
Diagnosis of whooping cough is confirmed by culture of the bacterium *Bordetella pertussis* on per nasal swabs. Since *B. pertussis* can take several days to grow, PCR assay is increasingly used to assist in diagnosis.

Management
Children should be prescribed oral erythromycin or the newer macrolides in order to eradicate organism carriage and reduce spread amongst other family members. Unfortunately macrolides do not alter the course of the illness in those with active infection;

Table 23.3 Important causes of stridor in children

Diagnosis	Feature
Croup	Most common cause of acute stridor Peak age 1–2 years old Barking cough, hoarse voice, low-grade fever Often mild illness, although can occasionally be severe and need referral to paediatric intensive care unit (PICU)
Epiglottitis	Rare since vaccination against *Haemophilus influenzae* type B Often 1–7 years old Toxic, drooling saliva, dysphagia, soft muffled voice, no cough and quiet stridor Paediatric emergency
Bacterial tracheitis	Uncommon Usual organism *Staph. aureus* Toxic sick child with stridor, often requires intubation and IV antibiotics
Anaphylaxis	Acute stridor with swollen lips and/or urticaria following allergen exposure
Inhaled foreign body	Toddlers with history of choking Sudden onset of symptoms
Laryngomalacia	Noted in first few weeks of life, often from birth Floppy larynx that collapses inwards on inspiration Chronic stridor worse with crying, feeding, lying supine and infection (acute on chronic) Often resolves spontaneously by 1–2 years
Structural abnormalities	Uncommon, often < 4 months of age Children with multiple cavernous haemangiomas may have subglottic lesions Ex-preterm infants may have subglottic stenosis from endotracheal intubation

therefore, the mainstay of treatment remains supportive. Hospitalization should be strongly considered in children younger than 6 months with severe symptoms or underlying diseases. Close contacts should also be given macrolides to limit secondary infection. Current vaccination programmes in Europe provide up to 90% protection against pertussis infection after all three primary immunizations. Vaccination does not provide complete long-term immunity.

Stridor

Problem-orientated topic:

13 **a child with a loud barking cough**

Ben is a 1-year-old boy with a 2-day history of cough and noisy breathing. On examination he has a loud barking cough. His respiratory rate is 34 breaths per minute. He has significant tracheal tug and inspiratory stridor at rest. His temperature is 38.1°C. His parents have tried steam but there has been no improvement.

Q1. What important causes must you consider?

Q2. What therapies do you think may be effective?

Q3. When should you refer to hospital?

Q1. What important causes must you consider?

See Table 23.3.

Viral croup (laryngotracheobronchitis)

Viral croup is the most common cause of acute stridor in children. The peak age is around 1–2 years of age. Common pathogens include parainfluenza virus, RSV and rhinovirus. Inflammation and partial obstruction of the upper airways (larynx, trachea and bronchi) result in stridor and cough. Small children are particularly at risk because of the relative small size of their upper airways.

Unlike the relatively rare conditions such as epiglottitis and bacterial tracheitis, croup has a more insidious onset over a few days. Systemic toxicity and fever are considerably less. Children with croup have a typical barking or seal-like cough, often associated with a hoarse voice, stridor and low-grade fever. Symptoms last 3 days on average and, as in many respiratory conditions, symptoms are often worse at night.

The majority of children with croup will have a mild illness that can be managed at home. Children with significant respiratory distress and stridor at rest will require treatment and reassessment. Those who show significant improvement following treatment may be considered for discharge home. There should be a low threshold for admission in children under the age of 12 months, all children with marked respiratory distress or oxygen requirement at presentation, and cases where parents remain concerned or anxious about discharge.

Parents of children not requiring admission should receive clear instructions when to return (chest wall recession, tracheal tug, tachypnoea, colour change, inability to feed and decreased level of consciousness).

Spasmodic croup

Some children can develop recurrent short-lived episodes of croup, particularly at night, without the typical coryzal prodrome that is seen in classical viral croup. A history of atopy and episodic stridor is common in children with spasmodic croup. However, there are large numbers of children who have recurrent episodes of croup with features of both viral and spasmodic croup. It is more likely that these two presentations are opposite ends of a spectrum of a single illness.

Q2. What therapies do you think may be effective?

Simple measures

In all cases of stridor, it is very important to keep the child and parents calm. Direct inspection of the throat can be dangerous and may result in complete obstruction of the airway. Likewise, routine lateral neck X-rays are no longer useful and carry the risk of further upset and deterioration.

Humidification

Steam inhalation for croup is widely used but of no proven benefit. The perceived benefit (placebo effect) reported by many families probably relates to the presence of the carer in a warm calming environment. Athough there is no reason to encourage the use of steam at home, some parents will continue to use it, therefore the physician must assure that it is done safely. A steamy bathroom with the hot water tap running and the plug open is acceptable, but any use of kettles or bowls of hot water should be discouraged because of the risk of scalding.

Adrenaline (epinephrine)

Nebulized adrenaline is very effective in severe croup; the alpha-mediated vasoconstriction results in decreased mucosal oedema. The duration of action is between 20 minutes and 3 hours. Adrenaline is used in the most severe cases when intubation is considered. The waning pharmacological effects of adrenaline result in a return to the pre-treatment baseline rather than a true rebound. For a considerable number of children with severe croup, the period of improvement on adrenaline is long enough to allow the steroid treatment to start working.

Steroids

Approximately 1–5% of croup cases required endotracheal intubation before the introduction of steroid therapy. The use of corticosteroids has been shown to

improve clinical parameters, decrease admission rate, decrease the duration of hospital stay, and reduce the need for rescue nebulized adrenaline in children with croup. Nebulized budesonide or oral dexamethasone have been shown to be equally effective in treating children with mild, moderate and severe croup. Studies comparing oral dexamethasone with nebulized budesonide showed no significant difference in duration of onset.

Intubation

A small number of children will still require endotracheal intubation for severe croup. The decision to intubate should be based on worsening airway obstruction with signs of exhaustion or impending respiratory failure. Children with epiglottitis and bacterial tracheitis require specialist care, with input from senior ENT and intensivist staff. Intravenous antibiotics and intubation are often required. Steroids and adrenaline have minimal effect on these conditions.

Q3. When should you refer to hospital?

Most children with acute stridor will have viral croup. Those with mild croup (no signs of respiratory distress at rest) may be managed at home, with parental observation. Children with significant respiratory distress or those showing atypical features should be referred for acute paediatric assessment.

Ben has a typical history suggestive of viral croup. His significant inspiratory stridor at rest with marked tracheal tug would require acute paediatric assessment.

Worrying signs in children with stridor are listed in Box 23.15.

Snoring

Problem-orientated topic:

a boy who snores ○ ○ ○ ○ ○

Lars is a 6-year-old boy who has been brought to the surgery by his mother. His

Continued overleaf

mum is concerned that he is difficult to wake in the morning and tires easily during the day. General physical examination is unremarkable apart from grossly enlarged tonsils.

On further questioning, his worried mum comments that he snores very loudly.

How would you assess this problem?

How would you assess this problem?

Sleep-disordered breathing is a spectrum of disorders ranging from primary snoring to obstructive sleep apnoea. Snoring can occur in as many as 10–25% of children. However, less than 10% of these may have obstructive episodes of apnoea during sleep. The prevalence of behavioural disorders (aggression and hyperactivity) and cognitive impairment is increased in children who have significant sleep-disordered breathing.

Children with a history of significant snoring or obstructive episodes during sleep should be screened using overnight oximetry or, preferably, an outpatient overnight polysomnographic study where available. Children who have obstructive sleep apnoea will often demonstrate significant periods of desaturation associated with periods of obstructed breathing (30–45 seconds). Adenotonsillectomy can often lead to a dramatic improvement in children with primary obstructive sleep apnoea.

Allergic rhinitis

Allergic rhinitis is a common paediatric problem that is often dismissed as trivial or minor. Sufferers may complain of nasal discharge, itchy nose, sniffling, nasal congestion and excessive sneezing. Postnasal drip and cough are common, as are nosebleeds and middle ear effusions (glue ear) with associated hearing loss. It is not unusual for parents and teachers to become annoyed by the child's symptoms. Mouth breathing and snoring are also common. Sleep disturbance and school absence trouble the more severely affected cases.

Inflammation of the nasal mucosa in allergic rhinitis is usually mediated through the IgE inflammatory response to inhaled allergens. Perennial (all-year-round) symptoms are often triggered by house dust mite and animal dander, whereas seasonal rhinitis is often associated with pollens. Chronic inflammation of the nasal mucosa results in increased reactivity to non-allergenic stimuli such as heat and cold.

Allergic rhinitis is more common in children with a history of asthma, eczema or food allergy. Rhinitis is occasionally a feature of other conditions. Nasal polyps are uncommon in allergic rhinitis, so their presence would raise the suspicion of an alternative cause.

Cystic fibrosis and primary ciliary dyskinesia (Ch. 41) are probably the most important disorders to consider when polyps are detected.

Investigations

Routine investigations are not always required. IgE and radioallergosorbence testing (RAST) to common allergens may be useful to identify triggers, although not essential.

Management

Inhaled nasal steroids are safe and effective in the treatment of children with allergic rhinitis. The newer non-sedating antihistamines are useful adjuncts. Topical and systemic decongestants are of limited use in allergic rhinitis and should be avoided. All children should be given routine advice regarding avoidance of trigger factors.

Epistaxis

Epistaxis or nosebleed is common in childhood. More than 90% of bleeds occur anteriorly and arise from Little's area, where the venous plexus forms on the septum. These bleeds often provide a constant ooze of blood loss. Bleeding is often associated with local trauma from nose picking.

Investigations

Children with a history of recurrent nosebleeds and abnormal bruising/bleeding or a significant family history of bleeding disorders should be screened for coagulation disorders, along with a full blood count to exclude thrombocytopenia (leukaemia).

Bleeding associated with an offensive discharge should raise the suspicion of retained foreign body. Systemic hypertension rarely causes nosebleeds in children.

Management

It is often easy to control bleeding by applying local pressure (5–30 minutes) over the soft part of the nose. A nasal pack can be inserted if this fails. Cauterization of a bleeding point may also be performed for recurrent significant bleeding.

 http://www.clinicalevidence.com

Follow the links to the child health section: asthma, acute otitis media, bronchiolitis, croup and nosebleeds in children

Lars Palm   Gillian Robinson   Arnab Seal

Brain and movement disorders

LEARNING OUTCOMES

By the end of this chapter you should:

- Know how to assess and manage pain in children
- Know how to assess a crying baby and be aware of common causes
- Know how to assess children with headaches, recognizing common causes and danger signs
- Know how to assess children with abnormalities of head shape and size and how to distinguish normal variants from pathological conditions
- Know how to evaluate the child with episodic strange movements
- Know how to differentiate epileptic disorders from other paroxysmal disorders
- Know how to assess febrile seizures and be able to counsel parents
- Know how to assess and manage a child with a limp and recognize underlying common causes
- Know how to assess and manage a child with back pain.

MODULE FIVE

Recognition, assessment and management of pain in children

Painful conditions and procedures are common in babies and children. Recognition, assessment and management of pain are important, as unrecognized and inadequately managed pain can have negative physical and psychological consequences. In children this is particularly challenging due to their difficulties in expressing their pain to adults in ways that are recognized and clearly understood. At different ages and from child to child, children vary greatly in their

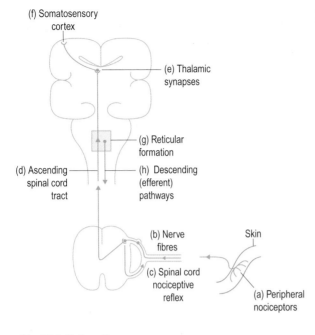

(f) Somatosensory cortex

(e) Thalamic synapses

(g) Reticular formation

(d) Ascending spinal cord tract

(h) Descending (efferent) pathways

(b) Nerve fibres

Skin

(c) Spinal cord nociceptive reflex

(a) Peripheral nociceptors

Fig. 24.1 Pain pathways

emotional and cognitive development, as well as their response to pain. It is also important to appreciate the effect of cultural factors, which may affect pain perception. This leads different children to prefer different strategies when managing their pain.

It is difficult to assess pain and distress separately. As pain perception increases with escalating distress, this also needs to be addressed. Measures include explanation to both the parents and the child, addressing their anxieties, comforting the child and providing distraction in addition to pain relief.

Basic science of pain

Pain evokes both a neurological and an emotional effect. The neurological pain pathways are shown in Figure 24.1. Pain is detected in peripheral nociceptors, or pain receptors (a), which are afferent nerve endings of myelinated A-delta and unmyelinated C nerve fibres (b). These synapse at the spinal cord, where a nociceptive reflex (c) exists that prompts withdrawal from painful stimuli before conscious perception of pain occurs. Pain impulses then ascend the spinal cord (d) to the somatosensory cortex (f) via subcortical connections in the thalamus (e).

Pain perception is modulated both in ascending pathways and in brainstem areas that affect descending (efferent) pathways (h) in the reticular formation (g) and inhibit pain stimuli, thus reducing pain perception and awareness in the injured tissue. Endogenous opioids such as endorphins and enkephalins have an important role in this effect.

Pain assessment

Pain needs to be assessed with techniques appropriate to the child's age and cognitive ability (see also p. 108). Pain can be assessed by:

- The child reporting pain
- The parent reporting pain on the child's behalf
- A change in a child's appearance, behaviour and activity level
- A change in physiological parameters: heart rate, blood pressure and respiratory rate
- Knowledge of the underlying medical condition and how it affects children.

There are a number of validated pain assessment and self-reporting tools available. Self-reporting tools can be reliably used for children over the age of 4 years. Pain assessment tools, which have a behavioural and a physiological basis, can be used from birth onwards. It is important to use a pain assessment tool that is appropriate to the child's developmental level, personality and condition. Examples include:

- Objective pain scale (OPS) for neonates and toddlers, which uses blood pressure, crying, movement, agitation and a verbal evaluation of body language indicators
- 'Faces' for 3–7-year-olds, which uses a set of cartoon-style faces in various stages of pain (Fig. 10.2, p. 108)
- Linear analogue scales for children over 3 years, which use a vertical or horizontal line with verbal, facial or numerical anchors on a continuum of pain intensity.

Holistic pain assessment should include the child's self-report using a validated pain assessment tool, and the parent or carer's report, together with the assessment of appropriately trained staff.

Pain management

Where pain is identified and its severity is assessed, measures are needed for its control. The management of pain involves identifying and addressing the cause of the pain, adequate analgesia and comfort. Children's distress may be helped by the presence of their usual carer, feeding, distraction or play therapy. The choice of analgesic and route of administration depends on the pain severity and cause. Opioids are of choice in severe pain, whilst paracetamol and ibuprofen are useful for mild to moderate pain. The route of administration and the dosage should be tailored to the needs of the individual child. There is little risk of adverse events if the correct dosage is used. Patient-controlled analgesia in children over 6 years and parent-controlled analgesia have been shown to be effective in the control of severe pain.

The use of local anaesthetic agents, either topically, e.g. local anaesthetic cream prior to venepuncture (p. 119), or by local infiltration or by regional techniques is a safe and effective method of controlling procedural pain in children. Topical anaesthetic cream (Emla, Amitop) needs to be applied under an occlusive dressing some 45–60 minutes before the painful procedure.

An accurate assessment of pain intensity, a combination of pharmacological and non-pharmacological measures to control pain and distress, and adequate counselling of the child and family are effective in pain management in babies and children.

Post-operative pain relief is discussed in Chapter 48.

🌐 http://www.rcn.org.uk/resources/guidelines.php

The recognition and assessment of acute pain in children

The crying baby

Problem-orientated topic:

a baby who will not stop crying

Mum brings Axel, a 3-month-old baby, to you, her primary care physician, as she is concerned that he has been crying and inconsolable for the last 18 hours. He has always been an unsettled baby, especially in the early evenings.

Q1. What is normal crying?

Q2. What is the most likely cause of Axel's crying?

Q3. What other causes should be considered?

Q4. What should you look for in your clinical evaluation?

Q5. Which investigations are useful?

Q6. When should referral to hospital be considered?

Q1. What is normal crying?

Babies cry to communicate their needs to their carers. Parents soon recognize different cries as signalling hunger, discomfort from a dirty nappy, a need for company and tiredness. Parents find the crying child that cannot be comforted stressful and worrying. A normal baby's crying increases from birth to a maximum at 2 months, averaging 2–2.5 hours a day, with a peak between 6 and 12 p.m. Excessive crying is most frequently a symptom of a problem with the child, but it may also reflect a problem within the environment being sensed by the baby; tense anxious parents will often have tense anxious babies.

Q2. What is the most likely cause of Axel's crying?

Three-month-old Axel's inconsolable crying, especially in the evenings, is likely to be a form of infantile colic. Colic is used to describe babies in the first months of life who have episodes of inconsolable crying, accompanied by drawing up of the knees, which occur a number of times a day, particularly in the evening. To date no cause has been identified. Useful strategies to manage this include:

• Providing a routine and avoiding over-stimulation
• Holding the baby and walking with him or her, or gently jogging the infant up and down
• White noise, such as the washing machine
• Visiting family and friends, and allowing trusted carers to help with the baby
• In the absence of a trusted carer and if the crying is intolerable, leaving the baby safely in cot or crib while the carer has some time away from the noise.

Q3. What other causes should be considered?

Abnormal or unusual crying in babies can be due to a variety of conditions. Asking parents about the nature of the cry and assessing whether the baby appears well or not help in diagnosis (Fig. 24.2).

Q4. What should you look for in your clinical evaluation?

A good history and physical examination will identify most pathological causes of excessive crying (Box 24.1).

History

Ask the carers about:

• Recent change in cry, feeding or general alertness (meningitis, sepsis, shaking injury)

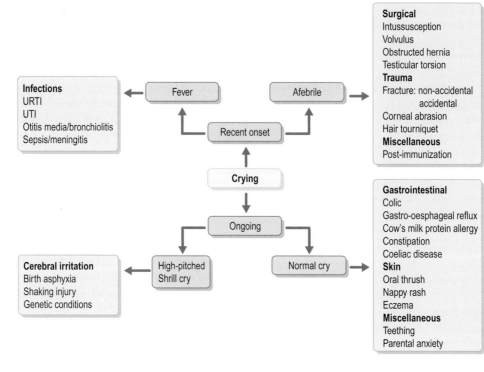

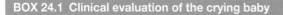

Fig. 24.2 **The crying baby: differential diagnosis.**
(URTI = upper respiratory tract infection; UTI = urinary tract infection.)

BOX 24.1 Clinical evaluation of the crying baby

Ask yourself:
- Does this baby 'handle well' or is it an unwell baby?
- Are the parents coping and is there enough support for them at home?

- Recent temperature (infections)
- Vomiting and whether bilious (bowel obstruction)
- Frequency and nature of baby's stool (constipation, gastroenteritis, intussusception)
- Timing of last immunization
- Whether the baby is moving all four limbs normally (trauma, non-accidental injury)
- Social history: how many other children there are in the family, social support available.

Examination

Assess the following:
- Temperature, perfusion, skin for rashes, including nappy area or bruising
- Coryzal symptoms: runny nose
- Respiratory system: respiratory rate, work of breathing
- Examination of ears and throat for signs of infection

- Abdominal examination: including mouth for thrush, any tenderness or masses, hernial orifices and testes
- Cardiovascular examination: including peripheral pulses
- Central nervous system examination: fontanelle, alertness, tone, ability to be comforted
- Limbs: swelling, localized tenderness, pain on limb movement
- Digits: ensure no hair or fabric tourniquet
- Eyes: fluoroscein — corneal abrasion; fundi — any retinal haemorrhages.

Q5. Which investigations are useful?

If the history and examination point to a particular cause, then specific investigation should be undertaken to confirm this, e.g. abdominal ultrasound for suspected intussusception.

Any irritable, unwell baby with fever needs to have clean-catch urine taken for urinalysis and microscopy culture and sensitivity. If this fails to demonstrate a cause, a septic screen should be considered, which could include full blood count (FBC), C-reactive protein (CRP), chest X-ray and lumbar puncture.

In the absence of any pointers in a well baby, reassurance with or without a period of observation is the correct management strategy. Always offer parents the opportunity to return if they have further concerns.

Q6. When should referral to hospital be considered?

- Baby appears systemically unwell
- Baby is febrile without a clinical focus
- Baby has bilious vomiting
- Baby cries, with episodes of pallor
- Baby has hernia or swollen testes
- Baby is of socially isolated carers
- Baby appears to have limb pain or there are concerns about child abuse (Ch. 21).

Headache

Problem-orientated topic:

a child with intermittent headache

Birgitta is a 12-year-old girl who, over the last 6 months, has been complaining of intermittent headache. She describes the headaches as being over both sides of her forehead, starting suddenly and being severe and throbbing. They make her feel sick. If she lies down in a dark room for a few hours the headache goes away. The headaches used to occur around once a month, but they are starting to become more frequent. Birgitta has been sent home early from school on a number of occasions due to her headaches. At school she is a popular girl and manages well with her school work. Apart from the headaches, she is in good health. Her mother remembers having similar headaches as a teenager. Birgitta is growing well and her examination is unremarkable.

Q1. What conditions should be considered?
Q2. What is the likely cause of Birgitta's headaches?
Q3. What are the important features to elicit in the clinical assessment?
Q4. When is referral indicated?
Q5. What investigations would you consider?
Q6. What management options should be considered?

Q1. What conditions should be considered?

Headache is a common symptom in school-age children. Severe acute headache can be a symptom of meningeal irritation or raised intracranial pressure, but it is more commonly associated with a viral 'flu-like illness. Recurrent and chronic headache can also stem from raised intracranial pressure, but is more commonly due to tension headache or migraine. Figure 24.3 is a simple clinical guide to approaching a child with headache.

Q2. What is the likely cause of Birgitta's headaches?

Intermittent severe frontal throbbing headaches associated with nausea suggest a diagnosis of migraine. This is supported by the absence of adverse social or academic factors, a positive family history, normal growth and clinical examination.

Q3. What are the important features to elicit in the clinical assessment?

A detailed history is key to identifying the cause of headaches.

History
- How often do the headaches happen? Is this changing?
- Onset of the headache: sudden or gradual?
- Is there any aura?
- Severity and duration of the headache
- Site of the headache
- Any pattern associated with the headaches
- Are there any associated features?
  - E.g. nausea, visual symptoms, weakness, seizures or altered behaviour
- Are there any precipitants?
  - E.g. foods, smells, stress or light
- Are there any factors that relieve the headache?
- Are there any other illnesses?
  - Does the child have a ventriculoperitoneal shunt in situ?
  - Any recent sinus, teeth, ear or visual problems?
- Is there any family history of note, particularly migraine?
- Psychosocial history:
  - What has been the impact of the headaches on the child at school and at home?

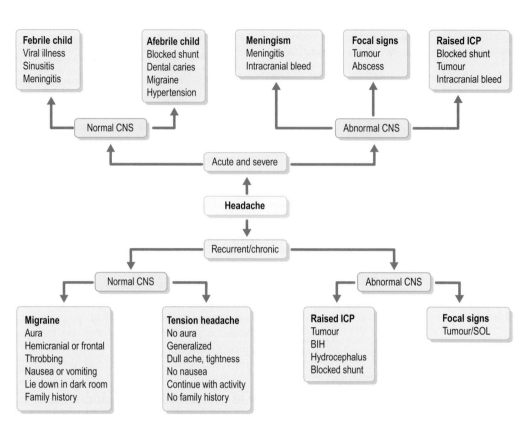

Fig. 24.3 A clinical approach to a child with headache.
(BIH = benign intracranial hypertension; ICP = intracranial pressure; SOL = space-occupying lesion.)

– Have there been any difficulties at home or school?
– How is the child managing with school work?
• Drug history.

Examination

What should you look for on examination? A thorough clinical examination focuses on:
• Growth, particularly short stature or falling off centiles
• Neurological examination, in particular fundi, coordination, gait
• Local causes, particularly ears, throat, teeth, sinus pain
• Blood pressure.

Q4. When is referral indicated?

Referral is indicated if there is:
• Acute severe headache with signs of meningeal irritation
• Acute or chronic headache in a child with an intracranial shunt
• Headache associated with altered consciousness, e.g. drowsiness
• Any of the danger signs shown in Box 24.2.

> **BOX 24.2 Danger signs associated with raised intracranial pressure**
>
> **Symptoms**
> • Morning headaches ± vomiting
> • Increasing frequency or severity
> • Recent onset or worsening seizures
> • Weakness
> • Diplopia
> • History of regression
> • Deteriorating school performance
>
> **Signs**
> • Papilloedema
> • Deteriorating coordination
> • VI nerve palsy
> • Decreased conscious level

Q5. What investigations would you consider?

There is no routine investigation indicated in the evaluation of recurrent headache. Neurological imaging should be considered in children with an abnormal

Table 24.1 Criteria of diagnosis of migraine (International Headache Society)

Type	Grade	Criteria
Migraine without aura	A	At least five attacks fulfilling B to D below
	B	Headache lasting 4–72 hours (2–48 hours in children)
	C	Headache characterized by at least two of the following:
		1. Unilateral location
		2. Pulsating quality
		3. Moderate or severe intensity (inhibits or prohibits daily activity)
		4. Aggravated by climbing stairs or similar routine physical activity
	D	Headache accompanied by at least one of the following:
		1. Nausea or vomiting, or both
		2. Photophobia and phonophobia
Migraine with aura	A	At least two attacks fulfilling B below
	B	Presence of at least three of the following:
		1. One or more fully reversible aura symptoms indicating focal cerebral cortical dysfunction or brainstem dysfunction or both
		2. At least one aura symptom develops gradually over more than 4 mins, or two or more symptoms occur in succession
		3. No aura symptom lasts more than 60 mins. When more than one aura symptom is present, accepted duration is proportionally increased
		4. Headache follows aura with a symptom-free interval of less than 60 mins (it may also begin before or simultaneously with aura)

neurological examination or other physical findings suggesting central nervous system disease.

Q6. What management options should be considered?

Acute treatment is adequate analgesia with paracetamol, ibuprofen and/or codeine. If vomiting is prominent, domperidone may be useful. For children over 12 years, sumatriptan nasal spray is effective if used at the onset of symptoms.

Preventative strategies should address avoidance of known precipitating factors. Drug therapy should be considered if there is social or academic disruption. Propranolol, clonidine or pizotifen may be tried, although results may be variable.

Common causes of chronic intermittent headache in childhood

Migraine

Migraine occurs in 10% of children aged 5–15 years. Migraines are slightly more common in boys during childhood, but in teenage years girls predominate with a ratio of 3:1. Menarche is associated with this increased prevalence and symptoms may relate to the menstrual cycle. The diagnosis of migraine is based on criteria set down by the International Headache Society, which have been modified for children (2nd edition, Table 24.1).

http://www.i-h-s.org

Follow the links to guidelines

Management

Most episodes of migraine can be managed with symptomatic treatment using paracetamol, ibuprofen and/or codeine. If vomiting is prominent, domperidone may be useful. For children over 12 years sumatriptan nasal spray is effective if used at the onset of symptoms.

Tension headaches

This is the most common type of primary headache. It was initially considered to be psychogenic in origin, but there is increasing evidence in adult studies of a neurological basis, especially in severe or chronic cases. Tension headaches are divided into episodic and chronic subtypes. The episodes of headache last minutes to days and the pain is bilateral with a pressing or tightening quality. It has a mild to moderate intensity and does not worsen with activity. There is no nausea but photophobia or phonophobia may be present. Physical and neurological examination are essentially normal, apart from pericranial tenderness in some cases. Investigations are not indicated; when performed, they are normal. Simple analgesia with paracetamol and ibuprofen, head massage and relaxation techniques are effective forms of treatment.

Local causes

Painful ears (otitis externa or otitis media), sinusitis, painful eyes (conjunctivitis, corneal abrasion, glau-

Table 24.2 Causes of abnormal head shape

Head abnormality	Definition	Causes
Microcephaly (p. 257)	Head circumference less than 2nd centile	Idiopathic Familial Infection — cytomegalovirus (CMV) Antenatal alcohol exposure After cerebral injury Associated with learning difficulties Craniosynostosis (p. 259)
Macrocephaly	Head circumference greater than 98th centile	Familial Increased fluid – Hydrocephalus (Ch. 28) – Subdural collections due to shaking injury (Ch. 36) Increased brain matter – Megencephaly, e.g. mucopolysaccharidoses, tumours Increased bone of skull – Syndromes, e.g. achondroplasia – Chronic haemolytic anaemias
Plagiocephaly	Normal head circumference, abnormal shape	Abnormal moulding Craniosynostosis (p. 259) Neuromuscular disorders Genetic disorders, e.g. Down syndrome

coma) and dental pain can all cause headache. This is best managed by addressing the primary cause and prescribing analgesia.

Raised intracranial pressure (ICP)

Raised ICP may present with one or a combination of the clinical features described in Box 24.2. Conditions presenting with raised ICP include blocked intracranial shunt, benign intracranial hypertension and space-occupying lesions; these are dealt with in detail in Chapter 28.

Hypertension

Hypertension (Ch. 39) is an important but uncommon cause of headache in children. In young children hypertension is usually secondary to acute or chronic renal disease. Primary hypertension becomes more common in obese adolescents, but is unlikely to be severe enough to cause headache or encephalopathy.

Abnormalities of head shape

Abnormalities of head shape and size are common. Many are benign or familial, but may reflect an underlying abnormality of cerebral ventricles, brain, dural collections or bone (Table 24.2).

Plagiocephaly

Asymmetric head shape or plagiocephaly is common after birth and is a consequence of moulding during delivery. Persistence of asymmetry may occur due to head positioning. Usually the asymmetry becomes less prominent as the child grows older and assumes a more upright posture. Babies born preterm may develop long heads with flattened sides (scaphocephaly). Some conditions have associated head shape abnormalities, e.g. flattened occiput (brachycephaly) in Down syndrome.

Abnormal head shape may also occur due to partial craniosynostosis. In this condition there is fusion of one or more of the skull sutures. If all sutures are involved, microcephaly results, with inadequate space for brain growth and consequent raised ICP. Clinically palpable ridges are felt over the fused suture lines and there may be signs of raised ICP such as papilloedema. Skull X-ray will identify premature fusion of one or more sutures. The child requires referral to a craniofacial team.

Microcephaly and macrocephaly

The causes are listed in Table 24.2. These children are approached by:
- Full developmental history and examination.
- Neurological examination, including fundoscopy.
- Measuring the head size using a non-expanding tape across the forehead, above the eyebrows and over the most prominent parietal and occipital areas. The largest of three measurements is taken as the true reading.
- Measuring parental head circumference and plotting the results on an appropriate chart.

- Assessing for:
  - Dysmorphic features
  - Congenital abnormalities
  - Palpable sutures.

Isolated postural, familial or idiopathic abnormalities of head shape without any neurodevelopmental features do not require specialist referral.

Hydrocephalus

Hydrocephalus is an important cause of large head and is discussed fully in Chapter 28. Hydrocephalus occurs when there is an imbalance between cerebrospinal fluid (CSF) production and absorption, leading to an increase in pressure and fluid volume within the ventricles. This may be due to obstructive hydrocephalus where CSF flow is obstructed within the ventricular systems, e.g. aqueduct stenosis, posterior fossa tumours. Alternatively, in non-obstructive hydrocephalus, it may be due to lack of free flow of CSF within the subarachnoid space, affecting CSF absorption. This is seen in premature babies following intraventricular haemorrhage. Rarely communicating hydrocephalus can occur due to increased CSF production.

Apart from a large head size, clinical signs include sunsetting eyes, a bulging anterior fontanelle, prominent scalp veins, and papilloedema progressing to optic atrophy. Where ICP is high, there may be a history of headache, vomiting, decreased conscious level or tonic seizures. Ominous signs are bradycardia, hypertension, VI nerve palsy, changing upper motor neuron signs and decerebrate or decorticate posturing. These suggest imminent coning. It is important to check for signs of raised ICP in children presenting with tonic seizures, as management of these seizures without addressing the primary cause can be fatal.

Investigation by CT or MRI scan usually establishes the diagnosis and identifies the specific cause. Management of hydrocephalus is usually with a ventriculoperitoneal shunt, together with appropriate treatment of any underlying cause.

Faints and funny turns

This condition is also discussed from the acute paediatric perspective in Chapter 28.

Problem-orientated topic:

a child who is blacking out ● ● ● ●

Karin, a 12-year-old girl, presents with a history of three episodes of loss of consciousness followed by twitching. On the first two occasions she was in school: once while standing in school assembly and the second in the toilet. The third episode was while standing in the supermarket with her mother. Her mother describes Karin as going limp and slumping to the floor. She was unresponsive and had jerking of her arms, but recovered within 5 minutes. Karin describes the episode as feeling lightheaded followed by blacking out. The next thing she remembers is finding herself on the floor. There was no associated incontinence of urine on any occasion. Karin felt tired after the episodes and slept for a short time. Karin's mother gives a history of seizures as a teenager, but says she grew out of them. She is worried that Karin may be epileptic.

Q1. What is the likely cause of Karin's paroxysmal events?

Q2. What other conditions should be considered?

Q3. What should you look for in your clinical evaluation?

Q4. When is referral indicated?

Q1. What is the likely cause of Karin's paroxysmal events?

The setting of the episodes, with the description of preceding lightheadedness and visual loss, is characteristic of syncope. Syncope occurs quite frequently in school, places of worship and hairdressers. Other triggers include minor injuries, immunization and venepuncture.

Syncope is caused by hypotension and bradycardia, resulting in cerebral anoxia. The twitching seen is of short duration, of decreasing amplitude and non-epileptic in origin.

Q2. What other conditions should be considered?

Reflex anoxic seizures

Reflex anoxic seizures are common in childhood. They are typically triggered by unpleasant events, e.g. emotional trauma, and result in vagal induced asystole of short duration with resulting cerebral anoxia. The onset is rapid and there is no preceding history of lightheadedness or visual loss. The child normally looks pale, loses consciousness and may have brief tonic or tonic–clonic seizures. These can be associated with

Table 24.3 Characteristics of epileptic seizures and psychogenic seizures

Feature	Seizure	Psychogenic seizure
Timing	Any — less frequent during activity	When many people around
Onset	Physiological spread Rhythmic movements	Non-physiological spread, non-rhythmic movement Movements in both limbs but conscious
Sound	Expiratory grunt on initiation Silent during tonic–clonic phase	Shout/groan throughout episode
Episodes	Each seizure type similar in different episodes Eyes — nystagmus Cyanosis may occur Incontinence may occur	Vary Bizarre eye movements may occur No cyanosis No incontinence
Recovery	Slow but orientated	Rapid, disorientated, amnesia

incontinence and tongue biting. Recognition that the attacks are triggered by an unpleasant event allows the correct diagnosis to be made. Management is by explanation and reassuring the family.

Beta-blockers or atropine may be helpful in recurrent and troublesome cases.

Psychogenic seizures/pseudoseizures

Psychogenic seizures are uncommon in children but increase during adolescence. The episodes occur more commonly in young people with true seizures but these episodes have different patterns, as detailed in Table 24.3. A detailed description of the episode and other behaviours, e.g. anxiety or panic attacks, or episodes of hyperventilation, is helpful in reaching a diagnosis. Emotional or sexual abuse can be a precipitant.

The features in Table 24.3 are only a guide. It is important to remember that not all of the features are present on every occasion.

Q3. What should you look for in your clinical evaluation?

Obtaining a detailed history with a careful clinical examination is time well spent. The diagnosis of paroxysmal events, whether epileptic or non-epileptic, is based on clinical assessment. Your diagnosis will be as good as your history. Video recordings of events, if available, are particularly useful and it is worth asking the families to obtain them in a child with frequent episodes.

History

Your history needs to focus on the exact sequence of events from before the episode up until complete recovery. History should be obtained both from observers and from the child, and should cover preceding events, where the event occurred, what the child was doing and whether the event was actually observed by the parents or the account is secondhand. It is common for parents to give a history of 'seizure' or 'fits' where a careful history can establish that the events are non-epileptic in origin. As mentioned earlier, even the occurrence of clonic movements does not automatically make the event epileptic. Asking the parent to mimic the episode can be helpful in diagnosis.

Symptoms suggesting an underlying condition, such as intracranial pathology, cardiac conditions, gastro-oesophageal reflux or chronic blood loss, should be obtained. A family history of similar episodes, along with an exploration of family dynamics, is important. The possibility of substance misuse, particularly in teenagers, needs to be considered.

Examination

A full physical examination, with a detailed cardiac and neurological examination including fundus examination and tests of coordination, is required. Remember to measure the head circumference.

Q4. When is referral indicated?

Non-epileptic disorders such as syncope and reflex anoxic seizures should be investigated with a 12-lead ECG for QTc measurement. An orthostatic test may be performed in older children. History of collapse during exercise or swimming, family history of sudden death, an abnormal cardiac examination or an abnormal ECG requires further cardiac evaluation. Referral is indicated for disorders thought to be epileptic in nature, and in children with neurological, cardiac or psychological difficulties.

Other non-epileptic paroxysmal disorders

Blue breath-holding spells

These occur in 4% of infants and toddlers and are precipitated by physical or emotional trauma. The child starts crying and holds the breath in a prolonged expiration, resulting in cyanosis. The resulting cerebral anoxia causes limpness and loss of consciousness for a short period of time. This may be followed by a small number of tonic–clonic jerks. The attacks last a few minutes and the child always recovers spontaneously. There is no need for any intervention, except reassuring the parents that the child will grow out of the episodes, usually by the age of 5 years.

Sleep phenomena

Night terrors

Night terrors occur in preschool children, usually in the early stages of sleep. Children are usually found sitting up in bed screaming and looking terrified. They do not recognize their parents and cannot be comforted. They have no memory of the episode.

Nightmares

Nightmares occur later in sleep. Children remain asleep but are distressed and, on wakening, have a good recall of the episode. They can be comforted by their parents.

Sleep myoclonus

Myoclonic jerking of the limbs or head is a common phenomenon and occurs most commonly in early phases of sleep in both neonates and children. It is important to check that it only occurs in sleep and it does not wake the child or cause any distress.

Daytime paroxysmal disorders

Day dreaming

Day dreaming involves episodes of vacant staring without any impairment of consciousness and is common in school-age children. It is a differential diagnosis of absence epilepsy and the key to differentiation is whether interacting with the child can interrupt the episodes.

Narcolepsy

Narcolepsy is the sudden onset of daytime sleep, often with cataplexies. It is uncommon but probably underdiagnosed.

Cataplexy

Cataplexy is the sudden onset of loss of tone, associated with laughter or excitement. It may occur with narcolepsy or alone.

Shuddering

Shuddering is common in infancy and is characterized by rapid shivering movements without loss of consciousness. This is a benign disorder, which resolves as the baby matures.

Benign paroxysmal vertigo

In benign paroxysmal vertigo the child stops suddenly and looks frightened for a few minutes, perhaps in association with nausea, vomiting and nystagmus.

Masturbation/self-gratification

This tends to be misunderstood for epilepsy. The child shows rocking, flush and staring. Masturbation can start from early infancy and is common in preschool children. It is managed by distracting the child and ignoring the behaviour. Masturbation with other sexualized behaviour raises concerns about sexual abuse.

Febrile convulsions

Problem-orientated topic:

a child with febrile convulsions

Two-year-old Erik presents with a history of episode of stiffness, followed by rhythmic jerking of all four limbs lasting 3 minutes, associated with a high fever. His parents feel that he was slightly drowsy after the seizure but is back to his normal self now, except for the fever.

Q1. What is the likely cause of Erik's symptoms?
Q2. What other conditions should be considered?
Q3. What should you look for in your clinical evaluation?
Q4. What investigations are appropriate?
Q5. When is referral indicated?
Q6. How should you counsel Erik's parents?

Q1. What is the likely cause of Erik's symptoms?

Erik has had a short generalized tonic–clonic seizure associated with fever, and has now made a full recovery apart from the underlying fever. The likely cause of his symptoms is a typical febrile convulsion.

A typical febrile convulsion is characterized by:
- Age 6 months to 5 years
- Generalized tonic–clonic seizure lasting less than 15 minutes
- Rapid and full neurological recovery
- Normal neurological examination including head circumference.

Q2. What other conditions should be considered?

- Central nervous system infections: meningitis, encephalitis or cerebral abscess
- Rigors and delirium associated with fever can mimic febrile convulsion
- True epileptic seizure: precipitated by fever, although within the typical age range this is rare.

Q3. What should you look for in your clinical evaluation?

History

A detailed history should be obtained from a witness of the event, and should cover:

- Child's health prior to onset of seizure
- Nature of onset of seizure, its progression and duration, whether any focal features were present at the start of the seizure
- How long it took for the child to recover after the seizure
- Enquiry into other symptoms that may explain the cause of the fever
- Family history of febrile convulsions
- History of developmental problems
- Immunization status.

Examination

Examination of the child at presentation should cover:

- Recording of body temperature
- Assessment of cardiorespiratory function
- Assessment of conscious level (*a*lert, responds to *v*oice, responds to *p*ain, *u*nresponsive — AVPU)
- Rashes, in particular petechial rash of meningococcal disease
- Signs of meningitis: neck stiffness, Kernig's sign
- Neurological examination, including fundoscopy and measurement of head circumference
- Ear, nose and throat examination.

A period of observation after a dose of antipyretics is helpful in assessment. With control of the fever the child often perks up and returns to his normal self, reassuring the parents and the doctor!

Q4. What investigations are appropriate?

A search for a focus of infection informs the choice of investigations to be performed. In the absence of any identified focus, urine should be collected for urinalysis, including nitrites and leucocytes as markers of infection. If any abnormality is shown, then the urine needs to be sent for microscopy and culture. If the child looks unwell or is under 18 months, then referral to hospital is indicated for septic screen, which could include full blood count, C-reactive protein, blood cultures and possibly chest X-ray and/or lumbar puncture.

An electroencephalogram (EEG) is not indicated for typical febrile convulsion. Neuroimaging is indicated for a focal seizure or if there are abnormalities on neurological examination. Neuroimaging may also be considered in children with previous developmental or neurological difficulties.

Q5. When is referral indicated?

Referral is indicated in the presence of any of the following:

- Focal seizure
- Prolonged seizure (urgent)
- Child with cardiorespiratory compromise (urgent)
- Presence of petechial rash (urgent)
- Presence of meningeal signs (urgent)
- Persistent altered consciousness (urgent)
- Abnormal neurological signs
- Child is under 18 months (urgent)
- Significant parental anxiety or inability to cope.

Parents find febrile fits terrifying, and most parents assume their child is dying during the seizure. It is often necessary to admit children with a first febrile convulsion for parental reassurance. Parents become more confident if the child has had a previous convulsion.

Q6. How should you counsel Erik's parents?

- What is a febrile convulsion?
  - Convulsion brought on by fever in a child aged 6 months to 5 years.
- What starts a febrile convulsion?
  - Any illness that causes high temperature, commonly cold viruses.
- Will it happen again?
  - Three out of 10 children who have a febrile convulsion will have a further convulsion.
- What should you do if it happens again?
  - If a child has a further seizure stay calm; you know what is happening.
  - Note the time so you know how long the seizure is lasting.
  - Only move the child if he or she is in a dangerous place.
  - Do not try to restrict the jerking movements.
  - Do not put anything into the child's mouth.
  - Call an ambulance if the seizure continues beyond 5 minutes.
  - As soon as the seizure ends, roll the child on to his or her side.

- Arrange for a doctor to see your child to look for a cause for the fever.
- Is this epilepsy?
  - No, this is not epilepsy.
- Will this lead to epilepsy?
  - Most children who have febrile convulsions do not go on to develop epilepsy.
- Do febrile convulsions cause brain damage?
  - Almost never, and only in children who have seizures lasting more than 30 minutes.

Epilepsy in primary care

(Hospital-based care of epilepsy is described in Chapter 28.)

Consider the following questions:
1. What is epilepsy?
2. Why do children develop epilepsy?
3. How is epilepsy classified?
4. What different seizure types are recognized?
5. How is epilepsy diagnosed?
6. How are paroxysmal episodes investigated?
7. What is an epileptic syndrome and why is it important?
8. How is epilepsy managed?
9. When is referral indicated?
10. What is the key information in counselling parents and children?

1. What is epilepsy?

An epileptic seizure is a transient clinical event that results from abnormal and excessive activity of a more or less extensive collection of neurons. If a person has more than one such seizure, he or she has epilepsy.

2. Why do children develop epilepsy?

Children develop epilepsy for different reasons:
- *Symptomatic epilepsy* occurs in children who have had their brain injured in some way, perhaps as the result of a severe head injury, perinatal hypoxic insult or meningitis.
- *Idiopathic epilepsy* has no demonstrable cause. This is the most common form of epilepsy.
- *Cryptogenic epilepsy* is where no cause can be found, although one is suspected: for example, in children with severe learning difficulties.

3. How is epilepsy classified?

Epilepsy is broadly classified into generalized and focal. Generalized seizures are caused by electrical disorder of both hemispheres of the brain and are associated with impaired consciousness. Focal seizures are caused by electrical discharges from one part of the brain and the person remains conscious. The electrical activity can spread to affect both sides of the brain and cause impairment of consciousness (secondary generalization).

The internationally accepted classification of epilepsy has been evolved by the International League Against Epilepsy.

 http://www.ilae-epilepsy.org

Follow the links to epilepsy classification and terminology

4. What different seizure types are recognized?

 See Table 24.4.

5. How is epilepsy diagnosed?

Your diagnosis is as good as your clinical assessment. Principles of diagnosis include:
- Determining whether the episode is epileptic or non-epileptic from the history of witness and child. Getting the witness to mimic the event can be helpful. Video recordings are also useful.
- Identifying different seizure types.
- Looking for a history of neurological, developmental and possible genetic difficulties.
- Taking a family history.

6. How are paroxysmal episodes investigated?

All acute seizures should be investigated with measurement of blood sugar. In infants other biochemical abnormalities, e.g. hypocalcaemia, should be checked.

An interictal EEG can be helpful if a specific pattern is recognized. A normal interictal EEG does not rule out epilepsy. Abnormal EEG findings are found in 5% of the normal population. EEG recording during a seizure is helpful in differentiating epileptic from non-epileptic paroxysmal disorders. It is also useful in identifying the origin of the seizure. Sleep deprivation, sleep itself, photic stimulation or hyperventilation can be used during an EEG in an attempt to induce a seizure or abnormal electrical brain activity. Where the nature of the attacks is unclear, a video EEG can be useful.

A CT scan, or preferably an MRI scan, of the brain can be useful in identifying structural lesions and is valuable in children with focal seizures or complex difficulties. Neuroimaging is not routinely indicated

Table 24.4 Seizure types and features

Seizure type	Features
Generalized	
Tonic–clonic	During the tonic phase there is loss of consciousness and the child will fall, which may be associated with an expiratory noise. The eyes roll back and the muscles undergo tonic contraction. There is sudden onset of cyanosis. During the following clonic phase there is rhythmic jerking in all limbs. Loss of sphincter control is common
Tonic	The muscles of the whole body become stiff and the child falls if standing. Recovery is usually rapid
Atonic, drop attacks	The muscles of the whole body lose their tone and the child falls to the ground
Typical absence	Abrupt onset of impaired conscious level with cessation of motor activity or speech, a blank facial expression and flickering of eyelids, which last less than 10 seconds. The child continues with previous activity after the seizure. The child never falls to the ground
Atypical absence	Abrupt or gradual onset of impaired conscious level with cessation of motor activity or speech. More complex automatism, including lip smacking and fumbling. May be associated autonomic features such as flushing or micturition. Absences are longer and can cause the child to fall down
Myoclonic jerk	Brief, often symmetrical muscle contracture. Myoclonic jerks often occur shortly after wakening
Spasm	Lightning flexion of trunk, arms extended, abducted or flexed. Often occur in runs and are followed by child crying. Spasms occur more commonly on falling asleep and wakening
Focal	
Temporal lobe	Child complains of unpleasant smells, abdominal sensations or déjà vu
Parietal lobe	Regular jerking (clonic movements) in one muscle group
Frontal lobe	Bizarre motor movements, e.g. thrashing, scratching genitals, vocalizations, dystonic movement. These may occur frequently
Occipital lobe	Crude visual distortions

in generalized seizures. Functional imaging with a positron emission tomography (PET) scan is only undertaken if epilepsy surgery is a possibility.

7. What is an epileptic syndrome and why is it important?

Children diagnosed with epilepsy syndromes have clinical and seizure characteristics that occur together. Seizures classified within a syndrome have a typical pattern and age when they start, and may produce specific EEG findings. The syndrome may follow a definite pattern of progression. Syndromes are important to recognize as they help the doctor to choose the most appropriate treatment and to be able to counsel the family accurately about the course of the condition, e.g. typical juvenile absence epilepsy, infantile spasms.

8. How is epilepsy managed?

Acute episode
- Note the time so you know how long the seizure is lasting.
- Only move the child if he or she is in a dangerous place.
- Do not try to restrict the jerking movements.
- Do not put anything into the child's mouth.
- Give oxygen if available.
- Check temperature and perform a blood sugar stick test.
- Give rectal diazepam if the seizure continues beyond 5 minutes and call an ambulance.

Table 24.5 Medications used for different seizure types

Seizure type	First-line agent	Second-line drug
Idiopathic generalized epilepsy	Lamotrigine	Sodium valproate or levetiracetam
Focal epilepsy	Oxcarbazepine	Sodium valproate or levetiracetam
Absence epilepsy	Lamotrigine	Sodium valproate or levetiracetam
Infantile spasm	Vigabatrin	ACTH/tetracosactide

- As soon as the seizure ends, place the child in the recovery position.

Ongoing management
Long-term management of primary epilepsy is with anti-epileptic medication. Table 24.5 lists medication used for different types of seizure. Although this area is controversial, the table is presented as a therapeutic orientation guide for the paediatrician but medication should be discussed with a paediatric neurologist. The use of medication is based around the risk of recurrent seizures, the seizure type and recognized seizure patterns or syndromes, together with the wishes of the child and family. Monotherapy is aimed for in all cases and the duration of treatment varies with response and recognized seizure patterns. The majority of anti-epileptic agents are started at a low dose, which is titrated up over the course of 2 months. The minimum dose that controls the seizures is used. Withdrawal of treatment is considered for most children who have been seizure-free for 2 years, except for lifelong epilepsy syndromes.

9. When is referral indicated?

All children with suspected epilepsy based on a detailed history should be referred to a paediatrician with an interest in epilepsy. For children with long-term epilepsy, care is usually shared between a general paediatrician and a paediatric neurologist (Ch. 28).

10. What is the key information in counselling parents and children?

- What epilepsy is
- Information regarding any underlying cause
- Benefits and side-effects of treatments
- Avoidance of precipitants where appropriate: sleep deprivation, drugs, alcohol, bright flashing lights
- How to manage a seizure episode
- Precautions; supervised bathing and swimming (in older children showering is safe), avoidance of climbing heights and cycling on busy roads
- Need for school to be informed and appropriate staff training in seizure management
- Allowing the child to live an otherwise normal life.

Absence epilepsy

> **Problem-orientated topic:**
>
> **a child with episodes of blankness**
>
> Eight-year-old Maia presents with a 3-month history of episodes when she becomes blank for a period of a few seconds. During these episodes she stands still, stares and flutters her eyelids.
>
> Q1. What is the likely diagnosis?
> Q2. What other conditions should be considered?
> Q3. How will you clinically evaluate this child?
> Q4. What investigations are indicated?
> Q5. When is referral indicated?
> Q6. What is the key information in counselling parents?

Q1. What is the likely diagnosis?

Staring episodes lasting for a few seconds with altered consciousness but no loss of postural tone constitute absence epilepsy. There may be associated fluttering of the eyelids, mouthing or minor twitching of the fingers. Episodes lasting more than 30 seconds are unlikely to be absence episodes.

Q2. What other conditions should be considered?

Day dreaming is common and is not associated with altered consciousness. Children can be made to 'snap out of it' if their attention is gained.

Complex partial seizures normally last longer and the child is drowsy afterwards. These seizures can have a premonition or aura and may involve automatisms (simple repetitive motor movements).

Atypical absence episodes are uncommon and mostly occur along with other seizure types. The onset and offset may be gradual, the duration is usually longer and changes in body tone are more pronounced, leading to a fall.

Q3. How will you clinically evaluate this child?

History

- A detailed description of the episodes from a witness and the child is key to the diagnosis. Asking the witness to act out the episode may be useful.
- Are there other types of seizure, especially myoclonic?
- Any history of neurological disorders?
- Any history of developmental difficulties? Has there been any recent loss of skills (regression)?

Examination

- Dysmorphic features
- Signs of neurocutaneous syndromes: unusual birth marks or rashes
- Abnormalities on neurological examination
- A timed 2-minute period of hyperventilation to evoke an absence seizure (ask the child to blow a piece of paper).

Q4. What investigations are indicated?

An EEG would be helpful in defining the epilepsy syndrome that is causing the absence seizures in Maia. The EEG classically shows 3 per second spike and wave discharges during a seizure in children with typical absence epilepsy of childhood.

Q5. When is referral indicated?

If a diagnosis of absence seizures is made, with or without other seizure types, a referral to a consultant paediatrician is indicated.

Q6. What is the key information in counselling parents?

- Absence epilepsy is a form of epilepsy, which does not cause children harm beyond losing part of their day.
- There is no underlying cause — not a tumour.
- Absence epilepsy usually responds well to treatment.
- The child will usually grow out of the absence seizures. Out of 10 children, two will go on to have generalized tonic–clonic seizures in adult life.

Limp

> **Problem-orientated topic:**
>
> ### a child who is limping ● ● ● ● ●
>
> Johan is a 5-year-old boy who is brought to see you by his Mum, as he has been miserable for 2 days and walking with a limp.
>
> Q1. What conditions should be considered?
>
> Q2. Which questions will be most helpful in determining the underlying cause?
>
> Q3. What signs are helpful in determining the underlying cause?
>
> Q4. What is the most likely cause of Johan's limp?
>
> Q5. Which investigations would be useful and why?
>
> Q6. What are the other common causes of an acute painful limp?
>
> Q7. What are the common causes of chronic gait abnormalities?

Q1. What conditions should be considered? (Fig. 24.4)

54–57

A limp can be painful or painless. With a painful limp the child spends a smaller proportion of time weight-bearing on the painful limb. In painless limp children will spend an equal time on both limbs, but may shift their centre of gravity over the affected limb to help with their balance.

Q2. Which questions will be most helpful in determining the underlying cause?

Ask yourself if there is any evidence of:
- Local trauma or painful condition
- Infection

- Joint disease
- Systemic illness
- Weakness and/or altered muscle tone
- Leg length discrepancy.

History
- Is there any history of trauma?
- Is it painful or painless to walk?
- Are the difficulties acute, intermittent or chronic?
- Is there a history of fever?
- Does the child have any other condition or receive any medication?

Q3. What signs are helpful in determining the underlying cause?

See Table 24.6.

Q4. What is the most likely cause of Johan's limp?

Your history and examination reveal that Johan has complained of sudden onset of pain in his right hip on walking for the last 2 days. The pain and walking improve with paracetamol. He has never had this problem before. He had a cold 5 days ago but has otherwise been well. On examination he is afebrile and has no signs of a systemic disorder. There is no local deformity or swelling and he has decreased abduction and internal rotation. Neurological examination is normal. With encouragement he walks with an antalgic (painful) gait. These features would suggest a transient synovitis, which is managed by rest and analgesia. Recovery would be expected within a week.

Q5. Which investigations are useful and why?

See Table 24.7.

Q6. What are the other common causes of an acute painful limp?

These include minor trauma, ill-fitting shoes or ingrowing toenail.

Septic arthritis
Septic arthritis must be considered in all children who have a history of fever, look unwell and have a painful joint. Local signs are only seen in superficial joints. Leucocytosis, raised CRP and joint ultrasound with aspiration will confirm the diagnosis. Management is with analgesia and antibiotics, initially intravenously and later as a 3–4-week oral course.

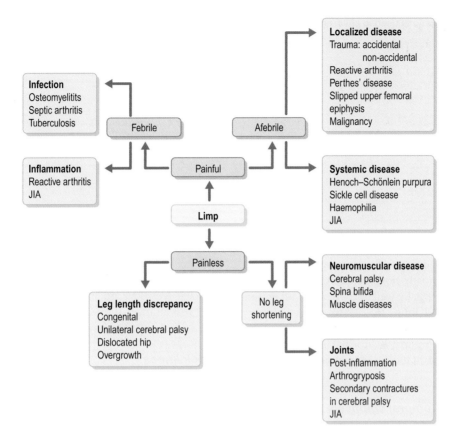

Fig. 24.4 The child with a limp.
(JIA = juvenile idiopathic arthritis.)

Table 24.6 Signs and diagnosis in children who limp

Approach		What to look for	Diagnostic relevance
General		Temperature	Evidence of infection
		Does the child look unwell?	
		Pallor, lymphadenopathy, splenomegaly	Disseminated malignancy: leukaemia, neuroblastoma
Look			
	Gait	Antalgic	Painful hip
		Hemiplegic	Cerebral palsy — hemiplegia
		Scissor gait	Cerebral palsy — diplegia
	Skin	Petechial/urticarial rash	Henoch–Schönlein purpura
		Signs of trauma	
		Blisters on feet	Poorly fitting shoes
		Widespread bruising	Non-accidental injury, coagulopathy
		Local painful conditions	Ingrowing toenail
	Leg length	See page 305	See page 305
Feel			
	Joint	Temperature, tenderness, effusion	Infected or inflamed joint
		Deformity	Chronic inflammatory changes
			Malignant bone disease
Move		Range of movement	Evidence of pain, contractures
	Neurological examination	Weakness with increased tone	Upper motor neuron disorder, e.g. cerebral palsy
		Weakness with decreased tone	Lower motor neuron or muscle disorder, e.g. spina bifida, muscular dystrophy

Table 24.7 Investigations used in children who limp

Investigation	Significance
X-ray of painful bone or joint	Identify bone and joint causes May be normal initially
FBC and film	Leucocytosis may indicate infection Sickle cell disease, leukaemia
ESR, CRP, plasma viscosity	Elevated in both local and systemic infective and inflammatory conditions
Clotting studies	Haemophilia Exclude other causes of purpura in Henoch–Schönlein purpura
Ultrasound of joint	Demonstrate effusion
Joint aspiration and culture	Septic arthritis
Technetium bone scan	Hot spots with infection, inflammation and malignancy

Perthes disease

Perthes disease is an avascular necrosis of the femoral head. It affects mostly boys between 3 and 10 years. The children are usually well and present with gradual onset of pain and limp. In 20% of cases Perthes is bilateral. Plain X-ray shows increase density within the femoral head but may be normal initially. Management is bed rest, pain relief and traction. Most children recover well.

Slipped upper femoral epiphysis

This is displacement of the femoral head. It occurs most commonly in overweight boys at the start of their pubertal growth spurt. They present with a limp and hip or knee pain, which may have been precipitated by minor trauma. In 20% the process is bilateral. On examination the leg may be 1–2 cm shorter and externally rotated. Internal rotation and abduction may be limited. The diagnosis is confirmed by X-ray of the affected joint. Management is surgical, usually with pin placement in situ and weight reduction.

Q7. What are the common causes of chronic gait abnormalities?

Intoeing

In-toe gait can be due to:

- *Metatarsus varus*: in-turning of the forefoot in babies. Provided this can be passively corrected with ease, no further action is required.
- *Medial tibial torsion*: the tibia is rotated inwards compared to the femur. This is seen in toddlers, often with bow legs, and corrects spontaneously.
- *Femoral anteversion*: the femoral neck is twisted forwards more than normal. This presents in children who 'W sit'. It usually corrects spontaneously by 8 years.

Flat feet

All toddlers have flat feet, and most children develop a medial longitudinal arch. This can be demonstrated by standing the child on tiptoe. Very flat feet may result from lax ligaments and rarely from a connective tissue disorder, e.g. Ehlers–Danlos syndrome. Most children with flat feet have no problems and management is with reassurance. If the child complains of painful feet, an arch support may help.

Knock knees

Knock-kneed preschool children are common and a normal variant. They usually correct spontaneously by 10 years, and persistence beyond this age warrants referral. In children with pigmented skin look for other signs of rickets: enlargement of costochondral junctions and wrists. This can be confirmed by plain X-ray showing 'splaying and fraying' of the metaphyses and by bone biochemistry with decreased serum calcium, increased alkaline phosphatase and low vitamin D levels.

Toe walking

Toe walking is very common in 1–3-year-olds. It may persist beyond this age, usually from habit. Spastic hemiplegia or diplegia and Duchenne muscular dystrophy can present with toe walking. It is important when examining these children to look at their tone and power as well as the range of ankle movement. A normal creatine kinase excludes Duchenne muscular dystrophy.

Cerebral palsy

54
55
○

Cerebral palsy (see also Ch. 29) is a cause of impaired motor function in children and can present with chronic abnormalities of gait as well as delayed gross motor development. Cerebral palsy is a persistent but not necessarily unchanging disorder of posture and/or movement due to a non-progressive defect or lesion in the brain in early life. Even though the condition affecting the brain is non-progressive, the clinical presentation can evolve and change. Children with cerebral palsy may have isolated motor difficulties or may have a number of comorbidities such as learning difficulties and epilepsy. The description of cerebral palsy can be based on distribution (unilateral, bilateral, either lower limb or whole body) or muscle tone (hypertonic, ataxic, dyskinetic).

Cerebral palsy is a clinical diagnosis with a number of different underlying causes. These may be:

- *Antenatal*, such as congenital malformations, antenatal stroke or congenital infection
- *Perinatal*, such as birth asphyxia, although this is a relatively unusual cause of cerebral palsy
- *Postnatal*, such as intraventricular haemorrhage in premature neonates or meningitis in the first year of life.

Cerebral palsy is discussed in detail in Chapter 29.

There will be a history of gross motor difficulties and on examination the child usually has altered tone and brisk reflexes. There may be tendon shortening, contractures, hip dislocation or leg length shortening, contributing to gait difficulties.

Talipes

- *Positional*. This is common and due to compression in utero. The foot is of normal size with a mild deformity, which can easily be corrected with passive manipulation. It resolves spontaneously over time and can be aided by corrective manipulation by parents.
- *Equinovarus*. This congenital malformation causes the foot to be inverted, supinated and adducted. The position of the foot is fixed and cannot be corrected by passive manipulation; the condition is frequently bilateral. It may occur spontaneously but is associated with neurological and muscle disorders. The treatment is commenced at birth with stretches, strapping and plaster casts. Surgery is necessary for significant abnormalities.
- *Calcaneovalgus*. This causes the foot to be dorsiflexed and everted. If the foot position can be passively corrected, then it usually corrects spontaneously with time.

Inequality of limb length

Causes may be:

- *Post-traumatic*: due to growth plate disturbance
- *Congenital*: developmental dysplasia of hip
- *Neurological*: unilateral cerebral palsy, poliomyelitis
- *Overgrowth*: arteriovenous malformation, syndromic.

History. Ask about a history of trauma or neurological disease.

Examination. Asymmetry can be judged by comparing the position of the patella when both hips and knees are flexed to 45 degrees. It is possible to identify

---

BOX 24.3 Causes of limb pain

Bone
- Trauma:
  - Accidental
  - Non-accidental
- Infection:
  - Osteomyelitis
- Tumours:
  - Local, e.g. osteosarcoma
  - Disseminated, e.g. leukaemia
- Metabolic:
  - Rickets
- Growing pains

Joints
- Hypermobile joints
- Infection
- Systemic disorders:
  - Vasculitis
  - Inflammatory bowel disease
  - Juvenile idiopathic arthritis
  - Systemic lupus erythematosus

Neuromuscular
- Referred pain
- Reflex sympathetic dystrophy: over-protection following minor injury

---

whether the femur or tibial component is short. It is also possible to measure leg length using the anterior superior iliac spine to medial malleolus as markers. Thigh length is measured from anterior superior iliac spine to tibial plateau. Look for skin abnormalities, e.g. haemangiomas. Assess for tone, moving the spine and lower limb joints through their full range of movement. Complete a neurological examination.

Management. Address the underlying cause and provide an orthosis where indicated, e.g. heel raise to shoe.

Limb pain

Limb pain in childhood is most commonly attributed to growing pains, where the aetiology of the pain is little understood. In the first instance it is important to exclude organic pathology, as listed in Box 24.3. The approach is the same as that for a child with a limp. A history compatible with growing pains, together with an examination failing to reveal any abnormality, is an adequate assessment in the first instance. Referral for investigation is indicated if there are any abnormal signs or the pain is always at one site or is severe or persistent.

Growing pains

These are episodes of pain in the lower limbs, which classically wake the pre-adolescent child at night. The

Spinal causes — central pain

- Discitis
- Tumour (benign tumours more common):
  - Bone, e.g. osteoid osteoma
  - Spinal cord, e.g. neurofibroma
  - Disseminated, e.g. leukaemia
- Diastematomyelia
- Epidural abscess
- Scheuermann disease
- Spondylolysis, spondylolisthesis

Muscular — localized to side pain ± scoliosis

- Poor posture:
  - Heavy school bags
- Trauma:
  - Muscle spasm
- Myalgia:
  - Secondary to viral or bacterial infection
- Urinary tract infection
- Stress-related

- Neurological symptoms or signs, including bladder or bowel dysfunction
- Persistent or increasing pain
- Systemic symptoms, particularly fever or weight loss

child is otherwise well and there are no abnormal findings on examination. The pain settles with massage, comforting or simple analgesia. Psychological factors have an association with limb pain and therefore it is important to enquire about possible predisposing, precipitating or perpetuating social factors.

Back problems

Back pain

Back pain is unusual in childhood and a cause needs to be sought (Box 24.4).

A careful history will help identify clues to the underlying cause. This includes the onset, duration of symptoms, the nature and site of the pain and any radiation (nerve root pain) or neurological symptoms such as weakness, or alteration of bladder or bowel function. Enquiry should be made into antecedent factors, general health and family history. Physical examination should cover spinal alignment, mobility, muscle spasm and areas of tenderness, together with a full neurological examination (Box 24.5).

Scoliosis

Scoliosis is lateral curvature of the spine, with resulting prominence of the posterior ribs. This is more obvious when children are asked to touch their toes. The most common cause is idiopathic scoliosis, but it is important to exclude other causes by clinical assessment (Table 24.8).

Clinical assessment includes a history of the age of onset and any associated pain or neurological symptoms, including difficulties with continence. This is followed by an enquiry into past history or family history of neuromuscular disorders or congenital malformations. Physical examination should start by excluding leg shortening as a cause of scoliosis; examine the child's spine sitting down and scoliosis due to leg shortening will resolve. Examination of the spine should record the site of the scoliosis, as well as any café au lait patches (neurofibromatosis), sacral dimpling or midline hairy patches associated with a spina bifida occulta. The forward bend test will reveal raised ribs on the convex side of the scoliosis. If no abnormalities are detected on this test, this suggests a positional scoliosis, which requires follow-up but no additional management apart from postural advice. Conclude with a neurological examination to exclude neuromuscular causes.

If an apparent scoliosis is identified due to leg length shortening, then this requires further evaluation along with a suitable orthosis such as a shoe raise. The remainder require X-ray to assess the scoliosis and exclude any underlying bony abnormality. The degree of scoliosis is assessed by Cobb's angle. This is formed by two perpendicular lines to the end plates of the superior and inferior ends of the vertebrae of the major curve on PA radiography.

If the Cobb's angle is:

- *Less than 20 degrees*, then observe 6–12-monthly, particularly during the adolescent growth spurt. Many mild idiopathic scolioses do not progress or resolve.
- *20–40 degrees or progressing rapidly*, consider bracing or a plaster jacket.
- *Greater than 40 degrees*, consider surgery to avoid respiratory compromise.

Torticollis

Torticollis is the term used for a twisted neck. It is a clinical sign that has a number of different causes (Box 24.6).

A clear history can help to elucidate the cause. For example, onset from birth would suggest a congenital abnormality or sternomastoid tumour. In later childhood the mode of onset, the presence of any

Table 24.8 Causes of scoliosis

Classification/subgroup	Features
Idiopathic	
Early onset	< 5 years, usually resolve
Later onset	Adolescent, mostly girls. Most common cause
Neuromuscular	
Neurological	E.g. cerebral palsy, neurofibromatosis
Muscular	E.g. Duchenne muscular dystrophy
Bony	
Congenital/infectious/malignant	Single vertebral anomaly or part of syndrome, e.g. VATER (*vertebral, anal, tracheo-oesophageal, renal*)
Ligamentous	E.g. Marfan syndrome
Apparent	Compensatory, e.g. due to leg length discrepancy

BOX 24.6 Causes of torticollis

Acute

- Inflammation:
  - Cervical lymphadenitis
  - Abscess: retropharyngeal, neck
  - Polyarticular juvenile arthritis
- Trauma:
  - Injury C1–C2 (associated with Down syndrome)
- Atlanto-axial subluxation/dislocation
- Oculogyric crises, e.g. phenothiazines
- Posterior fossa tumour

Chronic

- Congenital:
  - Sternomastoid tumour
  - Bony abnormality
- Compensatory due to ocular cause:
  - VI nerve palsy/squint
- Neurological:
  - Posterior fossa tumour
- Bony/ligamentous:
  - Vertebral anomalies, e.g. Klippel–Feil

neurological symptoms, general health and any history of recent trauma, together with the past medical history and any medication, help to identify the underlying cause. Physical examination includes an assessment of the child's systemic wellbeing, the presence of a sternomastoid swelling, and lymph glands, as well as any ear, nose and throat, eye or other neurological signs.

The most common cause of torticollis in a baby is a sternocleidomastoid tumour (congenital muscular torticollis) due to birth trauma to the sternocleidomastoid. It presents with restriction of head movement in the first months of life, with a palpable swelling within the sternocleidomastoid. Management involves passive stretches taught by physiotherapists.

Further reading

Royal College of Paediatrics and Child Health 1997 Prevention and control of pain in children: a manual for health care professionals. RCPCH, London

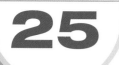
David Branski   Nigel Kennedy

Abdominal disorders

LEARNING OUTCOMES

By the end of this chapter you should:

● Know how to diagnose the common and important conditions responsible for symptoms and signs in young children with abdominal disorders
● Know the causes of these conditions and details of the important conditions
● Know the appropriate management at primary care level
● Know when to refer for further specialist investigation
● Know how to take a full clinical history and examine the child to formulate a management plan.

Introduction

Symptoms related to the child's abdominal disorders present commonly to physicians in paediatric primary care. Many of these disorders are self-limiting and require no treatment, but less frequently, serious disease may be present and urgent referral to hospital is required. This chapter discusses an approach to these common conditions.

Constipation

Problem-orientated topic:

a constipated child

Patrick is a 3-year-old who is brought to see you, his paediatrician, because his mother is

Continued overleaf

MODULE FIVE

concerned that he is constipated. She tells you that for the last 3 months he only has his bowels open every 4–5 days, and when he does, his stools are hard, small and pellet-like, and he often complains that passing the stool is painful. She has occasionally noticed red, streaky blood on the outside of the motion associated with some mucus. She is aware that he is constipated but wants help and advice to correct the problem.

Q1. What is constipation?

Q2. What are the common causes of this condition?

Q3. What would you look for in your clinical evaluation?

Q4. What investigations would be required?

Q5. How would you manage the situation at a primary care level?

Q6. When would you refer for specialist advice?

BOX 25.1 Causes of constipation

Infants
- Common:
  - Inadequate fluid or food intake
- Rare:
  - Food protein hypersensitivity
  - Hirschsprung disease
  - Hypothyroidism

Toddlers and children
- Common:
  - Secondary to minor illness
  - Anal fissure
  - Functional/psychological
  - No obvious cause
- Rare:
  - Anal stenosis
  - Hirschsprung disease
  - Hypothyroidism
  - Hypercalcaemia
  - Coeliac disease
  - Neurological problems/hypotonia

Q1. What is constipation?

Constipation is defined as pain, difficulty or delay in defaecation with stools that are hard and small. Parents have very different ideas about what constitutes constipation and some normal children may only have their bowels open 2–3 times a week. It is important to recognize that breastfed babies may only have a bowel motion every 7–10 days and this can be quite normal for them.

Q2. What are the common causes of this condition?

See Box 25.1.

Q3. What would you look for in your clinical evaluation?

History
In order to evaluate the problem, it is important to seek answers to certain questions. These include:
- Did the problem begin at birth, and if not, at what age? (Was there a delay in the passage of meconium at birth?)
- What does the parent/carer mean by constipation?
- Does the infant or child pass hard stools causing bleeding?
- What does the child eat?
- Is the child thriving?

Examination
The examination will need to focus on recording the child's growth, with height and weight plotted on a centile chart. Signs of anaemia should also be sought, with palpation of the abdomen for abdominal masses, and a gentle but careful rectal examination can be helpful to confirm a loaded rectum.

Patrick has a history of infrequent bowel motions occurring every 4–5 days, which are hard and associated with some blood. It is likely that he has developed an anal fissure as a consequence of the hard stools, and the pain associated with defaecation is likely to encourage him to suppress the urge to defaecate, in order to avoid a painful experience. This will compound the overall problem, causing him to become more constipated and exacerbating the original problem.

Other causes, such as Hirschprung disease or hypothyroidism, are unlikely in this case but must be considered if the problem is ongoing.

Q4. What investigations would be required?

As a rule, investigations are not required in the majority of children presenting with constipation. Rare causes, such as hypothyroidism and hypercalcaemia, will require thyroid function and serum calcium levels to be measured. When constipation presents in early infancy Hirschsprung disease should be ruled out.

Q5. How would you manage the situation at a primary care level?

- Give dietary advice to ensure that the child has an appropriate diet of cereals, fruit and vegetables, leading to a normal stool.
- Advise the use of stool softeners such as lactulose or unabsorsable polyethylene glycol.

There should be regular follow-up of the child by the physician to ensure the restoration of a normal bowel habit and normal motions once the problem has been addressed. A sympathetic and reassuring approach to the problem is essential in gaining and maintaining the confidence of the child and parents.

Early explanation of the problem to Patrick's parents, fluid and dietary advice, with increased cereal and fibre, may help to solve the problem. At times lactulose or polyethylene glycol may be prescribed. Left untreated, this may develop into a chronic situation such as encopresis requiring more intensive management such as enemas to empty the rectum and, in more severe cases, hospital admission.

Q6. When would you refer for specialist advice?

Specialist referral will be necessary for those children who do not respond to simple dietary measures or the introduction of faecal softeners and laxatives. For those children with gross constipation and impacted faeces, enemas to clear the rectum may be required; rarely, manual evacuation under anaesthetic may also be needed. For those children in whom an alternative diagnosis for the constipation, such as Hirschsprung, may be considered, referral to the specialist will be required for further investigation.

Causes of constipation in children

Common causes

Inadequate fluid

Young children may become fluid-depleted during a febrile illness, particularly if this is associated with vomiting. The constipation may resolve by the simple increase of fluids, but may also lead to later chronic constipation.

Anal fissure

A small tear in the anal mucosa can lead to painful defaecation associated with fresh rectal bleeding and may cause the child to suppress the desire to defaecate to avoid the painful experience. This itself may then lead on to the development of chronic constipation. Anal fissures heal spontaneously but symptomatic treatment to include faecal softeners and local anaesthetic jelly are useful.

Functional constipation

This is by far the most common cause of constipation seen by physicians. There may be an obvious precipitating cause in the history, such as an anal fissure or a febrile illness. The stools become hard, pellet-like and difficult to pass, and because of the pain the child is reluctant to attempt to pass them. Fresh blood may be present on the surface of the stools. The rectum becomes distended and loaded with faeces. It is particularly common in children with disability/immobility.

Less common causes

Food protein allergy, mainly cow's milk based protein, can present with constipation.

Coeliac disease may present with constipation.

Rare causes

Hirschsprung disease (Ch. 48)

Whilst this is a rare condition, with an incidence of 1 in 5000 live births, it must always be borne in mind in a child presenting with constipation. It is caused by an aganglionic segment of bowel and, while severe cases present in the neonatal period with delay in the passage of meconium or delay in the changing stool, less severe cases occur in infancy and rarely beyond. Abdominal distension with infrequent passage of stools in the first month of life as well as faecal explosion following rectal examination require a full investigation and referral to the specialist. It must also be borne in mind that older children may still have the condition in a milder form with short-segment Hirschsprung, and if the constipation does not respond to normal measures, Hirschsprung must still be considered and referral to a paediatric gastroenterologist made.

Anal stenosis

One other condition to consider is anal stenosis, which can be diagnosed by a rectal examination. The problem usually responds to anal dilatation.

Endocrine causes

These include hypothyroidism and hypercalcaemia (Ch. 35).

Neurological causes/hypotonia

These include cerebral palsy and spina bifida (Chs 28 and 29).

Soiling and encopresis

Soiling

This term is usually used to describe the situation when there is leakage of liquid stool around impacted faeces in a child with chronic constipation, leading to staining of the pants. Treatment is to correct the underlying problem of chronic constipation and faecal impaction.

It can also be used to describe the situation when a child has not developed bowel continence by an appropriate age (usually 4 years). Management of this situation requires a regular toilet training plan along with a sympathetic and supportive approach from the physician.

Encopresis

This describes a situation where a child who is not constipated passes stools in an inappropriate place. It indicates the presence of behavioural problems, sometimes severe. Referral to a child psychiatrist is usually necessary to explore the reasons behind the behaviour and to introduce behavioural management, along with providing a supportive attitude to overcome the problem. In most of the cases the therapeutic approach should be as outlined above for the treatment of soiling, as well as behavioural management.

Recurrent abdominal pain

Problem-orientated topic:

a child with recurrent abdominal pain ●●●●●

Cacey is an 11-year-old girl who presents to her physician with a 6-month history of recurrent abdominal pain. The pain originally began following an episode of chickenpox and has continued since then. She has only attended school intermittently since because of the pain, and her parents are becoming concerned about her. She describes the pain as being situated in the centre of her abdomen, around the umbilicus. There is no history of diarrhoea or vomiting but there is a family history of migraine.

Q1. What are the causes of recurrent abdominal pain?

Q2. What would you look for in your clinical evaluation?

Q3. When should you consider referral to the specialist (red flags)?

Q1. What are the causes of recurrent abdominal pain?

This is a common condition affecting 10–15% of schoolchildren, but only 1 in 10 has an organic problem. In

Table 25.1 Non-organic versus organic causes of abdominal pain

Non-organic pain (functional)	Organic pain
Periodicity	No periodicity
No constitutional upset	Associated with constitutional upset, e.g. weight loss, anorexia, fever
Periumbilical pain	Pain distant from umbilicus
Normal growth	Growth failure
Relationship to possible stress/domestic/school factors	Organ-specific symptoms, e.g. diarrhoea, polyuria, gastrointestinal bleeding

---

BOX 25.2 Causes of recurrent abdominal pain

- Idiopathic ⎫
- Psychogenic ⎭ (90%)
- Gastrointestinal:
  – Irritable bowel syndrome
  – Constipation
  – Oesophagitis
  – Peptic disease.
  – *Helicobacter pylori*
  – Inflammatory bowel disease
  – Coeliac disease
  – Other malabsorption syndromes
- Renal:
  – Urinary tract infection (UTI)
  – Renal calculus
- Hepatic:
  – Hepatitis
- Pancreatic:
  – Pancreatitis
- Gynaecological:
  – Dysmenorrhoea
  – Pelvic inflammatory disease
  – Ovarian cysts
  – Haematocolpos
- Others:
  – Lymphoma
  – Lead poisoning
  – Sickle cell disease
  – Abdominal migraine
  – Henoch–Schönlein purpura
  – Familial Mediterranean fever

these children, the skill is to distinguish those with an organic problem from those with a non-organic (functional) problem (Table 25.1).

Recurrent abdominal pain represents pain of 3 or more months' duration.

The causes of recurrent abdominal pain are shown in Box 25.2.

Q2. What would you look for in your clinical evaluation?

History

It is important in these cases to take a detailed history from the child and parents to determine the precise nature of the pain, its frequency, its site and whether or not it affects their daily activities. Constitutional symptoms such as weight loss, anorexia or fever should be asked for and organ-specific symptoms likewise, e.g. renal — dysuria, frequency, haematuria regarding UTI/renal calculus. Gentle exploration into any domestic, school or family stress factors should also be made.

Examination

A full physical examination should be undertaken, both to elicit any abdominal signs and also, more importantly, to reassure the child and parents that the symptom is being taken seriously. Growth measurements (height and weight) should be recorded and plotted on a centile chart. On general examination signs of anaemia and jaundice should be looked for. On abdominal examination evidence of organomegaly should be considered.

Q3. When should you consider referral to the specialist?

Referral to the specialist should be made if the child shows the following signs/symptoms (red flags):

- Constitutional symptoms/signs, e.g. poor appetite, weight loss, vomiting, diarrhoea, fever
- Growth failure
- Gastrointestinal bleeding
- Organ-specific symptoms/signs, e.g. dysuria/ haematuria (urinary tract)
- Hepato/splenomegaly
- Abdominal mass
- Pallor
- Jaundice
- Arthritis.

Causes of recurrent abdominal pain

Non-organic/functional causes

Idiopathic recurrent abdominal pain

These are children who present with recurrent abdominal pain, usually in the periumbilical T10 distribution, associated with periods free from abdominal pain and with good health between episodes. They are often children who are high achievers with a history of colic as a baby.

General examination shows no abnormality, and growth and routine investigations are normal.

Management of the condition is one of strong reassurance, both to the child and the parents, that there is no specific cause for this condition, whilst accepting that the child is suffering attacks of pain. These cases are best followed up on a regular basis for a variable period of time, depending on the symptoms, and it often helps for children to keep a diary of their symptoms, graded by severity and relating the pain to any potential environmental factor or stress.

Abdominal migraine

Abdominal migraine is the name given to a condition from which some children suffer that involves recurrent episodes of abdominal pain, often associated with nausea and vomiting. The term cyclical vomiting used to be used for this condition and often patients required admission for intravenous fluids to be given and for the vomiting to settle. As well as periumbilical abdominal pain, some also suffer from headaches or develop classical migraine later on in adolescence or as an adult. There is often a strong family history of migraine. The condition described as abdominal migraine can sometimes be treated with pizotifen or a trial of food exclusion.

Irritable bowel syndrome

Some children with recurrent abdominal pain have a pattern of symptoms associated with some minor gastrointestinal upsets such as short-lasting diarrhoea alternating with constipation. There is usually no psychological stress identifiable. There may be a history of bloating and a past history of colic as an infant. It is thought that dysfunction of the autonomic nervous system to the gut may be responsible. Reassurance is the order of the day and the symptoms resolve spontaneously over time.

Organic causes of pain

- Gastrointestinal (Ch. 38):
  - Peptic ulcer
  - Gastro-oesophageal reflux disease
  - Inflammatory bowel disease
  - Constipation
  - Pancreatitis
  - Cholecystitis/Cholelithiasis
- Urinary (Ch. 39):
  - Infection
  - Obstruction
  - Calculus
- Gynaecological:
  - Dysmenorrhoea
  - Ovarian cyst
- Others:
  - Henoch–Schönlein purpura
  - Lead poisoning

- Complete blood count (CBC) and erythrocyte sedimentation rate (ESR)/C-reactive protein (CRP), to exclude anaemia or chronic infection
- Liver function tests (+ hepatitis serology), to exclude hepatitis
- Urea and electrolytes, to exclude renal disease
- Serum amylase, to exclude pancreatitis
- A midstream urine sample (MSU), to check for urinary infection
- A stool sample, for microscopy, culture and sensitivity, to exclude parasites, e.g. *Giardia*
- Occult blood × 3, to exclude gastrointestinal bleeding from inflammatory bowel disease or peptic disease
- Abdominal and pelvic ultrasound
- Abdominal X-ray for constipation, lead poisoning, renal calculi

– Familial Mediterranean fever
– Porphyria.

In Carey's case, provided that the history and physical examination are in keeping with a non-organic (functional) cause, strong reassurance from the physician is satisfactory. In order to exclude the rarer causes of the condition, some investigations (Box 25.3) may be required, particularly if the pain is situated elsewhere in the abdomen or there are constitutional upsets.

Whilst the vast majority of these cases are functional in aetiology, organic causes must not be forgotten; in those cases that do not settle with reassurance, referral to the specialist after primary care investigations is then appropriate.

Acute abdominal pain

Problem-orientated topic:

a child with acute lower abdominal pain

Aiden, a 13-year-old boy, is brought to his physician by his parents with a 3-day history of lower abdominal pain associated with mild diarrhoea. He has a mild fever and has been off school. General examination shows some lower abdominal tenderness.

Q1. What are the causes of Aiden's acute abdominal pain?

Q2 What would you look for in your clinical evaluation?

Q3. What investigations would be required?

Q4. When should you consider hospital referral?

Q1. What are the causes of Aiden's acute abdominal pain?

Causes of acute abdominal pain in children are many and varied, and do not all lie within the abdomen (Boxes 25.4 and 25.5).

Surgical intra-abdominal
- Acute appendicitis
- Intestinal obstruction
- Intussusception
- Inguinal hernia
- Peritonitis
- Meckel diverticulum
- Cholecystitis/Cholelithiasis
- Pancreatitis
- Mesenteric adenitis
- Trauma

Medical
- Gastroenteritis (viral or bacterial, e.g. *Shigella*, *Campylobacter*)
- Renal (UTI, renal stones, hydronephrosis)
- Henoch–Schönlein purpura
- Diabetic ketoacidosis
- Sickle cell disease
- Hepatitis
- Irritable bowel disease
- Recurrent abdominal pain
- Gynaecological causes (dysmenorrhoea, pelvic inflammatory disease, haematocolpos)
- Constipation
- Psychological
- Lead poisoning
- Porphyria

Extra-abdominal
- Lower lobe pneumonia
- URTI
- Testicular torsion
- Referred pain from hip/spine
- Herpes zoster (shingles)

Infant
- Colic
- Gastroenteritis
- Constipation
- Intestinal obstruction (intussusception, volvulus, incarcerated hernia, Hirschsprung disease)

Preschool child
- Gastroenteritis
- Constipation
- Mesenteric adenitis
- UTI
- Trauma
- Sickle cell crisis
- Henoch–Schönlein purpura (HSP)

Schoolchild
- Gastroenteritis
- Appendicitis
- Constipation
- Functional abdominal pain syndromes
- UTI
- Mesenteric adenitis
- Pneumonia
- Sickle cell crisis
- HSP
- Inflammatory bowel disease

Adolescent
- Gastroenteritis
- Appendicitis
- Constipation
- Functional abdominal pain syndromes
- Inflammatory bowel disease
- Testicular torsion
- Ovarian torsion
- Threatened abortion
- Ectopic pregnancy
- Dysmenorrhoea

Q2. What would you look for in your clinical evaluation?

The assessment of a child with acute abdominal pain requires a detailed history, a full examination by the physician and a decision as to whether the child requires further tests, usually carried out in hospital, or whether he or she can be monitored at home, with a review should the symptoms change or not improve.

A high index of suspicion of organic disease should be the rule with any child presenting with acute abdominal pain. A low threshold for either regular review by the physician or hospital admission must be used.

The history given in Aiden's case should suggest the possibility of acute appendicitis, particularly associated with localized lower abdominal tenderness/pain and fever. A history of mild diarrhoea is not unusual. The pain is also situated in the lower abdomen and should raise suspicion of an organic cause.

Other causes to consider in his case would be urinary tract infection/renal calculus and referred pain, e.g. scrotum, hip and spine. The overriding decision in such a case is whether a surgical opinion is required, and if so, referral to the appropriate paediatric surgical department will be necessary.

History

The type of pain, its duration and its position are very important features to ascertain from the history. However, in very young children this is not possible. A significant feature associated with pain is intermittent bouts of screaming, particularly associated with pallor. This is an important feature of an intussusception. Older children are more able to give a history and may relate a pain initially to the periumbilical area, only later moving to the lower abdomen and the right iliac fossa: for instance, in appendicitis. In general, children are poor localizers and generally point to the whole of the abdomen when asked to describe where the pain is maximal.

A history of blood in the stool may occur with intussusception (red currant jelly stools) but may also be associated with an acute gastroenteritis (e.g. *Campylobacter* infection, with abdominal pain and a bloody characteristic diarrhoea).

Other features such as a skin rash or arthralgia should be enquired for in relation to Henoch–Schönlein purpura.

Examination

On physical examination the position of the child is important. The child who lies still and is not keen to move may well have peritoneal signs.

Localized tenderness is an important sign, as is tachycardia and/or fever. Examination of the throat or neck for signs of URTI may be relevant (mesenteric adenitis). Signs of peritonism, namely guarding and rigidity, will require a surgical follow-up and admission of the child to hospital. Rectal examination is indicated. In acute appendicitis it may be helpful in making a diagnosis of a pelvic appendix but it should not be a routine investigation.

Q3. What investigations would be required?

Investigations at primary care level may include CBC for leucocytosis, ESR and a urine culture to exclude a UTI, but generally investigations are performed by hospital paediatricians.

Q4. When should you consider hospital referral?

The most important question for the primary care physician to answer in a child with an acute abdomen is whether he or she will require a surgical opinion, and hospital admission is essential if this question is raised. Conditions such as lower lobe pneumonia and diabetic ketoacidosis as extra-abdominal causes of acute abdominal pain must be borne in mind. Again, they usually occur with an ill child who will require investigation and referral to the local paediatric department.

Causes of acute abdominal pain in children

Infantile colic

This commonly occurs around the age of 3 months in full-term infants. The incidence is equal for bottle-fed and breastfed babies. Parents are aware of the infant having paroxysmal episodes of crying, often later in the day. During these episodes infants draw up their legs, exhibit fisting and sometimes are puce in the face. Sometimes the problem is relieved by the passage of flatus or faeces. Possible theories as to causation suggest that certain infants are susceptible to colic and it may be associated with hunger, aerophagy and abdominal distension, and overfeeding.

Differential diagnoses include intussusception, a strangulated inguinal hernia and also infections such as otitis media or UTI, which can present in a similar way.

The management consists of a full history and examination of the child to exclude any obvious cause and then strong reassurance to the parents that there is no abnormality and that the problem will resolve. Additional sucrose has been suggested as a treatment. For some mothers who are breastfeeding, the exclusion of cows' milk sometimes improves the problem, but if these mothers are on a diet free of cows' milk, it is important for them to take additional calcium and vitamin D. It is known that prolonged colic can be one of the precipitating factors in non-accidental injury.

Acute appendicitis

This is the most common surgical cause of acute abdominal pain that a primary care physician will see. The frequency is 3 per 1000 children. It may occur in very young infants up to teenagers and beyond. It is more difficult to diagnose in very young children. The old adage of 'grumbling appendix' is no longer tenable.

The classical presentation is of initially mild periumbilical abdominal pain, often associated with a mild fever, one or two episodes of diarrhoea, and then movement of the pain to the right iliac fossa and an increase in severity; in the presence of peritoneal irritation, the pain causes the child to lie still, since movement will aggravate it.

Clinical signs will include localized tenderness in the right iliac fossa, guarding and rebound tenderness. Should perforation have occurred and peritonitis ensued, a rigid board-like abdomen may be found.

The child requires to be referred to hospital as soon as possible, having been seen by the primary care physician. Investigations in hospital are discussed in Chapter 38.

Treatment is appendicectomy.

Mesenteric adenitis

Children often present to their physician following a recent history of URTI with abdominal pain sometimes localized to the right iliac fossa. On examination there may be signs of residual infection in the throat or ears, possibly with cervical lymphadenopathy, but abdominal examination is entirely normal. It is thought that the condition is caused by acute enlargement of the abdominal lymph nodes that leads to the pain. Management is expectant and the condition resolves spontaneously.

Intussusception

This is a condition that commonly occurs between the ages of 3 months and 2 years, and is caused by invagination of one part of the bowel into another (see also Ch. 38). The most common site is the ileocaecal junction. It may follow an URTI or gastroenteritis such as rotavirus. It is thought that enlarged Peyer's patches may form the leading edge of the intussusception.

The child is often brought to the physician by the parents because of episodic screaming. This is characteristically associated with pallor. In between bouts of pain, the child may appear quite well. Passage of diarrhoea with blood ('red currant jelly') is an important but often late sign of intussusception and requires the child to be immediately referred to hospital.

- Diabetic ketoacidosis
- Lower lobe pneumonia
- Henoch–Schönlein purpura
- UTI
- Gynaecological causes, e.g. dysmenorrhoea
- Pancreatitis
- Gallbladder disorder

This is a diagnosis that should always be borne in mind with a child in this age group (3 months to 2 years), who has a history of episodic crying and associated pallor.

Management is discussed in Chapter 38.

Other causes

Other causes of acute abdominal pain that should be considered are shown in Box 25.6.

Vomiting in children

Problem-orientated topic:

a vomiting baby ● ● ● ● ●

Alana is a 9-month-old baby who has a history of vomiting after feeds over the last 3–4 months. Mother describes Alana as vomiting large quantities of food and is concerned that she is not getting adequate nourishment. She describes occasional small amounts of blood in the vomit. The child's weight chart appears to show static weight gain over the preceding 6 weeks. Vomiting appears to occur after both solid and liquid feeds. Up until recently Mother has not been concerned, but the onset of blood in the vomit and Alana's static weight have brought her to your attention.

Q1. What are the common causes of vomiting in infants?

Q2. What should you look for in your clinical evaluation?

Q3. What, if any, investigations would be appropriate and when is hospital referral indicated?

BOX 25.7 Causes of vomiting in children

Newborn and infants
- Common causes:
  - Regurgitation
  - Gastro-oesophageal reflux
  - Gastroenteritis
  - Overfeeding
- Less common causes:
  - Pyloric stenosis
  - Intussusception (Ch. 38)
  - Occult infection, e.g. UTI
  - Raised intracranial pressure (Ch. 28)

Young children
- Common causes:
  - Gastroenteritis
  - Systemic infection
- Less common causes:
  - Toxic ingestion

Adolescents
- Common causes:
  - Gastroenteritis
  - Systemic infection
- Less common causes:
  - Migraine
  - Pregnancy
  - Bulimia
  - Raised intracranial pressure

Q1. **What are the common causes of vomiting in infants?**

See Box 25.7.

Regurgitation

In the first 6 months of life it is normal for children to regurgitate small amounts of feed and this does not lead to any long-term problems. The condition usually rectifies itself once the child is sitting upright and particularly when he or she starts to walk. Sitting the child upright after a feed and not winding immediately after a feed can reduce the incidence of regurgitation. This is a common condition seen by primary care physicians, and requires only reassurance of the parents.

Gastro-oesophageal reflux

This condition (see also Ch. 38), an exaggerated form of regurgitation, is common in babies, in particular those with developmental disabilities such as severe cerebral palsy. It is caused by a lax gastro-oesophageal sphincter, which allows reflux of the stomach contents into the oesophagus. There are many degrees of the condition, from simple regurgitation to significant aspiration leading to oesophagitis, apnoea and recurrent chest infection. It is a possible cause of sudden unexplained death in infancy (SIDS). It is thought that up to 50% of newborns will suffer from some degree of reflux, almost all resolving within the first year. It may be associated with abnormal neck movement (Sandifer syndrome) and may lead to a number of complications, including bleeding/stricture from oesophagitis, failure to thrive, apnoea, hoarseness and Barrett ulcer. There is a possible association with apparent life-threatening events (ALTEs) and SIDS but these are controversial.

In its mildest form the condition can be managed in primary care with advice on thickening feeds for bottle-fed infants. The use of posture, i.e. sitting infants upright after feeds rather than laying them supine or to place them supine after 30 minutes, and the use of Gaviscon following each feed, often improve the condition. In the moderate and severe forms treatment with acid suppression medication such as histamine receptor antagonists or proton pump inhibitors is indicated. Should these not be effective, there is still a very small place for surgery with fundoplication. Careful growth monitoring to ensure that the infants thrive is also important.

If these measures are not successful, referral to the paediatric department for further investigation should be undertaken. Further investigations include barium swallow, oesophageal pH monitoring, 'milk scan' and endoscopy.

Pyloric stenosis

This occurs in 7 per 1000 live births and has a 6:1 male:female preponderance. It is due to hypertrophy of the circular muscle of the pylorus and usually occurs between the ages of 3 and 6 weeks, presenting with increasingly progressive forceful vomiting of non-bile-stained fluid. Following the vomit, the child is hungry and anxious to feed again, but over a short period of time may lose a considerable amount of weight and become dehydrated, with visible peristalsis seen in the left hypochondrium and associated pyloric tumour palpable between the umbilicus and the right costal margin. A history of projectile vomiting should alert the physician to this possible diagnosis. Even if a pyloric tumour is not palpable, a child should be referred to hospital for further investigations, which may include a test feed, ultrasound scan or barium studies to confirm the diagnosis.

Treatment is surgical (Ramstedt's operation, pyloro-myotomy). The surgery must be delayed until the child is biochemically normal, with correction of the metabolic alkalosis that can occur with this condition.

Postoperatively children do very well, resuming normal feeds within a few hours, and continue to thrive.

Bowel obstruction

There are four features of intestinal obstruction, which include:
- Bile-stained vomiting
- Failure to pass stool
- Abdominal distension
- Visible peristalsis.

Causes include:
- Hirschsprung disease
- Volvulus secondary to a malrotation
- An incarcerated inguinal hernia
- Intussusception.

Referral for a paediatric surgical opinion is essential in order to delineate cause and specific treatment.

Q2. What should you look for in your clinical evaluation?

History

A history of vomiting in a child of any age must be taken seriously and a full history and examination undertaken to ascertain the cause. Whilst the majority of these causes are minor and often self-limiting, there are major and serious causes that require hospital treatment and which need to be identified early to prevent any complications, e.g. meningitis, pyelonephritis, pyloric stenosis and intussusception.

From the history the physician should ascertain the duration of the vomiting, the state of health of the child and whether the vomiting is associated with loss of weight, fever or diarrhoea to suggest an infective cause. The type of vomit should be enquired about, first to differentiate regurgitation from true vomiting, and then to establish the presence of blood-stained vomit, which may suggest oesophagitis. Bile-stained vomit suggests intestinal obstruction. Projectile vomiting may suggest pyloric stenosis.

Examination

A physical examination will include examination of the abdomen and scrotum. A high suspicion of causes outside the abdomen must be borne in mind, e.g. meningitis or pyelonephritis, both of which may present with vomiting. Otitis media is commonly associated with vomiting. Examination of the throat and ears will be required as well.

Vomiting is a common complaint of children who are brought by their parents, particularly in those under

1 year of age. As can be seen from Box 25.7, many causes must be considered. Alana's vomiting suggests gastro-oesophageal reflux; in particular, traces of blood in the vomit suggest the development of oesophagitis. A static weight over the preceding 6 weeks poses the need for referral, investigation and treatment, while the majority of cases at this age can be dealt with by a primary care physician, who should give reassurance after a full examination and weight check, with advice on management as described previously (p. 316).

Q3. What, if any, investigations would be appropriate and when is hospital referral indicated?

Regurgitation

Although this condition usually just requires reassurance from the physician, it is helpful to keep a record of the child's growth to check this is proceeding along satisfactory lines. Growth failure would indicate a need for expert referral for further investigations.

Gastro-oesophageal reflux

Initial management (see also p. 316) is centred around posture after feeds, feed thickeners and use of Gaviscon. If these measures are not satisfactory, a hospital referral would be indicated for further investigations such as barium swallow, ultrasound and 24-hour pH intra-oesophageal monitoring.

Pyloric stenosis

A history of projectile vomiting requires hospital referral for further investigations by the paediatric department and probable referral to the surgeons for pyloromyotomy or Ramsted's procedure.

Bowel obstruction

If bowel obstruction is suspected, immediate referral to a paediatric surgeon is necessary in order for the problem to be further evaluated and, if necessary, for corrective measures to be undertaken surgically.

In Alana's case, referral to a paediatric gastroenterologist would be appropriate, where a full history and examination will be undertaken and further investigations considered, to include ultrasound, barium studies and possibly oesophageal pH monitoring. The use of histamin2 receptor blocker or proton pump inhibitors and prokinetic agents should also be considered when the child is not thriving. Surgery has a very small place if at all in the overall management.

Acute diarrhoea

Problem-orientated topic:

a child with diarrhoea

Liam is a 10-month-old child who returned home 2 days ago following a 4-week stay in Pakistan with his family. On the flight home he developed acute vomiting and diarrhoea. The diarrhoea has persisted on his return home, and his parents have brought him to the clinic because he is now reluctant to take his feeds and is drowsy.

Q1. What are the common causes of diarrhoea?
Q2. How would you assess the child in the clinic?
Q3. How would you manage this situation at home?
Q4. When would hospital referral be indicated?

Q1. What are the common causes of diarrhoea?

Acute diarrhoea is a common world-wide illness in young children under 5 and still has a significant morbidity and mortality. Whilst mortality has dropped significantly in the West, there is still significant morbidity and mortality in developing countries such as those in Africa, Asia and the Far East (Ch. 37). The majority of cases are caused by infectious agents but causes outside of the gastrointestinal tract must not be forgotten (Box 25.8).

Viral gastroenteritis

The most common viral agent is the rotavirus, which tends to cause outbreaks and epidemics in the winter months. It begins with a low-grade fever for 1–2 days, followed by the onset of vomiting and then watery diarrhoea, which usually lasts from 1 to 5 days. Recently an immunization against rotavirus strains has been introduced in some European countries. This

> **BOX 25.8 Causes of acute diarrhoea**
>
> - Viral gastroenteritis, e.g. rotavirus (common), echo and adenoviruses
> - Bacterial gastroenteritis, e.g. *Campylobacter*, *Shigella*, *Salmonella*, cholera, *Escherichia coli*
> - Protozoal, e.g. *Giardia*, *Cryptosporidium*
> - Others, e.g. otitis media, URTI, UTI, antibiotic-induced
> - Non-infectious gastrointestinal causes, e.g. intussusception ('red currant jelly diarrhoea')

will decrease the incidence of acute gastroenteritis in childhood. Other viral causes include the echo- and adenoviruses, which can produce a similar picture but are less common than rotavirus.

Bacterial gastroenteritis

The picture here is similar to viral cases but a history of overseas travel is important if present. In addition, *Campylobacter*, *Shigella*, *Salmonella* and *E. coli* are associated with bloody diarrhoeal stools and abdominal pain. *E. coli* strain O157:H7 may lead to haemolytic uraemic syndrome and acute renal failure.

Protozoal gastroenteritis

Causes include *Giardia lamblia*, *Cryptosporidium* and *Entamoeba histolytica*.

Other conditions to consider

- Otitis media
- URTI
- UTI
- Antibiotic associated diarrhoea, e.g. with amoxicillin.

Intussusception associated with blood-stained diarrhoea ('red currant jelly') is a late feature of this condition.

Q2. How would you assess the child in the clinic?

History

It is important to take a full history from the parents to determine the duration of the diarrhoea, frequency of stools and type of stool, i.e. soft, liquid and/or blood-stained. Recent overseas travel clearly is an important part of the history to determine.

Examination

On examination the abdomen is checked for tenderness or masses and the presence of bowel sounds. It is also important to consider systems outside of the abdomen. Complete physical examination including the ears, throat, chest and urine is indicated.

The history given for Liam is suggestive of acute gastroenteritis that began on his journey home, suggesting that the causative agent may have been acquired abroad. It is important to take a full history and perform a full examination, looking particularly for signs of dehydration and, if this is present, to assess the degree. Less than 5% dehydration may be managed at home, but 5–10% and certainly over 10% dehydration will require hospital referral. It is important to enquire about other family members to see if anyone else has been affected. Three stool cultures (Box 25.10 below) should be sent to the local

---

> **BOX 25.9 Degrees of dehydration**
>
> **Less than 5% (mild)**
> - Dry mouth and lips
>
> **5–10% (moderate)**
> - Dry tongue
> - Sunken eyes and fontanelle
> - Loss of skin turgor
> - Reduced urine output
> - Tachycardia
>
> **10% and above (severe)**
> - Poor peripheral perfusion
> - Drowsy
> - Urine output nil for 12 hours
> - Sunken eyes and fontanelle
> - Tachycardia and reduced blood pressure

---

laboratory and the child should be treated with oral rehydration fluid for the first 10 hours initially.

Important features of the history will include fever, the presence of vomiting associated with the diarrhoea, mucus and blood in the stool, both of which will raise the likelihood that the child may require paediatric hospital opinion.

Q3. How would you manage this situation at home?

The majority of these cases can be managed at home and will have negative stool cultures; they should be able to resume normal fluids and solids within 1 or 3 days of coming home. However, should they continue to have diarrhoea and vomiting, a hospital admission will become necessary and, depending on stool cultures and investigations such as blood tests, further treatment may be indicated.

The most important complication of acute diarrhoea is dehydration (Box 25.9). This is caused by the excess loss of water and sodium in the liquid stools, the loss not being compensated by oral intake. The presence of vomiting compounds the problem, but with acute diarrhoea and vomiting, as a rule, the emesis only lasts about 12 hours. Dehydration is assessed in three degrees by estimating the percentage of fluid loss: mild (less than 5%), moderate (5–10%) and severe (>10%). It is important to make an accurate assessment of the level of dehydration, as water makes up 80% of the body weight of infants.

Fluid deficit varies from 50 ml/kg (mild) in acute diarrhoea up to >100 ml/kg (severe) and can lead to dehydration ranging from mild to moderate/severe. It is important, if possible, to measure body weight when the child is first seen and to compare this with

- Blood-stained diarrhoea
- Diarrhoea for greater than 1 week
- History of overseas travel ⎫ Consider
- Ill child during epidemic ⎭ hospitalization

the most recent weight from the parent-held records in order to obtain an estimate of the volume of body water lost. (1 kg body weight is equivalent to 1 litre of fluid.) However, this is not always possible and a clinical estimate of fluid loss has to be made (<5%, 5–10% and >10% — Box 25.9).

Mild dehydration (< 5%)

This can be managed at home. Cows' milk is stopped and clear fluids are given for a few hours. Toddlers may be offered a flat cola drink or juices but young babies should be given oral rehydration fluids, which contain electrolytes and calories in the appropriate amounts: Na (45 mmol/l), K$^+$ (20 mmol/l), glucose (100 mmol/l). Breastfeeding should be continued throughout the illness.

Reintroduction of milk and solids can be started after a couple of hours to 1 day of clear fluids because there is no longer any evidence for regrading milk feeds. Milk and solids can be reintroduced at an earlier age than was previously advised. A small minority of infants may relapse with diarrhoea because of a temporary lactose intolerance or cows' milk protein intolerance and may take longer to resume normal feeds with normal stools. The majority of children will be able to tolerate cows' milk and solids within a few days of the onset of diarrhoea.

There is no place for antidiarrhoeal or antiemetic agents in the management of acute gastroenteritis in children. Antibiotics, however, may be considered in specific situations, e.g.:

- *Campylobacter* — erythromycin
- Dysentery — ciprofloxacin (in general do not treat *Salmonella* with antibiotics unless the patient is very young, immunocompromised or has systemic presentation suggesting sepsis)
- *Giardia lamblia* — metronidazole.

Stool cultures will need to be taken in order to confirm these bacterial causes (Box 25.10).

Q4. When would hospital referral be indicated?

Moderate (5–10%) to severe (> 10%) dehydration

If clinical assessment indicates that the child has a degree of dehydration of 5–10% or greater than 10%,

the child should be admitted to hospital for further assessment and investigation. Treatment will include intravenous fluids, assessment of urea and electrolytes, stool cultures and other investigations such as blood cultures, urine cultures and imaging as indicated.

Prolonged diarrhoea

This is discussed in more detail in Chapter 38.

Diarrhoea lasting for more than 14 days is defined as chronic and requires further investigation by a secondary care paediatrician or paediatric gastroenterologist if available.

Lactose intolerance (Ch. 38)

This is usually a secondary phenomenon following an episode of gastroenteritis. A primary form of lactose intolerance does exist but it is extremely rare and causes diarrhoea after the first milk feed. In non-Caucasian children, however, it is common to find no lactase in the brush border of the small intestine. The absence of the disaccharide lactase leads to watery stools due to osmotic diarrhoea. The stools have a low pH and positive reducing substances may be detected by using Clinitest tablets.

Management

Management involves stopping lactose-containing milk and substituting with soya milk or semi-elemental formula, for a period of time until the brush border lactase is reformed, following which the infant will again be able to tolerate lactose in the diet. In the primary form, lifelong avoidance of lactose may be required.

Cow's milk protein intolerance (Ch. 43)

This occurs in between 1 and 7.5% of infants. It tends to occur in the first 3 months of life in babies fed on formula milk. Breastfed babies may develop it if their mothers are drinking cows' milk. The symptoms that the infants exhibit are varied and may include vomiting, which is common, usually about an hour after ingestion of the milk, loose stools, which may sometimes be blood-stained with mucus, abdominal pain, discomfort, crying and irritability. In addition, some children develop wheezing, cough or rhinitis and those with an atopic background may develop eczema and urticaria on areas of skin with which the milk has been in contact. Angioedema, producing acute stridor, and anaphylaxis are rare but can be delayed phenomena. Around 50% of children with cows' milk protein intolerance have other food intolerances and most of them are intolerant to soya protein. Some infants may present with constipation.

Diagnosis

Skin prick and radioallergosorbence testing (RAST) is unreliable, as is jejunal biopsy. Elimination diets and later milk challenge are the best ways to determine diagnosis. Natural history suggests that the condition will last a few months and has usually resolved by the age of 1 year. However, it may last up to the age of 3. To assist mothers in maintaining a cows' milk-free diet, the help of the paediatric dietician is very useful. There are several substitute milks that can be used, including soya milk and semi-elemental formulae. In very rare situations the intolerance is severe enough to lead to intolerance even to extensively hydrolysed protein formulae, therefore elemental formulae (based on amino acids) are indicated.

Toddler diarrhoea (chronic non-specific diarrhoea — CNSD)

This condition, which occurs in infants from the age of 6 months to around 5 years, is sometimes described as irritable bowel syndrome of infancy. It is essentially diarrhoea without failure to thrive, and is associated with rapid gastrocolic transit time. It comes under the umbrella of the functional bowel disorders and is one of the spectrum of motility disorders of the gastrointestinal tract. An alternative name is 'peas and carrots diarrhoea' since the diarrhoea often contains undigested food particles. The incidence is greater in male infants.

It is known that the diarrhoea is made worse by a high-roughage diet, a diet with additional fruit and sugary drinks. An important factor on examination is that there is no failure to thrive. Growth charts must be checked and plotted in order to ensure that this is the case.

Management

Removal of excess fruit juices may help, and exploration of a possible food allergy can sometimes be useful. There is sometimes a history of atopy. Diets low in fat are known to increase intestinal transit time, and stress in the family or personal stress may be a factor. However, the prime feature of these infants is that they are healthy and thriving but have loose stools. Management is strong reassurance that the condition will improve spontaneously. Increasing the fat intake in the diet sometimes helps in decreasing the transit time. Loperamide may be used symptomatically. Stress management strategies have been employed. The condition resolves spontaneously by the age of 5.

Blood in the stool, rectal bleeding

Problem-orientated topic:

a child with blood in the stool

Aaron is a 3-year-old with a history of constipation. His mother reports that he only passes a motion once or twice a week and the stools are hard when passed. She has noticed some bright red bleeding on the outside of the stool recently when he has been straining for long periods. She also mentions that he cries with the passage of the stool.

Q1. What are the causes of blood in the stool?

Q2. What important features in the history and examination should you look for?

Q3. What is your management of this problem?

Q1. What are the causes of blood in the stool?

See Box 25.11.

BOX 25.11 Causes of blood in stool

Neonates
- Swallowed maternal blood
- Necrotizing enterocolitis
- Haemorrhagic disease of newborn
- Midgut volvulus
- Anal fissure

Well child
- Bright red blood:
  - Anal fissure, polyp or rectal prolapse
  - Milk allergy
- Large amount of blood:
  - Meckel diverticulum
  - Polyp
  - Peptic ulcer
  - Oesophageal varices

Sick child
- Gastroenteritis (*Campylobacter/Shigella/Salmonella*)
- Intussusception
- Henoch–Schönlein purpura
- Crohn disease
- Ulcerative colitis

Aaron's history is very typical of a child with constipation (infrequent stools that are hard when passed). The bright red blood is present as a result of straining and the development of an anal fissure, which also causes him to cry when passing the stool.

Q2. What important features in the history and examination should you look for?

History

A history of constipation is important and helpful, also the colour of the blood and whether the blood is on the outside of the stool or mixed with it. Red blood suggests bleeding from the lower bowel, a black stool (melaena) suggests bleeding from the upper gastrointestinal tract, and with an intussusception the associated diarrhoea is described as 'red currant jelly' with blood mixed with the motion.

A history of pain associated with constipation suggests an anal fissure. Inspection of the anus is important to identify this cause.

A history of bleeding from other sites, e.g. epistaxis/ urine, would suggest a generalized bleeding disorder rather than a local cause and would require further investigation.

Examination

On examination a history of diarrhoea, bleeding and associated fever suggests gastroenteritis. Henoch–Schönlein purpura — a combination of abdominal pain, arthralgia and characteristic rash on extensor surfaces — should be looked for (Ch. 33). Weight and height should be obtained especially in cases with bloody diarrhoea. Sexual abuse should also be considered (Ch. 36).

Q3. What is your management of this problem?

With constipation and anal fissure, investigations are not necessary at primary care level but advice is necessary about the management of the constipation with softeners and bowel stimulants.

With anal fissure stool softeners and anaesthetic jelly may relieve the symptoms while the fissure heals.

Specialist referral

- Intussusception requires surgical referral for further investigation.
- Recurrent red rectal bleeding requires specialist follow-up to exclude conditions such as a rectal polyp.
- Swallowed maternal blood can be differentiated using the APT test.

Scrotal swelling

Problem-orientated topic:

a child with a swollen scrotum

Na is a 5-year-old boy who is brought to see you with a 6-hour history of increasingly severe pain in the scrotum. His mother has noticed that the scrotum is swollen and is anxious to seek your advice.

Q1. What are the causes of scrotal swelling?
Q2. How do you manage these conditions?
Q3. What complications may arise?
Q4. When is hospital referral indicated?

Q1. What are the causes of scrotal swelling?

38
58

In evaluating the cause of a scrotal swelling (Box 25.12) there are important features in both the history and physical examination that will help to determine the diagnosis and the course of management.

Scrotal pain must always be considered seriously in a child of any age, as the possibility of a testicular torsion must not be missed. In Na's case, he should be seen as soon as possible by the physician and as far as possible the cause of the testicular pain and swelling should be ascertained. Conditions such as a hydrocele, which are painless, and an inguinal hernia, likewise painless unless it becomes incarcerated, are usually not difficult to establish. The differential diagnosis between testicular torsion and epididymo-orchitis may be difficult at times, and should not be made without a second opinion, which will require a hospital surgical referral to the paediatric team. With testicular torsion, time is paramount, and if delay occurs, the affected testis will become ischaemic and atrophy, and function will be lost.

BOX 25.12 Causes of scrotal swellings

Painful
- Testicular torsion
- Epididymo-orchitis

Usually painless
- Hydrocele
- Inguinal hernia (pain if incarcerated)

Q2. How do you manage these conditions?

Hydrocele

A hydrocele is a collection of fluid in the tunica vaginalis. It may communicate with the peritoneal cavity via a patent processus vaginalis, in which case it may vary in size. Most, however, do not fluctuate in size and are separate from the peritoneal cavity. They usually resolve by the age of 18 months but occasionally require surgical treatment. The development of a hydrocele in an older boy should raise the suspicion of testicular malignancy. Clinically, hydroceles are often present at birth. They do not extend into the groin unless there is a communication into the peritoneal cavity. The testis cannot be palpated through the fluid and they can be transilluminated. Treatment is surgical if the condition has not resolved by the age of 18 months.

Inguinal hernia

An inguinal hernia characteristically causes intermittent swelling in the scrotum and is particularly noted when the child is crying or straining. The swelling can be massaged out of the scrotum back into the abdomen through the inguinal ring. Inguinal hernias in childhood are indirect (associated with a patent processus vaginalis). Premature infants are more at risk of an inguinal hernia.

Management of an inguinal hernia is surgical, and referral to a paediatric surgeon is the preferred choice. The hernia may become incarcerated and irreducible. This is an acute surgical situation requiring immediate referral. Pressure on the testicular vessels produced by the incarcerated bowel within the confined inguinal canal may also lead to testicular necrosis and subsequent atrophy. An irreducible hernia may lead to abdominal distension resulting from bowel obstruction.

Testicular torsion

This occurs usually before the age of 6 years. The torsion occurs suddenly and is extremely painful. The testis and epididymis twist on the spermatic cord, usually within the tunica vaginalis. This is commonly associated with an abnormal attachment of the tunica (clapperbell testis) or an undescended testis.

Urgent surgical treatment is required to prevent ischaemic damage to the testis. At operation both the affected testis and the contralateral normal testis should be fixed in the scrotum (orchidopexy) to prevent recurrence of the torsion.

Torsion of a testicular appendage (hydatid of Morgani) can present with acute scrotal pain, usually on the upper pole of the testis, and may mimic testicular torsion. Treatment is surgical.

Epididymo-orchitis

Epididymo-orchitis in the absence of urinary tract abnormalities, e.g. a neuropathic bladder or reflux, is uncommon in young boys and a swollen tender testis and hemiscrotum must be assumed to be due to torsion until proved otherwise. The child must be referred for an immediate surgical opinion. Orchitis may occur with mumps and Henoch–Schönlein purpura. Epididymo-orchitis requires antibiotic treatment; the symptoms and signs may mimic testicular torsion and frequently require a surgical opinion first.

Q3. What complications may arise?

The hernia may become incarcerated and irreducible. This is an acute surgical situation requiring immediate referral. Pressure on the testicular vessels produced by the incarcerated bowel within the confined inguinal canal may also lead to testicular necrosis and subsequent atrophy. An irreducible hernia may lead to abdominal distension resulting from bowel obstruction.

Q4. When is hospital referral indicated?

The management of an inguinal hernia is surgical, and all patients with this condition should be referred to a paediatric surgeon.

Food allergy (see also Ch. 43)

Food allergy occurs in between 0.5 and 30% of infants. The common foods involved include milk, soy, egg, fish, wheat and peanuts. It is usually an IgE-mediated response. Histamine may also be involved in reactions to strawberries, egg white and cheese. Atopic individuals are more prone to food allergies.

Egg intolerance

This occurs in 1.6% of infants. It first appears around 6 months of age. Within 1 hour of ingestion of egg, a rash (erythema) appears around the mouth, associated with urticaria of the oral mucosa. Angioedema of the face may occur, with stridor and wheezing. Anaphylaxis is rare. Skin prick and RAST testing is unreliable. The treatment is to exclude egg. The prognosis is good. By the age of 3 years most children have lost the egg allergy and are able to eat egg without problems. A few cases have a lifelong allergy and are required to exclude egg permanently.

Peanut allergy

The prevalence of peanut allergy in the Western world is about 0.5%. Atopic children are more prone to this

323

condition. Commonly, ingestion of peanuts causes urticaria and may cause angioedema leading to wheeze, tightness of the chest, cough and breathlessness. Acute anaphylaxis is not uncommon. A lifelong allergy is common. Treatment consists of exclusion of peanuts, the use of antihistamines and subcutaneous injection of 1:1000 adrenaline (epinephrine) using Epipen. Skin testing under controlled conditions may also be appropriate to determine whether the allergy is present or not.

Food additives

Allergies occur to tartrazine (an azodye or yellow colouring agent), which can lead to urticaria, asthma and rhinitis. Sulfites are another food additive that can lead to wheezing, particularly in children with pre-existing asthma.

Iron deficiency anaemia

This is a very common problem seen by physicians in babies and toddlers and is due to a combination of rapid growth requiring extra iron, a diet deplete of iron-rich foods and, in some children, chronic blood loss and malabsorption syndromes such as coeliac disease. It is usually asymptomatic initially, but with falling haemoglobin levels the child may then suffer from lethargy and anorexia, and low levels of iron may affect intellectual function. Apart from pallor of mucous membranes, splenomegaly may be detectable in 10% of cases and systolic flow murmurs are frequently heard. Blood loss should always be considered a possibility, although dietary causes predominate.

Secondary causes (blood loss) include:
- Nose bleeds
- Meckel diverticulum
- Gastrointestinal polyps
- Peptic ulceration due to *Helicobacter pylori*.

Pica and breath-holding spells have also been shown to relate to low haemoglobin values.

The prevalence of iron deficiency anaemia ranges from 12 to 40% of 1–2-year-olds if deprived populations are included.

Investigation

The initial investigations at primary care level are haemoglobin, blood film, serum ferritin as well as the MCV value. In iron deficiency anaemia the haemoglobin is low (<10 g/l). The blood film shows microcytic hypochromic red blood cells and the serum ferritin is low, indicating iron deficiency.

BOX 25.13 Failure of iron therapy
- Non-compliance
- Wrong diagnosis, e.g. haemoglobinopathies, thalassaemia, chronic renal failure, chronic infection, myeloproliferative disorders
- Lead poisoning
- Chronic blood loss, e.g. cow's milk protein allergy, Meckel diverticulum, epistaxis

Management

Treatment is with iron supplements orally (ferrous sulphate/fumarate/gluconate) and measurement of the haemoglobin periodically. Parents should be encouraged to give a diet to the child containing iron-rich foods. On oral iron treatment haemoglobin should improve by approximately 1 g/dl per week. If the haemoglobin does not improve on iron therapy, consider the reasons shown in Box 25.13.

Failure of the haemoglobin to respond to iron therapy will require referral to a paediatric gastroenterologist or haematologist for further investigation.

Prevention

Breastfeeding protects against iron deficiency anaemia, as the iron is absorbed more effectively. Cow's milk should not be given to infants under 1 year, as this may cause blood loss from the gastrointestinal tract.

Bruising

Apart from bruising on the legs of toddlers, which is a common finding, and cough purpura on the face, which can occur with coughing and vomiting, bruising must always be taken seriously. A full assessment should be made, with referral for further investigations if appropriate (see also Ch. 42). Box 25.14 lists the common causes of bruising in the different ages but these will all require specialist referral for haematological and other paediatric investigations to ascertain the precise cause and management plan.

Neonatal jaundice

Problem-orientated topic:

a jaundiced baby

Faith is an 8-week-old breastfed baby born at term, who was noted to be jaundiced in the first week of life and remains jaundiced now. She is feeding well but the parents are concerned because the jaundice does

Continued overleaf

not appear to be clearing, as it has in other babies at the clinic. She is brought to see you for your advice.

Q1. What causes of jaundice must be considered at this age?

Q2. What is your clinical approach to this problem?

Q3. When is hospital referral indicated?

BOX 25.14 Causes of bruising in children

Neonates
- Birth trauma, e.g. cephalohaematoma and subconjunctival haemorrhage
- Coagulation disorders, e.g. haemorrhagic disease of the newborn (vitamin K-dependent factors), haemophilia, liver disease
- Thrombocytopenia: maternal autoimmune thrombocytopenia, maternal systemic lupus erythematosus
- Congenital infection, e.g. cytomegalovirus and rubella
- *Thrombocytopenia with absent radius* (TAR syndrome)

Infants
- Coagulation disorder:
  - Haemophilia
  - Late-onset haemorrhagic disease
  - Liver disease and enterohepatic circulation of bile salt disorders
- Thrombocytopenia:
  - TAR syndrome
  - Congenital infection
  - Idiopathic thrombocytopenic purpura (ITP)
  - Malignancy
  - Wiscott–Aldrich syndrome
- Trauma:
  - Accidental
  - Non-accidental injury (NAI, child abuse)

Older children
- Trauma, both accidental and NAI
- Bleeding disorders: ITP, haemophilia and von Willebrand disease
- Liver disease
- Bone marrow failure, e.g. leukaemia
- Infections, e.g. meningococcal sepsis
- Haemolytic uraemic syndrome
- Vasculitis, e.g. Henoch–Schönlein purpura
- Systemic lupus erythematosus (SLE)

BOX 25.15 Causes of jaundice

Less than 24 hours
- Haemolysis (unconjugated bilirubin)
- ABO/rhesus incompatibility
- Congenital infection
- Bleeding
- Excessive bruising
- Congenital spherocytosis
- Physiological

1 day to 2 weeks
- Physiological
- Breast milk jaundice
- Infection, e.g. UTI
- ABO/rhesus incompatibility
- Glucose-6-phosphate dehydrogenase (G6PD) deficiency
- Bruising
- Polycythaemia
- Crigler Najjar

Older than 2 weeks (prolonged jaundice)
- Unconjugated:
  - Physiological/breast milk jaundice
  - Infection
  - UTI
  - Hypothyroidism
  - Haemolytic
- Conjugated:
  - Neonatal hepatitis
  - Biliary atresia
  - Infection
  - Dubin Johnson

Q1. What causes of jaundice must be considered at this age?

Jaundice (see also Ch. 47) in the neonatal period is a common problem presenting to the physician. Around 60% of normal infants will show signs of jaundice in the first week but the majority will have resolved by the end of the second week. Persistence of the jaundice beyond this time must be considered to be pathological until proved otherwise and requires a very thorough assessment. There are several reasons why children are clinically jaundiced in the first week or so (Box 25.15) and these include:
- Haemolysis in the first days as the haemoglobin concentration falls
- Reduced lifespan initially of the red blood cells (70 days as opposed to 120)
- Liver immaturity with reduced glucuronyl transferase activity, leading to reduction in conjugation of bilirubin initially.

Unconjugated bilirubin is fat-soluble and bound to albumin. Unbound unconjugated bilirubin in excess may lead to the serious complication of kernicterus. This may lead in turn to the development of cerebral palsy, choreoathetosis, nerve deafness and mental retardation.

Breast milk jaundice (unconjugated form)

This occurs in breastfed babies who are thriving but remain jaundiced for a period longer than 2 weeks. The cause is unknown but breastfeeding may be allowed to continue quite safely for as long as the mother wishes. On cessation of breastfeeding the jaundice will disappear and there are no complications of the condition.

Hypothyroidism (unconjugated form)

This condition is now screened for using the neonatal (Guthrie) screening test. If jaundice continues for more than 2 weeks, however, thyroid function testing should be undertaken and hypothyroidism excluded. Very seldom conjugated hyperbilirubinaemia can also appear in hypothyroidism.

Faith presents with a typical history for a breastfed term baby. She is well and the jaundice generally does not fluctuate very much. Tests will show that the bilirubin is unconjugated, generally < 200 µmol/l, and it is quite safe to advise the mother to continue breastfeeding until she decides to stop or her milk becomes insufficient. There is no associated risk of the jaundice to the baby.

It is, however, important to investigate the jaundice with a full history and examination of the child, and with investigations to ascertain the level of serum bilirubin and the amount of conjugated and unconjugated bilirubin, in order to exclude the other conditions listed in Box 25.15. These will require hospital referral as appropriate and further investigations as outlined in the chapter.

Q2. What is your clinical approach to this problem?

The physician must take a careful history to ascertain when the jaundice started and the state of wellbeing of the infant. The colour of the stools and urine must be asked for. Pale stools and dark urine suggest conjugated hyperbilirubinaemia and require prompt early referral for further investigation.

Measurement of total and unconjugated levels of bilirubin must be made to determine the type of jaundice present. A level of bilirubin > 200 µmol/l requires hospital referral.

The common situation of physiological and breast milk jaundice, both of which are associated with an unconjugated hyperbilirubinaemia, are self-limiting, but raised levels of conjugated bilirubin suggest the possibility of either a hepatic or a post-hepatic cause for the jaundice and hospital referral is essential.

Prolonged jaundice lasting more than 2 weeks (Box 25.15) requires full explanation, in particular to rule out an infective cause such as a UTI or neonatal hepatitis and, most importantly, obstruction to biliary outflow from biliary atresia, which requires prompt surgical treatment to prevent complications. Potential complications include biliary cirrhosis and portal hypertension (Ch. 48).

Q3. When is hospital referral indicated?

Hospital referral is indicated in the following situations, to which the physician must be alert:
- Early onset of jaundice within the first 24 hours
- A serum bilirubin > 200 µmol/l
- Conjugated hyperbilirubinaemia (pale stools/dark urine)
- An ill baby who is jaundiced in whom the immediate cause is not apparent.

Lumps in the neck

Problem-orientated topic:

a child with swellings in the neck

Madeline is a 2½-year-old who is brought to see you because her parents have noticed swellings on either side of the neck following a series of upper respiratory infections that she has been experiencing over the last 2 months or so. They tell you that she is generally well, with a good appetite and full of energy, but appears to be prone to these recurrent infections. They are concerned that she has an underlying problem and seek your advice.

Q1. What are the important causes of cervical lymphadenopathy?
Q2. When should hospital referral be considered?

Q1. What are the important causes of cervical lymphadenopathy?

This is a common presentation to physicians and requires a careful assessment to determine the cause

More common

- Cervical adenitis, e.g. URTI, tonsillitis, otitis media, rubella
- Glandular fever (EBV), parotid enlargement, e.g. mumps
- Mastoid enlargement, e.g. mastoiditis
- Cervical abscess

Less common

- Thyroglossal cyst
- Branchial fistula remnant
- Thyroid enlargement (goitre)
- Tuberculosis (Ch. 43)
- Lymphoma (Ch. 50)
- Leukaemia (Ch. 50)

and reassure the parents and child. The most common neck swellings that a primary care physician will see are cervical lymph glands, usually in the anterior cervical chain, but posterior triangle cervical lymph nodes also occur (rubella, EBV).

See Box 25.16 for causes of cervical lymphadenopathy.

Cervical adenitis

Enlargement of the cervical glands in the anterior cervical chain commonly occurs with infections such as tonsillitis, pharyngitis and otitis media. The glands enlarge but remain discrete and are tender on palpation. Viral infections predominate as the cause of enlarged cervical lymph nodes but bacterial causes can occur and may require antibiotics. Spontaneous resolution of the underlying enlarged lymph nodes is the normal course of events, but in many children glands do not totally resolve and remain as a persisting cervical lymphadenopathy. This triggers attendance at the clinic and a request for the physician to examine the child.

A full history is obtained from the parent and child to determine the length of history, any preceding symptoms or signs to suggest viral infection, and whether antibiotics have been given already. Examination of the throat and ears is undertaken, along with examination of the neck to determine the site of the cervical swelling/lymphadenopathy. It is also important to examine other lymphatic areas such as the axillae and groin and to exclude enlargement of the liver and spleen. Specific clinical signs such as palatal petechial haemorrhages in glandular fever may be found, and in myeloproliferative disorders a bleeding tendency may also be found due to low platelets leading to purpuric rash.

Infectious mononucleosis (glandular fever) can lead to a severe exudative tonsillitis associated with generalized lymphadenopathy and splenomegaly and, in particular, large painful cervical lymph nodes. Palatal petechiae also occur. It is important to suspect this on clinical grounds and to arrange a specific test (EBV IgM antibodies) to confirm the diagnosis, as antibiotics play no part in the management; indeed, if these children are given amoxicillin they may develop a florid and extensive maculopapular rash.

Malignancy

A more serious cause of persistent cervical lymphadenopathy may be myeloproliferative disorders including leukaemia and lymphoma (Ch. 50). In these situations the nodes tend to be fixed — matted together and non-tender, and the child has constitutional symptoms including fever, night sweats, weight loss and malaise. There may also be hepatosplenomegaly and lymphadenopathy at other sites. These children require urgent referral to the hospital paediatric department for further assessment.

Thyroid swelling (goitre)

Here the swelling is anterior in the midline of the neck. A smooth diffuse swelling on both sides of the neck may be due to hypo- or hyperthyroidism. In addition, a pubertal goitre can occur, particularly in girls who have normal thyroid function tests. For Hashimoto thyroiditis antithyroid antibodies should be determined even if thyroid function tests are completely normal.

Mastoid swelling

This is a tender red swelling over the mastoid process behind the ear, with the ear displaced anteriorly, associated with the presence of otitis media; this requires immediate hospital referral for ENT assessment, intravenous antibiotics and possible surgery to drain the mastoid.

Midline swellings of the neck

These may be caused by:
- Submental lymph node.
- Dermoid cyst.
- Thyroglossal cyst. These cysts arise from the thyroglossal duct, which develops at the base of the tongue and migrates into the neck in the development of the thyroid gland. Cysts may become infected and cause a swelling in the anterior part of the neck. They characteristically move with the tongue and on swallowing. They require surgical excision following referral to a paediatric surgeon.

Table 25.2 Investigations for neck swellings

Test	Reason
CBC/film	To exclude anaemia and myeloproliferative disorder
White blood count (WBC)	Raised in bacterial infections
Atypical lymphocytes	Present in glandular fever
EBV IgM	Positive in glandular fever
CMV IgM	To exclude CMV infection and toxoplasmosis
Throat swab	Group A haemolytic *Streptococcus*

- Ectopic thyroid or goitre at the site of the normal thyroid.

Branchial fistulae/remnants

Persistence of the second branchial cleft may give rise to a blind-ending sinus or fistula between the tonsillar fossa and the skin overlying the anterior border of the sternomastoid muscle at the junction of its lower third and middle third. A mucous discharge may occur and occasionally the fistulae become infected. Treatment is by surgical excision after the first 6 months of life.

Investigations

See Table 25.2.

Madeline presents with a typical story of a child suffering from upper respiratory viral infections associated with cervical adenopathy. In between the episodes of infection she is well and thriving but continues to have bouts of infection that tend to make her unwell and produce concern in the parents. A full history and examination are essential for the aetiology, and rare causes such as tuberculosis, including atypical TB, lymphoma and leukaemia must not be forgotten. Investigations as listed will be necessary in order to establish the precise diagnosis.

Following investigation Madeline is found to have a normal blood count and a negative EBV, CMV and toxoplasmosis dye test; the most likely cause of her cervical lymphadenopathy is recurrent URTI, which will have no long-term detrimental effect. Parents are reassured and advised that no further investigation is necessary.

Q2. When should hospital referral be considered?

Hospital referral should be considered for all children in whom the cause of the cervical swelling is not apparent. In particular, initial investigations such as full blood count may lead to a diagnosis, e.g. myeloproliferative disorder, that requires immediate hospital referral. It may be possible for the physician to manage conditions in primary care such as throat and ear infections, glandular fever and other viral infections. The presence of goitre requires investigation with thyroid function tests and antithyroid antibodies ultrasound and hospital referral. Parotid enlargements may occur with mumps and be managed by the physician. Mastoid enlargements generally require assistance from the ENT department. Cervical abscess, thyroglossal cysts and branchial fistulae will all require the assistance of the paediatric surgeons in order to treat these problems.

Adamos Hadjipanayis   Ed Peile   Constantinos J. Stefanidis

CHAPTER

Disorders of the urinary tract

26

LEARNING OUTCOMES

By the end of this chapter you should:

- Know the basic anatomy and physiology of the urinary tract
- Recognize common and less common patterns of urinary incontinence in children and be able to offer appropriate treatments for enuresis
- Know the appropriate investigations for children with suspected and proven urinary tract infections
- Recognize normal and abnormal frequency of micturition, and know how to assess the child who appears to be passing excessive amounts of urine
- Be able to describe in detail the appropriate treatments for children with uncomfortable urination
- Know the likely causes of macroscopic and microscopic haematuria in children and the indications for referral
- Be able to discuss the psychosocial aspects of urinary dysfunction in children, and have an informed understanding of the relevance of possible sexual abuse to urogenital problems.

You should also take this opportunity to ensure that:

- You can take a proper history of voiding
- You know how to test urine accurately with commonly available dipsticks
- You can undertake simple microscopy of urine
- You can give detailed advice and support on the use of enuresis alarms
- You can examine the scrotum and external genitalia.

MODULE FIVE

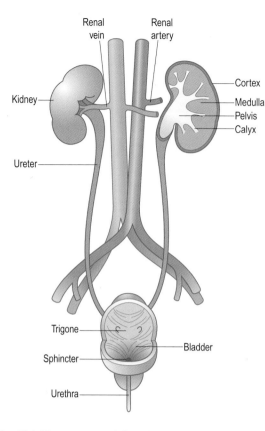

Fig. 26.1 The anatomy of the urinary tract.
(Adapted with permission from the Virtual Autopsy site of the Clinical Division of Pathology, University of Leicester.)

Basic science: the anatomy of the urinary tract

The renal system (Fig. 26.1)

The kidneys are essentially regulatory organs that maintain the volume and composition of body fluid by filtration of the blood and selective reabsorption or secretion of filtered solutes.

The kidneys are retroperitoneal organs (i.e. they are located behind the peritoneum) situated on the posterior wall of the abdomen on each side of the vertebral column, at about the level of the 12th rib. The left kidney is slightly higher in the abdomen than the right, due to the presence of the liver, which pushes the right kidney down.

The kidneys take their blood supply directly from the aorta via the renal arteries; blood is returned to the inferior vena cava via the renal veins. Urine excreted from the kidneys passes down the fibromuscular ureters and collects in the bladder. The bladder muscle (the detrusor muscle) is capable of distending to accept urine without increasing the pressure inside; this means that large volumes can be collected (700–1000 ml in older children) without high-pressure damage to the renal system occurring.

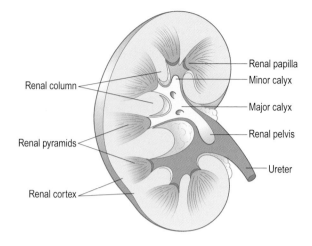

Fig. 26.2 Structure of the kidney

When urine is passed, the urethral sphincter at the base of the bladder relaxes, the detrusor contracts, and urine is voided via the urethra.

The structure of the kidney (Fig. 26.2)

On sectioning, the kidney has a pale outer region — the cortex — and a darker inner region — the medulla. The medulla is divided into 8–18 conical regions, called the renal pyramids; the base of each pyramid starts at the corticomedullary border, and the apex ends in the renal papilla, which merges to form the renal pelvis and continues to form the ureter. In humans, the renal pelvis is divided into two or three spaces — the major calyces — which in turn divide into further minor calyces. The walls of the calyces, pelvis and ureters are lined with smooth muscle that can contract to force urine towards the bladder by peristalsis.

The cortex and the medulla are made up of nephrons — the functional units of the kidney — and each kidney contains about 1 to 1.3 million of these. Each nephron is made up of:

- *A filtering unit: the glomerulus.* As blood is filtered through this sieve-like structure, 125 ml/min/1.73 m^2 of filtrate is formed by the kidneys of children older than 2 years. This filtration is uncontrolled.
- *The proximal convoluted tubule.* Controlled absorption of glucose, sodium, phosphate and other solutes goes on in this region.
- *The loop of Henle.* This region is responsible for concentration and dilution of urine by utilizing a counter-current multiplying mechanism; basically, it is water-impermeable but can pump sodium out, which in turn affects the osmolarity of the surrounding tissues and will affect the subsequent movement of water in or out of the water-permeable collecting duct.

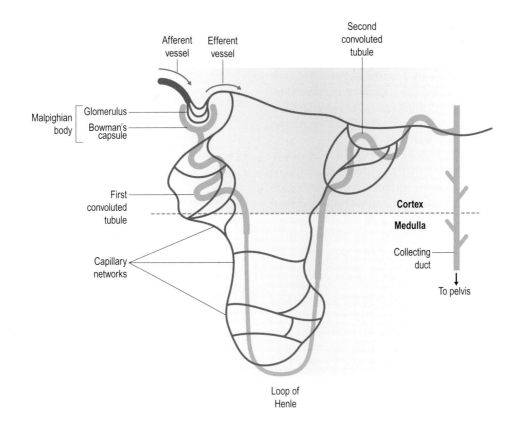

Fig. 26.3 Structure of the nephron

- *The distal convoluted tubule and collecting duct.* This region is responsible for absorbing water back into the body. Simple maths will tell you that the kidney does not produce 125 ml of urine every minute. Around 99% of the water is normally reabsorbed, leaving highly concentrated urine to flow into the collecting duct and then into the renal pelvis.

The structure of the nephron is shown in Figure 26.3.

Enuresis

Basic science of enuresis

Control of micturition

The human bladder has to manage the two associated functions of storing and emptying. To achieve dryness, children need a compliant bladder capable of expanding to adequate volume, and working detrusor and sphincter muscles. In addition, the autonomic control must be such as to manage appropriately coordinated contraction and relaxation.

The sympathetic nervous system releases noradrenaline (norepinephrine) to stimulate contraction of the bladder neck and posterior urethral sphincters, and simultaneously relax the detrusor muscle, so that urine storage

may take place. When it is time to empty the bladder, this is achieved by acetylcholine release from the preganglionic nerves (S2–S4) of the parasympathetic nervous system, stimulating detrusor contraction.

Any detrusor contraction in babies is accompanied by simultaneous sphincter relaxation, so that wetting results immediately. The process of potty training is thought to be one of recruiting supraspinal polysynaptic reflexes to bring the processes of inhibition and stimulation of detrusor contractions, as well as contraction and relaxation of the sphincters, under voluntary control.

Social and behavioural science

The stages of social development that underpin childhood emotions involve a progression from the realization of object permanence in the infant (required for trust in a parent's return, for example), through the egocentric stages of magical thinking in the toddler to the stages of logical thinking, conception of time and differentiation of self from others, which progress through childhood, leading to the establishment of independence and abstract thinking that characterize adolescence (Ch. 3).

Psychological distress, which can manifest as enuresis, can be interpreted against this developmental background.

Anxiety is a normal behavioural response to an event that is perceived as threatening or dangerous. Separation anxiety occurs when children are separated from their parents and is a normal reaction, which in some circumstances can become excessive. The majority of children rapidly reduce the onset and frequency of distress as they develop new social relationships and become confident that parents will reliably and predictably return.

Bullying and sexual abuse are examples of threats to the child's wellbeing that can result in disturbed behaviour patterns, including enuresis, regression, aggression or sexualized behaviour. Masturbation is a normal childhood behaviour from infancy onwards, and is usually devoid of ulterior significance. Healthy children may also experience sexual behaviour with their peers from the onset of puberty, but appropriate social support within the family, school and neighbourhood can help the child to avoid adverse consequences of exploratory behaviour. Sexual abuse happens to children of all ages and to both sexes, in all social classes.

Developmentally appropriate environmental challenges, such as change of school or teacher, may lead to transient emotional disturbances, including enuresis, as may the loss reactions that occur with family breakdown or bereavement.

Control of micturition requires attentional skills, which are closely dependent upon successful biological development. Difficulty with attention is a common impairment in many childhood developmental conditions. Attention is the process of focusing on relevant information and inhibiting responses to irrelevant stimuli — for example, prioritizing the bladder over playtime!

Problem-orientated topic:

a child with daytime and night-time wetting

Michal, who is 7 years old, attends the village primary school where he is doing well academically. He enjoys football and cub scouts, and has several good friends, but he avoids sleepovers because he is nervous about his bed-wetting. Several times a week he will also have slightly wet pants in the daytime, and this happens on holidays as well as at weekends. He says he does not know anything about it until he feels the dampness. Mum, who works in a supermarket, and Dad, who works for the council, are both supportive of Michal, and his older sister does not tease him about it.

Q1. When should one become concerned about wetting?

Q2. What is the likely cause of Michal's daytime wetting and bed-wetting?

Q3. What other conditions should be considered?

Q4. What should you look for in your clinical evaluation?

Q5. What investigations might be appropriate?

Q6. When is referral indicated?

Q1. When should one become concerned about wetting?

See Box 26.1.

> **BOX 26.1 Enuresis: guidelines for concern**
>
> - Daytime urinary symptoms accompanying bed-wetting in children older than 3 or 4 years suggest there may be an underlying bladder dysfunction
> - Between 2 and 4% of children are still enuretic at puberty, and although some will resolve in adolescence, others will turn out to have hereditary enuresis with a high chance of this persisting into adult life
> - Secondary bed-wetting after the child has been dry should prompt enquiry about emotional upset; in particular, bullying or sexual abuse should be considered as possibilities
> - Secondary bed-wetting may be a sign of urinary tract infection (UTI), particularly if accompanied by frequency or dysuria
> - Bed-wetting associated with chronic constipation or encopresis.

Q2. What is the likely cause of Michal's daytime wetting and bed-wetting?

Primary enuresis would be the most likely cause of bed-wetting, but the daytime wetting is a greater cause of concern.

Bladder dysfunction needs to be considered, particularly the urge syndrome, as well as simple inattention to the need to void. In urge syndrome, the volume of urine lost is usually very small, only enough to cause damp patches on the child's underwear.

Rarely, incontinence may be due to structural abnormalities of the urinary tract, such as posterior urethral valves, or abnormalities of the nervous system.

Q3. What other conditions should be considered?

See Box 26.2.

Physiological causes

- Maturation — primary enuresis
- Inattention to the need to void (much more common in boys)
- Giggle incontinence
- Constipation
- Hinman syndrome

Pathological causes

- Neurological:
  - Detrusor hyperreflexia
- Bladder dysfunction:
  - Primary detrusor instability
  - Secondary detrusor instability (can result from over-frequent voiding in an attempt to avoid incontinence)
  - Urge syndrome
  - Urge incontinence
- Congenital malformation:
  - Spinal dysraphism
  - Posterior urethral valves
- Genetic:
  - Hereditary enuresis persists into adulthood in 1–2% of cases
- Psychosocial:
  - Anxiety
  - Bullying
  - Sexual abuse

Q4. What should you look for in your clinical evaluation?

Key points

- A good history and physical examination will frequently help to distinguish children with neurological or bladder dysfunction from those with simple enuresis.
- It is also important to assess the psychosocial dimensions of the problem.
- It is vital to ascertain the child's and parents' views on desired approaches to the problem.

History

- Medical history:
  - Establish whether wetting is nocturnal or happens in the day.
  - Check bowel control and constipation.
  - How much wetness? How often? (In urge syndrome, the volume of urine lost is usually very small, causing only dampness on the underwear.)
  - What circumstances? Does this suggest inattention or a relation to stress?
  - Is there ever any pain? (Pain can be a feature of detrusor instability.)
  - Is the child aware when wetting?
  - Is there associated urgency? If so, is this primary or secondary to frequent micturition in an attempt to avoid incontinence?
  - Has the child ever been dry and for how long?
  - Potty-training attempts?
  - Previous treatment?
  - Other medical conditions, especially diabetes mellitus or insipidus?
  - How many times a day does the child void?
- Family history:
  - Who has had bed-wetting problems?
- Birth history:
  - Congenital malformations?
  - Good stream observed as neonate?
- Psychosocial history:
  - Personality — happy, easygoing, recent change?
  - Affect?
  - Family relationships?
  - Interests, sports, pastimes?
  - School performance? Any reluctance to attend, school refusal or truancy?
  - Peer relationships? Bullying?
  - Any sexualized behaviour?

Examination

Physical examination should include general inspection, looking particularly at the back for evidence of occult sacral and spinal anomalies (Ch. 28), such as unusual hairy patches, vascular malformations, asymmetry or dermal pits.

In the abdomen, inspect, palpate and percuss for a full bladder, and check for the faecal loading of constipation.

In appropriately chaperoned conditions, check the genitalia, looking for epispadias and any evidence of sexual abuse (p. 235). Ballooning of the foreskin is rarely of concern. Anal tone and sensation should be checked where there is any possibility of bladder dysfunction.

Neurological examination includes power, tone, and sensation in the lower limbs.

Q5. What investigations might be appropriate?

Your clinical evaluation should guide any investigations (Table 26.1).

Q6. When is referral indicated?

- May need psychology assessment
- Urological assessment for persistent primary daytime enuresis where a voiding problem is suggested by the voiding chart

Table 26.1 Investigations in a child with wetting

Investigation	Relevance
Blood count, haematocrit	Polyuria to assess plasma hydration
Urea, creatinine and electrolytes	Renal impairment or hyponatraemia
Urine dipstick for glucose	Mandatory to exclude diabetes in all cases of polyuria or secondary urinary incontinence Follow up positive tests with blood glucose test
Urine dipstick for blood and protein	If renal impairment suspected
Urine dipstick for protein, white cells and nitrite	To exclude urinary tract infection
Mid-stream urine culture and microscopy	If nitrites or pyuria
Urine concentration test	Polyuria to exclude diabetes insipidus N.B. Early morning specific gravity is not reliable
Urine acidification test	Polyuria in context of renal impairment
Urine plasma osmolality	Polyuria to exclude nephrogenic diabetes insipidus
Urodynamic studies	A bladder is defined as unstable if urodynamic investigation shows detrusor contractions during the filling phase while the patient is attempting to inhibit voiding

- May need cystoscopy or imaging if primary urethral valves are suspected
- May need urodynamic studies if proven neurological disorder or if history suggests detrusor instability.

Polyuria

Basic science of urine formation

The process of urine formation has three distinct parts: filtration, reabsorption and tubular excretion. During glomerular filtration, blood pressure forces all small molecular components of blood into the lumen of the nephron through the pores in the walls of the glomerular capillaries and pores in the wall of the Bowman's capsule. As the filtrate passes through the tubules of the nephron, up to 99% of the water is reabsorbed into the bloodstream, together with many solutes. A process of active tubular excretion supplements the initial glomerular filtration, and allows for some larger molecules to be excreted in urine.

In the younger child it may be difficult to distinguish polyuria from enuresis, as incontinence (the cardinal feature of enuresis) may accompany the frequent micturition that defines polyuria. The distinguishing feature is that polyuria involves the passage of abnormally large daily quantities of urine (over 50 ml/kg/24 hrs as a rough guide in the school-age child).

In the absence of dehydration, polyuria has to be accompanied by polydipsia — the drinking of excessively large or frequent amounts of fluid — and it is important to tease out whether the drinking is the primary phenomenon or is a response to involuntary polydipsia.

Problem-orientated topic:

a child with frequent urination ● ● ●

Monika, a 7-year-old girl, was referred by the school nurse because teachers have noticed over the past 6 months that she cannot last through a double class period (1 hour 20 minutes) without needing to go to the toilet. She is starting to get teased by the other children for this. She is always drinking large amounts of water, but appears to be embarrassed by her thirst rather than seeking to draw attention to herself. Her mother cannot recall a time in recent months when Monika has had less than about 15–20 drinks in a day. So long as she is allowed to go to the toilet on request and to get up as frequently as she needs to at night, Monika does not wet herself.

Q1. When should one become concerned about children who urinate often?

Q2. What is the likely cause of Monika's polyuria?

Q3. What other conditions should be considered?

Q4. What should you look for in your clinical evaluation?

Q5. What investigations might be appropriate?

Q6. When is referral indicated?

Q1. When should one become concerned about children who urinate often?

See Box 26.3.

Q2. What is the likely cause of Monika's polyuria?

As far as can be assessed from the history, Monika does not seem to have evidence of compulsive water drinking or to be attention-seeking.

There is a strong possibility that her thirst is secondary to excessive urine production, and the two likely causes are diabetes insipidus — a lack of antidiuretic hormone (ADH) — or a failure of the kidneys to respond to ADH. Such primary renal concentration defects are known as nephrogenic diabetes insipidus (Ch. 39).

Q3. What other conditions should be considered?

See Box 26.4.

Q4. What should you look for in your clinical evaluation?

Key points

- A good history is crucially important in helping to decide whether psychogenic polydipsia or attention-seeking behaviour is likely.
- Examination should firstly exclude signs of dehydration, and it is then important to look for the stigmata of chronic disease, including growth stunting.
- Features of chronic renal disease may include palpable kidneys in polycystic disease, pallor and anaemia.
- In thinking about diabetes insipidus, look for signs or symptoms of head injury or brain disease.

- Any child of Mediterranean or Afro-Caribbean origin should have sickle cell disease excluded (Ch. 42).

History
- Medical history:
  - When did the problem start?
  - Daily pattern of urination/drinking?
  - Any record of total input and output?
  - Fed well/grown well?
  - Brain injury or surgery?
  - Meningitis/encephalitis?
  - Tuberculosis/sarcoid?
- Family history:
  - Sickle cell trait/disease?
  - Polycystic kidneys?
  - Renal failure?
  - Diabetes mellitus or insipidus?
- Psychosocial history:
  - Family dynamics happy?
  - Other evidence of attention-seeking?

Examination
- Growth stunting?
- Pallor/anaemia?
- Signs of head injury?
- Palpable kidneys? Polycystic?

Q5. What investigations might be appropriate?

If urine Osm > 600 mOsm/kg or serum Osm < 270 mOsm/kg unlikely to be diabetes insipidus. If

Table 26.2 Investigations in a child with polyuria

Investigation	Relevance
Blood count, plasma viscosity or erythrocyte sedimentation rate	Excludes anaemia
Sickle cell screen	Sickle cell disease a common cause of nephrogenic diabetes insipidus in susceptible populations
Urea, creatinine and electrolytes	Chronic renal failure
Plasma glucose	Excludes diabetes mellitus
Formal water deprivation test (this should only be done in a hospital setting)	Osmolality of an early morning urine sample is often taken as a measure of urinary concentration in children with a history of polydipsia and polyuria, but studies have shown that only around 4 normal children out of 5 will have an osmolality of 600 mmol/kg or more in an early morning urine, making this test too non-specific for routine use
Magnetic resonance imaging (MRI)	Studies of posterior pituitary if diabetes insipidus suspected
Renal ultrasound	Polycystic disease and small shrunken kidneys of chronic renal failure

serum Osm: 270–300 mOsm/kg perform the urine deprivation test. See Table 26.2.

Q6. When is referral indicated?

All children with unexplained polyuria not responding to gently encouraged fluid restriction should be referred to hospital for further assessment.

Dysuria in girls

Problem-orientated topic:

a girl with painful urination

Zuzana is 8. She has not started her periods yet. She tells her mother that it hurts her whenever she passes urine. Sometimes it hurts so much that she cries. Her mother says Zuzana denies 'interfering with herself', yet it is getting to be so much of a problem that she is frightened of going to school. She is an only child and lives with her mother (a beauty therapist) and stepfather (a builder). She has no significant past illness. Zuzana feels the urge to pass urine a lot of the time, but tends to 'hang on' because it is so sore. She has sometimes had a little buff-coloured staining on her pants but has not noticed any blood in her urine. Initially, she got some relief from cool baths but this has not lasted.

Q1. When should one become concerned about uncomfortable urination?

Q2. What is the likely cause of Zuzana's dysuria?

Q3. What other conditions should be considered?

Q4. What should you look for in your clinical evaluation?

Q5. What investigations might be appropriate?

Q6. When is referral indicated?

BOX 26.5 Dysuria: guidelines for concern

- Dysuria that is persistent and troublesome should always be fully assessed
- Most often this distressing symptom is relievable
- A further concern about dysuria is that sometimes it may represent a child's distress following sexual abuse, or may even be a symptom of sexually transmitted disease

---

Q1. When should one become concerned about uncomfortable urination?

See Box 26.5.

Q2. What is the likely cause of Zuzana's dysuria?

Zuzana is most likely to have simple vulvovaginitis of childhood.

Q3. What other conditions should be considered?

See Box 26.6.

Q4. What should you look for in your clinical evaluation?

Key points

- Vulvovaginitis in prepubertal girls is common and the challenge for clinicians is to diagnose and treat

BOX 26.6 Causes of dysuria

Physiological causes
- Tight or nylon underwear causing excessive local warmth
- Masturbation
- Inexperienced tampon use

Pathological causes
- Dermatological:
  - Dermatitis, including the perineal dermatitis of gluten enteropathy and Crohn disease (Ch. 38)
  - Sensitivity to irritants like bubble bath or perfumed soap
  - Eczema (Ch. 27)
  - Psoriasis (Ch. 27)
- Infective:
  - Lower UTIs, most commonly due to faecal organisms
  - Candidal vulvovaginitis
  - Sexually transmitted disease, including *Chlamydia* and gonococcal disease
  - Threadworms
- Psychosocial:
  - Child sexual abuse (p. 235)

- Where there is any possibility of sexual abuse, the examination is best performed by someone with specialist expertise, and in all cases appropriate documentation should be done and swabs must be taken (Ch. 36).

History
- Medical history:
  - Clarify symptoms: genital pain, pruritus, dysuria/haematuria, frequency of micturition, vaginal discharge/vaginal bleeding?
  - Tampon use in the older child
  - When did symptoms start?
  - Were there any triggers to the symptoms?
  - Any history of a dermatological condition, e.g. eczema?
  - Bubble baths or perfumed soaps?
  - Enuresis or faecal soiling?
  - What type of underclothing is worn?
  - How does the child wipe to clean herself after using the toilet?
- Psychosocial history:
  - Sensitive enquiry around possibility of sexual abuse.
  - Enquire if caregiver has any concerns about sexual interference.
  - Ask directly about the possibility of a foreign body.
  - Normal masturbatory behaviour?

Examination
- Inflammation and excoriation of the labia majora, labia minora, clitoris and introitus
- Hymen intact?
- Vaginal discharge/stains on underwear.

Q5. What investigations might be appropriate?

Your clinical evaluation should guide any investigations (Table 26.3).

simple conditions with a minimum of fuss, whilst at the same time remaining vigilant about the possibility of sexual abuse and sexually transmitted disease.
- A good history and simple external physical examination, backed up by culture of a vulval swab and mid-stream urine (MSU), will generally be all that is needed to diagnose simple vulvovaginitis.
- Examination of external genitalia in children is a sensitive issue. Cultural norms must be respected and the examination must always be fully chaperoned by a nurse.

Table 26.3 Investigations in a child with dysuria

Investigation	Relevance
Mid-stream or clean-catch urine	Lower urinary tract infections commonly
Vulval swab (bacteriology and *Candida*)	If vaginal discharge detected
Full sexually transmitted infection (STI) screen, including swabs in specialist culture and transport media and rubbed on glass slides	Whenever STI is suspected, it is vital to avoid half-measures and ensure proper samples are taken. Positive results must be followed up by family screening
Full blood count	Chronic dermatitis (also consider checking serum zinc levels and excluding gluten enteropathy)
'Sellotape slide'	Threadworms are a common cause of vulvovaginitis in the younger child. More sensitive test than stool microscopy
Pelvic and renal ultrasound	Check for urinary tract abnormalities if UTI proven or any anomaly of external genitalia

Q6. When is referral indicated?

All children in whom sexual abuse is suspected should be referred for expert examination in accordance with local practice guidelines. Likewise, if there is a possibility of retained foreign body, children should be referred to a paediatric gynaecologist.

Prepubertal girls with simple vulvovaginitis can be satisfactorily treated in primary care. Simple clear advice to parents and child, backed up by leaflets, can be helpful. Children have a tendency to wipe their bottoms forwards, increasing the likelihood of faecal contamination of the vulva because of the proximity of the anus. Advice on wiping, improved hygiene practices, avoiding local irritants such as bubble baths, and possibly advising salt baths or showers after defaecation may be all that is needed

Some authors recommend the use of topical oestrogen creams for resistant cases, on the grounds that hypo-oestrogenization of childhood genitalia reduces introital protection against infection, as the mucosa is thin and alkaline and there is a paucity of the protective 'Doderlein's bacillus' (*Lactobacillus acidophilus*). However, this is not without hazard, as there is systemic absorption of topical oestrogens and repeated applications may lead to side-effects such as breast enlargement.

Another contentious point for primary care is the use of antifungal creams or steroid/antifungal combinations. Creams such as Canesten are best reserved for children in whom *Candida* has been isolated, and likewise Daktacort, although effective for mild dermatitis and some bacterial and fungal infection, risks masking other problems if used blindly.

Acute urinary tract infection

Problem-orientated topic:

a child with a urine infection

Ján is 4 and has been dry by day and by night since he was 2. Yesterday he was off-colour at the preschool playgroup, and was sick just before bedtime. He woke in the night having wet the bed, and Mum thought he was hot. He now complains of tummy ache and his urine has an offensive smell. Ján's parents are university teachers of Nigerian origin and he has two older brothers, both well. Ján was born by full-term normal delivery after an uneventful pregnancy and has thrived since. His urinary stream has always been good but he tends not to drink a lot of fluid. A dipstick shows no blood but +protein, +++ white blood cells and ++nitrite. His temperature is 38.2°C.

Q1. When should one become concerned about urine infections?

Q2. What is the likely cause of Ján's urine infection?

Q3. What other conditions should be considered?

Q4. What should you look for in your clinical evaluation?

Q5. What investigations might be appropriate?

Q6. When is referral indicated?

BOX 26.7 Acute urinary tract infection: guidelines for concern

- Earlier evidence about the risks of urine infections in the child under 5 years of age, causing scarring leading to chronic pyelonephritis has recently been challenged
- Nevertheless, it remains true that UTIs are under-diagnosed and it is particularly important to establish the diagnosis in infants and toddlers, in whom sample collection is the most difficult. Using syringes to collect fresh nappy urine where bags or clean-catch specimens are impractical is often possible in primary care. A fresh specimen should be sent for phase contrast microscopy or culture
- As in adults, the absence of proteinuria, and pyuria and nitrites on dipstick testing are strongly reassuring that infection is unlikely
- If infection is established, differentiate between lower UTIs in the child who is only mildly unwell, and acute pyelonephritis, which usually merits immediate intravenous therapy

---

Q1. When should one become concerned about urine infections?

See Box 26.7.

Upper urinary tract infections (acute pyelitis and pyelonephritis) are the more serious forms of UTI, both from the risk of septicaemia and on account of the complications of chronic permanent renal lesions. Upper UTIs are rarely accompanied by dysuria. Sometimes there is loin pain, or more usually in children, vague abdominal pain. This condition is discussed in Chapter 39. The child is usually febrile and may have systemic symptoms, e.g. vomiting.

Physiological causes

- Perineal hygiene problems include wet nappies being left too long and causing balanoposthitis in boys, as well as forwards wiping after defaecation in girls
- Poor fluid intake and infrequent voluntary voiding are predisposing factors for lower UTIs, as high urine throughput is an important protection against cystitis
- All ascending infection is much more common in girls than boys (5:1), as the direct short female urethra offers less protection than the male urethra
- Voiding dysfunction is a highly important contributing factor and raises the importance of avoiding constipation

Pathological causes

- Blood-borne:
  - The majority of acute renal infections are believed to be bacteraemic in origin. They are more common following acute gastroenteritis
- Genetic:
  - Structural anomalies of the urinary tract predispose to infection, and they are a particular problem for children with spina bifida
  - Vesico ureteric reflux has a strong familial component
- Instrumentation:
  - Ascending UTIs are an ever-present risk in children who have to be catheterized

Lower UTIs frequently cause dysuria. The child can have vague abdominal pain or even systemic symptoms of diarrhoea or vomiting. Children with lower UTIs are often afebrile.

Q2. What is the likely cause of Ján's urine infection?

Ján could have either an upper or a lower UTI, and the difficult decision here is whether to admit him to hospital for systemic therapy. Unless there are excellent facilities for specimen collection and transport in the practice, it seems reasonable to ask the local paediatric unit to obtain a high-quality urine specimen for culture and to guide on treatment.

Q3. What other conditions should be considered?

See Box 26.8.

Q4. What should you look for in your clinical evaluation?

Key points

- UTIs are often missed because they are not considered. In all febrile or unwell children, in whom a positive diagnosis has not been established, UTIs must be excluded.

History

- Medical history:
  - Previous infections?
  - Any known renal or urological problems?
- Psychosocial history:
  - Nappy changing practices
  - Perineal hygiene
  - Drinking and voiding habits.

Examination

- Temperature
- Hydration
- Capillary refill
- Pulse and blood pressure
- Abdominal tenderness
- Renal enlargement or tenderness
- Perineal soreness.

Q5. What investigations might be appropriate?

Your clinical evaluation should guide any investigations (Table 26.4).

The further investigation of UTI in hospital is discussed in more detail in Chapter 39.

Q6. When is referral indicated?

Most children with UTIs have an excellent prognosis. The greatest risk of renal involvement in febrile UTI is in newborn boys and pre-school-age girls.

Any child who is unwell, and most children under 6 months, should be admitted for intravenous antibiotics. The management of UTI in hospital is discussed in Chapter 39.

Haematuria

Haematuria is potentially a very serious symptom in children and urgent referral to hospital may be required (Ch. 39). The approach in primary care is described in this chapter.

Table 26.4 Investigations in a child with urinary tract infection

Investigation	Relevance
Dipstick urine tests	The presence of white cells and nitrites on dipstick testing is a strong pointer to UTI, and red cells or protein may also be found BUT absence of all of these does not exclude UTI in the unwell child, and other causes such as glomerulonephritis must be considered for haematuria and/or proteinuria
Blood count, with white cell differential	High neutrophilia a strong pointer to infection
Urea, creatinine and electrolytes	Renal function should be checked in any *unwell* child with UTI and in children with recurrent UTIs
Urine culture and phase contrast microscopy	Important in all children in whom UTI is suspected, as screening dipstick tests may miss important infection
Blood culture	Important for all potentially bacteraemic children, including infants under 1 year
Lumbar puncture	Should not be omitted in unwell infants just because a UTI has been diagnosed
Suprapubic aspiration	For children too young to obtain an MSU and with a high probability of UTI, or who are unwell and warrant more invasive investigation

Problem-orientated topic:

a boy with haematuria ●●●●●

Ladislav is 5 years old and in his first year at school. He drew his mother's attention to his dark urine ('coca-cola wee') and the sample that his mother brought to clinic tested +++blood and +protein on dipstick. He has never had any serious illness and there is no family history of haematuria or renal problems. Ladislav is well grown and energetic, and rarely misses school, though he did have a few days off recently with a cold. He has no pain on passing urine and has noticed no rashes or anything else out of the ordinary.

Q1. When should one become concerned about blood in urine?

Q2. What is the likely cause of Ladislav's haematuria?

Q3. What other conditions should be considered?

Q4. What should you look for in your clinical evaluation?

Q5. What investigations might be appropriate?

Q6. When is referral indicated?

BOX 26.9 Haematuria: guidelines for concern

● Significant haematuria is determined by finding more than 5 red blood cells per high-power field on a slide of fresh spun urine

● A dipstick test will detect red blood cells but in addition will detect myoglobin and haemoglobin, which are also clinically important findings

● After a positive dipstick, it is imperative to do a urine analysis. Other causes of red urine include dietary ingestion of beetroot or blackberries, treatment with rifampicin or sedimentation of urate crystals, which may cause red discoloration on a nappy

● Deformed red cells on phase contrast microscopy or casts in the urine usually indicate glomerular involvement, but the absence of casts does not rule out glomerular pathology

● Proteinuria accompanying microscopic haematuria makes significant renal pathology more likely, but small amounts of protein are usually detected when haematuria is macroscopic and do not have ominous significance

Q2. What is the likely cause of Ladislav's haematuria?

Ladislav is likely to have post-infective acute glomerulonephritis (Ch. 39), possibly post-streptococcal. It is essential to check for oedema and hypertension, and to arrange for baseline blood and urine investigations.

This condition will need careful monitoring until it has fully resolved, but in the majority of cases there are no long-term sequalae.

Q1. When should one become concerned about blood in urine?

See Box 26.9.

Q3. What other conditions should be considered?

See Box 26.10.

BOX 26.10 Causes of haematuria

Physiological causes

- Idiopathic transient haematuria is not uncommon
- Exercise haematuria resolves within 48 hours
- Familial benign haematuria is usually asymptomatic

Pathological causes

- Infective:
  - UTIs (Ch. 39)
- Traumatic:
  - Blunt abdominal trauma
  - Perineal trauma
- Immunological:
  - One of the most frequent causes for persistent or intermittent gross or microscopic haematuria during childhood is Berger disease (IgA/IgG nephropathy). It affects males:females (2:1). Progressive disease develops in 30% of patients. The development of hypertension, diminished renal function or proteinuria (>1 g/1.73 m^2/day) indicates a poor prognosis. There are many other rarer forms of glomerulonephritis
- Acute illness:
  - Renal vein thrombosis (Ch. 39)
  - Haemolytic uraemic syndrome (Ch. 39), though uncommon, is the most common cause of acute renal failure in young children and follows an acute gastroenteritis or upper respiratory tract infection (URTI)
  - Neonatal asphyxia
- Chronic illness:
  - Systemic lupus erythematosus (Ch. 33)
  - Chronic glomerulonephritis (Ch. 39)
  - Idiopathic hypercalciuria: excessive gastrointestinal absorption of normal dietary calcium intake or a defect in renal calcium reabsorption
- Haematological:
  - Bleeding diatheses and thrombocytopenias
- Genetic:
  - Alport syndrome (familial nephritis)
- Congenital:
  - Rare vascular abnormalities: haemangiomas, arteriovenous malformations
- Neoplastic:
  - Nephroblastoma (Ch. 50) and other rare tumours
- Drugs:
  - Heparin, warfarin, aspirin, penicillins, sulphonamides, cyclophosphamide
- Psychosocial:
  - Factitious bleeding (interference by child or carer, p. 234)

Q4. What should you look for in your clinical evaluation?

Key points

- As so often in paediatrics, the key question is 'Is this child unwell?'
- Haematuria, whether microscopic or gross, carries very different implications if the child is unwell.
- Look carefully for evidence of fever, poor feeding, dehydration or oedema, and always check the blood pressure and for coexistent proteinuria.

History

- Medical history:
  - Any symptoms of a UTI, such as dysuria and frequency? Any suprapubic pain?
  - Any recent URTI or sore throat?
  - Any skin rashes or vesicles?
  - Are the stools loose or bloody?
  - Any recent trauma?
  - Any joint pains or swellings?
  - What medications does the child take?
- Family history:
  - Sickle cell disease or trait?
  - Renal disease, nephrolithiasis, renal transplants or dialysis? Hearing deficits?
- Psychosocial history:
  - Any pointers to factitious illness?

Examination

- Anaemia or jaundice?
- Growth retardation?
- Oedema is a prominent finding in acute glomerulonephritis.
- Blood pressure recording is vital, as hypertension is a serious finding.
- Examine external genitalia for a local cause of bleeding (e.g. urethral caruncle).
- Look for any rashes, evidence of trauma and bruising, petechiae and purpura (look especially at feet, thighs and buttocks for Henoch–Schönlein purpura, Ch. 33).
- Examine all joints for signs of arthritis — red, warm or swollen.
- Abdominal masses or tenderness? Enlarged kidney(s)?

Q5. What investigations might be appropriate?

Your clinical evaluation should guide any investigations in primary care. Investigation of glomerulonephritis is discussed in Chapter 39.

Q6. When is referral indicated?

Until recently, all children with asymptomatic microscopic haematuria would have been referred for further investigation. It now seems that a reasonable policy in respect of the well child with no proteinuria, in whom an infection has been excluded, is to check and record the blood pressure and to monitor urine dipstick tests at intervals until blood is no longer detected, in order to check that proteinuria does not develop.

A reasonable policy for a well child reporting macroscopic (gross) haematuria is to recheck the urine in a few days if physical examination is normal and there is no family history of renal disease. Then, if the dipstick is still positive, obtain a fresh sample for phase contrast microscopy and to check the spun urine for blood, casts, protein, white blood cells and bacteria.

All infants and unwell children with haematuria should be referred for immediate investigation, as should any child with proteinuria (>1 g/1.73 m^2/day), hypertension, oedema or reduced urine output.

The management of glomerulonephritis is discussed in Chapter 39.

Painless scrotal swelling and maldescent of testis

Basic science of testicular descent

During fetal development, the testis is formed within the peritoneal cavity. As it descends through the inguinal canal and into the scrotum, the testis brings with it an extension of peritoneum, known as processus vaginalis (PV). After the testis has completed descent, the PV closes off and becomes a fibrous cord with no lumen. Once the duct connecting scrotum to abdomen has closed off, neither abdominal contents nor peritoneal fluid should gain access to the scrotum or inguinal canal. If the PV does not close, it is referred to as a patent processus vaginalis (PPV).

A communicating hydrocele occurs if the PPV is only large enough to allow fluid to pass. Herniation of other abdominal contents can occur if the PPV is larger.

At any point along its descent, the testis may become arrested, resulting in maldescent, with either an impalpable testis or one that is palpable at the inguinal ring.

Problem-orientated topic:

a baby with painless scrotal swelling ● ● ● ● ●

Jozef is 1 week old and is due to have a circumcision for religious reasons next week.

He is a healthy neonate, but his parents have noticed a unilateral painless swelling on the right side and are concerned.

Q1. When should one become concerned about painless scrotal swelling in infants?

Q2. What is the likely cause of Jozef's scrotal swelling?

Q3. What other conditions should be considered?

Q4. What should you look for in your clinical evaluation?

Q5. What investigations might be appropriate?

Q6. When is referral indicated?

Q1. When should one become concerned about painless scrotal swelling in infants?

See Box 26.11.

BOX 26.11 Painless scrotal swelling: guidelines for concern

- Infant hydroceles need no action, as the vast majority will have resolved within the first year of life as the patent processus vaginalis closes
- Inguinal hernias require surgical repair, and opinion differs as to how early this should be performed on infants. Seek local advice from a paediatric surgeon
- For older children and those awaiting routine surgery, parents should always be told to report any tenderness suggestive of incarceration
- In preterm babies, hernia is common and the timing of surgical repair is a matter of expert judgment, weighing risks of complication against those of intervention

Q2. What is the likely cause of Jozef's scrotal swelling?

He is likely to have an innocent infant hydrocele. You should examine him to ensure that he does not have an inguinal hernia and to check his testicular descent.

Q3. What other conditions should be considered?

See Box 26.12.

Physiological causes

- Neonatal hydrocele (80–90% of newborns have a patent processus vaginalis)
- Varicocele (uncommon in prepubertal children)

Pathological causes

- Developmental:
  - Inguinal hernia
- Trauma:
  - Post-traumatic hydrocele
- Neoplastic:
  - Tumours of the testis (benign or malignant) should be considered in the older child

Q4. What should you look for in your clinical evaluation?

Key points

- Clinicians will usually be able to reassure parents on the basis of a thorough examination.

History

- Medical history:
  - Check if the child is unwell.
- Birth history:
  - Hernias in preterm babies require very careful evaluation because of the risk of complication.

Examination

- Transillumination is useful to characterize hydroceles, but beware the hernia that transilluminates.
- Checking testicular descent is part of routine paediatric surveillance in boys. Warm hands and a gentle technique are needed to perform adequate examination in a calm child. If conditions are not ideal, the examination should be repeated.
- Check for inguinal lymphadenopathy.

Q5. What investigations might be appropriate?

Investigations play little part (Table 26.5).

Scrotal pain

Problem-orientated topic:

a boy with scrotal pain ○ ○ ○ ○ ○

Miroslav is 12 and over the past 24 hours he has noticed intermittent discomfort 'in the balls'. His scrotum has now become very uncomfortable, particularly on the left side where it is noticeably swollen. The pain radiates up into his abdomen, and it is so sore that it is difficult for him to walk. He feels sick and his temperature is 38.0°C.

Q1. When should one become concerned about scrotal pain?

Q2. What is the likely cause of Miroslav's scrotal pain?

Q3. What other conditions should be considered?

Q4. What should you look for in your clinical evaluation?

Q5. What investigations might be appropriate?

Q6. When is referral indicated?

Q1. When should one become concerned about scrotal pain?

See Box 26.13.

- Any acute scrotal pain needs careful evaluation
- To miss an acute torsion of the testis is to risk total unilateral loss of gonadal function through infarction
- Strangulated inguinal hernia is another surgical emergency
- Likewise, epididymo-orchitis merits prompt antibiotic therapy

Q2. What is the likely cause of Miroslav's scrotal pain?

The dilemma here is that Miroslav's history does not permit reliable distinction between testicular torsion, strangulated hernia and epididymo-orchitis.

Table 26.5 **Investigations in a boy with painless scrotal swelling or undescended testis**

Investigation	Relevance
Routine blood count and urinalysis	Routine preoperative checks for children having surgery are all that is needed

Physiological causes

- Idiopathic scrotal oedema

Pathological causes

- Trauma:
  - Scrotal injuries include sliding down banisters and handlebar injuries
  - Inconsistent or vague stories should raise concern about abuse
- Surgical emergency:
  - Torsion of the testis
  - Incarcerated hernia
  - Torsion of the appendix testis
- Infection:
  - Epididymo-orchitis
- Immunological:
  - Henoch–Schönlein purpura (Ch. 33)

Q3. What other conditions should be considered?

See Box 26.14.

Q4. What should you look for in your clinical evaluation?

Key points

- A good history and physical examination will establish the diagnosis in most cases.

History

- Medical history
- Family history
- Birth history
- Psychosocial history.

Examination

- Transillumination — classically hydroceles transilluminate but beware, so may hernias.
- Purpuric rash of Henoch–Schönlein purpura over scrotum (may have associated vasculitic rash of

buttocks and lower limbs, arthritis, abdominal pain with gastrointestinal bleeding, and nephritis.
- Haematoma to indicate trauma?

Q5. What investigations might be appropriate?

Your clinical evaluation should guide any investigations (Table 26.6).

Q6. When is referral indicated?

Early surgical consultation is vital, as delay in scrotal exploration and relief of torsion of a testis will result in testicular infarction within 8–12 hours. Keep the child fasted pending surgical review.

Epididymo-orchitis should be managed with antibiotics once a suitable urine sample has been sent. Young infants or systemically unwell children should be admitted for intravenous antibiotics.

Most patients can be successfully managed as outpatients. Adolescents with epididymo-orchitis should have sexually transmitted infection excluded.

Circumcision

Basic science of penis development

At birth, the shaft of the penis and the glans forming the rounded end are separated by a sulcus. The bilaminar foreskin covering the glans penis is called the prepuce. Before birth, prepuce and glans have developed as one tissue, and before a boy's foreskin can retract, the prepuce must separate from the glans, a process that may take several years. The prepuce has a protective function, shielding the delicate glans from faecal and urinary irritation.

Circumcisions are done for religious as well as medical reasons (Box 26.15). There is a wealth of information on the Circumcision Information and Resource Pages (CIRP), including factual descriptions of the procedure. However, there is a strong detectable bias on this site against subjecting children to the procedure, which

Table 26.6 Investigations in a boy with scrotal pain

Investigation	Relevance
Blood count	More important to exclude anaemia than to base decisions on white cell count, which can be misleading
Urine culture and microscopy	Obligatory for all
Meatal swab for *Chlamydia* and gonococcus	Adolescents with epididymo-orchitis must have STI excluded
Ultrasound and radiology	Rarely helpful here. Colour Doppler ultrasonography is useful in differentiating torsion of the testis from other causes but there are still some case reports of a missed diagnosis due to normal or increased testicular blood flow noted on colour Doppler.

BOX 26.15 Circumcision

- Religious circumcision is often practised by non-medically qualified practitioners. For this reason many paediatric surgeons prefer to offer the procedure in order to ensure that children receive the benefits of sterile procedures in clinical settings
- The procedure is often performed without anaesthesia, as some doctors prefer to avoid local anaesthesia, both on account of the local pain and transient swelling induced by the local anaesthetic, and because of the cardiovascular risks in small infants, risks that can also occur following systemic absorption of topical anaesthetic creams
- General anaesthesia is generally avoided in young babies and immobilization is crucial
- Circumcision involves removal of a considerable proportion of the preputial skin along with peripenic dartos muscle, the frenar band and part of the frenulum. This can make urethroplasty in later life more difficult for those men who are unfortunate enough to damage their urethra
- Cheesy smegma consists of the discarded epithelial layers of glans and inner foreskin. Adult smegma also contains a lubricating substance from Tyson's glands around the base of glans penis
- Hygiene in the infant involves cleaning around the meatus of the foreskin. It should not involve probing with cotton buds or attempts at retraction
- Retraction of the foreskin may not happen until school age in many boys. It is of no concern until the time the pubescent child starts to get erections, and then it is rare for non-retraction to be a problem. Retraction should never be forced
- Painless ballooning of the foreskin on micturition in children is not of concern, as it merely represents the separation of glans from prepuce in the prelude to the foreskin becoming retractile
- Penile cancer is a very rare cancer in adults, but used to be more common in uncircumcised men. However, since the present epidemic of human papillomavirus, causing penile warts (which are a risk factor for penile cancer), there is likely to be little protective advantage in circumcision
- STIs such as syphilis and herpes simplex may cause penile ulcers and are more common in uncircumcised men. Penile warts and gonococcal and non-gonococcal urethritis are, however, more common in circumcised men. Candidal balanitis may be asymptomatic in males and is equally common in circumcised and uncircumcised men, although those who are circumcised are more likely to notice visible signs of thrush
- Opinions differ on the effect of circumcision on the transmission of HIV infection and on cervical cancer. Any effect is now considered small, and unlikely to constitute an indication for circumcision
- Lower UTIs are up to ten times more common in uncircumcised male infants

many doctors perceive as cruel in the absence of strong medical indications. The religious and cultural drivers towards circumcision in some families are very strong, notwithstanding the secular and religious arguments reviewed on the CIRP website.

http://www.cirp.org/

BOX 26.16 Possible medical indications for circumcision in childhood

- Phimosis causing pain or urinary obstruction
- Painful erections due to non-retraction of foreskin in adolescence
- Irreducible paraphimosis

Phimosis

Phimosis is defined as constriction of the orifice of the prepuce so as to prevent the foreskin from being drawn back to uncover the glans penis. Non-retractile foreskins are common among young boys and are a normal part of preputial development. The foreskin is retractable in approximately 50% of cases at 1 year of age, 90% by 3 years of age, and 99% by age 17. With normal washing, using soap and water, and gentle retraction during urination and bathing, most foreskins will become retractile over time.

Balanoposthitis

This occurs when the phimotic foreskin becomes white, hard and scarred. Advanced changes in the prepuce are known as balanitis xerotica obliterans and can become cancerous if left untreated, which is why circumcision is usually advised for this condition.

Balanitis

This is irritation of the glans, and occurs under the same conditions as cause nappy rash, especially ammoniacal dermatitis. Balanitis can occur due to poor hygiene and is common among boys still wearing diapers (nappies). Rarely it can be a marker for diabetes if heavy glycosuria has stimulated candidiasis.

Paraphimosis

This occurs if the foreskin has been retracted past the sulcus and not replaced. If the retracted skin becomes swollen, it then forms a tight painful band around the penis. This surgical emergency can often be treated by skilled manipulation, but sometimes reduction under anaesthesia or emergency circumcision is needed (Box 26.16). The condition can always be avoided if the foreskin is never left retracted.

Ekaterine Chkhartishvili   Diego van Esso   Malcolm Levene
Alfred Tenore   Julian L. Verbov   Richard B. Warren

Skin disorders

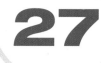

LEARNING OUTCOMES

By the end of this chapter you should:

- Be able to make an initial assessment of a child with a skin complaint
- Be able to describe skin lesions using the appropriate nomenclature
- Be able to recognize common birthmarks and give appropriate advice to the parents
- Know the common causes of pruritus (itching)
- Be able to recognize a number of common disorders of the skin
- Be able to construct a reasonable differential diagnosis
- Be able to implement a management plan.

MODULE FIVE

Introduction

In this chapter we will discuss commonly encountered conditions based on the very common symptom of itching, and will consider a chronic eruption. Important disorders not covered in this format will also be briefly discussed.

Basic science

A basic understanding of skin anatomy is desirable and is best understood from a cross-section (Fig. 27.1). The skin is the largest organ in the body and has a mean thickness of 2 mm, of which the outermost portion, the epidermis, is 0.2 mm thick and the dermis is 1.8 mm thick. The epidermis is mainly cellular whereas the dermis is vascular and contains collagen and elastic tissue, glands (sweat and sebaceous) and hair follicles. Beneath the skin lies the subcutaneous fat. Basic cells within the skin include keratinocytes (responsible for skin reproduction), melanocytes (for pigment production), Langerhans cells (with an immunological function) and numerous adnexal structures such as sweat and sebaceous glands. The

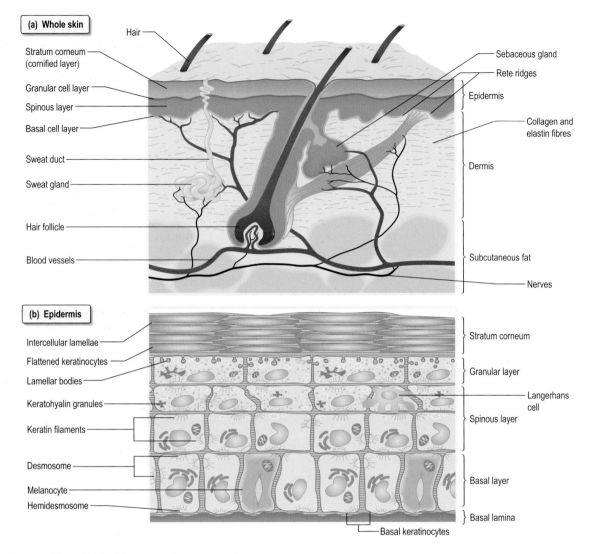

(a) Whole skin

- Hair
- Stratum corneum (cornified layer)
- Granular cell layer
- Spinous layer
- Basal cell layer
- Sweat duct
- Sweat gland
- Hair follicle
- Blood vessels
- Sebaceous gland
- Rete ridges
- Epidermis
- Collagen and elastin fibres
- Dermis
- Subcutaneous fat
- Nerves

(b) Epidermis

- Intercellular lamellae
- Flattened keratinocytes
- Lamellar bodies
- Keratohyalin granules
- Keratin filaments
- Desmosome
- Melanocyte
- Hemidesmosome
- Stratum corneum
- Granular layer
- Langerhans cell
- Spinous layer
- Basal layer
- Basal lamina
- Basal keratinocytes

Fig. 27.1 **Normal skin. Diagrammatic cross-section.**

epidermis originates from the ectoderm whereas the dermis originates from the mesoderm. Melanocytes originate from the neural crest. Fetal skin development occurs mainly between 4 and 6 months of gestation.

The skin has a number of basic functions (Box 27.1). It is important to appreciate the special needs of the preterm infant, who has high transepidermal fluid loss because the skin is very thin and poorly keratinized and lacks subcutaneous fat. This has clear implications for both fluid balance and temperature control (p. 684). Absorption of noxious substances across the skin is also possible in the preterm infant. To some extent this situation is replicated in diseased skin if there is epidermal loss.

Description of terminology

See Box 27.2.

BOX 27.1 Basic skin functions

- Protective barrier
- Temperature regulation and fluid regulation
- Immunological function

Birthmarks

Birthmarks may be divided into vascular and pigmented lesions (Box 27.3). Birthmarks are common and may affect 1 in 3 babies. The most common is the naevus flammeus. Apart from cosmetic concerns, birthmarks are usually benign. Pigmented birthmarks are less common than vascular marks, but if large may become malignant.

BOX 27.2 Glossary of basic dermatological terms

Macule	Indicates a change in colour of skin, either localized or widespread, e.g. freckles or measles
Papule	A circumscribed solid raised lesion less than 0.5 cm in diameter, e.g. molluscum contagiosum
Pustule	An elevated fluid-containing lesion, the fluid being pus, e.g. impetigo
Vesicle	An elevated fluid-containing lesion less than 0.5 cm in diameter, e.g. varicella
Bulla	An elevated fluid-containing lesion greater than 0.5 cm in diameter, e.g. epidermolysis bullosa
Weal	A localized area of dermal oedema, e.g. urticaria
Plaque	A well-defined elevated area of skin that may or may not show scaling, e.g. psoriasis
Purpura	Bleeding into the skin or a mucosal surface. Small areas of purpura are termed petechiae and larger areas ecchymoses, e.g. Henoch–Schönlein purpura
Naevus	A localized malformation of tissue structures, e.g. moles (pigmented naevi)
Erythema	Redness
Annular	Ring-shaped
Atrophy	Tissue loss that may affect all levels of skin and subcutaneous fat
Dermatitis/eczema	In general the terms can be considered synonymous – an inflammatory condition of the skin characterized by papules and vesicles on an erythematous (red) base. Because of the irritation, excoriations and secondary infection (impetiginization) are common
Lichenification	A peculiar skin change with accentuated markings, usually as a consequence of prolonged rubbing of the skin in localized areas of atopic eczema
Pruritus	Itching
Excoriation	Loss of the epidermal surface (partial or complete) due to scratching, e.g. in eczema
Ulcer	A break in the continuity of the skin that can involve loss of the whole thickness of the epidermis and upper dermis
Fissure	A small narrow ulcer, e.g. in the perianal region

BOX 27.3 Types of birthmark

- Vascular
  - Naevus flammeus
  - Strawberry naevus
  - Port-wine stain
- Pigmented
  - Mongolian blue spot
  - Café-au-lait spots
  - Moles

Naevus flammeus (stork beak mark)

These relatively small vascular naevi are extremely common and become more obvious when the baby cries (Fig. 27.2). They are most frequently seen on the nasal bridge or forehead in the midline, over the nape of the neck or on the eyelids. They usually fade as the baby gets older.

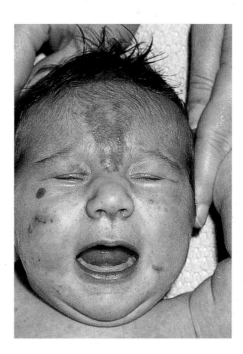

Fig. 27.2 **Stork beak mark. (Reproduced with permission from Blackwell Science.)**

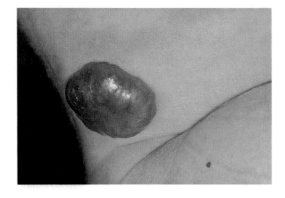

Fig. 27.3 Strawberry naevus in a 3-month-old baby.

Strawberry naevus (capillary haemangioma)

Capillary haemangiomas are common vascular naevi that may or may not present at birth but grow rapidly over the first few weeks and months to become raised red lobulated tumours, with capillaries sometimes visible over the surface (Fig. 27.3). They grow rapidly with the child in the first 8–18 months of life and then remain fixed in size, involuting over the subsequent 5–8 years. Around 95% disappear by the time the child is 9 years old.

Strawberry naevi most commonly occur on the face, scalp, back or chest. They may cause mechanical problems if they compromise the eye, mouth or nose as they grow. Rarely capillary haemangioma may occur in the upper respiratory tract, leading to life-threatening obstruction of the airway.

They may ooze blood if subject to constant rubbing, but serious haemorrhage is very rare.

A cavernous haemangioma refers to a deep capillary haemangioma that causes a lump and often a blue discoloration of the skin.

Treatment is rarely required, as the natural history is for them to regress spontaneously.

Port-wine stain

This is a flat capillary malformation, most commonly unilateral and found on the face in the trigeminal nerve distribution (Fig. 27.4). It has an incidence of 0.3% in newborn babies. It usually does not fade and may cause distressing facial disfigurement. There may be local tissue overgrowth in the region of the stain. Port-wine stains around the eye may be associated with glaucoma.

Port-wine stains involving the supraorbital region are particularly likely to be associated with similar lesions involving the meninges on the same side, con-

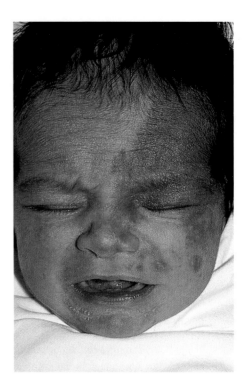

Fig. 27.4 Port-wine stain in the upper trigeminal area. (Reproduced with permission from Blackwell Science.)

stituting the Sturge–Weber syndrome, also characterized by the presence of intracranial calcification and clinical manifestations of convulsions and possibly hemiplegia.

Management is usually with cover-up cosmetics, but laser treatment may be effective in causing the lesion to fade. Best results are obtained when the laser treatment is started early in life.

Mongolian patches (blue spot)

These lesions are congenital macular slate-grey or black patches; they are generally found over the lumbosacral areas and buttocks but can occur anywhere (Fig. 27.5). Most black and oriental babies show them but they are present in less than 10% of white Caucasians. They may be mistaken for a bruise and child abuse may be suspected. They usually fade as the child gets older and tend to disappear by the end of the first decade. They are always benign and require no treatment.

Café-au-lait spots

These are light-brown pigmented lesions that usually develop in childhood. Six or more café-au-lait spots with regular margins, >5 mm in pre-pubertal, and >15 mm in post-pubertal children, may be a feature of neurofibromatosis (Ch. 28).

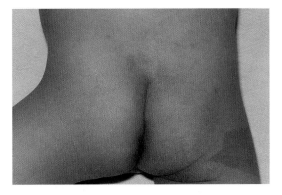

Fig. 27.5 Mongolian blue spot in gluteal cleft and café au lait lesion on thigh. (Reproduced with permission from Blackwell Science.)

Pigmented naevi (moles)

These are very common, benign lesions that are usually small but grow as the child grows. Rarely a large congenital pigmented naevus occurs and is very disfiguring. Change in shape, colour or size should raise the possibility of malignant melanoma, which, however, is rare in children under 14 years of age. Careful follow-up observation of the lesion should be arranged.

Itching (pruritus)

Problem-orientated topic:

a child with an itchy scalp

Helga is a 6-year-old girl whose mother has noticed that she has developed an itchy scalp over the last 2 weeks. Her 4-year-old sister has also started scratching in the last week.

Q1. What is the likely diagnosis?
Q2. What investigations are required?
Q3. How would you manage this condition?
Q4. When should a child with prolonged itchiness be referred to hospital?

Q1. What is the likely diagnosis?

A careful history and examination are essential in all cases. In particular, ask about the following:

- Is there a rash?
  - Atopic dermatitis (examine flexures and face)
  - Psoriasis (flexor surfaces)
  - Scabies (palms and soles)
  - Pityriasis rosea (trunk)
- Contacts?
  - Scabies
  - Head lice
  - Fungal infection (ringworm)
- Systemic upset?
  - Chickenpox
  - Infected atopic dermatitis
  - Allergic reaction.

Further history indicates that other children at Helga's school also have itchy scalps and examination reveals the characteristic egg cases of the lice on several of her hair shafts (see below).

Q2. What investigations are required?

Investigations into the cause of itching in primary care are limited, but the following should be considered:

Skin scrapings should be sent for mycological examination for confirmation of a ringworm fungal infection.

If scalp ringworm is considered, a plucked hair sample should be sent for examination.

Scraping of a scabietic burrow can isolate the mite, its larvae, empty egg cases or faecal material.

Patch testing of the skin for allergens in childhood eczema has limited value.

Q3. How would you manage this condition?

The management of head lice and other differential diagnoses is described below.

Q4. When should a child with prolonged itchiness be referred to hospital?

The most common causes of itching should be diagnosed and managed in a primary care setting. In this case the vignette suggests head lice infestation; this should be diagnosed by examination of the hair for egg cases and appropriate treatment prescribed. Scabies is another diagnosis that, if thought of, should be readily diagnosed and treated. Many cases of mild atopic dermatitis or other eczema can be managed at home, but children with more resistant cases should be referred to a dermatologist.

Head lice (*Pediculosis capitis*)

This is due to infestation by the human head louse (*Pediculus humanus capitis*) and is very common

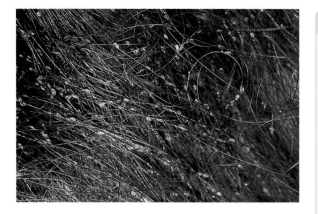

Fig. 27.6 Nits attached to hair shafts.

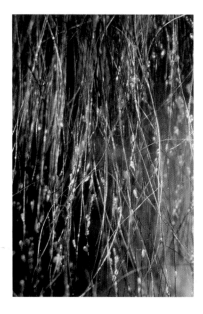

Fig. 27.7 Head lice infestation (pediculosis capitis). Numerous nits can be seen on hairs.

in school-age children (4–11 years). The louse is contracted through close head contact, often in classrooms or amongst siblings. Parents may also be infested.

The louse is 1–3 mm long and lives on blood sucked from the host's scalp. Females lay eggs on hair shafts close to the scalp (Fig. 27.6). These are light grey in colour and may be very extensive. The nymphs hatch in 7 days and mature in 10–14 days, when they mate and lay eggs. Nits (empty egg cases) and live lice should be looked for (Fig. 27.7).

Children usually present with scalp and nape irritation and secondary bacterial infection over the neck (impetiginization) is common.

Management strategies are summarized in Box 27.4.

Problem-orientated topic:

itching ● ● ● ● ●

Gunnar, a 1-year-old boy, attends clinic with a 12-week history of an increasingly itchy rash. The rash, which began over the face, is spreading over much of his body, including the antecubital and popliteal fossae, and is described by the physician as weeping around the neckline. He has been given 1% hydrocortisone cream by his physician with little effect. Gunnar has an older sister who has had mild itching over her arms.

Q1. What is your differential diagnosis of a child with pruritus?

Q2. What further history would you like to know?

Q3. On examining the child, what features may help you to decide on appropriate investigations?

Q4. What is the most likely diagnosis in this child?

BOX 27.4 Strategies for managing head lice

- Only treat if live lice are identified on fine combing to avoid drug resistance
- The most effective evidence-based lotions are permethrin, synergized pyrethrin or malathion 0.5%
- Apply an aqueous lotion to the whole scalp at night and wash out the following morning (leave for 12 hrs). Repeat application 7 days later
- Thorough daily combing with an appropriate fine comb helps control the infestation
- Resistance may be a problem in some areas and local information on best choice is recommended

Q1. What is your differential diagnosis of a child with pruritus?

See Box 27.5.

Q2. What further history would you like to know?

Commonly in a child with a rash the details are sparse with little history. It is, however, very important that due attention is applied to the history, as in any other medical case. A basic knowledge of descriptive terms for skin disorders is essential (Box 27.2). In this

- Eczema/dermatitis
- Psoriasis
- Scabies
- Varicella
- Head lice infestation
- Fungal infection
- Pityriasis rosea
- Urticaria
- Papular urticaria
- Urticaria pigmentosa
- Drug eruption

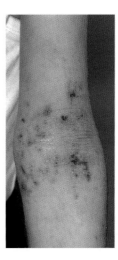

Fig. 27.9 **Atopic dermatitis. Left cubital fossa showing excoriated and infected eczema. Lichenification is also visible in this 5-year-old boy.**

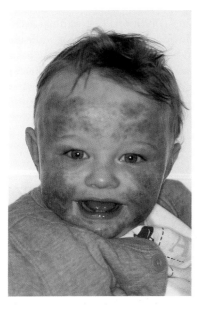

Fig. 27.8 **Atopic dermatitis. A 1-year-old boy with severe facial eczema. With treatment other affected body areas cleared rapidly but his face was slow to respond.**

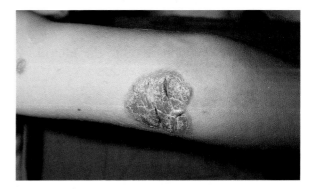

Fig. 27.10 **Psoriasis. Typical well-defined plaque over elbow.**

particular instance the differential diagnosis includes both inflammatory and infective conditions.

Distribution

Focusing on the distribution of the rash can be extremely helpful. Atopic dermatitis commonly affects the face or scalp initially (Fig. 27.8). Common eruptions, such as atopic dermatitis and psoriasis, are classically distributed on the flexor and extensor surface of the limbs respectively (Figs 27.9 and 27.10). Particular focus on the palms and soles may reveal scabietic burrows that can easily be missed and confused with eczema, as the itching invoked by the mite may cause eczema (and often bacterial infection) as a secondary phenomenon.

Duration

Duration of the rash may prove helpful; if the rash clears quickly within hours to days, this may for example suggest a diagnosis of urticaria. In addition, pityriasis rosea can be diagnosed from the history, as there may have been an initial lesion, known as the herald patch, prior to the evolution of a more widespread rash.

Family history/contacts

Scabies, lice infestation and fungal infection may all be spread by contact; others in close contact who itch should be actively sought. The genetics of atopic dermatitis and psoriasis is complex, but this clearly plays a role and knowledge of family history is essential. In this case we have details of another family member being itchy; examination of the second case would therefore be useful and desirable.

Systemic upset

In this history the neck has been described as weeping. An early sign of skin infection may be 'breaks' in the skin surface with weeping from the lesion. The child's general wellbeing should be established. If there is systemic upset a parenteral antibiotic may be indicated. In addition, rare conditions such as urticaria pigmentosa (a form of mast cell disorder) may be associated with systemic symptoms such as flushing or wheezing.

Compliance/understanding

Two of the major reasons for failure of therapy in eczema or psoriasis are lack of understanding of how and when to apply topical therapy, and fear of the consequences of topical steroids. It is extremely important that support is offered to parents and children, with initial practical supervision being invaluable.

Q3. On examining the child, which features may help you to decide on appropriate investigations?

Investigations will be guided by the appearance and history of the eruption but the following should be considered.

In the case of atopy, IgE level is often elevated. As patients with dermatitis are susceptible to infection, they may also have a neutrophilia.

Skin scrapings can be sent for mycological examination for confirmation of a ringworm fungal infection. If scalp ringworm is suspected, plucked scalp hairs can be sent for mycological analysis. Scraping of a scabietic burrow can isolate the mite (*Sarcoptes scabiei* var. *hominis*), larvae, empty egg cases or faecal material.

In most cases in children, skin biopsy can be avoided with an accurate history and examination. This investigation is usually reserved for, and is more appropriate to, the diagnosis of puzzling lesions.

Allergy testing can take several forms (Ch. 43) but is usually neither indicated nor useful in young children with atopic dermatitis. If a child appears to be reacting to a topical product, then patch-testing may be useful. This, however, is more often useful in adults. If the history has revealed urticaria/angioedema, then radioallergosorbent testing (RAST) against a diverse range of dietary products is available in some laboratories. These tests are of low specificity, however, and their role can be overstated. Anxious parents will express a desire for 'allergy' testing, believing that this holds the answers to their child's problems; it is very important to explain that there is little evidence for a role of dietary allergy in the pathogenesis of most dermatological conditions.

However, negative skin prick tests or RAST for food and environment allergens may sometimes be useful in older children with atopic dermatitis.

Q4. What is the most likely diagnosis in this child?

The vignette suggests that atopic dermatitis is the cause of the itching in this particular child. Atopy refers to an inherited tendency to develop one of several related conditions (asthma, eczema of atopic type, allergic rhinitis and urticaria of allergic type) but it is also subject to environmental influence. It is a very common condition, affecting up to 20% of children; in most cases onset is in the first year of life, but its severity varies widely. The skin is usually dry in atopic eczema. This condition, like asthma, has shown an increased incidence, with no clear indication of why this should be. In this child there may have been fear over the use of topical steroids by his physician, which allowed the condition to flare. In some instances a stronger steroid is required for a short time to regain control.

Management of atopic dermatitis is shown in Box 27.6.

Atopic dermatitis (atopic eczema)

Atopic dermatitis (also referred to as atopic eczema) is a very common skin disorder of children. It is estimated that 1 in 5 school-age children suffer from this condition. It is a polygenic disorder, with a strong family history of atopic disorders such as asthma and hay fever. It may also be worsened by contact with a variety of substances, including detergents and some metals (nickel is a common allergen). Exclusive breastfeeding for at least 6 months may delay the onset of atopic dermatitis.

The most common presenting feature is an itchy rash over the face or limb flexures (antecubital fossa, backs of knees). In infants evidence of scratching or rubbing the skin must be sought. The skin appears dry, red and inflamed, particularly in the flexures, neck or face. Prolonged rubbing or scratching of the affected lesions causes the outer layer of the skin to become hypertrophied, resulting in thickening of the skin and exaggeration of the normal skin markings (lichenification) with increased pigmentation in dark-skinned children.

Involvement of the face is common and particularly distressing for the child and family. The cheeks and forehead are frequently involved initially, with itching, dryness and inflammation. The eyelids may be involved (blepharitis) particularly, causing thickening of the lower eyelid in long-standing cases.

Children with moderate or severe forms or those not responding to basic management should be referred to a paediatric dermatologist.

Infantile seborrhoeic dermatititis (cradle cap)

Classically this self-limiting condition, found in infants in the first 3–4 months of life, involves the napkin (diaper) area, axillae and scalp, with erythema, maceration and scaling often confluent in the skin folds. When it affects the scalp it is often referred to as 'cradle cap' and is characterized by a yellowish greasy scalp with thick flakes on the head and behind the ears, but is not sore or itchy (Fig. 27.11).

It is usually self-limiting and disappears by the age of 1. Candida infection may sometimes complicate this eruption in the napkin area.

Basic management is with moisturizing (emollient) creams and bath oils.

http://www.eczema.org/

Atopic dermatitis is a chronic condition that is likely to relapse and remit during childhood. There is no cure but in many cases simple remedies will control the unpleasant symptoms of the condition. Around 50% of children with atopic dermatitis will clear by 12 years of age.

Management in primary care can be considered under several headings (Box 27.7).

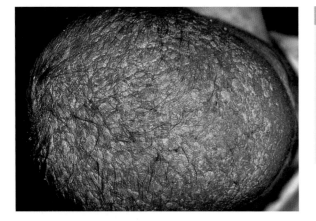

Fig. 27.11 **Severe cradle cap.**

BOX 27.8 Management of scabies

- Treat on clinical suspicion even if a mite is not identified
- Topical application of aqueous permethrin 5% is the treatment of choice. Apply twice, 1 week apart
- Alternative topical applications include malathion and lindane
- Resistance may become a problem

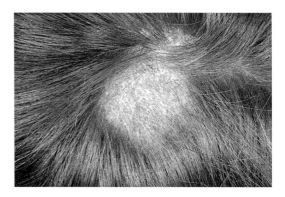

Fig. 27.13 **Scalp ringworm with a patch of hair loss. (Reproduced by permission from Blackwell Science.)**

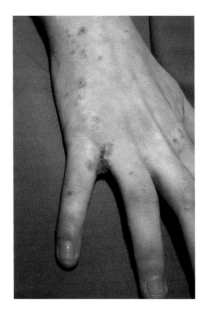

Fig. 27.12 **Scabies. Finger web involvement.**

Other pruritic conditions

Scabies (Fig 27.12)

This is due to infestation by the mite *Sarcoptes scabiei* var. *hominis*, which causes intense itchiness. The mite is acquired by direct skin-to-skin contact and is highly contagious. The adult female mite burrows into the skin and lays its eggs. The larvae mature and mate, and the cycle is repeated every 2 weeks. Itchiness is due to an allergic reaction to the mites and their products. Symptoms occur after 6 weeks of primary infection, but within 48 hours of reinfestation.

The diagnosis is suggested by itching in several family members at the same time and the definitive diagnosis is made on identification of the burrow (Fig 27.12). In older children the burrow is usually seen on the hands, but in younger children and babies scabies often affects the face, scalp, head, palms and soles. Longer-standing infestation can cause widespread eczematized lesions, particularly on the trunk. Very young babies do not scratch but appear miserable.

It affects areas below the neck, including finger and toe web spaces, palms, elbows, soles, wrists, breasts and penis. Severe irritation tends to be worse at night.

Treatment must include all family contacts, whether symptomatic or not. Options include application of permethrin cream (5%) from the neck down, with washing 8–12 hours later and malathion (0.5%) in an aqueous base.

Management is summarized in Box 27.8.

Tinea capitis (scalp ringworm)

Tinea capitis, also known as scalp 'ringworm' for its ring-shaped lesions, is a highly contagious fungal infection that particularly affects Afro-Caribbean children. It causes intense itchiness of the scalp and on examination there is usually patchy (ring-shaped) alopecia with scaling (Fig. 27.13). The scales may be confused with cradle cap. The infection can lead to marked inflammation with pustule formation, termed a kerion (Fig 27.14), often with lymphadenopathy of the neck.

Diagnosis is made by finding the fungus on a hair or scale sample. Treatment is with an oral antifungal agent such as griseofulvin until the fungus is eradicated.

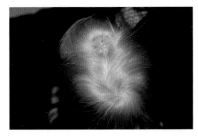

Fig. 27.14 **Scalp ringworm (tinea capitis). Kerion on scalp. The father had active ringworm over the neck.**

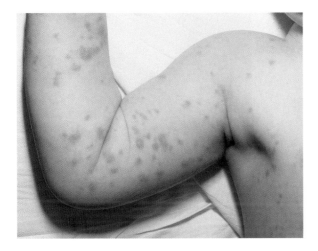

Fig. 27.15 **Urticaria. Typical pink wheals over an upper limb.**

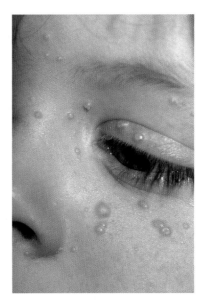

Fig. 27.16 **Molluscum contagiosum. Some of the pearly lesions show umbilication.**

Tinea corporis

Tinea corporis is common, especially among children. The ring-shaped rash is red coloured, with scaly borders, and usually occurs on the arms, legs, face or other exposed body area. Lesions are active at the periphery and 'heal' in the centre. Topical antifungals are the usual treatment. Oral antifungals may be indicated in severe or widespread lesions.

Urticaria

The lesions are characterized by an itchy erythematous eruption of flesh-coloured wheals that are due to local increased permeability of capillaries and small venules.

The lesions occur on any skin area and are usually transient (lasting only a few hours) and migratory. Urticaria may be due to contact with noxious plants (nettles) or be the result of allergy to some foods (e.g. strawberries). The lips may be affected as the result of food allergy and this is an IgE-mediated reaction. Rarely swelling of the tongue and glottis may occur, which may be life-threatening; this may result from nut allergy (Ch. 43).

Urticaria may be associated with angioedema, in which swelling of the lips, eyelids, genitalia, tongue or larynx can occur (Fig. 27.15).

Infections, drugs, inhalants and food allergies account for the most frequent known causes, although in more than 50% of the cases the cause remains unknown. Insect bites may cause a very itchy papular urticaria.

Papular urticaria

This represents a hypersensitivity reaction to a bite from a flea, bed bug, or mosquito. Irritation, vesicles, papules and wheals appear over buttocks and limbs but distribution can be wide in chronic cases.

Urticaria pigmentosa

This is the most common of a group of uncommon conditions in which there is accumulation of mast cells in the skin. It is, however, an important condition to recognize, as occasionally there may be involvement of other tissues, most notably the bone marrow. The initial presentation is a widespread orange-red maculopapular rash, some lesions of which may urticate with rubbing. The condition can appear in infancy and may occasionally be associated with severe itching, flushing and wheeze. Lesions tend to become pigmented with time. Treatment is with oral antihistamines and sometimes in severe disease sodium cromoglicate can be added as a mast cell stabilizer.

Molluscum contagiosum (Fig. 27.16)

This infection is caused by a poxvirus and it is contracted from affected children by direct contact.

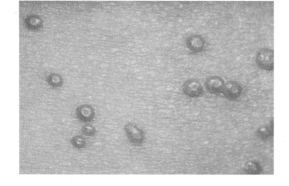

Fig. 27.17 **Molluscum contagiosum lesions. (Reproduced with permission from Blackwell Science.)**

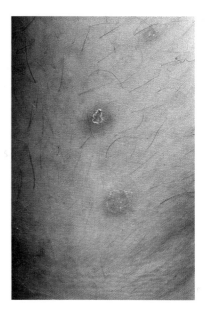

Fig. 27.18 **Pityriasis rosea. Close-up to show scaling lesions in the popliteal fossa.**

The lesions appear as discrete, multiple 1- to 10-mm, pearly dome-shaped papules with a central depression (umbilication), usually occurring on the trunk or limb flexures (Fig. 27.17). It is a common lesion in children 2 to 5 years old. It can be mildly itchy and may complicate atopic dermatitis, making treatment more difficult. Steroids used to suppress the dermatitis appear to encourage the lesions, so atopic dermatitis treatment should be restricted to emollients or other non-steroidal applications if these conditions occur together. Molluscum contagiosum is self-limiting. The natural history is for the lesions to resolve spontaneously within 8–12 months, but new ones can occur by autoinoculation. Secondarily infected lesions require topical antiseptic/antibiotic treatment. In view of their benign and self-limiting natural history, no treatment is generally recommended but in case treatment is required to avoid the spread to other children the lesions can be removed by curettage, or treated with cryotherapy using liquid nitrogen.

Varicella

This eruption can be itchy at the outset and, as it evolves, the diagnosis will become clear from the typical erythematous vesicular rash. Varicella is most common in young children and systemic symptoms are mild. Secondary bacterial infection of the lesions is the most frequent complication of varicella, occurring in 5–10% of children. Healthy children rarely develop more serious side-effects such as pneumonitis, encephalitis and cerebellar ataxia. In patients with atopic dermatitis the eruption may resemble eczema herpeticum.

Pityriasis rosea (Fig. 27.18)

In approximately 60% of patients, the initial lesion is a 'herald patch', a scaly patch that precedes the generalized eruption by 1–3 weeks. Lesions are concentrated on the trunk and spare the face and extremities. The rash is composed of small (1–2 cm in diameter), red, oval, scaling areas with the long axes parallel to lines of skin stress, often giving a Christmas-tree disposition over the back. The lesions are commonly mildly itchy, particularly after a bath, and can be mistaken for psoriasis. It is more common in the winter months (November to February) and affects adolescents more than infants. This condition is self-limiting and therefore requires non-specific treatment. The cause is unknown but it is thought to be due to an infective agent.

Pityriasis versicolor

Pityriasis versicolor is a common recurrent skin disease, seen mainly in older children or adolescents, in which discoloured or brown lesions forming patches appear mainly on the trunk, neck and arms. The skin lesions are usually asymptomatic but may be mildly itchy and are sometimes scaly . Pityriasis versicolor is more common in hot, humid climates or in individuals who sweat heavily.

Granuloma annulare

Granuloma annulare is a common condition of unknown cause that affects the skin of children, teenagers or young adults. Granuloma annulare can occur on any site of the body. The most common presentation is a skin-coloured annular lesion with a raised papular border and depressed centre, usually on the back of the hands, or on top of the foot or ankle, and over the elbows. Although the rash is usually asymptomatic, it may be slightly itchy. Granuloma annulare will disappear after a few weeks or months without leaving a scar, but it may recur at the same site or somewhere else at a later date.

Drug eruptions

Drug eruptions are uncommon in young children. However, widespread maculopapular eruptions and urticaria are the most frequently seen presentations. More extreme reactions with marked mucosal involvement and skin loss can occur as part of the Stevens–Johnson syndrome, in which drugs such as sulphonamides and anticonvulsants (carbamazepine and phenytoin) may be implicated.

Diaper (napkin or nappy) rash

Problem-orientated topic:

a baby with diaper rash ● ● ● ● ●

Jóhann is a 6-month-old baby who has developed a sore, red rash in the diaper area. He screams when he passes urine and his mother has noted that he has been febrile on occasions. Four weeks earlier he developed a less severe diaper rash, which improved spontaneously.

Q1. What is the differential diagnosis of this rash?
Q2. What is the management?

Q1. What is the differential diagnosis of this rash?

Diaper or nappy rash is a very common occurrence in babies and may be severe. Some babies develop repeated episodes of this condition. Table 27.1 lists the causes and distinguishing features of diaper rash.

Q2. What is the management?

The major points in the management are summarized in Box 27.9.

Contact (ammoniacal) diaper (nappy) rash

This is now a very uncommon condition, because of the widespread introduction of disposable absorbent

Table 27.1 Clinical assessment of a diaper rash

Cause	Distinguishing features
Contact (ammoniacal)	The whole of the diaper area is affected, but the skin creases are spared
Thrush	The skin in the diaper area is bright red and the skin creases are involved. Satellite lesions may extend beyond the napkin area.
Seborrhoeic dermatitis	Red rash with flakes and pustules. There are often eczematous patches elsewhere, particularly the scalp
Psoriasis	Rare. Red scaly rash often involving non-diaper areas

BOX 27.9 Management of diaper rash

- Keep the diaper area dry and clean by changing frequently
- Use disposable diapers, which absorb water, rather than towelling
- Leave the baby without a diaper whenever possible
- Use a barrier cream (e.g. zinc and castor oil, petroleum jelly, Sudocrem)
- If the skin is very inflamed, use a mild steroid cream (1% hydrocortisone) before applying the barrier cream
- If thrush is present, use an antifungal cream (see below)

diapers. The effect of bacteria on urine is to produce ammonia, which, if in contact with the skin for a prolonged time, leads to inflammation. Contact dermatitis in the diaper area also occurs rarely as few mothers wash towelling diapers in sensitizing biological washing powders.

The characteristic feature of contact diaper rash is that the skin creases are usually not red, as the diaper does not come in contact with the creases except if secondary fungal or bacterial infection occurs. Treatment is based on prevention of the skin being exposed to urine and faeces for a long time and use of a barrier cream.

If recovery does not occur rapidly with this treatment, secondary infection should be considered and an antifungal cream with 1% hydrocortisone used. Rarely secondary bacterial infection occurs and this is usually staphylococcal. Severe infection is associated with a fever and an oral antibiotic (flucloxacillin) should be given.

Once the diaper area has recovered, the mother should be advised on basic hygiene measures to prevent recurrence.

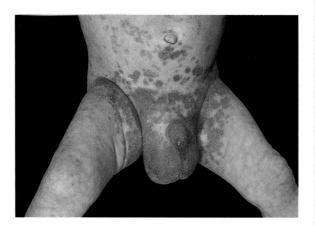

Fig. 27.19 **Candida rash in the diaper area. (Reproduced with permission from Blackwell Science.)**

Thrush (*Candida*) rash

Fungal infections cause a very red and sore diaper rash, with involvement of the skin creases. Sometimes small satellite lesions develop on the abdominal wall or thighs outside the diaper area (Fig. 27.19).

General treatment should be instituted, as outlined above, together with an antifungal cream or ointment (miconazole 2% or nystatin). If the skin is very sore, a combined antifungal and 1% hydrocortisone cream is recommended.

Oral candidiasis (oral thrush)

Oral candidiasis (oral thrush) is caused by *Candida albicans*. Cotton white lesions are present on the inner cheeks, lips and tongue, although they can spread to other parts of the oral cavity. It is more frequent in babies but can also be seen in patients on inhaled corticosteroids or as a sign of a compromised immune system. If oral thrush appears in older children investigate previous antibiotic treatments or immunodeficiency.

Treatment is with antifungals specially formulated to be used on oral mucosa.

Chronic eruptions

Problem-orientated topic:

chronic eruptions ● ● ● ●

An 11-year-old boy, Einar, is referred from his physician with a persistent rash consisting of discrete small reddish lesions, with scaling over much of the trunk. A week or two before the onset of the eruption he had a sore throat. The eruption has been treated with emollients but is unresponsive. It has now been present for over 3 months. All other family members are fit and well. Einar was treated for congenital hip dislocation in infancy, but otherwise is fit and well.

Q1. What is your differential diagnosis in this child?

Q2. What is the basic abnormality in the skin in psoriasis?

Q3. How would you manage this patient?

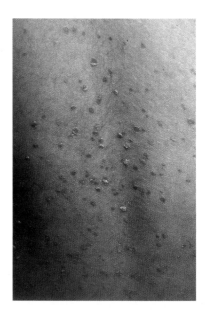

Fig. 27.20 **Psoriasis. A 5½-year-old boy with guttate psoriasis over the back. An attack of guttate psoriasis often follows a streptococcal tonsillitis or other infection.**

Q1. What is your differential diagnosis in this child?

Psoriasis seems the most likely diagnosis here. Psoriasis usually presents at a later age than eczema, with onset before the age of 2 years being rare. It is subject to exacerbations and remissions. The genetic links with this condition are stronger than with atopic dermatitis, and it is now clear that psoriasis is an immunologically driven disorder. This condition is not usually as pruritic as atopic dermatitis. The plaque type of psoriasis typically affects bony prominences but in children guttate (raindrop-like) lesions (Fig. 27.20) often follow a streptococcal or viral ear or throat infection. In both types the lesions show overlying silvery scales. In active psoriasis the Köbner phenomenon may be found, with lesions occurring at the sites of trauma. Nail changes such as pitting and separation of the free end of the nail from the nail bed (onycholysis) may also be seen. Psoriatic arthritis is uncommon in children.

Other chronic eruptions include eczema, of which there are many types, although in children atopic dermatitis is the most common. Eczema can be excluded by assessing the morphology of the rash, as can chronic urticaria. In some instances of chronic eruption a skin biopsy may be required, for example in suspected urticaria pigmentosa.

Q2. What is the basic abnormality of the skin in psoriasis?

Examination of a psoriatic plaque allows a basic understanding of the abnormalities that occur in psoriasis. There is increased thickness of the outer layer of the skin (the epidermis), resulting in a raised scaly surface. In addition gentle removal of superficial scale will often reveal visible pinpoint capillary bleeding (the Auspitz sign). Historically, psoriasis was thought to be due to an abnormality in keratinocytes (the reproductive cell in the skin), with division of these cells being too rapid and not allowing adequate differentiation of the skin. It is now clear that psoriasis is a T-cell-mediated condition, with the increased epidermal turnover being immunologically driven. In many ways it is analogous to other autoimmune diseases in which antibodies are interacting with a self-antigen leading to inflammation, the end result in this case being over-activity of the keratinocyte. What is not clear in psoriasis is what may be acting as the antigen.

Q3. How would you manage this patient?

See Box 27.10.

Other common skin lesions which may be seen in primary care

Warts

Viral warts, which are common in children, are caused by the human papillomavirus, of which there are many types. The virus is spread by direct contact from person to person. They may occur as common warts (usually on hands and feet) or plantar warts (verrucae). In the vast majority of cases the wart resolves spontaneously after a number of years. However, problem warts can be treated with a variety of topical treatments (e.g. salicylic acid-based preparations) and liquid nitrogen cryotherapy, which is painful and not advised in young children.

Genital warts are discussed in Chapter 19.

BOX 27.10 Management of psoriasis

Education
- Relapsing and remitting nature of the disorder

Emollients
- Liberal use of emollients, which minimizes skin scaling

Vitamin D analogues
- Calcipotriol is easy to apply and may sometimes be combined with a potent topical steroid

Coal tar preparations
- Safe but messy

Dithranol derivatives
- Effective but have the potential to burn the skin

Ultraviolet light
- Can be used in guttate flares that are slow to settle but long-term risk of skin cancer limits its use

Systemic treatment
- Methotrexate and ciclosporin are rarely used in children

Sunburn (acute solar dermatitis)

Sadly this is a very common entity. Proper preventive measures, such as covering up with loose cool clothing, hats and sunscreen lotion/cream of sun protection factor (SPF) 30 and above, are most important, particularly in infants and fair-skinned children. Parents must be educated.

Contact dermatitis

This is often due to an allergen causing a delayed hyper-sensitivity reaction. In children the most common sensitizing substance is nickel, used in cheap jewellery and studs. There is erythema and blistering at the contact site. The localization of the lesion usually suggests the cause. The allergen should be avoided and the lesions, if severe, respond rapidly to hydrocortisone 1% cream.

Cold sores

These are due to herpes simplex virus (HSV-1) infection and cold sores develop when the HSV is reactivated. The lesions usually affect the lips, but may also involve the mouth, and start with tingling followed by multiple vesicles erupting in a group (Fig. 27.21). It is self-limiting but tends to recur. Children with eczema may develop a more severe form of HSV-1 infection (eczema herpeticum), with multiple lesions, fever and malaise.

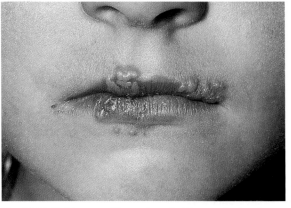

Fig. 27.21 **Cold sores. (Reproduced with permission from Blackwell Science.)**

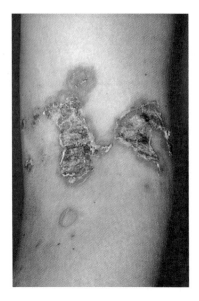

Fig. 27.23 **Lesions of impetigo with satellite lesions. (Reproduced with permission from Blackwell Science.)**

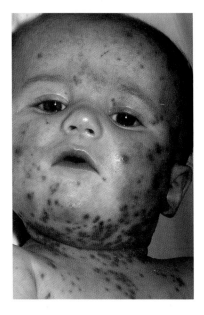

Fig. 27.22 **Eczema herpeticum. This 6-month-old infant with atopic eczema was admitted as an emergency. He was unwell with fever. He has primary herpes simplex with profuse lesions, some showing umbilication. He rapidly improved following administration of intravenous aciclovir.**

Treatment of cold sores is by topical aciclovir cream until the lesion resolves.

Eczema herpeticum

This acute, sometimes disseminated, herpes simplex infection appears most commonly against a background of atopic dermatitis (Fig. 27.22). Usually there will be a sudden decline in control of the child's eczema, with vesicles and oozing from the sites involved. Often the child will be systemically unwell. Treatment is usually with intravenous aciclovir and skin swabs should be taken to exclude the presence of a secondary bacterial infection. In practice, systemic antibiotic treatment for secondary bacterial infection is often required. Topical steroids should be discontinued because their use may encourage spread of the virus.

Impetigo

This is a highly contagious skin lesion caused by *Staphylococcus aureus* or *Streptococcus pyogenes* that is often associated with poor hygiene and overcrowding. It most commonly presents in young children (2–6 years) as multiple golden crusty lesions growing slowly in size and reaching 2 cm in diameter (Fig. 27.23). It is not usually painful or itchy and does not scar. In some cases the crusts develop following a bullous eruption (blistering). Impetigo may occur in already damaged skin, such as in atopic dermatitis or scabies.

A swab from the lesions should be taken, as methicillin-resistant strains (MRSA) are common. Topical mupirocin or fusidic acid cream is recommended in mild cases with few lesions, but topical antibiotics will not eradicate organisms on uninvolved skin. Oral flucloxacillin or erythromycin is recommended in more severe cases. Resistance is growing and microbiological sensitivities of the organism may guide the choice of antibiotics.

Epidermolysis bullosa (EB)

Epidermolysis bullosa (EB) indicates a group of inherited non-inflammatory disorders in which blisters and erosions occur with mechanical, often minor, trauma. There are both scarring and non-scarring types. Recessive forms tend to be much more severe.

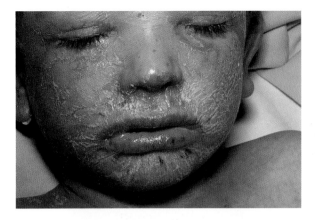

Fig. 27.24 Staphylococcal scalded skin syndrome. Close-up of face of a 4¹/₂-year-old boy admitted as an emergency, unwell with a widespread scalded skin appearance and crusting around the mouth. Four days later, following flucloxacillin, he was fine.

Staphylococcal scalded skin syndrome

This is due to a staphylococcal exotoxin and usually occurs in the under-5-year age-group. The scald-like appearance often involves much of the skin but not the mucosal surfaces. Crusting around the mouth is typical (Fig. 27.24). The condition is often preceded by a purulent conjunctivitis, otitis media or upper respiratory infection. Another family member, such as a sibling, may have ordinary impetigo. Treatment is with a penicillinase-resistant penicillin, fusidic acid, erythromycin or appropriate cephalosporin, with recovery in 5–7 days without scarring.

Cellulitis

Acute cellulitis (erysipelas) is due to group A haemolytic streptococci entering through a break in the skin, usually near the eye, ear, nostril or mouth. Treatment is with benzylpenicillin or oral phenoxymethylpenicillin (or erythromycin or other macrolide if child is penicillin-allergic). Low-grade cellulitis is more common and may be recurrent. Although usually due to haemolytic streptococcal infection, cellulitis can also be caused by other organisms such as *Staphylococcus aureus* (which can be treated with phenoxymethylpenicillin (or benzylpenicillin) plus flucloxacillin), *Streptococcus pneumoniae* and *Haemophilus influenzae*. Before young children began to be immunized with conjugate *H. influenzae* type b vaccine, buccal cellulitis, due to *H. influenzae* type b, was responsible for up to 25% of cases of facial cellulitis in children of 3–24 months of age. Now such cellulitis is rare. Infection originated in the upper respiratory tract.

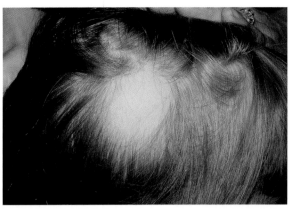

Fig. 27.25 Alopecia areata. Patch of scalp hair loss showing a well-defined area of complete hair loss without inflammation.

Perianal cellulitis

This occurs mainly in young children and is generally caused by group A streptococci. Manifestations include perianal pruritus and erythema, anal fissures, pus and rectal bleeding. Treatment is with oral phenoxymethylpenicillin. Child abuse may sometimes be suspected but can usually be excluded by history and clinical findings.

Alopecia

There are a number of causes of scalp hair loss, which in the child can cause significant concern. The four most common are discussed below.

Alopecia areata

This is a common cause of hair loss in childhood. Typically smooth areas of skin with exclamation mark hairs (broken hairs at the edge of active patches) occur (Fig. 27.25). Although most commonly seen as patches on the scalp, this condition can progress to involve the whole scalp or, more rarely, all body hair. The prognosis tends to be worse the more widespread the condition. It is linked to other autoimmune conditions such as vitiligo (a condition with primary loss of skin melanin pigment).

Traumatic alopecia

This can be intentional or unintentional. Typically traction from ponytails or other similar hairstyles may cause patchy alopecia. Intentional hair loss can be much more difficult to manage and used to be termed trichotillomania. Underlying triggers such as social deprivation in the home environment should be actively sought. In severe cases the appearance of the hair is often bizarre, with unusual patterns. It is interesting to note that trichotillomania may follow alopecia areata,

- Streptococcal infection
- Tuberculosis
- Sarcoidosis
- Drugs
- Inflammatory bowel disease
- Idiopathic

possibly as a consequence of the attention the child has been receiving for the original complaint.

Scarring alopecia

Any cause of scarring to the hair follicle will result in an area of alopecia. This can be difficult to distinguish from other causes.

Systemic disease

Endocrine abnormalities, such as hypothyroidism or diabetes, can produce hair loss.

Erythema nodosum

Typical erythema nodosum (EN) presents with discrete red painful nodules over the anterior shins that may later become confluent. In around 30% of cases no cause is found but the differential diagnosis is wide (Box 27.11). Lesions may involve other sites, including thighs, arms and even the face. Resolution takes around 5–6 weeks and typically the lesions become bluish in colour as they resolve.

Henoch–Schönlein purpura

This is the most common childhood vasculitis (Fig. 27.26) and is discussed in detail on page 623. In around one-third of children an upper respiratory infection precedes the eruption, with purpura predominantly over the extensor surfaces of the limbs. It is usually self-limiting but can involve gastrointestinal vessels, causing colic; although renal involvement is usually transient, glomerulonephritis can occasionally occur.

Problem-orientated topic:

an infant with flesh-coloured wheals

A 1-year-old boy suddenly develops a widespread irritant eruption consisting of flesh-coloured wheals. He had been eating strawberries just before the onset, a fruit that he had never eaten before.

What is the likely diagnosis?

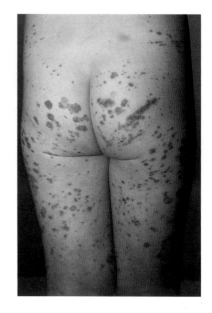

Fig. 27.26 Henoch–Schönlein purpura. A 6-year-old girl with purpura over buttocks and lower limbs.

What is the likely diagnosis?

Acute urticaria is most likely. Certain foods are one of the common causes of acute urticaria.

Problem-orientated topic:

a girl with scaling lesions

A 12-year-old girl developed a single scaling patch over the left upper chest a week ago. She had been well previously. Her family doctor diagnosed ringworm and prescribed a topical antifungal cream. The lesion has not altered. However, multiple smaller slightly scaling lesions are now appearing over the trunk and some seem to follow the line of the rib cage over the posterior chest.

What is your diagnosis?

What is your diagnosis?

Pityriasis rosea seems most likely. The description of the first or so-called herald patch and the trunk distribution is suggestive of this self-limiting condition.

Edited by Henry L. Halliday, Alfred Tenore

Childhood Disorders I

MODULE

SIX

Niamh Lynch   Paola Nicolaides   David W. Webb

CHAPTER

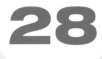

Central nervous system

LEARNING OUTCOMES

By the end of this chapter you should:

- Have an understanding of central nervous system embryology and brain development
- Be familiar with the principal disorders of brain development
- Be able to identify common episodic events in childhood
- Be familiar with the common epilepsy syndromes in children
- Be familiar with the common electroencephalogram patterns of childhood epilepsy
- Be aware of the common causes of epilepsy
- Know how to manage a child with status epilepticus
- Know how to assess and manage a child with hemiplegia
- Be familiar with the common childhood brain tumours and their presentation
- Know the causes of acute and chronic ataxia in childhood
- Be familiar with the common muscle diseases of childhood
- Know how to assess a child with neurodevelopmental regression
- Know how to evaluate a child with macrocephaly
- Have an understanding of neural tube defects and their management.

MODULE SIX

Basic science of brain development

Embryology of the central nervous system (Table 28.1)

In the third and fourth weeks of gestation the nervous system begins on the dorsal aspect of the embryo as a plate of tissue differentiating in the middle of the ectoderm. This differentiation results in formation of the neural plate and is induced by the underlying mesoderm at about 18 days of gestation. The lateral margins of this plate invaginate to form the neural tube, which in turn gives rise to the central nervous system (CNS); the cavity of this tube becomes the ventricular system. Neuralation, or fusion of the neural folds, begins at 22 days and is complete by 28 days. Neural tube defects arise as a result of the failure of the neural plate to form the neural tube during the first 28 days of gestation; they can vary in severity and occur at any level between the rostral and caudal ends.

Development of the prosencephalon (future brain) and its cleavage into two hemispheres (prosencephalic cleavage) occur in the second and third months and are induced by factors that influence development of the face; thus severe disorders of brain development at this time may result in facial anomalies.

The ventricular zone is the site of proliferation of neurons and glial cells, which occurs between 3 and 4 months. Neuronal cells migrate outwards from the area of the primitive ventricles and are guided as they travel by a network of glial fibres. This process ultimately results in the formation of the six-layered cerebral cortex. Subplate neurons are the first to migrate and act as the trigger for neuronal organization, which begins from the fifth month of gestation and continues into early childhood. During this phase there is glial differentiation and an orientation of neurons and their dendritic synaptic contacts, including a process of selective cell death and pruning. Myelination in the human nervous system begins in the peripheral nerves, where motor roots myelinate before sensory roots. Central brain myelination

begins to appear prior to birth and is most prominent in the major sensory systems of vision and hearing and in the major motor systems of the brainstem. Higher-level myelination progresses over decades.

Disorders of brain development and their consequences are listed in Table 28.2.

Neurons and synapses

Nervous tissue contains two distinct classes of cell: the neuron cell and the glial cell, both of which arise from the ectoderm. Neurons consist of a cell body, axon and dendrites that transmit impulses. Neurons are classified functionally as afferent (sensory), efferent (motor) and interneurons. The excitable nature of their resting membrane potential allows them to act as signalling units for behavioural responses.

The synapse is the point where neurons transmit signals between each other and consists of a presynaptic and post-synaptic membrane. Electrical synapses are extremely rapid and are facilitated by gap junction channels in the neuron membrane. Chemical synapse transmission is mediated by neurotransmitters that are stored in vesicles in the axon terminal. The main excitatory neurotransmitter in the brain and spinal cord is glutamate, while the major inhibitory neurotransmitters are gamma-aminobutyric acid (GABA) and glycine. To transmit impulses, neurotransmitters must attach to receptors, and it is the receptor and not the transmitter that decides whether the synaptic response is excitatory or inhibitory. Receptors are either ligand-gated ion channels or are coupled to an intracellular guanosine triphosphate (GTP) binding protein.

Table 28.1 Major events in human brain development and their timing

Event	Timing
Primary neuralation	Weeks 3–4
Prosencephalic development	Months 2–3
Neuronal proliferation	Months 3–4
Neuronal migration	Months 3–5
Neuronal organization	Month 5–years postnatal
Myelination	Birth–years postnatal

Source: Volpe 2001.

Table 28.2 Disorders of brain development and their consequences

Disorder	Consequence
Neuralation	Neural tube defects (spina bifida)
Prosencephalic development	Holoprosencephaly Agenesis of the corpus callosum Agenesis of the septum pellucidum Septo-optic dysplasia Fetal hydrocephalus (some cases)
Neuronal proliferation	Microencephaly Macroencephaly/cerebral gigantism Hemi-megaloencephaly
Neuronal migration	Schizencephaly Lissencephaly Polymicrogyria Heterotopias Focal cortical dysplasia ± Agenesis of the corpus callosum
Neuronal organization	Learning disability, autism and epilepsy

Neural pathways

The major functional systems in the human nervous system are the motor and sensory systems. The cortico-spinal (pyramidal) tract and corticonuclear fibres are the pathways of voluntary movement. These tracts arise in the primary and premotor cortex of the frontal lobe, travel down the posterior limb of the internal capsule, and then tightly bundle as they exit the cerebral hemispheres to form the cerebral peduncles. As they pass through the pons, the tracts rotate so that the corticonuclear fibres lie dorsally. In the medulla the corticonuclear fibres terminate on the cranial nerve nuclei, and the corticospinal fibres come together to form the pyramids. At the caudal end of the medulla 70–90% of the fibres decussate to form the lateral corticospinal tract, while the uncrossed fibres form the anterior corticospinal tract. Once in the ventral (or anterior) horn, fibres synapse with interneurons (most common) or directly with the α-motor neuron.

The two main sensory pathways in the spinal cord are the dorsal columns that carry the sensations of vibration, fine touch and proprioception, and the lateral spinal thalamic tracts that carry the more vaguely interpreted signals of pain, crude touch and temperature. The dorsal column fibres are well myelinated to transmit fast and accurate impulses. They travel up the cord without crossing until the medulla, and continue to the thalamus via the medial lemniscus and on to the post-central gyrus via the posterior limb of the internal capsule. The lateral spinal thalamic tracts cross over immediately on entering the cord and then follow a similar pathway.

Episodic events

Problem-orientated topic:

the child presenting with funny turns

(See also Chapter 24 for a more detailed description.)

Aurora is a 3-year-old girl who is brought to the accident and emergency department after a fall from her bike. After the fall she became extremely pale and floppy, then stiffened, extended her neck and jerked her arms and legs. She was incontinent. The episode lasted less than a minute and she was upset afterwards. She is otherwise a normal child.

Q1. Has this girl had an epileptic seizure?

Q2. What investigations are needed?

BOX 28.1 History-taking in the assessment of clinical events: the 'five Ss'	
Scene	What was the setting in which the event happened?
Start	How did it begin?
Sequence	What actually happened and in what order?
Stop	How did it stop?
Sequelae	Were there any after-effects?

Q1. Has this girl had an epileptic seizure?

This event involved truncal stiffening, limb jerking and incontinence, and on the surface might appear to be an epileptic seizure. However, there are several features that should raise suspicion of an alternative mechanism and the case highlights the importance of taking the whole event in context. The 'five Ss' will help with this (Box 28.1).

Q2. What investigations are needed?

This girl's episode occurred in the context of a minor injury, began with pallor and hypotonia and was brief. The history would be compatible with a reflex anoxic syncopal event (Ch. 24) and this should be considered. It would also be important to exclude a prolonged QT interval and electrocardiography (ECG) should be undertaken; electroencephalography (EEG) in this situation may be considered but may be misleading.

Other paroxysmal events seen in childhood

There are a number of non-epileptic paroxysmal conditions that occur in childhood. Those associated with anoxia/hypoxia and syncope are most likely to be confused with epilepsy (Box 28.2).

Epileptic seizures, epilepsy and status epilepticus

Problem-orientated topic:

the child with an epileptic seizure

Luca is a 2-year-old boy who is admitted following an episode of loss of consciousness associated with stiffening of his trunk, cyanosis, salivation, eye rolling and limb jerking for 4 minutes. Luca is febrile on admission. He is otherwise a normal child.

What is this clinical event?

BOX 28.2 Non-epileptic paroxysmal events

Anoxic syncope (Ch. 24)
- Blue breath-holding
- Pallid syncope (reflex anoxic syncope)
- Vasovagal syncope
- Cardiogenic syncope (prolonged QT interval)
- Obstructive syncope (Sandifer's syndrome, suffocation)

Involuntary movements
- Rigors, jitteriness, shuddering
- Paroxysmal dyskinesias
- Alternating hemiplegia of infancy

Migraine equivalents (Ch. 24)
- Benign paroxysmal vertigo
- Cyclical vomiting
- Paroxysmal torticollis

Behaviour
- Day-dreaming
- Hyperventilation
- Pseudoseizures
- Gratification phenomena

Sleep disorders (Ch. 24)
- Night terrors
- Sleep myoclonus
- Narcolepsy/cataplexy

What is this clinical event?

This boy has had a symptomatic seizure. The most common cause of this in his age group would be a 'febrile seizure'. Hypoglycaemia, electrolyte disturbances and intracranial infection or trauma may also cause symptomatic seizures and should be considered.

Precipitating factors to be considered
- Fever
- Meningo-encephalitis
- Head injury
- Hypoxic–ischaemic injury
- Toxin (endogenous/exogenous)
- Metabolic and electrolyte disturbance.

Febrile convulsions are considered in detail in Chapter 24.

Problem-orientated topic:

the child with epilepsy

Riccardo is seen in clinic with a history of events occurring in sleep. These began at the age of 7 years and cluster in the early morning. He comes to his parents' room and is upset. His face is twitching and he is salivating and cannot talk. He appears to remain awake throughout these events, which last 3–4 minutes.

Q1. Does this boy have epilepsy?

Q2. What type of epileptic seizure is Riccardo having?

Q3. What is the management?

Q4. What causes epilepsy?

Q1. Does this boy have epilepsy?

Epilepsy is the tendency to have recurrent unprovoked epileptic seizures. These are clinical events that arise from abnormal cerebral electrical activity. They are paroxysmal, stereotypical and unpredictable, and are characterized by their clinical manifestations and their effect on consciousness. Other non-epileptic causes of 'funny turns' must be considered (Ch. 24).

Q2. What type of epileptic seizure is Riccardo having?

See Box 28.3. See also International League Against Epilepsy.

 http://www.ilae-epilepsy.org/Visitors/Centre/ctf/ctfoverview.cfm

BOX 28.3 Classification of seizures

- Partial:
  - Simple
  - Complex partial
  - Secondary generalized
- Generalized:
  - Tonic–clonic, tonic, clonic
  - Absence
  - Atonic
  - Myoclonic
  - Infantile spasms
- Unclassifiable

Simple and complex partial seizures

Partial seizures have a focal onset. In a simple partial seizure the child remains fully aware and, if old enough, will recall the event in detail. In a complex partial seizure the child has altered consciousness with minimal recollection of the event. Both simple and complex partial seizures may progress to loss of consciousness. The typical simple partial seizure might involve a localized sensation, with associated motor or autonomic activity that the child is aware of and cannot suppress. The typical complex partial seizure might involve staring, confusion and automatic behaviours such as fumbling. Complex partial seizures of temporal lobe origin are often preceded by an aura of fear or an epigastric discomfort. Gustatory, visual or auditory hallucinations may occur.

Generalized seizures

Seizures without focal onset and with loss of consciousness from the onset are called primary generalized seizures:

- *Generalized tonic–clonic seizures*. The generalized tonic–clonic seizure is characterized by a sudden loss of consciousness, associated with stiffening of the trunk and limbs (tonic phase) that lasts about 10 seconds and is followed by rhythmic jerking of the limbs that is usually symmetrical (clonic phase). The patient may bite the tongue or be incontinent of urine and faeces. This phase usually lasts 2–5 minutes, and is followed by a post-ictal period of unconsciousness and confusion that can last up to 1 hour. The patient usually has no recollection of the seizure or the post-ictal period.

- *Absence seizures*. Absence seizures involve an abrupt brief cessation of activity, followed by a vacant stare and unresponsiveness. The child has no recollection of the event and will resume activity as if nothing has happened. There are no major motor phenomena, but the eyes may roll upwards and there may be automatisms such as lip smacking or picking at clothes. The events can be induced by hyperventilation and this can be a useful observation in the clinic.

- *Atonic, myoclonic and infantile spasms*. The atonic seizure involves an abrupt loss of tone usually associated with a head nod and/or fall. Myoclonic seizures involve single brief jerks. Infantile spasms, also known as 'salaam attacks', are brief forceful episodes of truncal flexion or extension, associated with elevations of the arms and legs. They typically occur in clusters on waking from sleep and appear to upset the child. Their usual age of onset is 3–12 months. Infantile spasms can be associated with prior brain injury, infection or cerebral malformation, but remain unexplained in about 25% of cases. Idiopathic cases and those with previously normal development have a better prognosis.

Epilepsy syndromes

The combination of seizure type, age, developmental profile, family history and EEG features is used to identify epilepsy syndromes (Box 28.4).

- *Childhood absence epilepsy*. Onset is between 3 and 12 years and is characterized by frequent brief absence seizures lasting 5–20 seconds. The child is developmentally normal and there is a

---

BOX 28.4 Epilepsy syndromes

Idiopathic

- Benign neonatal convulsions
- Benign infantile myoclonic epilepsy
- Childhood absence epilepsy
- Benign Rolandic epilepsy
- Juvenile myoclonic epilepsy

Cryptogenic/symptomatic

- West syndrome
- Lennox–Gastaut syndrome

Source: Roger et al 2005.

BOX 28.5 EEG findings in benign Rolandic epilepsy

- High-voltage diphasic centro-temporal spikes
- Unilateral or bilateral
- Activated by drowsiness and sleep
- Do not relate to seizure frequency or duration
- May be found in unaffected siblings

BOX 28.6 EEG findings in juvenile myoclonic epilepsy

- Polyspike and wave complexes
- Generalized discharges at > 3 Hz
- Photosensitivity is common

---

strong genetic predisposition. Seizures tend to remit in adolescence. EEG findings are bilateral, synchronous and symmetrical spike/wave discharges, at a frequency of 3 Hz.

- *Benign Rolandic epilepsy* (Box 28.5). Onset is at 3–13 years with a peak at 9 years and intelligence is normal. Seizures are typically nocturnal and begin with unilateral paraesthesia of the face, lips and tongue, associated with an ipsilateral motor seizure of the face. Awareness is maintained but the child is unable to speak and may salivate. Seizures last 1–2 minutes and nocturnal episodes may become generalized. Daytime seizures are rare and do not tend to result in loss of consciousness. Most children do not require treatment and the seizures typically resolve spontaneously during puberty.

- *Juvenile myoclonic epilepsy* (Box 28.6). Onset is between 8 and 26 years of age and intelligence is normal. Generalized tonic–clonic seizures provoked by sleep deprivation and brief absence seizures bring the child to medical attention. A specific enquiry about early morning brief extensor upper limb myoclonic jerks confirms the diagnosis.

- *West syndrome* (Box 28.7). A triad of infantile spasms, developmental arrest or regression and

- High-voltage disorganized and chaotic background
- High-voltage asynchronous spike/polyspike wave discharges
- A decremental (drop in voltage) seizure pattern

Table 28.3 Treatment of childhood seizures

Seizure type	First-line drug
Generalized tonic–clonic	Carbamazepine, sodium valproate, lamotrigine
Absence	Ethosuximade, lamotrigine, sodium valproate
Myoclonic	Sodium valproate
Tonic	Lamotrigine, sodium valproate
Atonic	Lamotrigine, sodium valproate
Partial	Carbamazepine, lamotrigine
Infantile spasms	Steroids, vigabatrin

a specific EEG pattern is the hallmark of this syndrome. The prognosis is poor and dependent on the aetiology. There is an associated mortality of 5%, with half of the survivors having severe developmental delay and half suffering from persistent seizures.

Q3. What is the management?

See Table 28.3.

http://www.nice.org.uk/CG020

NICE guidelines for epilepsy

Q4. What causes epilepsy?

See Box 28.8.

Neurofibromatosis

Neurofibromatosis type 1 (NF-1) accounts for 85% of all cases of neurofibromatosis. It has an incidence of 1/3000 to 1/4000, is dominantly inherited with 98% penetrance and approximately 30% of cases represent new mutations. It is linked to a gene on chromosome 17q11.2 that encodes a protein (neurofibromin) thought to act as a tumour suppressor gene.

Clinical features

The earliest features are multiple café au lait spots over the trunk and limbs, and freckling in the axilla (Fig. 28.1) and perineum. Pigmented hamartomas in the iris (Lisch nodules) may be visible with the assistance of a slit lamp and these increase in frequency through childhood. Neurofibromas are benign subcutaneous nodular tumours located along peripheral nerves. These increase with age and are rarely seen in childhood.

Idiopathic (genetic)	**80%**
Symptomatic	**20%**

- Acquired:
  - Post-infectious
  - Post-traumatic
  - Post-ischaemic
- Developmental:
  - Cerebral dysgenesis
  - Chromosomal
  - Neurocutaneous syndromes

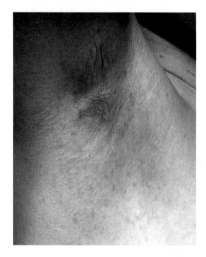

Fig. 28.1 Axillary freckling in neurofibromatosis type 1 (NF-1)

Plexiform neurofibromas represent a rare but serious and disfiguring complication of NF-1, particularly when they involve the head and neck. Bone involvement can lead to pseudoarthrosis and bowing of the long bones, and there is also an increased risk of scoliosis (present in 20%).

Complications

These include optic gliomas (15–20% of NF-1), which may be bilateral and tend to remain stable, particularly when located anterior to the optic chiasm. Other intracranial or intraspinal tumours (astrocytomas) are less common in NF-1 but there is an increased risk of malignancies in general. There is also a higher risk of mild learning difficulties and of hydrocephalus (as a consequence of aqueduct stenosis). There is an association with renal artery stenosis, systemic hypertension, a higher rate of vascular accidents and growth retardation.

Diagnosis

The diagnosis is clinical and based on the finding of two or more of the following:

- Six or more café au lait spots > 5 mm in diameter in prepubertal children or > 15 mm in diameter in post-pubertal children

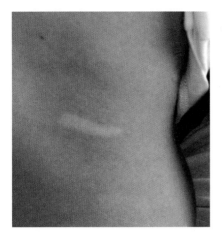

Fig. 28.2 **Depigmented ash-leaf macule in tuberous sclerosis**

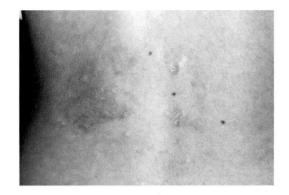

Fig. 28.3 **Shagreen patch**

- One plexiform neurofibroma or two or more neurofibromas of any type
- Axillary or inguinal freckling (Crowe sign)
- Optic gliomas
- Two or more Lisch nodules (iris hamartomas)
- Distinctive osseous lesion (e.g. sphenoid dysplasia or thinning of long bone cortex with or without pseudoarthritis)
- First degree relative with NF-1

Management

This includes genetic counselling and annual surveillance for complications. Some children with NF-1 will require neuroimaging with input from paediatric neurology and neurosurgery, orthopaedic and plastic surgery and ophthalmology.

Tuberous sclerosis

Tuberous sclerosis (TS) is a dominantly inherited neurocutaneous syndrome with a high spontaneous mutation rate (70%). Affected parents may not be aware that they have the condition and require careful examination and brain imaging before the risk of recurrence in future pregnancies can be given. The incidence is about 1/10 000. Gene loci have been identified on chromosomes 9q (TSC1 hamartin 25%) and 16p (TSC2 tuberin-more severe 75%), and are believed to represent 'tumour suppressor genes'. The condition is named after the cerebral 'potato-like' hamartomas (tubers) in the brain that become calcified (sclerosis).

Clinical features

The earliest cutaneous features of the condition are ash-leaf-shaped hypopigmented macules (Fig. 28.2), seen best with the aid of a Wood's lamp in a darkened room. These may be followed by the development of a shagreen patch (a roughened area of skin over the lumbar spine, Fig. 28.3), facial angiofibromas (adenoma sebaceum) over the nasolabial folds, cheeks and chin and periungual fibromas. The latter only become evident in late childhood and early puberty.

The majority of affected individuals (60%) develop epileptic seizures, infantile spasms being the most common, and onset usually before the age of 5 years. Cognitive difficulties are seen in 50% and are associated with infantile spasms, early onset of intractable seizures and multiple cerebral tubers. The condition is also associated with cardiac rhabdomyomas (fetal hydrops, neonatal heart failure), polycystic kidneys, renal and hepatic angiomyolipomas and retinal astrocytomas (and phakomas).

Diagnosis

Diagnosis is made on clinical and neuroradiological features and is based on the presence of two or more of the following:
- Facial angiofibromas or forehead plaque
- Non-traumatic ungual or periungual fibromas
- Hypomelanotic macules (≥ 3)
- Shagreen patch (connective tissue naevus)
- Retinal astrocytomas
- Cortical tuber
- Subependymal nodule
- Subependymal giant cell astrocytoma
- Cardiac rhabdomyoma, single or multiple
- Lymphangiomyomatosis
- Renal angiomyolipoma.

Management

This requires a multidisciplinary approach. Long term follow-up should include monitoring of lesion growth with periodic imaging of brain and abdomen. The major issues are control of seizures, surveillance for cognitive deficits and management of behavioural difficulties. There is a higher incidence of autistic behaviour. Vigabatrin for infantile spasms in children with TS has improved seizure control significantly, although this has to be weighed against the risk of potentially irreversible peripheral visual field defects with this drug. Facial angiofibromas may be disfiguring and may benefit from laser therapy.

Sturge–Weber syndrome

Sturge–Weber syndrome is the association between a flat facial angiomatous naevus (port-wine stain), venous angioma of the leptomeninges and choroidal angioma or glaucoma of the eye. Only 8% of all children with facial port-wine stains have the syndrome, but this increases to 25% of those with a port-wine stain in the ophthalmic division of the trigeminal nerve and 33% of children with bilateral facial angiomas. The disorder is sporadic.

Clinical features

The facial lesion is variable in size and does not correlate with the size of the intracranial angioma. Among children with Sturge–Weber syndrome 75–90% will develop seizures. The onset of epilepsy is usually in the first year of life and seizures are frequently resistant to anticonvulsant therapy. Cognitive difficulties occur in 80% and 30% have profound learning disability, most commonly in association with early onset resistant seizures and bilateral cerebral lesions. A hemiplegia develops in 50% of children on the contralateral side to the angioma which is often first noticed after a seizure and may progress in severity with subsequent events. Hemianopia is virtually constant and glaucoma is present in 50%.

Diagnosis

Children who present with focal seizures should have the eyelids and skin above the eye carefully examined for evidence of haemangiomas. Computed tomography (CT) of the brain may reveal 'railroad track' calcification of the cerebral cortex. Contrast-enhanced magnetic resonance imaging (MRI) will demonstrate the pial angioma and local cerebral atrophy.

Management

Among those with intractable epilepsy who fail to respond to standard anticonvulsant medication, a functional hemispherectomy or other resective surgery should be considered. Pulsed dye laser therapy for the facial lesion may be of cosmetic benefit. Regular ophthalmology review for glaucoma is also important.

Problem-orientated topic:

status epilepticus ● ● ● ●

Giulia is a 9-year-old girl with a previous history of epilepsy and mild learning difficulties. She presents to accident and emergency in a generalized tonic–clonic seizure that has lasted at least 35 minutes. You are called to the accident and emergency department to help control her seizures.

Q1. What is the emergency management of this clinical scenario?

Q2. What are the potential causes of this medical emergency?

Q3. What investigations should be undertaken?

Q4. What anticonvulsant drugs should be used?

Q5. What are the potential complications of status epilepticus?

Q1. What is the emergency management of this clinical scenario?

This girl is in status epilepticus. This is defined as a prolonged seizure lasting over 30 minutes or repeated seizures without inter-ictal recovery. Generalized tonic–clonic status is the most common neurological emergency in childhood that requires immediate action.

Management goals are:
- Maintain vital functions.
- Terminate the seizure.
- Identify and treat causal or precipitating factors.

Management protocol is:
- Place the child in lateral prone position.
- Secure airway with soft mouthpiece.
- Administer 100% oxygen.
- Obtain intravenous access.
- Administer emergency anticonvulsant therapy.
- Obtain urgent blood investigations.

Status epilepticus can occur as a consequence of an acute cerebral insult or may be provoked in a child with an underlying seizure tendency by factors such as intercurrent illness, sleep deprivation or anticonvulsant withdrawal.

Q2. What are the potential causes of this medical emergency?

See Box 28.9.

Q3. What investigations should be undertaken?

See Box 28.10.

Q4. What anticonvulsant drugs should be used?

See Table 28.4.

Q5. What are the potential complications of status epilepticus?

See Box 28.11.

Status epilepticus is a life-threatening event, with a mortality of 3–6% and a morbidity of 20%, depending on the aetiology of the seizures. Outcome is affected by duration of the seizure, age (worse under 3 years) and the cause of the status epilepticus.

Hemiplegia

Problem-orientated topic:

acute onset hemiplegia

Lorenzo is 7 years old and presents with a 6-hour history of right-sided weakness that seems to be getting worse. He can no longer stand unsupported and has stopped using his right hand.

Q1. What are the possible causes of Lorenzo's acute hemiplegia?

Q2. What investigations will you order?

Table 28.4 Drug management in status epilepticus

	Intravenous access	No intravenous access
Immediate	Lorazepam 0.1 mg/kg i.v. (give over 30–60 sec)	Diazepam 0.5 mg/kg PR
Seizure continuing at 10 minutes	Lorazepam 0.1 mg/kg i.v. (give over 30–60 sec) (if no pre-hospital benzodiazepine treatment)	Paraldehyde 0.4 ml/kg PR in same volume of olive oil
Seizure continuing at 20 minutes	*Call for senior help* Phenytoin 20 mg/kg i.v. (give over 20 min) OR (if already on phenytoin) Phenobarbital 20 mg/kg i.v. (give over 10 min) AND (if under 3 years with unexplained afebrile status) Pyridoxine 100 mg i.v.	*Call for senior help* Use intra-osseous route
Seizure continuing at 40 minutes	*Contact anaesthetist and paediatric ICU* Consider thiopental 4 mg/kg i.v.	*Contact anaesthetist and paediatric ICU*

PR = per rectum

- Epilepsy: Todd paresis
- Migraine: hemiplegic variant
- Stroke: ischaemic, haemorrhagic
- Tumour: brainstem in particular
- Trauma: extradural or subdural haematoma
- Infection: focal encephalitis, abscess
- Demyelination: acute disseminated encephalomyelitis, multiple sclerosis
- Diabetes: acute hypoglycaemia
- Metabolic: mitochondrial disorders

Q1. What are the possible causes of Lorenzo's acute hemiplegia?

(Box 28.12)

There is a broad differential diagnosis here and a child presenting with acute hemiplegia requires a careful history and examination. In the absence of a history of head trauma, headache, seizure activity or infection the most likely explanation is an acute ischaemic stroke.

Q2. What investigations will you order?

Ultimately the findings on brain imaging will guide further management. CT brain scan is usually the first form of brain imaging; an ischaemic lesion is seen as an area of low density that may not be visible in the first 24 hours post-insult but may with time enhance with intravenous contrast. The infarction is usually in the distribution of a single artery. MRI is preferred for imaging in childhood stroke; with an ischaemic lesion it will reveal an area of low density on T1-weighted images and high signal on T2-weighted images. Brain haemorrhage is seen as an area of increased density on a non-contrast CT scan and may be associated with significant oedema and midline shift. In addition transcranial and duplex/Doppler ultrasound examination, MRA and conventional angiography may be considered.

Stroke

Childhood stroke is rare, with an incidence of 2.6 and 3.1 per 100 000 white and black children per year, respectively. Ischaemic stroke usually presents as a sudden-onset hemiparesis or focal neurological disturbance in a previously well child. Additional clinical features vary and are related to the age of the child and location of the stroke. They may include hemisensory loss, hemianopia, dysphasia and ataxia. With involvement of the vertebrobasilar vessels (much rarer and caused by trauma-dissection, cervical spine abnormalities, vascular malformations), features may also include quadriplegia, vomiting, tremor, vertigo, ataxia, dysarthria, oculomotor palsies and lower cranial nerve involvement. Haemorrhagic stroke is most commonly seen with structural anomalies of the cerebral vasculature and disorders of coagulation. While hemiparesis is also common with haemorrhagic stroke, the dominant symptoms are often headache, vomiting and seizures. There may also be features of raised intracranial pressure.

Risk factors for childhood stroke

Risk factors for stroke in children are very different from those in adults (Table 28.5). With thorough evaluation, one or more risk factors can be identified in about 75% of children with ischaemic infarction and an even higher number of those with haemorrhagic stroke. Sickle cell disease is one of the most common causes world-wide and varicella infection is increasingly recognized as a risk factor.

Investigations in a child with ischaemic stroke

- ECG, echocardiography (cardiac consultation)
- MR angiography
- Carotid Doppler studies

Table 28.5 Conditions predisposing to stroke in children

Condition	Examples
Ischaemic stroke	
Congenital heart disease	Aortic lesions, complex congenital heart defect
Acquired heart disease	Endocarditis, cardiomyopathy
Vasculitis	Meningitis, varicella, HIV, Kawasaki disease
Vasculopathy	Moyamoya, fibromuscular dysplasia, Sturge–Weber syndrome
Vasospasm	Migraine
Haematological	Sickle cell anaemia, disseminated intravascular coagulation (DIC), thrombotic tendency
Metabolic	Homocystinuria, mitochondrial disorders
Trauma	Arterial dissection, child abuse
Haemorrhagic stroke	
Vascular lesions	Arteriovenous malformations, fistulas, aneurysm
Haematological	Haemophilia, thrombocytopenia, sickle cell anaemia
Lesional	Brain tumour, haemorrhagic infarction

- Ischaemic stroke: consider low-dose aspirin prophylaxis
- Ischaemic stroke in a hospital setting: consider tissue plasminogen activator
- Sickle cell disease: exchange transfusion
- Haemorrhagic stroke: immediate referral to unit with neurosurgical facilities
- Vascular (arterial) abnormalities -dissection-, or prothrombotic tendency: consider anticoagulation with low molecular weight heparin then warfarin

Source: Kirkham 1999.

- Thrombophilia screen (haematology consultation)
- Sickle screen
- Varicella serology
- Homocysteine levels
- ± Cerebrospinal fluid (CSF) lactate.

Management and prognosis (Box 28.13)

Treatment depends on the cause of the stroke and the underlying condition in the period immediately after the stroke. If the child is left with a persisting neurological deficit, multidisciplinary input is required, including physiotherapy, occupational therapy, speech therapy and psychological support. Adverse outcomes after childhood stroke include death in 10%, recurrence in 20%, and neurological deficits in two-thirds of survivors with epileptic seizures being relatively uncommon. A poor outcome can be predicted if the hemiplegia persists after a month, if the infarct is cortical and with bilateral disease.

Headaches

Problem-orientated topic:

the child with headaches

(See also Ch. 24.)

Mattia is 8 years old. For the past 2 months he has been complaining of headaches, which are particularly severe in the mornings. He was initially thought to have school refusal but recently has started to vomit. His examination appears normal.

Q1. What is the likely cause of Mattia's headache?

Q2. What is the most appropriate investigation?

- Cerebral tumour
- Hydrocephalus
- Cerebral oedema
- Cerebral abscess
- Idiopathic intracranial hypertension (pseudotumour)
- Cerebral venous obstruction (venous thrombosis)
- Intracranial haemorrhage
- Hypercarbia

Q1. What is the likely cause of Mattia's headache? (Box 28.14)

This is a sinister history and suggests raised intracranial pressure. The headache associated with raised intracranial pressure is worse when lying down, typically peaks in the early morning and may be associated with neck stiffness, vomiting and/or irritability. Mattia should be specifically questioned on the presence of diplopia and carefully examined for evidence of papilloedema.

Q2. What is the most appropriate investigation?

The absence of neurological findings is not reassuring and you need to image this boy immediately to rule out a space-occupying lesion or hydrocephalus. A posterior fossa tumour (infratentorial: 43–63% of all brain tumours) would be the most common cause of acquired hydrocephalus with raised intracranial pressure. CT scan with contrast will establish whether a lesion is present or not. If an abnormality is identified, one would proceed to further imaging with MRI (with and without contrast). Space-occupying lesions within the cerebral hemispheres in children will usually present with focal neurological deficits, seizures or signs and symptoms of raised intracranial pressure.

Brain tumours (Box 28.15) (see also p. 770)

Brain and spinal tumours are the most frequent solid tumour in children under 15 years of age. They are almost always primary as opposed to metastatic and the majority are infratentorial. Treatment options include surgery (often the primary treatment), radiation therapy and chemotherapy. The prognosis for brain tumours depends on the location and histology. Brainstem gliomas have a particularly poor prognosis.

- Astrocytomas (40%):
  - Juvenile cystic astrocytoma (Fig. 28.4) — cerebellar, slow-growing, good prognosis with surgery
  - Non-juvenile — often cerebral hemispheres, prognosis variable
- Embryonal tumours (25%):
  - Medulloblastoma — cerebellar, can have spinal metastases, prognosis poor
  - Primitive neuroectodermal tumour (PNET)
  - Atypical teratoid/rhabdoid
- Ependymoma (8%)
- Others:
  - Oligodendrogliomas
  - Glioneural/neuronal tumours
  - Choroid plexus tumours
  - Pineal tumours
  - Craniopharyngioma

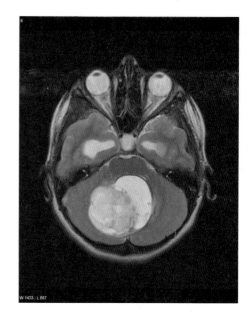

Fig. 28.4 MRI showing cystic astrocytoma in posterior fossa

Ataxia

Problem-orientated topic:

the child who goes off his feet

Alessandro, who is 18 months old and has been walking since the age of 1 year, is referred to the emergency department by his primary care physician because his mother reports that he is unable to stand up. She noticed some unsteadiness a week ago but he has deteriorated and now can no longer walk. He had an MMR vaccination 2 weeks previously but has been well since and there is no history of trauma.

Alessandro is irritable but afebrile. His balance is poor, even when sitting. When his mother hands him his pacifier (dummy), he has difficulty placing it in his mouth. He cannot stand or walk, but appears to have normal power in his limbs. Reflexes are normal. It looks as if he has nystagmus.

Q1. Why is Alessandro ataxic?

Q2. What investigations would you perform?

Q1. Why is Alessandro ataxic?

The term ataxia is used to imply a disturbance in gait. In its strictest sense, ataxia is caused by a dysfunction in the cerebellum or its major input systems from the frontal lobes or posterior columns of the spinal cord. The child with cerebellar ataxia will be unable to stand with two feet together and will have a broad-based and staggering gait. There may be associated limb ataxia, intention tremor, past pointing, bobbing of the head (titubation), dysarthria and/or nystagmus.

It is important to remember that an unsteady child may have pathology outside of the cerebellum, including:

- Peripheral weakness (myopathic-proximal; neuropathic-distal).
- Non-convulsive status epilepticus.
- Bifrontal white matter disease
- Vestibular or labyrinthine dysfunction
- Visual impairment, developmental coordination disorder (dyspraxia)

It can be difficult to distinguish between cerebellar, sensory, vestibular and other causes of acute ataxia, and other signs of CNS dysfunction need to be carefully sought.

The most common causes of acute ataxia in childhood are post-infection and drug ingestion. The differential diagnosis is outlined in Box 28.16. Brain tumours usually cause a slowly progressive ataxia but many slowly progressive ataxias may be noticed acutely to begin with (Box 28.17).

This boy could have post-infectious/vaccine-related ataxia but there are unusual features, including the subacute onset, marked irritability, nystagmus and upper limb signs. On closer inspection the boy's abnormal eye movements are not nystagmus but rather the jerky and chaotic movements of opsoclonus–myoclonus syndrome. This is associated with a significant risk of occult neuroblastoma and further investigation is

Ingestion of drugs or intoxication

- One of the most common causes in a previously healthy child
- Drug ingestion is usually associated with drowsiness and lethargy (onset over hours)

Acute post/para-infectious cerebellar ataxia

- Varicella is the most common association
- Ataxia is maximal at onset and settles spontaneously over 4–6 weeks

Encephalitis

- Ataxia can be the initial presentation of encephalitis, usually of the brainstem

Space-occupying lesion

- Posterior fossa tumours usually present with insidious onset but can present acutely if there is bleeding into the tumour, a sudden shift in position or rapid growth

Acute disseminating encephalomyelitis (ADEM)

- Usually affects cerebral hemispheres but can be confined to the cerebellum
- Usually preceded by a non-specific viral infection but can occur after vaccination

Basilar migraine

- Benign paroxysmal vertigo is probably a childhood variant of basilar migraine

Rare causes

- Familial episodic ataxia (type 1 and 2)
- Metabolic (mitochondrial, urea cycle disorders, organic acidaemias)
- Neuroblastoma (opsoclonus–myoclonus syndrome)
- Vertebrobasilar dissection (brainstem stroke)
- Multiple sclerosis

Brain tumours

- Cerebellar astrocytomas, embryonal tumours and ependymomas

Developmental malformations of the posterior fossa

- Cerebellar hypoplasias
- Dandy–Walker malformation
- Chiari malformation

Hereditary ataxias

- Friedreich ataxia
- Ataxia telangiectasia
- Ataxia oculomotor apraxia
- Mitochondrial disorders
- Hereditary spinocerebellar ataxias

Demyelination

- Multiple sclerosis

- Urine toxicology (if relevant blood alcohol or drug levels)
- Viral serology
- Brain imaging (CT/MRI brain)

needed, including urinary catecholamines and MRI of the thorax and abdomen. If these investigations are negative, an isotope MIBG scan should be considered.

Q2. What investigations would you perform?

See Box 28.18. In addition consider, where appropriate, the following tests: metabolic tests, cholesterol and lipid profile, Vit E, CK, LFTS, alpha fetoprotein, blood film, EMG/NCV.

Friedreich ataxia

Friedreich ataxia is an autosomal recessive disease with a prevalence of about 1/50 000 and accounts for half of all cases of hereditary ataxia. The gene protein known as 'Frataxin' includes a repeat GAA sequence on chromosome 9q13. It affects the central sensory pathways in the posterior columns and spinocerebellar tracts of the spinal cord and the efferent cerebellar and corticospinal tracts. Large myelinated peripheral sensory nerves are also affected.

Clinical features

Onset of symptoms is typically around puberty but early- and late-onset cases exist. Ataxia with a broad-based gait, pes cavus and clumsiness are among the first manifestations. Scoliosis and hypertrophic cardiomyopathy rarely precede neurological symptoms. Limb dysmetria, action tremor and dysarthria develop with time. Absent deep tendon reflexes and diminished joint position and vibration sensation, with extensor plantar responses and pes cavus, are typical findings. The eyes show abnormalities in smooth pursuit and saccadic movement. The majority of patients develop cardiac complications including a cardiomyopathy, cardiac failure and arrhythmias. A smaller proportion may develop optic atrophy, deafness and diabetes mellitus. The disease progresses throughout childhood and the patient is usually wheelchair-bound an average of 10–15 years after onset of symptoms. Cognitive function usually remains intact.

Diagnosis

MRI reveals atrophy of the spinal cord but cerebral imaging is usually normal until disease is advanced. Sensory nerve action potentials are severely reduced or absent, while sensory and motor nerve conduction velocities are normal. Most patients are homozygous for the expansion of a GAA triplet repeat sequence in the *Frataxin* gene on chromosome 9.

Management

There is no specific therapy. Coenzyme Q with Vitamin E, and Idebenone have been used recently with some beneficial effects. Multidisciplinary supportive care is helpful and surveillance for cardiac involvement, diabetes and scoliosis is important.

Ataxia telangiectasia

This is an autosomal recessive, progressive neurodegenerative disorder associated with significant immunodeficiency in most patients and a risk of malignancy. It is the most common recessive ataxic disorder in children under 5 years of age. The gene has been mapped to chromosome 11q22–23 and produces a protein, ATM, which has a role in DNA repair. Numerous mutations have been identified.

Clinical features

Truncal ataxia is usually evident before the age of 3 years, and choreoathetosis and oculomotor apraxia (limitation of ocular movement to command) are other prominent early neurological features. Telangiectasia usually develops after the onset of neurological symptoms and can be seen on the bulbar conjunctivae, neck and ears. Intelligence is usually normal but motor disability is progressive, with the typical child requiring a wheelchair by the age of 10 years. The leading causes of death are infection, malignancy and non-specific pulmonary failure.

Diagnosis

In infancy ataxia telangiectasia can be confused with mild cerebral palsy, acute infectious or episodic ataxia, ataxia with oculomotor apraxia or other rare genetic and mitochondrial disorders. By the age of 10 years a clinical diagnosis is usually readily apparent. Cerebellar atrophy is usually not seen on MRI in young patients. Three routine tests support a diagnosis: serum alpha-fetoprotein levels, karyotyping with special attention to inversions and translocations involving chromosomes 7 and 14, increased chromosome breakage points and B- and T-cell immune studies. Deficiencies in IgE, IgA and IgG2 may also be found. CT and brain MRI may show evidence of non-specific cerebellar atrophy.

BOX 28.19 Conditions associated with cerebellar hypoplasia

- Dandy–Walker malformation: agenesis of the cerebellar vermis, 4th ventricular cyst and hydrocephalus
- Joubert syndrome: vermis agenesis, neonatal breathing disturbance, abnormal eye movements
- Smith–Lemli–Opitz syndrome: dysmorphic syndrome, learning disability and low plasma cholesterol
- Fetal alcohol syndrome
- Trisomies 13 and 18, fragile X syndrome

BOX 28.20 Conditions associated with progressive cerebellar atrophy

- Pontocerebellar hypoplasia type I
- Carbohydrate-deficient glycoprotein syndrome
- Spinocerebellar degenerative conditions
- Mitochondrial disorders
- Tay–Sachs disease
- Menkes disease
- Joubert syndrome

Management

This is focused on neuro-rehabilitation and medical management of immunodeficiency (consider regular immunoglobulin infusions) and surveillance for malignancy. It is important to limit exposure to radiation and provide genetic counselling to the family.

Cerebellar hypoplasia (Box 28.19)

The cerebellar hypoplasias are a group of developmental disorders of the cerebellum arising during fetal life and diagnosed on brain MRI. They should be distinguished from acquired and especially progressive cerebellar atrophies (Box 28.20). The cerebellar hypoplasias may be isolated or seen in association with a more widespread CNS malformation, structural congenital myopathies or congenital muscular dystrophies. They present with gross motor developmental delay and truncal hypotonia that is usually moderate or severe. Titubation of the head usually predicts future ataxia when the child eventually walks at 2–3 years. More widespread CNS involvement is common and additional features may include epilepsy, language delay, learning disability, autism and other psychiatric disorders.

The weak child

Problem-orientated topic:

the weak child ● ● ● ● ●

Martina is 9 years old and has been referred with a 4-month history of generalized weakness and malaise. She had not been well since a bad cold last winter. Her teacher noticed that Martina has stopped running with her friends at break time and seems to have difficulty with physical activity. Martina's mother tells you that she is often too weak to climb the stairs at home and her father has to carry her to bed.

Martina is a polite, anxious little girl. She has subtle periorbital oedema and an erythematous rash on extensor surfaces of both elbows. There is proximal muscle weakness and she has difficulty in moving from lying prone to standing. There is some wasting of the shoulder girdle muscles. Reflexes, coordination and sensation are normal.

Q1. What are the causes of weakness in childhood?

Q2. How would you investigate Martina?

Q1. What are the causes of weakness in childhood?

- *Inflammatory muscle disease.* Dermatomyositis occurs in children and is associated with irritability and a rash. Viral myositis causes tender aching calves or thighs (elevated CK)
- *Limb girdle muscular dystrophies.* (genetically heterogeneous group related to structural proteins). Martina could have an inherited muscular dystrophy, although the subacute onset of symptoms and absence of a family history make this unlikely.
- *Myasthenia gravis.* Fatiguable ptosis is the most common presentation but more generalized weakness can occur.
- *Congenital myopathies.* Less likely, due to the subacute onset.
- *Peripheral neuropathy.* Normal reflexes and the presence of proximal weakness make this less likely.
- *Non-organic cause.* The presence of muscle wasting and definite weakness makes this untenable.

BOX 28.21 Investigations in a weak child

Serum creatine kinase (CK)
- Markedly elevated CK can be seen with muscular dystrophy, inflammatory muscle disease, hypothyroidism and defects of carnitine metabolism

C-reactive protein (CRP) and erythrocyte sedimentation rate (ESR)
- Elevated CRP and ESR would support an inflammatory process

Myositis-specific antibodies
- Antinuclear antibody (ANA), anti-Mi-2 antibodies and anti-Jo-1 antibodies may be elevated in inflammatory muscle disease but results will take some time to obtain

Nerve conduction studies
- Demyelination is associated with conduction block and slow nerve conduction velocities; in axonal neuropathy conduction is normal but amplitudes are reduced

Electromyography
- Low-amplitude short-duration muscle unit potentials support muscle pathology

Muscle biopsy
- In Martina's case, this showed perivascular and interfascicular inflammatory infiltrates with groups of muscle fibre degeneration and regeneration, confirming dermatomyositis

---

Q2. How would you investigate this child?

See Box 28.21.

Muscular dystrophies

These are a group of hereditary myopathies caused by defects in muscle structural proteins. The limb girdle muscular dystrophies (MDs) have onset after birth and present with slowly progressive weakness of predominantly proximal distribution. They are now known to be associated with defects in dystrophin, dystrophin-associated glycoproteins and other sarcolemmal proteins along the muscle membrane. There have been recent advances in understanding the basic biology and genetics of this group of disorders, which are now classified into defects of either sarcolemmal or nuclear envelope proteins.

Basic science

The sarcolemma is the microscopic sheath covering muscle fibres and is composed of the plasma membrane, basement membrane and the adjacent reticular lamina that also contains fibrillar collagens.

Duchenne and Becker muscular dystrophy

 Duchenne and Becker are the commonest limb girdle MDs and are X-linked recessive disorders resulting from a defect in the *dystrophin* gene at Xp21. This gene codes for dystrophin, a muscle membrane protein thought to strengthen muscle cells by anchoring elements of the internal cytoskeleton to the surface membrane. Dystrophin deficiency weakens the integrity of the muscle cell wall, leading to irreversible destruction of muscle cells. Duchenne MD is the more severe phenotype, with less than 3% of the normal dystrophin content present.

Clinical features

Duchenne MD affects 1 in 3500 boys and usually presents with delayed walking. There is hip girdle weakness leading to an inability to run, jump or climb stairs. The gait is characteristically 'waddling' due to hip muscle weakness and there is an associated lumbar lordosis and a tendency to toe-walk. With progressive weakness the child will have difficulty standing from the lying position and to do this will first turn prone, then raise the buttocks and, using the arms, climb up along the thighs until upright (Gower sign). In the calves, deltoids and buttocks, muscle fibres are replaced by fat and connective tissue, leading to pseudohypertrophy. Boys with Duchenne MD may also present with speech delay or early learning difficulties, and as a cohort have a lower than average IQ.

Diagnosis

Serum creatine kinase is markedly elevated before the age of 5 years. Following this, there is a decline in the level, due to loss of muscle. Genetic diagnosis is based on mutation analysis, and carrier detection and antenatal diagnosis is possible.

Clinical course

The ability to walk is usually lost between the ages of 9 and 12 years, with progressive weakness and limb contractures. Patients usually die in their late teens or early twenties due to progressive respiratory failure or associated cardiomyopathy. Boys with Becker MD have a later onset of symptoms, follow a more slowly progressive course and remain ambulant into their late teens. They survive into adult life.

Management

To date there is no cure for DMD. The use of oral steroids has been shown to delay functional deterioration in muscle strength, pulmonary function, and may prolong the ambulatory period. A multidisciplinary approach to management is needed.

Other limb girdle muscular dystrophies

The identification of the dystrophin-associated glycoproteins and other sarcolemmal proteins that are relevant to the functional integrity of the muscle membrane led to recognition of an increasing number of new genetic limb girdle MDs. These are predominantly autosomal dominant and recessive, and have varying ages of onset and rates of progression. There is considerable overlap in the clinical presentation of this group of disorders and specific diagnosis often requires histopathological and molecular analysis in a tertiary neuromuscular centre.

Myotonic dystrophy

This is an autosomal dominant disorder resulting from an unstable trinucleotide (CTG) repeat expansion on chromosome 19 resulting in anticipation. Myotonia refers to the failure of the muscle to relax after sustained contraction and can be demonstrated: for example, following a handshake. A severe neonatal presentation is recognized, with weakness, hypotonia, bulbar paresis and respiratory failure requiring ventilatory support and tube feeding. The mother is always affected.

Adolescents presenting with the condition may have a characteristic pattern of weakness involving the face and peripheries (hands and feet). There is typically ptosis and drooping of the corners of the mouth. Other features include premature frontal baldness, cataracts, cardiomyopathy, multiple endocrinopathies and, for some, significant learning difficulties. Weakness is progressive and disabling, with more than half of those developing symptoms in adolescence dying before the age of 50 years. Surveillance is important to detect cardiac conduction defects and screen for diabetes mellitus.

Dermatomyositis (see also p. 455)

Dermatomyositis is a symmetrical, rapidly progressive inflammatory disease of muscle with associated skin inflammation. Onset of symptoms may be insidious or fulminant, and typically there is a proximal weakness associated with marked pain, malaise, fatigue, fever, arthralgia and irritability. A heliotrope (violaceous) facial rash may be seen and in children is commonly associated with periorbital oedema. It may also affect the extensor surface of joints (Fig. 28.5), with the skin then becoming scaly and atrophic. Contractures and calcinosis of the skin can occur. Corticosteroids are the first line of treatment for this condition with slow tapering.

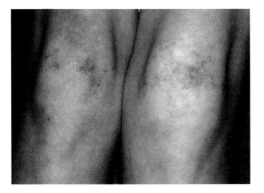

Fig. 28.5 **Skin lesions of dermatomyositis over knees**

Myasthenic syndromes

Myasthenia gravis is an acquired autoimmune disease that results from the formation of autoantibodies to acetylcholine receptors (AChR-MG) with the blockage of acetylcholine receptors on the post-synaptic membrane, leading to fatiguability with repeated muscle contractions. It is associated with abnormalities of the thymus but the exact nature of the autoimmune process remains unclear. Maternal transmission of acetylcholine receptor antibodies can result in a transient but severe neonatal myasthenia.

The child with prepubertal onset of myasthenia gravis is usually male and seronegative for acetylcholine receptor antibodies. Presentation is with ptosis and/or diplopia that affects both eyes, although not always equally. Ocular myasthenia can follow a relapsing and remitting course, with 20% having a complete remission. Post-pubertal onset of myasthenia is more common in girls and is associated with seropositivity and generalized myasthenia. This may also begin with ocular involvement but generalized weakness usually becomes apparent within a year of ocular symptoms. There may be bulbar involvement, with dysarthria, dysphagia and difficulty chewing. Limb fatiguability becomes evident with time and there is a risk of respiratory insufficiency and myasthenic crisis if not treated.

The edrophonium chloride (Tensilon) test is used as a standard of diagnosis for both ocular and generalized myasthenia gravis. This is an inhibitor of acetylcholinesterase. The endpoint should be measured objectively (resolution of ptosis or restoration of ocular motility). As some children are hypersensitive to edrophonium chloride, the test dose should be given and administered with the use of an oxygen saturation monitor. Atropine and ventilatory support should be readily available. Repetitive nerve stimulation (RNS) and single fibre EMG provide electrical evidence of neuromuscular blockade. In addition, measurement of the AChR and MuSK antibodies may be considered. Ocular myasthenia may resolve spontaneously.

Anticholinesterases (neostigmine) are usually the first-line symptomatic treatment, whilst corticosteroids may induce a remission although on occasion long-term immunotherapy may be required. In generalized myasthenia with acetylcholine receptor antibodies, thymectomy is considered as the main long-term strategy in moderately severe disease with good remission rates being achieved.

Peripheral neuropathies

Most neuropathies have a gradual onset and are slowly progressive, with symmetrical predominantly distal mixed sensory and motor manifestations. An acute onset of neuropathy is seen in a small number of conditions and in children is most commonly due to vincristine toxicity during chemotherapy, Guillain–Barré syndrome or a critical illness polyneuropathy.

Guillain–Barré syndrome

This is an acute inflammatory demyelinating polyneuropathy of autoimmune origin. The majority of cases present a few days to 1–2 weeks after an upper respiratory tract or gastrointestinal infection, or vaccination with an ascending weakness of the lower limbs associated with absent reflexes and sometimes sensory symptoms and signs with paraesthesia and pain. The weakness should have reached its peak within 4 weeks of onset. Progression to respiratory failure is associated with cranial nerve involvement and a short incubation period, and mechanical ventilation is required in 7–15% of cases.

CSF examination typically reveals a markedly elevated protein with normal white cell count, although protein elevation may not be apparent until week 2 of the illness. Nerve conduction studies show slowed conduction secondary to demyelination.

Treatment is supportive, with careful vigilance of vital functions. Steroids have not been shown to be beneficial. Intravenous immunoglobulins may be used particularly in moderate and severe, rapidly progressive disease (rapid extension or impending respiratory insufficiency). Virtually complete recovery is seen in two-thirds of patients and begins after a plateau of weakness.

Hereditary motor sensory neuropathies (HMSN)

56

This group of disorders leads to a slowly progressive muscular wasting that is distal and symmetrical. Inheritance can be autosomal dominant, recessive or X-linked. The most important assessment is to examine the child's siblings and parents. The most common condition in this group is HMSN type 1 (Charcot–Marie–Tooth disease). This is an autosomal dominant condition with a gene locus on chromosome 17p11.2 duplication; it initially presents with delay in motor milestones, toe-walking, frequent falling or foot deformity (pes cavus). There is progressive atrophy of the muscles supplied by the peroneal nerve, with weakness of ankle dorsiflexion resulting in foot drop and a high-stepping gait. Thigh muscles are spared in comparison with the wasted calf muscles, giving rise to an 'inverted champagne bottle' appearance. Deep tendon reflexes are present initially but disappear later. As the disease progresses, the distal muscles of the hands may become involved causing weakness, tremor and mild incoordination. Mild sensory deficit may be present and important to differentiate from motor disorders. Nerve conduction studies reveal a demyelinating neuropathy with a decrease in nerve conduction velocities.

Spinal muscular atrophy

See page 675.

Neurodevelopmental regression

Problem-orientated topic:

the child with neurological regression

Chiara is a previously healthy 10-year-old girl who has undergone a change in behaviour and deterioration in school work in the past 4 months. Her parents have also noted jerking movements of the arms. She was adopted from Nepal at the age of 3 years and did not have vaccinations prior to adoption.

Chiara is a quiet, small child with little spontaneous speech. She follows simple instructions but struggles with more complex commands and has difficulty reading. She has some cogwheel rigidity in her upper limbs and myoclonic jerks are noted. These do not appear to be associated with altered awareness.

Q1. What are the causes of regression in childhood?

Q2. What investigations would you undertake in a child who is regressing?

BOX 28.22 Causes of childhood regression	
Epilepsy	Non-convulsive status, Landau–Kleffner syndrome, epileptic encephalopathy
Increased intracranial pressure	Hydrocephalus, brain tumour
Endocrine	Hypothyroidism
Inflammatory	HIV, subacute sclerosing panencephalitis (SSPE), acute disseminating encephalomyelitis (ADEM), Creutzfeldt–Jakob disease (CJD)
Vascular	Moyamoya syndrome
Toxic	Lead poisoning, drug ingestion
Nutritional	Thiamine deficiency, B_{12} deficiency, pellagra
Psychiatric (Ch. 30)	
Inherited metabolic disorders (see Ch. 34)	

Q1. What are the causes of regression in childhood? (Box 28.22)

The two essential features in considering a child who has regressed are the observance of a 'free interval' or period where the child is not affected, followed by demonstration of a 'progressive loss of skills'. While we immediately associate childhood regression with inherited metabolic neurodegenerative disorders, there are a number of 'non-metabolic' causes of regression in childhood that should always be considered, as some of them are treatable.

Chiara was born in Nepal and did not have measles immunization. Asia has a higher incidence of subacute sclerosing panencephalitis (SSPE) than Europe. She may also have been exposed to HIV infection. Chronic lead ingestion through the chewing of leaded paint is a cause of toxic encephalopathy in childhood, but presents subacutely with vomiting, irritability and ataxia, usually in the under 3-year age group. Chiara may not have had screening for hypothyroidism and this should be excluded. Wilson disease is an autosomal recessive condition that can present with hepatic, neurological or haematological signs and is treatable. In the neurological form there is mental deterioration, and dystonic movements are common. Myoclonus is frequently observed. This child has SSPE.

Q2. What investigations would you undertake in a child who is regressing?

Precise investigations should be tailored to the individual case. Below is an outline in this child:

- Full blood count:
  - Lead poisoning can give rise to anaemia
  - Wilson disease can cause haemolytic anaemia
  - HIV infection is associated with a low CD4 count
- Toxicology:
  - Serum lead levels and urine toxicology
- Serum ceruloplasmin:
  - Serum ceruloplasmin levels will be low in Wilson disease
- Metabolic screen:
  - Serum amino acids, blood gas, lactate, ammonia and urinary organic acids
  - Metabolic consultation may also be needed
- Virology screening:
  - Measles antibody titres
- Ophthalmology review:
  - Wilson disease — Kaiser–Fleischer rings or metabolic retinopathy
- EEG:
  - SSPE — periodic bursts of spike/wave complexes with the myoclonic jerks
- MRI scan:
  - SSPE — can be normal or reveal patchy focal abnormalities
  - Wilson — symmetrical hypodensity in the thalami and basal ganglia
- CSF analysis:
  - Measles antibody titres and/or polymerase chain reaction (PCR).

Subacute sclerosing panencephalitis (SSPE)

This is due to chronic persistent measles infection of the CNS following exposure to the measles virus, typically in the first 2 years of life. It has become very rare in the developed world due to vaccination, although this may change with falling vaccination rates. Symptoms usually occur within 6 years of the initial infection and involve subtle personality change, intellectual decline and behaviour change which is often regarded as the child suffering from psychological problems. There is a progressive decline in cognitive function, and within months of onset of symptoms the patient develops involuntary movements including myoclonic jerks followed by dementia and pyramidal and extrapyramidal dysfunction. The majority of those affected die within 3 years of the onset of symptoms. CSF contain high IgG anti-measles antibodies. A characteristic EEG abnormality (with periodic complexes) may be observed before any clinical manifestation. There is no cure as yet although Isoprinosine and intraventricular Interferon and Ribavarin have been used with some limited success.

Acquired immune deficiency syndrome (AIDS) encephalopathy

AIDS-related encephalopathy is now the most common cause of neurodegenerative disease in childhood worldwide. Maternal intravenous drug abuse and prostitution are risk factors in the Western world. Antiretroviral drugs have greatly reduced the risk of an infant contracting HIV due to transplacental or perinatal transmission but are not readily available world-wide. Children with untreated HIV are likely to show evidence of infection within the first year of life. Neurological disease can arise from opportunistic infections in the brain or HIV encephalitis that causes a progressive loss of developmental milestones, microcephaly, dementia and spasticity, and is associated with an elevated CSF protein (0.5 to 1 g/l) and slightly reduced CSF glucose. Neuroimaging may reveal cortical atrophy, white matter high signal and calcification of the basal ganglia. HIV encephalopathy carries a very poor prognosis, although with the use of the combination antiretroviral therapy (ART) children are surviving longer.

Inherited metabolic neurodegenerative disorders
(See also Ch. 34.)

The inherited metabolic conditions associated with childhood regression are largely autosomal recessive, so that familial incidence or consanguinity may be important clinical clues. The clinical syndromes associated with these disorders presenting in the first few years are relatively non-specific, so that different diseases present in very similar ways. To complicate the situation further, the same disease can manifest differently at different ages. The most helpful approach is to classify the conditions clinically on the basis of age at onset of symptoms: during the neonatal period, during the first 2 years of life, or in the older child.

Presentation in the neonatal period is usually with reduced alertness, coma, seizures, hypotonia and feeding difficulties (Box 28.23).

In the infant and young child with neurological regression it is possible to distinguish disorders with predominant involvement of specific areas of the CNS (Boxes 28.24 and 28.25). Cerebral MRI, EEG,

- Amino acid disorders: galactosaemia, maple syrup urine disease
- Urea cycle disorders
- Peroxisomal disorders (p. 463): Zellweger syndrome, neonatal adrenoleucodystrophy
- Mitochondrial disorders (p. 463): Leigh disease
- Ketotic and non-ketotic hyperglycinaemia (p. 461)
- Sulphite oxidase deficiency

- Amino acid disorders: phenylketonuria (p. 463), homocystinuria
- Lysosomal disorders:
  - Sphingolipidoses (p. 463): GM1/GM2 gangliosidoses; Gaucher (type II), Niemann–Pick (type A); metachromatic leucodystrophy, Krabbe
  - Mucopolysaccharidoses (p. 463)
  - Mucolipidoses
  - Glycoproteinoses
- Neuronal ceroid lipofuscinoses
- Mitochondrial disorders (see below): Leigh, Alpers, Menkes
- Neuroaxonal dystrophy
- Lesch–Nyhan syndrome
- Rett syndrome
- Alexander disease (p. 387), Canavan disease
- Pelizaeus–Merzbacher disease

White matter disease

- Spastic paralysis ± ataxia
- Loss of tendon reflexes
- Blindness + optic atrophy (normal retina)

Grey matter disease

- Seizures, myoclonus
- Dementia
- Blindness with retinal changes

evoked potentials and peripheral nerve conduction studies can be helpful in localizing nervous system involvement. It is also helpful to establish whether there are features to suggest multi-organ involvement (organomegaly, skeletal and/or connective tissue involvement). The mucopolysaccharidoses are unique in having a characteristic phenotype that can be readily

Table 28.6 Enzyme deficiencies associated with specific lysosomal disorders

Disorder	Enzyme
GM1	Beta-galactosidase
GM2	Hexosaminidase
Gaucher	Glucocerebrosidase
Niemann–Pick	Sphingomyelinase
Metachromatic leucodystrophy	Arylsulphatase
Krabbe leucodystrophy	Galactosylceramidase
Mucopolysaccharidoses	Multiple enzymes
Mucolipidoses	Multiple enzymes
Glycoproteinoses	Multiple enzymes

recognized. This includes coarse facial features, visceromegaly, hernias and joint contractures.

Basic science

Lysosomes are cytoplasmic vesicles that contain enzymes responsible for degrading the products of cellular catabolism. When these enzymes are deficient, abnormal storage of material occurs. Each condition is associated with an enzyme deficiency (Table 28.6).

The neuronal ceroid lipofuscinoses are a group of genetically determined neurodegenerative disorders associated with the accumulation of autofluorescent lipopigment inclusions. Seizures, dementia and visual impairment are the prominent clinical features (Boxes 28.26 and 28.27).

The mitochondrial encephalomyopathies

These are a diverse group of disorders associated with defects in the oxidative metabolism of pyruvate or in the five respiratory chain complexes.

Leigh disease

This is characterized clinically by the combination of hypotonia and regression, with nystagmus or ophthalmoplegia and abnormal breathing. There may be evidence of a raised CSF lactate concentration and abnormalities on MRI in the deep grey nuclei and brainstem.

Menkes syndrome

This is an X-linked disorder of copper transport and metabolism, associated with early intractable seizures, dementia and abnormalities of scalp hair (sparse, poorly pigmented and wiry hair). Plasma copper concentrations and ceruloplasmin levels are decreased.

Lesch–Nyhan syndrome

This is an X-linked disorder caused by a deficiency of the enzyme hypoxanthine guanine phosphoribosyltransferase. It presents with motor delay followed by progressive limb rigidity, spasticity and chorea. Self-mutilation is a prominent feature and high uric acid levels are a marker.

Rett syndrome

Rett syndrome (see also p. 393) is an important cause of neurological regression in girls, with loss of language, gait ataxia and autistic features to begin with, followed by the loss of purposeful hand function associated with stereotypical hand movements (wringing and clasping). Breath-holding and hyperventilation may be prominent features and there is a fall-off in head growth with microcephaly. Diagnosis is confirmed by evidence of a mutation on the *MECP2* gene on the X-chromosome present in 70–80% of cases. The late stages are characterized by spasticity, dystonia and scoliosis. Cognitive function is severely diminished. Treatment is supportive.

Alexander disease

This is caused by a mutation in the gene for glial fibrillary acidic protein (GFAP), a component of the astrocyte intermediate filament structure, and is associated with the presence of Rosenthal fibres. Canavan disease is caused by a deficiency of the enzyme aspartoacylase, leading to tissue accumulation of N-acetylaspartic acid. Measurement of this metabolite in urine is a good marker of the condition. Both conditions present clinically with hypotonia and megalencephaly, with evidence of a leucodystrophy on MRI.

Pelizaeus–Merzbacher syndrome

This is an X-linked dysmyelinating encephalopathy caused by a defect in a structural protein of the myelin sheath. It is associated with mutations in the *PLP1* gene. The clinical features include early hypotonia, evolving spasticity, intermittent head-bobbing, nystagmus and stridor.

Huntington disease

This is an autosomal dominant disorder caused by an expanded trinucleotide repeat on chromosome 4. Symptoms begin before the age of 20 years in 10% and usually involve behavioural disturbance, cognitive decline, rigidity, lack of facial expression, and abnormal eye movements (oculomotor apraxia). Imaging reveals ventricular dilatation with atrophy of the head of the caudate. Death usually occurs within 8 years of onset of symptoms. Preclinical and prenatal DNA diagnosis is possible.

Adrenoleucodystrophy

This is an X-linked recessive condition resulting in the accumulation of saturated very long chain fatty acids (VLCFAs) in all tissues of the body. The cerebral form of the disease usually has its onset between the ages of 5 and 10 years, with deterioration in behaviour and school work, followed by a disturbance of coordination and gait and a decline into a persistent vegetative state within 3 years of the onset of symptoms. CSF protein is increased and MRI reveals high-signal intensity in the periventricular white matter. Analysis of VLCFAs provides the definitive diagnosis. Bone marrow transplant has been shown to be beneficial in some isolated presymptomatic cases.

Macrocephaly

Basic science

Cerebrospinal fluid (CSF) is produced in the choroid plexus of the lateral, third and fourth ventricles. From the lateral ventricles it flows through the foramen of Munro to the third ventricle, and into the fourth ventricle via the aqueduct of Sylvius. From there it flows through the foramina of Luschka and Magendie into the basal cisterns, out over the surface of the brain and down the spinal cord. It is reabsorbed into the blood stream in the superior sagittal sinus through the arachnoid villi. This circulation occurs 6–7 times per day.

Problem-orientated topic:

the child with a large head ● ● ● ●

Matteo is referred by his primary physician at the age of 8 months because of concerns about the size of his head. Having started on the 50th centile, his occipito-frontal head circumference is now above the 98th centile. His anterior fontanelle is large and pulsatile but not bulging. He is well and appears to be developing normally. His height and weight are on the 50th centile.

Q1. What is the likely cause of Matteo's macrocephaly?

Q2. What investigations would you undertake?

Q1. What is the likely cause of Matteo's macrocephaly? (Box 28.28)

This is a common clinical scenario. The child is well and does not have symptoms or signs of raised intracranial pressure. The most helpful assessment is measurement of the parents' head circumferences, as the likely aetiology is benign familial macrocephaly. This is commonly associated with a benign enlargement of the subarachnoid spaces (communicating hydrocephalus) in the first 2 years of life.

BOX 28.28 Causes of macrocephaly in childhood

- Large baby
- Benign familial macrocephaly
- Hydrocephalus
- Subdural effusions
- Megaloencephaly:
  - Anatomical — Soto, Weaver, neurocutaneous syndromes
  - Metabolic — Alexander, Canavan, glutaric aciduria type 1, storage disorders, leucodystrophies
- Skull vault disorders

BOX 28.29 Causes of hydrocephalus

Communicating hydrocephalus

- Benign enlargement of subarachnoid spaces (Fig. 28.6)
- Post-haemorrhagic
- Post-meningitic
- Achondroplasia
- Sagittal sinus thrombosis
- Venous obstruction

Non-communicating hydrocephalus

- Aqueduct stenosis: genetic/acquired
- Dandy–Walker malformation
- Arnold–Chiari malformation
- Mass lesions: tumour, haematoma, abscess, vein of Galen malformation

---

Q2. What investigations would you undertake?

Hydrocephalus (Boxes 28.29 and 28.30)
Obstruction of CSF flow or failure of CSF reabsorption gives rise to hydrocephalus (an excess of CSF in the ventricular system). Non-communicating hydrocephalus results from obstruction in the ventricular system at a point at or above the level of the fourth ventricular outflow. Communicating hydrocephalus occurs as a result of failure to reabsorb CSF.

Treatment of hydrocephalus associated with raised intracranial pressure requires placement of a shunt from one of the ventricles to the peritoneum (ventriculoperitoneal shunt). The catheter in the peritoneum is coiled to allow for growth. Shunt drainage can become ineffective because of infection (typically *Staphylococcus aureus*), obstruction or breakage. In cases where surgery is not possible or must be delayed, e.g. in premature neonates, repeated aspiration of CSF may be helpful as a temporary measure.

Infant

- Increase in the rate of head growth
- Macrocephaly
- Splaying of the sutures
- Tense anterior fontanelle
- Dilated scalp veins
- Vertical gaze paresis (sun-setting eyes)

Older child

- More typical features of raised intracranial pressure
- Headache, vomiting, irritability
- Papilloedema and bilateral abducens paresis
- Lower limb spasticity and ataxia

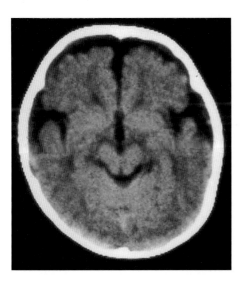

Fig. 28.6 CT scan showing benign external hydrocephalus

Table 28.7 Head shapes associated with suture synostosis

Head shape	Suture involved
Scaphocephaly	Sagittal suture
Brachycephaly	Both coronal sutures
Plagiocephaly	One coronal or lambdoid suture
Trigonocephaly	Metopic suture
Oxencephaly	All sutures

Craniosynostosis

Craniosynostosis (Table 28.7) is a skull vault abnormality associated with premature closure of one or more cranial sutures. If multiple sutures are involved, raised intracranial pressure is a complication. Skull X-ray reveals increased density along the prematurely fused suture. Referral should be made to a craniofacial surgeon.

Spina bifida

Problem-orientated topic:

the child with spina bifida

You are asked to see a term infant in the neonatal unit who has just been born. She has a congenital anomaly of her back with a large defect in the spinal column and is not moving her legs. She has evidence on examination of a myelomeningocele at L3 and has a flaccid paraparesis. Her parents have a number of questions.

Q1. How common is this and what are the risk factors?

Q2. What other associated problems should be investigated?

Q3. What is the likelihood of future disability?

Q4. What are the important points of management?

Q1. How common is this and what are the risk factors? (Boxes 28.31 and 28.32)

The incidence of neural tube defects (NTDs) varies widely; in continental Europe it is about 1/1000 live births, compared with 0.5/1000 in the USA. The causes of NTDs are multifactorial, with both genetic and environmental factors being important. The use of preconceptual supplementary folic acid (0.4 mg/day) reduces the risk by 70%.

An encephalocele is a sac-like protrusion of brain and meninges through a midline skull defect anywhere from between the nose and forehead to the back of

- Maternal diabetes
- Sodium valproate in pregnancy
- Previously affected child (recurrence risk = 5%)

- Anencephaly
- Encephalocele
- Meningocele
- Myelomeningocele

MODULE SIX

389

Table 28.8 **Neurological outcomes of myelomeningocele**

Type	Level	Effect
Non-ambulant	Low thoracic/high lumbar	Flaccid complete lower limb paresis Absent reflexes and sensation Retained upper limb movement Normal head/neck movement Varying truncal control
	High lumbar (L1–L3)	Hip flexion/adduction preserved Hip extension/abduction absent No knee or ankle movements
Usually ambulant	Low lumbar (L3 or lower)	Hip/knee movements present but variable strength Ankle movement variable

the skull, and is often associated with other cerebral malformations or craniofacial abnormalities. Posterior lumbosacral area defects are more common. Small frontal encephaloceles in the nasal or forehead regions can go unnoticed and may present with rhinorrhoea and/or intracranial infection. Treatment of the defect is surgical.

A meningocele is the protrusion of meninges and CSF through a vertebral defect without neural tissue. It is covered by skin and usually has a good prognosis following surgery. A myelomeningocele is a complex NTD with involvement of the spinal cord, meninges, nerve roots, vertebral bodies and overlying skin. Neural tissue develops abnormally (myelodysplasia) and results in neurological deficits that correspond to the level of the lesion. There may be additional developmental anomalies in the brain and there is a strong association with the Arnold–Chiari type II malformation, characterized by cerebellar hypoplasia and associated displacement of the hindbrain through the foramen magnum. The result is an obstruction of CSF flow causing hydrocephalus in 90% of children with a myelomeningocele.

Q2. What other associated problems should be investigated?

See Box 28.33.

Q3. What is the likelihood of future disability? (Table 28.8)

Most infants will have surgery to repair the skin defect soon after birth. The majority will have a neuropathic bladder and are usually incontinent, with impaired emptying and high voiding pressures. Recurrent urinary tract infections, impaired renal function and hypertension are potential complications. Neuropathic bowel with constipation and faecal impaction may also be a problem. Cognitive problems occur in 25% of children with myelomeningocele, and up to 15% of children with ventriculoperitoneal shunts for hydrocephalus develop epilepsy.

> **BOX 28.33 Anomalies associated with neural tube defects**
>
> - Cerebral malformations
> - Brainstem dysfunction
> - Hydrocephalus
> - Neurological deficits
> - Cardiac malformations
> - Genitourinary tract malformations
> - Orthopaedic deformities

The spinal cord lesion leads to paraplegia, the severity of which is dependent on the level of the lesion (Table 28.8). Children with thoracic or high lumbar lesions will be confined to a wheelchair, with no lower limb function. Children with low lumbar or sacral lesions may walk with the assistance of devices such as splints and walking aids. Many children develop joint contractures and scoliosis.

Q4. What are the important points of management?

- A multidisciplinary team approach
- Closure of skin defect
- Shunt insertion for associated hydrocephalus
- Surveillance for brainstem dysfunction
- Orthopaedic intervention
- Management of neuropathic bladder/bowel.

References

Engel J Jr, ILAE 2001 A proposed diagnostic scheme for people with epileptic seizures and with epilepsy: report of the ILAE Task Force on Classification and Terminology. Epilepsia 42:796–803.

Kirkham FJ 1999 Stroke in childhood. Archives of Disease in Childhood 81:85–89

Roger J, Bureau M, Dravet C et al 2005 Epileptic syndromes in infancy, childhood and adolescence, 4th edn. John Libbey Eurotext

Volpe JJ 2001 Neurology of the newborn. W.B. Saunders, Philadelphia

Susan M. Gentle   Valerie A. Harpin   Hojka G. Kumperscak
Marta Macedoni-Luksic   David Neubauer

Neurodevelopmental disability

LEARNING OUTCOMES

By the end of this chapter you should:

- Understand the causes of intellectual disability, hyperkinetic disorder or attention deficit/hyperactivity disorder (HKD/ADHD), cerebral palsy and communication disorders
- Understand the principles of management of intellectual disability, hyperkinetic disorder (HKD/ADHD), cerebral palsy and the different types of language impairment and communication disorders
- Understand the concept of the autism spectrum and what it includes.

You should also take the opportunity to ensure that:

- You can make an initial assessment of a child with intellectual difficulties, hyperkinetic disorder (HKD/ADHD), delayed walking and cerebral palsy, and delayed language development
- You are aware of the different ways of assessing of language impairment and communication disorder
- You are aware of appropriate management.

MODULE SIX

Introduction

The prevalence of physical and multiple disabilities in children is estimated to be approximately 10–20 per 1000. Chapter 18 describes the concepts and causes of disability, and emphasizes that its management requires a multidisciplinary approach, often focused on a Child Development Centre. This chapter concentrates on the causes, investigation and management of common specific neurodisabilities of childhood. Although each disability is considered separately, multiple disabilities in the same child are common.

Intellectual disability

Problem-orientated topic:

the slow learning child

Pavel is a 3-year-old boy who is referred because of suspected developmental delay. His vision and hearing are normal. There is no family history of intellectual disability, fits or serious illness. His parents are not

Continued overleaf

related. Pavel was born at term weighing 3.5 kg, following a normal pregnancy. He had no neonatal problems. There is no relevant past medical history and no evidence of fits. He smiled at 8 weeks, sat by 8 months and walked at 15 months. He has had no feeding difficulties. His early social interaction was normal. On examination he is not dysmorphic. His head circumference is on the 70% centile. He has no neurocutaneous lesions; his gait, fundi and deep-tendon reflexes are normal, and his plantar reflexes are down-going. Arm and leg tone is normal and symmetrical. He shows good eye contact, early turn-taking and uses his index finger to point for a drink or food. The only word he uses is 'Mum', with some other early babble.

Q1. What is the definition of intellectual disability?

Q2. How do you make the diagnosis of intellectual disability?

Q3. What are the pros and cons of investigating a child with an intellectual disability?

Q4. What investigations would you perform, if any?

Q5. How would you manage this child and family?

Q1. What is the definition of intellectual disability?

A child or young person has an intellectual disability when an individual's intellectual ability and his/her adjustment abilities do not reach the level expected for their age and when this global developmental deficit becomes apparent prior to age 18 (Box 29.1).

The International Statistical Classification of Diseases–10th revision (ICD-10) defines it as 'a condition of arrested or incomplete development of the mind which is especially characterized by impairment of skills manifested during the developmental period contributing to the overall level of intelligence, i.e. cognitive, motor and social abilities'. This is not a helpful definition for parents.

For research and study it is sometimes necessary to have a definition that can be measured. Average intelligence quotient (IQ) is 100, with a standard deviation (SD) of 15. Intellectual disability may then be defined as > 2 SD below the mean or the ICD-10 definitions:

- Mild   IQ 50–69
- Moderate   IQ 35–49
- Severe   IQ 20–34
- Profound   IQ < 20.

In practice, the definitions shown in Table 29.1 are often used.

> **BOX 29.1 Definitions of learning/Intellectual disability**
>
> In the UK, the term 'learning disability' is currently used in preference to intellectual disability or 'mental retardation', whereas in the USA the term 'learning disability' means 'specific learning disability'. If only the IQ criterion is used, the expectation, based on a normal distribution curve, would be that about 2.3% of the population should exhibit the condition.

Table 29.1 Definitions and incidence

Definition	IQ	Incidence (per 1000)	Cause identified*
Mild/moderate	50–70	5	68%
Severe	< 50	3.8	96%
Severe (developing countries)		9.3	

* This is higher, however, than in routine clinical practice (Whiting K 2001 Investigating the child with learning difficulty. Current Paediatrics 11:240–247).

We will use the abbreviations SL/ID for severe learning/intellectual disability and 'ML/ID' for mild/moderate learning/intellectual disability.

Some psychometric tests
The following two tests are commonly used by paediatricians. Both require training and special equipment:
- *Griffiths*. This has been standardized on 0–8-year-old British children but relies on parental reporting; many items are timed. It has recently been updated.
- *Bayley III*. This scale (age range 0–42 months) is used to assess developmental age and has been standardized on American children as well as on children in some EU countries.

Q2. How do you make the diagnosis of intellectual disability? (Box 29.2)

Mild/moderate intellectual disability
While children with SL/ID often have associated problems such as cerebral palsy, those with ML/ID often have no other problems. Many will be the tail-end of the normal distribution; others will have learning difficulties as a result of environmental factors (lack of early oppor-

> **BOX 29.2 A point to remember**
>
> History and examination are the main ways in which a diagnosis is made. Investigations are most useful in confirming or clarifying a diagnosis. When the cause is genetic (hereditary), identifying the precise defect is crucial for assessing the risk of having other affected children.

tunities or iron deficiency) and be functioning below their genetic potential; some will have an identifiable remediable cause such as vision or hearing problems; some will have an intrinsic problem such as neurofibromatosis or a chromosome abnormality.

All children with significant intellectual difficulties should have at least some paediatric assessment to contribute to identification of special educational needs.

When seeing a child referred from school with ML/ID enquire about:

- History
- Birth
- Progress from birth
- Family
- Other concerns
- Hearing and vision
- Behaviour
- Poor general health
- Time off school, leading to under-achievement
- Whether children are working at their best in school
- Epilepsy (absences, minor status).

Look for dysmorphism or other clues to aetiology.

Severe intellectual disability

It is important to ask or examine for:
- Genetic abnormalities:
  – Dysmorphism
  – Malformations
- Metabolic defects:
  – Failure to thrive
  – Hypotonia
  – Consanguinity
  – Recurrent unexplained illness (especially anorexia and vomiting)
  – Loss of skills
  – Coarse facies
  – Ocular abnormalities
  – Macro- or microcephaly
  – Family history of unexplained illness or death
- Brain malformation:
  – Abnormal skull
  – Focal deficit
  – Loss of skills
  – Micro- or macrocephaly
  – Seizures
  – Visual abnormality.

Syndromes

These are more likely in children with SLD but should be considered in all children with learning difficulties. In children with SLD, about one-quarter have a chromosomal disorder; 80–90% of these have Down syndrome. The next most common disorder is fragile X syndrome (p. 396).

There are now over 2000 syndromes and the number continues to increase. From a practical day-to-day perspective they fall into two broad groups: the more common or easily recognized syndromes, such as Down, Edward and Sturge–Weber; and others with a number of abnormal features not immediately recognizable as a syndrome but in whom it is possible to make a diagnosis.

 http://www.ncbi.nlm.nih.gov/Omim/

OMIM (Online Mendelian Inheritance in Man) dysmorphology database

Developmental regression

If there is progressive loss of skills (Ch. 28) it is important to consider:
- Hydrocephalus
- Poorly controlled epilepsy
- Metabolic disorder/neurodegenerative disorder
- Pervasive developmental disorders (Rett syndrome) and childhood disintegrative disorder
- Infection, particularly in an immunocompromised host (e.g. AIDS)
- Vascular problem, e.g. repeated minor strokes from moyamoya or sickle cell disease; malformations causing vascular 'steal'.

True regression can be hard to ascertain because development is taking place at the same time. All children, and particularly those with an intellectual disability, will sometimes learn something new and then appear to forget it for a while.

Reasons to ask for further assessment

- To obtain an objective assessment of abilities
- To identify strengths and weaknesses that may help with management
- To assess progress
- For the court, such as in cases of neglect
- For research.

Q3. What are the pros and cons of investigating a child with an intellectual disability?

Pros

- Treatable cause, e.g. hypothyroidism
- Genetic counselling may be useful
- For prognosis
- The parents may be helped by knowing the cause.

Cons

- False positives and false negatives
- Pain and complications of investigations (especially anaesthesia)
- Financial cost.

Q4. What investigations would you perform, if any? (Box 29.3)

Investigations should be performed on the basis of clues from the history and examination. The following investigations may be indicated, particularly in children with SL/ID:

- Chromosome analysis
- Brain imaging
- Metabolic investigations.

Q5. How would you manage this child and family?

The neurodevelopmental paediatrician's role is:

- *Establishing whether there is an intellectual disability* (usually done with a multidisciplinary team). In younger children it is the health services that are primarily involved in this. In older children it is primarily school-based.
- *Identifying the cause.* This may be from the history and examination or may include investigation.
- *Referral to other professionals as appropriate.* These may include:
  - Speech and language therapy (SLT), occupational therapy (OT), physiotherapy
  - Psychology, child and adolescent psychiatry
  - Other medical specialties
  - Education
  - Social services.
- *Looking for and managing associated difficulties.* There may be problems with hearing, vision, motor function, behaviour or epilepsy. Some are specific, e.g. hypothyroidism in Down syndrome.
- *Counselling parents.* The neurodevelopmental paediatrician may be the initial person to do this, although others may take up the role later.
- *Liaison with education.*
- *Explanation to child and parents of the likely effects of the disabilities.*
- *Responding to concerns.*

In metabolic disorders some pharmacological treatments may have an effect on progress. This is a very specialized area and one that is constantly changing, but it is a good reason for trying to make a specific diagnosis.

Down syndrome (Tables 29.2 and 29.3)

Incidence is approximately 1 in 1000 live births. The risk of having a child with Down syndrome increases with maternal age, so that for a mother in her twenties the risk is less than 1 in 1000, but greater than 1 in 100 in mothers over 40. However, most babies are born to mothers in their twenties and thirties.

Almost everyone can recognize a child or adult with Down syndrome. One of the problems with a well-recognized syndrome is that people can have preconceived ideas about what a child with Down syndrome is like. Children with Down syndrome can be as different from each other as any other group of children in the population. Some children are able to follow a mainstream curriculum and achieve GCSE passes. Others may never develop language. Some have very limited exercise tolerance, while others achieve sporting excellence.

Genetic types (see also Ch. 9)

Most are caused by non-disjunction in meiosis, resulting in an additional chromosome 21 (47 XY with additional chromosome 21). In 20–25% the extra chromosome is paternal. When Down syndrome is caused by trisomy 21, the recurrence risk is about double that of a woman of the same age without a previous history.

Three to four percent result from translocation of material from chromosome 21 on to another chromosome. A parent may often have a balanced translocation (one of their chromosome 21s is attached to another chromosome), but this causes no problem because they have a normal total amount of chromosome material. However, this tagged-on chromosome may be present in a gamete in addition to a normal chromosome 21, giving rise to extra chromosome material in the offspring. There is a greatly increased risk of a couple having a second affected child.

Mosaicism accounts for 2–6% and such individuals are usually affected to a lesser degree.

Diagnosis

If the diagnosis is not made on antenatal screening, it is usually made early in the neonatal period by recognition of the typical features of Down syndrome. It may be a midwife, a paediatrician or the parents who first recognize that there is a problem with the baby. There is strong evidence from parents to suggest that disclosure should be made as soon as the diagnosis is suspected, preferably with both parents present. The diagnosis is confirmed by chromosome analysis.

Management

Down syndrome has possible effects on all body systems. Management of children therefore needs

Table 29.2 Down syndrome

Feature	Comments

Facial features
    Prominent epicanthic folds
    Flat nasal bridge
    Small nose
    Protrusion of tongue
	
	This is not a large tongue but poor tone/micrognathia

Brachycephaly	
Wide hands, short fingers Distal tri-radius, clinodactyly Single palmar crease Wide gap between first and second toes	 Simian crease may be present in normal individuals
Brushfield spots	Spots on iris
Fine soft hair Dry, hyperkeratotic skin Other skin problems	Can have alopecia Helped by simple emulsifying cream and appropriate bath oil Such as vitiligo, papular erythema, mottled skin (cutis marmorata)
Hypotonia	Prominent in the neonatal period. Influences motor development. May result in joint dislocation
Orthopaedic problems	Atlanto-axial instability (see below) Hip dysplasia/dislocation Dislocation/displacement of other joints
Cardiac problems	See below
Bowel problems	Duodenal atresia presents neonatally Also look out for constipation (Hirschsprung disease, hypothyroidism) and malabsorption
Infections	More prone to infections, e.g. bacterial pneumonia, otitis media
Hypothyroidism	Higher incidence of autoimmune hypothyroidism; important to screen for this
Leukaemia	About a 10–20-fold increase. Children may cope badly with intensive treatment
Low fertility	Females are fertile Males often have undescended testes and hypogonadism
Behaviour difficulties	Management should be appropriate to developmental age
Poor growth and weight problems	Frequently poor feeders in infancy. Later a tendency to become overweight and attention to diet and activity levels is needed N.B. Use growth charts for children with Down syndrome
Presenile dementia	Important for long-term support, as carers may be elderly with an affected young adult

Table 29.3 Average milestones for children with Down syndrome

Milestone	Mean age	Range
Sitting	13 months	6–30 months
Standing	22 months	9–48 months
Walking	30 months	12–60 months
Single words	34 months	12–72 months
40% of children with Down syndrome are able to learn to read		

a multidisciplinary approach. Of the many other potential problems in a child with Down syndrome, there are two that deserve particular mention:

- *Congenital heart disease.* This occurs in 40–50% of babies with Down syndrome. All newborn babies should be evaluated, with observation (of feeding etc.), physical examination, electrocardiogram (ECG), chest X-ray (CXR) and echocardiogram.

Atrioventricular (AV) canal defects (endocardial cushion defects) occur very specifically in children with Down syndrome (p. 571). Any newborn found to have an AV canal defect should have chromosomal analysis.

Patent ductus arteriosus (PDA), ventricular septal defect (VSD) and atrial septal defect (ASD) are also more common in children with Down syndrome.

Damage to pulmonary vasculature with irreversible pulmonary hypertension can occur much earlier in children with Down syndrome than expected from the size of the shunt alone. PDA, ASD, VSD and AV canal defects should be considered for early surgical intervention.

- *Atlanto-axial instability.* Routine cervical spine X-ray used to be recommended but review of X-rays of the same child taken minutes apart could give rise to completely different advice. Spinal cord damage in Down syndrome is rare and usually insidious rather than acute. It is important not to frighten parents and cause children to be wrapped in cotton wool and prevented from joining in appropriate activities; however, parents do need relevant information to enable them to recognize symptoms that should be reported. The three most common symptoms are:

- Deterioration/change in gait or manipulation skills
- Neck pain/stiffness
- Difficulties with sphincter control.

Children with any of these should be investigated urgently.

Advice should be given to other regular carers of children with Down syndrome and included in medical advice for assessment of special educational needs.

http://www.edsa.info

http://www.dsmig.org.uk

Guidelines on surveillance for people with Down syndrome. For patients' organizations throughout Europe go to: http://www.orpha.net

Fragile X syndrome

This is probably the second most common known syndromic cause of global learning disability (about 1 in 1360 males and 1 in 2000 females; a further 1 in 1000 females are asymptomatic carriers). The degree varies from mild to severe in boys, and mild to moderate in girls. The defect in fragile X is now known to be an expansion in a specific DNA triplet repeat (CGG) on the X chromosome.

Physical features include:

- Long face and slightly increased head circumference
- Macrognathia
- Large protuberant ears
- Flattened nasal bridge
- Abnormal dermatoglyphics
- Macro-orchidism
- Infantile hypotonia
- Connective tissue dysplasia (joint laxity and soft velvety skin)
- Aortic dilatation and mitral valve prolapse
- Recurrent otitis media
- Failure to thrive in infancy
- Tonic–clonic or partial epilepsy, temporal spikes on electroencephalogram (EEG)
- MRI scan abnormalities (especially cerebellum).

Psychological features include:

- Variable intellectual impairment
- Language delay

- Social impairments, such as those seen in autism
- Attention and concentration difficulties.

Features are very variable and some are only evident in adolescent or adult life. Clinical diagnosis in a young child is difficult.

Families need careful genetic advice.

Other sex chromosome abnormalities in which learning disability may occur are discussed in Chapter 9.

Neurocutaneous syndromes

These may also cause learning disability (pp. 372–4).

Rett syndrome

This presents as a neurodegenerative disorder but is probably a neurodevelopmental disorder. It is sometimes classified with the pervasive development disorders such as autism. Milder cases and cases in boys are being described. It constitutes about 10% of SL/ID in girls. Most common cause is a de novo mutation in the MECP2 gene located on the X chromosome.

Specific learning difficulties

The Education Code of Practice defines children as having specific learning difficulties when they have 'significantly' more difficulty in a specific area than most children of the same age that is not due to general learning disabilities.

ICD and DSM (*Diagnostic and Statistical Manual of Mental Disorders*) definitions depend on the child having a normal IQ and no other problems, but there is no reason why a child with generalized learning difficulties cannot have specific difficulties in one particular area, over and above their general level of difficulty.

Specific reading disorder

The term 'dyslexia' is used, but very loosely, for a wide variety of difficulties at school.

Writing disorder

There is a lot of overlap between reading and writing problems (dysgraphia).

Mathematics disorder (dyscalculia)

Incidence is probably similar to dyslexia and dysgraphia but there are interesting differences:

- Dyscalculia is seen equally in boys and girls (though recent work suggests that dyslexia may also be equally represented).

- It is seen more in fragile X carriers, Turner syndrome, phenylketonuria (PKU) and ADHD.
- It is the most common learning difficulty in epilepsy.

Developmental coordination disorder (DCD)

Currently, this is the term used most commonly for children with motor coordination problems. A number of conditions can present with clumsiness other than DCD and these need to be excluded because management is different. Evidence of deterioration should be sought at presentation and at reviews.

Differential diagnosis includes especially
- Neuromuscular diseases
- Cerebral palsies
- Brain tumours
- Brain injury
- Ataxias, such as Friedreich ataxia (p. 378)
- Metabolic disorders
- Vestibular disease
- Tremors and other involuntary movements.

History, examination and, if appropriate, investigation should exclude these diagnoses.

Presentation
Developmental coordination disorder (DCD) is defined, using the Diagnostic and Statistical Manual of Mental Disorders, Fourth Edition (DSM-IV), as a condition marked by significant impairment in the development of motor coordination, which interferes with academic achievement and/or activities of daily living. The calculated prevalence of DCD ranges from 1.4% to 19%, depending on case definition. Children presenting with DCD or clumsiness often exhibit signs of minor neurological dysfunction (MND). Two basic forms of MND can be distinguished: simple and complex MND. During school age children with simple MND are characterized by one or two dysfunctional clusters of MND while those with complex MND will have at least three. In adolescence they present with choreiform dyskinesia or hypotonia (simple MND) or problems in fine manipulation or coordination (complex MND). Clusters are: posture and tone, reflexes, choreiform dyskinesia, coordination and balance, fine manipulative ability and, less frequently, cranial nerve dysfunctions (e.g. 6th or 7th nerve palsy).

Secondary problems include:
- Behaviour problems
- Poor self-esteem
- School failure.

When a child first presents at the clinic, a general paediatric and neurological assessment is needed, particularly to exclude other causes. There are no specific signs on neurological examination. Assessments specifically for DCD are best carried out by an occupational therapist, but the paediatrician should perform some initial screening.

Management
The mainstay of treatment is occupational therapy and physiotherapy. Management can be considered under the following headings:
- Explanation to child, parent and teacher
- Specific advice to parents and teachers to help in specific areas such as handwriting and dressing
- Improving self-esteem
- Specific therapy.

Hyperkinetic disorder (HKD)

Problem-orientated topic:

disruptive behaviour HKD/ADHD

Vladimir is 7 years old. His mother, a single parent to Vladimir and his 4-year-old sister, has always struggled with his behaviour. Now things are going very badly at school. Vladimir has barely started to acquire literacy skills, although he seems a bright child. His disruptive behaviour in class is now such a problem that he is frequently sent home. He often fails to pay close attention to details, does not listen to what is being said, leaves his seat in the classroom and is often noisy. He was initially slow to acquire language but other milestones were normal. Last week he set fire to his bedroom carpet.

Q1. What is hyperkinetic disorder or ADHD?
Q2. How would you assess Vladimir for this condition?
Q3. How should you manage Vladimir and his family?
Q4. What is Vladimir's prognosis?

Q1. What is hyperkinetic disorder or ADHD?

This is not a new disorder explained by environmental pollutants or 'made up' to explain away naughty children. Subjects with symptoms of HKD/ADHD were already described in the late 19th century.

Individuals with HKD/ADHD have:
- Inattention
- Hyperactivity
- Impulsivity: excessive in the context of age, sex and cognitive ability.

For a diagnosis to be made these symptoms should be:
- Present in more than one situation
- Present before the age of 7 years
- Impairing the child's educational or social functioning.

Inattention
There is poor regulation of attention and this is manifest particularly in difficult, imposed tasks that are not immediately rewarding. A child may attend to a video game or watch a TV programme with sustained attention but be unable to concentrate in school.

Hyperactivity
This is manifest differently at different ages:
- The preschool child will rush around, jumping and climbing noisily and being unable to settle in play.
- The school-age child may be fidgety, squirming and having difficulty remaining seated.
- The adolescent is restless, with foot-tapping and twiddling, and is unable to sit quietly.

Impulsivity
Impulsivity means not thinking before acting; it often results in getting into trouble for being cheeky or reckless. The child may have frequent accidents.

Secondary problems
Most children have secondary problems, including:
- Poor self-esteem
- Poor peer relationships
- Poor relationship with parents
- Sleep/wake problems
- Dietary problems (will not settle to eat).

Epidemiology
HKD/ADHD has a prevalence of about 1.5% in the primary school age population. The rate at which the problem is in practice recognized varies greatly between different European countries, from approximately zero to nearly 2.5%. The prevalence of the broader category of HKD/ADHD symptoms, namely Attention-Deficit/Hyperactivity Disorder (ADHD) is higher (from 4.5 to 19%). Obviously ADHD is a more common diagnosis. All studies show a predominance of boys, but this may be over-estimated because boys show more obvious aggressive behaviour and girls have more inattention.

The underlying problem
This appears to be an executive function deficit. Executive functions include:
- Self-regulation
- Sequencing of behaviour
- Flexibility in response
- Response inhibition
- Planning
- Organization.

Pathology
Development of the frontal lobes is relatively late and myelination is not complete until adolescence. Neuroimaging studies have been inconsistent but the frontal cortex and its connections, as well as intracerebral connections via the corpus callosum, have abnormal activity. There may be differences in brain volume and size of the cerebellum. Functional magnetic resonance imaging (MRI) shows diffuse and decreased activity when individuals with HKD/ADHD undertake tasks requiring concentration. There is abnormal handling of noradrenaline (norepinephrine) and dopamine in the brain. This theory is supported by response to treatment with drugs affecting these neurotransmitters.

Aetiology
- *Genetics.* Genetics is the major factor governing whether or not a child has HKD/ADHD. It has been estimated that there is between 54% and 98% heritability.
- *Environment.* This also plays a part, particularly maternal depression and/or smoking. It is likely that there is an interplay of genetics and environment, with environmental factors maintaining or exacerbating HKD/ADHD rather than causing it.
- *Central nervous system damage.* HKD/ADHD is also more frequent following:
  - Perinatal problems and prematurity
  - Antenatal insults, such as fetal alcohol syndrome or maternal smoking
  - Head injury, especially frontal lobe damage
  - Encephalitis and meningitis
  - Hypoxic episodes, such as drowning and strangling
  - Cerebrovascular accidents
  - Chronic neurological illness, such as epilepsy, metabolic problems (e.g. PKU)
  - Medical treatments, such as cerebral irradiation, anticonvulsants
  - Certain conditions such as William syndrome, hypothyroidism, tuberous sclerosis, XYY, XXY and fragile X syndrome.

Q2. How would you assess Vladimir for this condition?

Diagnosis is made by assessing information from a variety of sources. This is time-consuming and more than one clinic visit is usually needed.

History
- Current concerns, with specific examples, onset of problems and situation
- Antenatal and perinatal history for possible risk factors
- Early development: babies may be hyperactive with sleep problems, feeding difficulties, colic, waking early
- Medical problems for risk factors and differential diagnosis
- Educational problems for difficulties in different environments
- Relationships with parents and peers
- Family history
- Social situation, looking for other causes of difficulties
- Possible comorbidities (see below).

Examination
- Physical and neurological examination for associated problems (e.g. clumsiness), other problems (e.g. hearing, vision) and other diagnoses putting the child at risk (e.g. dysmorphism, tuberous sclerosis)
- Mental state looking for poor self-esteem, depression, anxiety
- Developmental assessment: behaviour inappropriate for developmental age.

    Observation in different settings is vital:
- During the initial assessment
- In school/playground/nursery/playgroup
- At home (parental report may be adequate).

    Structured questionnaires, e.g. Conner's Scales, play an important role in the screening and diagnosis of ADHD.

    Psychometric testing is helpful in identifying those children whose primary problem is a learning difficulty and comorbid specific learning difficulties.

Differential diagnosis
- Physical illness
- Drugs (either prescribed or of abuse)
- Attachment difficulties
- Social issues (e.g. family break-up)
- Child abuse (especially if change in behaviour)
- Depression/anxiety
- Hearing problems

- Unrealistic expectations on the part of parents or teachers
- Poor parenting
- Bullying
- Bored bright child
- Learning difficulties
- Sleep problems
- Conduct disorder.

Investigations
These are rarely indicated but you may need to exclude other causes of hyperactivity or inattention, such as hearing loss, epilepsy, thyroid disorders, side-effects of drugs:
- Request chromosomes if the child is unusually tall (XYY) or has learning difficulties (fragile X) or dysmorphism.
- Order an EEG if there is suspicion of subclinical epilepsy or absence epilepsy (poor concentration rarely is absence epilepsy).

Comorbidities
Comorbidity appears to be the rule rather than the exception in HKD/ADHD. The common additional problems are:
- Specific learning difficulties (particularly in reading)
- Delayed language development and poor language skills
- Developmental coordination difficulties (DCD)
- Oppositional/defiant disorder and conduct disorder (ODD/CD)
- Mood disorders (anxiety, depression, bipolar disorder)
- Obsessive–compulsive disorders (OCD)
- Tourette syndrome
- Autism spectrum disorders, substance abuse (children/adolescents with HKD abuse drugs earlier, more frequently and more intensively than controls).

    It is important to identify the most severe disorder and treat it first or together with HKD.

Q3. How should you manage Vladimir and his family?

Information is an important aspect of management. Making the diagnosis and making this known to all involved may, in itself, help the child, parent and teachers to cope with the HKD/ADHD:
- Oral and written information should be made available.
- The child should be informed as well as the parents.
- Teachers should be informed about the diagnosis and, if necessary, about what it means.

Support groups

These can be very helpful to parents and child.

Educational measures

Simple suggestions can be very helpful such as:

- Having the child sit near the teacher
- Removing distractions where possible
- Clear, frequent and small rewards and discipline
- Working alone or in small groups
- Addressing any learning difficulties.

Behaviour modification

Positive reinforcement is very important. Children with ADHD often have low self-esteem. Children respond best to a well-structured, predictable environment where expectations and rules are clear and consistent, and consequences are set down ahead of time and delivered immediately.

Medication

Medication is the single most effective approach in severe HKD/ADHD.

Stimulant medications (methylphenidate, dexamphetamine) affect the dopamine pathways in the brain but the exact mechanism of action is unclear. They may stimulate areas of the brain that are not functioning properly. They do not affect the underlying pathology but control some symptoms, so that behavioural management can be more effective, school work can progress and social relationships can develop better. They work best in controlling hyperactivity and impulsivity but are less effective in controlling inattention. Methylphenidate, the most frequently used medication, is usually started at a dose of 2.5–5 mg twice or three times a day, increasing by 2.5–5 mg weekly until the desired effect is achieved. A maximum of 20 mg per dose, or 45–60 mg per day, should be used. If there is no effect after 3 weeks at maximum dose, it should be stopped.

Sustained-release products are now available. These have a lower incidence of side-effects and, as they are long-acting, do not need to be given in school.

Between 60 and 80% of children are helped by stimulant medication. Side-effects occur but are not usually severe and include:

- Stomach ache and headache
- Decreased appetite
- Sleep disturbance
- Cardiovascular effects (blood pressure should be checked before starting treatment and at follow-up)
- Unhappiness/withdrawal
- Growth suppression (0.5–1.0 cm if treatment is continued throughout puberty)
- Rebound behaviour difficulties

- Tics, although it is not certain that these are a true side-effect or constitute a coexistent tic disorder
- Marrow aplasia (very rare).

Atomoxetine is a non-stimulant selective noradrenergic reuptake inhibitor, which was licensed for use in HKD/ADHD in almost all European countries in recent years. It is used in patients who failed to respond to a stimulant, or where a stimulant has been used but side-effects were a problem. Atomoxetine may be preferred as a first choice in patients with risk of substance abuse, comorbid tics or anxiety. It is used as a once- or twice-daily medication (and therefore does not need to be given in school). Side-effects may include somnolence, gastrointestinal effects and rarely liver problems.

http://www.nice.org.uk//page.aspx?o=TA098guidance

Diet

There is limited evidence from clinical trials that only a few children with HKD/ADHD react badly to some foods (cow's milk, wheat flour, citrus fruits and food dyes); therefore, an elimination diet might only be helpful to a minority of patients. The diets are troublesome to apply and could easily become an unnecessary battlefield between child and parents. European clinical guidelines conclude that at the present time there is not enough scientific evidence for dietary treatment.

Sleep

Many children and young people with HKD/ADHD have poor sleep patterns and cannot usually stop themselves waking others when they are awake. It is seldom safe to leave such a child unattended for long and families are often very sleep-deprived. This may greatly limit their capacity to cope with their constantly active offspring in the daytime! Although stimulants may cause insomnia in some children, a teatime dose may actually help a child to get off to sleep by calming a racing mind. In other children, the use of melatonin to regulate sleep patterns and quality is very useful.

Q4. What is Vladimir's prognosis?

Some children continue to have difficulties in adult life. Various groups have reported similar findings, with approximately 30% within the normal range as adults, 50–60% continuing to have problems with concentration, impulsivity and social interaction, and 10–15% having significant psychiatric or antisocial problems (depressed, suicidal, drug and alcohol abuse, convictions for assault, armed robbery etc.).

The prognosis is best for those children with only hyperactive symptoms, which are most likely to subside

Have a go at defining these commonly used terms:

- Tone
- Spasticity
- Ataxia
- Athetosis
- Chorea
- Dystonia
- Rigidity

with puberty and adulthood. The prognosis is worse for those with severe symptoms, comorbidities, and poor family and educational support.

The cerebral palsies

Several definitions of cerebral palsy (CP) exist in the literature; however, although these may vary in their wording, they are broadly similar, and can be summarized as follows:

CP is a group of permanent, but not unchanging, disorders of movement and/or posture and of motor function which are due to non-progressive interference, lesion or abnormality of the developing/immature brain (Surveillance of Cerebral Palsy in Europe — SCPE definition). This definition specifically excludes progressive disorders of motor function, defined as loss of previously acquired skills in the first 5 years of life.

There are three main types:
- *Spastic* CP, which can be divided into diplegia, hemiplegia and bilateral hemiplegia or quadriplegia depending on areas affected
- *Ataxic* CP
- *Dyskinetic* CP which can be either dystonic or choreo-athetotic.

Terminology
See Boxes 29.4 and 29.5.

Classification
CP refers to a group of disorders. Classification is based upon clinical descriptions of neurological signs. It is commonplace to find mixed patterns with one predominant aspect, e.g. hemiplegia with some involvement of the good side, diplegia with asymmetry in the upper limbs etc.:

- 27 55 63 *Spastic diplegia.* Recent magnetic resonance studies show that the underlying lesion in most cases of spastic diplegia is periventricular leucomalacia (p. 724).
- 54 *Spastic hemiplegia.* Spastic hemiplegia constitutes about 25% of all cases of CP. The cause is usually an infarction within the distribution of the middle cerebral artery (p. 724).

- *Tone* is the resistance of a muscle to passive stretch (hypertonia — increased resistance, hypotonia — reduced resistance)
- *Spasticity* is a velocity-dependent increase in resistance to passive stretch. The key is the velocity dependency; spasticity is an abnormal response to rapid stretch. Often there is a "clasp-knife" release, in which there is a sudden reduction in resistance following the catch. Usual associated features are clonus, increased deep tendon reflexes and extensor plantar responses
- *Ataxia* is a condition characterized by impaired ability to coordinate voluntary movements. Ataxia may result from damage to the cerebellum, cerebellar pathway or the spinal cord. In relation to gait, ataxic means broad-based, poorly coordinated
- *Athetosis* is the characteristic of slow writhing movement, usually seen in the distal part of the limb during voluntary activity
- *Chorea* is rapid, high-amplitude, sudden and irregular involuntary movement that primarily involves head and extremities
- *Dystonia* usually refers to abnormal sustained contractions of agonists and antagonists resulting in an unusual and abnormal posture e.g. inversion of foot, retraction of shoulders, twisting or writhing movements etc.
- *Rigidity* is stiffness or resistance to movement. There are different types: cogwheel rigidity (jerky resistance) and lead-pipe rigidity (continuous rigidity).

- 12 64 *Total body involvement CP.* In these cases the brain pathology most commonly originates in the prenatal period and may be due to a variety of abnormalities such as primary cerebral dysgenesis (lissencephaly/pachygyria), early pregnancy infections (e.g. cytomegalovirus (CMV), toxoplasmosis), or vascular malformations and vascular accidents (e.g. hydranencephaly). *Spastic tetraplegia* with bilateral cerebral hemisphere infarction, sometimes with extensive cyst formation (multicystic encephalomalacia) and severe intellectual disability, may occur as a result of brain injury in late third trimester. Prolonged partial asphyxia in a term infant may be the cause (p. 722). The contribution of perinatal asphyxia to the overall prevalence of CP is debatable, but most agree an estimate of about 10% of all cases. *Dyskinetic CP* may also arise due to bilirubin encephalopathy in the neonatal period. These cases were more common in the past, but prevention and improved management of rhesus iso-immunization have resulted in a dramatic fall in the number of cases.

Ataxic CP (about 5% of CP) is mainly of prenatal origin. There may be strong familial patterns, with autosomal dominant, X-linked and autosomal recessive modes of inheritance. Sporadic cases are also seen. Children show ataxia, intention tremor and dyskinesia, usually before 2 years of age. Some may achieve independent walking by 4–6 years, although in these cases handwriting remains problematic and, in more severe cases, learning difficulties and seizures may complicate the presentation. About 30% show normal or borderline intellectual function. A magnetic resonance study of ataxic CP showed that over 50% were unclassifiable, 23% were genetic, and only 4% (3 cases) may have had a perinatal cause.

Epidemiology

Prevalence of the cerebral palsies is about 1.7–3 cases/1000 live births. There may have been a trend of increase in the overall prevalence of CP in children born in the 1970s and 1980s. The main area of increase has been in the most immature babies weighing under 1 kg. The reasons for this increase are unclear but probably relate to dramatic changes in survival of very immature infants.

Another important aspect of epidemiology is survival. Most children with CP now survive to adult life, even when disease is severe. This is having an impact on services for adults as well as children.

Problem-orientated topic:

delay in walking ● ● ● ● ●

Stefan is 18 months old and his mother is concerned that he is not yet walking. He is a bright, sociable child, who has several single words. He was born at 27 weeks' gestation and had a difficult neonatal course.

Q1. What questions would you ask to elucidate a cause?

Q2. What are the possible diagnoses?

Q3. What are the principles of management?

Q1. What questions would you ask to elucidate a cause?

An underlying cause may not be apparent, but the following should be considered in history-taking:

- Prenatal:
  - Genetic
  - Infection (e.g. CMV, rubella, chorioamnionitis)

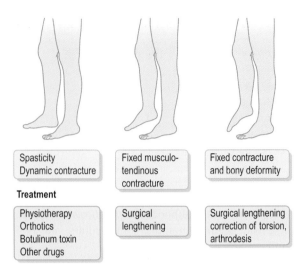

Fig. 29.1 **Spasticity: management**

Spasticity Dynamic contracture	Fixed musculo-tendinous contracture	Fixed contracture and bony deformity
Treatment		
Physiotherapy Orthotics Botulinum toxin Other drugs	Surgical lengthening	Surgical lengthening correction of torsion, arthrodesis

  - Toxins (e.g. drugs)
  - Trauma
  - Nutritional ('placental insufficiency')
- Perinatal:
  - Prematurity (intraventricular haemorrhage/periventricular haemorrhage/periventricular leucomalacia)
  - Infection (e.g. meningitis)
  - Toxins (e.g. hyperbilirubinaemia)
  - Perinatal asphyxia
- Postnatal:
  - Infection
  - Vascular accidents
  - Head injury (accidental or non-accidental)
  - Encephalopathy
  - Anoxic event.

Q2. What are the possible diagnoses?

The most likely cause for this history is CP (spastic diplegia) and this should be confirmed by abnormal neurological signs. A familial delay in walking should also be considered, as well as rarer causes such as Duchenne muscular dystrophy (p. 382) in boys.

It is important to remember that everything that looks like CP may not be. Many infants with complex congenital abnormalities may display central motor impairment. Such children will require similar services.

Q3. What are the principles of management?

This depends upon the stage of the disorder (Fig. 29.1).

Different approaches to treatment have, from time to time, attracted considerable interest and enthusiasm, as well as opposition. Only recently have attempts been made to study the relative merits of each in objective ways. No single approach will suit all children with a particular form of CP. No study has convincingly shown benefits of one approach over another.

Management involves regular assessment of the child (with parent/carer involvement) and close multi-disciplinary working.

Key professionals

- *The physiotherapist* is responsible for development of motor skills, and assessment for lower limb orthoses and specialized supportive equipment, such as standers and mobility aids. In the early stages physiotherapy is aimed at interrupting the circle of malachievement caused by abnormal muscle tone. The child's carers are shown methods of handling and carrying out everyday tasks that help this.
- *The speech and language therapist* plays these key roles in CP:
  - Most importantly, helping with feeding early in life
  - Helping early communication development
  - Help with speech, which may be severely impaired
  - Management of dribbling
  - Provision of communication aids.
- *The occupational therapist* will assess the need for equipment to facilitate aspects of daily living, e.g. bathing, toileting, static seating, feeding etc., and fine motor skill function, perceptual skills and the use of upper limb orthoses. Adaptations may also be required in the home.

Specialized equipment

- *Orthoses.* The purpose of an orthosis is to restore the normal distribution of forces acting through the limb, thereby normalizing musculoskeletal relationships and establishing a normal pattern of motion and/or prevention of progressive deformity. Hence children with a persistently equinus foot may wear an ankle orthosis. Other orthoses facilitate hand function. A night resting splint will hold the hand in a neutral position in children, thus optimizing functional use during the day.
- *Special seating, standing and lying frames.* These are used to try to maintain good posture and to give the child optimal positioning and support for feeding and play.
- *Supportive bracing.* This may be needed in some quadriplegic patients to prevent progression of spinal deformity.

Specific drug treatment

Drugs are now being used more widely in CP:

- *Botulinum toxin A (BT A).* This works by chemically denervating the muscle, allowing it to relax,

which may enable improved gait or easier care, for example. Relaxation of the muscle may also enable it to grow better by allowing stretching and thereby reducing contractures. The duration of effect is usually 10–14 weeks, and measurable effects may persist for up to 26 weeks.
- *Baclofen.* This analogue of gamma-aminobutyric acid (GABA) impedes excitatory neurotransmission at a spinal level. Oral baclofen is rapidly absorbed, but is protein-bound and has poor penetration into CSF because of poor lipid solubility. The half-life is 3–4 hours, requiring regular dosing (3 times daily). Response to oral baclofen is unpredictable; a number of children will show a satisfactory response, with reduction in muscle tone, but others will develop unacceptable side-effects, including somnolence, confusion, difficulties with oral control, ataxia and increased frequency of micturition. Recently, baclofen by continuous infusion has been given by an intrathecal catheter and pump delivery system to achieve higher and continuous CSF baclofen levels. Baclofen is perhaps most useful when there is generalized increase in tone, which would require multiple injections of botulinum toxin, e.g. in the child with severe spastic tetraplegia.
- Other medications (Table 29.4).

Surgery

The orthopaedic surgeon has a major role to play in management of CP. Orthopaedic surgery may be indicated to improve function, to prevent deterioration, to relieve pain and to facilitate care.

There are two surgical aspects to the management of CP:

- *Selective posterior rhizotomy.* Two groups of patients are most suitable: children who are of good intelligence, well motivated and sufficiently strong to achieve walking after spasticity is reduced, and severely affected, non-ambulant patients in whom painful spasm can be reduced.

Table 29.4 Medications used for the treatment of different forms of tone abnormalities

SPASTICITY	diazepam, nitrazepam, klorazepat, baclofen, tiagabine, tizanidine, dantrolene, piracetam, clonidine, cannabinoids
DYSTONIA	trihexyfenidil, L-Dopa, procyclidine, tetrabenazine (for dyskinesia)
CHOREO-ATHETOSIS	valproate, haloperidol, benztropine, procyclidine, tetrabenazine, levetiracetam
RIGIDITY	biperidene, benztropine, procyclidine, rotigotine transdermal.

- *Single event multilevel surgery with associated gait analysis*. When fixed contracture of muscles occurs, surgical release has been required to correct the deformity. The traditional approach has been to undertake soft tissue surgery in a 'phased' manner, dealing with one area at a time. Techniques for thorough pre- and post-operative assessment have been developed, in particular gait analysis. The latter has led to a better understanding of normal gait in children and hence the abnormal gait of the child with CP. Detailed surgical planning is based upon objective rather than subjective information. Gait analysis also allows proper objective review after surgery.
- *Deep brain stimulation (DBS)*. DBS involves surgical implantation of brain pacemaker which sends electrical impulses to the brain. DBS may relieve symptoms like dyskinesias (especially dystonia), stiffness and to a lesser extent also spasticity. Throughout Europe there are several specialized centres for DBS surgical procedures.

Associated problems

Difficulty may arise from motor problems:

- *Feeding difficulties*. Feeding may be a considerable problem, leading to inadequate quantity and quality of intake. Children with spastic quadriplegia or athetoid CP may have such severe feeding difficulties that they fail to thrive. Recurrent aspiration during feeding may lead to serious chest complications, and children with severe CP commonly suffer from significant gastro-oesophageal reflux (up to 70% having oesophagitis). It is important to address positioning and consistency of food, and to consider the need for gastrostomy feeding. A multidisciplinary approach is essential for significant feeding problems and many places will have a 'feeding clinic'.
- *Drooling*. This is associated with speech and feeding problems and can be a significant cosmetic handicap, as well as being very messy and affecting the skin around the mouth and neck. It is usually due to a problem with swallowing saliva rather than excessive production. Techniques used to help it are:
  - Prompting and rewards for swallowing
  - Positioning and exercises to improve oro-motor function and sensory awareness, now sometimes aided by intra-oral training appliances
  - Medication with anticholinergics to reduce secretions (especially helpful are scopolamin transdermal preparations)
  - Surgery to direct the ducts further towards the back of the mouth
  - Occasionally, removal of salivary glands
  - Intraglandular botulinum toxin injections.

- *Dislocated hips*. These are an important complication in CP and routine screening by X-ray is needed. Good postural management will help to prevent dislocation.
- *Bowel and bladder problems*. Incontinence may result from intellectual disability, but may be a problem of not being able to get to the toilet in time or undress quickly enough. Constipation is common, particularly in the immobile child and those with restricted diets. It may also be associated with abnormal gut sensitivity and motility. It is important to try to prevent problems by explaining to the parents and child about normal bowel function and giving dietary advice. If constipation occurs, the earlier it is treated, the better.
- *Osteopenia*. The increased risk of bone fractures in children with motor disabilities is linked to reduced bone density. Measures such as weight-bearing, particularly ambulation, good nutrition (especially calcium, vitamin D and magnesium) and sunlight will help.

Other associated problems include:

- *Vision problems*. These are common (50%), particularly myopia, cortical visual impairment and squint.
- *Hearing problems*. These occur in 20–30%, particularly sensorineural deafness. It is also important to look for conductive problems.
- *Intellectual disabilities*. These are found in all types of CP. Generalized intellectual difficulties tend to be related to severity of physical problems; however, children with relatively mild motor problems may have significant intellectual difficulties and vice versa, but all children will need early psychological evaluation and follow-up.
- *Specific learning difficulties*. These are also seen more frequently in CP and can easily be overlooked. Assessment can be very difficult if there are severe motor problems.
- *Epilepsy*. Around 21% of children with CP develop epilepsy, which may be difficult to control.
- *Psychological problems*. These may be due to physical difficulties, or children may have problems directly related to the underlying brain disorder.
- *Educational issues*. Most children will go to mainstream school and need a minimum of help. Some adaptations may be necessary, e.g. ramps, handrails, lifts, special toilet facilities and adapted working surfaces in the classroom.

http://www-rheop.ujf-grenoble.fr/scpe2/site_scpe/index.php

Communication and its disorders

Basic science

When thinking about speech and language development, you must address the different skills necessary for communication. These include the following.

Attention control
The child must have adequate listening skills and attention.

Symbolic understanding
Words are symbols, so unless children can understand the concept of symbols, they will not understand speech.

Comprehension
Does the child understand spoken language?

Expressive speech
This is the area of communication most easily identified by both parents and professionals, and so tends to be what people concentrate on in the early stages.

Phonology
The development of sounds proceeds largely in the same order in all children, the easier sounds being acquired earlier.

Oromotor skills
These depend on normal orofacial development and functioning bulbar innervation.

Grammar/syntax
The rules of language (e.g. plurals, tenses, word order) need to be acquired.

Semantics
Semantics is about the meaning of words. Children can just learn words by rote and not be able to use them appropriately in context.

Pragmatics
Pragmatics is the way in which language is used in the social context. It includes turn-taking, keeping to the subject, selection, context, verbal jokes and negotiation. This is an area that children with developmental language difficulties, and in particular autism, find hard to learn.

Non-verbal communication

A lot of non-verbal communication occurs without thought, but in children with autism it has to be taught. It includes:

- Tone of voice, pauses etc.
- Facial expression, including eye contact
- Body posture
- Gesture and signing
- Physical contact.

These become more important in children with speech problems and may be the predominant form of communication in some, such as those with profound deafness.

Problem-orientated topic:

delay in speaking

Stanko is 2¹/₂ years old. His parents are concerned that he is still only using a few single words. He has achieved his motor milestones within the average range and has no significant previous medical history.

Q1. How would you assess this child?
Q2. What other information would you seek?
Q3. What investigations would you perform?
Q4. How would you manage this child?

Q1.   How would you assess this child?

History
Ask in particular about:
- *Pregnancy and birth history.*
- *Family history of language problems or learning difficulties.* There is certainly a strong genetic component in language disorder and possibly in the normal range of language acquisition.
- *Early input.* Carer/child interaction is clearly vital.
- *Bilingualism.* This was thought to be a problem for children first learning language but there is no evidence for this.
- *General development.* Language delay is often a marker for general delay.
- *Any worry about hearing?* Has the hearing been checked? Is there intermittent hearing loss or high-frequency loss? Profoundly deaf children will not learn spoken language without considerable help. Some children with mild hearing losses are delayed in their language development.
- *Any feeding problems in early life?*
- *Any problems now with chewing or dribbling?*
- *Any difficulties with social relationships?*

Observation
- Is there any clumsiness?
- Observe the child's attention span.

- Watch children in a free play situation. Do they make good eye contact with their parent and with other people in the room? Do they turn to share enjoyment of a toy with their parent? How does the parent respond? Is there imaginative play?
- What spontaneous sounds, words or phrases do they use?
- Is there good non-verbal communication?

Examination

- Do the ears look normal? Undertake a full ear, nose and throat examination (Ch. 5).
- Are there local problems in the mouth? Submucous cleft or problems with tongue movements?
- Assess hearing in your clinic (Ch. 5).
- Associated disorder. Any evidence of a movement disorder, e.g. CP?
- Try to engage the child in some one-to-one activities. Some children may appear to have poor auditory attention. Does this improve when you work one-to-one with the child (as in a child with an attention disorder) or is the child unable to tolerate this one-to-one direction (raises the possibility of autistic spectrum disorder)?

These factors may interplay.

Q2. What other information would you seek?

There are a number of aspects of language that need to be addressed separately.

Listening and attention

Can the child attend to language?

Verbal comprehension

What level of verbal comprehension has the child developed?

- From the history, get particular examples and make sure that they show verbal rather than non-verbal comprehension. Beware the child understanding from context alone. Can the child identify single objects (from objects or pictures)?
- Can the child understand prepositions (in/on/under/behind) and concepts (big/little)?
- How many key words can the child follow? For example:
  - 'Put the *big* pencil in the box' — 1 key word. There are only pencils and a box and it is automatic to put things in boxes.
  - 'Put the *cat under* the *chair*' — 3 key words.

> **BOX 29.6 Pitfalls in assessing verbal competence**
>
> Beware of the echolalic child or the child using chunks of 'late echoing', which will give the impression of a verbally competent child. This may indicate delayed verbal comprehension or semantic–pragmatic problems.
>
> Beware of children who initially appear to have good expressive language using appropriate social phrases but who demonstrate a lack of variety or range in their speech. These may be children with general delay or with very little language stimulation.

Non-verbal strategies

What non-verbal strategies does the child use to communicate, both for comprehension and expression?

- Pointing and facial expression plus non-speech sound to indicate needs?
- Common gestures, such as pointing, arms up for wanting to be lifted up and waving bye-bye?
- More complex gestures as a means of self-expression?

Verbal expression (Box 29.6)

- Pre-speech babbling or only open vowel sounds?
- Some symbolic noise or word approximations: e.g. 'hiya' (for 'here you are') or 'brrmm brrmm' (for car play)?
- How many single words is the child using that Mother understands (not necessarily other people)?
- Are there some learned phrases that are two- or three-word combinations learned together, e.g. 'all gone', or has the child started flexible word joining, e.g. 'teddy gone' or 'daddy car'?
- Are longer structures used, e.g. 'my teddy gone' or 'my teddy's called Joe and he's going to bed now'?
- Does the child ask questions?
- Can the child tell you what he or she has been doing?
- Does he or she tend to copy what you say?

Phonology

This is an area that parents often get worried about, but which has the best prognosis:

- Is it dysarthria (due to abnormal neurology, e.g. CP)?
- Is it dysphonia (e.g. hoarseness due to disorder of the voice box)?
- Is it delay (the way a younger child would talk) or deviance?

Semantics and pragmatics (Box 29.7)

This is an area of difficulty that may only become evident as the child develops more language. It is rare for children to have semantic or pragmatic disorders with completely normal early language development:

- Does the child have difficulties following instructions, particularly complicated ones?
- Does the child understand tenses?
- Are conversational skills age-appropriate? Can the child turn-take? Is the content of speech pertinent?

Q3. What investigations would you perform?

- Hearing should be tested in all children.
- Test chromosomes only if there are other indications.
- Order an EEG if there is loss of language or some other reason to suspect epilepsy.

Any child with severe language impairment or complex problems should be seen by a paediatrician.

Q4. How would you manage this child?

The role of the doctor in the management of language difficulties is:

- To identify and address any possible causes (e.g. hearing loss, submucous cleft)
- To identify and address associated difficulties (e.g. epilepsy).

Management of language impairments lies predominantly with the speech and language therapist (SLT), whose role is:

- To advise parents on how they can help the child
- To monitor young children or those with mild delay
- To work with nursery or school, advising how to help language development
- To work with groups of children who have similar problems, to encourage language development
- To work with individual children, usually for short intensive bursts of speech therapy
- To advise on and implement alternative communication systems.

Education

Fortunately, most language difficulties have resolved by school age or soon after. Some children will go on to have reading difficulties.

A small number of children need specialist educational input, which may be available locally at nursery or primary school, but by secondary school age the numbers are so small that the child may need to travel some distance and occasionally even board at a special school to obtain this level of specialist education.

English as a second language

Special problems may arise for children whose maternal language is not English. These include:

- *Late recognition*. People assume that there are no problems, or that any difficulties in English result from it being the child's second language.
- *Assessment*. Is there a problem in the first language or is the problem only in English? Trying to assess this means having an interpreter.
- *Treatment*. Should this be in the first language? Can this be achieved?

Children with profound and multiple learning difficulties

The SLT will be part of a team caring for these children. He or she may be involved initially with feeding difficulties and can anticipate language problems.

Key elements for aiding communication in children with profound and multiple difficulties are:

- Using all senses to give messages about the child's world: hearing, vision, touch, taste, smell
- Helping the child to learn to control the environment at a basic level: making simple choices, turn-taking
- Helping the child to develop relationships: limiting numbers of professionals involved directly with the child and working through other people
- Using augmentative communication systems.

Language disorders

Definitions

The terms 'communication' and 'language' are sometimes used interchangeably. Communication problems encompass a wider range of disorders, including difficulties in non-verbal communication and ability to use language (as in autism). We will discuss language problems other than autism here, although this is not always a simple distinction:

- *Delay* implies that language is slow to develop; it is progressing in a normal pattern but is like that of a younger child.
- *Disorder* implies that language contains elements that are not part of normal development.

- *Impairment* is the term that is currently preferred and encompasses both delay and deviance. Specific language impairment is used for children who have isolated language impairment with non-verbal learning skills at a higher level. However, studies show that children with 'specific' language impairment have a high incidence of other neurodevelopmental disorders.

Prevalence

Studies on prevalence vary, depending on definition and whether children with intellectual difficulties are included. About 5–7% of children have significant language difficulties without other learning difficulties. Around 1% have severe persisting difficulties.

There is a wide variation in normal development of language. This can make it hard to decide when there is an abnormality, particularly when there is delay rather than deviance and it affects verbal expression and phonology. Many (though not all) of these children will have corrected themselves by school age or soon after.

Classification

There are problems with classification of communication disorders; children often overlap categories or change from one to another. There is also difficulty because of the wide spectrum of normal development.

A practical classification can be used to assist assessment and investigation:

- Disorders affecting speech production:
  - Neurological problems, e.g. CP
  - Structural problems, e.g. cleft lip and palate ('tongue-tie' rarely, if ever, causes speech problems)
  - Dysphonia, e.g. abnormalities of the vocal cords
  - Dysfluency (stammering), a frequently normal stage of development between 2 and 4 years
  - Elective (or selective) mutism
- Specific language impairments:
  - Expressive language delay
  - Articulatory dyspraxia, possibly associated with feeding difficulties
  - Difficulties in producing sounds accurately, in comprehension or in finding a word
  - Semantic–pragmatic difficulties. These children may have had normal early development of language but often have had delay or deviance that resolved. Difficulties become apparent later with inability to maintain a conversation, 'getting the wrong end of the stick', going off at a tangent, misunderstanding rules of conversation, or difficulty with puns and jokes. There are often problems with social interaction, which may overlap with the autistic spectrum.

- Children who stop talking:
  - Usually associated with loss of other skills, e.g. neurodegenerative disorders
- Impaired language and social interaction:
  - These are considered in the section on autistic spectrum disorders.

http://www.afasic.org.uk

The Afasic website has information sheets on different types of disorder

Aetiology

Most children with language difficulties not linked with other major disabilities have no identifiable cause for their problems.

Children with language disorders are known to have an increased family history of language disorders and twin studies suggest strong heritability.

Associated problems

- *Epilepsy* has a higher incidence in children with language disorders. This supports the idea that language disorders are due to problems with brain development.
- *Left-handedness* (especially in girls) is often noted but not always confirmed. The significance is unclear; it may sometimes be a pathological left-handedness.
- *Clumsiness* is found in 90% of children with severe language disorder. Studies and clinical observation confirm this link.
- *Educational difficulties* are complicated and depend on the type of language impairment.

Autism spectrum disorders

Problem-orientated topic:

the isolated child ○ ○ ○ ○ ○

Blaz is 3 years of age and has been referred by his primary care physician because he has recently started nursery school and his teacher has expressed concern that he may be autistic. Blaz is his mother's third child and he has always acted differently to the other two. Since the age of 6 months he stopped making eye contact and is now a very solitary child, preferring his own company to that of his family. He spends hours spinning a toy top and becomes inconsolable if interrupted. His speech development is immature and he tends to echo phrases made by his brothers.

Q1. What are the three core impairments seen in autism spectrum disorders?

Q2. How would you assess this child?

Q3. What alternative conditions do you need to consider?

Q4. What investigations should be considered?

Q5. What are the advantages/disadvantages of finding a diagnostic label for Blaz and his family?

Q6. What are your management options?

Q7. What is the prognosis for this condition?

Q1. What are the three core impairments seen in autism spectrum disorders?

Autism is a specific type of communication disorder, which has some overlap with semantic–pragmatic disorders of language (p. 405) and also with other types of neurodevelopmental disorder. The present concept is of an 'autistic spectrum', in which the three core features are:

- Impairment of social interaction
- Impairment of communication
- Restricted interests and activities

It can be useful within this spectrum to define the type (autism, Asperger syndrome and pervasive developmental disorder-not otherwise specified (PDD-NOS), while accepting that some children do not fit any one of these labels but still show significant features within the spectrum.

Impaired social interaction

Eye contact may be present but is abnormal in its nature (fixed and staring, held too long). However, there may be good reasons for a child to have poor eye contact in the clinic, such as shyness, embarrassment, wilfulness.

Lack of cuddliness is another popular concept, but autistic children may be willing to be cuddled and even give cuddles back, especially with their parents, though the parents may describe it as 'on the child's terms' or 'too intense'.

Key indicators of impaired social interaction are:

- Lack of sharing and directing attention
- Poor recognition of others' affect
- Poor understanding of social situations.

Impaired communication

In classic autism there will be delayed development of communication, though many autistic children develop some language. About 33% of children with autism develop some early words and then lose them. It is often apparent that they had social interactional problems from the outset and/or never used their words

really communicatively. Only 7–8% of autistic children have a setback in language development following completely normal development in the first couple of years with acquisition of two-word phrases. Children with Asperger syndrome may have normal language development, but content and use of language may be unusual.

Rigidity/stereotyped thought and behaviour

These include the hand flapping and turning in circles seen in autism and the intense narrow interests of children with Asperger syndrome. Some children have no imaginative play; others will have restricted imaginative play, such as going through the same routine, probably copied from a video.

Q2. How would you assess this child?

With practice it becomes relatively easy to identify most children within the spectrum in the informal clinic situation and many parents have already suspected the diagnosis. In some children it is less easy, and it is important to have reliable methods of assessment so that the diagnosis can be made or excluded with confidence and backed up with evidence.

History

Diagnosis depends greatly on history, so it is important to have a framework that will cover the triad of impairments. In addition a standard medical, developmental and family history may indicate a different diagnosis, associated problems or a possible cause for the autism.

There are formal scored interviews for the autistic spectrum, which have diagnostic cutoff points and may also give an indication of where in the spectrum the child lies.

Examination

This may identify possible causes, including:

- Dysmorphism
- Neurological abnormality, including head size
- Skin markers (should include examination under Wood's light for depigmented patches, p. 373).

Informal observation in the clinic setting will often give clues as to diagnosis, but children may act fairly normally in this structured one-to-one situation, so it is helpful to observe them in different settings and over time.

Assessing where on the spectrum a child lies

The formal scored tools will help with this. Beware of being too precise early on because this may change as time goes by and as you obtain more information about the child.

Assessing the child's strengths and weaknesses

Each aspect of the child's difficulties is assessed:
- Its nature
- Its degree
- Whether it is primary or secondary
- Whether it is changing over time.

Other aspects can be assessed, such as:
- Rigidity/routines
- Motor abilities
- 'Dangers' of special interests
- Motivation/reliability
- Obsessional–compulsive behaviours
- Insight
- Depression/anxiety
- Temperament
- Support systems.

Children are presenting younger with possible autistic spectrum disorder and this may present difficulties around stability of the diagnostic label over time.

Q3. What alternative conditions do you need to consider?

Social impairment may be secondary to other disorders:
- Learning difficulties, leading to social immaturity
- Dyspraxia, leading to invasion of other people's social space
- Psychopathy (p. 417)
- Shyness, leading to social awkwardness
- Conduct disorder, bullying, abuse, depression, which may all lead to abnormal social relationships
- Semantic–pragmatic disorders (p. 405), leading to abnormalities in social relationships; there is overlap between these and autism
- Secondary social impairment, which may occur as a result of HKD/ADHD (p. 397), depression, bullying or abuse
- Rett syndrome (p. 387), but the relationship to autism is debatable; certainly, these children develop features of severe autism but also tend to lose them as the condition progresses.

Comorbidity

Children with an autistic spectrum disorder have a greater incidence of other developmental and psychiatric disorders and these should be sought:
- Learning difficulty is the most common associated problem in classic autism (70–75%). Also, children with learning disorders may show features of autism and it is important to ascertain whether this is sufficient to give an additional diagnosis of autism.

- HKD/ADHD.
- Depression.
- Affective disorder.
- Anxiety disorder.

Q4. What investigations should be considered?

Children with autism find investigations very difficult to cope with; therefore consider the reasons for ordering them. These reasons are:
- To identify a treatable cause
- To identify genetic implications
- Parental 'need to know'
- Research.

Investigations are most likely to be positive in children with a severe cognitive impairment.

Cytogenetics

Around 3% of children with autism have an abnormal karyotype. This figure is higher in children with dysmorphisms, severe learning difficulties and identifiable syndromes.

Imaging

Most common abnormalities are of the cerebellum but the significance of this is unknown. Cortical migration anomalies may sometimes be seen, but they are non-specific and will not help in diagnosis of autism or discovery of the cause. Features of tuberous sclerosis and neurofibromatosis may be recognized. Routine imaging is not recommended.

EEG

Between 21 and 43% of children with autism have an abnormal EEG. The longer the EEG, the more likely it is to reveal abnormalities, but these do not necessarily have implications for clinical care.

Q5. What are the advantages/disadvantages of finding a diagnostic label for Blaz and his family?

Advantages
- Changes attitudes towards the child positively (more understanding and appropriate responses)
- Mobilizes resources
- Indicates type of management for specific problems
- Gives an explanation to the child and parents
- Gives access to support networks.

Disadvantages
- Changes attitudes towards the child negatively (inappropriate lowering of expectations, assumptions about what diagnosis means)

- A label for life
- The label may need to change with passage of time.

Q6. What are your management options?

These include:
- Management of the child:
  - Medical and psychological
  - Social skills (group work)
  - Educational
- Management of the family:
  - Parent courses
  - Parent support
- Information/education about the condition:
  - For the parent
  - For the child.

Goals for management include:
- Fostering of development
- Promotion of learning
- Reduction of stereotypy
- Elimination of maladaptive behaviours
- Alleviation of family distress.

There are different approaches to management, which will be used in conjunction with each other.

Pharmacotherapy

In the US 30% of children with autism and 55% of children with high-functioning autism and Asperger are on medication. The corresponding figures in the UK are only 5% and 10%.

Drugs will not generally affect the core symptoms of autism (and there is no evidence at present of long-term benefits) but they can ameliorate symptoms. It is important when considering medication that you are clear about the specific symptoms you are targeting and that ongoing behavioural and educational management is continued. Ensuring safe and consistent administration and monitoring for side-effects is essential. You also need to consider who you are treating (child, parent, doctor, teacher) and make sure you have informed consent as far as you are able. Substances suggested as a general treatment for autism are:
- *Secretin.* There is no evidence from randomized controlled trials of any benefit.
- *Vitamins, minerals, essential fatty acids and metals.* No studies have shown any effect.
- *Gluten- and casein-free diets.* These have their supporters but robust evidence is not yet available. Some children with autism have distressing bowel problems and a gluten- or casein-free diet may decrease bowel symptoms and greatly improve general wellbeing.

Family support

This is important from the start. Some support will come from the medical and educational teams but families should also be made aware of local and national parent groups. There are practical issues that can be addressed and which will make life easier.

Behaviour management

Difficult behaviours can be analysed as follows:
- Instrumental: in order to get something
- Social: in order to get attention
- Self-stimulatory.

The first two types of behaviour are most amenable to behaviour therapy and the last type to drug treatment.

Educational management

Many educational intervention programmes are advocated in autism; some claim to provide a 'cure' but most claim only improvement. Most approaches have in common a high degree of one-to-one intervention, often with highly structured activities. Some focus on parent intervention and some use professionals or trained workers.

Multidisciplinary teams

Many children will benefit from going through a formal multidisciplinary assessment and management. This may be at the local Child Development Centre or may be within the community.

http://www.autismeurope.org

Q7. What is the prognosis for this condition?

The degree of independence reached by a child within the autistic spectrum depends to a major extent not only on the degree of intellectual impairment, but also on severity of the autism. Parents have a real anxiety that some children with high-functioning autism and Asperger syndrome will find it hard to manage on their own. Undoubtedly some people with autism do very well, and there are a number of accounts written by autistic people about their experiences that give an insight into what autism is like from the inside.

Autism

Autism has a prevalence of about 0.5/1000. This rate has remained fairly steady over the years. The corresponding figure for Asperger syndrome is around 0.25/1000.

Autistic spectrum disorder prevalence is between 3 and 6/1000, rising to nearly 1 in 100 in studies seeking out the whole range of disorders. It appears to be rising but this is likely to be because the diagnosis is being more readily recognized.

Aetiology of autism

A long list of associated conditions have been found in studies of children with autistic spectrum disorder:

- Fragile X syndrome (p. 396; either some autistic impairments or full autism)
- Tuberous sclerosis (p. 373; 43–60% of children with tuberous sclerosis will have autism or pervasive developmental disorder)
- Phenylketonuria (p. 463)
- Neurofibromatosis (p. 372)
- Down syndrome (p. 394)
- Williams syndrome
- Duchenne muscular dystrophy (p. 382)
- Non-specific dysmorphisms and other chromosomal abnormalities
- West syndrome (p. 371)
- Hydrocephalus (p. 388; 23% have autism)
- Severe sensory deficits
- Congenital infections
- Encephalitis (p. 648)
- Hypothyroidism (p. 475)
- Fetal alcohol syndrome
- Neurometabolic disorders (p. 460).

Autism is probably under-diagnosed in many of these conditions because, once a child has a label, there may be reluctance to pursue an additional label.

A variety of possible aetiological agents have been proposed, but convincing evidence for any of these is not available. There is no evidence linking measles/mumps/rubella (MMR) vaccination to autism.

High-functioning autism and Asperger syndrome

These are not 'mild' autism! The distress caused to the child can be greater than with 'classic' autism because of the awareness the child has of the difficulties without the ability to understand them.

What worries me is that when Jonathan leaves school he'll have 6 or 7 GCSEs (General Certificate of Secondary Education) but he won't be able to go out and buy himself a shirt. (Parent of a boy aged 15 years)

David knows that when he walks into the tennis club he 'gets it wrong', whilst his younger brother Peter is fine. He doesn't understand why this is and he gets very depressed. (Parent of a boy aged 11 years)

The characteristics are as follows:
- Presentation is usually after 3 years of age but, with hindsight, indicators can be identified in the first 3 years of life.
- Language may be normal, at least superficially.
- Presentation is often via the school with behavioural difficulties, school failure and 'oddness'. The difficulties become apparent with the pressures for social conformity at school.

The terms high-functioning autism and Asperger syndrome are sometimes used interchangeably but there are differences.

Asperger syndrome is characterized by:
- Highly developed special interests
- Verbal IQ being greater than performance IQ
- Frequent clumsiness
- More social interest than in high-functioning autism
- Socially approaching (but may be unusual or inappropriate)
- More insight into own thoughts and feelings
- Greater desire to fit in
- Cognitive (but not empathic) understanding of social rules.

These difficulties can give rise to:
- High levels of anxiety
- Psychiatric morbidity
- Socially manipulative behaviour, such as school exclusion
- Problems gaining independence
- Vulnerability, both socially and practically.

Acknowledgement

We would like to thank the Sheffield Distance Learning Programme for Paediatric Neurodisability and in particular Dr Hilary Cass, Professor David Hall, Dr Mike Smith, Dr Connie Pullon, Dr Peter Baxter, Sian Bell and Dr Karen Whiting for their kind permission to use materials they have written.

Wolf-Rüdiger Horn   Neil Kennedy

Child and adolescent mental health

LEARNING OUTCOMES

By the end of this chapter you should:

- Know the diagnostic criteria of somatoform disorders (SFD)
- Know the basic investigations that are necessary in cases of possible SFD
- Know the principles of management of SFD
- Know the diagnostic criteria of chronic fatigue syndrome (CFS)
- Know the basic investigations that are necessary in cases of possible CFS
- Know the principles of management of CFS
- Be able to recognize children and adolescents at risk of suicide
- Know the principles of management of self-harm
- Know how to assess suicide intent in adolescents
- Know the differential diagnosis of acute psychosis in children and adolescents.

MODULE SIX

Introduction

Children and adolescents with symptoms of a severe emotional or apparent psychiatric nature are usually first seen by their primary care physician who will in most cases refer the young person to a child and adolescent psychiatrist. Most young people with not so severe emotional-based problems are managed by primary care physicians and are discussed in Chapter 20. Sometimes children with more serious psychiatric problems present directly to an ambulatory child and adolescent psychiatrist or to the paediatric accident and emergency department. It is important that paediatric trainees develop a knowledge of psychiatric problems in children and adolescents in order to decide when referral to a mental health professional is appropriate.

Somatoform disorders

Problem-orientated topic:

An adolescent with aching testicles

Karl is a 15-year-old boy who is brought to your paediatric practice because of an 8-week history of recurring nagging and increasingly tearing pain at the base of his penis and extending into both testicles. The pain began after an episode of frequent urination during a common cold. Since then he has missed 4 weeks of school because of being increasingly

Continued overleaf

unable to sit on a chair for more than a few minutes.

Some years ago Karl had suffered from recurrent tension headaches and because of school problems you had referred him to a child psychiatrist. On examination, the boy appears rather shy and anxious. Physically you do not find any abnormalities, his pubertal maturity is normally developed (Tanner PH4 G4).

His father hands over reports from an urologist and an orthopaedic surgeon whom he consulted before. These specialists did not find any pathology. Now the father asks you to arrange for further investigations like more blood tests (i.e. for Lyme disease etc.) and MRI: 'There must be a cause for his pain!'

Q1. Could Karl be suffering from somatoform disorder?

Q2. What further investigations should be done?

Q3. What are the principles of management?

BOX 30.1 Diagnosis of somatoform disorders (SFD)

Somatization disorder (rare in young people)
- Multiple, recurrent and frequently changing physical symptoms of at least two years' duration
- Long and complicated history of contact with both primary and specialist medical care services, during which many negative investigations or fruitless exploratory operations may have been carried out
- Symptoms may be referred to any part or system of the body
- Chronic and fluctuating course of the disorder, often associated with disruption of social, interpersonal, and family behaviour.

Undifferentiated somatoform disorder
- Short-lived (less than two years) and less striking symptom patterns

Hypochondriacal disorder

Somatoform autonomic dysfunction

Persistent somatoform pain disorder

Other somatoform disorder, unspecified

lead to costly and potentially dangerous medical investigations and treatments.

Q1. Could Karl be suffering from a somatoform disorder?

Epidemiology
- Prevalence of medically unexplained recurrent pain in children is estimated to be about 10%.
- In a representative survey in Germany the prevalence of somatization disorders amongst adolescents was 2.7%, another 11% showed an incomplete clinical picture of somatization. Thus, these disorders seem to belong to the most frequent chronic conditions in adolescence.

Pathogenesis
Headaches (Ch. 24), recurrent abdominal pain (Ch. 25) or fatigue are very common complaints in childhood and adolescence. These functional disorders may develop into somatoform disorders especially in the presence of co-morbid mental disorders like anxiety or depression and of different catastrophic thoughts. Somatization has been defined as the tendency to experience and communicate somatic distress and symptoms not accounted for by pathologic findings, to attribute them to physical illness and to seek medical help for them. This may

Diagnosis
The first step in the diagnostic algorithm in somatoform disorders (see Box 30.1) is a careful history and clinical examination in order to rule out any underlying medical condition that may explain the symptoms and signs.

The second step should be a cautious exploration of whether unconscious, unresolved conflicts or stress may be related to the pattern of symptoms. Keep in mind that about one fifth of all children and adolescents suffer from one or more moderate-to-severe mental health problems, often presented as physical symptoms.

The third step is to evaluate the environmental factors such as family, siblings, peers, school, and cultural norms and expectations.

Q2. What further investigations should be done?

Not doing enough diagnostic testing may lead to 'doctor shopping' and negative test results may disappoint the patient and his family. So from the very beginning you should establish good rapport and try to begin an effective and symptom-relieving treatment.

Q3. What are the principles of management?

The key components of management have to include:
- Acceptance of the pain as 'real' and assurance that the illness is the result of a complex interplay of several factors. Avoid discrediting or trivializing the symptoms ('it is all in your head')
- Application of the principles of the bio-psycho-social approach and incorporation of psychological health aspects to the problem
- Psycho-education of parents and children
- Individual cognitive-behavioural therapy
- Treatment of specific co-morbid psychiatric conditions, considering psychopharmacologic treatment with selective serotonin-reuptake inhibitors
- Reconnection to school where necessary.

Chronic fatigue syndrome

Problem-orientated topic:

a child with chronic fatigue

Lea is a 13-year-old girl who is referred to your outpatient clinic because of a 2-month history of tiredness which began after an episode of 'possible glandular fever'. Lea is 'exhausted all the time' but finds sleep at night difficult. She regularly complains of limb pain, headache and poor concentration. She has missed 4 weeks of school. Prior to this episode she was well, lively and active. On examination you find some small cervical lymph nodes but otherwise no abnormality.

Q1. Could this child be suffering from chronic fatigue syndrome?

Q2. What is the differential diagnosis and what investigations should be done?

Q3. What are the principles of management?

Q1. Could this child be suffering from chronic fatigue syndrome?

Epidemiology
- Prevalence is estimated at 0.5–1% in 12–16-year-olds.
- It is perhaps the most common cause of long-term school absence through illness in UK adolescents.

BOX 30.2 RCPCH diagnostic criteria for chronic fatigue syndrome

- Persisting debilitating generalized fatigue, for which no other cause can be found
- (RCPCH criteria do not prescribe a minimum duration of fatigue prior to diagnosis in children; adult criteria require fatigue > 6 months)
- Fatigue exacerbated by effort

Common associated symptoms
- Headache/myalgia
- Sleep disturbance
- Memory impairment/concentration difficulties
- Sore throat/tender lymph nodes
- Depressed mood
- Nausea/abdominal pain

Rarer associated symptoms
- Dizziness
- Hyperacusis/sensitivity to light
- Weight loss/gain
- Diarrhoea

- Female:male ratio in some studies is 3:1.
- Mean duration of symptoms is 3–4 years.

Pathophysiology
- This is unknown but many theories exist.
- Slightly higher rates are reported in monozygotic than in dizygotic twins.
- Inconsistent findings of immune system abnormalities have been reported. Subtle defects in the hypothalamic–pituitary axis and muscle pathology are detected in some studies.
- Recent viral infection is common, particularly with Epstein–Barr virus (EBV), but the significance of this is uncertain given the ubiquitous nature of this infection in this age group.

Diagnosis
The first step is a careful history and thorough examination. Pay particular attention to the fundi, muscle bulk, lymph nodes, presence of hepatosplenomegaly, and lying and standing blood pressure.

There is no single diagnostic feature in this condition. The Royal College of Paediatrics and Child Health (RCPCH) has published diagnostic criteria (Box 30.2).

http://www.rcpch.ac.uk/publications/clinical_docs/cfs.pdf

Table 30.1 Differential diagnosis and *minimum* investigation required in chronic fatigue syndrome

Test	Aims to exclude
Full blood count (FBC)/film	Anaemia, iron deficiency, leukaemia
Erythrocyte sedimentation rate (ESR)/C-reactive protein (CRP)	Autoimmune disorder, chronic infection
Urea and electrolytes (U&Es), glucose	Renal impairment, Addison disease, diabetes
Thyroid function	Hypothyroidism (increasingly common in this age group)
Liver function	Hepatitis
Viral serology (EBV, IgM, IgG)	Recent viral illness
Urinalysis (glucose, white blood cells (WBC), protein)	Urinary tract infection (UTI), renal disease, diabetes

Q2. What is the differential diagnosis and what investigations should be done?

(Table 30.1)

Secondary investigations may be required if symptoms or signs suggest an alternative diagnosis.

Q3. What are the principles of management?

The key components of management are likely to include:

- *A multidisciplinary approach.* Involve the child and parents at every stage.
- *Graded exercise therapy (GET).* Using a detailed diary, establish a baseline of activity. Gradually increase activity levels in partnership with the patient.
- *Sleep hygiene.* (Advice on establishing a helpful sleep pattern).
- *Cognitive behavioural therapy (CBT).*
- *Pain management.* Simple analgesics for most cases. Amitriptyline may be necessary.
- *Treat accompanying mood disorders.* Referral to the CAMHS team may be necessary if there is significant evidence of low mood.
- *Liaison with education services.* For home tuition and gradual reintegration into school.

Attempted suicide

Problem-orientated topic:

an adolescent who has attempted suicide

Emilie is 13 years old and presents to the accident and emergency department with her older sister (aged 18). She reports that she took six paracetamol tablets 2 hours ago 'because I was so fed up I wanted to kill myself'. She has never attempted suicide in the past. You note (a) several old transverse scars and (b) a 3 cm long superficial abrasion on the anterior aspect of her left forearm. Her paracetamol levels 2 hours later are below the treatment threshold for N-acetylcysteine.

Q1. How do you assess suicidal intent in children and adolescents such as Emilie?

Q2. What are the principles of management of self-harm in children and adolescents?

Q1. How do you assess suicidal intent in children and adolescents such as Emilie?

- Actual suicide is rare in children < 12 years old.
- Age-specific mortality from suicide rises from 1.6/100 000 per year in 10–14-year-olds to 9.5/100 000 in 15–19-year-olds in the USA.
- It is more common in males and there is no trend in social class.
- Methods of suicide in males differ from those in females (for example, violent methods such as hanging in males, self-poisoning in females).
- There is evidence for a pre-existing mental illness in ~90% (mood disorder (depression) or anxiety disorder). A previous suicide attempt is common.
- Suicide is precipitated by common, 'minor' stressful events: e.g. trouble at school, argument with parents/friends/boyfriend or girlfriend.

http://www.surgeongeneral.gov/library/mentalhealth/chapter3/sec5.html

More information on suicide

Attempted suicide is common (4/1000 per year in 15–19-year-olds), and more common in females and lower socioeconomic groups. Mental illness is found in ~50% (depression), and alcohol and drug misuse are common.

Q2. What are the principles of management of self-harm in children and adolescents?

Medical/surgical management (see also Ch. 49)

- Consider activated charcoal if the patient presents within 2 hours of ingestion of a poison, is conscious and is able to maintain an airway (see also p. 754).
- Obtain samples for toxicology (blood, urine, vomitus). Measure paracetamol levels in all children with suspected overdose or self-harm.
- Do *not* use cathartics (ipecac) or laxatives, unless directed by a poison information centre.
- Consult a poison information centre and manage accordingly.
- Treat superficial wounds with tissue adhesive or skin closure strips.

Further management of acute episode

- Admit to hospital overnight and ensure full mental health assessment the next day.
- Arrange a multidisciplinary child and adolescent psychiatric assessment of needs and risks.
- Check to see if there are youth protection issues.

Assessing suicidal intent in adolescents

Circumstances of the attempt

- Precipitating factors
- Did you actually want to die?
- Detailed history of the attempt: where, when, how, who else was around?
- Was there any planning?
- Was anyone else told?
- Was help sought, and if so, when?

Current mental state

- Evidence of depression/anxiety
- Do you still want to die?

Attitude towards the future

- Has the attempt changed your attitude to the future or the attitude of your carers?
- How do you feel about the future? Do you feel hopeless?

 http://www.rcpch.ac.uk/publications/clinical_docs/self_harm.pdf

RCPCH appraisal of NICE guidelines

http://www.rcpsych.ac.uk/mentalhealthinformation/mentalhealthandgrowingup.aspx

Royal College of Psychiatrists: Mental Health and Growing Up. Sheet 25 Suicide and attempted suicide; sheet 26 Deliberate self-harm in young people

Acute psychosis

Problem-orientated topic:

a boy with acute psychosis

Daerik is urgently referred to you by his primary care physician. He is 12 years old and has mild learning difficulties. He attended speech therapy until he was 7 years old. He goes to a mainstream school. He has always been a quiet boy with few friends, but over the last 3 months his mother has noticed him becoming increasingly withdrawn. She wonders if he is depressed because he 'doesn't seem to react to anything'. Two days ago she found a collection of canned food and biscuits in Daerik's bedroom. When questioned, he told her he was keeping them because a ghost had been telling him to.

Q1. How do you clinically assess Daerik?
Q2. What investigations should be ordered?

Q1. How do you clinically assess Daerik?

- Obtain a detailed history, paying particular attention to behaviour, emotions, relationships, family history, developmental progress and recent loss of skills.
- Perform a detailed neurological examination.
- Perform a mental state examination. You may consider using a standardized instrument such as the 'Kiddie Schedule for Affective Disorders and Schizophrenia' (KSADS, see below).
- Request an urgent psychiatric opinion.
- Consider and test for differential diagnoses (Table 30.2 below).

http://www.wpic.pitt.edu/ksads/ksads-pl.pdf

KSADS

Table 30.2 Differential diagnosis and investigation of psychotic symptoms in children

Diagnosis	Test
Schizophrenia	Clinical diagnosis
Psychosis associated with bipolar/mood disorder	Clinical diagnosis
Drug misuse (especially hallucinogens)	Toxicology
Brain tumour (p. 770)	MRI brain scan
Late-onset neurodegenerative disorder (e.g. metachromatic leucodystrophy)	MRI brain scan
Wilson disease (p. 544)	Copper/ceruloplasmin
Porphyria	Urinary porphobilinogen
Subacute sclerosing panencephalitis (p. 385)	EEG/CSF measles titres

Q2. What investigations should be ordered?

See Table 30.2.

Schizophrenia in childhood/ adolescence (Box 30.3)

- This is a rare disorder affecting 3/10 000 adolescents; it is much rarer before puberty.
- There is a large genetic component in the aetiology; 20% have a first-degree affected relative.
- One-third have a long-standing history of difficulty in making and keeping friends.
- Mean IQ of patients at initial presentation is 80–85.
- Insidious onset is common, with gradual social withdrawal.

Management

Treatment is generally with newer antipsychotic drugs (risperidone, olanzapine), as these have fewer side-effects (extrapyramidal effects and drowsiness) than traditional antipsychotics.

BOX 30.3 Symptoms of childhood/adolescent schizophrenia

Positive ('florid')
- Delusions
- Hallucinations (auditory > visual)
- Distortions of thinking (thought insertion)

Negative
- Social withdrawal
- Lack of motivation
- Poverty of speech
- Slowness of thought

Prognosis is probably worse than in those who present as adults. Poor premorbid functioning, predominance of negative symptoms and a long period of untreated illness are associated with a poor prognosis.

Further reading

Kreipe RE 2006 The biopsychosocial approach to adolescents with somatoform disorders. Adolesc Med 17: 1-24

Mario Angi   Vernon Long

The eye and vision

LEARNING OUTCOMES

By the end of this chapter you should:

- Be able to undertake a fundoscopic examination
- Be able to assess a child for a squint
- Know the common causes of a red eye
- Understand the causes of visual impairment
- Know how to examine for a cataract and its common causes.

MODULE SIX

Basic science

The eye is the organ of vision and is highly specialized in its structure and function. Many disorders of vision can be explained by understanding the embryology of the eye and visual development.

Normal visual development depends on normal structure of the eyes and an intact visual system to the striate cortex in the occipital lobe. Also, the midbrain and cerebellum play an important role in eye movements.

The eye is the sensory organ of vision. It focuses light on the retina, which is able to change light energy into nerve signals. These signals are sent along the optic nerves to the occipital lobe of the brain. For an image to be in focus on the retina, the cornea and lens bend the light, a process called refraction. The refractive power of the lens (measured in dioptres) is altered by changes in its shape effected by the ciliary muscles. This process of the lens changing shape to focus light on the retina is described as accommodation.

Visual disturbance as a result of ocular problems can be described as:

- *Myopia* (near-sightedness), in which images are focused in front of the retina because the eye is too long for the refractive process
- *Hypermetropia* (long-sightedness), in which images are focused behind the retina because the eye is relatively short

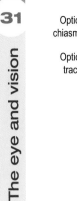

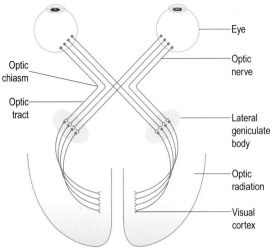

Fig. 31.1 **Visual pathways**

Labels on figure: Eye, Optic nerve, Optic chiasm, Optic tract, Lateral geniculate body, Optic radiation, Visual cortex

- *Astigmatism*, in which there is asymmetrical focusing mainly due to corneal distortion of refraction.

The retina is the most metabolically active tissue in the body for its size and depends on many biochemical reactions for its normal function. It contains different photoreceptor cells called rods and cones. Both types of cell contain a photosensitive pigment called rhodopsin, which is dependent on normal levels of vitamin A. The rods are particularly sensitive to light (photons) and the cones provide the ability to discriminate colours. Colour blindness, a genetic disorder, results from the loss of one or more of the cone cell types.

The optic nerves take visual impulses from the retina to the central visual projections in the brain (Fig. 31.1). The optic nerves decussate at the optic chiasm into optic tracts, which then synapse at the lateral geniculate body and project to the visual cortex via the optic radiation. The lateral geniculate body is the first level of elaboration of visual information before being processed by the visual system: more than 30 specialized areas located in the occipital and parietal lobes of the brain.

Interruption to the visual pathway at different points will result in different types of visual field defect. A lesion affecting the optic chiasm causes loss of vision in both temporal fields and is referred to as bitemporal hemianopia. Damage to an optic tract causes loss of vision in the contralateral half of the visual field of each eye, a condition referred to as homonymous hemianopia.

The processing of visual information in the visual system is a complicated process that needs to be learned by visual stimulation. Amblyopia (see below) occurs as a result of failure to stimulate the visual system at a critical phase of development in early postnatal life.

Strabismus

Problem-orientated topic:

a child with a squint ○ ○ ○ ○ ○

Stefan, a 4-year-old boy, has been identified by the school nurse as having a possible squint. His vision appears to be normal on gross testing in the primary care surgery, and the primary care physician is not certain whether Stefan has a squint or not. He refers the child to the paediatric department for advice.

Q1. How would you assess whether Stefan has a squint?

Q2. How would you classify squints?

Q3. What is the management of a definite squint?

Q1. How would you assess whether Stefan has a squint?

Assessment includes all of the following:
- Corneal light reflex
- Ocular movements (is there an increasing angle of squint with different eye movements?)
- Visual acuity (each eye separately)
- The cover test (Box 31.1)
- Fundoscopy (Box 31.2).

Q2. How would you classify squints?

Strabismus (squint) is defined as a misalignment of one eye in relation to the other. It may have its onset in

---

BOX 31.1 Skill: cover test

26 See also Chapter 5

BOX 31.2 Skill: fundoscopy

Take an ophthalmoscope and set the lens dial to zero. From an arm's distance, look through the eyehole towards the patient's pupils. Note the presence and relative brightness of the red reflex (reflection). Use your right eye and right hand to look at the subject's right eye. Change your hand and eye to view the subject's other eye. Looking through the eyepiece, move towards the red reflex of the right eye. Move the lens dial to focus on a blood vessel. Follow the blood vessel to find the optic disc.

infancy or in later childhood. It is a common disorder in childhood.

Some young children with a prominent nasal bridge give the appearance of a squint. On testing with a penlight (Hirschberg test) if the corneal reflexes look symmetrical in the pupils, the child is said to have a 'pseudostrabismus'.

Most true strabismus in childhood is inturning (esotropia). Exotropia is less common in childhood, although children with neurological problems may have a tendency to develop it. The strabismus may be present some of the time (latent) or all of the time (constant). A latent squint is the most likely cause in Stefan's case.

The most common childhood strabismus is an accommodative esotropia. This is usually seen in hypermetropia (all images focused behind the retina). Without glasses, the child can still see by using a lot of accommodative effort to focus distant or near images. This excess accommodative effort causes the eyes to converge and gives an esotropia. Continuous wearing of the correct glasses can improve the angle of strabismus, and in some cases can cause the eyes to straighten completely.

Sudden onset of strabismus in childhood should be referred to the eye department. If the findings are consistent with an accommodative esotropia, then corrective glasses may be given and no other investigations may be required. Sudden onset of esotropia can sometimes be a manifestation of a sixth nerve palsy (e.g. raised intracranial pressure) and this needs urgent investigation.

Q3. What is the management of a definite squint?

Binocular vision cannot develop while the visual axes are not aligned.

Management of a squint is as follows:
- Testing for amblyopia and patching of the good eye to stimulate visual input into the affected eye
- Assessment for refractive errors, as glasses may be required
- Strabismus surgery, often carried out early to help in the development of binocular vision by aligning the eyes.

Ptosis

This is the term given to the lowering of the upper eyelid.

The upper lid is normally elevated by the levator muscle that is innervated by the third cranial nerve, which also innervates most of the ocular movements and constricts the pupil. It also receives a contribution from the sympathetic system, which dilates the pupil.

Ptosis may be congenital (structural disinsertion of levator into eyelid) or caused by the following problems:
- lesions in the central nervous system
- sympathetic chain (e.g. neuroblastoma)
- muscular (myasthenia gravis).

Horner syndrome

Horner syndrome is the term given to ptosis caused by a lesion of the sympathetic system. The main signs are ptosis (about 2 mm) and a constricted pupil. The lesion may be anywhere along the sympathetic system, e.g. along the carotid artery or in the lung apex.

Proptosis

This term refers to forward displacement of the eye due to the presence of a mass behind the eye. The most common primary malignant tumour that can cause this is a rhabdomyosarcoma. The most common secondary tumour is a neuroblastoma. Other conditions that can give rise to proptosis in childhood include capillary haemangioma, lymphangioma, orbital pseudotumour (idiopathic orbital inflammation) and, rarely, thyroid eye disease.

Orbital imaging is required and prompt biopsy may be indicated if rhabdomyosarcoma is suspected.

Amblyopia

Amblyopia (lazy eye) is caused by a lack of visual experience on the part of one or both eyes during the developmental stages of vision. Binocular stimulation of cells of the visual cortex is required from birth in order to develop normal and stereoptic vision. It is the most common cause of visual loss in childhood and in young adults.

The amount of amblyopia a child experiences depends on its time of onset, duration and severity of the amblyopic factor. Different types of amblyopic factors include refractive (light not focused on the retina), strabismic (eyes misaligned; see below) and sensory deprivation (light blocked from entering the eye, e.g. cataracts or ptosis). So a cataract that affects a child at 7 years of age is less likely to be as amblyogenic as a congenital one. This is why all babies must have their red reflex tested as part of their first-day check.

Amblyopia is treatable by clearing the visual axis, prescribing glasses if required and encouraging the child to use the amblyopic eye. Patching or atropine drops to the fellow eye will improve visual acuity of the amblyopic eye in most cases.

Children affected by amblyogenic factors early in their development should be urgently referred to the ophthalmology department for optimization of their vision. This may require early cataract surgery, with visual rehabilitation and close follow-up throughout childhood.

Nystagmus

This is a rhythmic to-and-fro movement of the eyes, a disorder of fixation of vision. There is usually slow movement, as fixation is lost with a rapid refixation movement. It is rarely seen from birth but becomes more apparent after about 2 months of age.

Nystagmus may be caused by a problem in the anterior visual system affecting vision or by a central motor problem causing fixation to be lost (e.g. in the midbrain or cerebellum). Nystagmus may result from poor vision, and may be the reason for presentation. Ocular albinism is a common cause of nystagmus. If the eye examination is otherwise normal, a retinal dystrophy should be considered.

In many cases, there is no obvious cause and this may be congenital idiopathic motor nystagmus. New onset of nystagmus may sometimes herald an optic nerve glioma; intracranial imaging should be considered, along with early referral to ophthalmology.

Infantile glaucoma

Glaucoma is a condition that results in optic nerve damage from increased intra-ocular pressure. It can rarely present in the first years of life. It is a serious problem because, without treatment, severe irreversible visual loss would be expected.

The most common symptoms are an aversion to lights (photophobia) and watering eyes (epiphora).

Because the intra-ocular pressure is raised during a period in which the eye would be enlarging, the most noticeable sign of infantile glaucoma is enlarged corneal diameter. The cornea is noted to be cloudy, which may give a reduction in the red reflex.

The most common cause of infantile glaucoma is a congenital abnormality in the formation of the anterior chamber angle that normally removes aqueous fluid from the eye. This results in an increase in intra-ocular pressure. Generally speaking, an operation is required to overcome this drainage problem.

Cataract

Problem-orientated topic:

a child with cataract ● ● ● ● ●

Ioana, a 2-year-old child, is referred because she is thought by her parents to have impaired vision in her left eye. On examination she has an obvious opacity in her left eye, which you think might be a cataract.

Q1. Why is evaluation urgently required?

Q2. What are the important causes to consider?

Q3. What would you look for in your clinical examination?

Q4. What investigations are required?

Q5. What is the management of cataract?

Q1. Why is evaluation urgently required?

Cataracts that cause reduced vision in childhood can result in permanent blindness due to amblyopia if not removed promptly. Adult-onset cataracts can be removed years after their onset with a complete return of vision. This is because normal visual development will have occurred during childhood. Normal development requires the exposure of neurons in the visual system to stimulation from visual experience during the development of the visual system.

Childhood cataracts (Fig. 31.2) are a very potent amblyopic stimulus. They should be operated on appropriately and early. Significant cataracts at birth are generally operated on in the first few weeks of life to allow visual development to occur.

Q2. What are the important causes to consider?

The causes of cataracts in childhood are many. Some may be related to systemic conditions (Box 31.3).

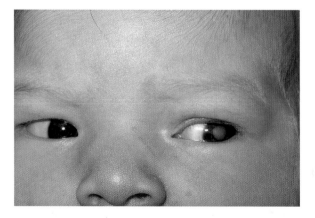

Fig. 31.2 **Cataract of left lens in a 3-month-old baby**

baby definitely fixes on a face intermittently. Examination of the eyes is unremarkable. There is no history of any other medical problems.

Q1.   What is the likely cause of reduced vision?
Q2.   What should be noted on clinical examination?
Q3.   What investigations should be considered?

Q3. What would you look for in your clinical examination?

Most congenital cataracts will be picked up on the first-day examination by the paediatrician checking the red reflex. Developmental cataracts that are not present at birth will be picked up later due to reduced vision. Very advanced cataracts may present when the parent notices a white pupil (leucocoria). This is also a presentation of retinoblastoma and should always be promptly referred to the ophthalmology service.

Q4. What investigations are required?

A complete physical examination is recommended but further investigations are usually not required unless some other abnormality is detected. Often, examination of the parents and the history will reveal an autosomal dominant isolated cataract that requires no further investigation. Investigations that are worth considering include urine for reducing substances, amino acids and organic acids. Rubella, calcium and glucose may also be considered.

Q5. What is the management of cataract?

Cataract surgery involves removing the cataract and either placing an intra-ocular lens or fitting the child with contact lenses if a lens cannot be placed inside the eye. Frequent follow-up in the eye clinic is needed, as visual development must be carefully monitored.

Reduced vision

Problem-orientated topic:

the child who appears not to see

Denisa, a 4-month-old baby, was noticed not to be making eye contact from birth. The parents say that her vision has improved in the past week. Vision testing shows that the

Q1. What is the likely cause of reduced vision?

In this case of reduced vision from birth in the absence of any other medical problems, delayed visual maturation is most likely.

Conditions affecting the apparently blind child with a normal eye examination can generally be divided into those affecting the anterior visual pathway and those affecting the posterior visual pathway (see below).

Q2. What should be noted on clinical examination?

Each child with visual loss should have a careful examination to detect any other physical signs that may be associated with the condition.

Q3. What investigations should be considered?

Any eye abnormality should initially be ruled out. Presence or absence of nystagmus and pupil reactions to light are important to note.

In Denisa's case, where the vision is improving, no further testing is required. Tests that would otherwise be considered include visual electrophysiology and brain imaging.

Anterior visual pathway problems

These can be located anywhere from the eye to behind the optic chiasm. While other causes of reduced vision, like corneal opacities and cataracts, are also anterior visual pathway problems, they are not included in this section because they are easily detected on clinical examination. This section will deal with the child who has reduced vision due to an anterior visual pathway problem with an apparently normal eye examination.

Anterior visual pathway disorders in infancy are associated with nystagmus (see above), whereas posterior visual pathway disorders are not.

Table 31.1 Examples of systemic conditions associated with retinal dystrophies

Condition	Other systems/organs affected
Isolated retinal dystrophy	None
Leber congenital amaurosis	None
Senior–Loken syndrome	Renal
Usher syndrome	Hearing and balance
Kearns–Sayre syndrome	Central nervous system (CNS), skeletal muscle, cardiac and endocrine
Batten disease	CNS
Alstrom syndrome	Cardiac, endocrine and hearing

Retinal dystrophies (Table 31.1)

Retinal dystrophies involve a progressive inherited reduction in retinal function. This usually results from reduced cone and/or rod retinal function. With a cone dystrophy, the person will prefer dark conditions to optimize rod function; with a rod dystrophy, the converse is true. In some retinal dystrophies, and especially in childhood, the retina may have a relatively normal appearance. Electrophysiology may be useful in identifying retinal dysfunction.

Retinitis pigmentosa (RP) is a form of retinal dystrophy that may present in childhood. There are various forms of RP, which affects the rods more than the cones. Visual function is affected in dark conditions more than in light conditions. RP is usually associated with relatively good central vision. While progression may occur, it is unlikely that all vision would be lost.

Retinal dystrophies have a typical appearance of pigmentary changes in the retina, narrowing of the retinal vessels and a pale optic disc. They may be inherited as an isolated disease or may be associated with other systemic conditions.

Optic nerve

Optic nerve disorders can also cause reduced vision. Some examples of causes are:

- Congenital
- Inherited
- Neoplastic
- Toxic
- Metabolic
- Traumatic.

Raised intracranial pressure from any cause, e.g. hydrocephalus or idiopathic intracranial hypertension, may result in reduced optic nerve function. Treatment is to normalize the raised intracranial pressure. Optic nerve function in these cases should be followed by assessing visual acuity and visual fields and monitoring

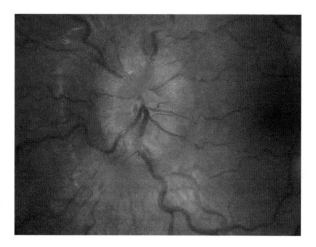

Fig. 31.3 Papilloedema

the optic disc appearance. Papilloedema is shown in Figure 31.3.

Posterior visual pathway problems

Children who do not appear to see due to a posterior visual pathway problem may have cortical visual impairment or delayed visual maturation.

Cortical visual impairment

Cortical visual impairment is reduced vision from a posterior visual pathway problem that results from a neurological cause. Causes of this condition may include:

- Seizures
- Metabolic
- Ischaemic
- Neuronal migration disorders.

Generally speaking, some improvement in visual performance occurs as the child gets older. The amount of improvement can range from a small change to full development of normal visual function. The timing of return of vision can be only a few days or it may take several weeks or months, depending on the cause and severity of injury. Treatment of the underlying cause is paramount to helping visual outcome to improve. Visual electrophysiology is useful in these cases. An electroretinogram measures function of the retinal layers and should be normal in this condition. A visual evoked potential will usually be reduced and delayed. Improvement in the visual evoked potential may precede clinical visual improvement.

Delayed visual maturation

Delayed visual maturation is usually a retrospective diagnosis. It is a congenital condition whereby the timing of myelination of the posterior visual pathway neurons is delayed but will develop fully with time. This may take 3–6 months to occur. Full visual function is expected with this condition. A comprehensive ophthalmology clinical examination is mandatory to rule out treatable ocular causes of reduced vision such as congenital high refractive errors or other amblyogenic factors.

Retinopathy of prematurity

Some premature infants are vulnerable to the development of retinopathy of prematurity (ROP). The normal retina begins vascularization from the optic disc towards the periphery after the ninth week post-conception. The entire surface area of the retina should be vascularized by term. Premature birth exposes the infant to higher oxygen tensions than would have been experienced in utero. This creates a relative ischaemia between the better-oxygenated, vascularized retina and its less oxygenated, non-vascularized periphery. This results in the non-vascularized retina releasing various angiogenic factors that cause the changes seen in ROP. ROP can cause retinal detachment and severe visual loss in its severest form.

Factors that seem to predispose infants to ROP include prematurity, low birth weight, chronic lung disease, intraventricular haemorrhage and necrotizing enterocolitis. It is important that all infants who are at risk of developing ROP are screened by an ophthalmologist. Children born at less than 32 weeks' gestation or weighing less than 1.5 kg at birth are usually screened. Screening usually commences 4–6 weeks after birth.

> http://www.site4sight.org.uk/Quality/RGov/
> Guidelines/Retinop.htm

Treatment of infants who are deemed to have sufficient ROP (stage 3 plus) are treated by laser. The aim of treatment is to destroy the ischaemic retina in an attempt to stop the liberation of further ischaemic products. This usually results in resolution of the condition.

The red eye

Problem-orientated topic:

a child with a red eye ● ● ● ● ●

Andrei, a 3-week-old term baby, presents with a 1-week history of bilateral red sticky eyes. On examination, there is a conjunctivitis. The child is otherwise clinically well.

Q1. What is the likely diagnosis?
Q2. What investigations would you perform?
Q3. Is treatment required, and if so, when?
Q4. What follow-up may be required?

Q1. What is the likely diagnosis?

The most likely diagnosis in this case is neonatal conjunctivitis (ophthalmia neonatorum). This may be caused by various organisms and may have been picked up during delivery. Organisms that may be implicated include *Chlamydia trachomatis*, *Neisseria gonorrhoeae* and herpes simplex.

Infection of a blocked nasolacrimal duct may present in a similar manner. Corneal ulcers (caused, for example, by *Pseudomonas aeruginosa*) may present in the neonatal period.

Silver nitrate drops are sometimes routinely instilled in the eyes of newborns at birth to reduce the risk of infectious conjunctivitis. The silver nitrate itself can sometimes cause conjunctival irritation and redness.

Q2. What investigations would you perform?

Conjunctival swabs or scrapes should be taken for Gram stain, *Chlamydia* polymerase chain reaction (PCR) and culture.

Q3. Is treatment required, and if so, when?

Immediate treatment of suspected neonatal conjunctivitis is indicated because there is a risk to vision and to the child. Systemic therapy is usually required because neonatal conjunctivitis is considered to be a systemic condition.

Q4. What follow-up may be required?

Follow-up is needed to check for resolution of the signs in the baby. The results of laboratory investigations should be checked. The parents should be informed of the results, as sometimes they may also require treatment.

Uveitis

The most common uveitis in childhood is iritis due to juvenile idiopathic arthritis (JIA). A characteristic feature of the ocular inflammation is that there are no symptoms. Also, the eye may remain white. Similar iritis in an adult would be expected to cause photophobia and a red eye. For this reason, the eyes of children with JIA should be checked for the presence of iritis (p. 453).

Visual loss may occur due to glaucoma, cataract or swelling of the central vision part of the retina.

Treatment involves frequent steroid eye drops. If this is insufficient, then commencement or alteration of systemic immunosuppressive medications should be considered to control the iritis.

Congenital nasolacrimal duct obstruction

At birth, a substantial number of infants do not have patency of the nasolacrimal duct. A 'sticky eye' is often indicative of congenital dacriostenosis. The symptoms associated with this condition are epiphora (excessive tears), recurrent conjunctivitis and discharge; photophobia is absent. The diagnosis can be confirmed by expressing mucopus from the punctae with the application of gentle pressure. The management depends on the severity of the symptoms and age of the child. Before the age of 6 months, parents should be instructed to massage the nasolacrimal sac region 3–4 times a day first with upward motion to free the canaliculi from any discharge, then with downward pressure to help the opening of the passage to the nose. Antibiotic eye drops should be prescribed only when there is evidence of purulent conjunctivitis. Within the age of 9–12 months, 80% of the obstructions have a spontaneous resolution. The decision to proceed with nasolacrimal probing is based on the severity of discharge, age, and standard practice in the community.

Neil Kennedy   Florence McDonagh   Eva Orzan   Mary O'Sullivan

CHAPTER

32

Disorders of hearing, the ear and throat

LEARNING OUTCOMES

By the end of this chapter you should:

- Know when to be concerned about a child's hearing and refer appropriately
- Understand the implications of a report on a hearing assessment
- Know the causes of children's hearing difficulties
- Know what difficulties a deaf child may encounter
- Understand the implications of communication difficulties
- Understand the importance of working closely with other agencies
- Understand screening of children's hearing and its limitations
- Understand the natural history of adenotonsillar enlargement
- Know the indications for adenoidectomy and tonsillectomy
- Know when to use antibiotics for tonsillar exudate and sinusitis.

MODULE SIX

Basic science

Hearing and its disorders are intimately connected with the anatomy and physiology of the auditory system, which consists of the ear and its neurological pathways. The greatest impact of hearing loss upon a child is on development of speech and language. The weight of this impact highly depends, among other factors, on the site of the lesion and the degree of impairment.

Embryology

A basic knowledge of the embryology of the ear is helpful in understanding those hearing problems that are a result of trauma or teratogenic agents at specific stages of embryonic development.

Inner ear

Early in week 4 of embryonic development, a thickening (the otic placode) forms on each side of the head.

427

The gross structures of the inner ear develop from the otic placode at between 5 and 8 weeks of embryonic life and continue to mature until between 25 weeks and term.

Middle ear

Around 32 days the middle ear begins to develop from the first pharyngeal pouch, which expands to form the middle ear cavity. Medially it forms the Eustachian (auditory) tube. Later the middle ear cavity expands by programmed cell death (apoptosis) and the ossicles become suspended in the cavity.

External ear

The external ear develops from the first pharyngeal groove, from three pairs of auricular hillocks that fuse to form the pinna. The cartilage of the otic capsule begins to ossify in the sixth month.

Physics of sound

Sound is the pattern of changes in pressure caused by movement or vibration of an object. From a central source it travels outwards in all directions in waves like ripples on a pond. The frequency of a sound, which allows differentiation of pitch, is the number of waves that pass in 1 second (known as cycles). The more cycles per second, the higher the pitch. Cycles per second are called Hertz (Hz). Most sounds, including speech, are a mixture of frequencies. A drum makes a low-frequency sound and a whistle is a high-frequency sound. A sound of a single frequency is called a pure tone.

In general, the closer one is to a sound source, the louder the sound. Sound levels are quantified in decibels (dB). The lowest intensity of a sound that a person needs to detect its presence is called threshold, and the reference dB for normal human hearing is called dB HL (Hearing Level). Therefore, the normal threshold value at each frequency is said to be 0 dB HL. Figure 32.1 shows examples of everyday sounds, with their frequency and intensity plotted on an audiogram. An audiogram is a chart used to record the patient's thresholds at each frequency. Thresholds can be measured with headphones, inserts, bone vibrators or in the sound field. Hearing is considered normal if threshold is within 15–20 dB HL.

How does the ear work? (Fig. 32.2)

The ear is the organ of hearing and balance. It receives sound, amplifies it, converts it into neural impulses and sends it to the brain. The pinna funnels sound waves into the ear canal. Air vibrations are converted into vibrations of the tympanic membrane and ossicles of the middle ear. These, in turn, create vibrations in the fluid within the cochlea. Cochlear fluid waves stimulate hair cells which transduce movements into electrical

---

BOX 32.1 Skill: otoscopy

Otoscopy is an important part of paediatric assessment. It should be carried out methodically in order that important information is not missed. An adequate otoscope is essential. It may be helpful and less frightening (especially for the child with speech difficulties) to look in Teddy's ears first! It is helpful if babies, small children and toddlers are appropriately cuddled and restrained. In babies, the pinna should be gently pulled upwards and backwards to straighten the ear canal. First the external auditory meatus is examined, looking out in particular for foreign bodies. Then the handle of the malleus is identified, with the pars flaccida above and the pars tensa below. In the normal eardrum a 'cone of light' can be observed. The colour and appearance of the tympanic membrane are noted, as well as the presence of any effusion beyond. Any tympanosclerosis, perforation or retraction is looked for and noted. Tympanometry can be carried out while the child is in the parent's arms. The findings can then be related to the hearing thresholds obtained.

---

signals that are transmitted via the eighth nerve to the brainstem and, after extensive processing, to the cerebral cortex.

Hearing loss can be classified according to the site of lesion in:

- *Conductive*, i.e. there is a problem in the external or middle ear
- *Sensorineural*, i.e. there is a problem with the inner ear structures (cochlea)
- *Mixed*, i.e. is a combination of conductive and sensorineural hearing loss
- *Central auditory dysfunction*, results from damage or dysfunction at the level of the eight nerve, auditory brainstem or cerebral cortex.

Clinical assessment of hearing

The purpose of audiological assessment is to measure hearing thresholds, and if a hearing loss is present, to establish its type, configuration and severity.

Observation of the child's play and communicative behaviour is very important not only because most objective and behavioural strategies for audiological assessment are chosen as a function of child's age and development but also because it helps to orient a clinical suspicion of hearing impairment.

Routine hearing assessment is usually accompanied by:

- *Otoscopy* (Box 32.1): aids clinical decision-making (see above)

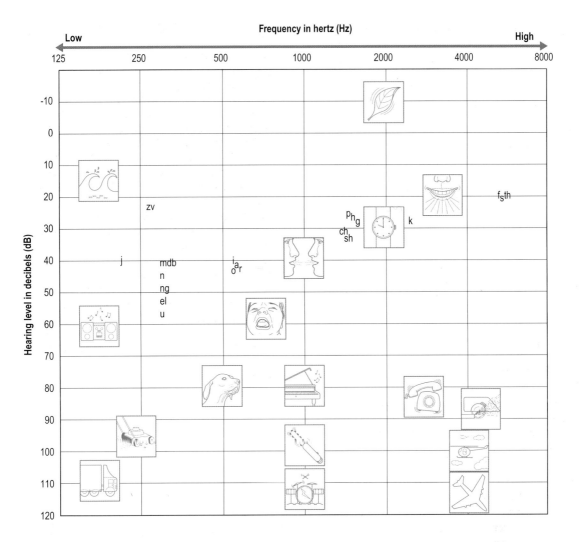

Fig. 32.1 Frequency and intensity of some everyday sounds plotted on an audiogram. Vowels and consonants used in human voice perception are also shown. When hearing loss affects this area, communication is altered
(Source: Deafness. HMSO. This figure is reproduced under the terms of the click-use licence.)

- *Tympanometry* (Box 32.2, Fig. 32.3): gives an indication of middle ear function.

A test-battery approach is essential in the evaluation of hearing in children at any age. A full assessment by an audiologist may include:

- *Evoked oto-acoustic emissions (EOAEs)*, are sounds originating within the cochlea that can be used to assess cochlear function when middle ear function is normal.
- *Auditory brainstem response (ABR)*, or *brainstem auditory evoked potentials (BAEPs)* uses a stimulus (click) to evoke electrophysiological responses that originate in the eighth nerve and auditory brainstem. This technique is essential if behavioural audiometry findings are inconsistent, incomplete or inconclusive.
- *Visual reinforcement audiometry (VRA)*, can be used from 5 months of age once a child can turn the head in response to hearing a sound.

- *Performance testing or conditioned play audiometry*, can usually be used by 2½ years when a child can be conditioned to reliably respond with a play action (i.e. put a ring on a stick).
- *Conventional pure-tone audiometry*, is the 'adult' technique for obtaining thresholds. Generally recommended for 5–7 years and older (Fig. 32.4).

Hearing assessments should be carried out in a child- and family-friendly environment. Parents can be included in 'playing the games' in clinic, and can observe when the child responds to a sound. The hearing thresholds at each frequency are discussed and related to the loudness of certain sounds in running speech. Some parents will welcome confirmation of a hearing loss they have suspected, while others will be shocked to find their child is hearing impaired. For some parents there is only one interpretation of the word 'deaf', so it is important to explain carefully the degree of hearing loss and the implications in relation to specific speech sounds.

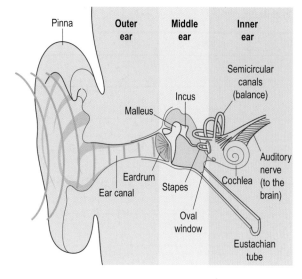

Fig. 32.2 Diagram of the ear
(Source: Deafness. HMSO. This figure is reproduced under the terms of the click-use licence.)

BOX 32.2 Skill: tympanometry

Middle ear problems are very common in childhood and tympanometry is a quick and reliable indicator of middle ear function. The assessment of middle ear function is an essential part of the test battery so that hearing thresholds are correctly interpreted. Before commencing, the audiologist will check for contraindications such as tenderness or the presence of discharge. After the procedure is explained to the parent, the child should be seated sideways on the parent's knee; the pinna is pulled gently backwards and an appropriately sized probe tip is placed at the entrance to the child's ear canal. Movement and excess noise can give spurious or inconclusive results. If abnormal shapes are obtained, the test should be repeated.

Figure 32.3 shows the most common types of tympanogram in paediatric practice.

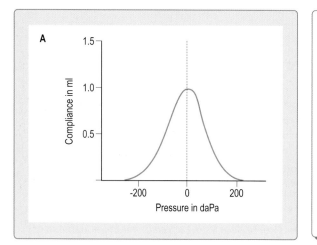

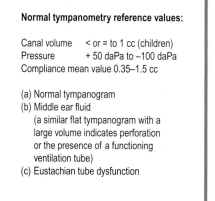

Normal tympanometry reference values:

Canal volume — < or = to 1 cc (children)
Pressure — + 50 daPa to −100 daPa
Compliance mean value 0.35–1.5 cc

(a) Normal tympanogram
(b) Middle ear fluid
(a similar flat tympanogram with a large volume indicates perforation or the presence of a functioning ventilation tube)
(c) Eustachian tube dysfunction

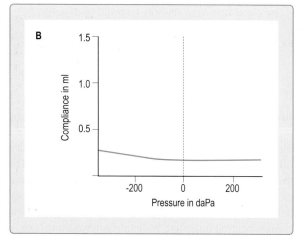

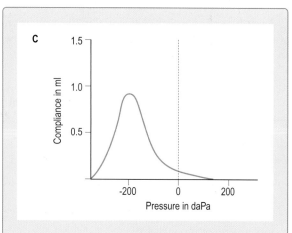

Fig. 32.3 Tympanometry

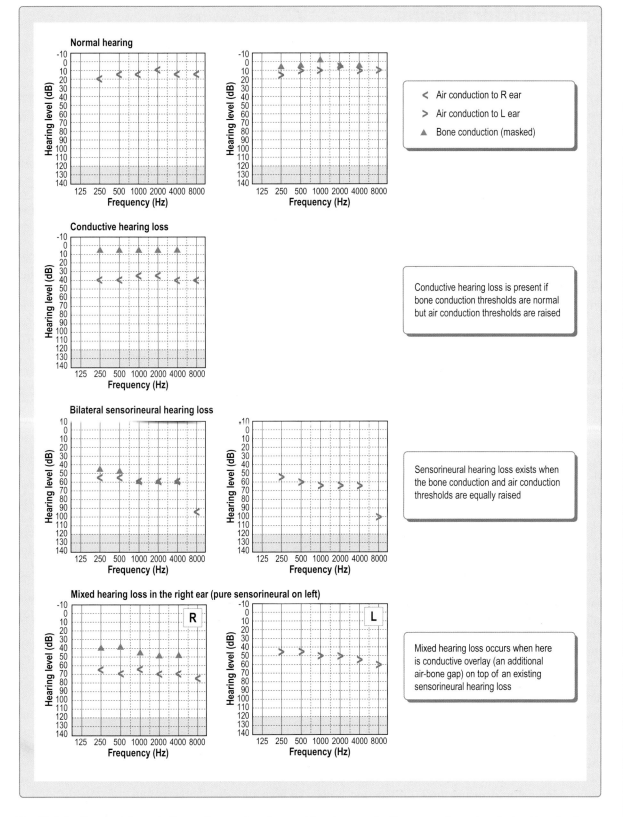

Fig. 32.4 Audiogram interpretation and examples of normal hearing, conductive, sensorineural and mixed hearing loss

Screening for hearing impairment

The term deaf (with small 'd') should be considered a colloquial term that implies hearing thresholds in the severe-to-profound range. Hearing impairment can affect the linguistic, social, emotional and educational development of a child and is the most common birth defect, having a greater incidence than cystic fibrosis and hypothyroidism. Significant hearing loss (>40 dB in the better ear) affects about 1 in 1000 children born in developed countries. The prevalence is higher in the developing world. Acquired and late-onset cases add to this number. Over 50% of these children will have a moderate hearing loss, with approximately equal numbers of children having severe and profound deafness. More than 30% of hearing impaired children have no known history of risk factors for hearing impairment.

Neonatal screening

A universal newborn hearing screening programme has been recommended in international consensus statements and is now available in several European countries. Although neonatal screening will detect children with hearing loss at birth, professionals need to continue to be vigilant regarding the possibility of acquired, progressive and late-onset hearing impairment.

The aim of a universal newborn hearing screen is the early identification of children who have a significant permanent hearing impairment in the neonatal period. Early detection of hearing impairment and early intervention lessen the impact of significant hearing loss on the child, the child's family and society. Studies have highlighted the importance of diagnosis and introduction of early support programmes before 6 months of age for the future speech and language abilities of the child.

Two non-invasive, quick and reliable screening tests are available for screening for hearing impairment in the newborn period. Specific screening protocols may vary but more frequently a two-stage process is adopted with otoacoustic emissions (OAE) being used in all babies and automated brainstem response (A-ABR) being used only in those babies who do not pass OAE. A separate protocol is generally adopted for babies admitted to neonatal units, carrying out both screening tests in all babies. The baby who fails the screening is referred for audiological evaluation before 3 months of age. Intervention should initiate before 6 months of age in case of ascertained significant permanent hearing loss.

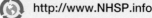

http://www.NHSP.info

Oto-acoustic emissions

OAEs are tiny sounds that can be evoked and measured in the ear canal in 98% of normally hearing people by placing a small probe in the ear. They originate in the inner ear and are thought to be produced as a by-product of the amplification action of the outer hair cells (OHCs). They are only present in ears with normal OHCs and correlate highly with normal hearing. Since the vast majority of hearing impairment is due to OHC damage, recording an OAE provides a sensitive and accurate means of identification of cochlear hearing impairment. Since the test is robust and easy to perform, it is an excellent screening test. OAEs are not normally present when the hearing loss is greater than 30 dB. The presence of a clear response on OAE testing suggests normal cochlear function in an ear. An automated OAE system has been designed for screening and indicates the presence or absence of a clear response.

Auditory brainstem response test

ABR records the electrical activity in the auditory nerve and in the brainstem when sounds are presented in the ear. An automated ABR system has been designed for screening. A click stimulus at 35 dBnHL (n = normal) is presented into the ear via a probe or ear cuffs, and the machine automatically records with surface electrodes the presence or absence of a clear response. Some infants are at greater risk of damage to the auditory pathway. ABR is the test of choice for these infants, as it tests the integrity of the auditory pathway as well as the cochlea. For this reason babies admitted to neonatal units will have an OAE test and an AABR test as routine, as these infants are at greater risk of developing retrocochlear hearing problems.

Surveillance and later screening

Some babies are at risk of developing late onset or progressive hearing problems, other children meet one or more of the criteria specified in Box 32.2. These risk factors should be identified (at birth and later) and the children should be included in an audiological surveillance program which usually consists of an audiometric evaluation before 12 months and a follow-up until 3 years of age. Intermediate screening between the newborn screen and school entry is no longer recommended in many countries, but it is important to ask parents about hearing concerns and speech and language development at routine health

- Parental or professional concern
- Meningitis, chronic middle ear effusion and craniofacial abnormalities
- Family history of prelingual sensorineural hearing loss (SNHL) in parents or siblings
- Special care baby unit (SCBU)/neonatal intensive care unit (NICU) child with no clear responses on OAEs despite clear responses on ABR
- SCBU/NICU child who had intermittent positive pressure ventilation (IPPV) for more than 5 days
- Jaundice, where bilirubin levels indicate a need for exchange transfusion
- Congenital TORCH (*t*oxoplasmosis, *r*ubella, *c*ytomegalovirus, *h*erpes simplex) infection
- Neurodegenerative or neurodevelopmental disorders
- Confirmed syndromes related to hearing loss, e.g. Down syndrome (see Box 32.4)

BOX 32.4 Hearing surveillance for children with Down syndrome

Over 50% of people with Down syndrome have hearing loss of a mild/moderate/profound degree.

- Newborn hearing screen
- Full audiological assessment between 6 and 10 months
- Review audiological assessment at 18 months
- Yearly audiological assessment until 5 years old
- Thereafter, 2-yearly review for life
- Assessment should include 8 kHz in view of early onset of presbycousis

checks. A test of hearing at school entry can pick up late and acquired losses not present at the time of the previous screening test.

Babies who are found to have permanent congenital or prelingual hearing loss as a result of neonatal screening and subsequent evaluation require early intervention. Developments that may improve speech and language and communication are shown in Box 32.5.

BOX 32.5 Developments in the management of permanent congenital and prelingual hearing loss

- Newborn hearing screening and targeted follow-up
- Early cochlear implantation
- Guidelines on support in the early years
- Digital signal processing hearing aids

Hearing loss

Problem-orientated topic:

poor speech development

Oliver, aged 18 months, has been referred by his health visitor because he is not making progress with his speech. The referral indicates that he had started to babble but this has ceased. His mum gives a history of bilateral ear infection with discharge at age 1 year. Oliver had a 'pass' result at the neonatal hearing screening test.

Hearing assessment with visual reinforcement audiometry indicates a flat loss across the thresholds of 50–60 dBHL at 500–4000 Hz. Otoscopy and tympanometry indicate middle ear effusions (MEE) bilaterally.

Q1. What are the possible causes of Oliver's hearing loss?

Q2. How would you manage this condition?

Q3. What factors in Oliver's history would contraindicate the normal practice of watching and waiting for improvement?

Q1. What are the possible causes of Oliver's hearing loss?

Conductive hearing loss occurs when sound transmission through the outer or middle ear is not efficient. The causes of conductive loss include:

- Blockage of the ear canal (atresia, wax, foreign body)
- Perforation of the tympanic membrane
- Otitis media with effusion (OME), also called middle ear effusion (MEE) or 'glue ear' (by far the most common cause in children)
- Ossicular problems: e.g. disarticulation or necrosis
- Otosclerosis: i.e. bridge formation from footplate to oval window (unlikely in young children).

Oliver has MEE.

Q2. How would you manage this condition?

Initial management, in the absence of significantly raised hearing thresholds or indicators of persistence or other causes for concern, will be watching and waiting for spontaneous resolution. Arrangements should be made to reassess the hearing in 3 months. Meanwhile, advice with regard to risk factors is given to parents/carers and information can be gathered about school progress and speech and language development, which will be useful for the review appointment. If there is a significant hearing loss, advice to school is useful, once parental consent is obtained. Balance may be affected temporarily.

Early referral to an ear, nose and throat (ENT) surgeon is prompted by:

- The possibility of a mixed hearing loss
- Significantly raised hearing thresholds (> 35 dB)
- Speech and language difficulties
- Educational difficulties
- Recurrent ear infections
- Persistent snoring or sleep apnoea syndrome
- Behavioural difficulties linked to hearing.

Q3. What factors in Oliver's history would contraindicate the normal practice of watching and waiting for improvement?

Concerns in Oliver's case include:

- Lack of progress with speech
- Likely duration of condition (6 months)
- Significantly raised hearing thresholds.

The latter raises the possibility of a mixed hearing loss.

With children like Oliver, it is important to assess their hearing after intervention or resolution of glue ear (MEE, OME) in order to rule out a sensorineural hearing loss. Children who have a first episode of glue ear in their first 18 months are more prone to recurrence.

Otitis media with effusion (OME)

OME is an accumulation of fluid behind an intact tympanic membrane in the absence of acute infection. It is the most common cause of hearing difficulty in childhood, with peak prevalence at around 1 year of age, rising again around the age of 3–5 years. Spontaneous resolution occurs in most cases in about 3 months. Persistence is more likely in children who first present early in life. Most children with conductive hearing loss have a mild loss (< 45 dBHL). Even mild losses, however, can have an effect on speech discrimination and hence on language acquisition. The duration of the loss is important, as is adequate exposure to language. There is an increasing body of evidence to suggest that OME puts children at risk with regard to language acquisition and subsequent schooling.

Risk factors for OME include:

- Age
- Season (more likely in winter)
- Sibling history
- Group childcare (possibly due to cross-infection)
- Environmental smoke exposure
- Bottle feeding (breastfeeding is protective in the first year)
- Allergy
- Anatomical predisposition (including cleft palate, craniofacial abnormalities, Down syndrome).

The infant's Eustachian tube is more horizontal than that of the adult. Eustachian tube dysfunction is causally linked to OME. Microorganisms have been cultured in the effusion in a significant proportion of cases. OME is associated with adenoidal hypertrophy (p. 439) and adenoidectomy is a treatment option. When OME is suspected, it is obviously important to assess the child's hearing. If there are no signs of acute infection (pain or signs of inflammation, red and bulging tympanic membrane), antibiotics are not indicated.

Management decisions then depend on:

- Hearing levels
- Whether there are indicators of persistence
- Whether there is parental, carer or professional concern
- Presence of other symptoms and signs, e.g. recurrent ear infections, snoring
- Presence of other issues, e.g. learning difficulties.

The hearing levels in OME are prone to fluctuate. This has been linked to the poor listening skills that are evident in some of these children. It is also helpful to consider whether hearing difficulties are having an adverse effect on the parent–child relationship. If hearing difficulties persist after a period of watching and waiting, treatment options such as ventilation tube insertion or trial of hearing aids need to be considered and this usually necessitates a referral to ENT. Close liaison with ENT is helpful, especially for children with particularly poor speech or where there are learning difficulties and complex needs that are associated with more adverse outcomes.

It is helpful for children who have been adversely affected by OME to be followed up, and this can sometimes be usefully done by the family doctor, who can monitor for recurrence, persistent perforation, significant tympanic membrane retraction and cholesteatoma. Certain groups are at particular risk, e.g. children with Down syndrome or cleft palate (see also Boxes 32.3 and 32.4). Thus there is a need for vigilance and routine review in these groups. Surveillance guidelines are helpful. Parents are often unaware of children's hearing difficulties and notice a difference only after intervention.

Acute otitis media (OM)

Acute OM is a common infection in childhood and usually presents with pain in the ear, fever and hearing loss. The diagnosis is made by otoscopy, when a red, bulging tympanic membrane is seen. An effusion may be evident behind the membrane.

Bacteria cause the majority of cases of acute OM and the most common are:

- *Streptococcus pneumoniae*
- *Haemophilus influenzae*
- *Moraxella catarrhalis*
- Group A streptococcus
- *Staphylococcus aureus*.

Viruses cause a minority of infections in the middle ear.

Acute OM is generally treated with antibiotics, but antibiotic management remains controversial. In fact, spontaneous recovery occurs in 80% of cases and there is a small risk of serious complications (mastoiditis, meningitis). Most guidelines recommend treating after a period of 48–72 hours in older children with non-severe symptoms, whereas immediate amoxicillin as a first line of treatment should be provided to a younger infant.

> http://www.cochrane.org/reviews/en/ab000019.html

Problem-orientated topic:

failed hearing screening test at 8 months ● ● ● ● ●

Jessica, aged 10 months, has been referred by her health visitor because she did not pass her hearing screen at 8 months of age. On testing, Jessica responds at 75 dB throughout the frequencies tested. On examination she has middle ear effusions bilaterally. She is referred immediately to a joint clinic with an ENT surgeon, who agrees to see her urgently in view of the severity of her hearing loss. He confirms middle ear effusions and Jessica is listed for ventilation tube insertion within the week. On retesting afterwards she has a 60 dB loss.

Q1. What type of hearing loss does Jessica have?

Q2. What are the most likely causes of Jessica's sensorineural hearing loss?

Q3. How should a deaf child be managed?

Q4. What is Jessica's prognosis?

Q1. What type of hearing loss does Jessica have?

Jessica has mixed hearing loss and has been urgently referred to ENT services because of the severity of her hearing loss. Although her long-term prognosis is expected to be reasonably good, she requires to be carefully followed up to manage her sensorineural hearing loss (SNHL) and to detect any recurrence of middle ear effusion.

Mixed hearing loss occurs when a conductive loss is superimposed on a sensorineural loss. Hearing assessment shows air conduction (AC) thresholds to be poorer than the (abnormal) bone conduction (BC) thresholds. When the conductive element is treated or disappears, AC thresholds revert to BC levels. When a hearing loss is purely sensorineural, AC and BC thresholds are the same, i.e. there is no air bone gap (Fig. 32.4).

SNHL is caused by abnormality of the cochlea or ascending neural pathways. Most often it is due to hair cell damage in the cochlea. SNHL is less common than conductive loss, with a prevalence of about 1.2 per 1000 live births for moderate loss and above. Most SNHL is congenital and is usually permanent. The prevalence of SNHL increases with increasing age due to acquired and progressive losses. Hearing loss is described as unilateral or bilateral and also by the degree of the impairment, as follows:

- Mild hearing loss: < 40 dBHL
- Moderate: 41–70 dBHL
- Severe: 71–95 dBHL
- Profound: > 95 dBHL.

When children are able to cooperate with pure-tone audiometry, the presence of the mixed loss is shown by a gap between the AC threshold and the BC threshold (Fig. 32.4). If the conductive element is due to OME, it is important to remedy this as soon as possible with a referral to an ENT specialist. It has been shown, however, that the necessity for an ENT operation can significantly delay the age of identification and hearing aid fitting in children with severe hearing loss. Thus there is a need for clear communication and urgency in liaison between professionals and departments. Not all conductive components are due to effusions, however. Permanent conductive losses occur infrequently but are more likely in certain syndromes, e.g. Treacher Collins syndrome.

Q2. What are the most likely causes of Jessica's sensorineural hearing loss?

Investigation of the cause of SNHL is important because:

- Parents want to know why their child is hearing impaired.
- They may want to know about the risk of hearing loss in further siblings.
- Hearing loss may be associated with medical problems that need to be identified.
- The cause of hearing loss may influence management.

The causes of childhood sensorineural hearing loss include both environmental and genetic conditions:

- Neonatal problems (asphyxia, prematurity)
- Toxicity (aminoglycosides, Ch. 10; hyperbilirubinaemia, p. 730)
- Genetic (see below)
- Craniofacial abnormality
- Infection (post-meningitis, p. 643)
- Trauma.

Post-meningitis (bacterial) deafness

This remains an important cause of severe acquired hearing loss. The important points are as follows:

- Hearing loss of any degree follows bacterial meningitis in 10% of children.
- The onset of hearing loss may occur late after the infection has been treated.
- Optimum time for assessment of hearing is 4–6 weeks post-infection.
- 1–4% have bilateral profound deafness.
- The hearing loss may be progressive.
- There is a risk of cochlear ossification.

With the advent of universal neonatal screening, which has led to earlier identification of childhood hearing impairment, it is likely that more precise diagnosis will be achieved; for example, congenital infection may be identified with greater certainty.

http://www.nhsp.info

Medical Management of Infants with Significant Congenital Hearing Loss Identified

Vestibular investigations should be performed on all children with permanent sensorineural hearing loss.

Progressive hearing loss can be familial but can also be due to viral infections (e.g. rubella, cytomegalovirus), metabolic causes or bacterial meningitis.

Genetic considerations

A genetic referral is suggested in most cases of permanent prelingual hearing loss but is particularly indicated if:

- There is a positive family history
- There are complex needs, learning difficulties or other medical problems
- There are dysmorphic features
- The family request it.

In most cases sensorineural hearing loss is nonsyndromic, i.e. not associated with other congenital features and the child is otherwise healthy. About 50 genes have been associated with nonsyndromic hearing loss. Most of these are recessive, some dominant. Among the genetic causes, by far the most frequent are mutations in GJB2 (Connexin 26) gene which account for up to 30% of prelingual hearing loss in many populations. Other genetic causes include syndromic disorders such as Pendred syndrome, Waardenburg syndrome and Usher syndrome.

The most common acquired cause is congenital cytomegalovirus infection. Congenital rubella syndrome, ototoxicity, neonatal asphyxia, prematurity and meningitis are other common causes.

Q3. How should a hearing impaired child be managed?

Professionals involved in the management of hearing impaired children want the best outcome for the child and family, i.e. a well-rounded individual who communicates well, is healthy and happy, is learning appropriately in school, and has good relationships with peer groups and family alike. Specific goals include:

- Early identification of hearing loss
- Optimal habilitation, i.e. appropriate aiding and family support
- Appropriate communication strategies and support.

The multidisciplinary team management of a hearing imparied child may include:

- Audiologist: hearing assessment, hearing aid work
- Parent
- Doctor: examines, treats, investigates, refers, advocacy work
- Teacher: with a special qualification for teaching the deaf
- Speech and language therapist
- Nurse (health visitor, school nurse)
- Social worker (may be a 'specialist' working with deaf children only).

How confirmation of hearing loss is imparted to the family, the language used by professionals, good listening skills and treating parents as partners all play an important part in managing the stress and anxiety for the family around the time of identification of hearing loss. Confident parental involvement will facilitate successful hearing aid use, encourage successful communication and enable the child to reach his or her potential.

Once the degree and nature of the hearing loss is apparent, the team, together with the parents, can meet and plan intervention. Initial work will include:

- Fitting of appropriate hearing aids
- Supply of information about voluntary organizations
- Ongoing recursive assessment (to verify hearing aid fitting)
- Involvement of the early intervention team
- ENT and paediatric assessment
- Aetiological assessment and investigation
- Communication assessment and input as needed
- Referral for ophthalmological assessment.

The degree and configuration of the loss will determine hearing aid fit. It is important that parents understand the potential effect of the hearing loss on the child's ability to communicate and thus accept the need to wear hearing aids. If the child shows no benefit after 3 months of hearing aid wear and the child has been confirmed as being affected by a severe-profound hearing loss, consideration should be given to referral with a view to cochlear implantation if appropriate.

As the child approaches 2 years of age, there needs to be consideration of schooling options in consultation with parents. When a deaf child is born to hearing parents, there is a sense of loss and grief. This may show as anger against professionals and parents may seek alternative opinions. While parents are working through these emotions, they will not be able to take in all the information given to them by professionals. Thus they need time and space to talk about their feelings and a sympathetic and supportive attitude from the multidisciplinary support team. Some parents may need psychological counselling or intervention. Meanwhile, they need to be encouraged to work with their child to improve communication and may themselves need to consider alternative strategies, e.g. learning sign language so they can begin to communicate appropriately with their child.

There is a higher prevalence of child abuse in deaf children, and it is more difficult for the deaf child to disclose abuse. Mental health problems are more prevalent in deaf children, and mental health services with appropriate communication and professional skills should be available as necessary.

Q4. What is Jessica's prognosis?

When children are learning to talk they need to be able to hear all of the individual sounds of speech in order to reproduce them properly. Some speech sounds are significantly quieter than others: for example, 's', 'f' and 'th' (Fig. 32.1). Therefore even mild hearing losses make it difficult for children to hear plurals, tenses and voiceless consonants. Children with moderate losses cannot hear most of conversational speech sounds.

Children with SNHL need to be monitored in case the loss progresses, i.e. hearing gets worse.

Children with SNHL are more dependent on their vision to access the environment and education. They are more likely to have visual problems. Aetiological clues may sometimes be evident to the ophthalmologist. Thus ophthalmological assessment and oversight is essential for hearing impaired children.

'Deaf' awareness

Hearing impaired children need to understand and communicate as hearing children do. Going to the doctor or into hospital can be a frightening experience. Paediatricians need to understand the implications of a child's hearing loss for communication (see p. 435 for definitions):

- A child with mild hearing loss may find it difficult to understand quiet speech, particularly in background noise, and the use of a sound field system in the classroom may need to be considered.
- A child with moderate hearing loss will find it difficult to follow conversational speech without the use of a hearing aid.
- A child with severe hearing loss will not be able to follow conversational speech without the use of a hearing aid.
- A child who is profoundly deaf will be unable to hear speech, and will only hear loud environmental sounds without amplification or cochlear implant.

Professionals need to be aware of and sensitive to the child's preferred communication mode, and to make sure children understand planned investigations and treatment. An interpreter should be available for the child who signs. Communication should be effective, i.e. the speaker should avoid jargon, explain clearly, write things down as necessary, and be aware that hearing impaired children's literacy skills may be limited.

Minimizing the effects of permanent hearing impairment in children

Until the introduction of the NHSP, identification of hearing impaired children was significantly delayed. They were deprived of much auditory experience during the first year(s) of life at a stage when environmental stimulation is necessary for the development of neuronal connections in the auditory nervous system. Even though it may not be obvious to the casual observer, receptive language is developing in the first year of life, leading to understanding and production of first words at around 1 year of age.

It is anticipated that early identification through NHSP and early intervention, including an early support programme, will facilitate language acquisition in this group and improve outcomes, i.e. will reduce the linguistic, social, educational and cognitive sequelae as well as the mental health implications of deafness for this group.

It has been shown that approximately 40% of hearing impaired children have another disability in addition to their deafness and over 60% of these will have more than one additional disability. Visual problems are four times as common in deaf children, who depend largely on their vision to access the environment.

Children with complex needs are more likely to have hearing difficulties. They are also more likely to be adversely affected by hearing difficulties, either permanent or temporary. Children with unilateral hearing loss have problems with learning and with discriminating speech in noisy environments.

Even children with mild hearing loss that may not be considered to be 'significant' in terms of need for support or who would not be fitted with hearing aids may be at risk of 'academic failure'. There are links between minor hearing difficulties and self-esteem and peer status, and thus it becomes clear that the management of the child with even minor hearing difficulties needs to involve many disciplines working together.

Cochlear implantation

Cochlear implantation aims to provide hearing sensation for children who are severely and profoundly deaf and derive no useful benefit from conventional hearing aids. A cochlear implant bypasses cochlear function by directly stimulating the auditory nerve and has the potential to deliver hearing sensation at levels of 30–45 dB across speech frequencies. Sound is received by an external microphone, analysed by a speech processor and sent to the internal receiver. Acoustic input is now represented in electrical pulses and delivered by electrodes surgically inserted in the cochlea in order to stimulate the auditory nerve. Each Cochlear Implant Centre conducts a detailed multidisciplinary assessment to determine cochlear implant candidacy and identifies factors that can affect outcomes after implantation. The device is switched on about 3–4 weeks after surgery when the incision behind the ear has healed. The stimulation levels of each implanted electrode needs to be customized for each child and several adjustments are required on follow-up sessions.

Pre-lingually and post-lingually deaf children will derive benefit from a cochlear implant. Children with profound deafness who receive a cochlear implant early on derive most benefit from it. Cochlear implantation is also an option for children who have progressive hearing loss or who suddenly become deaf, e.g. post-meningitis. Post-meningitis patients need to be fast-tracked. Around 40% of deaf children have additional complex needs and cochlear implantation will offer an important management adjunct for some of these children. Cochlear implantation is usually carried out on one side only, although there is increasing interest in bilateral implantation.

Every child's experience with a cochlear implant is unique. Cochlear implantation does not restore hearing but it does provide an auditory sensation that has been described by some people who were hearing previously as mechanical or synthetic. With support over time, children will hear and understand everyday environmental and speech sounds through their cochlear implant, which means they may develop speech themselves. Some users may advance to understand speech without the help of lip reading and go on to use the telephone.

http://www.bcig.org

Criteria for referral for cochlear implantation

- Bilateral severe/profound sensorineural hearing impairment ($\geq$ 90 dBHL at 2 kHz and 4 kHz in the better ear)
- Clinical ABR thresholds $\geq$ 90 dBHL
- No minimum age for referral
- Children with additional needs should be referred
- Post-meningitis patients need to be fast-tracked
- Children of any age who fulfil the audiological criteria should be discussed with the cochlear implant team.

Factors that influence outcome of cochlear implantation

- Age of the child and duration of deafness at time of implantation
- Aetiology of deafness
- Type of device implanted
- Educational setting and auditory environment post-implantation, i.e. rich in spoken language
- Degree of engagement in the habilitative process
- Consistent use of the cochlear implant over time.

Balance disorders

Balance problems and hearing problems often coexist. Delay in establishing head control, sitting and walking can indicate vestibular dysfunction. A history of ototoxic medication or meningitis (or both) may be significant aetiological factors in the genesis of vestibular dysfunction. Children with vestibular areflexia do not suffer from motion sickness. Walking is delayed until after 18 months of age in children with bilateral vestibular areflexia.

Children may not complain of vertigo; therefore it is important to elicit from parents whether the child has signs or symptoms suggestive of vestibular dysfunction. These may include sudden onset of nystagmus, vomiting, pallor and falling without loss of consciousness, or the older child may complain that the environment is moving.

Afferent information from the vestibular system, visual information and proprioceptive information are integrated in the brainstem, pons and cerebellum. This generates efferent signals that facilitate coordinated movement. Vestibular assessment aims to isolate these components. Teamwork by paediatricians, neurologists, audiological physicians and others may be needed in individual cases.

The presence or absence of vestibular dysfunction can be helpful in separating genetic syndromes. Rehabilitation (which may simply include playing and sport) facilitates central compensation.

Tonsillar and adenoidal hypertrophy

Problem-orientated topic:

tonsillar and adenoidal hypertrophy ● ● ● ● ●

Ruby, a 4-year-old, is brought to her primary care physician by her mother. She is having frequent episodes of tonsillitis, which cause her to miss school. She is chronically tired, sleeps poorly and snores loudly.

On examination Ruby is thriving. She is a persistent mouth breather. Her tonsils are non-inflamed but large enough to obstruct over 60% of her airway.

Q1. What features in the history suggest that she should be referred to an ENT surgeon?

Q2. What are the indications for adenoidectomy/tonsillectomy?

Q1. What features in the history suggest that she should be referred to an ENT surgeon?

The tonsils and adenoids begin to develop in the third month of gestation. Their maximal period of enlargement is in the first and second years of life. They continue to grow until, at around 8 or 9 years, they begin a slow process of involution. Only a remnant remains by early adulthood. Some genetic disorders predispose to adenoidal airway obstruction, e.g. trisomy 21.

Obstructive sleep apnoea syndrome is an increasingly common indication for surgery.

Adenoidal obstruction of the nasopharynx (Fig. 32.5) can present as:

- Prolonged (3–4 weeks) upper respiratory tract infections, with purulent rhinorrhoea
- Persistent mouth breathing with hyponasal ('adenoidal') speech
- Recurrent otitis media/otitis media with effusion
- Obstructive sleep apnoea syndrome.

Obstructive sleep apnoea syndrome (OSAS)

Symptoms of OSAS include noisy breathing at night and/or loud snoring accompanied by nocturnal apnoeic pauses, poor sleep quality and daytime somnolence. In contrast to adults, episodes of airway obstruction in children usually occur in rapid eye movement (REM) sleep. A reduction of time in REM sleep can lead to cognitive or behavioural disorders. Untreated, OSAS is associated with chronic hypoxia, secondary pulmonary hypertension, cor pulmonale and failure to thrive.

OSAS can be confirmed by a 'sleep study'. The gold standard is polysomnography: continuous concurrent recording of oxygen saturation, heart rate, end-tidal CO_2, abdominal and thoracic breathing movements, nasal airflow, oculograms and electroencephalogram (EEG). This is rarely available in practice and overnight oxygen saturation monitoring is substituted. Compared with polysomnography, oximetry has a positive predictive value (PPV) of 97% and a negative predictive value (NPV) of 47%, i.e. it has a high false negative rate. The American Academy of Pediatrics has published evidence-based guidelines for the diagnosis and management of OSAS.

> http://aappolicy.aappublications.org/cgi/ reprint/pediatrics;109/4/704.pdf

Q2. What are the indications for adenoidectomy/tonsillectomy? (Box 32.6)

Reasonable evidence exists for adenoidectomy/tonsillectomy in the treatment of OSAS. There is some evidence for adenoidectomy as a treatment for OME if there are signs of recurrent upper respiratory tract infections and adenoidal symptoms and signs.

Enlargement of the tonsils alone is not an indication for surgery. Clear criteria exist for referral to ENT services for recurrent tonsillitis (Box 32.7).

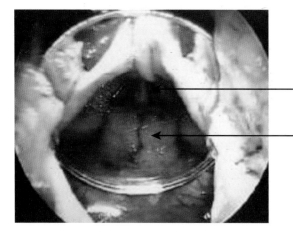

Fig. 32.5 **Adenoidal obstruction of the nasopharynx**

Nasal airway

Adenoid

BOX 32.6 Relative indications for adenoidectomy

- Obstructive sleep apnoea syndrome (often with tonsillectomy)
- Recurrent acute otitis media
- Otitis media with effusion and hearing loss
- Severe persistent nasal obstruction

BOX 32.7 Referral criteria for recurrent tonsillitis in children

All the following criteria should be met:
- Five or more definite episodes of tonsillitis per year
- Symptoms for at least 1 year
- Episodes of tonsillitis that are disabling and prevent normal functioning, e.g. school attendance

 http://www.cochrane.org/reviews/en/ab001802.html

Following referral, a 6-month period of 'watchful waiting' is recommended to establish the symptom pattern and to allow time to consider the implications of surgery (Box 32.8).

Complications of adenotonsillectomy

Post-operative bleeding occurs in 0.5–1.5%. Treatment of primary post-operative haemorrhage (within the first 24 hours) consists of local pressure, fluid or blood replacement, and return to theatre for diathermy/ligature of the bleeding vessel. Secondary haemorrhage (usually day 6–10) is associated with wound infection.

Rare complications include damage to the soft palate or Eustachian tube.

The effects of adenotonsillectomy on the immune system have been debated. Most studies do not show

BOX 32.8 Indications for tonsillectomy

- Recurrent tonsillitis (see above)
- One or two episodes of quinsy
- Obstructive sleep apnoea syndrome
- Suspicion of other pathology, e.g. lymphoma

any significant alteration in immune function following surgery.

Tonsillar exudates

Problem-orientated topic:

the child with tonsillar exudate

Ethan, a 5-year-old, is brought to the accident and emergency department by his mother, who is concerned about his high temperature. On examination, temperature is 38.9°C. He has bilateral red swollen tonsils with exudate. His superior cervical lymph nodes are swollen and tender. He has no rash and appears systemically 'well'.

Q1. What are the causes of tonsillitis with exudate?
Q2. What investigations (if any) should be done?
Q3. Should Ethan be treated with antibiotics?

Q1. What are the causes of tonsillitis with exudate?

The palatine tonsils and adenoids are part of a protective ring of lymphoid tissue in the oropharynx and nasopharynx. A surface lining of stratified squamous epithelium is invaginated by 15–20 deep grooves or crypts. Deeper lie multiple lymphatic nodules, several of which coalesce and contain germinal centres. The crypts frequently contain 'cheesy' debris consisting of food particles, mucus, neutrophils and lymphocytes. A dense connective tissue capsule separates the tonsil bed from the pharyngeal wall. Efferent lymphatics drain to the jugulodigastric (behind the angle of the mandible) and upper cervical lymph nodes. Sensation is supplied by the glossopharyngeal and vagus nerves.

Functionally, both tonsils and adenoids serve to detect and defend against oral or inhaled pathogens. Antigens presented to T-helper cells are in turn presented to B cells within the germinal matrix of a lymphoid nodule. IgA is secreted as a result.

In cases of tonsillitis with exudates consider:

- Bacterial infection
- Epstein–Barr virus infection (glandular fever)
- Diphtheria.

Q2. What investigations (if any) should be done?

Organisms cultured from the tonsils are listed in Box 32.9. Most episodes of tonsillitis are caused by viral infection. Group A β-haemolytic streptococci (GABHS) are isolated in approximately 30% of people with a sore throat. However, GABHS is also isolated in 5–40% of asymptomatic carriers.

BOX 32.9 Organisms cultured from the tonsils

Viruses
- Epstein–Barr (EBV)
- Adenovirus
- Respiratory syncytial virus (RSV)
- Influenza A and B
- Parainfluenza
- Herpes simplex
- Coxsackie A

Bacteria
- Group A β-haemolytic streptococci
- Other β-haemolytic streptococci
- *Streptococcus pneumoniae*
- *Haemophilus influenzae*
- *Moraxella catarrhalis*
- *Staphylococcus aureus*
- Anaerobes (*Bacteroides* spp, peptostreptococci etc.)
- Occasionally, *Mycobacteria* spp, *Neisseria* spp, *Corynebacterium diphtheriae*

BOX 32.10 Differential diagnosis of tonsillitis: non-specific features suggesting viral infection

- Age < 3 years (GABHS unusual in this age group)
- Extrapharyngeal signs and symptoms (rhinorrhoea, cough, hoarseness)
- Conjunctivitis (exudative tonsillitis and conjunctivitis suggest adenovirus)
- Fatigue, generalized lymphadenopathy, splenomegaly (suggest EBV)
- Vesicular/ulcerative lesions (suggest Coxsackie A: herpangina or herpes simplex)

It is not possible to distinguish bacterial from viral infection reliably by clinical examination. Tonsil exudate is not specific for bacterial infection. Other non-specific features suggesting a viral origin are listed in Box 32.10.

Throat swab culture cannot reliably distinguish streptococcal disease from carriage. Furthermore, swabs have low sensitivity and take 48 hours to be reported. Rapid antigen tests also have poor sensitivity.

Current guidelines suggest that throat swabs or rapid tests should not be carried out routinely in children with tonsillitis. Further research into the role of rapid tests is required.

http://www.sign.ac.uk/pdf/qrg34.pdf

Group A β-haemolytic streptococcal (GABHS) throat infection

GABHS species, which include *Streptococcus pyogenes*, can cause disease by direct invasion or toxin production. Several strains produce an erythrogenic toxin responsible for the rash of scarlet fever. Complications are listed in Box 32.11.

GABHS infection is the most common bacterial cause of tonsillitis. It is usually a self-limiting illness, resolving in 90% of patients within 1 week regardless of whether or not antibiotics are used.

BOX 32.11 Complications of streptococcal tonsillitis

- Otitis media
- Sinusitis
- Cervical adenitis
- Peritonsillitis or abscess (quinsy)
- Scarlet fever
- Streptococcal toxic shock syndrome
- Rheumatic fever (p. 454)
- Post-streptococcal glomerulonephritis (PSGN, p. 557)

- Marked systemic upset with sore throat: scarlet fever, streptococcal toxic shock syndrome
- Peritonsillitis or abscess (quinsy)
- History of rheumatic fever
- Increased risk from acute infection: e.g. child with diabetes, immunodeficiency, congenital heart disease

Q3. Should Ethan be treated with antibiotics?

A Cochrane review concluded that antibiotics confer only modest benefit, reducing symptom duration by an average of only 16 hours. Over-prescribing risks the harms of antibiotic resistance, diarrhoea and rash. Current guidelines therefore do not recommend 'routine' antibiotic treatment. This raises several questions:

- *Should antibiotics be prescribed to prevent complications?* Not in countries with a low incidence of complications. Although the complication rate is reduced by antibiotics, the absolute risk of secondary otitis media, quinsy, sinusitis, rheumatic fever or glomerulonephritis is low in Europe. For instance, the number needed to treat for benefit (NNT_B) to prevent one case of otitis media is approximately 200. However, in developing countries, where complication rates are significantly higher, antibiotics may be indicated.
- *Should antibiotics be prescribed to prevent cross-infection?* Yes, if the index case is returning to a closed institution, e.g. boarding school. No, for children from the general community.
- *Should antibiotics ever be prescribed?* Yes, in the specific situations listed in Box 32.12. Antibiotics should not be withheld if the clinical condition of the patient is causing concern.

http://www.cochrane.org/reviews/en/ab000023.html
http://www.sign.ac.uk/pdf/qrg34.pdf

Choice of antibiotic
Penicillin for 10 days is still the drug of choice (erythromycin if allergic to penicillin).

Scarlet fever

See page 648.

Quinsy

This is uncommon in children. Infection spreads into the surrounding pharynx and soft palate (peritonsillitis).

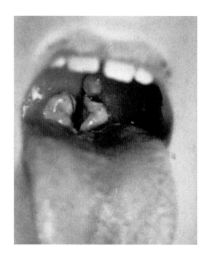

Fig. 32.6 Diphtheria pseudomembrane
(Courtesy of Centers for Disease Control, Atlanta)

Untreated, an abscess may form (quinsy). The child with quinsy usually presents with unilateral marked pain and swelling, dysphagia and otalgia. Trismus may make examination difficult. The affected tonsil is inflamed and displaced medially by a swelling in the lateral pharyngeal wall, which can occasionally cause airway obstruction. Treatment is by surgical drainage and antibiotics.

Diphtheria

Corynebacterium diphtheriae (a Gram-positive bacillus) infection is rare in western Europe but should be considered in the differential diagnosis of children recently in Eastern Europe, Russia or South-East Asia. After 1–2 days of malaise, fever and sore throat, a 'pseudomembrane' (Fig. 32.6) forms over the tonsils, palate or larynx. The grey–green membrane adheres firmly to underlying tissues. Significant soft tissue swelling and cervical lymphadenopathy ('bull neck') occur. Mortality without treatment (diphtheria antitoxin and penicillin) is high.

Sinusitis

Problem-orientated topic:

sinusitis

Alfie is 5 years old. Last week he developed a 'viral upper respiratory tract infection', which has not resolved. Yesterday he developed poorly localized facial pain and fever. His father has brought him to the accident and emergency department of his local hospital because his right eye seems swollen. On

Continued overleaf

examination, temperature is 39.4°C. There is a non-tender boggy swelling around his right eye. The periorbital skin is not inflamed. On rhinoscopy he has a thick purulent nasal discharge, with inflamed nasal mucosa. He is alert, without any meningism.

Q1. What is the differential/most likely diagnosis?
Q2. What are the factors predisposing to sinusitis?
Q3. What investigations and treatment are required?
Q4. What are the major complications of sinusitis?

Q1. What is the differential/most likely diagnosis?

The four paranasal sinuses (ethmoid, mastoid, frontal and sphenoid) are air spaces within the anterior skull, draining via narrow openings (ostia) into the middle or superior meatus of the nasal cavity (Fig. 32.7). They are lined by pseudostratified ciliated columnar epithelium. Mucus produced within the sinuses is continually moved towards the ostia by ciliary action.

The maxillary and ethmoid sinuses are present at birth, and are the main site of sinusitis in young children over 3 years old. The frontal sinuses develop from the anterior ethmoid sinus in mid-childhood. Although difficult to see on X-ray before the age of 12 years, the frontal sinuses can cause symptoms after the age of 10 years.

Symptoms
- Prolonged upper respiratory tract infection associated with fever and purulent nasal discharge

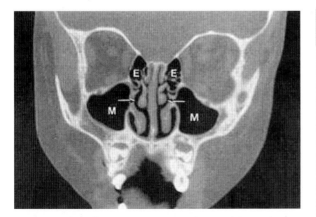

Fig. 32.7 Coronal CT of normal sinuses (maxillary ostia arrowed)
(M = maxillary; E = ethmoid)
(© Texas Tech University)

Table 32.1 Differential diagnosis of sinusitis

Condition	Distinguishing features from sinusitis
URTI	Discharge less purulent, less systemic upset
Allergic rhinitis	Watery discharge, repeated episodes, seasonal variation
Periorbital cellulitis	Tenderness, fewer nasal symptoms

- Cough
- Malodorous breath
- Less commonly:
  - Facial pain/headache
  - Painless periorbital swelling due to ethmoid sinusitis.

Signs
- Thick mucopurulent nasal discharge
- Inflamed nasal mucosa
- Pyrexia
- Occasionally:
  - Non-tender periorbital swelling (particularly young child with ethmoid sinusitis)
- Rarely:
  - Tenderness on palpation or percussion of sinuses.

Differential diagnosis
See Table 32.1.

Q2. What are the factors predisposing to sinusitis?

Sinusitis is a result of ostial obstruction, defective ciliary function or abnormal mucus production (Box 32.13), leading to poor drainage and subsequent infection. Typical organisms recovered include *Haemophilus influenzae*, *Streptococcus pneumoniae* and *Moraxella catarrhalis*.

BOX 32.13 Pathophysiology of sinusitis in children

Ostial obstruction
- Viral URTI*
- Allergic rhinitis*
- Nasal polyps
- Foreign body
- Trauma
- Unilateral choanal atresia

Defective cilia
- Ciliary dyskinesia (e.g. Kartagener syndrome)

Abnormal mucus
- Cystic fibrosis

* Common cause.

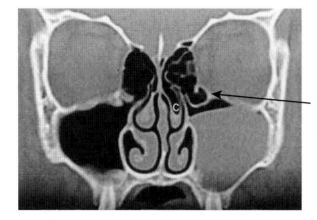

Fig. 32.8 **Maxillary sinusitis with visible air/fluid level on coronal CT**

Maxillary sinusitis with visible air/fluid level on coronal CT

Q3. What investigations and treatment are required?

Investigations include:
- Culture of nasopharyngeal secretions
- X-rays ('sinus views' must be requested); false negatives are common
- CT scan (Fig. 32.8): the gold standard, particularly if orbital involvement is suspected.

Treatment is:
- Antibiotic for 10–14 days: oral amoxicillin or erythromycin if mild disease; cefuroxime or co-amoxiclav i.v. if more severe
- Topical ephedrine (to reduce mucosal oedema blocking ostia)
- Surgery if local abscess formation.

Q4. What are the major complications of sinusitis?

Important complications include:
- Orbital:
  - Periorbital oedema
  - Orbital abscess, subperiosteal abscess: may cause proptosis
  - Periorbital cellulitis
- Intracranial:
  - Cavernous sinus thrombosis
  - Meningitis
  - Intracranial abscess.

Mastoiditis

Problem-orientated topic:

mastoiditis ● ● ● ● ●

A 21-month-old girl, Emily, is referred by her primary care physician. She developed otitis media 1 week ago. Her fever has

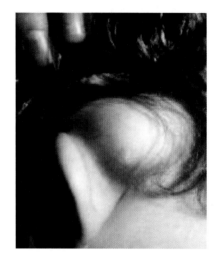

Fig. 32.9 **Mastoiditis**

persisted despite 5 days of amoxicillin. She has developed a tender swelling behind her left ear. On examination, she has a swelling, as shown in Figure 32.9. Her temperature is 39.4°C. The left tympanic membrane is inflamed and bulging.

Q1. What is the most likely diagnosis?
Q2. What else could it be and how will you confirm the diagnosis?
Q3. How should Emily be treated?
Q4. What complications should you look out for?

Q1. What is the most likely diagnosis?

Mastoid pneumatization occurs shortly after birth and is complete by age of 10 years. The mastoid air-cell system communicates with the posterior aspect of the middle ear through the narrow aditus ad antrum.

Acute mastoiditis is a result of infection spreading from the middle ear. The antrum is blocked by inflamed mucosa, inhibiting drainage and triggering mastoid empyema. Bacteria causing otitis media are usually responsible: *Streptococcus pneumoniae*, *Haemophilus influenzae*, group A streptococci (rarely *Moraxella catarrhalis*, *Mycoplasma*, *Pseudomonas* or anaerobes).

Mastoiditis is usually a disease of young children. It is uncommon. Symptoms include:
- Recent otitis media
- Fever despite adequate antibiotic treatment
- Pain located in or behind the ear
- Less commonly: purulent otorrhoea, hearing loss.

On examination there is:
- Pyrexia
- Otitis media with or without tympanic perforation
- Tender swelling behind the ear, which displaces the auricle laterally and obliterates the post-auricular skin crease (Fig. 32.9).

Q2. What else could it be and how will you confirm the diagnosis?

The differential diagnosis includes:
- *Otitis externa*: less systemic upset, no post-auricular swelling
- *Post-auricular lymph node abscess*: post-auricular skin crease is preserved.

Investigations are directed towards identifying the responsible organism, monitoring the response to treatment and detecting spread outside the mastoid. Therefore:
- Culture any discharge (some surgeons suggest myringotomy to obtain a sample).
- Order blood culture, full blood count, erythrocyte sedimentation rate/C-reactive protein.
- Organize a CT scan if there is evidence of complications, i.e:
  – Facial palsy
  – Persistent fever despite parenteral antibiotics
  – Reduced level of consciousness
  – Recurrent vomiting with headache
  – Signs of meningism.

BOX 32.14 Complications of mastoiditis
- Subperiosteal abscess
- Meningitis
- Facial (seventh nerve) palsy
- Cavernous/sigmoid sinus thrombosis
- Osteomyelitis of the petrous temporal bone
- Intracranial abscess
- Labyrinthitis

Q3. How should Emily be treated?

- *Antibiotics.* Prescribe a parenteral third-generation cephalosporin. Consider adding vancomycin or clindamycin and/or anaerobic cover. Oral antibiotics may be substituted after 18–72 hours if the temperature settles. Give 14 days of antibiotics.
- *Obtain an ENT opinion.* Surgery (myringotomy and/or mastoidectomy) becomes necessary in approximately 25% of children. Indications for surgery include failure to respond to medical treatment or complications.

Q4. What complications should you look out for?

Complications (Box 32.14) arise when infection spreads beyond the mastoid into local structures.

Further reading

Bamiou DE, Macardle B, Bitner-Glindzicz M et al 2000 Aetiological investigations of hearing loss in childhood: a review. Clinical Otolaryngology 25:98–106

Fortnum HM 1992 Hearing impairment after bacterial meningitis: a review. Archives of Disease in Childhood 67:1128–1133

Hall DMB, Elliman D 2003 Health for all children, 4th edn. Oxford University Press, Oxford

Medical Research Council Multi-centre Otitis Study Group 2001 Risk factors for persistence of bilateral otitis media with effusion. Clinical Otolaryngology 26:147–156

MODULE SIX

Neil Kennedy   Malcolm Levene   Rotraud K. Saurenmann

Disorders of bones, joints and connective tissue

LEARNING OUTCOMES

By the end of this chapter you should:

- Be able to screen a child for joint disorders
- Be able to undertake an examination of the major joints
- Be able to undertake a screening test for neonatal development dysplasia of the hip
- Know the common causes of limp
- Know the presentation and management of bone and joint infection
- Know the common causes of joint swelling
- Know the presentation, classification and management of juvenile idiopathic arthritis.

Clinical assessment

Examination of the joints should always be a part of a routine clinical examination (Ch. 5). If a child presents with joint or bone pain, then more careful history and examination are required.

History

Important questions in the history include:

- *What is the nature of the pain (arthralgia)?* Ask about location, exacerbating and relieving factors, radiation and timing of onset of the pain (whether it is related to times of the day). Pain or immobility (stiffness) first thing in the morning is suggestive of an inflammatory cause. Pain caused by a mechanical problem will usually be exacerbated by exercise and resolve with a period of rest.
- *Are there constitutional symptoms?* These include fever, fatigue, anorexia, weight loss and rashes.

- *Are there emotional, family or school-related problems?* Non-organic causes of limb pain are common and are discussed in Chapter 24.

Examination

- *Gait.* With an antalgic (painful) gait the child spends as little time as possible during the walking cycle on the painful leg. Important points include the ability to weight-bear on a joint.
- *Rash.* Look carefully for rashes (in particular on the face, eyelids, flexor surfaces of joints and knuckles).
- *Muscle tenderness or wasting.* Assess muscle strength.
- *Joint examination.* Look for:
  - Evidence of wasting or limb length differences
  - Redness of the joint
  - Swelling
  - Range of movements (are there joint contractures?).
  - Pain on motion, especially towards the end of the normal range of movement of a joint.

It may be useful to perform a screening musculoskeletal examination if in doubt as to whether the child has an organic cause for the joint pain (Box 33.1). A child who can perform all these functions without difficulty is unlikely to have a significant musculoskeletal problem.

Developmental dysplasia of the hip

This refers to a disorder of hip development that may predispose to dislocation either at birth or later. Hip instability is present in 1:60 neonates and, before the introduction of widespread clinical neonatal hip screening, late dislocation occurred in 1–2 per 1000 live births. This incidence has fallen with routine screening but the condition still occurs in 0.8 per 1000 live births.

Risk factors for developmental dysplasia include:

- Gender: it is six times more common in girls than boys
- First-born children

- Breech position in utero
- Maternal oligohydramnios
- Family history of developmental dysplasia of the hip.

Screening

All newborn infants should be routinely examined for hip dysplasia. Screening should be performed by ultrasound wherever available. Mechanical testing of the hip joint by the Barlow and Ortolani test is less specific and should only be used when routine ultrasound screening is not available. Repeat screening is recommended at 6 weeks and 6 months of age by the primary care physician or health visitor.

Newborn screening involves the following elements.

Is the hip in joint?

Inspect gluteal folds. Are they symmetrical? Are the legs of equal length? If either of these is abnormal, it suggests the hip may be dislocated.

Test hip abduction. If the hip abducts fully, it is not dislocated.

Is the hip stable?

If the hip is not dislocated, then its stability should be tested by Barlow's test. The essence of this test is to exert downward pressure through the femur to see whether the hip can be dislocated backwards. If the hip is unstable, a 'clunk' is felt as the head of the femur is pushed over the lip of the acetabulum.

Can a dislocated hip be relocated?

If the hip cannot be fully abducted and dislocation is suspected, then the Ortolani test is used to attempt to relocate the hip into joint. Upward traction on the femur is used to relocate the hip in the acetabulum. Relocation is accompanied by a 'clunk' sensation. Once the hip is relocated, then the hip can be gently abducted.

Ultrasound assessment

Ultrasound examination of the hips is a very useful way of determining hip architecture and is widely used to assess the child who is at high risk of hip dysplasia or where there is an equivocal screening test. In some countries the hip joints of all newborns are routinely screened by ultrasound for developmental dysplasia.

Management

The dislocated or dislocatable hip should be reduced into the acetabulum and maintained in the position of flexion and abduction until it becomes stable. A variety of harnesses are used to maintain stability, including the Pavlick harness, the most widely used. The hips are located into the harness under the supervision of an orthopaedic surgeon and the harness is worn continuously for 12–16 weeks. Regular adjustments to ensure appropriate fitting of the harness are required.

Dislocation diagnosed after 4 months of age will require specialist orthopaedic attention. Initially a 2-week period of traction is initiated, followed by surgical intervention to ensure the hip is relocated and remains stable.

Complications

Avascular necrosis of the femoral head is the most important serious complication. This may arise as the result of forceful reduction or immobilizing the hip too fully in an abduction harness or splint.

Arthritis

Problem-orientated topic:

the child with a limp (see also Ch. 24)

Tim is 4. He is brought to the accident and emergency department having developed a right-sided limp a day ago. He has had a recent 'cold'. His mother tells you that he fell off his scooter 4 days ago, but other than cutting his knee, he had no major injury. On examination, Tim is pyrexial (38.3°C) and appears mildly unwell. He has a healing abrasion on the right knee, which does not appear to be infected. When asked to stand, he will weight-bear only on his left leg and holds his right leg flexed at the hip. When lying down, he will allow you to flex, extend, adduct and abduct his hips. However, passive internal flexion of the right hip causes him pain.

Q1. What is the differential diagnosis of a child with a limp?

Q2. How can you differentiate septic arthritis from 'irritable hip'?

Q3. What are the causative organisms of septic arthritis?

Q1. What is the differential diagnosis of a child with a limp?

These are listed in Box 33.2.

BOX 33.2 Causes of acute limp in children

- Transient synovitis (sometimes known as 'irritable hip')*
- Septic arthritis/osteomyelitis of hip, femur or knee*
- Trauma*
- Perthes disease
- Slipped capital femoral epiphysis
- Juvenile idiopathic arthritis
- Idiopathic chondrolysis
- Neoplastic: osteosarcoma/bony infiltrate of other malignancy

* Common cause.

Table 33.1 **Features differentiating septic arthritis from irritable hip**

Feature	Irritable hip	Septic arthritis
Fever	None/mild	Moderate/high
Systemic upset?	None/mild	Moderate/severe
White cell count (WCC)	Mild ↑	↑↑ – ↑↑↑
Erythrocyte sedimentation rate (ESR)	Mild ↑	↑↑
Ultrasound	Effusion	Effusion
Improves with rest?	Yes	No

Q2. How can you differentiate septic arthritis from 'irritable hip'?

'Irritable hip' occurs in up to 3% of children between 3 and 8 years, more commonly in boys. Typically a child will develop a limp a few days after an upper respiratory tract infection. The child remains systemically well. On examination, internal rotation of the hip may be limited. The child rests with the hip held in flexion and external rotation. Ultrasound will often show an effusion of the hip. The syndrome is probably caused by a transient reactive hip synovitis. Most cases settle in 5–10 days, with symptomatic treatment only. The important differential diagnosis is septic arthritis and the main distinguishing features are shown in Table 33.1. Be aware that, depending on the virulence of the pathogen, septic arthritis may occasionally present with very mild constitutional features.

Tim probably has 'irritable hip'.

Q3. What are the causative organisms of septic arthritis?

- *Staphylococcus aureus* (75% of cases)
- Group A β-haemolytic streptococcus (*Strep. pyogenes*)

- *Strep. pneumoniae*
- Occasionally: Salmonellae species, Mycobacterium tuberculosis
- In neonates the spectrum of pathogens is the same as for neonatal sepsis (see Chapter 47)

Osteomyelitis and septic arthritis

In this condition there is infection in the bone. It most commonly arises as the result of haematogenous spread and rarely following trauma. Septic arthritis may develop as a result of direct spread from adjacent osteomyelitis, especially in younger children and neonates. The most common site of involvement is the metaphysis of long bones or vertebral bodies.

Osteomyelitis may be acute, subacute or chronic. Subacute is usually the result of less virulent organisms and chronic usually arises as a result of inadequately treated infection.

Presentation

Pain and loss of function are the most common presenting features. The pain can usually be localized by the child, and if a lower limb is involved, limp or refusal to walk is common. Hip infection results in the child lying with the hip flexed and in internal rotation, with the knee in flexion. Localizing signs are less obvious when the primary infection arises in pelvis or spine.

Neonates present with non-specific signs, including unstable temperature, poor feeding, pallor, recurrent apnoea and pseudoparalysis (maintaining the limb completely immobile). The affected limb may be swollen and tender to touch. Diagnosis requires awareness of osteomyelitis as a cause of severe infection in a non-specifically unwell baby.

Infecting organisms

In Europe *Staph. aureus* causes 75% of osteomyelitis infection. Other infecting organisms include group A β-haemolytic streptococcus (*Strep. pyogenes*) and *Strep. pneumoniae*. In the neonate, group B β-haemolytic streptococcus is relatively common. *Haemophilus influenzae* type b (Hib) is now very rare due to widespread immunization. Other organisms to be considered include tuberculosis (usually insidious in onset), brucellosis, salmonellae and *Mycoplasma pneumoniae* (these latter three may cause low-grade septic arthritis).

Investigations

Full blood count, ESR and C-reactive protein (CRP) usually suggest infection. Blood cultures should be taken prior to starting antibiotics. Culture from bone or a joint effusion may identify the organism, together with a marked pleocytosis in the synovial fluid.

The first X-ray change is periosteal reaction (Fig. 33.1) and is seen within a few days of infection with bone

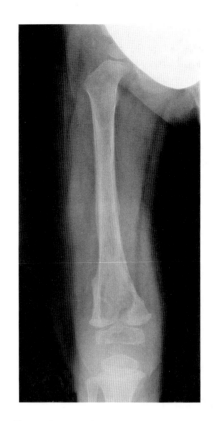

Fig. 33.1 **X-ray of femur showing periosteal reaction in acute osteomyelitis**

changes later. Radionuclide bone scanning may reveal areas of multiple infection. In septic arthritis the early radiological features are osteopenia of the epiphysis, increased joint space and soft tissue swelling. Ultrasound imaging may reveal fluid in the joint.

Management

Early administration of antistaphylococcal antibiotics (flucloxacillin and cefotaxime in a neonate or child below 2 years; flucloxacillin and ampicillin in an older child) in appropriate dosage is essential. A broader-spectrum choice is recommended in immunosuppressed children until the organism has been identified. It is recommended that intravenous antibiotics are used for at least 3 days, followed by an oral course for 3–4 weeks if the fever has settled. Neonates require a longer intravenous course.

The role of bone drilling in the management of this condition is controversial. Biopsy for microbiological diagnosis may be useful.

Aspiration of a septic joint is always recommended for diagnostic purposes. Surgical drainage is necessary for septic arthritis to eliminate effectively the pathogens from the joint space and in the hip to minimize risk of avascular necrosis of the femoral head.

An ill child will require supportive c... intensive care unit.

Complications

Outcome is usually good with early treatment. Disturbance of bone growth may occur following septic arthritis or if osteomyelitis involves the epiphysis. Chronic osteomyelitis may lead to bone necrosis and sequestration.

Reactive arthritis

Arthralgia and joint swelling may occur directly or indirectly as a result of a number of infections. Viruses such as rubella, parvovirus (erythrovirus) and varicella commonly cause a short period of arthralgia.

True 'reactive' arthritis occurs after enteric infection with *Salmonella*, *Shigella*, *Yersinia* and *Campylobacter* and is often associated with the child expressing the HLA B27 antigen. Joint(s) of the lower limb are usually involved in an asymmetrical manner. Dactylitis (swelling and pain of interphalangeal joints) may also occur. Non-steroidal anti-inflammatory drugs (NSAIDs) are indicated until pain and swelling regress.

Swollen joints

Problem-orientated topic:

swollen joints ● ● ● ● ● ●

Lara (3 years old) presents in the outpatient department. She has been complaining of pain in her knee on and off for several weeks. The pain is mainly in the morning, and gets better over the day. In the last 10 days, her left knee has swollen. Lara is otherwise well. On examination she has an effusion of the left knee. There is mild pain when you passively flex the knee by more than 60°.

Q1. What is the differential diagnosis for inflammatory arthritis in children?

Q2. What is the classification of juvenile idiopathic arthritis (JIA)?

Q3. What type of JIA does Lara have?

Q4. What are the principles of treatment of JIA?

Q1. What is the differential diagnosis for inflammatory arthritis in children?

The differential diagnosis is listed in Box 33.3.

Q2. What is the classification of juvenile idiopathic arthritis (JIA)?

...fication proposes the following

- Infection
  - Viral arthritis
  - Septic arthritis
  - Reactive arthritis transient para-/post-infectious arthritis
- Juvenile idiopathic arthritis (JIA)
- Vasculitis
  - Henoch–Schönlein purpura (HSP)
  - Kawasaki disease (p. 642)
  - Polyarteritis nodosa
- Trauma
- Autoimmune disorders
  - Systemic lupus erythematosus
  - Juvenile dermatomyositis
- Malignancy
  - Leukaemia (p. 775)
  - Neuroblastoma (p. 778)
- Blood disorders
  - Sickle cell disease (p. 619)
  - Haemophilia (p. 624)
- Drug reactions

1. Systemic arthritis
2. Oligoarticular arthritis
   (a) Persistent
   (b) Extended
3. Polyarthritis: rheumatoid factor (RF) negative
4. Polyarthritis: RF positive
5. Enthesitis-related arthritis (inflammation at insertion of tendons into bones)
6. Psoriatic arthritis
7. Undifferentiated arthritis.

http://www.medscape.com/viewarticle/520063

Juvenile Idiopathic Arthritis: Insights into Classification, Outcomes and Treatment

Q3. What type of JIA does Lara have?

Lara probably has the oligoarthritis form of JIA (see below for a description of this condition).

Q4. What are the principles of treatment of JIA?

These are summarized as follows:
- An NSAID is the first-line drug.
- Intra-articular corticosteroids are very effective at relieving pain.
- Methotrexate is indicated for persistent synovitis.
- There is only a very limited role for systemic corticosteroids.

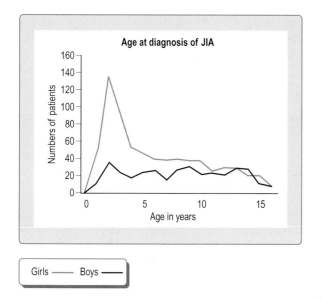

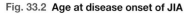

Fig. 33.2 **Age at disease onset of JIA**

- Management must be within a multidisciplinary team under the supervision of a paediatric rheumatologist.

More details of management are discussed below in the section on JIA.

Juvenile idiopathic arthritis (JIA)

This represents a spectrum of disorders most recently classified as JIA. It is a disease of children with onset below 16 years of age and presents as synovitis (joint swelling, limitation of movement, or pain) persisting for at least 6 weeks. In addition, varieties of JIA include different distributions of synovitis and sometimes other clinical involvement such as skin, eyes and heart.

The annual incidence of JIA is 10–20 per 100 000 children in Europe and the USA. Twice the number of girls as boys are affected. There are two peak ages of onset: early and late. In the early group presentation is at 1–3 years and is mainly of the oligoarthritis form, affecting girls. The second age peak is at 9 years, and boys and girls are equally affected (Fig. 33.2 and Fig. 33.3).

Basic science

The genetic susceptibility to JIA is multifactorial. A variety of single nucleotide polymorphisms (SNPs, Ch. 9) have been found to be associated with either a general risk for autoimmune diseases or a more specific risk for joint inflammation. The human leucocyte antigen (HLA) genes comprise an important

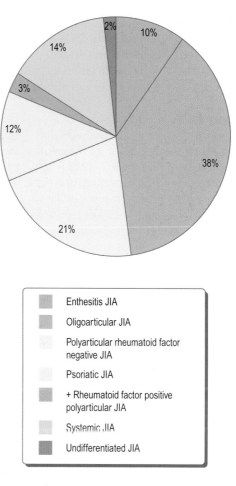

Fig. 33.3 **Subtype distribution in a cohort of over 1000 JIA patients**

part of the MHC and susceptibility to JIA is particularly associated with HLA A2, DR5, DR8 and DPB1*0201. In older boys, oligoarthritis is associated with HLA B27. Genetic susceptibility may require a second environmental trigger to induce disease. Triggers such as infective agents may account for seasonal variations in the onset of this disease.

Inflammation is mediated through expression of cytokines, a family of soluble proteins that exert either pro-inflammatory or anti-inflammatory activity. In JIA certain pro-inflammatory cytokines, such as tumour necrosis factor-alpha (TNF-α) induce release of tissue-destroying metalloproteinases and stimulate release of other members of the pro-inflammatory cytokine cascade. TNF-α is produced by activated macrophages, T-lymphocytes and synovial cells, and contributes to joint destruction.

Clinical features

The classical presentation of redness, pain or tenderness and limitation of joint mo stiffness is a common complaint in children. The presentation may be dramatic or protean, and systemic features are seen in systemic arthritis.

The form of JIA can be defined on the basis of joint involvement as well as involvement of other organs.

Oligoarthritis

Oligoarthritis refers to disease affecting 1–4 joints during the first 6 months of the illness. It is the most common form of JIA and accounts for 50% of affected children: mainly girls, with peak age of onset at 1–3 years. It most commonly presents insidiously with isolated joint involvement, particularly of knee or ankle, or more rarely an upper limb joint. Eye involvement (uveitis) may occur and because it is often asymptomatic all affected children should be regularly screened by an ophthalmologist.

The child may present with a limp but rarely complains of severe pain. On examination the joint is hot and swollen and an effusion may be present. Clinical signs include reduction in passive movement, which may result in contractures in long-standing disease.

Affected children often have positive antinuclear antibodies (ANA). The presence of these auto-antibodies is associated with an increased risk for uveitis.

Polyarthritis

This refers to disease affecting five or more joints during the first 6 months of illness, and occurs in about 25% of children with JIA. It usually involves joints symmetrically. The polyarthritis can be further subdivided into rheumatoid factor positive and negative subtype of JIA, based on whether or not IgM rheumatoid factor is present. Rheumatoid factor negative disease is much more common than rheumatoid factor positive disease in children.

Rheumatoid factor negative polyarthritis has a peak incidence at 6–7 years and may be insidious or more aggressive in some children. Rheumatoid factor positive disease starts later in late childhood or adolescence and affects smaller joints of hands and feet.

Systemic arthritis

In this form, joint involvement is accompanied by fever and other systemic features. It accounts for about 10% of cases of JIA and occurs at a peak age of 5 years. The fever usually follows a characteristic pattern, being present for at least 2 weeks, and spiking once or twice a day, usually in the evening, and returning to normal between spikes (Fig. 33.2). A pale pink macular rash and malaise are particularly common when the child is pyrexial. Lymphadenopathy, hepatomegaly or spleno-megaly is also commonly present. Because of the similarity to infections and malignancy in the way this disease presents, other conditions must be carefully excluded (Ch. 50).

Joint manifestation is variable and may only present weeks or months after the onset of fever but is most commonly of the polyarthritis form. Some children have a very aggressive form, with joint destruction within 2 years.

Investigations

The presence of antinuclear antibodies (ANA) and rheumatoid factor (RF) is important in classifying the disease. A positive ANA in oligoarthritis is a risk factor for uveitis.

Ultrasound is a sensitive investigation for joint effusions and may help guide needle aspiration of fluid.

Radiology is most important to exclude other causes of joint swelling and may show the following features:
- *Early signs*: periarticular osteopenia (Fig. 33.5)
- *Intermediate signs*: cortical erosions (Fig. 33.6), advanced bone maturation, joint space narrowing and subchondral cysts
- *Late signs*: destructive changes with ankylosis and growth anomalies.

Management

The management of children with chronic disorders must be within a multidisciplinary team (Ch. 18) and under the supervision of a paediatric rheumatologist. Physiotherapy aims to maintain joint function, with an occupational therapist to facilitate normal living skills and provision of aids to overcome impairment. Well-fitting splints to support acutely inflamed joints are of particular importance.

NSAIDs are the first-line drug at diagnosis. Intra-articular corticosteroids are very effective at relieving pain and may prevent or reduce synovial damage and disability. Methotrexate is indicated for persistent synovitis and has been shown to be effective for all types of JIA.

Recently, anti-TNF therapy has been shown to give significant benefit to children with polyarticular JIA who failed to respond to methotrexate. It has been shown that 60–70% of children who fail to respond to methotrexate show some improvement with anti-TNF therapy. Long-term safety of these agents has not been fully assessed in children. Further drug management schedules depend on the type of JIA that the child shows. The role of systemic corticosteroids in JIA has reduced in recent years with the introduction of more effective drugs such as methotrexate. It may be valuable for inducing remission in particularly aggressive forms of the disease.

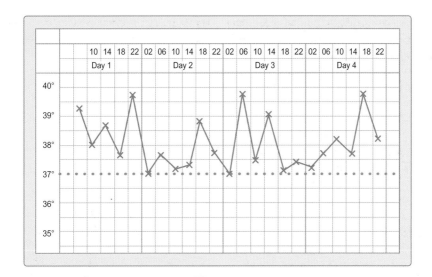

Fig. 33.4 **Typical temperature chart of a child with acute-onset systemic rheumatoid arthritis**

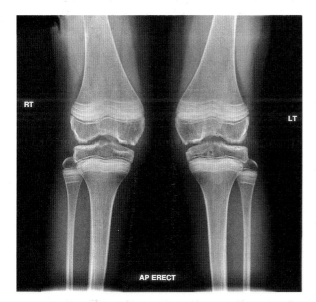

Fig. 33.5 **X-ray of knees showing periosteal osteopenia in a child with rheumatoid factor positive JIA**

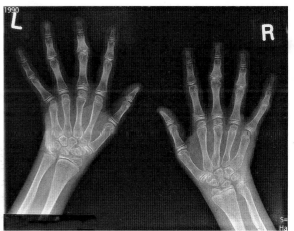

Fig. 33.6 **X-ray showing destructive changes of carpal bones in a child with polyarthritis**

Complications

Uveitis occurs in 15% of all children with JIA but in up to 30% of children with early onset oligoarticular JIA. Acute painful iritis is rare but is seen particularly in children with enthesitis. Painless anterior uveitis is more insidious, and if unrecognized, may cause severe visual impairment, particularly in pre-school-age children with oligoarthritis; it is strongly associated with ANA. Regular ophthalmological assessments are necessary for recognizing and treating this condition.

The major complications of JIA are bone erosion leading to disfigurement, joint destruction and major mobility problems. A multiprofessional approach is required to minimize the destructive potential of this condition.

Henoch–Schönlein purpura

Henoch–Schönlein purpura (HSP, see also pp. 364 and 623) is an IgA mediated vasculitis affecting skin, joints, bowel and kidneys (p. 563). The cause is unknown but most probably HSP is an immunologic reaction triggered by an upper respiratory tract infection. It has an incidence of 10–15 per 100 000 children and although it may occur at any age it usually presents in children below the age of 10 years, with a peak at 5 years.

Children present most commonly with a palpable (raised) purpuric rash characteristically involving

453

buttocks, lower limbs and elbows and/or arthralgia with joint swelling (see DVD 28). Abdominal pain occurs commonly with blood in the stool, but serious bleeding, intussusception and bowel perforation, although recognized, are rare. Renal involvement (haematuria/proteinuria, rarely hypertension) occurs in 50% of cases, but persisting renal disease is rare and is seen in only 1% of cases. Urinalysis for proteinuria should be undertaken regularly throughout the course of the illness to identify renal involvement.

HSP is usually a relatively mild and benign condition that resolves fully within a couple of weeks of its onset. Recurrent episodes may occur over the next few weeks or months. In rare cases a more aggressive, even life threatening course of the disease has been reported.

Management is symptomatic, with simple analgesics for pain relief. Corticosteroids are very effective but should be restricted to severe cases requiring hospitalization. The management of renal involvement is discussed on page 565.

Rheumatic fever

Rheumatic fever (see also p. 585) is now rarely seen in Western Europe but remains common in the developing world. It is due to a complication of infection with group A β-haemolytic *Strep. pyogenes*. The organism induces an immune-mediated reaction, resulting in vasculitis. Affected organs include joints, heart (pancarditis, arrhythmias), skin (erythema marginatum, subcutaneous nodules) and brain (Sydenham chorea).

Clinical features

There are no specific markers of rheumatic fever, but the diagnosis is made on the basis of the presence of a number of clinical features that are described as the modified Jones criteria (Box 33.4). The diagnosis is made on the presence of two major criteria or one major and two minor criteria, together with evidence of recent group A streptococcal infection (positive throat swab, elevated antistreptolysin O titre (ASOT) or other antistreptococcal antibodies).

http://www.arthritis.org/conditions/
DiseaseCenter/jra.asp

Management

- Eradication of streptococcus with penicillin for 10 days
- Symptomatic relief of arthralgia with NSAIDs
- Steroids: reserved for pancarditis

BOX 33.4 Modified Jones criteria for the diagnosis of rheumatic fever

Major criteria
- Polyarthritis involving large joints and flitting*
- Carditis*
- Chorea (Sydenham)
- Erythema marginatum
- Subcutaneous nodules on extensor surfaces

Minor criteria
- Fever
- Arthralgia
- Prolonged P–R interval
- Elevated ESR/CRP, leucocytosis
- Previous rheumatic fever
- Common.

* Common feature.

- Prophylactic penicillin against further streptococcal infection for 5 years or until adulthood, depending on the severity of the cardiac involvement.

Polyarteritis nodosa (PAN)

This rare vasculitic condition in children affects medium-sized arteries and presents with non-specific symptoms including fever, malaise, rashes, and joint or muscle pain. Investigation findings are also non-specific and diagnosis is made on abnormal biopsy appearance. Management should be under the supervision of a paediatric rheumatologist.

Systemic lupus erythematosus (SLE)

This is rare in children but more common in adolescent and young female adults. The hallmark of this autoimmune condition is the production of auto-antibodies directed against a variety of organs and tissues. The resulting inflammation leads to non-specific constitutional signs and symptoms such as fever, weight loss, arthralgias and fatigue. Common presenting symptoms are facial (butterfly) rash (Fig. 33.7), thrombocytopenia, anemia and lymphopenia. Renal and CNS involvement are common and of importance for the prognosis. Rarely severe renal or neurological SLE may be life-threatening. The ESR is usually elevated and positive ANA is found in all cases, although these findings are non-specific as they may also be positive in the presence of other diagnoses. Management should be under the supervision of a paediatric rheumatologist.

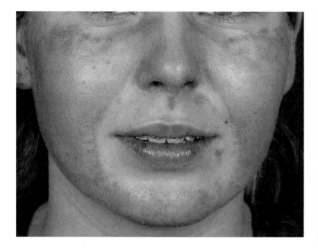

Fig. 33.7 Typical 'butterfly' rash in a 14-year-old girl with systemic lupus erythematosus (SLE). Note that the rash bridges the nose but usually spares the nasolabial folds and the perioral area.

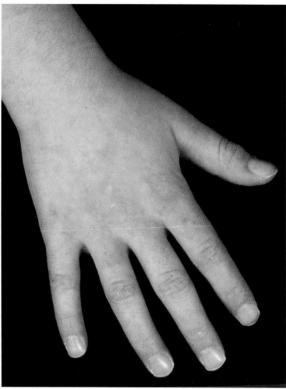

Fig. 33.9 JDM Gottron rash: Gottron papules are typically located over the knuckles and look like irritated skin with some scaling. They heal leaving superficial atrophic scars.

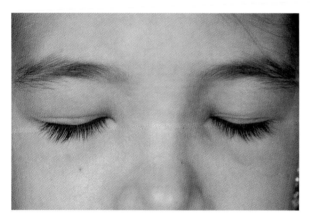

Fig. 33.8 Heliotrope rash: pinkish, slightly swollen appearance of the face and especially the eyelids in juvenile dermatomyositis.

Dermatomyositis (see also p. 282)

This is a rare autoimmune disorder in children with a peak of onset between 4–8 years of age. The diagnosis is made on the basis of a characteristic rash together with:

- Symmetrical proximal muscle weakness
- Abnormal muscle biopsy
- Elevated muscle enzymes
- Changes on electromyography.

The rash is the first feature in about 50% of cases, affecting eyelids (heliotropic rash), knuckles (Gottron papules) (Figs 33.8 and 33.9) and extensor surfaces of the elbows and knees (Fig. 28.5). Erythema of the nailfolds is a particular feature (Fig. 33.10).

Often the muscle weakness first becomes obvious when difficulty climbing stairs or brushing hair is noticed. Muscle pain is frequently a feature at onset,

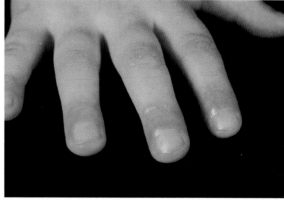

Fig. 33.10 Periungual oedema: swelling and redness of the nailfold area with cuticle overgrowth and visible anomalies of the nailfold capillaries (giant loops, drop-outs) are typically found in juvenile dermatomyositis.

whereas calcinosis of the skin and muscle is a well recognized complication occuring after longstanding uncontrolled inflammation. Myositis is confirmed by elevated muscle enzymes.

The mainstay of management is corticosteroid therapy in combination with immunosuppressants. Early aggressive treatment is necessary to control the inflammatory process and prevent complications and long-term disability. Management should be under the supervision of a paediatric rheumatologist.

Acknowledgement

We are grateful to Dr R. Arthur for permission to use the radiographs.

Further Reading

Saurenmann RK, Levin AV, Feldman BM et al. 2007 — Prevalence, Risk Factors and Outcome of Uveitis in Juvenile Idiopathic Arthritis — A Long-term Follow up Study. Arthritis Rheum Feb 56(2): 647–57

Carl J. Harvey   Chris J. Hendriksz   Saikat Santra   Flemming Skovby

Inborn errors of metabolism

LEARNING OUTCOMES

By the end of this chapter you should:

- Understand the clinical presentation of metabolic disorders in the newborn
- Know the clinical features of metabolic disease in the older child
- Be able to administer and interpret tests of common metabolic disorders in conjunction with a specialist metabolic laboratory
- Be able to recognize, initiate diagnostic tests for and outline the management of hypoglycaemia, persistent or recurrent episodes of metabolic acidosis (including lactic acidosis), acute encephalopathy (including intractable seizures) and neurodevelopmental regression/dysmorphism.

Basic science and cell function

At a cellular level the nucleus is the centre of or major contributor to gene expression. Enzymes are proteins that are produced according to the genetic information provided by the nucleus. This production process is supported by other organelles that play a crucial part in the final functioning of the enzyme. Knowledge of the supporting organelles that are associated with disease is increasing but for simplicity the following model may help understanding.

The nucleus holds the genetic material of the ovum and sperm from the point of conception. The genetic material represents an equal contribution by both parents in most circumstances. This equal contribution explains why in most metabolic conditions carriers are not affected, as although enzyme activity will be reduced

in carriers, it would still be sufficient to prevent disease. The exceptions are some X-linked diseases, in which the majority of patients will be males.

The mitochondrion has its own genetic material and is referred to as the mitochondrial genome; it represents only 1% of cellular nucleic acid material. This genome consists of 37 genes and has been fully sequenced. The mitochondria contain about 1000 proteins, of which only 13 are encoded by mitochondrial DNA; the rest are imported but under control of nuclear encoded DNA. Mitochondria are derived from maternal origin only, as the sperm does not contribute to the mitochondrial pool. Defects in the mitochondrial gene are inherited in a maternal inheritance pattern also called cytoplasmic inheritance. Great variability within families with maternally inherited mitochondrial disease can be explained by the principle of heteroplasmy. Heteroplasmy is the unequal division of mitochondria in the early developmental phase, meaning that cells and

Normal enzyme function depends on:

- Normal genetic material in the nucleus
- Adequate energy supplied by the mitochondria
- Functioning Golgi apparatus and endoplasmic reticulum
- Housekeeping organelles, like lysosomes and peroxisomes
- Vitamins that are frequently used as co-factors and enhance enzymatic function.

Abnormalities of these systems form the basis of the common inborn errors of metabolism.

different tissues can get variable amounts of affected mitochondria. It is important to realize that not all mitochondrial disorders are maternally inherited, and each and every form of inheritance has been associated with mitochondrial disease. The unifying principle is that mitochondrial dysfunction is associated with energy deficiency and that is the cause of disease manifestations.

The lysosomes are intracellular organelles that are produced by the Golgi apparatus and are filled by enzymes (Box 34.1). These nuclear encoded enzymes that are produced in the endoplasmic reticulum only function at low pH and this is only found inside the lysosomes. They have a housekeeping function and, together with the peroxisomes, digest organisms, defective organelles or foreign particles.

Presentation of inborn errors of metabolism (IEMs) in the neonate

Problem-orientated topic:

metabolic disease in the newborn ● ● ● ● ●

Mikkel is a 5-day-old baby who has been rushed to hospital acutely unwell. He was born at term and has been exclusively breastfeeding well. He is the second child of consanguineous Asian parents who lost their first child last year from cot death. Over the last 24 hours, Mikkel has been feeding less well, has become less responsive and now looks pale and mottled, his skin is cold to the touch. He is floppy and tachypnoeic with a respiratory rate of 82 breaths per minute but has only mild subcostal recession. A

capillary blood gas taken by the admitting nurse shows pH 7.07, base excess −15 mmol/l, PCO_2 4.35 kPa, PO_2 3.85 kPa and blood glucose 1.2 mmol/l.

Q1. What are the three important groups of disorders in the differential diagnosis?

Q2. What features make an inborn error of metabolism more likely?

Q3. What further investigations are indicated?

Q4. What are the main principles of emergency management?

Q1. What are the three important groups of disorders in the differential diagnosis?

Neonates present with non-specific symptoms and hence the differential diagnosis is always wide. For an acutely acidotic neonate the three most common problems are:

- Sepsis
- Congenital heart disease
- IEMs.

Although IEMs are individually rare, they are collectively not uncommon and hence the possibility of an IEM should be considered, as many cases are amenable to early treatment that improves mortality and long-term neurological morbidity.

Q2. What features make an inborn error of metabolism more likely?

A number of factors in the history and examination may raise the suspicion of an IEM. These include:

- Parental consanguinity
- A family history of unexplained deaths in infancy
- Maternal history of HELLP syndrome (*h*aemolysis, *e*levated *l*iver enzymes and *l*ow *p*latelets) or acute fatty liver of pregnancy
- Previous miscarriages or non-immune hydrops fetalis
- Well period before deterioration (effectively dialysed by placenta)
- Encephalopathy ± seizures
- Metabolic acidosis with raised anion gap
- Raised blood ammonia
- Hypoglycaemia
- Urinary ketones
- Dysmorphic features
- Unusual odours.

Types of IEM that present in the neonate

These fall broadly into five clinical 'syndromes', as shown in Box 34.2.

BOX 34.2 Types of IEM that present in the neonate

1. Acute intoxication picture
- Organic acidaemias like propionic acidaemia, methylmalonic acidaemia and isovaleric acidaemia
- Maple syrup urine disease
- Urea cycle defects
- Fatty acid oxidation defects
- Transient hyperammonaemia of the newborn

2. Encephalopathy with seizures
- Non-ketotic hyperglycinaemia or other neurotransmitter defects
- Sulphite oxidase deficiency
- Pyridoxine- or folinic acid-dependent seizures
- Urea cycle disorders and maple syrup urine disease
- Congenital lactic acidosis

3. Neonatal liver disease and/or multi-organ failure
- Galactosaemia
- Tyrosinaemia
- Neonatal haemochromatosis
- Fatty acid oxidation disorders
- Mitochondrial disease
- Organomegaly: glycogen storage diseases and Niemann–Pick type C

4. Non-immune hydrops and/or dysmorphism
- Lysosomal storage disorders
- Sterol metabolism defects like Smith–Lemli–Opitz syndrome
- Peroxisomal disorders (can have Down-like features)
- Red cell enzyme defects

5. Neurological deterioration and/or energy deficiency
- Mitochondrial disease
- Peroxisomal disorders

Q3. What further investigations are indicated?

Using the numbered categories shown in Box 34.2, investigations can be planned as most appropriate. Table 34.1 will provide the best-guess investigations in a neonate.

Table 34.1 Further investigations in IEM in the neonate

Investigation	Most helpful	Possibly helpful	Non-specific
Blood ammonia	1	2, 3, 5	4
Plasma lactate			1–5
CSF lactate		2, 5	1, 3, 4
Acyl-carnitine profile	1	2, 3, 5	4
CSF amino acids	2		1, 3, 4, 5
Plasma amino acids	1	2	3, 4, 5
Urine organic acids	1–3	5	4
Urine amino acids	2	1	3–5
Urine oligo- and polysaccharides	4		1, 2, 3, 5

(CSF = cerebrospinal fluid, see Box 34.2 for number explanation)

Q4. What are the main principles of emergency management?

Obviously each IEM has its own specific management plan, but even before a specific diagnosis is made there are several generic approaches to management that can be used:
- *Eliminate toxic precursors* likely to be protein, fats or some carbohydrates: therefore stop feeds
- *Ensure anabolic state*: maintain hydration and supply sufficient calories in a simple form such as intravenous 10% dextrose or glucose polymer solution
- *Remove toxic metabolites*: may need dialysis or alternative pathway stimulation. For hyperammonaemia use sodium benzoate and sodium phenylbutyrate as well as arginine. Choose carnitine in organic acidemias
- *Give supportive treatment*: correction of hypoglycaemia with dextrose and acidosis with bicarbonate if needed. Treat shock and coagulopathy. Treat concomitant or suspected sepsis with broad-spectrum antibiotics
- *Reintroduce appropriate feed* when diagnosis is confirmed: will need metabolic dietician's input.

Presentation of inborn errors of metabolism in the older child

It is important to consider inherited metabolic diseases in your differential diagnosis when presented with a child in the following clinical scenarios:
- Unexplained acute or chronic encephalopathy
- Progressive neurological disease or regression
- Dysmorphism
- Hypoglycaemia.

Many inherited metabolic diseases are exacerbated by metabolic stress such as a prolonged fast or intercurrent illness and so, when presented with a child who is disproportionately unwell with some of the above features, the diagnosis of a metabolic disease must be considered.

Problem-orientated topic:

acute encephalopathy ● ● ● ● ●

Freja, a 6-year-old girl who is known to have been previously well, is admitted to the ward with a 3-day history of diarrhoea and vomiting. Her parents have been increasingly concerned about her because she has been increasingly lethargic, although she has been able to drink some fluids. On examination she appears 5–10% dehydrated and seems to be drowsy and confused. She is tachypnoeic and tachycardic, and has a capillary refill time of 3 seconds. She has developed some unusual movements over the last few hours.

Q1. What would your initial management be?

Q2. What is your initial differential diagnosis?

Q3. What investigations would be appropriate?

Q4. What features of this presentation should make you suspect a potential inherited metabolic disease?

Q5. What conditions cause hypoglycaemia?

Q6. What investigations should be performed before children are fasted for diagnostic purposes?

Q1. What would your initial management be?

The initial management of this girl should be as outlined in Advanced Paediatric Life Support (APLS, see also Ch. 44), with a primary survey addressing airway, breathing, circulation, disability (Glasgow Coma Score, pupils, posture) and exposure. These should then be addressed before going on to complete a secondary survey. Freja has signs of respiratory distress and shock. Her airway is stable but she should be given facial oxygen and an intravenous cannula should be inserted, with blood being taken for initial investigations (including blood glucose). She will then require a bolus of 0.9% saline and the response should be assessed. It is also important to correct hypoglycaemia and start some intravenous 10%

dextrose to try to reverse the catabolic state, which may make any underlying metabolic disorder worse.

Q2. What is your initial differential diagnosis?

See Box 34.3.

Early identification of encephalopathy is often difficult, and signs such as drowsiness, altered behaviour or unsteadiness of gait/ataxia should alert you to the fact that a child is encephalopathic. Associated with vomiting, this is a strong indication for investigation into an inherited metabolic disease.

Q3. What investigations would be appropriate?

First-line investigations into a child with acute encephalopathy should include those shown in Table 34.2.

Many of these investigations are also useful in identifying the cause of hypoglycaemia, but in addition blood should be taken for insulin, C-peptide, growth hormone (GH), cortisol, 3-hydroxybutyrate and free fatty acids.

BOX 34.3 Differential diagnosis for acute encephalopathy due to an IEM

- Hyperammonaemia: late-onset urea cycle disorders, organic acidaemias, liver failure
- Fatty acid oxidation defects: cause encephalopathy before hypoglycaemia in older children
- Late-onset/intermittent maple syrup urine disease
- Porphyria
- Mitochondrial disease

Table 34.2 First-line investigations in acute encephalopathy

Test	To detect
Blood gases	Metabolic or respiratory acidosis
Blood glucose	Hypoglycaemia
Electrolytes	Increased anion gap
Liver function tests	Raised transaminases
Urinalysis	Ketones and reducing substances
CSF lactate	
Blood ammonia	Hyperammonaemia
Urinary organic and amino acids	
Plasma amino acids	
Plasma carnitine and acyl-carnitines	

Results of investigations in Freja are:

- pH   7.1
- PCO_2 3.0 kPa
- HCO_3^- 16.2 mmol/l
- Lactate   2.8 mmol/l
- NH_4^+ 116 umol/l
- Na^+ 132 mmol/l
- K^+ 3.8 mmol/l
- Urea   6.8 mmol/l
- Cl^- 92 mmol/l
- Glucose   2.2 mmol/l.

There are a number of abnormalities in these results and this can sometimes cause some confusion. This child has a metabolic acidosis, with decreased bicarbonate, raised ammonia and hypoglycaemia. At this stage it is helpful to calculate the anion gap, as the pH is low and you do not know whether this is because the bicarbonate buffer is saturated due to reduced bicarbonate with increased renal or gastrointestinal losses (i.e. renal tubular acidosis or gastrointestinal losses with diarrhoea), or whether other unmeasured anions are contributing. Albumin is a major anion (buffer) but unmeasured anions, such as lactate, ketones (aceto-acetate, β-hydroxybutyrate), phosphate, sulphate or other organic acids, may contribute. The anion gap can be calculated as follows:

$$\text{Anion gap} = [Na^+] - ([Cl^-] + [HCO_3^-])$$
normally 10–15 mmol/l
$$= 132 - (92 + 16.2)$$
$$= 23.8 \text{ mmol/l}$$

In this case there was an increased anion gap and this was due to a previously undiagnosed organic acidaemia. Freja's condition decompensated at this time of metabolic stress when she had an intercurrent illness and entered a catabolic state.

Q4. What features of this presentation should make you suspect a potential inherited metabolic disease?

- Inappropriately ill for history given
- Unexplained acidosis with increased anion gap
- Hypoglycaemia
- Abnormal movements, which may point towards involvement of the basal ganglia that is frequently associated with IEMs.

Q5. What conditions cause hypoglycaemia?

Although hypoglycaemia is frequently associated with IEMs, it is infrequently the presenting sign. The following conditions may present with hypoglycaemia:

Ketotic hypoglycaemia

This is the collective term for the most frequently seen cause of hypoglycaemia. It is a poorly understood condition but seems to represent decreasing fasting tolerance in the young child. It is frequently associated with babies who were intrauterine growth retarded or small for dates. This diagnosis is made by exclusion of other causes and children should never be fasted to make this diagnosis before other causes have been excluded. Treatment is by use of an emergency feeding plan during episodes of illness and prevention of prolonged fasting. Use of a glucose polymer is encouraged, and when vomiting is present, there should be early use of intravenous 10% dextrose with added electrolytes.

Medium-chain acyl-CoA dehydrogenase deficiency (MCADD) and other disorders of fatty acid oxidation

These are usually preceded by encephalopathy, and hypoglycaemia is a late sign of decompensation. The most common disorder in this group is MCADD. It is possible to screen for this condition in the neonatal period by either cord blood analysis or blood collected to measure carnitine and acyl-carnitines. Typical abnormalities of urine organic acids are also seen and are more pronounced during times of intercurrent illness or fasting. Management is by emergency feeding plan. This is a condition with a very good outcome if managed correctly, but a very poor outcome if missed in the presenting phase. Adolescents may present with acute encephalopathy after experimenting with alcohol.

Glycogen storage disorders

These can present at any age but the most common form usually presents within a few months of life with severe hypoglycaemia, high plasma lactate, urate and palpable liver. Milder variants may present with hypoglycaemia only but hepatomegaly is fairly universal.

Hyperinsulinism and hyperammonaemia

These are rare metabolic causes of hypoglycaemia but can be treated easily. This is the reason for measuring ammonia in children during episodes of hypoglycaemia. It is due to a defect of the glutamate dehydrogenase enzyme.

Multi-organ failure

This causes hypoglycaemia and is associated with tyrosinaemia, galactosaemia and mitochondrial disorders.

Q6. What investigations should be performed before children are fasted for diagnostic purposes?

- Measurement of glucose by laboratory method, as glucose meters are poor at recording hypoglycaemia
- Good clinical history and examination
- Plasma carnitine and acyl-carnitines
- Plasma lactate and uric acid
- Urine for organic acids and amino acids
- Pre- and postprandial 3-hydroxybutyrate and free fatty acids.

A fasting test is generally more useful to diagnose endocrine abnormalities. It should be done by professionals who are experienced in performing it and have access to a specialized laboratory.

Presentation of dysmorphism and IEM

Problem-orientated topic:

dysmorphism and progressive neurological disease (neurodevelopmental regression)

Emil, a 4-year-old boy, presents with a history of global developmental delay and aggressive challenging behaviour. His parents report that he had apparently normal development and behaviour up until 18 months of age, but they then became concerned that his developmental progress slowed and he even lost some skills that he previously had. His parents are double first cousins and they have one other normal child. On examination Emil has soft dysmorphic features with mild coarsening of his facial features. He has chronic diarrhoea and has been diagnosed with Perthes disease of his left hip.

Q1. What features in the history and examination might suggest an inherited metabolic disease?

Q2. In what types of inherited metabolic diseases would you expect dysmorphism to be present?

Q3. What metabolic studies would you carry out to investigate this child's condition?

Q4. What other features should you look for on examination?

Q1. What features in the history and examination might suggest an inherited metabolic disease?

The history of a period of normal development followed by later onset of neurodevelopmental regression or slowing associated with facial coarsening/dysmorphism and skeletal abnormalities should alert you to the fact that this boy may have an inherited metabolic disease.

Q2. In what types of inherited metabolic disease would you expect dysmorphism to be present?

- Abnormalities of protein glycosylation
- Lysosomal storage disorders
  - Mucopolysaccharidoses
  - Mucolipidoses
  - Sphingolipidoses
- Peroxisomal disorders
- Mitochondrial disorders
- Abnormalities of sterol metabolism.

Q3. What metabolic studies would you carry out to investigate this young man's condition?

Often clinicians talk about doing a metabolic screen, but this is not useful and the investigations that are performed need to be carefully chosen depending on the most likely diagnosis based on the clinical picture. It is thus important to discuss the most appropriate investigations with your local laboratory.

For this child an initial list of investigations might include:
- Serum transferrins: disorders of protein glycosylation
- Urine glycosaminoglycans: mucopolysaccharidoses
- Urine oligosaccharides: oligosaccharidoses
- Very long chain fatty acids (VLCFA): peroxisomal disorders
- MRI brain: distinguish between grey and white matter disease
- Skeletal survey: dysostosis multiplex
- Ophthalmology review: clouding/cherry-red spot
- Electroretinogram: retinopathy
- Visual evoked potentials: brainstem dysfunction.

Q4. What other features should you look for on examination?

- Eyes: corneal clouding, cataract
- Skin: abnormal fat distribution
- Skeletal deformity: gibbus, kyphosis, macrocephaly

- ENT: recurrent otitis media, persistent nasal discharge
- Face: puffiness of eyelids, coarsening of features, broad nasal bridge and prominence of brow/tongue
- Teeth: small, widely spaced teeth
- Abdomen: umbilical/inguinal hernia and hepatosplenomegaly.

Peroxisomal disorders

Although there are many varied disorders in this group (e.g. Zellweger spectrum disorders), they have very similar presentations, including dysmorphism (characteristic facies), psychomotor retardation, profound hypotonia/weakness, intractable seizures, leucodystrophy (on MRI), impairments of vision and hearing and hepatocellular dysfunction. They represent a spectrum of disease from an early-onset severe disorder to milder older-onset disease.

Lysosomal storage disorders

Broadly speaking, this group of disorders presents with a number of similar features, although they may vary slightly for each individual group:
- Severe hyperactivity and poor sleeping pattern
- Skeletal abnormalities: gibbus and kyphosis
- Recurrent hernias
- Disproportionate or dysmorphic dwarfism (skeletal dysplasia)
- Increasing hepatosplenomegaly
- Gingival hypertrophy
- Degenerative disease of the central nervous system
- Clouding of the cornea
- Changes in retinal pigmentation.

Mucopolysaccharidoses

Mucopolysaccharidoses are caused by a deficiency of lysosomal enzymes that degrade glycosaminoglycans, with a variable degree of progressive mental and physical deterioration. The clinical features of these individual conditions vary depending on the normal rate of enzymatic activity within each tissue. All are inherited in an autosomal recessive manner, except Hunter syndrome, which is X-linked.

Oligosaccharidoses

These resemble the mucopolysaccharidoses but are less common and the age of presentation tends to be earlier. Main features are skeletal dysplasia, developmental delay, coarse facial features and progressive neurological deterioration. Examples are fucosidosis, alpha-mannosidosis and sialidosis.

Sphingolipidoses

Sphingolipids are present throughout the body but are particularly important in nervous tissue, where they are components of myelin sheaths. Abnormal sphingolipids frequently accumulate in the reticuloendothelial system. They are commonly diagnosed after an incidental finding of an enlarged liver or spleen. Examples are Gaucher disease, Fabry disease and Niemann–Pick type A and B. Others present with severe developmental regression, a leucodystrophy picture and cherry-red spot of retina.

Mucolipidoses

These have a combination of features of the mucopolysaccharidoses and sphingolipidoses.

Lipidoses (e.g. Niemann–Pick type C)

The lipidoses or lysosomal lipid storage diseases are a diverse group of conditions that lead to accumulation of the enzyme's substrate. Presentation is either as neonatal cholestasis, as splenomegaly or with ataxia and vertical gaze palsy.

Mitochondrial respiratory chain disorders

Mitochondrial disorders can also present in a very non-specific manner affecting any organ in the body (see Box 9.7). The classical clinical picture is of failure to thrive, associated with renal tubular leak or specific constellations that give raise to the names: e.g. MELAS — *m*yoclonic *e*pilepsy, *l*actic *a*cidosis and *s*troke-like episodes, or MERRF — *m*yoclonic *e*pilepsy and *r*agged *r*ed *f*ibres.

Specific disorders

There are many IEMs that present in childhood, most of which are very rare. Only the more classical disorders are discussed here.

Phenylketonuria

This is a disorder of amino acid metabolism where deficiency of the phenylalanine hydroxylase enzyme causes a deficiency of tyrosine and an increase in phenylalanine. Its incidence is 1:10 000–20 000. Persistently elevated levels of phenylalanine are associated with microcephaly and mental retardation. Acute elevations are not significant and no special precautions are needed during illness or surgery.

Presentation

Presentation is normal at birth and the condition should be diagnosed from screening:

- Measurement of phenylalanine from blood collected within the first days of life is part of most neonatal screening programmes in Europe (see Tables 9.4 and 9.5)
- Children arriving from other parts of the world may not have been screened and may present with developmental delay, eczema and microcephaly.

Diagnosis

- There is an elevated level of phenylalanine but decreased tyrosine
- Biopterin metabolism is normal
- Enzyme activity can be measured from liver tissue but is hardly ever justified
- Mutational analysis is possible but expensive and is unlikely to influence management.

Management

- Phenylalanine-restricted diet
- Supplementation of tyrosine and other essential amino acids with special protein substitutes
- Monitoring blood levels and checking for nutritional deficiencies
- Avoidance of aspartame-containing foods
- Pregnancy counselling for adolescents, as control needs to be much tighter during pregnancy. Uncontrolled phenylalanine levels in pregnancy are associated with a high incidence of fetal abnormalities.

The organic acidurias

The organic acidaemias are a group of conditions arising from defects in the breakdown of amino acids further down the pathway from that seen in maple syrup urine disease. They include:

- Propionic acidaemia
- Methylmalonic acidaemia
- Isovaleric acidaemia (rarer than the two above).

All three conditions present and are broadly managed in similar ways.

Presentation

Children are normal at birth but usually present in the first week with:

- Acute encephalopathy
- Marked metabolic acidosis: raised lactate
- Hyperammonaemia (organic acids inhibit urea cycle)
- Dehydration/shock
- Bone marrow suppression: neutropenia, thrombocytopenia
- Sweaty odour (isovaleric acidaemia)
- Neurological complications: metabolic stroke, basal ganglia involvement
- Cardiomyopathy (propionic acidaemia)
- Pancreatitis.

These disorders are triggered by sepsis, fasting or surgery.

Diagnosis

These disorders are included in extended neonatal screening programmes (see Tables 9.4 and 9.5). Diagnosis can be made by the following findings:

- Marked metabolic acidosis with ketosis
- Hyperammonaemia
- Urinary organic acid pattern is usually diagnostic and supported by acyl-carnitine profile
- Confirmation by enzyme analysis on fibroblasts.

Management

- Acute management is as described above, including stopping protein feeds and using 10% dextrose to prevent catabolism
- Correct dehydration with intravenous fluids
- Correct acidosis with sodium bicarbonate

Table 34.3 Conditions in which raised lactate is seen

Condition	Defect	Examples
Hypoxia	Increased pyruvate production	Poor perfusion, systemic disease, cardiac disease
Impaired glucose production	Increased pyruvate production	Glycogen storage disease I, hereditary fructose intolerance
Impaired NADH metabolism		Mitochondrial disorders of electron transport chain
Impaired pyruvate breakdown		Pyruvate dehydrogenase deficiency, pyruvate carboxylase deficiency, biotinidase deficiency
Impaired acetyl-CoA production	Impaired pyruvate breakdown	Fatty acid oxidation disorders
Other		Organic acidaemias

NADH = nicotinamide adenine dinucleoide.

- Remove ammonia; may need dialysis
- Remove organic acids:
  - Supplement with oral carnitine
  - Glycine for isovaleric acidaemia
- Metronidazole reduces gut bacterial production of propionic acid (for propionic and methylmalonic acidaemia)
- Co-factor supplementation (biotin for propionic acidaemia and vitamin B_{12} for methylmalonic acidaemia); some variants may be due to co-factor deficiency alone
- Long-term treatment involves low-protein diet with long-term oral bicarbonate, carnitine, metronidazole and co-factor, if needed.

Lactic acidosis

Lactic acid is produced by the anaerobic respiratory pathways and can be raised in two general situations. By far the most common of these (type A) is in states of tissue hypoxia that can arise from shock, cardiac failure or other organ failure or from severe disease. A raised lactate is also seen in some metabolic conditions. Lactate is formed from the reduction of pyruvate. Therefore a raised lactate can be seen in the conditions listed in Table 34.3.

Sabah Alvi   Paul Arundel   Carine E. de Beaufort
Gun Forsander   Ragnar Hanas   Stefan Riedl

CHAPTER

35

Endocrinology and diabetes

MODULE SIX

LEARNING OUTCOMES

By the end of this chapter you should:

- Understand the basic physiology of the endocrine system
- Know what constitutes normal growth and puberty
- Be able to recognize when patterns of growth and puberty are abnormal, and construct a differential diagnosis for the child with short stature
- Be able to plan investigations of disorders of growth and puberty
- Know the common causes of thyroid and adrenal abnormalities
- Know the pathophysiology of diabetes mellitus and its long-term complications
- Understand the principles of management of diabetes, including diet, insulin regimens and home monitoring
- Understand the pathophysiology of diabetic ketoacidosis and its acute management.

Introduction

An understanding of normal growth and development is fundamental to the concept of paediatric medicine. Poor growth can be the first sign of a significant clinical problem and in most instances will not be due to an endocrine abnormality. However, to recognize abnormal growth, it is essential to understand what constitutes normal growth with its variants and determinants. Growth and its disorders are discussed fully in Chapter 22. The aim of this chapter is not to provide a comprehensive text on endocrinology and diabetes, but to focus on the essentials of hormone disorders along with the basic science underlying the physiology and pathology of the endocrine system.

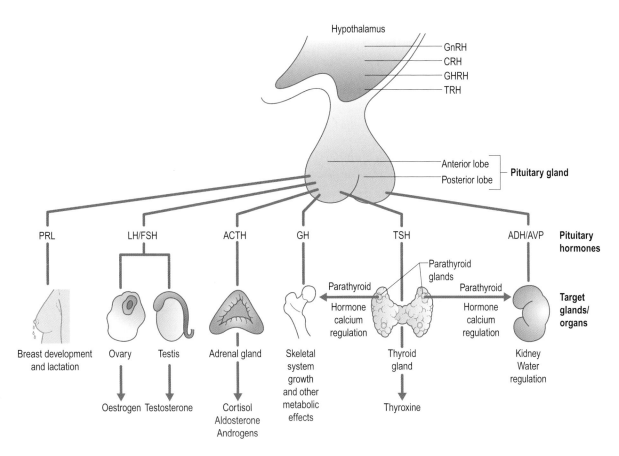

Fig. 35.1 Endocrine regulation.
(ACTH = adrenocorticotrophin; ADH/AVP = antidiuretic hormone/arginine vasopressin; CRH = corticotrophin-releasing hormone; FSH = follicle-stimulating hormone; GH = growth hormone; GHRH = growth hormone-releasing hormone; GnRH = gonadotrophin-releasing hormone; LH = luteinizing hormone; PRL = prolactin; TRH = thyrotrophin-releasing hormone; TSH = thyroid-stimulating hormone)

The endocrine axis and hormonal regulation (Fig. 35.1)

Basic science

The hypothalamo-pituitary axis is fundamental to the exchange of hormonal information. Hormonal control is dependent upon pulsatility of secretion and responds to circadian rhythms, as well as to environmental factors and higher neural centres. Knowledge of the structure and function of this intricate communication system is essential to the understanding of endocrine function, investigation and treatment. Faults at any level can disrupt the finely balanced feedback system.

The hypothalamus

The hypothalamus lies above the pituitary gland and has connections with other parts of the brain, such as the cerebral cortex, as well as the pituitary itself. The hypothalamus secretes corticotrophin-releasing hormone (CRH), thyrotrophin-releasing hormone (TRH), gonadotrophin-releasing hormone (GnRH) and growth hormone-releasing hormone (GHRH), all of which act on their corresponding pituitary hormones. Somatostatin and dopamine, which have inhibitory effects, are also secreted by the hypothalamus. All these hypothalamic hormones are carried to the anterior pituitary by the portal blood system.

The pituitary

The pituitary gland plays a critical role in growth, reproduction and homeostasis. It integrates complex feedback mechanisms, receiving information from the brain via the hypothalamus and signalling to peripheral endocrine organs such as the adrenals, thyroid and gonads. The pituitary gland lies within the sella turcica at the base of the brain and consists of two main lobes. The anterior lobe, the adenohypophysis, develops from the oral ectoderm, whilst the posterior lobe, the neurohypophysis, develops from the neural ectoderm.

The anterior pituitary produces six main hormones: growth hormone (GH), thyroid-stimulating hormone (TSH), adrenocorticotrophin (ACTH), luteinizing hormone (LH), follicle-stimulating hormone (FSH) and prolactin (PRL). The posterior pituitary is responsible for release of the antidiuretic hormone, vasopressin, which regulates water balance, and oxytocin, which is instrumental at parturition and lactation.

The stimulatory and inhibitory releasing hormones that are secreted by the hypothalamus regulate the hypothalamo-pituitary axis via the pituitary stalk.

Disorders of the pituitary gland and growth

Disorders of growth are the most common presenting problem in a general endocrine clinic. To recognize normal and abnormal growth you must be able firstly to measure and plot accurately on the most up-to-date centile charts, calculate mid-parental heights and then recognize when to be concerned. This topic is discussed in detail in Chapter 22 and only aspects of growth that may be referred to a more specialist clinic are discussed here.

Problem-orientated topic:

short stature ○ ○ ○ ○ ○

Lena, a 6-year-old girl, is brought to clinic by her mother who is concerned that her 4-year-old sister is almost as tall as Lena. The child is wearing out all her clothes and shoes, rather than outgrowing them. She has never been to the hospital before, but she has had several ear infections and glue ear. She has mild asthma and has been on treatment with 'a brown and a blue inhaler when she needs them', but she has not been using either recently.

Q1. What are the possible causes of this problem?
Q2. How would you assess this child?
Q3. How would you manage this condition?

Q1. What are the possible causes of this problem?

There are many reasons a child may be short (Box 35.1), but to determine which of these is the cause it is essential to take a systematic history and have a sensible differential diagnosis and investigation plan. Always remember that there may not be an endocrine cause and you must not

---

BOX 35.1 Causes of short stature

Normal variation
- Familial
- Idiopathic

Intrauterine growth retardation
- Infections
- Poor placental function

Genetic/congenital/chromosomal conditions
- Turner syndrome, Noonan syndrome, Down syndrome
- Septo-optic dysplasia
- Skeletal dysplasias

Chronic systemic disorders
For example:
- Gastrointestinal disorders: inflammatory bowel disease, coeliac disease
- Respiratory diseases: cystic fibrosis, severe asthma
- Chronic renal failure

Endocrine abnormalities
- Hypopituitarism
- Hypothyroidism
- Cushing syndrome

Emotional/psychosocial
- Can result in reversible growth hormone deficiency

---

miss other problems, especially chronic illnesses or their treatments. Familial and idiopathic short stature are very common, and it is essential to recognize this fact so that parents and children can be appropriately reassured and not inappropriately investigated.

Hypopituitarism
- *Congenital.* Growth hormone deficiency (GHD) can be inherited due to mutations in the genes responsible for regulating growth, or may be due to developmental defects in the pituitary gland (pituitary aplasia or hypoplasia). It can occur in isolation or combined with other pituitary hormone deficiencies (ACTH, TSH etc.) and may present with hypoglycaemia or jaundice in the neonate.
- *Acquired.* This is due to damage to the pituitary or hypothalamus, e.g. intracranial tumours, surgery, radiotherapy, infections or trauma.

Q2. How would you assess this child?

History
- Gestation, birth weight, perinatal problems
- Duration of concern: always been short or recently falling away from centiles?

- Family history, consanguinity, growth problems in family, (biological) parental heights
- Past medical history: chronic illnesses/operations
- Medication: corticosteroids can cause significant growth suppression
- Full systems enquiry.

Measurements
- Parental heights where possible
- Accurate measurements of height and weight
- Accurate plotting of all measurements on decimal centile charts
- Past measurements, e.g. from the child's health record booklet
- Repeated measurements, height velocity calculated over 6–12 months
- In specialist clinics, sitting height and span should also be measured.

Examination
- Any dysmorphic features, e.g. neck webbing
- Signs of chronic illness, e.g. abdominal distension, buttock wasting, pectus excavatum
- Nutritional status
- Systematic examination
- Pubertal staging (p. 472).

Investigations: blood tests
- Haematology: iron deficiency, erythrocyte sedimentation rate (ESR)
- Biochemistry: urea and electrolytes (U&E), calcium and bone profile, liver function
- Immunology: coeliac, thyroid antibodies
- Karyotype: Turner, Down, Klinefelter syndromes
- Specific endocrine tests: thyroid function tests, IGF 1, IGFBP3, dynamic GH secretion tests, LHRH, TRH tests.

Investigations: radiology
- X-rays:
  - Bone age (Ch. 22): this is *not* a diagnostic tool; it helps you to assess growth reserve (or limitation) by scoring the maturity of certain bones of the hand and wrist. You would not be expected to know how to calculate a bone age.
  - Skeletal survey: if considering a skeletal dysplasia such as achondroplasia.
- Ultrasound scans: renal, if any suggestion of renal disease; pelvic, e.g. ovaries for Turner syndrome.
- Echocardiogram: heart symptoms/signs.
- CT/MRI scans: brain (intracranial space-occupying lesions, structural abnormalities of hypothalamus or pituitary); adrenal (tumours of the adrenal gland).

Of these radiological investigations, only a wrist X-ray for assessment of skeletal maturity (bone age) should be considered a baseline test.

Q3. How would you manage this condition?

For familial short stature or constitutional delay of growth, only reassurance is required. For underlying diseases, these must be corrected first; adverse psychosocial conditions may need to be addressed by removing the child from the inappropriate environment. Recombinant human growth hormone is available as a daily subcutaneous injection and this is currently licensed for use in children with:
- GH deficiency
- Turner syndrome
- Chronic renal failure
- Prader–Willi syndrome
- Intrauterine growth restriction (small for gestational age), without catch-up growth.

Growth hormone will not usually make children grow taller than they are genetically programmed to be; however, it will help children to catch up much of their lost growth and will enable them to attain a normal growth velocity.

Septo-optic dysplasia

This is a congenital condition comprising:
- Absent septum pellucidum
- Optic nerve aplasia/hypoplasia
- Pituitary gland hypoplasia dysfunction.

Children with this condition may be visually impaired and have multiple pituitary hormone deficiencies.

Growth hormone insensitivity syndrome (GHIS; Laron syndrome)

Children with GHIS have a genetic defect of the growth hormone receptor, which means that they cannot respond to growth hormone. Endogenous levels of GH are frequently very high. Currently, these children can be treated with IGF1 (mecasermin) to improve their adult height. If untreated, they have an adult height of about 120–130 cm. This condition is very rare.

Hypothyroidism (p. 475)

Slowing of growth rate may be the only sign.

Cushing disease or syndrome (p. 477)

Along with obesity, poor growth is the most consistent feature in paediatric Cushing, and helps differentiate

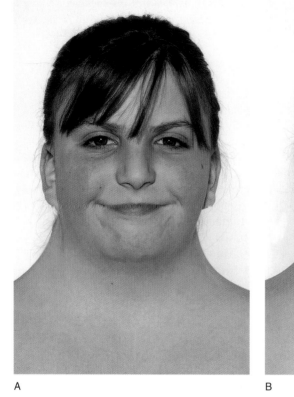
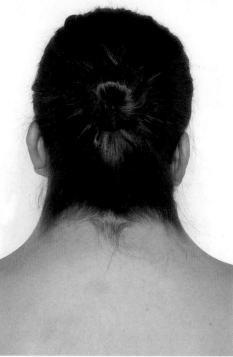

A

B

Fig. 35.2 **Turner syndrome.**
(A) Note the neck webbing and low-set ears; (B) low posterior hairline.

the weight gain of exogenous obesity from that seen in conditions of excess glucocorticoids.

Turner syndrome (Fig. 35.2)

Turner syndrome results from a chromosome anomaly that affects expression and/or regulation of genes located on the X chromosome (Ch. 9). It arises in 1 in 2500 live-born girls but many affected pregnancies do not reach term. The most common karyotype is 45X but variants such as 45X/46XX, 45X/46XY or 45X/47XXX can all occur (mosaicism). The most consistent features of Turner syndrome are short stature (structural X abnormalities) and gonadal dysgenesis (failure of development of the ovaries, which may be completely absent, or present just as 'streaks' of tissue), resulting in absence of secondary sex characteristics (Box 35.2). All short girls should have their karyotype checked, even if no other clinical features are present.

Although they are not GH-deficient, girls with Turner syndrome are usually treated with GH, as untreated adult height is in the range of 142–147 cm. Almost all girls will require induction of puberty with oestrogen.

Any girl whose karyotype contains Y material must have a gonadectomy, as there is a small risk of developing a gonadoblastoma.

BOX 35.2 Clinical findings in Turner syndrome

- Short stature
- Cubitus valgus
- Hypertelorism
- Low-set ears
- Low posterior hairline
- Multiple naevi
- Lymphoedema
- Dysplastic nails
- Broad chest
- Inverted nipples
- Neck webbing
- High-arched palate

Associated features
- Hypertension
- Renal anomalies (horseshoe kidney)
- Cardiovascular abnormalities (e.g. aortic coarctation or stenosis)
- Recurrent ear infections
- Autoimmune thyroiditis

Noonan syndrome

This is usually an autosomal dominant condition, with short stature, cardiac abnormalities (usually pulmonary stenosis) and cryptorchidism.

Key points: short stature

- Not everything that is short is abnormal.
- The most common causes of short stature are non-endocrine in nature.
- All girls with short stature should have a karyotype, as many girls with Turner syndrome do not have the classical phenotype.
- Chronic disease can cause severe growth failure and only appropriate management of the underlying disease will resolve the growth problem.
- Always measure and plot accurately.
- Always obtain parental heights and calculate the mid-parental height centile (Ch. 22).
- Height velocity over at least a 6-month period is of greater value than a single height measurement.
- Random GH levels are of no value in assessment of short stature.

Tall stature

This is described in Chapter 22.

Disorders of the posterior pituitary

The posterior pituitary gland secretes the antidiuretic hormone vasopressin (to regulate salt and water balance) and oxytocin. For all practical purposes in paediatrics, you need only know about disturbances in the secretion of vasopressin.

Diabetes insipidus (DI)

This results from either lack of vasopressin (cranial DI) or renal tubular unresponsiveness to vasopressin (nephrogenic DI). It must be differentiated from habitual water drinking, which will also present with polyuria and polydipsia.

Cranial DI

Congenital absence of the posterior pituitary (e.g. septo-optic dysplasia) is rare. Cranial DI usually results from mechanical damage such as surgery or radiation to the pituitary stalk, or is due to infiltrative disease such as histiocytosis. Children develop polyuria and intense polydipsia, and become dehydrated. Treatment is with the antidiuretic hormone analogue, DDAVP.

Nephrogenic DI

This is usually genetic (X-linked or autosomal recessive).

Disorders of puberty

Basic science

Normal puberty

- Follows a set sequence of hormonal and clinical events but tempo varies.
- Centrally initiated by pulsatile release of hypothalamic hormone (GnRH).
- Acts on anterior pituitary to produce luteinizing and follicle-stimulating hormones (LH and FSH).
- LH/FSH stimulate oestrogen and testosterone production; assisted by adrenal steroids, these stimulate development of physical sex characteristics and follicular maturation/spermatogenesis.

Physical changes of puberty (see also Ch. 5)

In girls
- Pubertal growth acceleration is the first evidence of the beginning of puberty.
- Breast budding is the first clinical sign of puberty occurring after growth velocity has begun to accelerate.
- Periods start after breast stage 3 has been reached.
- Peak height velocity occurs relatively early in puberty, approximately 1 year before menarche.
- Menarche is the last event of puberty.
- After menarche there is very little growth left (average 7–8 cm).

In boys
- The first sign of puberty is enlargement of the testes (4 ml).
- Pubertal growth acceleration begins after testes have reached 4 ml volume.
- Peak pubertal growth velocity occurs about 2 years later than in girls (~13.5 years vs ~11.5 years).
- Peak height velocity occurs in mid-puberty.

Effects of pubertal hormones
- Testosterone:
  - Penile enlargement
  - Pubic and axillary hair
  - Development of a male body habitus and voice change
- Oestrogen:
  - Breast development
  - Uterine enlargement
  - Endometrial thickening

Table 35.1 Staging of pubic hair, breast and genital development (see also Fig. 5.5)

Stage	Girls		Boys	
	Pubic hair	Breasts	Pubic hair	Genitalia
1	None	Pre-adolescent, elevation of papilla only	None	Pre-adolescent; testes, scrotum and penis are about same size and proportion as early childhood
2	Sparse growth of long, slightly pigmented, downy straight hair, chiefly along labia	Breast bud stage; elevation of breast and papilla as a small mound, enlargement of areolar diameter	Sparse growth of long, slightly pigmented, downy straight hair, chiefly at base of penis	Scrotum and testes have enlarged, with reddening and change of texture of scrotal skin
3	Considerably darker, coarser and more curled. The hair, spreads sparsely over the junction of the pubes	Further enlargement of breast and areola, with no separation of their contours	Considerably darker, coarser and more curled. The hair spreads sparsely over the junction of the pubes	Growth of penis in length and breadth; further growth of testes and scrotum
4	Hair adult in type, but smaller area covered; no spread to medial surface of thighs	Projection of areola and papilla to form a secondary mound above the level of the breast	Hair adult in type, but smaller area covered; no spread to medial surface of thighs	Further enlargement of penis with development of glans. Further growth of scrotum and testes
5	Adult in quantity and type, forms inverse triangle and spreads to medial surface of thighs	Mature stage; projection of papilla only, due to recession of the areola to the general contour of the breast	Adult in quantity and type, forms inverse triangle and spreads to medial surface of thighs	Adult in size and shape

Source: after Marshall and Tanner, with permission from the BMJ Publishing Group.

BOX 35.3 Constitutional delay of growth and puberty

- Most common cause of delayed puberty
- Affects boys more than girls
- Usually long history of short stature
- Often a family history of delayed puberty
- Delayed bone age
- No associated features to suggest pathology
- No investigations required except bone age
- Reassurance
- Can give small dose of testosterone to initiate puberty if distress/embarrassment

---

- Adrenal hormones:
  - Acne/greasy skin
  - Body odour
  - Pubic and axillary hair.

Puberty is staged using the Tanner system (Table 35.1).

Normal variants (Box 35.3)

Tempo

This is the timing of puberty. It can be slower or faster than the average in certain groups, e.g.:
- *Familial*: children with delayed or early puberty often have parents with the same.
- *Ethnicity*: earlier in Asian and African–Caribbean girls.

- *Psychosocial*: e.g. adopted girls may have early puberty.
- *Secular trends*: trend towards earlier age of onset since war years — probably related to better nutrition.

Premature adrenarche
- Pubic and axillary hair
- Body odour
- Acne
- No other signs of puberty.

Premature thelarche
- Isolated breast development
- Commonly infants/pre-school children
- No other signs of precocity.

Problem-orientated topic:

disorders of puberty

A mother brings her 7-year-old son, Yann, to see you, worried that he has developed pubic hair and has a strong body odour. He has been a bit more aggressive lately and seems to be going through a growth spurt; he is the tallest in the class but 6 months ago, when a class photograph was taken, he was about average height.

Continued overleaf

Table 35.2 Investigations in disorders of puberty

Test	Significance
Bone age	Usually advanced because of effect of high oestrogen and androgens
GnRH test	Will show rise in gonadotrophins if puberty imminent
Thyroid function tests	Hypothyroidism will cause elevated TSH levels which may cross-react with FSH receptors and stimulate gonadal activity
Adrenal androgens	Very high if pubertal signs are due to an adrenal tumour
Synacthen test	To exclude congenital adrenal hyperplasia
Pelvic ultrasound scan	To look for ovarian cysts and maturation of the uterus and ovaries
Adrenal scan	Adrenal tumours
Cranial MRI	Intracranial tumours or malformations: mandatory in all boys with central precocious puberty

(FSH = follicle-stimulating hormone; GnRH = gonadotrophin-releasing hormone; TSH = thyroid-stimulating hormone)

Q1. What further information do you require?

Q2. What investigations will you request?

Q3. What is your management plan?

Q1. What further information do you require?

When you are presented with a child who displays symptoms or signs of puberty, ask yourself the following questions:

▪ Is this a normal sequence of puberty but happening at an abnormally early age, i.e. is it consonant? This is true or central precocious puberty and is gonadotrophin-dependent.
OR
• Is the normal sequence disrupted and are there signs of peripheral development without activation of the hypothalamus and pituitary, i.e. is it non-consonant? This is peripheral or pseudo-precocious puberty and is gonadotrophin-independent.

As with assessment of stature, when possible disorders of puberty are presented to the clinician, it is essential to know the normal sequence of pubertal changes.

Q2. What investigations will you request?

See Table 35.2. Not all of these will be necessary; the tests selected will depend on the clinical picture Baseline investigations usually will include bone age, FSH, LH, testosterone, DHEA-sulfate and 17-OH-progesterone.

Q3. What is your management plan?

Medical treatment is available to arrest idiopathic central precocious puberty and ameliorate the psychosocial problems that often accompany it. Rapid progression through puberty can cause early epiphyseal fusion and arresting precocious puberty may prevent height limitation.

Treatment for puberty that is not idiopathic (e.g. adrenal tumour) is directed at the underlying cause.

Central precocious puberty: gonadotrophin-dependent

Definition
Central precocious puberty is the onset of pubertal signs before age of 8 years in girls and 9 years in boys. It is often accompanied by rapid growth and skeletal maturation. LH, FSH and oestradiol/testosterone levels are raised. In girls, precocious puberty is usually idiopathic. In boys, it is usually pathological and must always be fully investigated.

Causes
• Idiopathic — majority in girls:
• Central nervous system lesions:
  – Tumours
  – Hamartoma of hypothalamus
  – Infections
  – Vascular lesions
  – Hydrocephalus
  – Trauma
  – Irradiation or surgery
• Hypothyroidism
• Following pseudo-precocious puberty, e.g. in congenital adrenal hyperplasia.

Peripheral (pseudo-)precocious puberty: gonadotrophin-independent

In this there will be changes of puberty but they are not consonant, i.e. there will be no central activation, so that in a boy you may see pubic hair and enlargement of genitalia, but no enlargement of testes, which would

473

normally be the first sign of onset of true puberty. Gonadotrophins are not raised.

Causes

- Tumours:
  - Adrenal
  - Gonadal
- Congenital adrenal hyperplasia
- Hypothyroidism
- McCune–Albright syndrome:
  - Usually affects girls
  - Non-consonant puberty — often due to ovarian cysts
  - Autonomous endocrine hyperfunction, most commonly causing precocious puberty
  - Bony dysplasia, seen on X-rays (polyostotic fibrous dysplasia)
  - Café-au-lait skin pigmentation with jagged borders.

Delayed puberty (Box 35.4)

Delayed puberty is the absence of secondary sex characteristics at the age of 13 years in girls or 14 years in boys.

Causes

See Box 35.5.

Klinefelter syndrome

- Most common cause of male hypogonadism.
- Between 1 in 300 and 1 in 1000 male births.

BOX 35.4 Causes of delayed puberty

With low gonadotrophins
- Constitutional (p. 472):
  - Often familial
- Hypothalamo-pituitary problems:
  - Panhypopituitarism
  - Tumours: e.g. craniopharyngioma; prolactinoma
  - Hypothyroidism
  - Kallmann syndrome (anosmia, hypogonadism, colour blindness)
- Systemic disease:
  - Severe chronic illness, e.g. Crohn disease, renal failure
  - Malnutrition/anorexia/nervosa athleticism

With high gonadotrophins
- Gonadal dysgenesis:
  - Turner syndrome
  - Klinefelter syndrome
- Primary gonadal failure:
  - Testicular torsion
  - Gonadal irradiation

BOX 35.5 Causes of abnormal pubertal development

- Familial/constitutional
- Chronic ill health
- Intracranial lesions: germinoma, prolactinoma
- Adrenal/gonadal abnormalities: congenital adrenal hyperplasia (CAH), tumours
- Undernutrition: anorexia, athleticism
- Iatrogenic: surgery/radiotherapy to pituitary
- Syndromes: Turner, Klinefelter

- Most common karyotype 47XXY, but variants reported.
- There may not be any problems before puberty, which may be delayed.
- At puberty, pubic hair is usually normal but testes remain small.
- Child is often tall; may develop gynaecomastia.
- Infertile.

Amenorrhoea

Primary: never had periods

- Anatomical abnormalities, e.g. absence of uterus/ovaries
- Turner syndrome
- Androgen insensitivity syndrome (46XY girl).

Secondary: cessation of established periods

- Can be due to anorexia, systemic disease or damage to hypothalamo-pituitary-ovarian axis after puberty is complete.

Remember, even in paediatric medicine, pregnancy can be a cause of secondary amenorrhoea.

Disorders of the thyroid gland

Basic science

The function of the thyroid gland is to concentrate iodide from the blood and to return it to peripheral tissues via the thyroid hormones, thyroxine (T_4) and tri-iodothyronine (T_3). These hormones play a vital role in cellular metabolism and have profound effects on growth and differentiation of most organs, including the brain. Consequently a deficit in thyroid hormones and/or iodine during early life will result not only in general reduction in metabolism, but also in severe intellectual deterioration.

The human fetal thyroid gland develops in two parts. A midline out-pouching of the endoderm in the floor of the primitive buccal cavity is first visible by

16–17 days of gestation. At the same time two lateral structures derived from the fourth pharyngeal pouches appear and develop. By 24 days the gland is still attached to the buccal cavity. By 50 days of gestation the gland descends to the lower part of the neck. It is able to accumulate iodine by 10–12 weeks of gestation. T_4 and T_3 are present at the end of the first trimester.

The thyroid gland grows progressively and thyroid hormones accumulate during the second and third trimesters.

Regulation of thyroid hormones

- Thyrotrophin-releasing hormone (TRH) is secreted by the hypothalamus.
- This stimulates the anterior pituitary to secrete thyroid-stimulating hormone (TSH). TSH binds to its specific receptor on the thyroid cell and triggers off intracellular processes that result in the synthesis of thyroid hormones.
- Iodine is essential in the synthesis of thyroid hormones and this is actively taken up from dietary sources.
- Formed thyroid hormones are released into the circulation, mainly bound to thyroid-binding globulin (TBG).
- Free hormone is released at target tissues.

Classification of thyroid disorders (Box 35.9)

Congenital hypothyroidism (CHT)

- Incidence is 1 in 3500–4500 births.
- Children in developed countries have been screened since the early 1980s.
- Thyroid dysgenesis is the most common cause.
- Heel prick sample at day 2–7 (Guthrie card) measures TSH (or FT4).
- It is easy to treat with daily oral thyroxine.
- It is essential to start treatment as soon as diagnosis is made (and definitely within 2 weeks) to prevent/minimize developmental delay.
- Treatment required is life-long.
- There is a good long-term prognosis if treatment is started early enough, if there is good compliance and if the appropriate dose is given.
- Higher doses are required in infancy and puberty.

Clinical features (Box 35.6)

As the neonatal screening system is so successful, it is rare to see the developed picture of congenital hypothyroidism, but in a sleepy lethargic baby with a history of poor feeding and prolonged jaundice, you should always consider a missed diagnosis.

BOX 35.6 Presentation of congenital hypothyroidism

Signs
- Jaundice
- Macroglossia
- Umbilical hernia
- Wide posterior fontanelle
- Hypotonia

Symptoms
- Poor feeding
- Lethargy
- Sleepiness
- Constipation

Screening for congenital hypothyroidism

Screening for this condition started in most European countries in the early 1980s. Congenital hypothyroidism fulfils all the characteristics of a disease for which screening is justified:

1. It is a common condition.
2. Serious problems (neurodevelopmental delay) can only be prevented when the diagnosis is made very early, ideally during the first few days of life.
3. Clinical recognition of the disease at that early age is difficult as the signs and symptoms are non-specific.
4. Screening tests are available with high sensitivity and specificity.
5. Cost-effective treatment is readily available.

Acquired hypothyroidism (Box 35.7)

- Iodine deficiency most common reason world-wide.

BOX 35.7 Main features of acquired hypothyroidism

Signs
- Full, puffy face
- Short stature
- Dry skin
- Obesity
- Goitre

Symptoms
- Fatigue
- Weight gain despite reduced appetite
- Poor growth
- Cold intolerance
- Constipation

- Autoimmunity (Hashimoto thyroiditis) most common in the West.
- More common in girls.
- Can present at any age but most commonly does so in adolescence.
- Often there is a family history of autoimmune thyroid disease or other autoimmune conditions.
- Can be secondary to pituitary or hypothalamic disease/damage.
- Treatment is with thyroxine.

Hyperthyroidism

Problem-orientated topic:

goitre ●●●●●

Mara, a 14-year-old girl, presents with a neck swelling and a history of weight loss and restlessness.

Q1. What features of her history do you want to explore?

Q2. What other clinical features will you look for on examination?

Q3. How would you manage this problem?

Q1. What features of her history do you want to explore?

A goitre is an enlargement of the thyroid gland and is not indicative of aetiology. The child/adolescent with a goitre may be euthyroid, hypothyroid or hyperthyroid (see Box 35.9 below).

The main causes are:

- Simple colloid goitre: usually pubertal, euthyroid
- Hashimoto thyroiditis: hypothyroid
- Graves disease: hyperthyroid
- Viral thyroiditis
- Congenital hypothyroidism due to inborn errors of thyroid hormone metabolism (dyshormonogenesis).

In this case the most likely cause is Graves disease, which accounts for more than 90% of childhood hyperthyroidism. The main features of Graves disease are:

- Autoimmune condition in genetically susceptible individuals.
- Affects girls about seven times more often than boys.
- Can develop at any age but adolescence most common time for presentation.
- Presentation often insidious (see below).
- Caused by TSH receptor antibodies that mimic action of TSH.

BOX 35.8 Main features of Graves' disease

Signs
- Diffusely enlarged thyroid gland
- Thyroid and/or carotid bruits
- Tachycardia
- Ophthalmopathy: often 'staring' eyes rather than ophthalmoplegia
- Warm moist hands with fine tremor
- Restlessness

Symptoms
- Heat intolerance
- Anxiety and palpitations
- Diarrhoea
- Weight loss despite increased appetite
- Deteriorating school performance and behaviour
- Menstrual irregularities
- Rapid growth

- Diagnosis made on history, examination and raised T_4 and T_3 but suppressed TSH levels.

Q2. What other clinical features will you look for on examination?

See Box 35.8.

Q3. How would you manage this problem?

There are three therapeutic options:
1. *Medical*: with carbimazole or propylthiouracil (PTU), usually for 2–3 years; beware of idiosyncratic bone marrow suppression. High rate of relapse on discontinuing treatment.
2. *Radioactive iodine ablation*: increasing experience in children; fear of inducing malignancy. Permanent ablation, lifelong thyroxine required.
3. *Surgery*: should only be performed by experienced surgeons: risk to recurrent laryngeal nerve. If total thyroidectomy, will require lifelong thyroxine replacement and may result in hypoparathyroidism.

Neonatal thyrotoxicosis

This is a rare condition but can be an emergency when it arises. It occurs because of transplacental transfer of maternal antibodies — from a mother with Graves disease — which stimulate the fetal thyroid gland, and symptoms will often develop in the first few days of life. It is a self-limiting condition, as the antibodies will clear from the infant circulation by about 3 months of age. Goitre, irritability, weight loss, tachycardia, arrhythmias and heart failure are features of neonatal thyrotoxicosis. Treatment is with antithyroid drugs (carbimazole or PTU), and may also require iodine and propranolol until symptoms have diminished. The condition will usually respond to these manoeuvres within a week to 10 days, but antithyroid drugs may be necessary for up to 3 months.

Disorders of the adrenal gland

Basic science

The adrenal gland is encapsulated and developed by the ninth week of gestation and is clearly associated with the upper pole of the kidney, which is much smaller at this stage. It is composed of an outer cortex that accounts for about 90% of the gland and is derived from the mesodermal urogenital ridge; this synthesizes steroid hormones. The inner medulla is derived from the neural crest, from ectodermal tissue, and synthesizes catecholamines.

The adrenal cortex is divided into three zones (Fig. 35.3):
- *The zona glomerulosa*, the outer zone, produces aldosterone and is under control of the renin–angiotensin system
- *The zona fasciculata* secretes glucocorticoids under hypothalamo-pituitary control via corticotrophin-releasing hormone (CRH) and ACTH (adrenocorticotrophin).
- *The zona reticularis* is largely inactive until puberty and secretes predominantly adrenal androgens (dihydroepiandrosterone, DHEAS).

These three types of steroid are synthesized from a common precursor, cholesterol, and there are many pathways involved in their production. In practice you will need to know about the effects of too much or too little corticosteroid and about the most common problem of steroid synthesis, congenital adrenal hyperplasia.

Glucocorticoid excess: Cushing syndrome

Primary Cushing disease, caused by an ACTH-secreting pituitary adenoma (Fig. 35.4), is very rare in childhood, but Cushing syndrome is more commonly seen and most often will be iatrogenic in origin.

Causes of Cushing syndrome
The main causes are:
- Iatrogenic : oral, inhaled or topical steroids
- Adrenal adenoma.

Clinical features of Cushing syndrome
- Central obesity
- Moon face
- Poor growth/short stature

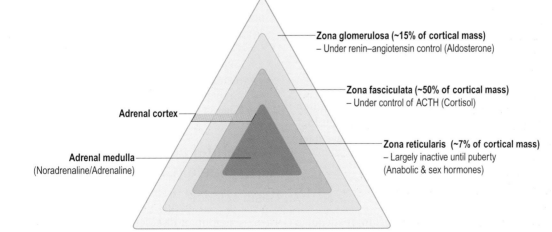

Zona glomerulosa (~15% of cortical mass)
– Under renin–angiotensin control (Aldosterone)

Zona fasciculata (~50% of cortical mass)
– Under control of ACTH (Cortisol)

Zona reticularis (~7% of cortical mass)
– Largely inactive until puberty
(Anabolic & sex hormones)

Adrenal cortex

Adrenal medulla
(Noradrenaline/Adrenaline)

Fig. 35.3 Structure of the adrenal glands

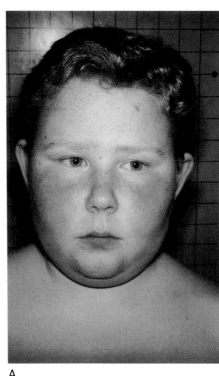
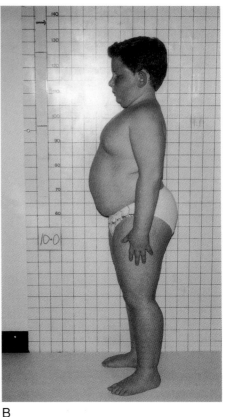

A   B

Fig. 35.4 Cushing disease.
(A) Note the central obesity, striae and plethoric facies; (B) this boy is also short.

- Hirsutism
- Striae
- Acne
- Hypertension
- Thin skin.

The history of poor growth in the presence of obesity is fundamental in this diagnosis, as exogenous obesity is almost never accompanied by slowing of linear growth; indeed, these children are usually tall compared with their peers. Always ensure you have a couple of measurements so that you can assess the child's height velocity. If this is normal and there are no other worrying features, Cushing is highly unlikely.

In paediatrics, you are more likely to see children with iatrogenic Cushing in respiratory, rheumatology and renal clinics, when high-dose steroids have been used for their immunosuppressive activity.

Adrenal insufficiency

Primary adrenal insufficiency is due to inadequate secretion of adrenal steroids; secondary deficiency is usually due to lack of ACTH (Box 35.10).

BOX 35.10 Some causes of adrenal insufficiency

Primary
- Congenital:
  - Congenital adrenal hyperplasia
  - Adrenal hypoplasia congenita
- Acquired:
  - Autoimmune: Addison disease
  - Adrenoleucodystrophy

Secondary
- Congenital:
  - Congenital hypopituitarism
  - Septo-optic dysplasia
- Acquired:
  - Cranial surgery or irradiation
  - Steroid therapy/withdrawal

Congenital adrenal hyperplasia (CAH)

Basic science

There is a group of disorders of steroid synthesis collectively called the adrenal hyperplasias, and each is caused by a particular enzyme defect. The resultant clinical picture

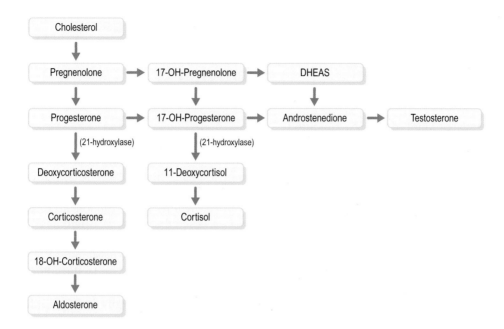

Fig. 35.5 **Deficiency of the 21-hydroxylase enzyme**

depends on the specific enzyme deficiency. Although the biochemical pathways are quite complicated, the simplified summary in Figure 35.5 can help you to understand the most common enzyme problem, deficiency of the 21-hydroxylase enzyme (Box 35.11).

This single enzyme defect results in three major (and potentially fatal) clinical problems:

1. Block in the mineralocorticoid pathway means the child is unable to synthesize aldosterone, which helps to conserve sodium. Absence of this hormone results in renal salt-wasting (salt-losing crisis) and retention of potassium.

2. Block in production of cortisol causes hypoglycaemia and a classical 'adrenal crisis'. The child therefore typically presents with a short history of lethargy, poor feeding, abdominal pain and vomiting, and is usually found to be dehydrated and hypotensive. There is hyponatraemia, hyperkalaemia and hypoglycaemia, and there may be a profound metabolic acidosis if the process continues unchecked. (This situation can be fatal; it is necessary to recognize it as an acute medical emergency. Intravenous access should be obtained at once; the child should be resuscitated with saline and dextrose and given intravenous hydrocortisone.)

3. There is a build-up of precursors proximal to the block, i.e. 17-hydroxyprogesterone. As this cannot be converted to the next stage in the glucocorticoid pathway, it is diverted into an alternative pathway

BOX 35.11 21-hydroxylase deficiency

- Most common adrenal disorder in childhood
- Approximately 1 in 15 000 births (ethnic dependent variability)
- Causes ~90% of all CAH
- Autosomal recessive: gene mutation on chromosome 6

Presentation
- Females: virilized; genital ambiguity at birth
- Males: salt-losing/adrenal crisis at age 7–14 days

Investigations
- Neonatal screening programmes are ongoing in several EU countries
- Day 1: karyotype, pelvic ultrasound scan
- Day 3: 17-hydroxyprogesterone/urea and electrolytes

Management
- Hydrocortisone (glucocorticoid replacement)
- Fludrocortisone (mineralocorticoid replacement)
- Salt supplements in infancy
- Virilized female may require surgery

Long-term problems (often relate to level of compliance)
- Short final height, due to early bone maturation
- Virilization
- Precocious puberty
- Subfertility

  Antenatal diagnosis and treatment (dexamethasone) possible in subsequent pregnancies.

and is converted into androstenedione and testosterone. It is these androgens that cause virilization.

Congenital adrenal hypoplasia

- Rare autosomal or X-linked recessive condition.
- Presentation may be with an adrenal crisis, similar to CAH, but 17-hydroxyprogesterone levels will be low or normal.
- Treatment identical to CAH, but virilization not an issue.
- Can be associated with hypogonadism in some boys.

Acquired adrenal deficiency

- Most common cause is autoimmune: Addison disease.
- Can be isolated or found in association with other autoimmune disorders such as Hashimoto thyroiditis, or diabetes mellitus.
- Can be part of autoimmune polyglandular syndromes.

Features of Addison disease

- Pigmentation in areas not exposed to sun
- Lethargy
- Weakness
- Weight loss
- Abdominal pain
- Vomiting.

Other causes of adrenal insufficiency

Although the development of Cushing syndrome is a possibility in children who have been on long-term steroid therapy, adrenal deficiency can result from prolonged suppression of endogenous cortisol production, and therefore sudden withdrawal of therapy can result in an adrenal crisis. Although this usually occurs in those who have been on prolonged courses of oral steroids, more cases are coming to light in children who have been on high doses of inhaled steroids and therefore it is vital to remember *all* forms of steroid treatment when faced with a possible adrenal crisis.

All children who are dependent on steroid treatment must carry steroid cards, wear some form of SOS talisman and be given instructions to double their maintenance dose of oral hydrocortisone during intercurrent illness. If they are unable to tolerate oral medication, they must seek immediate medical help, as they may need parenteral treatment. Patients undergoing surgery must be given intravenous steroid cover.

Disorders of sexual development/genital ambiguity

Basic science

Sexual determination and differentiation are quite complicated and are set early in life. It is important to have a basic understanding of the processes involved, as occasionally children will be born whose sex is not immediately clear.

There are three main components to gender:
- *Genetic sex*: the genotype, determined at the time of conception
- *Sex differentiation*: the development of the internal and external genitalia under the influence of genes and hormones
- *Sexuality*: gender identity under the influence of genes, hormones and psychological/environmental factors.

Fetal sex differentiation

Basic science of embryology (Fig. 35.6)

The main events are as follow:
- Gonadal development is apparent from week 5 of gestation.
- The thickened area of the genital ridge develops into an undifferentiated (bipotential) gonad.
- Under the influence of a Y chromosome, the gonad develops into a testis and secretes testosterone and a substance called anti-Müllerian hormone. These cause regression of the female system, and the Wolffian ducts develop into epididymis, vas deferens and seminal vesicles.
- In the absence of a Y chromosome, a testis is not formed, the gonad develops into an ovary, the Wolffian ducts involute and the Müllerian system develops into the Fallopian tubes, uterus and upper third of the vagina. The urogenital sinus develops into the lower two-thirds of the vagina and urethra.

Genital ambiguity

This is a very traumatic situation for both parents and professionals and must be handled with extreme sensitivity. Always ask for senior help immediately. Explain to parents that, although there is something the matter with the way the baby's genitals have developed, this does arise from time to time, and some tests will need to be done before it will be possible to say whether baby will be brought up as a boy or girl. Reassure the

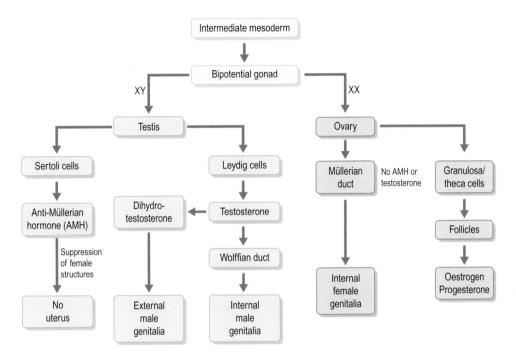

Fig. 35.6 **Sex differentiation**

parents that the baby will be assigned the appropriate gender and will not be 'something in between'.

The vignette below shows how to manage a newborn baby with genital ambiguity.

Q1. What are the causes of genital ambiguity?

- Virilized female (karyotype 46XX, ovaries present on pelvic ultrasound):
  - Almost always will be a girl with CAH.
- Undervirilized male (karyotype 46XY, testes present):
  - Defective testis differentiation: agenesis or dysgenesis
  - Defective testosterone synthesis: e.g. rare forms of CAH; 5-alpha-reductase deficiency (very rare)
  - Defective response to male hormones: partial androgen insensitivity syndrome

Q2. How do you approach this problem?

- Seek senior help.
- Do not refer to the baby as 'he', 'she' or 'it'.
- Reassure parents that gender will be assigned but tests will be necessary and results may take some time.

History
- Obstetric history
- Maternal virilization
- Family history (e.g. androgen insensitivity syndrome).

Examination
- Virilized female or undervirilized male?
- Are gonads present? Appearance of labioscrotal folds
- Size of clitoris/phallus; how many urogenital openings?
- Other abnormalities/recognizable syndrome?

Investigations
- Cord or venous blood for karyotype and DNA
- Pelvic and abdominal ultrasound:
  - Internal structures, gonads

- After 72 hours:
  - U&E
  - 17-hydroxyprogesterone
  - Urine for steroid profile
- Further investigations:
  - Discuss with paediatric endocrinologists, surgeons, geneticists, radiologists and psychologists.

Disorders of calcium and bone

Basic science of calcium homeostasis

Normal total serum calcium is 2.2–2.6 mmol/l. The vast majority of body calcium is found in bone and is fundamental to maintaining skeletal integrity. In blood, it is found in three forms: ionized, bound to proteins and as complexes with substances such as citrate. In its ionized (biologically active) form, calcium is vital to nerve conduction, muscle contraction and blood coagulation. Complexed calcium is largely insignificant, but protein-bound calcium is affected by albumin concentration and this must be taken into consideration when interpreting results. Extracellular calcium homeostasis is maintained by two main factors: vitamin D and parathyroid hormone.

Vitamin D

Vitamin D is obtained either from the diet (animal or vegetable sterols) or from the action of sunlight on skin. This circulating vitamin D is then metabolized in the liver to 25-hydroxyvitamin D, which is further hydroxylated in the kidney to the active 1,25-dihydroxyvitamin D. Vitamin D acts on intestinal epithelium to increase calcium and phosphate absorption, and increases skeletal mineralization and bone formation. Any problems in obtaining vitamin D (dietary deficiency) or metabolizing it (liver or renal disease) will therefore have consequences for calcium and bone regulation.

Parathyroid hormone

The four parathyroid glands, found behind the thyroid gland, develop from the third and fourth branchial pouches. They secrete parathyroid hormone (PTH) in response to low circulating ionized calcium. PTH regulates extracellular calcium by increasing renal calcium absorption and mobilizing calcium and phosphate from bone.

Hypocalcaemia

Problem-orientated topic:

tingling and spasms of the hands ● ● ● ● ●

Eva, a 14-year-old Asian girl, presents with a 6-week history of intermittent tingling and spasm of her hands. She is on the 25th centile for height and 10th centile for weight, and is in puberty. There are no abnormal findings on examination.

Q1. What is your differential diagnosis?
Q2. What investigations would you undertake?
Q3. How would you treat Eva?

Q1. What is your differential diagnosis?

In a teenager such as Eva, tetany due to hypocalcaemia is the most likely diagnosis. In practice you may also come across a baby with seizures who is found to have low calcium, or an infant with failure to thrive and features of rickets.

Clinical features of hypocalcaemia

- Infants:
  - Jitteriness
  - Poor appetite
  - Vomiting
  - Seizures
  - Apnoeic episodes
  - Stridor
  - Proximal myopathy with delayed motor development
- Older children/adolescents:
  - Tingling: fingers, perioral
  - Tetany: carpal/pedal spasm
  - Latent tetany: Chvostek/Trousseau signs.

Causes of hypocalcaemia

- In neonates:
  - Prematurity
  - Maternal vitamin D deficiency
  - Maternal hyperparathyroidism
  - Hypomagnesaemia
  - High milk phosphate
  - Congenital hypoparathyroidism
- In childhood:
  - Vitamin D deficiency
  - Hypoparathyroidism
  - Renal disease.

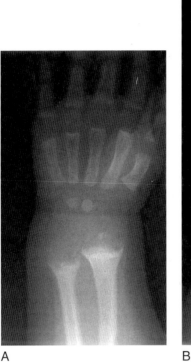 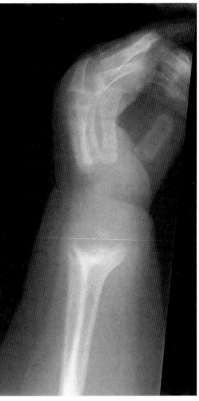

A   B

Fig. 35.7 Wrist X-rays showing changes of rickets – metaphyseal cupping and splaying. (A) Straight view; (B) lateral view.

Hypoparathyroidism
- *Congenital*: due to aplasia of the glands as part of the Di George spectrum of anomalies
- *Acquired*: can be isolated or in association with other autoimmune conditions, e.g. polyglandular syndrome 1.

Rickets
This describes the clinical picture resulting from defective mineralization of osteoid in the growing skeleton. There is a resurgence of rickets, especially in infants who are exclusively breastfed or from certain ethnic minority groups. It is imperative therefore that all babies at high risk of vitamin D deficiency should have feeds supplemented with vitamin D for at least the first 2 years of life. Pregnant women (especially those of Asian origin, as they are particularly susceptible) should also receive supplements. The most common cause of rickets is vitamin D deficiency, although rarer forms are also seen.

Causes of vitamin D deficiency
- *Inadequate sunshine*: most vitamin D is converted from sterols in the skin by the action of sunlight.
- *Dietary insufficiency*.
- *Malabsorption*: as vitamin D is fat-soluble, conditions such as coeliac disease can be a cause.

- *Hepatic/renal disease*: vitamin D is converted in both liver and kidney.

Clinical features of rickets
- Craniotabes: softening of skull with delayed closure of fontanelles
- Rachitic rosary: enlargement of costochondral junctions
- Delayed dentition
- Bowing of legs
- Tetany: usually adolescents.

Q2. What investigations would you undertake?

Biochemistry
- Alkaline phosphatase: high
- PTH: high
- Calcium: low or normal
- Phosphate: low or normal
- Vitamin D: low.

X-rays
These show widening of the growth spaces between metaphyses and ossification centres, with cupping and splaying of the metaphyses (Fig. 35.7).

483

Q3. How would you treat Eva?

- Give oral vitamin D supplementation (ergocalciferol or cholecalciferol).
- Calcium supplements may also be required if there is hypocalcaemia.

Hypercalcaemia

This is much less common than hypocalcaemia.

Causes

- Iatrogenic: hypervitaminosis D
- Williams syndrome:
  - 'Elfin' features
  - Supravalvular aortic stenosis
- Hyperparathyroidism.

Hypoglycaemia

Hypoglycaemia (plasma glucose below 2.6 mmol/l) occurs when glucose uptake exceeds supply. Especially in the neonatal period, this can cause seizures and severe neurodevelopmental or cognitive defects if it is persistent and profound. Hypoglycaemia can be the presenting feature of hypopituitarism, and therefore it is vital that it is fully investigated before it is corrected.

Causes

(Hypoglycaemia in diabetes is discussed in the next section.)

- *Hyperinsulinism*: Persistent hyperinsulinism of infancy (PHI) (previously known as nesidio-blastosis), Beckwith–Wiedemann syndrome (p. 745), insulinoma (very rare)
- *Hormone deficiency*: isolated or combined growth hormone/ACTH/cortisol
- *Metabolic conditions*: e.g. glycogen storage diseases, fatty acid oxidation defects (Ch. 34)
- *Miscellaneous*: aspirin, liver failure, Reye syndrome.

Investigations

Hypoglycaemia must be confirmed with a laboratory glucose level and the following blood tests taken before any glucose is given:

- Lactate
- Ammonia
- Insulin/C-peptide
- Growth hormone
- Cortisol
- Free fatty acids
- Beta-hydroxybutyrate/aceto-acetate
- Organic acids
- Acyl-carnitine.

Insulin should be undetectable in the presence of hypoglycaemia, and if measurable, confirms hyperinsulinism.

Medical (diazoxide) or surgical (pancreatectomy) treatment may be required. Deficiency of GH or cortisol calls for replacement of these hormones. Metabolic and hepatic causes of hypoglycaemia are discussed in Chapter 34.

Diabetes mellitus

Definition

Diabetes mellitus is a chronic disorder caused by an absolute or relative deficiency of (resistance to) insulin that is characterized by hyperglycaemia.

Basic science

Pathophysiology

Insulin is an anabolic hormone that has a central role in the metabolism of carbohydrate, fat and protein. It is produced in the pancreas by the beta cells of the islets of Langerhans. It reduces plasma glucose levels by stimulating the conversion of glucose to glycogen and enabling glucose to enter cells. It also inhibits the breakdown of glycogen, protein and fat.

The symptoms of diabetes mellitus at presentation depend upon the degree of metabolic decompensation and are generally secondary to hyperglycaemia, glyco-suria and ketoacidosis. Hyperglycaemia leads to glycosuria and an osmotic diuresis. This in turn causes polyuria (often worse at night and can therefore cause enuresis in a previously continent child), increased thirst and dehydration. Other symptoms at presentation include non-specific malaise and weight loss. The latter is due to the uninhibited breakdown of fat and protein that occurs in the absence of sufficient circulating levels of insulin. Uninhibited breakdown of fat leads to the generation of ketones. At high levels these cause nausea and vomiting that can further exacerbate the dehydration, leading to shock. This is the phenomenon of diabetic ketoacidosis (DKA), which is discussed in more detail later. Other clinical signs in DKA include an abnormal pattern of breathing due to the acidosis (Kussmaul breathing) that can mimic asthma or pneumonia, and abdominal pain that can mimic an acute surgical abdomen.

Classification and aetiology of diabetes mellitus

Type 1

Most diabetes developing in childhood is classified as type 1 diabetes, a term that encompasses cases of diabetes that are due to the destruction of pancreatic beta cells (usually leading to absolute insulin deficiency):

- Beta cell destruction is almost always caused by an environmental trigger in a genetically susceptible person (mainly linked with chromosome 6).
- HLA DR3 and DR4 are associated with type 1 diabetes.
- Monozygotic twins have up to a 60% lifetime concordance for the development of type 1 diabetes.
- Viral infections (with the enteroviruses as most diabetogenic) may be the most important environmental trigger, probably initiating or modifying an autoimmune process.
- Autoantibodies such as islet cell, glutamic acid decarboxylase (GAD) and insulin antibodies, are nearly always present at the time of presentation.
- Dietary factors are also relevant. Early introduction of cow's milk has been associated with an increased risk of diabetes.

According to the most recent 'Eurodiab' study, there is a wide geographical variation in the incidence and prevalence of type 1 diabetes throughout Europe:

- The incidence in Finland remains the highest with 52.6 per 100 000 children aged 0–14 years, whereas Lithuania with 10.3 per 100 000 appears the lowest. The overall annual increase is the highest in the younger age group (<5 years) with 5.4% per year.

Type 2

Type 2 diabetes mellitus is a heterogeneous condition characterized by variable degrees of insulin resistance and beta cell secretory failure. Although it is predominantly a condition of the over-40 age group, it has now been described in children, and the increasing prevalence of obesity in children and adolescents means that it is becoming more common, mainly in adolescents.

Common characteristics
- Overweight
- Strong family history of type 2 diabetes
- Female preponderance
- African, Hispanic, Afro-American, Asian or Arabic origin.

Management
Management of type 2 diabetes involves the introduction of oral hypoglycaemic agents in parallel with lifestyle intervention (dietary and exercise promotion) and, if necessary, insulin therapy.

Maturity-onset diabetes of the young (MODY)

- Autosomal dominant inheritance
- Strong family history of early-onset diabetes (< 25 years)

- Rare (only 1–2% of cases of diabetes mellitus in childhood)
- Mild presentation.

A number of specific genetic defects in beta cell function have been identified that explain most cases of MODY. One important reason for making the diagnosis is that some forms of MODY will not require treatment with insulin. Fifty percent of diabetes with an onset before 6 months has a genetic explanation (mutation in Kir6.2 or SUR).

Other types of diabetes mellitus

Diseases of the exocrine pancreas
- Cystic fibrosis
- Pancreatectomy, e.g. for PHI (p. 484)
- Pancreatitis
- Trauma
- Haemochromatosis.

Genetic syndromes associated with diabetes
- Turner syndrome
- Bardet–Biedl syndrome
- Prader–Willi syndrome
- Wolfram syndrome — *diabetes insipidus, diabetes mellitus, optic atrophy, deafness* (DIDMOAD).

Problem-orientated topic:

diabetes mellitus

Fynn, a 4-year-old boy, is referred urgently to the accident and emergency department by his primary care physician with a provisional diagnosis of diabetes mellitus. He has a 2-week history of weight loss and polyuria. The primary care physician had tested the boy's urine and found it to contain large amounts of glucose and a small amount of ketones.

Q1. How do you establish whether this child has diabetes mellitus?

Q2. What are the principles of management?

Q1. How do you establish whether this child has diabetes mellitus?

The diagnosis of type 1 diabetes in children is usually straightforward and made on the basis of:

- A typical history of polyuria, polydipsia, weight loss
- Hyperglycaemia
- Marked glycosuria
- Ketonuria.

- Paediatrician specialized in diabetes
- Children's diabetes nurse specialist
- Specialist dietitian
- Psychologist or psychiatrist
- Social worker

Two plasma glucose measurements in excess of 11 mmol/l (200 mg/dl) establish the diagnosis in such cases.

The World Health Organization (WHO) diagnostic criteria for diabetes mellitus are:

- Fasting plasma glucose ≥7.0 mmol/l (126 mg/dl); whole blood glucose ≥6.1 mmol/l
  or
- A plasma glucose level taken 2 hours following an oral glucose tolerance test (OGTT) ≥11.1 mmol/l (200 mg/dl).

An OGTT is rarely required in childhood.

Once the diagnosis of diabetes mellitus has been made, care and education of the child and family by a specialist multidisciplinary team must begin immediately.

Q2. What are the principles of management?

The long-term successful management of a child and the family with diabetes depends on effective team work (Box 35.12)

The majority of children who present with diabetes mellitus will be hospitalized, although they may not be acutely unwell. Much of the initial management and education in diabetes mellitus will be started in the clinic. Some teams do not routinely admit children to hospital to initiate insulin therapy unless they are unwell. It is essential to have a clear understanding of the principles underpinning the management of diabetes mellitus and the skills required.

Principles and practice of insulin therapy

Starting treatment

The first subcutaneous injection can have tremendous significance for children and their families. It should be taught or administered by someone experienced and confident with injections. Subcutaneous indwelling catheters (e.g. Insuflon) inserted using a local anaesthetic cream may be useful to overcome problems with injection pain. A dose of 0.5–0.7 units of insulin per kilogram body weight per day is usually required but will be tailored to individual needs. At diagnosis the need for insulin is often much higher, and may be as much as 1.5 U/kg. Insulin injection sites must be varied because repeated injections into the same site can cause lipohypertrophy; as well as being unsightly, this can lead to poor glycaemic control, as absorption from such sites is unpredictable.

Remission ('honeymoon') phase

Type 1 diabetes presents with symptoms when approximately 90% of the beta cells have been destroyed. This means that most children will still have some functioning beta cell mass for a period after the time of diagnosis. This is reflected in the low insulin requirements from a short time after diagnosis and during the remission phase. This phase usually lasts only a few months but can last for a few years.

Insulin types

Basic science

Insulin is a protein consisting of two peptide chains linked by two disulphide bonds. It cannot be absorbed intact (in its bioactive form) from the gastrointestinal tract and therefore at present is only routinely administered via subcutaneous injection. However, this suboptimal simulation of physiology results in many of the difficulties and complications of diabetes.

Until recently, most prescribed insulin was human insulin produced by recombinant technology. Pure insulin is short-acting and appears clear in solution. Various additives prolong the release of insulin into the blood stream (e.g. NPH) and produce intermediate or long-acting insulins. A number of so-called insulin analogues have also become available. These are modified forms of human insulin that have a more favourable profile than the traditionally used insulins. Now both rapid-acting and long-acting (or basal) insulin analogues are widely used in paediatric practice.

Insulin regimens

Traditionally children have most commonly been managed on twice-daily injections combining short- and intermediate-acting insulins (e.g. 1/3 short-acting and 2/3 intermediate-acting): one before breakfast and one before the evening meal. Typically around two-thirds of the total daily dose is given as the morning dose. Glycaemic control, however, is often limited by disabling hypoglycaemia. There are three main problems with this regimen:

1. Control of postprandial hyperglycaemia is difficult without a short-acting insulin bolus at lunchtime.
2. 'The dawn phenomenon' — the profile of the intermediate-acting component of the evening insulin results in a decline in insulin levels in

the early hours before breakfast, leading to hyperglycaemia that is exacerbated (particularly in adolescents) by the coincident surge in hormones that oppose the effects of insulin.

3. A snack is usually necessary to avoid hypoglycaemia mid-morning due to the profile of the intermediate-acting insulin.

Multiple daily injection (MDI) regimens using insulin analogues can overcome some of the above problems and this has led to their increasingly widespread adoption in paediatric practice. Such regimens usually consist of the administration of a dose of a long-acting insulin analogue either once daily (usually at night) or twice and doses of a rapid-acting insulin analogue to cover mealtimes (Fig. 35.8). The required dose of mealtime insulin depends on the carbohydrate content of a meal and the individual's sensitivity to insulin. Dose adequacy (and also sensitivity to insulin) can be judged by checking plasma glucose levels before and between 2–3 hours after a meal whose carbohydrate content is known.

Continuous subcutaneous infusion of rapid-acting insulin ('the insulin pump') may offer the possibility to provide an even more physiological profile of insulin delivery. Continuous infusion of rapid-acting insulin at an individualized rate covers basal insulin needs which can be adjusted percentage-wise to increased (illness) or decreased (physical activity) demands. At meal or snack times, the patient/parents administer(s) extra insulin, a 'bolus' which should cover the food intake. The subcutaneously placed cannula has to be changed every 2–3 days. Pump therapy should only be initiated by a trained specialist team. Patients with the required training and commitment to use this therapy effectively may benefit from it. It is recommended as an option for people with type 1 diabetes in the following situations:

- If MDI therapy has failed — meaning that it has been impossible to obtain/maintain an HbA$_{1c}$ level at less than 7.5% without major hypoglycaemia, despite a high level of self-care
- In those who are motivated to use this type of therapy
- In preschool children with fluctuating plasma glucose due to age-specific characteristics (e.g. unpredictable eating pattern, long overnight periods, frequent intercurrent infections etc)
- To improve quality of life.

http://www.ispad.org

Patient and parent education

An understanding of insulin therapy is crucial to the management of diabetes mellitus. But in order to maintain good glycaemic control without problematic

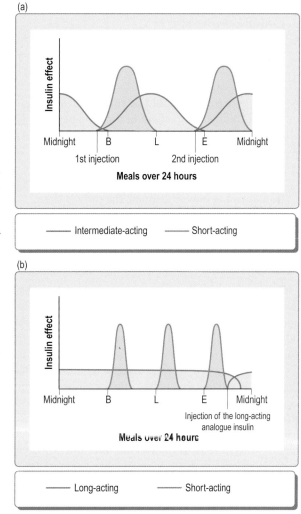

Fig. 35.8 Insulin action.
(a) Insulin effect of traditional regimen of twice-daily combination of short- and intermediate-acting insulin; (b) Insulin effect of multiple daily injection regimen of once-daily long-acting analogue insulin with rapid-acting insulin given at mealtimes. (B = breakfast; L = lunch; E = evening meal)

BOX 35.13 Distribution of total daily energy intake

- 50–55% carbohydrate, moderate sucrose intake (up to 10% of the total energy)
- 10–15% protein
- 30–35% fat

hypoglycaemia, children and their families must understand the effect of diet and exercise and be able to monitor plasma glucose levels.

Diet

The emphasis is on 'healthy eating'. Any diet should provide sufficient energy and nutrients to allow optimal growth and development (Box 35.13):

- Total energy intake depends on the individual's particular needs.
- The appropriateness of giving snacks can only be defined based on the insulin regimen being used. Taking insulin analogues (short acting) frequently does **not** require evening snacks.
- The dose of insulin should be adjusted according to the carbohydrate content of the food being consumed.
- The increased use of MDI regimens and pumps (e.g. the more physiological insulin replacement therapy) means that many individuals will benefit from learning how to estimate the carbohydrate content of their meals.

Exercise

Children with diabetes should be encouraged to undertake regular exercise and understand how to adjust diet and insulin in order to maintain good glycaemic control both during and after different types of exercise. In particular, children should be aware that exercise can lead to hypoglycaemia, sometimes several hours after the exercise, and that they will require extra carbohydrate before and after a bout of intensive exercise. They also should be encouraged to monitor their plasma glucose levels before and after exercise. Nighttime basal insulin often needs to be lowered after afternoon or evening exercise to avoid hypoglycaemia, especially if the exercise level is irregular.

Education

The amount of explanation required at diagnosis will vary according to the circumstances of the admission and the family involved. Prior to discharge there are several areas that ought to be covered in discussion with the family:
- Pathophysiology, including explanation of symptoms
- Lifelong need for insulin
- Methods of insulin administration
- Hypoglycaemia: how to identify and treat
- Importance of good control
- Details of support groups (e.g. http://www.IDF.org).

Education of the child and family is an ongoing process involving all members of the multidisciplinary team. Education should also be offered to other carers, such as teachers. It is particularly important that these people be able to recognize and manage hypoglycaemia.

http://www.ispad.org
http://www.idf.org

Plasma glucose monitoring

Monitoring of plasma glucose levels at home with hand-held meters allows short-term monitoring of glycaemic control and is associated with reduced levels of HbA_{1c}. HbA_{1c} is a derivative of glycosylated haemoglobin. It correlates well with average glucose concentrations over the preceding 6–8 (12) weeks and thereby provides an important measure of glycaemic control. The Diabetes Control and Complications Trial (1993) clearly showed a direct correlation between HbA_{1c} and long-term complications. The aim of treatment is to achieve an HbA_{1c} of less than 7.5% but this may not always be easy, especially because of fear of hypoglycaemia. HbA_{1c} should be checked at least every 3 months. Optimal targets for short-term glycaemic control are a preprandial plasma glucose level of 4–6 mmol/l and an ideal postprandial rise of 2 mmol/l but an absolute level which should be more than 10 mmol/l.

Hypoglycaemia

Hypoglycaemia is commonly due to inadequate carbohydrate intake, too much insulin or physical activity. It is a particular concern in preschool children because repeated episodes of hypoglycaemia may lead to intellectual impairment. This must be balanced against chronic hyperglycaemia, which also carries a risk of cognitive impairment in this age group.

For diabetes control hypoglycaemia is generally defined as plasma glucose below 4 mmol/l. Symptoms depend on the absolute plasma glucose value, the rate of fall of glucose levels and the background glycaemic control. Early (autonomic) symptoms include:
- Hunger
- Feeling shaky
- Sweating
- Pallor.

If these are ignored, or if no adrenergic symptoms are present, then more profound symptoms of neuroglycopenia may develop, including:
- Disorientation
- Aggression
- Difficulty with speech
- Poor concentration
- Changes in vision
- Loss of consciousness
- Seizures

At clinic visits it is important to enquire about hypoglycaemia unawareness, i.e. the onset of neuroglycopenic symptoms without the warning of autonomic symptoms.

Children should be encouraged always to have access to an immediate source of carbohydrate (glucose or sucrose) and to wear some form of medical identification.

Symptomatic proven hypoglycaemia, or low plasma glucose values without symptoms, should always be treated immediately. Parents should know how and when to administer oral glucose gel or glucagon. All families with a child with diabetes should be able to give glucagon in situations where a state of unconsciousness prevents the oral intake of rapid-acting carbohydrates. Other well-informed adults (e.g. at school or day care centres) could also be taught how to inject glucagon by training with expired injection tools. The dose could be individualized (0.1–0.2 mg/kg) to minimize the nausea that often follows the injection.

In hospital, intravenous treatment with 5 ml/kg 10% dextrose is usually sufficient to correct hypoglycaemia. There is no place for high-concentration glucose solutions.

Illness and hyperglycaemia

During periods of illness it is essential that insulin therapy is not interrupted and that plasma glucose is checked frequently. It is often necessary to increase the insulin dose during these periods. Only during gastro-enteritis should the dose be reduced (due to reduced caloric intake). Urine or blood should be regularly tested for ketones. The child should be encouraged to drink, and if food cannot be tolerated, then it should be replaced by small amounts of sugar-containing fluids. If the child is vomiting, develops ketones or otherwise deteriorates, then the family should seek medical help.

Long-term complications

Long-term complications such as nephropathy and retinopathy arise as a result of chronic hyperglycaemia. Their incidence is related to the duration of diabetes and the level of glycaemic control. Such complications are rare in childhood, but a young adult who was diagnosed in childhood will have already been exposed to the effects of hyperglycaemia for long enough to develop complications. There is therefore a particular obligation on the paediatric diabetes team to enable the family to achieve sustained good control of their child's diabetes. Screening for complications should begin from 10 years of age onwards.

Clinics and screening

Clinic visits are a convenient vehicle for the diabetes team to be able to review a child's insulin therapy, blood glucose control and diet. They also allow regular screening for complications and associations of diabetes mellitus to take place.

Finally, the annual review is an opportunity to consider aims and objectives for the 12 months ahead (Box 35.14).

Immunizations

Some countries in Europe recommend immunization against influenza for children over the age of 6 months.

Problem-orientated topic:

diabetic ketoacidosis

Sara, a 15-year-old girl, presents to the accident and emergency department with a history of abdominal pain and vomiting. She has a reduced level of consciousness and her breathing is laboured. Her capillary blood sugar is 35 mmol/l (630 mg/dl) and blood gas analysis shows: pH 7.09, base excess –17 mmol/l. This is the third time that she has presented to hospital in a similar way over the last 12 months.

Q1. What is the diagnosis?
Q2. How would you approach Sara's management?
Q3. Why do you think this has happened?
Q4. What are the complications of this condition?

Q1. What is the diagnosis?

This is a typical picture of DKA and is caused by insufficient circulating insulin associated with increases in counter-regulatory hormones. It has been reported to be present at diagnosis in 15–67% of new cases. The risk in established cases of type 1 diabetes is 1–10% per patient per year.

Q2. How would you approach Sara's management?

The International Study Group for Pediatric and Adolescent Diabetes has produced detailed guidelines for the management of DKA. Any prospective European certified paediatrician candidate should be familiar with these and have some practical experience of managing DKA. Therefore only the basic principles that underpin the management of DKA and the potential pitfalls have been highlighted.

Initial management consists of assessing and providing support to the airway, breathing and circulation. A naso-

At diagnosis (and every 5 years)
- Screen lipids
- Screen for coeliac disease

At every clinic visit
- Height and weight
- HbA_{1c}
- Check injection sites

Once a year
- Check for retinopathy, microalbuminuria and blood pressure from 10 years
- Screen for thyroid disease
- Review foot care
- Screen for coeliac disease (during the first 5 years after diagnosis)

gastric tube should be used to decompress the stomach and reduce the risk of aspiration in the unconscious or severly obtunded patient. Administer 100% oxygen and place the patient on a cardiac monitor. If the child is shocked, or has a decreased peripheral circulation, restore volume with normal saline, then rehydrate slowly over 48 hours. Start an intravenous infusion of short- or rapid-acting insulin to switch off ketogenesis and aim to achieve normoglycaemia gradually.

http://www.ispad.org

Q3. Why do you think this has happened?

Major reasons for recurrent DKA are insulin omission and acute illness. Education and other steps such as adult supervision of insulin administration have been shown to help prevent DKA.

Q4. What are the complications of this condition?

DKA has reported mortality rates of 0.15–0.30%. Be aware that some of the risks of DKA are associated with the period of stabilization when treatment has already begun. Although serum potassium levels are often high at presentation, they will fall once insulin has been started and this must be taken into consideration during the prescription of fluids and electrolytes as the consequent hypokalaemia may result in dangerous cardiac dysrhythmias. Hypoglycaemia can occur if glucose is not added to the intravenous fluids in a timely fashion. Cerebral oedema (which accounts for 60–90% of all DKA deaths) may develop as a result of rapid fluid replacement with hypotonic fluids, but

can occur even before the initiation of any treatment and up to 48 hours after admission. Therefore, once the patient is no longer in shock, it is important that fluid and electrolyte replacement is carried out in a well-balanced fashion, in accordance with established protocols and under supervision of a senior paediatrician, experienced in the treatment of DKA.

Monitoring to prevent further episodes of DKA

One of the key messages about the management of DKA is the importance of monitoring and frequent review:
- Frequent blood gases and electrolytes
- Cardiac monitoring
- Regular assessment of the Glasgow Coma Score
- Prompt reporting of any symptoms or signs that might indicate cerebral oedema.

Social and psychological aspects of diabetes

Type 1 diabetes is a lifelong condition. The implications of the diagnosis affect the entire family, as well as the child or young person. Anxiety, depression and eating disorders are well described in children and young people with diabetes. Good psychosocial support is vital if young people are to comply with treatment and maintain high self-esteem. In particular specific support strategies should be offered that reduce conflict within the family. In some cases child mental health teams may need to be involved. It is important to remember that a child's level of understanding changes with time and the condition and treatment must be explained regularly in terms that are age-appropriate.

Adolescence

During puberty, changes in GH and sex steroid secretion necessitate an increase in insulin requirements and make good glycaemic control more difficult to achieve. However, a major cause of poor glycaemic control in adolescence is poor compliance. Young people must be clearly but sensitively informed of the dangers of administering inadequate amounts of insulin, as the relationship between an individual and the diabetes team must not break down.

Adolescents should be warned of the specific effects of alcohol on glycaemic control, in particular the risk of nocturnal hypoglycaemia. They should be discouraged from cigarette smoking and be warned of the health problems associated with it, especially the risks of developing vascular complications. They should also receive education about sexual health and pregnancy planning.

Disability Living Allowance

Whether families can apply for a Disability Living Allowance differs between countries.

Driving

The Driver and Vehicle Licensing Agency (DVLA) must be informed of the diagnosis of diabetes. If the individual is considered safe to drive (well-controlled without frequent, unexpected hypoglycaemic episodes), a licence can be issued, but only for a limited period at a time.

Employment

People with diabetes cannot enter certain occupations due to the risk of hypoglycaemia endangering both the person with diabetes and others. The restrictions to employment faced by individuals with diabetes may vary between countries.

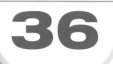

Malcolm Levene   Raisa H. K. Lounamaa   Martin Samuels   Neela Shabde

Child abuse and neglect: the hospital perspective

LEARNING OUTCOMES

By the end of this chapter you should:

- Know and understand the role and responsibilities of the paediatrician in recognizing and managing abuse and neglect
- Know and understand the importance of awareness of abuse and neglect
- Know and understand which children and families are most at risk of abuse and neglect
- Understand the importance of and threshold for reporting concerns
- Know and understand the legal aspects and the rights of the child
- Understand multi-agency working and confidentiality
- Know and understand the diagnosis of physical and child sexual abuse and appreciate that a multi-agency approach is essential
- Know and understand the importance of discharging the child to a safe place.

Table 36.1 Types of ill treatment and examples

Form of abuse	Example
Physical abuse	Fractures, burns, cerebral and abdominal injuries, bruises
Sexual abuse	Unlawful sexual intercourse, buggery, inappropriate touching and kissing, exposure to sexual acts between adults, participation in pornographic media
Emotional abuse and emotional neglect (Ch. 21)	Demeaning, critical and unloving behaviour, verbal abuse
Neglect (physical and emotional) (Ch. 21)	Failure to thrive, missed healthcare and/or educational opportunities, neglect of physical needs, clothing, hygiene, neglect of dental care
Induced illness (Ch. 21)	Suffocation, poisoning, inappropriate interference with feeding tubes and intravenous lines
Fabricated illness (Ch. 21)	Falsifying histories, exaggerating handicap, interfering with tests

Introduction

Protecting children from intentional and indeed unintentional harm is the role and duty of every paediatrician. There is a basic level of knowledge that all such doctors must possess in order to be able to fulfil this function. This chapter describes the basis of child protection from the point of view of a trainee in paediatrics in a hospital setting and Chapter 21 describes child protection in the community from a primary care doctor's perspective, a view which a paediatrician and a paediatric trainee should of course also be familiar with.

The basic principles involved in child protection are:

- Recognition of the problem
- Reporting the doctor's suspicions
- Investigation and management of the problem
- Multi-agency approach (essential).

These two chapters give an overview of child protection. As an example, in the UK it is a requirement that all paediatric trainees undergo a formal child protection educational programme for doctors, including a training day developed by the Royal College of Paediatrics and Child Health (RCPCH) in conjunction with the National Society for Prevention of Cruelty to Children (NSPCC) and the Advanced Life Support Group (ALSG).

Child abuse can be defined under various categories, which are not mutually exclusive and often form a spectrum of abuse (Table 36.1). A child suffering one form of abuse is often subjected to other forms as well.

Many of these forms of maltreatment present to healthcare providers in either primary, secondary or even tertiary care, usually in the form of apparently accidental injury or genuine illness. The health professional has the opportunity to recognize these forms of maltreatment, and in so doing, will have to document why maltreatment explains the child's condition. This may need further investigation and the opinions of other medical specialties, e.g. in radiology, ophthalmology, orthopaedics, neurosurgery or child and adolescent (forensic) psychiatry. It is important to note that a child with chronic illness or disability can also be subjected to fabricated and induced illness so there is a need for awareness and recognition of this form of abuse.

Child abuse is commonly considered to result from a pattern of behaviour by an adult that is apart from other human behaviour. Whilst the most severe abuse results from behaviour that is clearly abnormal (cigarette burns, sadistic beatings, sexual abuse and physical isolation), there is some behaviour where the definition of abuse is dependent on the culture in which it occurs. The whole range of maltreatment of children, therefore, is best considered part of a spectrum of behaviour, ranging from that which is often part of normal behaviour (the 'reflex' smack, frustrated aggressive shout or derogatory remark; conscious 'disciplinary' acts accepted in some societies) through to very disturbed patterns of behaviour that result in conscious sadistic acts by an adult.

Role of the paediatrician

Paediatricians are *not* expected to deal with the maltreatment of children and young people alone; their role is to recognize and report when abuse may be occurring in the many different clinical presentations and to assist statutory agencies in the investigation of possible significant harm to a child. This would include establishing the likelihood of non-intentional injury or organic disease versus deliberate harm to the child. Such distinction is not often easy or possible, as some children with chronic disease or disability may also be subjected to child abuse and neglect; indeed, research confirms that they are at increased risk. The paediatrician therefore must liaise with the statutory agencies for child protection. It is the statutory agencies, including social services and the police, that have a legal responsibility for protecting children and investigating child protection concerns. In most countries government guidance and law places professional responsibility on health professionals to recognize and respond to child protection concerns and work within an inter-agency framework (colleagues), cooperating with statutory agencies in the best interest of the child. Paediatricians usually refer to social services in keeping with the local procedures and protocols.

Thus the key tasks of the paediatrician are to (see also Key points p. 505):

- Take a detailed history and perform a full physical examination
- Document the findings accurately and legibly in the medical records
- Consider whether child protection concerns exist*
- Check whether the child is the subject of a child protection plan (held by the local social services or a similar agency where it exists)
- Communicate with other professionals who have seen the child
- Undertake further medical investigation or obtain specialist opinion, where appropriate*
- Decide on the likelihood of accidental versus non-accidental injury, or organic versus non-organic illness*
- Report any child protection concerns to the statutory agencies for child protection, both verbally and in writing
- Carefully and contemporaneously document what actions are being taken, including discussions with social services/police and the plan arising from these
- Explain any findings and concerns to the parents (unless to do so would increase the risk to the child). Parents should be shown respect.*

(* These tasks should be undertaken in consultation with senior colleagues, including the named or designated doctor or nurse for child protection.)

The investigation and management of a case of maltreatment of a child must be approached in the same systematic and rigorous manner as would be appropriate to the investigation and management of any other serious and potentially fatal disease (as suggested by Lord Laming in the Victoria Climbié inquiry). When a child is admitted to hospital, a clear decision must always be made and documented as to which senior paediatrician is responsible for the child protection aspects of the child's care. The child must *not* be discharged from hospital until child protection concerns have been resolved.

Importance of awareness of abuse

In cases where professionals who deal with children know of or suspect abuse there is the opportunity

> ### BOX 36.1 Examples of severe or life-threatening child abuse
>
> **Direct**
> - Asphyxia or suffocation
> - Non-accidental head injury
> - Poisoning and other induced illness, e.g. septicaemia
> - Abdominal injury
> - Spinal injury, including cervical spine
> - Rib cage and long bone fractures
> - Drowning
> - Burns
>
> **Indirect**
> - Sexual abuse
> - Severe emotional abuse (through later deliberate self-harm or other suicidal acts)
> - Neglect, e.g. accidents, lack of supervision, severe untreated infections, malnutrition, severe anaemia (secondary to scratching from head lice)

for intervention, including either family support or protection of the child by removal from home, but only if this is reported to child protection agencies. Failure to report concerns or knowledge of maltreatment can have substantial long-term consequences for the child, who may remain the victim of abuse.

The long-term effects of child abuse and neglect include:

- *Emotional harm*, e.g. low self-esteem, depression, unresolved anger and aggression, anorexia, self-harm and suicide
- *Physical harm*, e.g. brain injury, organ damage, deformities, scars (e.g. burns) and handicap
- *Educational problems*, e.g. learning difficulties, failed schooling, employment difficulties
- *Social and relationship difficulties*, e.g. family violence, promiscuity and prostitution, drug and alcohol abuse, parenting difficulties.

Each year, substantial numbers of children suffer long-term morbidity or death (in the UK, 50–100 cases per year) as a result of maltreatment. In large numbers of these cases, earlier detection and intervention can avoid the serious consequences of abuse. Some of the most serious abusive injuries, including those that are life-threatening, are listed in Box 36.1.

Children at risk of abuse

Following any childhood injury, it is important to consider the circumstances of the injury and to obtain a clear history of what is alleged to have happened.

If an explanation is absent, inconsistent or otherwise unsatisfactory, then the possibility of maltreatment must be considered. The same applies to illness that persistently defies explanation or is not consistent with usual medical experience. Child abuse/maltreatment occurs in all social classes. However, features that are known to occur more frequently in families who abuse their children, in comparison to families who do not, include:

- Where the relationship between the parent and child does not appear loving and caring
- Where one or both parents have been abused themselves as children
- Parents who are young, single, unsupported or substitutive
- Parents with learning difficulties
- Parents who have a poor or unstable relationship
- Situations where there is domestic violence
- Parents who have problems with drug or alcohol dependence/misuse
- Parents who have mental illness or personality disorders
- Situations of poverty and deprivation, although most poor families do not abuse their children.

Factors in the child that are associated with vulnerability to abuse and neglect include:
- Prematurity and/or separation in the neonatal period
- Chronic illness, with frequent or prolonged hospitalizations
- Physical or mental handicap
- Poor maternal attachment
- Behavioural problems, e.g. soiling and wetting, challenging behaviour and hyperactivity (often more consequences than primary risk factors)
- Difficult temperament
- Screaming, crying interminably and inconsolably
- Looked-after children, (i.e. children in the care of the local authority because they are often already traumatized by abuse and/or neglect)

The above may reflect both an increased susceptibility to and a consequence of maltreatment, but their presence does not mean abuse has occurred. Children in all circumstances may be subjected to abuse and have a right to be protected from it.

Legal aspects and rights of the child

The United Nations Convention on the Rights of the Child (1989) provides an internationally accepted set of principles and standards to ensure that children everywhere — without discrimination — have the right to survival; to develop to the fullest; to protection from harmful influences, abuse and exploitation; and to participate fully in family, cultural and social life. The rights apply to the practice of children's healthcare for all children and young people up to the age of 18 years. All but two countries in the world (USA and Somalia) have ratified the Convention.

Article 3 provides that any decision or action affecting children either as individuals or as a group should be taken with 'their best interest' as the most important consideration.

Article 9 holds that children have a right not to be separated from their parents or carers unless it is judged to be in the child's best interest.

Article 12 places an obligation on health professionals to seek a child's opinion before taking decisions that affect her or his future.

Article 19 states that legislative, administrative, social and educational measures should be taken to protect children from all forms of physical or mental violence, injury or abuse, neglect or negligent treatment, maltreatment or exploitation, including sexual abuse, while in the care of parent(s), legal guardian(s) or any other person who has the care of the child.

Article 37 states that no child shall be subjected to torture or other cruel, inhuman or degrading treatment or punishment.

Child protection in Britain is guided by a legal framework set out in the Children Act (1989). The new Children Act (2004) incorporates principles within the United Nations Convention on the Rights of the Child and the European Convention on Human Rights. Children are protected from abuse and neglect by multi-agency working and by both voluntary and legal intervention. The new act also emphasizes the promotion of children's welfare and their protection from abuse and neglect. The Department of Health (1999) and new Working Together (2006) document, 'Working Together to Safeguard Children', incorporates all the legislation and sets out principles for professionals working with children. In all European countries guidelines are likely to include and take into account the following principles:
- The welfare of children is paramount.
- Children must be listened to.
- Children should have the right to grow up within their families in an environment that promotes their health and safety.
- Look at the child and family rather than the injury.
- Describes roles and responsibilities of different agencies and practitioners.
- Places child protection procedures within the remit of local, regional or national safeguarding structures (e.g. local safeguarding children boards [LSCB] in the UK).

- Describes the agencies with child protection responsibilities
- Describes processes to be followed when there are concerns about a child and actions to be taken to safeguard and promote the welfare of children suffering, or at risk of suffering, significant harm.
- Provides guidance on child protection for 'looked-after' children who are in care of the local authority.

Reporting of child protection concerns

Any person who has knowledge or a suspicion that a child is suffering significant harm, or is at risk of significant harm, should refer that concern to one or more of the agencies with statutory duties and/ or powers to investigate and intervene: the social services department, the police or other relevant agency. All referrals to statutory authorities should be taken seriously and considered with an open mind. Professionals should be able to refer to child protection agencies in good faith without fear that this will lead to uncoordinated and/or premature action or any adverse consequences to themselves.

In many countries there is a mandatory requirement for all healthcare professionals to report suspicions of child maltreatment to the statutory agencies. However, there is always a professional and ethical duty to do so. In the UK, the General Medical Council (GMC) stipulates:

If you believe a patient to be a victim of neglect or physical, sexual or emotional abuse and that the patient cannot give or withhold consent to disclosure, you must give information promptly to an appropriate responsible person or statutory agency, where you believe that the disclosure is in the patient's best interest. If, for any reason, you believe that disclosure of information is not in the best interest of an abused or neglected patient, you must discuss the issues with an experienced colleague. If you decide not to disclose information, you must be prepared to justify your decision.

Whilst any health professional may report concerns or suspicions of child abuse to the statutory child protection agencies, more commonly general practitioners, community nursing staff and doctors in accident and emergency departments choose in the first place to refer such cases to paediatricians (either community or hospital-based paediatricians). In these circumstances, it is often the senior paediatrician who will then decide whether or not to refer a child to the statutory agencies. However, since it is recognized that 'health care is increasingly provided by multi-disciplinary teams', the UK GMC gives the following good general advice:

if you disagree with your team's decision, you may be able to persuade other team members to change their minds. If not, and you believe that the decision would harm the patient, tell someone who can take action. If there are difficulties or disagreements about if and when to refer a child, then discussion with a named or designated doctor or nurse (or other professional in the position to advise and bring the case forward) is strongly advised.

Critical threshold

Professionals need to be aware of the manifestations of maltreatment or abuse to ensure children are protected from harm. However, the detection of abuse is sometimes far from simple and requires the building up of a jigsaw of information; some of the pieces may be from a medical assessment (history, examination, investigations, subspecialty opinions) and some from information from other professionals or agencies. Sometimes the critical information — for example, a parent's past history of abusing a child — is held by the statutory agency and failure to share information with that agency may delay protection of the child. The clinician must make a decision when to liaise or refer to the statutory agencies. This is usually when the case has reached the 'critical threshold' (Boxes 36.2 and 36.3).

BOX 36.2 The child at risk of significant harm

In the UK, the Children Act 1989 (together with Children Act 2004) introduced the concept of 'significant harm' as the legal threshold for compulsory intervention in child protection cases. Where social services have reasonable cause to suspect that a child is suffering or is likely to suffer significant harm, they are under a duty to investigate the claim. Furthermore, courts can only make a care or supervision order if they are satisfied that:

- The child is suffering, or is likely to suffer, significant harm, and
- The harm or likelihood of harm is attributable to a lack of adequate parental care or control.

There are no absolute criteria by which significant harm can be judged; decisions take into consideration the effect of any ill treatment on the child's overall physical and psychological health and development. The Children Act 1989 introduced the concept of significant harm as the threshold that justifies compulsory intervention in family life in the best interests of children, and gives local authorities a duty to make enquiries to decide whether they should take action to safeguard or promote the welfare of a child who is suffering or is likely to suffer significant harm.

The 'critical threshold' is the point where the professional's concerns that the child may be being harmed cannot be satisfactorily resolved. Certainly in some cases it may fall short of clinical certainty or confirmation of diagnosis. Sometimes this critical threshold may be immediately apparent, e.g. an infant who has suffered a skull fracture and intracranial haemorrhage without adequate explanation. In other circumstances, a combination of history and non-specific signs suggests that there may be a problem. If there is any doubt about whether to report, consultation with a senior colleague or the named/designated doctor for child protection is recommended. As a rule, if in doubt after appropriate discussion and consultation, it is better for a report to be made to social services so that an assessment of the child and family can be made. This may identify that the child either is 'at risk' of significant harm, or may still be 'in need of services'. Both approaches should allow for the institution of appropriate family support and/or protection for the child and other measures as considered appropriate.

Inter-agency working/ working together

Child protection mostly involves working in partnership with the family and with professionals from other agencies. With regard to the former, there are some essential principles that the clinician should be aware of:

- Treat all family members as you would wish to be treated — with dignity and respect.
- Ensure family members know that the child's safety and welfare must be given first priority.
- Be clear with yourself and family members about the purpose of your professional involvement.
- Listen to the concerns of the child and his or her family.
- Respect confidentiality.

- Be open and honest about your concerns and responsibilities.
- Take care to distinguish between your professional role and responsibilities and your personal feelings, values, prejudices and beliefs.

It is not always possible to work in partnership with parents. In these circumstances, the best you can do is to keep the parents informed, whilst liaising with senior colleagues and the statutory authorities. If there is an immediate danger to the child's life, the police should be called.

Inter-agency working demands that agencies and professionals:

- Share information
- Collaborate and understand each other's position
- Work in partnership with each other and children and their families to plan comprehensive and coordinated services
- Recognize those most vulnerable children and coordinate services from various appropriate agencies, including the voluntary sector
- Work with adult services, particularly mental health
- Participate in joint working to safeguard children and where necessary to help bring to justice the perpetrators of crime against children.

In the UK all hospital trusts, be they primary, secondary or tertiary care providers, should have a named doctor and a named nurse for child protection, who take a professional lead within the trust on child protection matters. Their responsibilities include education, support and supervision. Each local area must have a designated doctor and nurse for child protection who work closely with the named professionals in supporting activities within trusts. Health professionals are expected to work in partnership with local authorities following government guidelines identifying clear roles and responsibilities for commissioners and providers within the health service.

Confidentiality

Issues around confidentiality often appear to be more complicated in child protection than in other areas, but it should always be recognized that the needs and the welfare of the child are paramount. Key issues for medical professionals and paediatricians to keep in mind are:

- The doctor's primary duty is to act in the child's best interest. If there is conflict between the doctor and parents or parents and child, then the child's needs are paramount.

- When there are reasonable grounds to believe a child is at risk of significant harm, the facts should be reported to a relevant agency with the duty and powers to investigate and act to protect the child. In many countries like England, Wales, Northern Ireland and the Nordic Countries, the agency is the Social Services. It is the duty of the paediatrician to be familiar with the reporting practices in the community where he practises.
- In general, healthcare professionals have a statutory duty to assist social services departments or other relevant agencies in undertaking investigations to evaluate the need for child protection measures to be taken.
- Consent to disclosure of relevant information about the child and other family members as a result of these enquiries should normally be sought from a competent child and carer, unless doing so would place the child or a sibling at greater risk or hinder enquiries by provoking interference with verbal evidence.
- Medical practitioners should disclose information about a non-competent child if they can justify doing so as essential to their patient's medical interest. Disclosure without consent may also take place where failure to do so may place a child at risk of death or serious harm, or where the information would help prevent, detect or prosecute a serious crime.
- Where there is uncertainty as to whether there is a risk of death or serious harm and an apparently competent child or parent refuses permission for disclosure, the doctor is obliged to act when a child is in danger.
- The doctor should document thoroughly all decisions and the reasoning behind them and should always separate details of fact from those of speculation and opinion.

The doctor–parent–child relationship is founded on mutual trust and respect, as well as a common aim to benefit the child. Where the child presents with symptoms or signs suggesting he or she has been a subject of abuse, it may no longer be possible to regard parent and child as a single unit. In this situation, it is the moral duty of the doctor to act in the best interest of the child.

The UK Department of Health best practice guidance (May 2003) states:

A decision whether to disclose information may be particularly difficult if you think it may damage the trust between you and your patient or client. Wherever possible you should explain the problem, seek agreement and explain the reasons if you decide to act against a parent or the child's agreement.

A sensible safeguard, before dispensing with parental consent, is to seek advice and a further opinion from a more experienced colleague.

Lord Laming chaired a major inquiry following the death of Victoria Climbié. Amongst his wide-ranging recommendations he stated that difficulties in seeking or refusal of parental permission must not restrict the initial information gathering and sharing, e.g. between health and social services, and this should if necessary include talking to the child. He stated:

When the deliberate harm of a child is identified as a possibility, the examining doctor should consider whether taking a history directly from the child is in that child's best interests. When that is so, the history should be taken even when the consent of the carer has not been obtained, with the reason for dispensing with consent recorded by the examining doctor. In those cases in which English is not the first language of the child concerned, the use of an interpreter should be considered.

Civil and criminal proceedings

Significant harm to children gives rise to both child welfare concerns, dealt with in civil proceedings by social services (local authorities), and law enforcement issues, dealt with in criminal proceedings. The police have a duty to carry out thorough and professional investigations into allegations of crime, and the obtaining of good evidence is often in the best interests of a child, as it may make it less likely that a child will have to give evidence in court. It also contributes to the development of a good evidence base upon which to develop future support and help for the child and family.

Health professionals need to keep in mind that child protection work can lead to criminal proceedings. In these situations it is of vital importance that the doctor and other healthcare professionals know their role and responsibility within the legal framework of the country where they work. The guidelines may vary significantly between countries as to who should take the lead reponsibility of interviewing the child and the family. Not following the set rules may harm the legal process. However, as a general rule irrespective of the set legal and procedural framework children should not be exposed to multiple intimate examinations simply to provide evidence for court proceedings. Furthermore, leading or suggestive communication with children or other members of the family should always be avoided. When in doubt it is good practice to seek further advice from either the law enforcement agency (the police) or legal advisors when a doctor believes that criminal offences may have been committed.

Physical abuse

Although serious cases of physical abuse may be obvious, the range and incidence of physical abuse varies depending on cultural practices. In some countries legislation has been established against smacking, which is considered abusive, but this is not the case in the UK and it remains legal to use reasonable force to discipline a child. Most people would, however, agree that any force that causes an injury to a child, such as bruising, represents unacceptable force. Bullying at school may also be a cause of physical or emotional abuse and it is estimated that 450 000 children are bullied at school at least once per week.

It has been shown that 14% of children in the UK suffered the effects of physical punishment, including babies who are regularly smacked or hit. Mothers hit their children more often than fathers, but severe injury is most commonly inflicted by a man in the household.

Abuse may be severe and result in the child's death. Fatal outcome may be due to:
- Shaking injury
- Blunt injury causing severe damage to brain or abdominal organs
- Suffocation (may present as recurrent apnoea or sudden unexplained death in infancy)
- Poisoning (see also Ch. 21).

Box 36.4 lists the more common types of injury that result from physical abuse.

The doctor must be alert to the varied ways in which physical abuse may present. Important features are listed in Box 36.5. A thorough medical examination (top-to-toe surface examination), including assessment of growth and development, is essential in all cases of suspected child abuse.

Bruising

There is no pathognomonic site of bruising that indicates child abuse. It is essential to document the number, distribution and pattern of all bruising carefully. Up to a half of all mobile children have at least one bruise and many have more than one, although more than ten are suspicious. An important clue to a potentially abusing family is if consent is not given to undress and examine the whole child. Describe how many bruises and illustrate distribution with a simple diagram on the body chart. (Those on shins, bony prominences and forehead are more likely to be accidental.) Attempting to age bruises is unreliable and should not be done. Is there a consistent history for the site of the bruising?

Particularly suspicious bruising includes:

BOX 36.4 Common types of injury that result from physical abuse

- Bruising from blows
- Fractures from grabbing limbs and direct blows
- Bites (distinguish between dog and human dental patterns)
- Burns from being held in direct contact with hot objects or scalds from forced immersion
- Intra-oral injuries suggesting forcible insertion of bottles or spoons

---

BOX 36.5 Features that should arouse suspicion of physical abuse

- Repeated injuries
- No consistent explanation for how the injury occurred
- Patterns of injury
- Evasive or uncooperative history from a parent or caregiver
- Inappropriate child response (e.g. 'didn't cry', 'felt no pain')
- Signs of other abuse (neglect, failure to thrive, sexual abuse)
- The child's age too young to be consistent with the history of how injury occurred (e.g. fracture in a child that is not yet cruising or fracture in a child under 1 year of age)
- Unreasonable delay in presentation
- Parental aggression

- Unusual sites such as ears, cheeks (Fig. 36.1), eyes, mouth, trunk, genitalia, upper or unexposed parts of limbs, buttocks and neck
- Unusual patterns suggestive of grip marks, bites (Fig. 36.2), marks consistent with a stick, belt (Fig. 36.3), buckle or shoe
- Injuries in the mouth (Fig. 36.4)
- Two black eyes.

The differential diagnosis of excessive bruising includes:
- Coagulation disorders
- Henoch–Schönlein purpura (p. 623)
- Collagen disorders (rare)
- Asphyxia
- Mongolian blue spots (p. 350)
- Artefacts such as dirt, felt tip marks or dye from clothes.

Fractures

Fractures due to child abuse are most common in babies below the age of 2 years. In the first 18 months

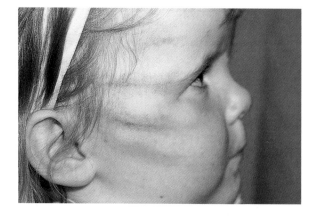

Fig. 36.1 **Bruising to cheek — adult hand slap in a female aged 3 years**
(Courtesy of Dr C Hobbs)

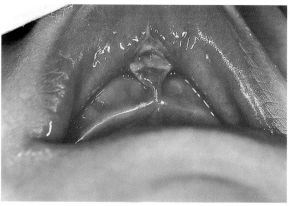

Fig. 36.4 **Torn frenulum in a male aged 3 months**
(Courtesy of Dr C Hobbs)

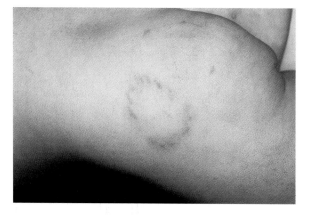

Fig 36.2 **Bite marks in a male aged 3 years**
(Courtesy of Dr C Hobbs)

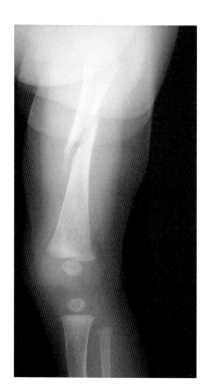

Fig. 36.5 **Femoral shaft fracture in a girl of 6 months**
(Courtesy of Dr C Hobbs)

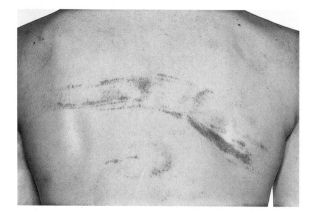

Fig. 36.3 **Bruising to back as a result of belt marks in a male child aged 13 years**
(Courtesy of Dr C Hobbs)

85% of fractures are due to abuse and in premobile children (<9 months) fractures should always be treated as highly suspicious.

In all children certain fractures should lead to suspicion of abuse. These include:

- Rib fractures, which are highly specific for abuse (fresh fractures may be difficult to recognize on X-ray). Cardiopulmonary resuscitation rarely causes rib fracture and does not cause posterior rib fractures.
- Fractures involving a long bone metaphysis (Fig. 36.5).
- Any fracture of femur or humerus in infants.
- Multiple fracture sites.
- Evidence of fractures of different ages on X-ray examination.

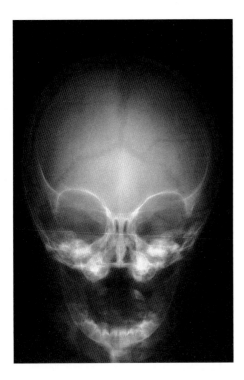

Fig. 36.6 **Bilateral linear parietal skull fractures in a girl of 6 months**
(Courtesy of Dr C Hobbs)

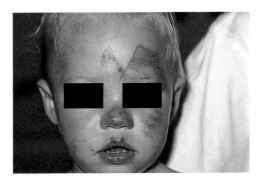

Fig. 36.7 **Contact burns from an iron in an 18-month old girl)**
(Courtesy of Dr C Hobbs)

- An inadequate or absent explanation for how the fracture occurred.
- A fracture that occurs as the result of minor trauma, e.g. an infant falling off a sofa.
- Skull fractures, which do not occur without considerable force. Is the explanation appropriate? Particularly concerning are those involving the occipital bone, depressed fractures, wide (> 3 mm) fractures and multiple fractures, particularly if crossing a suture line (Fig. 36.6).
- Spinal fractures. Cervical fractures occasionally occur with non-accidental shaking injury.

Differential diagnoses for the cause of fractures include:
- Accident
- Abuse
- Birth injury (e.g. clavicle, humerus)
- Osteopenia (rickets) of prematurity (p. 732)
- Osteogenesis imperfecta
- Copper deficiency (very rare)
- Structural variant, e.g. aberrant cranial suture.

Investigations

A skeletal survey is mandatory when there is a fracture suggestive of abuse. It is also recommended for any child under the age of 2 years who is suspected of being physically abused. Repeating the survey (a chest X-ray and films of other suspicious areas) after 2 weeks may reveal previously undiagnosed fractures and can help in the dating of the onset of the fracture. Computed tomography (CT) head scans and bone scans may be indicated but require discussion with a senior colleague. For more detailed instructions on radiological investigations, see the recent guidelines 'Standards for radiological investigations of suspected non-accidental injury' (March 2008).

 http://www.rcpch.ac.uk

Thermal injuries

These occur commonly in childhood and often present to primary care doctors. A relatively small number are due to child abuse but are known to be under-recognized. Thermal injuries include burns and scalds. These include scalds from hot water, food or steam. Burns may follow contact from hot metal objects such as an iron or radiator, cigarettes, matches or flames, friction from being dragged across a carpet, and from electrical and chemical sources.

In evaluating a burn the following features are important:
- Inconsistent history as to how the injury occurred
- Denial that the injury is a burn
- Repeated burns
- Site or multiple sites (lesions on the feet and backs of hands are commonly due to abuse)
- Shape:
  - Is it consistent with the history?
  - Are demarcation lines suggestive of a particular object (Fig. 36.7)?
  - Cigarette burns cause deep circular craters 0.5–1 cm in diameter, which scar (Fig. 36.8). Accidental brushed contact causes superficial injury roughly circular but with a tail.

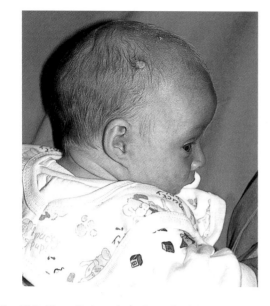

Fig. 36.8 **Cigarette burn in an 8-week-old male**
(Courtesy of Dr C Hobbs)

Immersion scalds should be particularly evaluated for evidence of:

- Tide marks indicating that limb or buttocks were forcibly immersed (Fig. 36.9)
- Absent splash marks suggestive of removal from the hot water.

The differential diagnosis of burns includes:

- Impetigo (p. 362)
- Diaper (nappy) rash (Ch. 27)
- Staphylococcal scalded skin (p. 363)
- Ringworm infection (p. 356).

Head injury

This form of abuse carries the highest mortality rates and is particularly common in infants. Isolated severe head injury suggests either shaking or impact injury or both. Shaking injury resulting in combinations of subdural haemorrhage, brain injury and retinal haemorrhage is most common at around 3–6 months of age. Subdural haemorrhage may follow birth or accidental trauma. Small asymptomatic bleeds may be seen with imaging performed after birth, but resolve within the first 4 weeks of life.

The main clinical features of non-accidental head injury (NAHI) include:

- *Delay in presentation*: e.g. child may be well with enlarging head
- *Inconsistent explanation*: e.g. history of a minor fall, severe injury
- *Sudden collapse* in an otherwise well child
- Presentation with or history of general symptoms: irritability, nausea, poor feeding, minor or vague neurological symptoms
- *Presence of other injuries* (bruises, skull, rib or long bone fractures)
- *Retinal haemorrhages* in one or both eyes.

N.B. The absence of one or more of fractures, bruises or retinal haemorrhages does not exclude abuse.

All children suspected of having non-accidental or other head injury should have a magnetic resonance (MR) or CT head scan to confirm the presence of subdural haemorrhage. Skeletal survey may reveal other bony injuries. An experienced ophthalmologist should be asked to examine the child's eyes as soon as possible after admission to look for retinal haemorrhages. These are a common feature after birth but usually disappear within days. They may occur after severe accidental injury (e.g. car accident).

Child sexual abuse

Sexual abuse in children will not be recognized if it is not considered by the clinician. A high index of

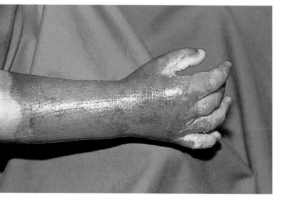

A

B

Fig. 36.9 **Forced immersion scalds in male 18 months old**
(A and B) (Courtesy of Dr C Hobbs)

suspicion must exist and healthcare professionals must acknowledge that child sexual abuse may occur in any family. One study found that in the UK 12% of girls and 8% of boys have suffered sexual abuse at some time in their childhood. Other studies have suggested higher figures. Boys are less likely to disclose abuse than girls. The abuser is most commonly a member of the household or an extended family member or friend. In the vast majority of cases the child knows the abuser, who may be either a man or a woman. Sexual abuse of children by strangers is much less common.

Abusers usually groom and manipulate children into silence over a period of time. A child who is abused by a close family member may adapt psychologically, a process that has been termed 'the child sexual abuse accommodation syndrome'. The components of this comprise:

- Secrecy
- Entrapment and helplessness
- Accommodation, in which the child takes responsibility and feelings of guilt for the abuse
- Delayed unconvincing disclosure and later retraction of disclosure.

Child sexual abuse has both short- and long-term effects. Short-term (childhood) effects include:

- Emotional, behavioural and psychosomatic disorder
- Difficulties forming friendships and trusting relationships
- School underachievement and truancy or excellent school performance and attendance
- Pregnancy, sexually transmitted infection (STI)
- Abusive behaviour towards younger children.

Long-term effects include:

- Sexual relationship difficulties
- Mental health problems, e.g. depression, eating disorder
- Social dysfunction
- May become a perpetrator
- May not be able to protect their own children from being sexually abused (studies have shown that mothers of sexually abused children are more likely to have been sexually abused themselves).

Problem-orientated topic:

a girl with blood-stained underwear

Irem is 3 years old and her preschool teacher has noted blood staining on her knickers three times in the last month. Irem is an aggressive child who frequently hits other children in the nursery. She uses swear words, which the teacher thinks she can only have heard at home. Her teacher is concerned but does not want to upset Irem's mother and notifies the health visitor, who in turn informs the primary care physician. The primary care physician refers the case to hospital.

Q1. What should the paediatrician do?
Q2. What investigations should be performed?
Q3. How should the child and family be managed?

Q1. What should the paediatrician do?

There are very few signs that are diagnostic of sexual abuse in themselves. The diagnosis is usually made by piecing together a jigsaw of information from many sources. The major clues to diagnosis are as follows.

Disclosure

This is the most common way in which sexual abuse is diagnosed. Children rarely fabricate disclosure of sexual abuse and their account should always be taken seriously and investigated. The child should be told that the disclosure will be passed on to social services and the police. The doctor to whom the child discloses should not interrogate the child, as this may compromise the subsequent legal process. The doctor may, however, gently question the child in open and non-leading ways to find out, for example, what it is that makes them sore between their legs. If a child discloses in confidence he or she must be told that the information will be passed on for his or her protection, as well as for the protection of other children. The doctor should have no ethical dilemma as to whether this information should be disclosed, as the GMC acknowledges that protection of the patient overrides the duty of confidentiality to the patient.

Never promise to keep a child's secret, especially in advance of knowing what it is.

Vaginal discharge or urinary symptoms

These are non-specific symptoms in prepubertal girls but should arouse suspicion of sexual abuse. Many girls who have been rubbed or fondled may develop vulvovaginitis, but only a proportion of girls with vulvovaginitis have been sexually abused. Vaginal discharge in one case control study was found significantly more often than in non-abused controls. The differential diagnosis of vulvovaginitis is discussed on page 336.

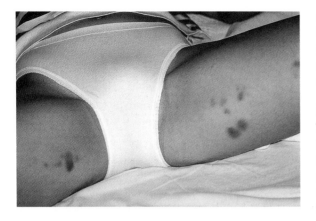

Fig. 36.10 Fingertip thigh bruises in sexual assault in female aged 9 years
(Courtesy of Dr C Hobbs)

A vulval swab and urine culture should be taken. Do not insert the swab into the vagina but take the specimen from the labia.

Rectal or vaginal bleeding

Vaginal bleeding in a prepubertal child is usually due to trauma and as such is strongly linked to sexual abuse. Differentiating abuse from non-abusive genital trauma, such as a straddle injury, is not always simple. Even with a clear history, repeated by the child, caution is required. Injury to the hymen, posterior genital injury and bruising elsewhere should raise concerns and prompt a thorough assessment and referral to social services. Rectal bleeding may occur as the result of a fissure, rectal polyp, inflammatory bowel disease or gastroenteritis. The presence of either of these symptoms in a prepubertal child without an obvious unambiguous history demands rapid referral to a child protection team (Fig. 36.10).

Behavioural disturbance

Emotional and behavioural disturbance following child sexual abuse is common and may include self-harm, mutilation, aggression and sexualized behaviours. More often, however, the parents describe non-specific symptoms including anxiety, interrupted sleep, bad dreams, naughtiness, disobedience or just a non-specific subtle change in the child's behaviour. Psychosomatic symptoms are common and include abdominal pains and headaches. Secondary wetting and soiling are also important symptoms.

Pregnancy

This is clear evidence of sexual activity! It is obviously important to distinguish between consensual intercourse with a teenage boyfriend, which is not abusive, and pregnancy resulting from an abusive exploitative

relationship with an older adult. The issue of consent in the latter situation is one of whether this can in reality be meaningful and given on an equitable basis or whether the girl has been groomed and exploited/corrupted.

Examination

There may be evidence of force during the assault, as seen in physical injuries such as bruising of the lower abdomen, genital area, thighs, buttocks, breasts and grip mark bruising around the knees or on the upper arms. Examination of the genitalia may reveal either supportive or diagnostic findings of abuse. For example, a fresh tear of the hymen with fresh bleeding or an old healed transaction of the hymen are both strong evidence of penetrating trauma. An anal laceration or scar is a diagnostic sign of anal penetration and reflex anal dilatation is one of a number of other findings supportive of anal abuse.

Q2. What investigations should be performed?

If a vulval swab identifies a sexually transmitted infection (STI), immediate referral to a child protection team should be made. The incidence of STI in abused children is about 5% and the most commonly encountered are gonorrhoea, genital or anal warts and chlamydia. *Trichomonas vaginalis* infection (usually asymptomatic) in a child over 12 months suggests recent sexual contact. Other infections that can be sexually transmitted include genital herpes simplex, human immunodeficiency virus (HIV), syphilis and pubic lice. Very often children with STI show no sign of injury to the genital or anal areas.

Q3. How should the child and family be managed?

If a doctor has evidence causing him or her to suspect child sexual abuse, this information must be passed on to the social services. Discussion with a named or designated paediatrician may be useful if further advice is required. The primary caregiver should be informed of the referral unless there is any concern that the abuser may be warned and evidence may be destroyed or pressure put on the child to withdraw the disclosure or change the story.

The doctor must keep careful and accurate contemporaneous notes of the interview, including who said what to whom and any examination findings. An excellent publication for all paediatricians to be familiar with is 'The Physical Signs of Child Sexual Abuse' (March 2008), which is a revision of a 1997 publication. It is an evidence-based review and guidance for best practice produced by the Royal College of Paediatrics and Child Health (RCPCH) in collaboration with the Royal College of Physicians (RCP) of London and its Faculty of Forensic and Legal Medicine.

Once the social services have been informed, a child protection investigation occurs. If the child is making a disclosure or allegation of abuse, he or she is usually interviewed jointly by an experienced social worker and police officer and the interview is videotaped as evidence for any later court hearing.

The child should be examined by a paediatrician or another specialist (in some settings a gynecologist) trained in examination and assessment of child sexual abuse either alone or jointly with an experienced police surgeon (forensic doctor). The key issue is whether the doctor has the necessary skills. Remember that no physical evidence may be found (which is most often the case), even in cases with a clear allegation of penetrative sexual abuse. The purpose of this examination is to:

- Assess the nature of any abuse
- Collect forensic evidence of sexual abuse (e.g. semen or spermatozoa in the vagina, rectum, mouth or elsewhere)
- Screen for STIs and pregnancy as required (taking into account the history and findings)
- Provide reassurance that there is no permanent physical damage
- Arrange a treatment plan for identified medical, psychological and emotional problems
- Offer emergency contraception to postmenarchal girls presenting within 72 hours of a sexually abusive event.

The main aim of management is to prevent further abuse and provide support for the child and family as necessary. Referral to a therapeutic service, e.g. Child and Adolescent Mental Health, may be required.

Neglect and the chronically ill child

The problem of recognizing and intervening with physical and emotional neglect is dealt with in more detail in Chapter 21. In the hospital setting it has to be emphasized that any chronically ill child may be at particular risk should his parents and carers not have the full capability to look after and support the child. It is well recognized that this can be a serious problem for a child with a chronic condition who lives in a severely neglectful or chaotic home with parents who may themselves have problems with mental health or

substance abuse. A parent may also cope and be a good enough parent for a healthy child but may not be able to provide adequate care and support for a child with asthma, diabetes or a mental or physical disability. The parental capacity and need of additional support must always be weighed against the child's needs.

It is of vital importance that a child with a chronic condition will be given the same prospect for good care and opportunity to learn to take care of himself, and as far as possible, to lead a healthy life despite the condition and irrespective of the parent's capacity to learn to look after and treat a chronic disorder (e.g. diabetes). This emphasizes the need to be able to assess potential and relative neglect and need for support with an open mind and without even unintentionally raising blame — and potentially opposition to treatment. In such a situation it is also important to keep in mind that all solutions are not medical and that the paediatrician is not required to deal with the problem alone but involve the multidisciplinary team and statutory agencies as required.

KEY POINTS

- Be aware of the range of presentations of child maltreatment/abuse.
- Take a detailed history and perform a full physical examination.
- Document your findings accurately in the medical records; note what was explained to the parents and what actions you are taking.
- If there are child protection concerns, try to find out if there have been previous concerns with the child or the family (this may mean a need to contact the primary care services for which you may need parental consent — care must be taken to always follow the national guidelines and work within the legal framework).
- Discuss your concerns with senior colleagues or the named/designated doctor/nurse for child protection.
- Consider the need to communicate with other health professionals who have seen the child.
- Undertake further investigation or obtain specialist opinion, where appropriate.
- Explain any concerns to the parents and what you intend to do as a result.
- Refer child protection concerns to the statutory agencies for child protection.
- Document any discussions, including referrals to social services and what actions will be taken.
- Do not discharge home until child protection concerns have been resolved.
- Always involve a senior colleague who will ultimately have responsibility for the patient.

http://www.bma.org.uk/images/
childprotectiontoolkitmay2009_
tcm41-184943.pdf

A tool kit on child protection for doctors, May 2009

http://www.gmc-uk.org/guidance/good_
medical_practice/index.asp

General Medical Council: advice on good medical
practice and confidentiality

Acknowledgments

We are very grateful to Dr Chris Hobbs for advice
about the manuscript and for allowing us to use his
illustrations.

Further reading

Finkel MA, Giardino AP (eds), 2009. Medical Evaluation of
   Child Sexual Abuse. A Practical Guide, 3rd edn. American
   Academy of Pediatrics, Elk Grove Village, IL.

Hobbs CJ, Wynne JM 2001 Physical signs of child abuse: a
   colour atlas, 2nd edn. WB Saunders, Philadelphia.
Intercollegiate Report from the Royal College of Radiologists
   and Royal College of Paediatricians, March 2008, 'Standards
   for Radiological Investigations of Suspected Non-accidental
   injury' (http://www.rcpch.ac.uk).
Reece RM, Christian CW (eds), 2009. Child Abuse. Medical
   Diagnosis & Management, 3rd edn. American Academy of
   Pediatrics, Elk Grove Village, IL.
Roesler TA, Jenny C. Medical Child Abuse. Beyond Munchausen
   Syndrome by Proxy (2009). American Academy of Pediatrics,
   Elk Grove Village, IL.
The Royal College of Paediatrics and Child Health 2006. Child
   Protection Companion. RCPCH London.
The Royal College of Paediatrics and Child Health 2008. The
   Physical Signs of Child Sexual Abuse. An evidence based
   review and guidance for best practice. RCPCH London.

Per Ashorn   Anthony Costello   Therese Hesketh
David Osrin   Andrew Tomkins

CHAPTER

Child health in developing countries

MODULE SIX

LEARNING OUTCOMES

By the end of this chapter you should:

- Know and understand definitions of key statistics
- Know and understand the UN Millennium Development Goals
- Be familiar with the major infectious illnesses of developing countries: malaria, HIV/AIDS and tuberculosis
- Understand why neonatal mortality is so high in developing countries and methods to reduce it
- Understand malnutrition: its dietary, social, environmental and disease causes; diagnosis — clinical and biochemical; its impact on child health; prevention and treatment
- Understand the concept and the global importance of children in difficult circumstances.

Introduction

A third of the world's 57 million deaths/year occur in children under 5 years. This equates to almost 18 million deaths per annum, of which almost all (98%) take place in developing countries.

Beneath the classification of cause of death lies a raft of influences, in which poverty, gender, governance, macroeconomics and malnutrition all play a part. It remains a fact that, of the 4.4 billion people living in developing countries, 60% lack access to sanitation, 33% lack clean water, 20% have no healthcare, and 20% do not have enough dietary energy and protein.

Child international health

Problem-orientated topic:

a presentation on child public health

You are invited to make a presentation on child public health in your area of Europe at an international meeting. The audience will include health professionals from a number of countries, with representation from Africa and South Asia. You feel that it would

507

be productive to set your discussion in the context of global child health, and to highlight the areas in which your practice is similar to and differs from that of your international colleagues. You will have to deal with questions about common international child health concerns.

Q1. Which child survival statistics will you use in the introductory discussion?

Q2. Against which international goals might you frame the discussion?

Q3. What are the world's top three causes of child mortality?

Q4. Can you name and summarize three international child health programmes that are relevant to both your practice in your own country and your colleagues' practice in low-income developing countries?

Q5. What are the immunization schedules likely to be in your colleagues' countries?

Q6. What is your opinion of the WHO strategy for the Integrated Management of Childhood Illness (IMCI) as a model for ambulatory paediatric clinics in Europe?

Q1. Which child survival statistics will you use in the introductory discussion?

Although rough figures are available, we do not have accurate data on the numbers and causes of child deaths in developing countries, particularly at the younger end of the scale. Ideally, statistics would be based on vital registration — as they are in many European countries — and death certification would be used to monitor mortality patterns and document leading causes of death. Unfortunately, vital registration systems are not fully functional in most poor countries, and we have to rely on either small sentinel registration initiatives or sample surveys. One well-known source of figures is the Demographic and Health Survey (DHS), which collects information on a range of family issues from a national sample and is organized to be comparable between countries.

The most common child health indices used to compare different areas or progress over time are the under-5 mortality rate and the infant mortality rate. Although child mortality does have a technical meaning, it is often used as shorthand for under-5 mortality.

Definitions

Definitions of terms are given in Table 37.1 and Figure 37.1.

Q2. Against which international goals might you frame the discussion?

Child survival is addressed in the Millennium Development Goals set by the UN. Although there is a specific

Table 37.1 **Definitions**

Term	Definition	Related term	Definition
Stillbirth*	A fetus born after 28 complete weeks of gestation, who has died before delivery	Stillbirth rate (SBR)	Stillbirths per 1000 births, live and still
Early neonatal death	Death of a live-born infant within 7 complete days postpartum	Early neonatal mortality rate (ENMR)	Early neonatal deaths per 1000 live births
Late neonatal death	Death of a live-born infant between 8 and 28 complete days postpartum	Late neonatal mortality rate (LNMR)	Late neonatal deaths per 1000 live births
Perinatal death	Stillbirth or early neonatal death	Perinatal mortality rate (PMR)	Stillbirths and early neonatal deaths per 1000 births, live and still
Neonatal death	Early or late neonatal death	Neonatal mortality rate (NMR)	Early and late neonatal deaths per 1000 live births
Post-neonatal death	Death of a live-born infant between 28 days and 12 complete months postpartum	Post-neonatal mortality rate (PNMR)	Post-neonatal deaths per 1000 live births
Infant death	Neonatal or post-neonatal death	Infant mortality rate (IMR)	Infant deaths per 1000 live births
Under-5 death	Death of a live-born infant within 5 complete years postpartum	Under-5 mortality rate (U5MR)	Under-5 deaths per 1000 live births

* This is a working definition, which accords with the International Statistical Classification of Diseases — 9th revision (ICD-9). In view of the fact that newborn infants of lower gestations now routinely survive in industrialized countries, the definition has been revised in ICD-10 to take in gestations as low as 22 complete weeks.

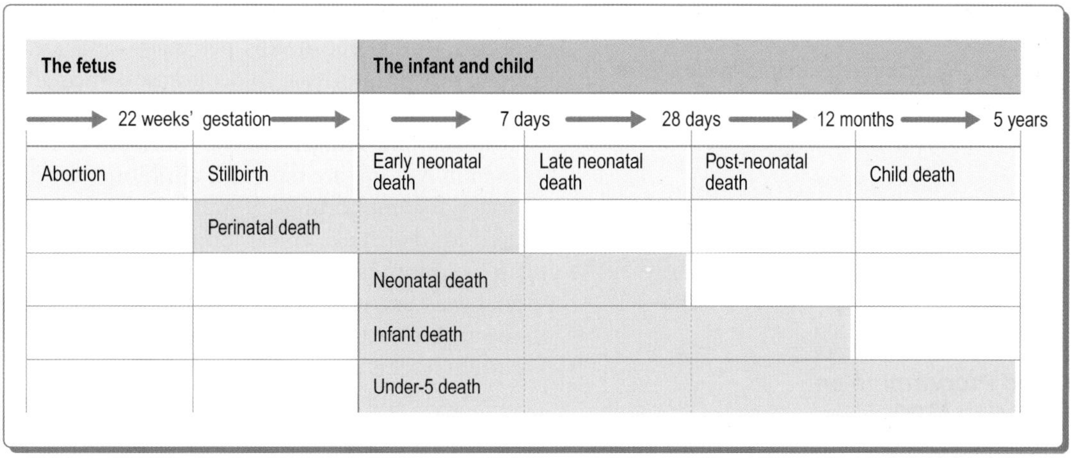

The fetus		The infant and child			
→ 22 weeks' gestation →		→ 7 days → 28 days → 12 months → 5 years			
Abortion	Stillbirth	Early neonatal death	Late neonatal death	Post-neonatal death	Child death
	Perinatal death				
		Neonatal death			
		Infant death			
		Under-5 death			

Fig. 37.1 **Definitions**

Table 37.2 **Millennium Development Goals**

Goal/target	Description
Goal 1	**Eradicate extreme poverty and hunger**
Target 1	Halve, between 1990 and 2015, the proportion of people whose income is less than US $1 a day
Target 2	Halve, between 1990 and 2015, the proportion of people who suffer from hunger
Goal 2	**Achieve universal primary education**
Target 3	Ensure that, by 2015, children everywhere, boys and girls alike, will be able to complete a full course of primary education
Goal 3	**Promote gender equality and empower women**
Target 4	Eliminate gender disparity in primary and secondary education, preferably by 2005 and to all levels of education no later than 2015
Goal 4	**Reduce child mortality**
Target 5	Reduce by two-thirds, between 1990 and 2015, the under-5 mortality rate
Goal 5	**Improve maternal health**
Target 6	Reduce by three-quarters, between 1990 and 2015, the maternal mortality ratio
Goal 6	**Combat HIV/AIDS, malaria and other diseases**
Target 7	Have halted by 2015, and begun to reverse, the spread of HIV/AIDS
Target 8	Have halted by 2015, and begun to reverse, the incidence of malaria and other major diseases
Goal 7	**Ensure environmental sustainability**
Target 9	Integrate the principles of sustainable development into country policies and programmes and reverse the loss of environmental resources
Target 10	Halve, by 2015, the proportion of people without sustainable access to safe drinking water
Target 11	By 2020, to have achieved a significant improvement in the lives of at least 100 million slum dwellers

goal for improving child survival, all the goals are intimately linked with child health (Table 37.2).

Q3. What are the world's top three causes of child mortality?

Global causes of childhood death, in order of magnitude, are:

- Perinatal and neonatal disorders
- Diarrhoeal disease
- Respiratory infection
- Malaria
- Human immunodeficiency virus/acquired immune deficiency syndrome (HIV/AIDS)
- Measles.

Q4. Can you name and summarize three international child health programmes that are relevant to both your practice in your own country and your colleagues' practice in developing countries?

Child health is affected by improvements in education, infrastructure, health service systems, sanitation and nutrition. However, a number of programmes specifically target health issues. Some of these programmes are limited to one type of disease (vertical) and some attempt to address a range of problems (integrated).

Three international programmes that are directly relevant to developing countries are discussed below (Box 37.1). These also have relevance in Europe.

- Expanded Programme on Immunization (EPI)
- Control of Diarrhoeal Disease (CDD)
- Acute Respiratory Infection (ARI)

Q5. What are the immunization schedules likely to be in your colleagues' countries?

Expanded Programme on Immunization (EPI)

The EPI is the basis for all global immunization programmes (Table 37.3), with varying support from international organizations depending on a country's needs. World-wide coverage is roughly 80% overall, but there are wide variations, especially in receipt of all three diphtheria/tetanus/pertussis (DTP) doses.

The campaign to eradicate polio began in 1988 and has achieved over 99% reduction in disease incidence through a strategy based on:

- High routine infant immunization
- Supplementary doses to all children under 5 years during national immunization days
- Surveillance for wild poliovirus through reporting and testing of all cases of acute flaccid paralysis in children under 15 years
- Targeted mop-up campaigns once wild poliovirus transmission is focal.

As of 2008, polio remains endemic in four countries (Afghanistan, India, Nigeria and Pakistan). In order to be certified polio-free, a country must have had at least 3 years of no cases of wild polio, demonstrate a capacity to detect, report and respond to imported cases, and have contained laboratory virus stocks. Likewise, sufficient stocks of vaccine must exist to cover potential outbreaks and routine immunization programmes must be strong. Because of the proportionately growing incidence of vaccine-derived polio, many countries are switching from oral to injectable polio vaccine.

Measles is responsible for about 10% of under-5 deaths — 800 000 deaths per year — 85% of which occur in Africa and Asia. Epidemics are particularly severe in crowded conditions such as urban slums, schools, hospitals and refugee camps. Mortality is reduced if vitamin A stores are replete, if antibiotics are given for bacterial complications, if oral rehydration therapy is used for diarrhoea, and if food intake is increased for up to 2 months after the illness. A measles eradication goal was set in 1997. Unfortunately, the necessary coverage to achieve eradication is over 90% and the current level is on average about 70%. Eradication will therefore require a series of national and local catch-up rounds of immunization, as well as very good routine immunization systems.

Control of Diarrhoeal Disease (CDD)

The discovery that oral water, salt and sugar repletion (oral rehydration solution, ORS) was a powerful tool for treating the dehydration caused by diarrhoea led to the institutionalization of oral rehydration therapy (ORT) and its inclusion in the child survival initiatives of the 1980s. Many healthcare facilities now have ORT areas, and outreach workers are routinely trained to assess degrees of dehydration and manage diarrhoea at home or refer appropriately.

Acute Respiratory Infection (ARI)

Outreach workers are also central to efforts to reduce the toll of lower respiratory tract infection. Pneumonia is responsible for 20% of child deaths, about 2 million annually. Current initiatives are based on the idea that:

- Most fatal pneumonias are bacterial (particularly *Streptococcus pneumoniae* and *Haemophilus influenzae*).
- Timely antibiotic treatment reduces case fatality.
- Simple algorithms based on counting respiratory rates are sensitive and adequately specific to identify children who require antibiotics.
- Health workers can use the algorithms, select appropriate treatment, administer antibiotics in

Table 37.3 Immunization programmes

Age	Vaccines	Where hepatitis B transmission common	Where hepatitis B transmission less common
Birth	BCG	HB1	
6 weeks	DTP1, OPV1	HB2	HB1
10 weeks	DTP2, OPV2		HB2
14 weeks	DTP3, OPV3	HB3	HB3
9 months	Measles, yellow fever*		

* Where yellow fever is a risk.
(BCG = bacille Calmette–Guérin; DTP = diphtheria, tetanus and pertussis vaccine; OPV = oral polio vaccine; HB = hepatitis B)

the community, counsel parents, follow children up and refer in case of complications. The World Health Organization (WHO) algorithm classifies a respiratory illness as pneumonia if the respiratory rate is greater than 50 per minute in a child older than 3 months. This model is being introduced in a number of countries but has yet to be rolled out world-wide.

Q6. What is your opinion of the WHO strategy for the Integrated Management of Childhood Illness (IMCI) as a model for ambulatory paediatric clinics in the UK?

A strategy adopted by the WHO, IMCI grew out of the knowledge that most childhood deaths occurred as a result of five conditions: pneumonia, diarrhoea, measles, malnutrition and malaria. A sick child may be suffering from more than one condition, individual symptoms and signs can arise from a number of conditions, and there is an opportunity to integrate programmes such as CDD and ARI into a more holistic package. The IMCI strategy has three components:

- Improving the skills of health personnel in the prevention and treatment of childhood illness
- Improving health systems to deliver quality care
- Improving family and community practices in relation to child health.

The introductory phase involves orientation of country decision-makers, creation of the necessary management structure, and extensive discussions with ministries of health. A national strategy is devised, IMCI guidelines are adapted for local use, and activities begin in a number of districts. These activities generally involve training of healthcare workers, health system strengthening and dialogue with communities about child health problems.

From a clinical point of view, health workers are trained to approach the sick child systematically: to check initially for danger signs, assess the main symptoms, assess nutrition and immunization status and feeding problems, and check for other problems. This allows classification into one of three groups: children who need urgent referral, children who can be managed at an outpatient health facility and children who can be managed at home. The first dose of treatment is given on site and the health worker counsels the family on subsequent treatment and follow-up. This systematic approach improves the quality of care, provider morale and client satisfaction. It also leads to more rational drug use.

http://www.who.int/child-adolescent-health/integr.htm

IMCI integrated approach to the management of childhood illness

Major infections

Malaria

Around 90% of the 1 million annual deaths from malaria occur in sub-Saharan Africa, mostly in pregnant women and children under 5. Malaria morbidity and mortality have actually increased over the last decade. In areas of low endemicity where immunity is not usually acquired, malaria during pregnancy doubles or triples the risk of death. In areas of high endemicity, infection during pregnancy tends to exacerbate anaemia and is associated with low birth weight in infants. About 500 000 African children develop cerebral malaria each year, of whom up to 20% die and about 7% are left with permanent neurological damage.

The 'Roll Back Malaria' campaign, launched in 1998, aims to halve the deaths from malaria by 2010. The key interventions for reducing malarial deaths are preventive — bed nets, particularly when treated with insecticides, household insecticide spraying — and therapeutic — treatment with standard drugs, and particularly artemisinin derivatives for resistant strains of *Plasmodium falciparum*. Although insecticide-treated bed nets are effective, increasing their usage has been problematic. At present, less than a fifth of children in Africa sleep under a net and as few as 2% sleep under a net that has been impregnated with insecticide. A growing threat is that of resistance in the *P. falciparum* parasite. Chloroquine resistance is now the norm in much of Africa and resistance to sulfadoxine–pyrimethamine is increasing. Combination therapy, including artemisinin derivatives, is now widely recommended but there are serious cost issues unless it is subsidized. Pregnant women can be offered intermittent preventive treatment with at least two doses of antimalarial to reduce the burden of placental infection and low birth weight.

HIV/AIDS (see also p. 633)

About 2 million children are currently living with HIV, 1.9 million of them in Africa. About half a million children die each year from complications of HIV/AIDS. Around 90% of HIV infections in children are acquired perinatally. About a third of perinatally infected children do not reach 1 year of age, and over half die before the age of 2. Progression is generally more rapid in children than in adults. Recurrent bacterial infections are common, HIV viral loads tend to be higher and opportunistic infections tend to be more aggressive. HIV/AIDS is cutting a swathe through the developing world, decimating the population of working age — including healthcare workers and schoolteachers — and leaving a growing pool of orphans in the care of overstretched communities and the elderly. Current initiatives include a drive towards having one agreed national HIV/AIDS action framework, one national AIDS authority and one country-level monitoring system.

Voluntary counselling and testing (VCT) acts as an entry point for HIV prevention and care, and is particularly important so that women can be offered treatment to prevent perinatal mother-to-child transmission (PMTCT). Untreated, the transmission rate of HIV-1 is about 35%. About half of this is explained by breastfeeding, another tranche by perinatal transmission and a smaller proportion by transmission in utero. Risk factors for PMTCT include new infection in mothers, high plasma viral loads, advanced disease, breast problems and prolonged breastfeeding. It is also possible that exclusive breastfeeding poses less of a risk than mixed feeding with breast milk and other liquids or solids.

There are four important ways to prevent MTCT. The first is to prevent a woman from ever acquiring the virus, through self-determination and safe sex. In the event of infection, MTCT can be reduced by operative delivery, by prophylactic antiretroviral therapy, and by changes in breastfeeding practice. In places where a woman receives zidovudine from 28 weeks' gestation onward, both mother and baby receive one dose of oral nevirapine and breastfeeding is avoided, transmission rates are as low as 1%.

Breastfeeding is the most controversial current issue. Attitudes vary since, on the one hand, breastfeeding may lead to around 300 000 HIV infections each year, and on the other hand, breastfeeding may prevent up to 1.5 million child deaths each year. The best analyses suggest that the risk of transmission increases by about 4% for every 6 months of breastfeeding.

Strategies to reduce PMTCT of HIV through breastfeeding in poor settings

- Exclusive breastfeeding during the first 6 months
- Shortening the duration of breastfeeding to about 6 months
- Good lactation management to avoid problems such as cracked nipples, engorgement and mastitis
- If a mother develops mastitis or abscesses, frequent expression of milk from the affected side (the mother should discard this milk, continuing feeding from the unaffected side)
- Use of condoms throughout the lactation period

- Encouragement of mothers with AIDS or low CD4 counts to replacement-feed
- Support for replacement feeding, if it is chosen.

Tuberculosis (see also p. 640)

Someone in the world is infected with *Mycobacterium tuberculosis* every second, someone dies from tuberculosis every 15 seconds and a third of all deaths are in children. The WHO declared tuberculosis a global emergency in 1993. Around 3.6 million cases are notified annually but the true incidence may reach 10 million.

Tuberculosis is difficult to diagnose in children; symptoms and signs are less specific, sputum samples are hard to get, and tuberculin test responsiveness is diminished with malnutrition and HIV/AIDS. Induced sputum may be useful and rapid T cell antigen tests are under trial. BCG vaccine is of variable utility. It reduces the incidence of meningeal and miliary tuberculosis by about 75% in infants and children and probably protects against *M. leprae*, but does not reduce the population prevalence of infection.

The current aim is therefore to treat infected people through case-finding and treatment, which will in turn protect children from exposure. The WHO strategy relies on diagnosis via sputum smear microscopy and short-course directly observed therapy (DOTS) with a standardized regimen. In a typical case, therapy would last for 6 months: 2 months of a daily four-drug regimen followed by 4 months of a thrice-weekly two-drug regimen. Presently, about 30% of people diagnosed with tuberculosis receive DOTS management.

Two major concerns for tuberculosis control are HIV/AIDS and the development of multidrug-resistant tuberculosis (MDR-TB). Development of active tuberculosis is anything from six to 100 times more likely in the presence of HIV infection. In sub-Saharan Africa, 70% of people with AIDS develop tuberculosis, and — conversely — progression of HIV/AIDS accelerates in the presence of tuberculosis. HIV/AIDS also modifies the clinical picture of tuberculosis (the 'new tuberculosis'). Extrapulmonary disease is more common, sputum smear microscopy and tuberculin tests are more often negative, and chest X-rays often atypical. Although treatment regimens are similar, case fatality rates are higher, and drug interactions and adverse effects are more common. The rise of MDR-TB has been mapped to a number of global hot spots in which its prevalence is over 3%, although in some areas it reaches 30%. Standardization of treatment is recommended in order to:

- Reduce the exposure of *M. tuberculosis* to a wide range of drugs
- Ensure drugs are used in combination and not singly
- Optimize cure rates.

Neonatal health

Problem-orientated topic:

neonatal health and care outside Europe ● ● ● ● ●

You are representing your department at an international meeting on newborn health and care at the WHO in Geneva. Before attending the meeting, you are keen to find out more about the problems of neonatal health outside Europe.

Q1. What is the burden of neonatal disease in the developing world?

Q2. What are the major causes of global newborn mortality?

Q3. What are the causes and consequences of being born with a low birth weight? What risks does a low birth weight present to an infant?

Q4. What are the essential principles of newborn care worldwide?

Q5. How might neonatal mortality be reduced in settings where resources are extremely limited and there is no access to neonatal units in hospitals? What is meant by 'levels of care'?

Q1. What is the burden of neonatal disease in the developing world?

Of the 130 million babies born every year, about 4 million die in the first 4 weeks of life: the neonatal period. A similar number of babies are stillborn, i.e. they die in the last 4 months of pregnancy. About half a million mothers also die from the complications of pregnancy and childbirth. Almost all maternal and neonatal deaths (99%) occur in low- or middle-income countries rather than the wealthy industrialized world, and about half occur at home. Three-quarters of deaths occur in the first week, and the highest risk is on the first day after birth.

Q2. What are the major causes of global newborn mortality?

Globally the three main causes of death are estimated to be preterm birth (28%), severe infections (26%) and asphyxia (23%). Neonatal tetanus accounts for a much smaller proportion of deaths but is easily preventable through maternal vaccination. Other infections include newborn septicaemia resulting from an unhygienic delivery or poor cord care, and pneumonia. Malaria exerts a more indirect effect in pregnancy by increasing the risk of low birth weight and stillbirth.

Asphyxia refers to an impairment of exchange of respiratory gases (oxygen and carbon dioxide), leading to neurological impairment in the newborn infant. Most commonly asphyxia results from a delayed or obstructed labour, or from failure of a birth attendant to resuscitate or assist breathing adequately after birth. The best way of assessing the severity of birth asphyxia in a newborn infant is to use a clinical scoring method to grade the severity of neonatal encephalopathy (grade 1, mild; grade 2, moderate; and grade 3, severe). There have been few studies on the epidemiology of asphyxia and encephalopathy in the developing world, but these show fresh stillbirth rates are 10–20 times higher than in rich countries, that encephalopathy rates are 2–3 times higher, and that survival of moderately or severely encephalopathic infants is poor.

Preterm birth rather than growth retardation, is probably the biggest risk to a newborn infant. Being born 1 or 2 months before the due date hugely increases the risk of newborn death in communities where special nursing care for low-birth weight babies is not available. Another indirect cause of neonatal deaths is hypothermia, which occurs throughout the world and in all climates, and is due to lack of knowledge rather than lack of equipment. Less than 5% die from other causes such as jaundice and haemolytic disease of the newborn. It is important to appreciate that a death may result from multiple causes, and the assignment of cause of death in the neonatal period is extremely difficult.

Direct causes of stillbirths include hypoxia during labour, asphyxia during delivery, infections such as HIV, malaria, maternal syphilis and chorioamnionitis, and congenital anomalies.

Q3. What are the causes and consequences of being born with a low birth weight? What risks does a low birth weight present to an infant?

Amongst the indirect causes of neonatal and perinatal death low birth weight, a weight of less than 2.5 kg at birth is the most important. Causes of low birth weight are complex and often stem from the effects of poverty in past generations. An important factor is the health and nutrition of the mother and other risk factors include untreated maternal infections, demanding physical work, the use of smoking, alcohol and drugs, and short inter-pregnancy intervals.

Low birth weight increases the risk of neonatal death and also the risk of complications later in pregnancy. More recently, researchers have identified a link between fetal and infant growth and the risk of diseases in adult life such as hypertension, ischaemic heart disease and diabetes. Programming of fetal physiology such as cortisol secretion in response to stress, insulin resistance and vascular responsiveness are thought to be some of the underlying mechanisms.

Q5. How might neonatal mortality be reduced in settings where resources are extremely limited and there is no access to neonatal units in hospitals? What is meant by 'levels of care'?

It is often believed, mistakenly, that good newborn care requires specialist units, high technology and expensive resources. In fact the principles of essential newborn care were laid down by Pierre Budin, a French obstetrician, in 1905 (Box 37.2). These principles can be implemented by mothers or health workers in the home or health centre, without access to expensive technology.

The top priority is to maintain an airway through clearance of secretions or by lying the baby on his or her side or in a prone position. Gentle stimulation of the baby may initiate breathing if there is apnoea. Some programmes have shown that primary care workers or even traditional birth attendants can be trained to conduct resuscitation of an apnoeic infant using a tube and mask or a bag and mask.

The most effective and reliable way to maintain body temperature and prevent hypothermia is to nurse the baby, skin-to-skin, on the mother's chest, the warmest part of her body. This has the added advantage of improving the chance of early breastfeeding. Skin-to-skin nursing has been shown to be more effective than incubator management in maintaining a steady body temperature, except in situations where the baby is sick or unstable.

Exclusive breastfeeding provides all nutritional needs, protects against infection, boosts passive immunity through immunoglobulins in colostrum, promotes thermal care and bonding with the mother as well as excellent growth in infancy. There are serious risks in

BOX 37.2 Principles of essential newborn care

Air	Maintain airway
Warmth	Keep warm
Love	Keep with mother
Food	Feed frequently, breastfeed immediately, avoid pre-lacteals
Hygiene	Avoid infection
Illness	Treat promptly

BOX 37.3 Interventions to reduce neonatal mortality

During pregnancy
- Tetanus toxoid
- Iron and folate supplementation
- Insecticide-treated bed nets and intermittent treatment for malaria
- Dietary supplements
- Birth preparedness
- Screening for and treatment of sexually transmitted infections (STIs) and HIV
- Antiretroviral treatment to prevent mother-to-child transmission (MTCT) of HIV

During childbirth
- A companion
- A skilled attendant
- Caesarean for obstructed labour
- Safe delivery kits
- Tube and mask resuscitation using air not oxygen
- Nevirapine to reduce MTCT

During the newborn period
- Drying and wrapping; skin-to-skin 'kangaroo care'; avoidance of early baths
- Early breastfeeding and colostrum
- Clean cord care
- Antibiotics for infants with signs of sepsis
- Avoid separation from mother

formula feeding in poor communities where water supplies are unsafe and illiteracy high. Failure to thrive, gastroenteritis and death are markedly increased in non-breastfed infants.

Hygiene is a critical element in reducing perinatal sepsis for both mothers and infants. A clean surface for delivery, hand-washing by birth attendants and clean cutting of the cord will prevent a large number of unnecessary deaths. A recent cluster randomized controlled trial of training traditional birth attendants in Pakistan showed a reduction in perinatal mortality and a large diminution in perinatal sepsis.

There are many potential low-cost and evidence-based interventions available to reduce newborn mortality. The challenge is how to implement these interventions on a large scale, reaching out to the families who are most at risk, particularly those where home delivery is the norm and access to obstetric and medical services is difficult (Box 37.3).

Levels of perinatal care (Box 37.4)

It is important to establish what should be the minimum standards of care at each level of a health system.

World Bank studies show that, in most developing countries, more than 90% of women living in the poorest quintile of households deliver their babies at home, usually with only a relative or a traditional birth attendant. The care provided at level 1 is therefore extremely important if neonatal mortality rates are to be reduced. In India a controlled, though not randomized, trial showed that mortality fell by 62% in villages where a home-based care package was introduced involving traditional birth attendant training, health education and the use of village women trained to detect and manage neonatal sepsis using injectable antibiotics in the home. In Nepal, a cluster randomized controlled trial of a participatory intervention involving women's groups addressed maternal and newborn health problems in a large rural population. The women's groups showed astonishing creativity and self-organizing capacity. They developed their own delivery kits, stretcher schemes, emergency funds and discussion groups using picture cards for illiterate women. After 2 years, even though health services remained weak, newborn mortality fell by one-third and maternal deaths by three-quarters. The cost of this demand-side intervention was just $0.75 per head.

http://www.child.ich.ucl.ac.uk

UCL Centre for International Health and Development

Nutrition and malnutrition

Causes of malnutrition

Malnutrition is essentially the end result of the interaction of three factors: diet, diseases and care.

Diet

Dietary intake should be assessed for macronutrient and micronutrient content and quality. Macronutrient intake comes from carbohydrate, fat and protein; the protein:energy ratio should exceed 15%. Micronutrients come from specific foods such as green leafy vegetables and carotene-containing fruits for vitamin A, meat for iron and fish for zinc. Poor dietary intake is caused by:

- *Inadequate nutritional knowledge*: parents/carers may not know what foods children need. Peer culture and food taboos are affected by commercial pressures/advertising.
- *Poverty*: nutritional knowledge may be adequate but poverty prevents parents/carers from purchasing foods that enable satisfactory growth and health of children.
- *Political factors*: wars prevent access to food.
- *Psychological factors*: anorexia nervosa.

http://ivacg.ilsi.org/

International Vitamin A Consultative Group

http://www.sphereproject.org/

Sphere Project Training of Trainers courses

Disease

Illnesses such as pertussis, otitis media, inflammatory bowel disease and cystic fibrosis and infections such as tuberculosis, HIV and persistent diarrhoea are often complicated by or contribute to malnutrition. There are several mechanisms:

- *Poor dietary intake*: painful mouth, cough and systemic infection (leading to elevated inflammatory cytokines that cause anorexia) prevent adequate food intake.
- *Malabsorption*: persistent diarrhoea (e.g. in coeliac disease and *Giardia* infection) causes malabsorption of fat and fat-soluble vitamins. High-lactose diets contribute to diarrhoea in clinical lactase deficiency.
- *Increased nutrient requirements*: energy expenditure is increased in systemic infection by around 10% for each degree Celsius rise in body temperature.
- *Metabolic responses*: inflammatory response causes reduction of plasma levels of micronutrients including vitamin A and zinc, and liver transport proteins such as albumin and retinol binding protein. Catabolic responses cause muscle breakdown and increased urinary nutrient loss.

Care

Lack of time and/or compassion lead to inadequate nutritional intake. A poor social environment at home where nurturing is absent, or an unsupportive feeding/nutrition culture in hospital/clinic causes malnutrition, especially if the patient has anorexia.

Diagnosis

Certain malnutrition syndromes have specific clinical signs such as severe malnutrition (previously called protein energy malnutrition) or deficiency of vitamin A, iodine or vitamin D. However, the majority of children have subclinical malnutrition.

http://indorgs.virginia.edu/iccidd/

International Council for the Control of Iodine Deficiency Disorders

Subclinical malnutrition

Diagnosing this form of malnutrition requires the use of anthropometric measurements and blood assays. Interpretation of blood assays in subclinical micronutrient malnutrition is difficult because of the variation in plasma levels of micronutrients such as retinol or zinc that occurs in inflammation. Evidence that a micronutrient deficiency is present in a population comes mainly from trials of micronutrient interventions, which have shown the impact of vitamin A deficiency on eye disease and mortality and the impact of zinc deficiency on diarrhoeal disease and mortality. Even children with satisfactory anthropometric indices (weight and height against international standards for their age) may have subclinical micronutrient malnutrition.

Severe acute malnutrition (SAM)

SAM is defined as the presence of pedal oedema or severe wasting (below 3 SD weight for height standard or below 70% median weight/height standard). There are several clinical syndromes:

- *Marasmus* is characterized by severe visible wasting with lack of body fat and loss of muscle mass around the arms, buttocks and thighs.
- *Kwashiorkor* involves severe pedal oedema, sometimes spreading all over the body and often associated with cracking of the skin; there may be discoloration of the hair in kwashiorkor. Plasma albumin is lower in kwashiorkor than in marasmus.

Causes

- Poor dietary intake of energy, protein and micronutrients
- Precipitating infection such as measles, persistent diarrhoea, tuberculosis and HIV
- Early cessation of breastfeeding
- Psychosocial stress within family.

Clinical features

- Poor resistance to infection, especially pneumonia, diarrhoea and tuberculosis

- Hypothermia
- Hypoglycaemia
- Dehydration: often under-diagnosed in kwashiorkor because of interstitial fluid and over-diagnosed in marasmus because of loss of skin elasticity
- Metabolic problems: decreased inability to excrete sodium adequately and tendency to develop fluid overload, leading to cardiac failure.

Prevention

Improving household food security, nutrition knowledge and care in poor communities is vital, as are promoting family hygiene and sanitation, ensuring immunizations and deworming, encouraging early treatment for childhood illnesses and protecting children in adverse circumstances, including political crises, wars and famines.

Management

1. *Initial stabilization phase* (1–7 days). This involves treatment of fluid and electrolyte imbalance and sepsis, corneal ulceration due to vitamin A deficiency, severe anaemia, hypoglycaemia, hypothermia and infection. Infections are difficult to diagnose on clinical grounds, as signs are less striking in SAM. All children with SAM should receive a broad-spectrum antibiotic. Refeeding starts with small frequent meals of low osmolality and low lactose providing around 75 kcal/kg body weight/day until oedema clears.

2. *Catch-up growth*. This requires at least 100 kcal/kg body weight/day for at least 2–6 weeks. Avoid over-feeding, which may precipitate cardiac failure. Use low-sodium rehydration solutions (60 mmol). Home treatment with micronutrient-fortified ready-to-use therapeutic foods, such as Plumpy'nut®, is nowadays recommended by WHO and several other UN organizations.

3. *Follow-up*. It is important to maintain an adequate dietary intake once the child is at home. Ready-to-use therapeutic feeds can be made up using local mixes of groundnuts, sugar, oil and micronutrients in heat-sealed bags, which can be given to mothers during regular visits to the nutrition unit for checking that weight gain is maintained. Sensory stimulation and emotional support are important to ensure recovery of child development. Rates of weight gain during the rehabilitation phase can exceed the normal (1 g/kg body weight/day) for children between 1 and 5 years. Weight gain of at least 5–10 g/kg body weight/day should be achieved. SAM is increasingly precipitated by HIV and antiretroviral drugs may be used.

Table 37.4 Deficiency syndromes, their causes and management

Deficiency	Clinical features	Prevention/treatment
Vitamin A	Xerophthalmia in severe cases Night blindness Reduced immunity	Mango, papaya, yellow sweet potatoes, carrots, palm oil
Zinc	Subclinical deficiency common Acrodermatitis enteropathica	Fish and meat Attention to cooking methods to reduce phytate levels
Thiamine	Beri-beri (peripheral neuropathy and cardiac failure)	Thiamine i.m. for beri-beri
Riboflavin	Angular stomatitis Anaemia	Avoid over-reliance on cereals Riboflavin orally
Niacin	Diarrhoea, dermatitis and dementia	Varied diet Thiamine orally
Vitamin C	Clinical signs rare (scurvy)	Ensure fruit in diet and avoid excessive boiling of vegetables
Iodine	Goitre, intellectual loss Poor growth	Supplement with iodine to combat deficiency in soil Treat with iodized salt
Iron	Anaemia in severe cases Impaired psychomotor development	Meat eating
Vitamin D	Rickets	Ensure adequate exposure to light
Folic acid	Megaloblastic anaemia Atrophic glossitis	Treat with folic acid

Deficiency syndromes

Disease or disability may arise as a result of a number of specific deficiency syndromes or a combination of multiple deficiency disorders. Table 37.4 lists the major features of deficiency syndromes.

 http://www.ennonline.net

Emergency Nutrition Network

http://www.who.int/child-adolescent-health/publications/CHILD_HEALTH/WHO_FCH_CAH_00.1.htm

Management of the child with a serious infection or severe malnutrition

Children in difficult circumstances (CDCs)

Who are CDCs?

The term 'children in difficult circumstances' describes a number of different categories of children who, as the name implies, live in difficult or extreme situations. The terminology in this area varies between countries and organizations, something you need to be aware of for Web searches. The other names frequently used for CDCs are shown in Box 37.5.

The major groups generally classified as CDCs are:
- Children living and working on the street
- Child workers

BOX 37.5 Other names for children in difficult circumstances

- Children in especially difficult circumstances (CEDCs)
- Children in special circumstances (CSCs)
- Children in need of special protection (CNSP)
- Children at risk
- Vulnerable children
- Orphans and vulnerable children, made vulnerable through HIV (OVC)

- Orphans (usually now defined as having lost one or both parents)
- Children living with HIV
- Refugees and migrants
- Child soldiers
- Sexually abused and exploited children (including those involved in prostitution and pornography).

Some countries and organizations would also include:
- Children in custodial care
- Children of imprisoned mothers
- Child/adolescent mothers
- Child carers
- Children of substance-abusing parents
- Children of parents with learning difficulties.

There is, however, considerable overlap between many of these groups. For example, nearly all street children are also working children and being in one group makes a child vulnerable to other forms of exploitation. For example, orphans are more likely to end up living and working on the street or in child labour, and girls in domestic service are particularly vulnerable to physical and sexual abuse.

We should not assume, however, that difficult circumstances are always harmful to children. Children respond very differently to adverse circumstances. Some children gain strength and resilience as a result of adverse situations. For many the circumstances will be the norm in their experience. For example, many children in poor communities would expect to work throughout childhood alongside their peers.

How many children are involved?

We know that huge numbers of children around the world can be classified as CDCs but it is very difficult to estimate actual figures for several reasons:

- In the countries where the numbers are greatest, information collection systems are usually very poor.
- Many of the activities of CDCs are illegal and hence hidden.
- Governments are not motivated to reveal real figures, even if they had them, for fear of criticism.

Furthermore, where figures are available, they are rarely disaggregated by age and sex, which are both key determinants in terms of vulnerability, exploitation and risk of long-term damage. For example, it may be quite acceptable for a 16-year-old to work on a plantation, but it is certainly not acceptable for a 6-year-old.

So, although global and national estimates should be treated with caution, they do give some indication of the magnitude of the problems. Some official estimates, mainly sourced from UN organizations, are shown in Box 37.6.

An influential UNICEF report has helped us to understand the impact on children of war alone. The report (UNICEF 2000) looked at the effect of wars from 1986 to 1996 and found that:

- 2 million children were killed
- 6 million children were injured
- 12 million children were made homeless
- > 1 million children were orphaned or separated from their parents.

What are the causes of difficult circumstances?

Clearly the causes are multifactorial and will vary by situation and country. The major causes are:

BOX 37.6 Some global estimates for children in difficult circumstances

- 210 million children aged 5–14 economically active (International Labour Organization (ILO) 2004)
- 110 million children aged 5–14 involved in hazardous or intolerable labour (ILO 2004)
- 10 million–100 million street children (depending on definition) (United Nations Children's Fund (UNICEF) 1998)
- 10 million children involved in the sex industry (UNICEF 2003)
- 300 000 children used in armed conflict (ILO 2003)
- 14 million children have lost one or both parents to HIV/AIDS (Joint United Nations Programme on HIV/AIDS (UNAIDS) 2004)

- Poverty
- Disruption of family and support systems:
  - Conflict
  - Urbanization (rural to urban migration)
  - Children separated from families to seek work
- Deficiencies in the educational system: inaccessible, unaffordable and poor-quality schooling
- Ineffective enforcement of relevant legislation.

What is the relevant legislation?

In most countries this is based on the UN Convention on the Rights of the Child (UNCRC, 1989). This has been a highly influential document in defining rights of all children (defined as under the age of 18) around the world. All but two countries (the US and Somalia) have ratified the Convention and most have incorporated much of the content into national legislature.

The UNCRC has 41 articles, which set standards for the rights of all children to survive, develop, be protected and participate fully in society. Articles include guarantees of:

- Health, education and care
- Protection from violence
- Protection from economic exploitation.

There are also important optional protocols on involvement of children in armed conflict and the sale of children for prostitution and pornography.

Clearly many governments cannot guarantee these rights, partly because of resource constraints, but all signatory countries report to the UN Committee on the Rights of the Child and they need to demonstrate progress at least towards meeting the obligations and standards in UNCRC.

http://www.unicef.org/crc

Full text of the UNCRC

Examples of CDCs

There are clearly many CDCs in Europe, but here we are going to focus on the two largest groups from a global perspective: working children, and children who live and work on the street.

Working children

Child labour is defined by the ILO as all economic activities carried out by persons less than 15 regardless of their occupational status, except household work in the parents' or carers' home. An estimated 210 million children under the age of 15 (or 20% of all children in the age group) are involved in some form of economic activity. Around 120 million work full-time while the rest combine work with some form of education. The highest prevalence of child work is in sub-Saharan Africa, where around 40% of all children are primarily involved in work. This compares with around 25% in Asia and 12% in Latin America.

What work do children do?

The major categories of child work are shown in Box 37.7.

Agriculture is clearly by far the most common form of child work, and children in rural areas are twice as likely to be working than children in urban areas. Agricultural work ranges from (usually unpaid) work on family land to plantation work within the formal sector.

Child labour is a necessity for many poor families, who rely on the income or help provided by their children to survive. This fact is acknowledged in the legislative framework for child labour, which is based on the UNCRC. What the legislation now recognizes is that abolition of child labour is not realistic in the foreseeable future, but that policy approaches should instead target work that is harmful to children for early

BOX 37.7 Types of child work	
Agriculture	70%
Domestic work	15%
Manufacturing	8%
Transport	4%
Construction	2%
Mining and quarrying	1%

(Data from 26 countries, ILO 2003)

BOX 37.8 Potential health hazards of child labour

General
- Exhaustion, abuse, loss of educational opportunity*

Agricultural work
- Injuries, pesticides, parasitic diseases, heat

Mining/construction
- Accidents, respiratory illness, musculoskeletal problems

Manufacturing
- Injuries, hearing loss, exposure to toxins/solvents

Domestic service
- Physical/sexual abuse

Street work
- Road traffic injuries, violence, substance abuse

Sex work
- STIs/HIV, violence

* Loss of educational opportunity leads indirectly to poor long-term health, partly through lower earning power, lower socioeconomic status and lower health knowledge. This health disadvantage is now known to extend to the next generation. The education of women is particularly important in improving health outcomes for children.

intervention. Harmful in this context means work that is likely to harm the health, safety or morals of children. Clearly the health of children is crucial to this definition

What are the health effects of child labour?

There is poor evidence of harm to health in many sectors of child labour (partly because of lack of systematic rigorous studies) but we can make certain assumptions (Box 37.8).

http://www.ilo.org/public/english/support/publ/chilwork.pdf

'Children at Work: Health and Safety Risks': a good summary of the potential health hazards

Three final points demonstrate the difficulties in trying to improve conditions for children who have to work:
- Workplace regulations often apply only to employees in the formal sector and most children work in the informal sector.
- Because children are 'not allowed' to work there is often no legislation to protect them from the more hazardous tasks.

Children *of* the streets
- Street is the child's home
- Seek shelter, food, companionship among other street dwellers
- Abandoned, orphaned, runaways
- Relatively small numbers, probably less than 10% of the total

Children *on* the streets
- Have family connections
- Go home (family/extended family/caring adult) to sleep
- Just work on the street

- For the same reason protective clothing and devices are often simply not made in child sizes.

Children who live and work on the street

This is the preferred term for what used to be known as street children (although street children is still used as a shorthand). They are defined as children who live or spend time on the streets, supporting themselves and/ or their families through various occupations, and who are inadequately cared for/supervised by caring adults.

The reason that the estimates of their numbers vary hugely (from 10 million to 100 million) is partly because of the different classifications used. They are usually divided into two categories: children of the streets and children on the streets. The characteristics of the two groups are shown in Box 37.9.

The largest numbers of street children are in Latin America (an estimated 40 million), followed by Asia with 30 million and Africa with 10 million. Boys outnumber girls by a factor of around 10 to 1.

What jobs do street children do?
- Begging
- Hawking to pedestrians, motorists
- Directing vehicles to parking areas for a tip
- Guarding vehicles for a tip
- Selling drugs
- Petty crime
- Collecting paper/rubbish
- Shoe shining
- Girls: mostly begging and prostitution.

What are the health risks for street children?
- Infectious disease, especially gastrointestinal disorders and skin conditions

- Population c. 87 million
- 2.4 million children on the streets
- 70% go home every night
- 5% completely abandoned
- 25% intermittent home support
- 5.5 million children (aged 5–14) in the labour market
- At least 500 000 girls under 15 in domestic service (ILO 2000)
- 60% exposed to hazardous work: 20% biological, 26% chemical, 51% environmental

- Substance misuse: alcohol, tobacco, cannabis, cocaine and especially solvents
- Mental disorders
- Violence
- Poor nutrition
- Limited access to healthcare
- STIs/HIV
- Pregnancy.

Pregnancy has led to the phenomenon of a second generation on the streets of many cities.

A country example

The Philippines is an example of a country with large numbers of working and street children (Box 37.10).

http://www.ilo.org

ILO: International Programme for the Elimination of Child Labour (IPEC)

http://www.streetchildren.org.uk/

An excellent starting point for information on street children

http://www.ucw-project.org

The Understanding Children's Work group, a collaboration of the ILO, UNICEF and the World Bank

http://www.unicef.org

Useful information about all types of CDC; now UNICEF collects specific data on child protection

Edited by Martin Ward Platt, Alfred Tenore

Childhood Disorders II

MODULE SEVEN

David Branski   Susan Bunn   Stephen Hodges

Gastroenterology and hepatology

LEARNING OUTCOMES

By the end of this chapter you should:

- Know and understand the basic science of bowel function
- Know and understand the common methods for investigating the gastrointestinal tract
- Know and understand the causes and management of common paediatric disorders affecting the bowel
- Know and understand the investigation and management of the common liver disorders.

Diagnostic investigations

In assessing a child for gastrointestinal conditions a careful and thorough history and examination are crucial (Ch. 5).

The tests undertaken can then be approached systematically. Blood tests may be helpful, but abnormalities are usually non-specific and not diagnostic. A diagnosis will generally be confirmed by a series of relevant tests or targeted therapeutic trials.

An ideal test is sensitive, specific, simple, inexpensive, safe, non-invasive, convenient, acceptable to patients and staff, objective, reliable and amenable to serial measurements to permit the assessment of therapeutic interventions. There are no such tests in paediatric gastroenterology, so a number of tests are often used and those chosen for a specific clinical scenario may differ between centres. General principles and applications are discussed below.

Oesophageal pH monitoring

Oesophageal pH monitoring permits the assessment of the frequency and duration of oesophageal acid exposure and its relationship to symptoms. A pH study monitors intra-oesophageal pH, usually over a period of 24 hours. It can be combined with heart rate and saturation monitoring in a young child to investigate whether respiratory events are associated with gastro-oesophageal reflux (GOR).

A pH study is a safe test, but it is invasive and keeping the probe in place may be difficult in toddlers and uncooperative children. It should therefore only be undertaken if the results will influence management.

The test is performed by the transnasal passage of a microelectrode containing a pH sensor into the lower oesophagus. Its position is usually confirmed radiologically. The child is encouraged to eat, drink and continue as near normal activities as possible during the study. The time of any drinks or meals is recorded so that their effect on the study can be assessed. If the study is being performed to see if other clinical features are associated with GOR (coughing, abnormal movements, crying, pain etc.), then the child or carer is asked to record the time of any of these events during the study. The pH data are recorded on to a portable recording device, from which they are downloaded on to a computer and analysed by software programmes. Usually a graph of intra-oesophageal pH against time is produced, on which meals and 'clinical events' can be shown (Fig. 38.1). The 'reflux index' (the percentage of the study in which intra-oesophageal pH is < 4) estimates the total acid exposure time and is considered the most sensitive and specific measure. A reflux index of up to 12% in the first year of life and up to 6% thereafter is considered normal. An abnormal reflux index is found in 95% of children with oesophagitis but the reflux index does not correlate with the severity of oesophagitis. Additionally, it should be remembered that not all children with significant GOR have oesophagitis. The time taken for acid to be cleared from the oesophagus after a reflux episode can also be assessed by a pH study as a proxy for oesophageal motility.

Limitations of the pH study

It is not a diagnostic test for GOR, as any cause of vomiting can cause an abnormal study. Likewise, a negative test does not exclude GOR, as only acid reflux episodes are detected. Postprandial GOR in particular is missed, as the gastric acid is buffered by foodstuffs and the refluxate tends to have a neutral pH. This can be overcome somewhat by using a dual probe technique (a lower and upper pH probe, the lower probe being placed in the stomach and the upper in the lower oesophagus — hence times can be identified when the intragastric pH is neutral and GOR would not be detected). Some centres also advocate that one feed with a relatively low pH (usually apple juice) is given over the study period so that an increase in postprandial reflux can be identified. Another option to overcome these problems is by using multichannel intraluminal impedance and pH monitoring, which detects non-acid reflux as well.

Situations in which a pH study is most helpful

A pH study is useful in determining whether symptoms such as pain, crying and abnormal movements (Sandifer

syndrome) are associated with acid reflux or whether GOR could be contributing to airway complications. It also has a place in assessing the adequacy of acid suppression in children who remain symptomatic despite being treated with a proton pump inhibitor (PPI).

Radiological contrast studies of the gastrointestinal tract

Radiological contrast studies of the gastrointestinal tract play an important role in assessing a child with gastrointestinal symptoms, but like the pH study they also have their limitations. All involve a significant radiation exposure, and some are invasive and unpleasant for the child. Before requesting a contrast study consideration has to be given as to whether it is the best test available to answer the clinical question posed. Contrast studies are particularly good at assessing for anatomical abnormalities causing symptoms. The commonly used contrast studies and their more usual indications are summarized in Table 38.1.

Hydrogen breath tests

The principle of the H_2 breath test is that any undigested/malabsorbed sugar that reaches a part of the gastrointestinal tract that has organisms within the lumen (most usually the colon but also the small bowel in small bowel overgrowth) is then fermented by the organisms, producing H_2, which is excreted in the breath. The breath H_2 monitor is a small hand-held device into which the older child simply exhales. In a younger child breath can be collected by the use of a face mask. Breath H_2 is plotted against time from carbohydrate ingestion on a graph. The normal small bowel transit time is considered to be approximately 2 hours, such that an increase in breath H_2 at baseline or before 2 hours suggests small bowel fermentation and overgrowth, and after 2 hours colonic fermentation due to sugar maldigestion/malabsorption.

If sugar maldigestion/malabsorption is suspected (for example, lactose), then the candidate sugar is given as an oral bolus after fasting. The study would start with two baseline readings at −30 mins and 0 mins, and then the sugar is administrated at time 0. Breath H_2 is measured every 30 minutes for 3 hours. Figure 38.2A shows a normal H_2 breath test in red, where there is no increase in breath H_2, as no significant amount of sugar has reached the colon. The results shown in blue are an abnormal H_2 breath test that suggests sugar malabsorption/maldigestion, as there is an increase in breath H_2 after 2 hours when the malabsorbed/maldigested sugar is fermented by colonic bacteria. Figure 38.2B shows a lactulose H_2 breath test, which is the preferred test for small bowel overgrowth. As lactulose

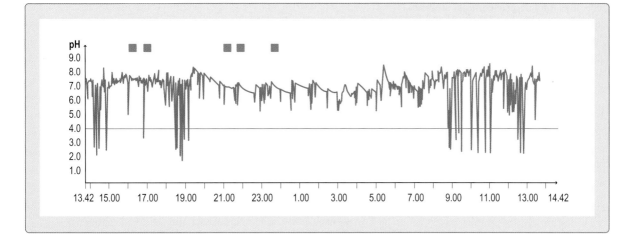

Period table			
Item		Total	Upright
Duration of period	(HH:MM)	24:00	24:00
Number of acid refluxes	(#)	31	31
Number of long acid refluxes	(#)	0	0
Longest acid reflux	(min)	1	1
Total time pH below 4.00	(min)	12	12
Fraction time pH below 4.00	(%)	0.8	0.8

■ Episodes of chest pain
(chest pain not related to
reflux events)

A

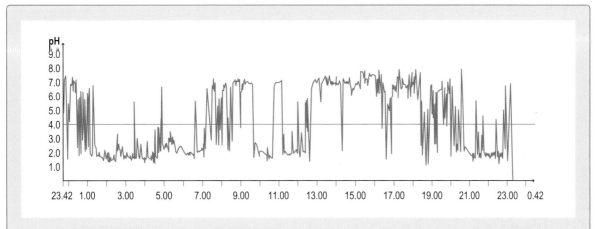

Period table		
Item		Total
Duration of period	(HH:MM)	23:40
Number of acid refluxes	(#)	392
Number of long acid refluxes	(#)	28
Longest acid reflux	(min)	37
Total time pH below 4.00	(min)	603
Fraction time pH below 4.00	(%)	42.4

B

Fig. 38.1 Results of a pH probe.
(A) Normal pH study in a 12-year-old boy with episodic chest pain. His chest pain is not associated with his (normal) reflux events; (B) pH study in an 8-year-old child with neurodevelopmental delay, showing severe gastro-oesophageal reflux (GOR). She has a reflux index of 42.4% and poor oesophageal clearance of acid, shown by numerous long acid reflux events, the longest being 32 minutes.

Table 38.1 **Radiological contrast studies**

Contrast study	Part of GI tract examined	Indications for use	Conditions identified
Videofluoroscopy	Oropharynx	Concerns regarding aspiration on swallowing Assessment of child's ability to swallow different consistencies of fluid/food safely	Bulbar palsy Pseudo-bulbar palsy
Barium swallow	Oesophagus	Dysphagia To investigate tracheo-oesophageal fistula	Oesophageal pouches/webs/strictures/fistulae
Barium meal	Oesophagus, stomach and duodenum	Recurrent vomiting	Hiatus hernia Gastric outflow obstruction Malrotation (if duodenal–jejunal flexure to right of midline)
Barium meal and follow-through	Oesophagus, stomach, duodenum, jejunum and ileum	To identify presence of small bowel Crohn disease Partial small bowel obstructive symptoms Note: images are not as good as with small-bowel contrast study	Small bowel Crohn disease Small bowel strictures due to Crohn disease or post-surgery
Small-bowel study (requires duodenal intubation)	Duodenum, jejunum and ileum	To identify small bowel Crohn disease Partial small bowel obstructive symptoms	Small bowel Crohn disease Small bowel strictures due to Crohn disease or post-surgery
Contrast enema	Rectum and colon	To reduce intussusception (therapeutic) Very rarely used diagnostically in children	

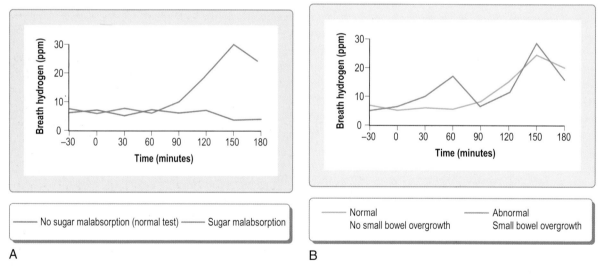

A   B

Fig. 38.2 **Hydrogen breath tests.**
(A) A normal test (red) with no sugar malabsorption, and an abnormal test (blue) when malabsorbed sugar is fermented by colonic bacteria, increasing breath hydrogen; (B) lactulose hydrogen breath test showing a normal test (green) when the non-absorbable sugar is fermented by colonic bacteria, increasing breath hydrogen, and an abnormal test (purple) when small bowel organisms ferment the lactulose, producing an increase in breath hydrogen prior to sugar arriving in the colon (double peak sign).

is a non-absorbable sugar, in a normal child the pattern is as shown in Figure 38.2A; the green line is seen as the non-absorbed lactulose is fermented in the colon. However, in Figure 38.2B the purple line shows an abnormal lactulose hydrogen breath test with an early peak, suggesting that the sugar is being fermented by organisms in the small bowel, and the second peak when the lactulose reaches the colon.

Both false positive and false negative hydrogen breath test results can occur. False positive results are seen with inadequate pretest fasting or recent smoking; false negative results can be seen after the recent use

Table 38.2 Serological studies

Antibody	Sensitivity	Specificity
IgA endomysial antibody (IgA EMA)	85–98%	97–100%
IgA tissue transglutaminase antibody (IgA tTG)	90–98%	95–97%
IgA antigliadin antibody (IgA AGA)	80–90%	85–95%
IgG antigliadin antibody (IgG AGA)	75–85%	75–90%

of antibiotics, in patients with lung disorders or in the approximately 1% of children who are 'non-hydrogen producers'. Oral bacteria may lead to an early hydrogen peak and pretest mouth-washing with an antiseptic is advocated by some units. The H_2 peak occurring from bacterial overgrowth in the distal small intestine may be difficult to discriminate from the normal peak seen when the test sugar reaches the colon. Additionally, rapid delivery of the test sugar to the colon in patients with short bowel syndrome may lead to false positive results.

'Coeliac antibodies'

Four serological studies have been described to aid the diagnosis of coeliac disease (Table 38.2).

Serum IgA endomysial and tissue transglutaminase antibody testing have the highest diagnostic accuracy. The IgA and IgG antigliadin antibody tests have lower diagnostic accuracy, with frequent false positive results, and are therefore no longer recommended for initial diagnostic evaluation or screening. All are less accurate in children under 2 years of age.

The serum antibodies commonly used in testing for coeliac disease are IgA and therefore all have high false negative rates in IgA deficiency. It should be remembered that the coeliac population has a higher rate of IgA deficiency than the non-coeliac population. Thus if coeliac disease is clinically suspected and serum antibodies are checked, IgA deficiency also needs to be excluded. None of the serum antibody tests has 100% sensitivity and specificity and therefore a small bowel biopsy is always needed for a definitive diagnosis. Likewise, when there is a high degree of clinical suspicion a small bowel biopsy needs to be performed, even with negative serological testing. Recently a new serological test for anti IgA and IgG deamidated gliadin peptides (DGP) has been shown to have high sensitivity and specificity rates, even in cases of IgA deficiency.

IgA endomysial antibodies

Endomysial antibodies bind to connective tissue surrounding smooth muscle cells. Serum IgA endomysial antibodies produce a characteristic staining pattern, which is visualized by indirect immunofluorescence. The test

result is reported simply as positive or negative, since even low titres of serum IgA endomysial antibodies are specific for coeliac disease. The target antigen has been identified as a tissue transglutaminase.

IgA tissue transglutaminase antibodies

Enzyme-linked immunosorbent assay (ELISA) tests for IgA tissue transglutaminase antibodies are now widely available and are easier to perform and less costly than the immunofluorescence assay used to detect IgA endomysial antibodies.

IgA EMA, IgA tTG, IgA and IgG DGP and IgA AGA levels fall with treatment; as a result, these assays can be used as a non-invasive means of monitoring the response and adherence to a gluten-free diet.

Testing for *Helicobacter pylori*

H. pylori can be identified by histological examination or on *Campylobacter*-like organism (CLO) testing of mucosal biopsies collected at upper gastrointestinal endoscopy. However, non-invasive tests have a role in diagnosing *H. pylori* infection and confirming eradication after treatment.

Urea breath testing

H. pylori has the enzyme urease, which converts urea to ammonia and bicarbonate and then carbon dioxide. The presence of this enzyme in the stomach in a child with *H. pylori* infection can be used diagnostically via a stable isotope breath test. In children, urea labelled with C^{13} (non-radioactive) is administered after fasting, usually with fresh orange juice to delay gastric emptying. If *H. pylori* is present the urea is hydrolysed, releasing C^{13}-tagged CO_2, which can be detected in breath samples. Breath is collected and analysed by mass spectrometry. C^{13} is a naturally occurring stable isotope, so it is present in small quantities in the breath, but there is an increase if *H. pylori* infection is present in the stomach. The test is both highly sensitive (> 90%) and specific (> 95%). However, the test becomes less sensitive (has a high rate of false negatives) if used within a month of antibiotic therapy or while the child is taking H_2-blocking agents or PPIs. To prevent false negative results, the child should not have taken antibiotics for at least 4 weeks and antisecretory agents for at least 2 weeks.

H. pylori serology

Laboratory-based serological testing using ELISA to detect IgG or IgA antibodies is inexpensive and widely available. Large studies have found uniformly high

Table 38.3 Common indications for upper gastrointestinal endoscopy and colonoscopy in children

	To diagnose macroscopically or histologically	Therapeutic procedures
Upper GI endoscopy	Reflux oesophagitis Oesophageal/gastric varices Gastritis/gastric ulcer (GU) Duodenitis/duodenal ulcer (DU) *H. pylori* infection Crohn disease of upper GI tract Enteropathies including coeliac disease (Fig. 38.3)	Dilatation of peptic stricture Sclerotherapy/banding of bleeding varices Bleeding control in bleeding GU/DU Insertion of feeding gastrostomy Passage of nasojejunal tube
Lower GI endoscopy	Polyps Inflammatory bowel disease	Removal of polyps

sensitivity (90–100%) but variable specificity (76–96%). However, the positive and negative predictive values of the test relate to the pretest probability of *H. pylori* in the population being studied. Generally, in children from countries where the prevalence of *H. pylori* is low, a negative test is helpful to exclude infection, but a positive serological test is more likely to be a false positive. As a result, it is recommended that secondary testing (urea breath test, stool antigen testing, endoscopy) is used to confirm the initial result before initiating treatment. *H. pylori* serology does usually become negative after successful eradication treatment but seroconversion is slow. Serological testing is therefore not useful for follow-up since many patients continue to have antibodies for months or even years after successful eradication therapy.

Stool antigen assay

The presence of *H. pylori* in the stool of infected patients has led to the development of faecal assays. A commercial enzyme immunoassay is available. The sensitivity and specificity of this test are 94% and 90% respectively, when compared to endoscopy and urea breath testing. The stool assay has the same limitations as the urea breath test regarding false negatives after antibiotic use and acid-suppressing drugs, and it can replace urea breath testing in an uncooperative young child.

Confirmation of eradication after treatment

Confirmation of eradication is required after treatment for *H. pylori* and is facilitated by the availability of accurate, relatively inexpensive non-invasive tests. Urea breath testing is the test of choice to confirm eradication of infection. Stool antigen testing is an alternative when urea breath testing is not available, but it is less accurate.

Upper gastrointestinal endoscopy and colonoscopy

These are important tests that are useful both diagnostically and therapeutically. However, they are invasive and in most centres are performed under general anaesthetic. Complications are rare but colonic perforation can occur at colonoscopy. Additionally, colono-

scopy requires bowel preparation with laxatives, which most children find unpleasant. Hence, they are only used in selected cases when the symptoms are sufficiently severe, a tissue diagnosis is needed or a therapeutic procedure is indicated.

Common indications for upper gastrointestinal endoscopy and colonoscopy in children are listed in Table 38.3.

Pancreatic function testing

Pancreatic function tests can be either direct or indirect. Direct pancreatic function testing is considered the 'gold standard' but is rarely performed, as it is invasive and requires intubation of the duodenum. Duodenal secretions are aspirated after pancreatic stimulation by intravenous cholecystokinin and secretin or a Lundh test meal (meal composed of standardized nutrients). It allows bicarbonate, amylase, trypsin and lipase to be assayed separately and there are clear normal ranges for comparison.

Several indirect (non-invasive) tests of pancreatic exocrine insufficiency have been developed. Of the available tests, the most commonly used are faecal chymotrypsin and faecal elastase measurements.

Faecal chymotrypsin

Faecal chymotrypsin is easy to measure and levels are stable in stools for several days. Measurement was frequently used in the past as a screening test for pancreatic insufficiency. However, levels are usually low only in advanced pancreatic disease and the sensitivity for pancreatic insufficiency is therefore only 50–60%. Additionally the test cannot be performed when the child is taking pancreatic enzyme replacement therapy.

Faecal pancreatic elastase

Faecal pancreatic elastase estimation is now the most widely used test for pancreatic exocrine insufficiency. The pancreatic enzyme, *elastase 1*, is stable during intestinal transit and is measurable as faecal elastase. After 2 weeks of age it has a high sensitivity in the diagnosis of moderate and severe pancreatic insufficiency. The test has a sensitivity and specificity of 93%

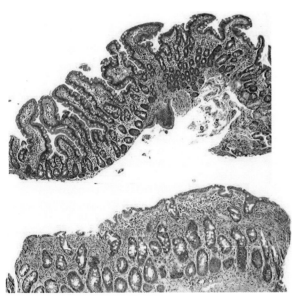

Fig. 38.3 **Endoscopic duodenal mucosal biopsies**

Normal duodenal mucosa with tall, finger-like villi and crypts of normal length

Almost total villous atrophy in a child with coeliac disease with elongation of the crypts, increased infiltration of intra-epithelial lymphocytes and disorganization of the enterocyte layer.

for pancreatic insufficiency. In addition, its values are independent of pancreatic enzyme replacement therapy and can therefore be used while the child is taking pancreatic enzyme supplements.

Tests of fat malabsorption

If the clinical history suggests significant fat malabsorption (steatorrhoea), then a variety of tests can be employed to identify whether steatorrhoea is present. However, all the tests have limitations and are not universally available.

Currently, the gold standard for diagnosis of steatorrhoea is quantitative estimation of stool fat. The method most commonly used for the measurement of faecal fat is the titrimetric Van de Kamer method. In adults, the test involves a diet containing 100 g of fat for 3–5 days. Stools collected over 72–96 hours are pooled and refrigerated. In children, the collection period is usually 3 days. Children find it difficult to adhere to a strictly regimented diet and therefore a careful dietary record is required to calculate the mean daily fat intake. Steatorrhoea is present if more than 7% of ingested fat is excreted, though infants under 6 months can excrete up to 15% of dietary fat due to the physiological immaturity of the pancreatic and biliary secretions. Despite it being the only quantitative test of fat excretion, 72-hour stool collection is rarely used in children, as it is cumbersome and unpopular with families and laboratory staff. Qualitative (subjective) tests are more commonly used and faecal Sudan III staining/microscopy and faecal acid steatocrits are the most widely available. Sudan III stain on a spot sample of stool can detect more than 90% of patients with clinically significant steatorrhoea, but it needs to be properly performed and interpreted by an experienced assessor. The acid steatocrit is performed rather like a haematocrit on a spot stool sample and gives the percentage of the stool that is composed of fat. It has a sensitivity of 100%, specificity of 95% and positive predictive value of 90%, as compared to the gold standard 72-hour faecal fat collection.

Tests of protein malabsorption

Alpha-1-antitrypsin is used for documenting creatorrhoea either due to protein losing enteropathy or exocrine pancreatic insufficiency. Alpha-1-antitrypsin is a stable protein which does not undergo digestion in the intestinal lumen; therefore, an elevated faecal alpha-1-antitrypsin level indicates creatorrhoea.

Enteral and parenteral nutrition

Total or supplementary nutrition can be given via different routes. These routes and their advantages, disadvantages and indications are shown in Table 38.4.

Acute diarrhoea

Diarrhoea is one of the most common causes of morbidity and mortality in children world-wide. World-wide childhood death secondary to diarrhoea declined from an estimated 5 million per year in 1980 to less than 2 million in 1999. The decline is attributed to global improvements in sanitation and the use of oral rehydration therapy (Ch. 37).

Basic science

Gut immunity

The gastrointestinal mucosal immune system protects the mucosal surfaces (400 m^2 surface area in adults)

Table 38.4 Enteral and parenteral routes of nutrition

Route of feed	'Anatomy' of feeding route	Advantages	Disadvantages	Common indications
Oral sip feeds	Drunk by child	No tube	Compliance Needs to like taste When child is nauseated/vomiting	As a supplement when high requirements or poor appetite, e.g. cystic fibrosis, Crohn disease As therapy in Crohn disease
Nasogastric	Tube passed via nose to stomach	Easy to place and to remove Can bolus-feed for convenience Can continuously feed	Placement uncomfortable Visible on face Easy to displace or remove accidentally Have to check position before using Blocks easily	Child cannot take full requirements due to problems sucking/swallowing, e.g. cleft palate, neurodisability Child cannot take full requirements due to illness or high requirements, e.g. bronchiolitis, cardiac disease Child needs continuous feeding, e.g. severe GOR, short gut
Nasojejunal	Tube passed via nose to jejunum	Relatively easy to place	Placement uncomfortable Difficult to place and often has to be passed under X-ray screening Position checked by X-ray Easy to remove	Child excessively vomits gastric contents, e.g. severe GOR or gastroduodenal dysmotility Child has pancreatitis (intragastric feeding causes stimulation of pancreas)
Gastrostomy	Tube inserted at endoscopy or surgically into stomach through abdominal wall	Discreet Difficult to pull out accidentally Position does not need to be checked	Needs general anaesthetic for initial insertion Risks of initial surgery Local infections	Child requiring medium- to long-term nutritional support
Jejunostomy	Tube placed surgically into jejunum via abdominal wall	Discreet Difficult to pull out accidentally Position does not need to be checked	Needs general anaesthetic for initial insertion Risks of initial surgery Local infections	Unusual feeding route usually used in child with gastroduodenal dysmotility requiring medium- to long-term nutritional support
Parenteral Peripheral	Intravenous nutrition given via peripheral cannula	Easy to place	Short-term as thrombophlebitis common Have to limit osmolality (and therefore glucose content) of parenteral nutrition Usually inadequate for full nutritional requirements	Child whose gut cannot be used for full nutritional requirements, e.g. post-surgery, during chemotherapy, short gut Short-term nutritional support while awaiting CVL placement
Central	Intravenous nutrition given via central venous line (CVL)	Secure access Can give high glucose concentrations and full nutritional requirements	Needs to be placed under general anaesthetic CVL sepsis a major risk	Child whose gut cannot be used for full nutritional requirements, e.g. post-surgery, during chemotherapy, short gut Can be used long-term

from harmful invasive organisms, but also has to suppress immune responses to food antigens (up to several hundred grams per day, depending on age) and commensal bacteria. Therefore, even under completely physiological conditions, the gastrointestinal tract contains enormous numbers of leucocytes diffusely scattered in the lamina propria and the intraepithelial compartment, or organized in the Peyer patches and isolated lymphoid follicles of the colon. Combined, they form the gut-associated lymphoid tissue (GALT). In health 40% of lymphocytes in the body are present in the gastrointestinal mucosa and GALT. The majority of them produce dimeric IgA antibodies. At birth, the gut-associated lymphoid tissue possesses the necessary cells with which to serve its function, but having never met foreign antigens, it lacks certain elements found in later life. Full maturity is not achieved for up to 2 years.

Water and electrolyte absorption

In healthy adults the small intestine is presented with approximately 8 litres of fluid each day. This amount includes both ingested liquids and gastrointestinal secretions. By the time the initial 8 litres of fluid reaches the ileocaecal valve, only about 600 ml remains and by the time this reaches the anus, only about 100 ml of fluid

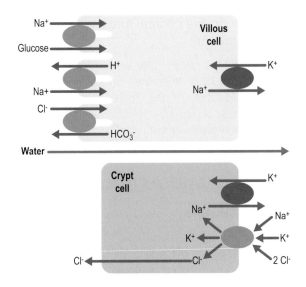

Fig. 38.4 Main intestinal absorptive/secretory processes for electrolytes and glucose

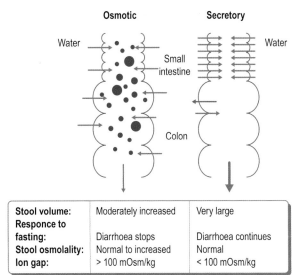

	Osmotic	Secretory
Stool volume:	Moderately increased	Very large
Responce to fasting:	Diarrhoea stops	Diarrhoea continues
Stool osmolality:	Normal to increased	Normal
Ion gap:	> 100 mOsm/kg	< 100 mOsm/kg

Fig. 38.5 Summary of features of osmotic and secretory diarrhoea

remains. The efficiency of water absorption in the small and large intestine combined is approximately 99%.

The normal absorption of electrolytes, glucose and water is shown in Figure 38.4.

In the villous cell Na/K adenosine triphosphatase (ATPase) maintains a low intracellular Na concentration, thus allowing the 'downhill' entry of Na, coupled Cl and nutrients. In the crypt cell the low Na concentration drives a carrier in the basolateral membrane coupling the flow of one Na, two Cl and one K from the serosal compartment into the crypt cell. As a result, Cl accumulates above its electrochemical equilibrium and under physiological circumstances leaks into the gastrointestinal lumen across a semipermeable apical membrane. In health the absorptive activity in the villous cell far exceeds the minor secretion from the crypts and the net result is absorption of electrolytes and nutrients. Water absorption then passively follows, mainly through the intercellular tight junctions.

Acute diarrhoea is the abrupt onset of increased fluid content of the stool above the normal value of approximately 10 ml/kg/day. Diarrhoea is the reversal of the normal net absorptive state. This can be due to an osmotic force acting in the lumen to pull water into the gut, as seen in sugar malabsorption (Fig. 38.5). This diarrhoea will stop on fasting. It can also be due to an active secretory state induced in the enterocytes. Secretory diarrhoea continues on fasting. The most common cause of secretory diarrhoea is infection, and different enterotoxins and inflammatory processes affect the transport of electrolytes in different ways. The classic example is cholera enterotoxin-induced diarrhoea, in which there is enhanced anion secretion by the crypt cell and an inhibition of the Na/Cl channels in the

apical cell. The consequential increase in electrolytes in the gastrointestinal lumen not only prevents passive water absorption but also reverses water transport, causing water loss into the gastrointestinal tract and profuse watery diarrhoea. The glucose/Na transporter is usually unaffected in infectious secretory diarrhoea, explaining the efficacy of oral rehydration solution.

Infective diarrhoea in the developed world

Approximately 1 in 50 children in developed nations are hospitalized for acute gastroenteritis some time during childhood. More than 95% of this risk occurs in the first 5 years of life.

Viral infections are most common between 6 and 24 months of age, after transplacental antibody is cleared and breastfeeding has stopped and before full acquisition of protective immunity.

Bacterial gastroenteritis is more common in the first few months of life and then again in school-age children. Most bacterial gastroenteritis is due to food-borne pathogens.

Problem-orientated topic:

acute diarrhoea ● ● ● ● ●

Lisette, an 18-month-old girl, presents with a 2-day history of non-bloody diarrhoea. She is passing more than 8 stools per day. She is pyrexial and vomiting but drinking well and not dehydrated.

Continued overleaf

Q1. What is the likely diagnosis and the most likely pathogen?

Q2. How do the clinical features help with diagnosis?

Q1. What is the likely diagnosis and the most likely pathogen?

The frequency of pathogens isolated in cases of childhood sporadic diarrhoea in developed countries is shown in Table 38.5.

Table 38.5 Frequency of pathogens in acute diarrhoea

Pathogen	Frequency
Viruses	
Rotavirus (more during winter months)	25–40%
Calicivirus	1–20%
Astrovirus	4–9%
Adenovirus	2–4%
Norovirus (Norwalk-like virus)	Unknown
Bacteria	
Campylobacter jejuni	6–8%
Salmonella	3–7%
Escherichia coli	3–5%
Shigella	0–3%
Yersinia enterocolitica	1–2%
Clostridium difficile	0–2%
Parasites	
Cryptosporidium	1–3%
Giardia lamblia	1–3%

Q2. How do the clinical features help with diagnosis?

See Table 38.6. With the recent availability of vaccination against Rotavirus strains, we expect a significant decline in the incidence of Rotavirus gastroenteritis. It remains to be seen whether the incidence of intussusception, attributed at least in part to Rotavirus infection, will also decline.

Vomiting and regurgitation

Basic science

Though vomiting can occur due to a wide range of stimuli and causes, regardless of the initiation, the complex vomiting 'reflex' is identical. There are three stages to vomiting:

- *Nausea*: a feeling of wanting to vomit, often associated with autonomic effects including hypersalivation, pallor and sweating. This phase is associated with decreased gastric motility and retrograde propulsion of duodenal contents into the stomach.
- *Retching*: a strong involuntary effort to vomit during which the glottis remains closed and there is contraction of the diaphragm and abdominal muscles.
- *Vomiting*: the expulsion of gastric contents through the mouth after relaxation of the cardia and lower oesophageal sphincter and sustained contraction of the abdominal muscles.

The mechanisms of provocation of vomiting are summarized in Figure 38.6. It should be noted that the

Table 38.6 Clinical features of pathogens

Pathogenesis	Predominant site of action	Infective agents	Clinical presentation
Direct cytopathic effect	Proximal small intestine	Rotavirus Adenovirus Calicivirus Norovirus (Norwalk-like virus) Enteropathogenic *E. coli* Giardia	Copious watery diarrhoea, vomiting, mild to severe dehydration; frequent lactose malabsorption; no blood in stools
Enterotoxigenicity	Small intestine	*Vibrio cholerae* Enterotoxigenic *E. coli* (ETEC) Entero-aggregative *E. coli* *Cryptosporidium*	Watery diarrhoea (can be copious in cholera or ETEC); no blood in stools
Invasiveness	Distal ileum and colon	*Salmonella* *Shigella* *Yersinia* *Campylobacter* Entero-invasive *E. coli* *Amoeba*	Dysentery: very frequent stools, cramps, pain, fever and often blood in stools. Variable dehydration. Course may be protracted
Cytotoxicity	Colon	*Clostridium difficile* Enterohaemorrhagic *E. coli* (EHEC) *Shigella*	Dysentery: abdominal cramps, fever, blood in stools. EHEC or *Shigella* may be followed by haemolytic–uraemic syndrome

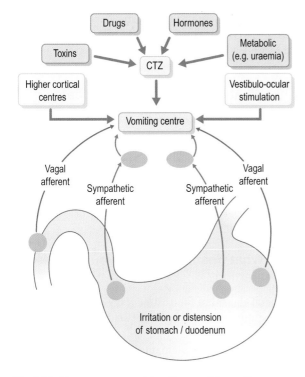

Fig. 38.6 Diagram summarizing the vomiting reflex (CTZ = chemoreceptor trigger zone)

Problem-orientated topic:

regurgitation

Rasmus, a 4-month-old boy, presents with regurgitation of small volumes of his milk feeds over 20 times per day, particularly in the hour after his feed. He is otherwise well and thriving.

Q1. What is the most likely diagnosis?
Q2. What investigations are indicated?
Q3. What treatment would you consider starting?

presence of an anatomically discrete 'vomiting centre' in the lateral reticular formation of the medulla is now questioned, but there is certainly a central process that functions as a vomiting centre.

The chemoreceptor trigger zone (CTZ) lies outside the blood–brain barrier in the floor of the fourth ventricle. It is stimulated by proemetic agents in the blood or cerebrospinal fluid. Table 38.7 summarizes the effects of antiemetic medication.

Q1. What is the most likely diagnosis?

Gastro-oesophageal reflux (GOR) is the involuntary retrograde flow of gastric contents proximally into the oesophagus. When the gastric contents reach the mouth, this is termed regurgitation. Both are commonly seen in infants. Both regurgitation and GOR are effortless and are not preceded by nausea and retching. The physiology of GOR is summarized in Figure 38.7. Infants and children with GOR have normal resting lower oesophageal sphincter pressures but demonstrate spontaneous relaxation of the lower oesophageal sphincter. It is not clear whether this is a local or centrally mediated process. The drop in the sphincter pressure precedes a drop in intra-oesophageal pH, indicating reflux of gastric contents into the oesophagus (p. 523). The reflux of gastric contents into the distal oesophagus is not caused by an increase in gastric pressure (as in vomiting), as the intragastric pressure remains unchanged.

Table 38.7 Drugs used to control emesis and their mechanism of action

Drug group	Indication	Mechanism
Antihistamines	Motion sickness and mild chemotherapy-induced vomiting	Labyrinthine suppression via anticholinergic effect H_1-receptor antagonism in vomiting centre
Substituted benzamides e.g. Metoclopramide	Chemotherapy, gastroparesis	D_2-receptor blockade at the CTZ. In high dose has $5-HT_3$ activity in the gut
$5-HT_3$ receptor antagonists e.g. Ondansetron	Chemotherapy Postoperative nausea and vomiting	$5-HT_3$-receptor blockade most important in the gut, but possibly some effect in CTZ and vomiting centre
Benzodiazepines e.g. Lorazepam	Chemotherapy	Central GABA inhibition, producing sedation and anxiolysis
Phenothiazides	Rarely used in children because of extrapyramidal side-effects	D_2-receptor blockade at the CTZ
Butyrophenones e.g. Domperidone	Chemotherapy, gastroparesis, GOR	D_2-receptor blockade at the enteric nervous system

(CTZ = chemoreceptor trigger zone; GABA = gamma-aminobutyric acid; GOR = gastro-oesophageal reflux)

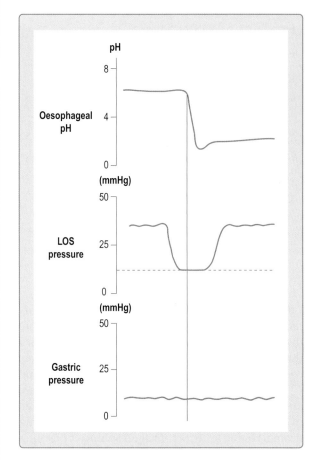

pH

Oesophageal pH

(mmHg)

LOS pressure

(mmHg)

Gastric pressure

Fig. 38.7 Simultaneous measurements of intra-oesophageal pH, lower oesophageal sphincter (LOS) pressure and intragastric pressure during an episode of gastro-oesophageal reflux

Features of excessive 'physiological' regurgitation in infants

- Natural history: improves with age
- Improves on weaning and on becoming more upright when walking
- Resolution in 80% by 18 months, and in 90–95% by 2 years.

Clinical presentation of gastro-oesophageal reflux disease (GORD) in infants and children is shown in Table 38.8.

Q2. What investigations are indicated?

Many clinicians recommend a therapeutic trial of treatment, rather than investigation. If GOR is clinically suspected and treatment will be implemented, even with a negative test, then the test should not usually be performed. If investigations are indicated, then the investigation chosen depends on the clinical question asked (Table 38.9).

Q3. What treatment would you consider starting?

A general algorithm for treatment is given in Figure 38.8 and a summary of the action of acid-blocking drugs in Box 38.1.

N.B. Cow's milk protein intolerance may mimic GOR and a trial of hypoallergenic formula may be helpful, particularly when there is a strong family history of atopy. Even in families without atopy it is usually recommended, especially before surgical intervention.

Specific management of clinical scenarios

An infant with uncomplicated reflux ('happy puker')

Diagnosis is made on history and examination. No investigations are indicated.

Reassurance without any other specific intervention is usually sufficient. Other treatment options include feed thickeners and positioning. Re-evaluation should take place if symptoms worsen or do not improve by the time the child begins to walk.

Table 38.8 Clinical presentation of gastro-oesophageal reflux disease

	Infants	Children
Excessive regurgitation	Vomiting Growth faltering	Vomiting Growth faltering
Oesophagitis	Irritability with feedings Feeding refusal Arching Haematemesis, anaemia	Heartburn Chest or abdominal pain Dysphagia, odynophagia Haematemesis, anaemia Sandifer syndrome
Respiratory disorders	Apnoea/stridor Aspiration pneumonia Laryngospasm (apnoea, stridor) Apparent life-threatening events Sudden unexpected death in infancy	Aspiration pneumonia Bronchospasm (asthma) Laryngospasm (apnoea, stridor) Hoarseness

Table 38.9 Regurgitation: investigations based on questions

Question to ask	Test performed
Are there structural abnormalities in the upper GI tract?	Barium meal
Is there a delay in gastric emptying?	Radionucleotide gastric emptying study
Does aspiration occur?	Chest X-ray, videofluoroscopy/barium swallow, bronchoscopy, radionucleotide 'milk scan'
Is oesophagitis present?	Endoscopy and biopsy
Are specific symptoms causally related to GOR?	pH monitoring with event recording, impedance
Is a hiatus hernia present?	Barium swallow, endoscopy
Is the quantity of acid GOR abnormal?	pH monitoring
Is there an oesophageal motility disorder?	Barium swallow, oesophageal manometry

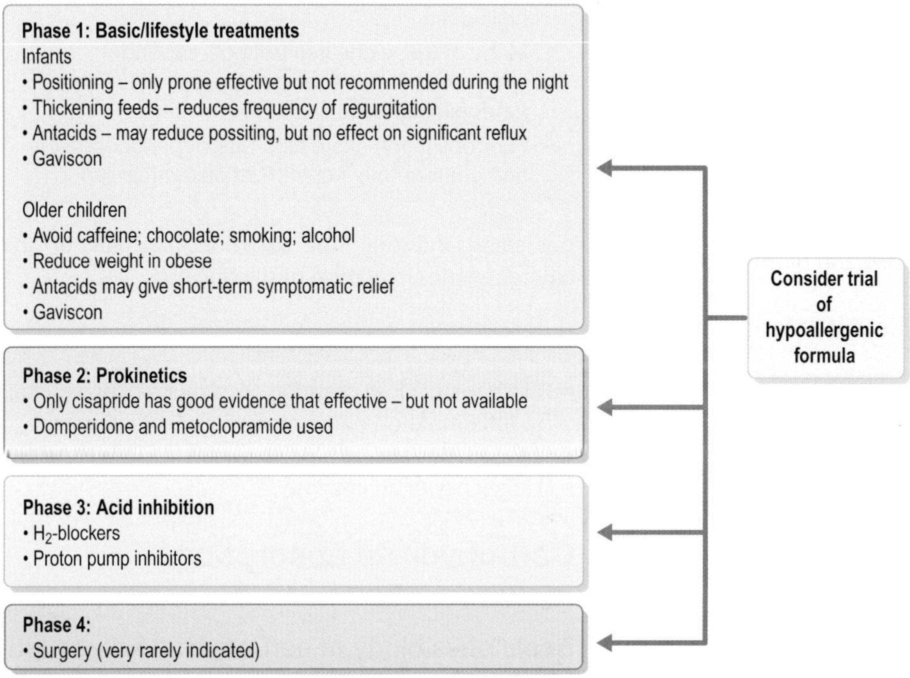

Phase 1: Basic/lifestyle treatments
Infants
• Positioning – only prone effective but not recommended during the night
• Thickening feeds – reduces frequency of regurgitation
• Antacids – may reduce possiting, but no effect on significant reflux
• Gaviscon

Older children
• Avoid caffeine; chocolate; smoking; alcohol
• Reduce weight in obese
• Antacids may give short-term symptomatic relief
• Gaviscon

Phase 2: Prokinetics
• Only cisapride has good evidence that effective – but not available
• Domperidone and metoclopramide used

Phase 3: Acid inhibition
• H_2-blockers
• Proton pump inhibitors

Phase 4:
• Surgery (very rarely indicated)

Consider trial of hypoallergenic formula

Fig. 38.8 Algorithm for treatment of regurgitation

BOX 38.1 Summary of action of acid-blocking drugs

Histamine type 2 receptor antagonists
• Ranitidine, cimetidine
• Inhibit acid secretion by blocking histamine H_2-receptors on the parietal cell

Proton pump inhibitors (PPIs)
• Omeprazole, lansoprazole etc.
• Block acid secretion by irreversibly binding to and inhibiting the hydrogen–potassium ATPase pump on the luminal surface of the parietal cell membrane

---

An infant with recurrent vomiting and poor weight gain

Dietetic assessment is indicated. Poor weight gain despite an adequate intake of calories should prompt evaluation for causes of vomiting and weight loss other than GOR; investigations should include a full blood count, electrolytes, liver and kidney function tests, blood gases, serum lactate and ammonia, glucose, urinalysis, urine ketones, reducing substances in the stool and a review of newborn screening tests.

Barium meal is usually required to exclude anatomical abnormalities. An upper endoscopy with biopsy may also be required in selected patients to exclude, among other things, a diagnosis of eosinophilic oesophagitis.

If GORD continues to be suspected after the above evaluation, treatment options include:
• Thickening the formula
• Positioning
• Trial of hypoallergenic formula
• Increasing the caloric density of the formula
• Prokinetic therapy, e.g. domperidone (though no evidence in this situation)
• Gaviscon
• H2 — blockers/PPIs
• Implementing continuous nasogastric feeding.

An infant with discomfort on feeding

If oesophagitis is suspected, endoscopy with biopsy is the investigation of choice, though a therapeutic trial may be carried out. The best treatment option is as described above.

A child or adolescent with recurrent vomiting or regurgitation

Otherwise healthy children with recurrent vomiting or regurgitation after the age of 2 years usually require evaluation, typically with a barium meal and/or upper endoscopy with biopsy. Treatment should be based upon the findings.

A child or adolescent with heartburn

These patients are usually treated empirically with lifestyle changes accompanied by a 4-week trial of an H_2-blocker or PPI.

Persistent or recurrent symptoms require investigation with an upper endoscopy and biopsy.

Apnoea or apparent life-threatening events

Recurrent vomiting or regurgitation occurs commonly in patients with apparent life-threatening events (ALTE, p. 756). However, an association between reflux and apnoea or bradycardia has not been convincingly demonstrated. In the evaluation of such patients pH monitoring may be useful to link intra-oesophageal acid with events. Infants with ALTE may be more likely to respond to antireflux therapy when:

- Vomiting or oral regurgitation occurs at the time of the ALTE
- Episodes occur while the infant is awake
- ALTE is characterized by obstructive apnoea.

Most infants respond to maximal medical therapy with formula thickening, prokinetic agents, Gaviscon and acid suppression. Only a minority require antireflux surgery.

GOR in children with neurodisability

Key points are given in Box 38.2.

Chronic diarrhoea and malabsorption

Basic science

Malabsorption syndromes are characterized by the association of chronic diarrhoea and failure to thrive. The disorders involve inadequate absorption of one or more of the major nutrients and primarily involve

---

BOX 38.2 GOR in children with neurodisability

- One-third of children with severe psychomotor retardation have significant GOR
- It is exacerbated in many by the presence of large hiatal hernias and diffuse foregut dysmotility
- Growth faltering and dental erosions are a frequent problem
- All severe sequelae of GOR have a higher incidence in children with neurodisability (recurrent aspiration pneumonia, blood loss from oesophagitis, stricture formation etc.)
- Oesophagitis can respond to H_2-antagonists, but most require 'maximum medical therapy' with high-dose PPIs
- Many of these children will not respond adequately to medical therapy and will require fundoplication
- Fundoplication has a high rate of perioperative and postoperative complications in this group

---

the small intestine, the exocrine pancreas or the enterohepatic circulation of the bile salts.

Causes of malabsorption

- Enteropathy: loss of surface area in small bowel due to inflammation of the mucosa and villi damage
- Defect in a transport mechanism
- Deficiency of an enzyme.

Carbohydrate absorption/ malabsorption

Basic physiology of carbohydrate digestion
(Box 38.3)

Carbohydrates in food comprise starch, disaccharides, sucrose and lactose. Starch molecules (amylase

---

BOX 38.3 Basic physiology of carbohydrate digestion

Starch 50–60%

- Digestion by salivary/pancreatic amylase to maltose and maltotriose
- Maltose and maltotriose:
    - ~80% hydrolysed by   →   glucose sucrase–isomaltase
    - ~20% glucoamylase

Sucrose 30–40%

- Hydrolysis by   →   glucose
  sucrase–isomaltase   fructose

Lactose 0–20% adults, 40–100% infants

- Hydrolysis by lactase   →   glucose
  galactose

---

and amylopectin) and glucose polymers require preliminary intraluminal digestion by amylase, releasing maltose and maltotriose. The final hydrolysis of di- and oligosaccharides occurs at the brush border. Glucose and galactose enter the enterocyte via a sodium-linked carrier (p. 531) and fructose via an energy-independent 'pore'.

Malabsorption of carbohydrate leads to osmotic diarrhoea. The undigested sugar is then fermented in the colon, producing excessive flatus and acidic stools.

Characteristic stools of sugar malabsorption

- Osmotic diarrhoea (stops on fasting)
- Very watery
- Acidic
- Passed with excessive flatus (explosive)
- Contains reducing substances.

Lactose malabsorption

The most common form of carbohydrate malabsorption is lactase malabsorption. Lactase is found on the brush border in the small bowel. Any mechanism causing damage to the mucosa and villi of the small bowel (enteropathy) will cause secondary lactase deficiency. This can be managed with a lactose-free formula or diet, but resolves spontaneously as the enteropathy resolves.

In all humans the amount of lactase present per area of small bowel reduces towards the middle of the first decade, but in some ethnic groups it falls to a level where symptoms will occur when even a small amount of lactose is ingested. This is termed congenital 'adult' type lactase deficiency and is very common. It is simply managed by consuming low lactose milk and adding lactase to dairy products.

Congenital glucose–galactose malabsorption

This is an extremely rare autosomal recessive condition due to the absence of the sodium, glucose–galactose co-transporter in the enterocyte. The newborn baby cannot tolerate lactose or glucose polymer-based feeds. Presentation is with life threatening osmotic diarrhoea. Fructose is the only dietary carbohydrate tolerated and treatment is with a fructose-based formula.

Sucrase–isomaltase deficiency

This is a rare autosomal recessive condition with variable presentation. Watery diarrhoea follows ingestion of sucrose and to a lesser extent starch. It therefore may present at the time of the introduction of solids and may be confused with toddler diarrhoea. Diagnosis is usually by sucrose hydrogen breath test or a sucrose challenge where explosive watery diarrhoea occurs after ingestion of sucrose, the stools testing positive for sucrose. Treatment is with dietary exclusion of sucrose and to a lesser extent starch.

Protein absorption/malabsorption

Initial digestion of protein is performed by gastric pepsin and pancreatic enzymes. Further hydrolysis of peptides takes place at the brush border of the intestine, where a mixture of peptides and amino acids are absorbed.

Protein-losing enteropathy (Box 38.4)

Loss of serum proteins across the gut mucosa may occur either because of abnormal or inflamed mucosal surface, from abnormal intestinal lymphatics or disturbed protein digestion. Methods for documenting enteric loss of protein are available but, in paediatric practice, are rarely used. The serum albumin is low. Alpha$_1$-antitrypsin can be measured in the stool and will be elevated.

Fat absorption/malabsorption

Fat digestion and absorption take place mainly in the duodenum and upper jejunum. The fat content of a normal diet is predominantly insoluble long-chain triglycerides. Digestion begins in the stomach with lipase produced in the gastric fundus. The fat is then emulsified by bile salts in the small intestine. Pancreatic lipase

---

BOX 38.4 Diseases associated with excessive enteric protein loss

Loss from abnormal/damaged small intestinal mucosa
- Coeliac disease (Fig. 38.3)
- Cow's milk protein enteropathy
- Tropical sprue
- Crohn disease
- Giardiasis
- Graft versus host disease
- Abetalipoproteinaemia

Loss from intestinal lymphatics
- Primary intestinal lymphangiectasia
- Secondary intestinal lymphangiectasia: obstructed lymphatics from lymphoma, malrotation or heart disease/failure

Maldigestion of proteins
- Exocrine pancreatic insufficiency: congenital enzyme deficiency such as enterokinase and trypsinogen deficiency
- Cystic fibrosis

Table 38.10 Presentation of coeliac disease

	Classical	Atypical
Stools	Pale, loose, offensive, sometimes watery, 'oat porridge'	Constipated
Weight	Weight loss/failure to thrive	Weight gain/growth failure
Personality	Fretful, clingy, withdrawn	
Anaemia	++	Iron resistant
Abnormal LFTs		Increased alanine/aspartate aminotransferase (ALT/AST)
Skin		Dermatitis herpetiformis
Bone/teeth		Dental hypoplasia Osteoporosis

then hydrolyses the triglycerides to monoglycerides and fatty acids. Pancreatic bicarbonate is required to maintain optimum pH for hydrolysis for the next step in fat absorption: the conjugation of monoglycerides and fatty acids by bile acids. This consists of their incorporation into aggregates called micelles that are absorbed by the intestinal mucosa cell. The monoglycerides and fatty acids are then re-esterified into triglycerides, which coalesce into chylomicrons. The chylomicrons pass out of the cell and are transported by the lymphatic system into the blood.

Steatorrhoea

Steatorrhoea results from the impaired digestion and absorption of fat due to exocrine pancreatic deficiency, lack of bile salts or damage to the small intestinal mucosa.

Causes of steatorrhoea
- Exocrine pancreatic insufficiency:
  - Cystic fibrosis (p. 608)
  - Shwachman–Diamond syndrome
  - Lipase/co-lipase deficiency
- Lack of bile salts:
  - Primary: Byler disease
  - Secondary: obstructive jaundice, ileal resection (due to impaired enterohepatic circulation), small bowel bacterial overgrowth
- Mucosal pathology:
  - Enteropathy (loss of surface area): coeliac disease, cow's milk protein intolerance, giardiasis, tropical sprue, autoimmune enteropathy
- Failure of chylomicron formation:
  - abetalipoproteinaemia
- Damage to intestinal lymphatics:
  - intestinal lymphangiectasia.

Coeliac disease

This is a disease of proximal small intestine characterized by abnormal small intestine mucosa, associated with a permanent intolerance to gluten (Table 38.10). Removal of gluten from the diet leads to full clinical remission with restoration to normal of small intestinal mucosa. The condition may present at any age and diagnosis is for life.

Coeliac disease is due to T lymphocyte-mediated small intestinal enteropathy induced by gluten in a genetically predisposed individual. There is increased incidence with HLA-DQ2 and -DQ8. Incidence is 1 in 100–200.

Associations include diabetes mellitus, thyroid disease, autoimmune hepatitis and arthritis and IgA deficiency.

Diagnosis
- Screening: page 527.
- Definitive: abnormal small intestinal biopsy with subtotal villous atrophy (Fig. 38.3), crypt hyperplasia, increased intraepithelial lymphocyte infiltration (CD8) and increased inflammatory cells in lamina propria.

When biopsy is abnormal, antibodies are positive and the patient is clinically responding to a gluten-free diet, the diagnosis is straightforward. Abnormal small bowel biopsy by itself is not enough for the diagnosis of coeliac disease, as there are other conditions that can cause a similar histological appearance, such as cow's milk hypersensitivity and giardiasis.

Management
Management involves withdrawal of gluten from the diet (wheat/rye/barley-free) under the supervision of a dietician.

Complications
Apart from anaemia and bone disorder there is an increased risk of developing small bowel lymphoma and carcinoma of the oesophagus in adult life. Strict compliance with a gluten-free diet reduces risk to that of the normal population. Autoimmune disorders can also complicate untreated coeliac disease.

Shwachman–Diamond syndrome

This rare autosomal recessive cause of pancreatic insufficiency is associated with cyclical neutropenia and other haematological abnormalities. Patients may be developmentally delayed, and have an enlarged liver with abnormal liver function tests. There are associated skeletal abnormalities and patients are at risk of developing haematological malignancies.

Treatment is with pancreatic supplements.

Cow's milk protein intolerance

(Box 38.5)

This is due to an intolerance to cow's milk protein, which is usually transient. The symptoms may be confined to the gastrointestinal tract or there may be other manifestations of atopy: cow's milk protein allergy.

There is a 30–50% cross-sensitivity between cow's milk and soya protein. In children with gastrointestinal manifestations changes in the small intestinal mucosa may vary from normal to patchy to partial to subtotal villous atrophy (Fig. 38.3).

Cow's milk protein colitis

This occurs in children less than 2 years of age, who present with bloody diarrhoea. Often there is a family history of atopy. At sigmoidoscopy there is a colitic appearance and biopsies show an increase in eosinophils in the lamina propria (eosinophilic colitis).

Investigations

There may be an increase in eosinophils in the peripheral blood film. IgE may be elevated. Patients may have a positive radioallergosorbence test (RAST) to cow's milk protein and a positive skin prick to cow's milk. However, cow's milk protein intolerance is often present when all these tests are negative, so a therapeutic trial is indicated when there is sufficient clinical suspicion.

BOX 38.5 Manifestations of cow's milk intolerance

Gastrointestinal manifestations
- Diarrhoea
- Vomiting
- Failure to thrive
- Acute colitis
- Constipation

Non-gastrointestinal manifestations
- Migraine
- Eczema
- Asthma
- Anaphylaxis

Management

Treatment is with a cows' milk protein-free diet, using a casein hydrolysate as a milk substitute. The child should be challenged at the age of 2 years, as most will have outgrown the condition by this age. Whilst anaphylaxis is rare, challenge should usually be carried out in hospital.

Short gut syndrome

This is a problem seen mainly in a small number of surgically treated infants when a large segment of gangrenous small intestine is resected as a result of necrotizing enterocolitis or midgut volvulus. These infants are dependent on parenteral nutrition (PN) following surgery and are prone to fluid and electrolyte disturbance, sepsis from central venous catheters and liver damage (PN cholestasis). They require 40–60 cm of non-dilated upper small intestine, preferably with an intact ileocaecal valve and a colon, to have enough bowel to sustain nutrition without PN in the long term. This length of bowel will not be sufficient initially, as it needs to undergo adaptation to increase its surface area. This process can take up to 1 year.

Acute abdominal pain

Abdominal pain of recent onset should trigger prompt diagnosis and active treatment. While most children with acute abdominal pain have a self-limiting condition, the pain may herald a serious medical or surgical emergency. Primary care aspects are discussed in Chapter 25.

Problem-orientated topic:

acute abdominal pain ●●●●●●

A 4-year-old boy, Markus, is admitted to the acute assessment unit with a 24-hour history of right upper quadrant pain that is worse on movement. On examination he has a temperature of $39°C$ and is grunting. He is tender in the right upper quadrant but has no signs of peritonism. His haemoglobin is 11.6 g/dl, white blood count $23 \times 10^9/l$, neutrophils $18 \times 10^9/l$, platelets $465 \times 10^9/l$, C-reactive protein 135 mg/l and serum amylase 90 IU/l.

Q1. How would you assess this child?

Q2. What is the most likely diagnosis?

History

- Pain:
  - Site, characteristics, exaggerating and relieving factors
  - Young child: unexplained screaming
- Associated symptoms:
  - Diarrhoea, vomiting, urinary, menstrual, rectal bleeding
- Trauma?
- Past medical history

Examination

- General:
  - Temperature, signs of cardiovascular instability, respiratory rate, rash, joints, lymph nodes
- Abdomen:
  - Signs of peritonitis, abdominal mass, intestinal obstruction

Investigations

- Blood:
  - Full blood count, urea and electrolytes, liver function tests, amylase
- Urine:
  - Urinalysis for blood, protein and glucose; microscopy and culture
- Radiological:
  - Plain abdominal X-ray, chest X-ray, ultrasound and CT of abdomen

Q1. How would you assess this child?

See Box 38.6.

Q2. What is the most likely diagnosis?

The clinical algorithm shown in Figure 38.9 is helpful in the diagnosis of acute abdominal pain. Markus suffered from lobar pneumonia.

Acute appendicitis (Ch. 25)

Initial symptoms are periumbilical pain, nausea, vomiting and anorexia. There may be associated frequency of micturition. Classically the pain then radiates to the right iliac fossa, though with a retrocaecal appendix the pain may be more lateral and in the flank. The patient will have a low-grade temperature and localized peritoneal signs in the right iliac fossa. Once the appendix has perforated, there is a high fever, grunting respiration and generalized signs of peritonitis. The appendix may perforate to form a localized abscess when a mass is palpable in the right iliac fossa. The diagnosis is usually based on the clinical presentation, though an elevated neutrophil white count and C-reactive protein may be helpful in supporting the diagnosis. The diagnosis can be difficult in younger children, who are usually more ill and have generalized peritonitis at presentation as a result of perforation. Treatment is surgical.

Acute pancreatitis

Acute pancreatitis results from autodigestion of the pancreas.

Causes of acute pancreatitis in childhood are:

- Trauma
- Gallstones
- Congenital abnormalities of the pancreas: pancreatic divisum
- Cystic fibrosis
- Hereditary (autosomal dominant, incomplete penetration)
- Hypercalcaemia
- Hyperlipidaemia.

Clinical features

- *Pain*: upper abdominal, sudden onset, continuous and intense, radiates to back and flank. The severity is related to the degree of peritoneal signs and is caused by liberation of enzymes and haemorrhage.

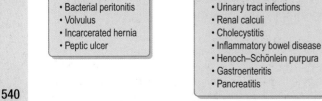

Fig. 38.9 Diagnosis of acute abdominal pain

Peritoneal signs / Mass / Signs of obstruction

Yes — No

Surgical
- Appendicitis
- Intussusception
- Bacterial peritonitis
- Volvulus
- Incarcerated hernia
- Peptic ulcer

Intra-abdominal
- Mesenteric adenitis
- Pelvic inflammatory disease
- Urinary tract infections
- Renal calculi
- Cholecystitis
- Inflammatory bowel disease
- Henoch–Schönlein purpura
- Gastroenteritis
- Pancreatitis

Systemic
- Pneumonia
- Diabetic ketoacidosis
- Sickle cell disease

- *Vomiting*: severe, bilious and may be faeculent as a result of paralytic ileus.
- *Clinical findings*: fever, signs of cardiovascular instability (tachycardia, hypotension), peritonism, ileus; there may be an epigastric mass.

The diagnosis is confirmed by an elevated serum amylase. Hypocalcaemia may accompany acute pancreatitis.

Management
- Resuscitation
- Nil by mouth
- Nasogastric aspiration
- Intravenous fluids
- Analgesia: pethidine
- Antibiotics
- Nutritional support: total parenteral nutrition or jejunal feeding.

Once the patient has recovered, the child should be investigated for an underlying cause. If the patient has gallstones, cholecystectomy should be undertaken when the patient is well.

Chronic pancreatitis

Repeated attacks of pancreatitis cause the pancreas to become atrophic and fibrotic. The ducts are obstructed and dilated and cyst-like cavities develop. Exocrine pancreatic insufficiency may occur. In children, this is usually due to hereditary pancreatitis. They either have recurrent bouts of acute pancreatitis or may develop intractable pain. Acute episodes are managed with analgesia and intravenous fluids. Attacks may be prevented with antioxidants and pancreatic supplements.

Pancreatic pleural fistula is a rare complication. The child will develop a pleural effusion that has a high amylase content.

Intussusception

This results from the invagination of one part of the bowel into another (usually the terminal ileum into the caecum). This results in the blood supply to that part of the bowel being severely compromised. It can occur at any time in childhood but the peak incidence is between 3 and 6 months of age following either an upper respiratory infection or gastroenteritis, or coinciding with the introduction of solids when the Peyer patches become enlarged and act as a lead point. The child has episodes of pain followed by pallor and may pass blood in the stools (redcurrant jelly). A mass is usually palpable though the diagnosis can be confirmed with an ultrasound scan (doughnut sign). Treatment is with either an air or a barium enema.

If this fails or the child has had symptoms for more than 24 hours, a laparotomy plus surgical reduction is indicated. Intussusception may be recurrent. Intussusception in children older than 2 years should alert the physician to the possibility of a polyp, cystic fibrosis or coeliac disease as contributing factors.

Volvulus

Volvulus or twisting occurs when a long mobile loop of bowel revolves around its own mesentery. Volvulus of the midgut from malrotation is most common during infancy but may occur at any time in childhood. It may be intermittent or may cause ischaemia and infarction of the gut. The symptoms are abdominal pain and bilious vomiting and there may be associated fullness/abdominal distension. A plain abdominal X-ray may show a double bubble appearance due to air proximal to the obstruction, though there is usually a small amount of distal air. The diagnosis is confirmed with an upper gastrointestinal contrast study, which will demonstrate the ligament of Treitz to be abnormally placed (it should lie to the left of the midline and above the duodenal bulb). Treatment is surgical.

Blood in the stool

(See also Ch. 25.)

Problem-orientated topic:

bloody diarrhoea ○ ○ ○ ○

Oskar, a 2-month-old boy, presents with bloody diarrhoea present for 2 weeks. His mother is well except for poorly controlled asthma. He is formula-fed and thriving.

Q1. What diagnoses would you consider?

Q1. What diagnoses would you consider?

Lower gastrointestinal bleeding (originating distal to the duodenum) is a common problem in paediatrics and, although most causes are self-limiting and benign, serious pathology can present this way. The most likely diagnoses based on history of the bleeding and age of the child are shown in Table 38.11.

Anal fissure

Anal fissure causes bright red blood on the outside of stool, sometimes dripping into the toilet and on the toilet tissue. Usually there is a history of passage

Table 38.11 Common causes of blood in the stool

Description of bleeding per rectum	Likely anatomical source/cause	Most likely diagnoses			
		Birth–1 month	1 month–2 years	2–10 years	10–16 years
Bright red blood coating formed stool	Anus or rectum	Vitamin K deficiency Anal fissure	Anal fissure	Anal fissure Polyp	Polyp Anal fissure Haemorrhoids
Bloody diarrhoea	Colonic/colitis	Food-allergic colitis Vitamin K deficiency Necrotizing enterocolitis Hirschsprung enterocolitis Intussusception	Food-allergic colitis Infectious enterocolitis Hirschsprung enterocolitis Necrotizing enterocolitis	Infectious enterocolitis Inflammatory bowel disease	Infectious enterocolitis Inflammatory bowel disease
Large-volume dark-red blood	'Surgical cause', distal small bowel/ proximal colon	Duplication cyst Volvulus	Meckel diverticulum Duplication cyst Volvulus	Meckel diverticulum Angiodysplasia	Angiodysplasia

of large constipated stool and pain on defaecation. The fissure is generally posterior and obvious on anal inspection. Treatment is usually by stool-softening agents.

Food allergy

Bloody diarrhoea can be the presenting feature of allergic enterocolitis, most commonly due to cow's milk and/or soy protein. The child is usually less than 3 months old and, though the infant can have associated vomiting and become dehydrated, the bloody stools are often the isolated concern in an otherwise well baby with normal weight gain. The child should be given a hypoallergenic formula, usually a hydrolysate.

Infectious enterocolitis

Bloody stools can occur in infections due to *Salmonella*, *Shigella*, *Campylobacter jejuni*, *Yersinia enterocolitica*, *Escherichia coli* 057 and *Entamoeba histolytica*. Pseudomembranous colitis due to *Clostridium difficile* should be considered in any child having received broad-spectrum antibiotics. Stool cultures and 'hot' stools for ova, cysts and parasite examination (and *Cl. difficile* toxin, if indicated) are mandatory in any child with bloody diarrhoea.

Meckel diverticulum

This typically presents before 2 years of age with the painless passage of a large volume of dark red blood in an otherwise healthy child. It is twice as common in boys as girls.

Intussusception

See page 541.

Polyps

Polyps are a relatively common cause of per rectum bleeding in children over 2 years. Bleeding is typically bright red, often on the surface of the stools, small in amount and painless. Ninety percent of childhood polyps are hamartomatous juvenile polyps, which are benign, generally singular and situated in the left colon. They are confirmed and removed at colonoscopy.

Haemorrhoids

Haemorrhoids are rare in infants and children, and if present, are usually due to portal hypertension. They do occur in constipated adolescents, causing bleeding during defaecation with blood on the surface of the stool or the toilet paper or dripping into the toilet bowl. The child may describe something 'coming out' from their anus during defaecation and the pain is typically aching in nature rather than sharp as described with fissures. Parents sometimes wrongly describe haemorrhoids when the child actually has rectal prolapse.

Inflammatory bowel disease: Crohn disease and ulcerative colitis

Crohn disease is an inflammatory condition affecting any part of the digestive tract and involving the entire thickness of the bowel wall. Isolated ileal disease is less common in children and Crohn colitis is the commonest distribution. Symptoms include abdominal pain, anorexia, weight loss, poor growth, diarrhoea (which may contain blood and mucus) and fever. Positive physical findings may include anorexia, thickening and fissuring of the lips (oro-facial granulomatosis),

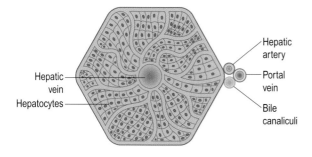

Fig. 38.10 **The anatomy of the liver lobule**

clubbing, abdominal masses, peri-anal fissures and skin tags. Blood tests reveal evidence of chronic inflammation (elevated ESR, CRP and platelet count and hypoalbuminaemia). Definite diagnosis is based an upper GI endoscopy, ileo-colonoscopy and biopsies. Treatments include dietary measures (elemental and polymeric diet), steroids and immunosuppressive agents. Surgery and resection of the affected areas may be needed particularly in severe growth failure or stricturing disease.

Ulcerative colitis is confined to the large bowel. Symptoms include abdominal pain, diarrhoea with mucus, rectal bleeding, tenesmus and fever. Diagnosis is based on colonoscopy and biopsies. Treatment is initially with steroids (systemic and local) and 5 aminosalicylic acid. Colectomy +/– ileal pouch is reserved for failure of medical treatment.

Liver disease

Basic science

The liver is divided into the right and left lobe, which are in turn divided into eight segments. Each segment is divided into lobules with a central vein. In the spaces between the lobules are branches of the portal vein, hepatic artery and bile duct canaliculi (Fig. 38.10).

The functions of the liver include formation and secretion of bile, glycogen storage and metabolism, ketone body formation, detoxification of toxins and drugs, and manufacture of plasma proteins and coagulation factors. Whilst biochemical liver function tests reflect the severity of hepatic dysfunction, they rarely provide diagnostic information of individual disease.

Baseline investigations

Bilirubin is nearly always elevated in liver disease; when detected in urine it is always abnormal. It may also be elevated in any condition causing haemolysis. Causes of elevated serum bilirubin are shown in Box 38.7.

BOX 38.7 Causes of an elevated bilirubin

Unconjugated
- Increased production of bilirubin:
  - Haemolysis
- Failure of transport of bilirubin to site of conjugation within the liver cell:
  - Gilbert disease: autosomal dominant, mild jaundice, increased with intercurrent illness, dehydration and exercise; often vague abdominal pain and general malaise
- Defective glucuronyl transferase activity:
  - Crigler–Najjar syndrome types 1 and 2:
    Type 1: no bilirubin uridine diphosphate glucuronyl transferase (UDPGT); risk of kernicterus; treatment with phototherapy/ liver transplant/auxiliary transplant
    Type 2: partial defect; treatment not usually required

Conjugated
- Failure to transport conjugated bilirubin to bile canaliculi:
  - Dubin–Johnson syndrome, Rotor syndrome: both autosomal recessive
- Intrahepatic and extrahepatic obstruction of bile flow:
  - Intrahepatic: drugs, viral and autoimmune hepatitis etc.
  - Extrahepatic: mechanical obstruction (gallstones, extrahepatic biliary atresia and choledochal cysts)

Other indices of liver function

(Table 38.12)

Aminotransferases

- Aspartate (AST)
- Alanine (ALT).

These are present in liver, heart and skeletal muscle, and are elevated if there is hepatocyte damage.

Alkaline phosphatase (ALP)

ALP is found in liver, kidney, bone, placenta and intestine. Elevation of this enzyme in liver disease indicates biliary epithelial damage, cirrhosis, rejection or osteopenia secondary to vitamin D deficiency/malabsorption.

Gamma-glutamyl transpeptidases (GGT)

GGT is present in biliary epithelium and hepatocytes, and increased in many forms of liver disease.

Table 38.12 Significance of abnormal investigations in the jaundiced child/child with abnormal liver function tests

Investigation	Significance
Haemoglobin	Low with elevated reticulocytes indicates haemolysis
Bilirubin	Unconjugated increase suggests haemolysis Conjugated increase suggests hepatic or post-hepatic disease
AST/ALT/gamma-glutamyl transferase (GGT)	Elevated with liver damage
Albumin/total proteins	Albumin low in chronic liver disease, globulin elevated in autoimmune hepatitis
Serology	Identification of virus causing hepatitis
Immunology	Increased IgG, +ve antinuclear antibodies (ANA) (type 1), +ve liver, kidney, microsomal antibodies (LKM) (type 2) in autoimmune chronic active hepatitis
Copper studies	Ceruloplasmin decreased, 24-hour urinary copper pre- and post-penicillamine increased in Wilson disease

Synthetic function of the liver

- *Albumin*. If decreased, indicates chronic liver disease.
- *Coagulation*. If abnormal, indicates significant hepatic dysfunction, either acute or chronic.
- *Blood glucose*. A finding of fasting hypoglycaemia in absence of other causes suggests poor hepatic function, particularly in acute hepatic failure.

Infectious hepatitis

Causes

- Acute viral:
  - Hepatitis A, B, C (D and E) (Table 38.13)
  - Measles
  - Rubella
  - Erythrovirus 19 (parvovirus B19)
  - Herpes simplex types I and II
  - Varicella zoster
  - Cytomegalovirus
  - Epstein–Barr virus
  - Human herpes virus type 6
  - Yellow fever
- Non-viral:
  - Leptospirosis
  - *Listeria monocytogenes*
  - Toxoplasmosis
  - Hydatid disease.

Hydatid disease

This is caused by *Echinococcus* (tapeworm), whose intermediate host is sheep and dogs. Following ingestion of ova by humans, the embryo develops and penetrates the stomach wall, reaching the liver via the portal vein. Cysts develop in the liver and lungs. Liver cysts are slow-growing, giving asymptomatic hepatomegaly.

Treatment is either by surgical excision, or with mebendazole for 3 months.

Autoimmune liver disease

Autoimmune chronic active hepatitis is a chronic inflammatory disorder affecting the liver, responding to immunosuppression. It may coexist with other autoimmune disorders and the male:female ratio is 1:3. It may present as hepatitis, fulminant liver failure or chronic liver disease (often despite a short history). The diagnosis is confirmed on liver biopsy (interface hepatitis). Investigations typically show raised total proteins and IgG, antinuclear antibody (ANA) and smooth muscle antibody positive (classed as type 1), and liver kidney microsomal (LKM) antibody positive (type 2). Treatment is immunosuppressive, with steroids and azathioprine.

Sclerosing cholangitis is an autoimmune condition predominantly affecting intra- and extrahepatic bile ducts, leading to fibrosis and usually associated with ulcerative colitis. As there are similar autoantibody features to type 1 autoimmune hepatitis, there is probably some overlap between the two conditions.

Wilson disease

This is a rare autosomal recessive disorder. There is an accumulation of copper in liver, brain (causing behavioural changes and extrapyramidal problems), cornea (Kayser–Fleischer rings) and kidneys (renal tubular problems, vitamin D-resistant rickets). The genetic defect results in decreased synthesis of copper-binding protein ceruloplasmin and defective copper excretion in bile. Children present mostly under 12 years with any form of liver disease or occasionally with haemolytic anaemia.

The diagnosis is based on measurement of serum copper, but this can be unreliable (usually decreased, occasionally normal or increased); decreased ceruloplasmin; increased 24-hour urinary copper after D-penicillamine; and increased liver copper.

Treatment is with penicillamine to chelate and excrete excess copper, and zinc to decrease absorption.

Table 38.13 Clinical features of hepatitis A, B and C

Type	Virus	Incubation period	Transmission	Clinical presentation	Treatment
Hepatitis A	RNA	30 days	Faecal–oral	Acute illness with nausea, abdominal pain, jaundice and hepatomegaly +ve IgM Very rare cause of acute liver failure, rare persistent cholestasis	Supportive, as normally self-limiting illness Vaccination available
Hepatitis B	DNA	30–180 days (mean 100)	Transfusion blood/blood products Needlestick injury Lateral spread in families Perinatal	May be asymptomatic, classical features of acute hepatitis, fulminant hepatic failure 1–2% +ve serology 30–50% chronic carriage 10% will develop cirrhosis with risk of hepatocellular carcinoma in later life	Interferon and lamivudine may be of benefit Prevention: pregnant women screened for hepatitis B surface antigen (HBsAg) Babies of all HBsAg +ve mothers receive vaccination If mother has hepatitis B e antigen, +ve baby receives immunoglobulin at birth Vaccination available
Hepatitis C	RNA	40–80 days	Transfusion blood/blood products Vertical transmission 7%	Rarely acute infection 50% will develop chronic liver disease, despite many having normal liver function tests, and progress to cirrhosis with risk of hepatocellular carcinoma in later life	Interferon and ribavirin in combination may be of benefit

Liver transplantation is reserved for acute liver failure and decompensated liver disease.

Acute liver failure

Acute liver failure is rare in childhood and has a high mortality. It is defined as onset of encephalopathy and coagulopathy within 8 weeks of the onset of liver disease. The most common causes are viral hepatitis, undefined metabolic conditions and, in the older child, deliberate overdosage of paracetamol and Wilson disease.

The child presents with jaundice, encephalopathy and hypoglycaemia. The signs of encephalopathy may initially be subtle and include drowsiness, night-time wakefulness and periods of irritability and aggression. Initially, the bilirubin may not be elevated but transaminases are very high, coagulation is abnormal and ammonia is elevated.

Principles of management of acute liver failure
- *Hypoglycaemia*: maintain blood glucose > 4 mmol/l with 10% dextrose.
- *Prevent sepsis*: broad-spectrum antibiotics/antifungals.
- *Coagulopathy*: correct with vitamin K and fresh frozen plasma.
- *Cerebral oedema*: nurse head up, restrict fluid to 60% maintenance, ventilation for encephalopathy.

- *Prevent gastrointestinal bleeding*: H$_2$-blockers/PPIs.
- *Liver protection*: N-acetylcysteine 150 mg/kg/24 hr.
- *Transfer when stabilized*: to liver transplant unit.

Cirrhosis and portal hypertension

Cirrhosis is a pathological diagnosis that includes the combination of fibrosis and regenerative nodules. It is the end result of many forms of liver disease and causes portal hypertension, ascites, distended veins on the abdominal wall and oesophageal varices.

Complications of portal hypertension
- *Ascites*: results from decreased albumin and sodium retention; treated with diuretics and albumin infusion
- *Hypersplenism*: decreased white cell count and platelet count
- *Oesophageal varices*: may bleed
- *Encephalopathy*: often precipitated by gastrointestinal bleed/sepsis/renal failure.

Management of bleeding oesophageal varices
- *Resuscitation*: blood transfusion, aiming for haemoglobin of 10 g/dl
- *Acid suppression*: H$_2$-blockers/PPIs

- *Lowering portal blood pressure*: octreotide (vasopressin analogue)
- *Endoscopy*: sclerotherapy or banding of varices
- *Resistant bleeding*: liver transplantation/shunt operations.

Extrahepatic portal hypertension/ portal vein thrombosis

Blockage of the portal vein may result from a congenital abnormality of the portal vein, blockage following umbilical venous catheterization, omphalitis and infiltration with tumour. The portal vein is not seen on ultrasound and is replaced by tangled enlarged venous collaterals: cavernous transformation of the portal vein/portal cavernoma. Presentation may be with haemorrhage from oesophageal varices, an enlarged spleen or hypersplenism. If gastrointestinal haemorrhage cannot be controlled endoscopically, blockage can be bypassed by a graft, usually taken from the external jugular vein: mesorex shunt.

Peter Hoyer   Heather Lambert

Urinary system

LEARNING OUTCOMES

By the end of this chapter you should:
- Know the common presentations of renal disease
- Understand the appropriate choice of investigations
- Know how to assess and manage the dehydrated child
- Understand the investigation and management of urinary tract infection
- Understand the causes and management of hypertension
- Understand the investigation, management and common presenting symptoms of diseases of the urinary tract.

Introduction

The kidneys have a wide range of functions. They are responsible for the control of the volume and electrolyte composition of extracellular fluid by a combination of glomerular filtration and tubular reabsorption. They play a role in maintenance of acid–base status through reabsorption of filtered bicarbonate and regeneration of bicarbonate. The kidney plays a role in the formation of red blood cells through production of erythropoietin; bone biochemistry through generation of 1,25-dihydroxycholecalciferol; and the regulation of blood pressure through the renin–angiotensin system.

Disorders of the urinary tract presenting in primary care are discussed in Chapter 26.

Investigating renal function

Serum creatinine

Serum creatinine is the best clinically useful and available guide in evaluating the filtering function of the kidney. It is easily, quickly and cheaply measured on a small blood sample. Individual measurements are of use in determining whether renal function is within the normal range. Sequential measurements are useful to follow deterioration or improvements of renal function over a short timescale of hours and days or over a long timescale of months and years. Serum creatinine varies with height, sex and muscle mass.

Concept of fractional excretion

Clearance of any substance that is filtered by the glomerulus and then reabsorbed by the tubule can be compared to the clearance of creatinine, which is filtered and then excreted largely unmodified by the tubule. The fractional excretion is that fraction of substance X that has been filtered at the glomerulus that actually reaches the urine.

$$\text{Fractional excretion (FE) } X\% = \frac{\text{urine } X}{\text{filtered } X} \times 100$$

Fractional excretion of sodium

Normally most of the filtered sodium (Na) is reabsorbed; the majority of this happens in the proximal tubule. When serum sodium is normal and the patient is not in circulatory failure or shock, fractional excretion of sodium can vary physiologically. However, calculating FE Na can give useful clues in pathological states.

The normal renal response to intravascular fluid volume reduction is to excrete urine with low sodium content. The kidney does this via a number of mechanisms, including reduction of glomerular filtration rate (GFR) and aldosterone-stimulated sodium reabsorption, which requires intact tubular function and transport systems.

Calculation of fractional excretion

See Box 39.1.

Table 39.1 shows the clinical picture.

BOX 39.1 Calculation of fractional excretion

Fractional excretion Na %	=	$\dfrac{\text{urine Na} \times 100}{\text{filtered Na}}$
Urine Na	=	UNa × V
and filtered Na	=	GFR × S Na
and GFR	=	$\dfrac{\text{UCr} \times \text{V}}{\text{SCr}}$
so **FE Na %**	=	$\dfrac{\text{UNa} \times \text{V} \times \text{SCr}}{\text{SNa} \times \text{UCr} \times \text{V}}$ *or* **U/S sodium ×** **S/U creatinine**

N.B. When calculating, remember to ensure urine (U) and serum (S) units are the same.

Table 39.1 Clinical picture from equation

Clinical picture	FE Na	Clinical significance
Shock	< 1%	= Tubules functioning = pre-renal failure
	> 1%	= Acute tubular necrosis (ATN)
Hyponatraemia	< 1%	= Salt loss or water overload (appropriate renal response)
	> 1%	= Renal salt wasting
Hypernatraemia	< 1%	= Renal concentration defect
	> 1%	= Salt overload

Table 39.2 Requirements for 24-hour water, sodium and potassium on average caloric expenditure

Age	Preterm	Term	1 year	5 years	12 years
Sodium (mmol/kg)	5	3	2	2	1
Potassium (mmol/kg)	5	3	2	2	1
Water (ml/kg)	200	150	100	75	50
Easy hourly rate (ml/kg/hr)	8	6	4	3	2

Water and electrolyte imbalance

Problems with fluid and electrolyte balance are common in ill children. They can occur in a wide variety of clinical situations and with a wide range of underlying diagnoses. A methodical approach to history-taking and clinical examination is therefore essential and interpretation of biochemical results must always be done in the context of the clinical situation.

Maintenance water, sodium and potassium requirements per 24 hours are shown in Table 39.2.

Dehydration and hypovolaemia

Dehydration represents a deficit between fluid and electrolyte intake and losses. Fluid within the body is normally distributed between the intracellular fluid (ICF) and extracellular fluid (ECF) compartments; the ECF is composed of intravascular and interstitial components. Differential solute composition of ICF and ECF compartments is maintained by cell membrane pump activity and solute size and electrical charge. Fluid movement is regulated by a balance between osmotically active solutes and hydrostatic pressure. It is useful when clinically assessing the fluid volume status of a patient to try to consider which compartment has insufficient or excess volume.

The effects of ECF volume depletion are usually shared between the intravascular and interstitial compartments and are seen as hypovolaemia and dehydration respectively. Assessment can be complex. For example, in a situation like nephrotic syndrome, there may be weight gain and oedema on examination. However, since there is hypoalbuminaemia and albumin is the primary intravascular osmotic component, the intravascular fluid volume may be low but the total ECF volume high. Conversely, in acute renal failure there can be weight gain and oedema in a situation where both the total ECF and the intravascular volume are high. Oedema can therefore occur with high or low intravascular fluid volume.

In a complex situation like intensive care, where there may be multi-organ failure and multiple drug therapies, clinical assessment of fluid status is very difficult and invasive monitoring becomes essential.

Clinical estimation of ECF volume deficit

This is based on symptoms and signs (Boxes 39.2 and 39.3), as well as weight on admission compared with an expected weight.

Often in dehydration, sodium and water have been lost in approximately normal ratio and therefore the deficit should be replaced as normal saline (Box 39.4).

Aim to treat cardiovascular collapse or 'shock' quickly over the first 1–2 hours. Infuse Ringer lactate solution or isotonic NaCl solution (note: high chloride content may aggravate hyperchloraemic acidosis) to restore circulating blood volume and thereafter slow the replacement rate so that total deficit is replaced over 24 hours. In hypernatraemic dehydration, after an acceptable cardiovascular state has been restored, aim

---

BOX 39.3 Practical point: clinical assessment of volume status

Good clinical assessment of volume status comes with experience. A good way of improving those skills is whenever a judgment of reduced ECF is made (for example, when admitting a toddler with dehydration from acute gastroenteritis), note the percentage deficit assessed and the weight of the child and compare this with the percentage gain in weight of the child once he or she is fully rehydrated (e.g. 48 hours later). This gives an indication, in retrospect, of the accuracy of the initial assessment.

BOX 39.4 Practical point: prescribing rehydration fluids

When prescribing rehydration fluids:

1. Make an assessment of volume deficit and replace this as normal saline (or sometimes human albumin solution in shock)
2. Calculate maintenance fluids and insensible losses
3. Initially estimate and then measure ongoing losses and replace appropriately in volume and composition.

   Fluid prescription should consist of 1 + 2 + 3.

---

to reduce plasma sodium slowly over 24–48 hours by altering the sodium concentration of the infusion fluid appropriately and repeatedly monitoring the rate of fall of serum sodium, which should not be more than 10–12 mmol/day to prevent cerebral oedema.

Management of fluid and electrolyte disorders depends on measurement of input and output plus *serial*:

- Clinical examination
- Biochemical data on urine and blood
- Weight measurements.

Hyponatraemia

Hyponatraemia is defined as a serum sodium of less than 130 mmol/l and occurs when there is:

- Sodium loss in excess of water loss
  or
- Water gain in excess of sodium gain.

The total body sodium may be high, low or normal and therefore clinical assessment of ECF volume is essential.

Hypernatraemia

Hypernatraemia is defined as a serum sodium greater than 150 mmol/l and occurs when there is:

BOX 39.2 Symptoms and signs of ECF volume deficit

	% weight loss	loss of water/kg
Minimal	(<3%)	30 ml
– Thirst		
Mild	(3–5%)	30–50 ml
– Dry mucous membranes		
Moderate	(5–7%)	50–70 ml
– Sunken eyes		
– Depressed fotanelle		
Moderate—Severe	(7–12%)	70–120 ml
– Decreased skin turgor		
– Cold periphery		
– Prolonged capillary refill time		
– Tachycardia		
Severe	(>12%)	>120 ml
– Hypotension		
– Drowsiness, confusion or coma		
– Shock		

- Water loss in excess of sodium loss

  or

- Sodium gain in excess of water gain.

Again, the total body sodium may be high, low or normal.

In hypernatraemic dehydration the water loss exceeds sodium loss. Because sodium is the principle ECF osmole, the ECF volume is relatively well maintained and signs of dehydration and hypovolaemia are less apparent.

Urinary tract infection

Urinary tract infection (UTI) is an important and common cause of acute illness in children, may be a marker of an underlying urinary tract abnormality and may cause significant long-term morbidity, particularly renal scarring, hypertension and renal impairment, which may not present until adult life (Box 39.5). There is good evidence that UTI in childhood is associated with renal scarring, the risk seems to be highest in the youngest infants. This is the very group in whom diagnosis is often overlooked or delayed because clinical features are frequently non-specific. Thus diagnosis of UTI requires a very high index of suspicion, particularly in the youngest. Accurate diagnosis is essential because of the need for prompt treatment, imaging and the risks associated with over- or under-investigation. UTI may be recurrent, about one-third of girls having a further UTI within a year. The recurrence rate in boys is much lower.

BOX 39.5 Clinical features of urinary tract infection

- Affects many children
- May be difficult to diagnose
- May cause acute illness and symptoms
- Is frequently over- or under-diagnosed
- May have long-term sequelae: hypertension, renal scarring, renal failure

---

Problem-orientated topic:

dysuria ● ● ● ● ●

Whilst away on holiday, Milica, a 5-year-old girl, complained of soreness and stinging on passing urine for 24 hours. She was taken to see the local doctor, who treated her with a 5-day course of antibiotics. Two weeks after return from holiday the symptoms recur and the girl is taken to see her primary care physician, who telephones you asking for advice.

Q1. Did Milica have a urinary tract infection?

Q2. What is the differential diagnosis of dysuria?

Q3. How would you assess Milica?

Q4. What would be your management?

Q5. Does Milica require further investigation?

Q1. Did Milica have a urinary tract infection?

Clinical features of UTI in childhood are often different to those found in adults and are frequently non-specific. Without a high index of suspicion many UTIs, especially in the very young, will be missed. Classical symptoms of lower UTI (dysuria, frequency and incontinence) and upper UTI (fever, systemic upset, loin pain and renal tenderness) are frequently not seen in paediatric practice. Attempts to distinguish between upper and lower UTI on clinical grounds are unreliable and clinical history is not closely related to findings on imaging. UTI can occasionally produce life-threatening illness, especially in very young infants, who may present severely unwell with shock or septicaemia. Boys and girls are equally affected in infancy but after that the ratio of girls to boys progressively rises. After puberty the incidence of UTI is low in both sexes but rises in females who are sexually active. Renal scarring may occur in association with few or no symptoms.

Preschool children

In general terms, the younger the child, the more diverse and less specific the symptoms and signs. Thus evaluation of any unwell or febrile young child must include examination of urine. Sometimes there is a history of smelly urine or of crying on passing urine. Children may have an altered pattern of micturition and day- or night-time wetting may recur. Non-specific manifestations, such as poor feeding, vomiting, irritability, abdominal pain, failure to thrive, lethargy and restlessness, should always lead to a suspicion of UTI.

Older children

Older children may have more typical signs and symptoms localizing to the urinary tract, including dysuria, frequency, urgency, hesitation and enuresis. Some may have loin pain but absence of loin pain does not exclude upper urinary tract involvement. Generalized symptoms are common and include fever, lethargy, anorexia, abdominal pain, nausea and vomiting.

From the information given by the primary care physician, it is not possible to be sure whether Milica had a UTI.

BOX 39.6 Methods of collecting urine in children

- Clean catch
- Pads
- Sterile adhesive bags
- Suprapubic aspiration (SPA)
- Potty (washed up)
- Midstream urine (MSU)
- Urethral catheterization

Q2. What is the differential diagnosis of dysuria?

Not all children with dysuria have a UTI. Dysuria may be associated with localized skin conditions, such as candidiasis, vulvitis or excoriation secondary to threadworms or other irritation. Febrile or mildly dehydrated children may complain of pain, stinging or discomfort on passing concentrated or what they term 'strong' urine. Children with quite minor degrees of haematuria — for example, from glomerulonephritis — may present with dysuria.

Q3. How would you assess Milica?

(Boxes 39.7 and 39.8)

Details should be sought of family history of urinary infection, vesico-ureteric reflux (VUR), renal disease or hypertension; antenatal and perinatal history; and drinking, voiding pattern and bowel habits. Examination should include examination of the urine; measurement of blood pressure; abdominal palpation for masses (bladder, kidney); inspection of external genitalia and lower back; and assessment of lower limb sensation and reflexes. When UTI is recurrent, it is particularly important that bladder and bowel habits are evaluated, as UTI may be associated with dysfunctional voiding, bladder instability and constipation.

Making the diagnosis of UTI: urine collection and testing (Boxes 39.6 and 39.8)

Infants with UTI but only non-specific symptoms are frequently under-diagnosed, whereas girls with vulvitis and febrile anorexic children who produce a highly concentrated urine and complain of dysuria are often falsely diagnosed as having a UTI.

Unfortunately, it is common for some children to receive an antibiotic for a presumed UTI without a urine sample being either collected or tested. Once this has happened, it is not possible to reach a certain diagnosis and the decision whether to investigate the child is very difficult.

BOX 39.7 Summary of UTI

- Evaluation of any sick child must include examination of urine
- Every young child with unexplained fever should have urine examined
- Clinical features of UTI are often non-specific
- Boys seldom get recurrent UTI in the absence of urinary tract abnormalities

BOX 39.8 Key points: urine collection and testing

- Accurate diagnosis of UTI is vital to appropriate subsequent management
- Antibiotic treatment should be started as soon as a suitable sample has been collected
- Urine can be collected in any setting by pad or bag, or by clean catch into a bottle or washed potty
- All urine collecting methods may fail or result in contamination
- All methods result in some false positives
- Phase-contrast microscopy is easy to learn and quick to perform
- Microscopy can immediately identify and prevent false positives
- Positive nitrite stick tests diagnose UTI but negative ones do not exclude UTI
- Urine white cell counts are unreliable in diagnosis of UTI
- Urine samples that cannot be transported to the laboratory quickly should be refrigerated or inoculated on to a dipslide
- Boric acid bottles are outdated, as they may produce false negative results

Organisms that cause UTI

About 85% of urine samples from boys and girls with a first UTI grow *Escherichia coli* on culture. *Klebsiella*, *Proteus* and *Streptococcus faecalis* are responsible for most of the rest. Children with abnormal urinary tracts are much more likely to have UTI due to less virulent organisms such as *Pseudomonas* or *Staphylococcus aureus*.

Laboratory culture for bacteria

There may be problems with over-diagnosis if organisms $>10^5$/ml are used. Using $>10^8$/ml would reduce false positives but would require special handling by laboratories. Refrigeration is highly effective for minimizing the overgrowth of contaminating organisms during storage and transfer to the laboratory.

Bacterial culture on dipslides

Urine can be cultured at any time and anywhere, and can be posted to the laboratory.

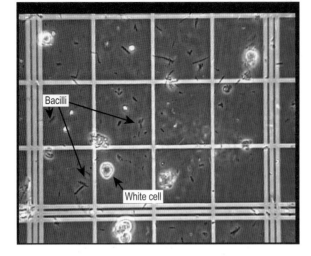

Fig. 39.1 **Phase-contrast microscopy of urine**

Bacilli

White cell

BOX 39.9 Treatment of UTI

- Treatment goal is prevention of renal injury and symptoms associated with UTI
- Start 'best guess' antibiotic as soon as urine obtained
- Change antibiotic if culture result indicates
- If clinical condition does not improve after 48 hours repeat urine culture and request urgent investigations to exclude urological problems
- Give prophylactic antibiotics until investigations complete
- Clinical experience suggests benefit from increasing fluid intake and treatment of constipation

Phase-contrast microscopy (Fig. 39.1)

Bacteria can be identified very easily in unprepared urine by phase-contrast microscopy. Therefore, phase-contrast microscopy can provide a fast, reliable, efficient and economic near-patient UTI diagnostic service.

When infected urine is examined by phase-contrast microscopy there will typically be tens, hundreds or thousands of identical rods per high-power field, equivalent to bacterial counts of between 10^6 and 10^9/ml. Uninfected urine simply has no organisms to see at all. The urine from a child with a UTI will almost invariably have many rods visible per high-power field, so a completely empty field virtually guarantees an uninfected sample.

Some urine samples will give uncertain results because either just one or two bacteria are seen, or rods and streptococci are present together, or there is amorphous debris, cotton strands etc. present. If these urine samples are cultured, they are likely to give uncertain results several days later. If microscopy is used, a repeat sample can be collected at once.

Identifying bacteria with nitrite stick tests

Most uropathogens produce nitrite as a result of their metabolism. Uninfected urine samples do not contain nitrite, so the specificity is about 100%. A positive test is diagnostic. However, it often takes hours for the bacteria to produce detectable quantities of nitrite and children with UTI tend to void frequently so the test sensitivity is low (53%, range 15–82). If samples test negative for nitrite this must be ignored since we may be dealing with non-urea splitting organisms.

Urinary white blood cells in UTI

White blood cells in the urine are essentially required for the diagnosis of urinary tract infection, whether detected by sticks or microscopy. However, it should be kept in mind that they may represent a false positive indicator because other conditions are also associated with leukocyturia.

Q4. What would be your management?
(Box 39.9)

Cefalexin, cefaclor, trimethoprim or nitrofurantoin is frequently used but discussion with the local microbiologist should help guide general advice about resistance patterns. Children, particularly infants, who are clinically dehydrated, toxic or unlikely to retain oral fluids, should be given parenteral antibiotics initially. There is no clear evidence about the ideal length of therapy to eradicate acute infection in children, but most recommend at least 7 days.

Asymptomatic bacteriuria in girls with normal urinary tracts should not be regarded as UTI and therefore needs no treatment.

Q5. Does Milica require further investigation?

The aims of investigation are to identify children:
- With an underlying renal tract abnormality or predisposition to UTI:
  - Structural abnormality of urinary tract
  - Urinary tract obstruction
  - VUR
  - Abnormal bladder emptying
- Who have already sustained damage to their kidneys
- Who are likely to sustain damage to their kidneys.

Investigation of UTI
- All children should have some investigation after a proven UTI.
- Unnecessary investigations should be avoided.

- VUR is found in up to 30% of children with UTI (see below).
- Babies with antenatal diagnosed hydronephrosis have increased risk of VUR.
- There is a 20 to 50% chance of VUR if there is a family history of VUR.
- There is an association between abnormal urodynamic variables and VUR.
- The relationship between VUR, renal scarring and reflux nephropathy is not clear.
- Renal scarring can occur without VUR.
- Young children and infants warrant intensive investigation.

Which investigations after UTI?

- Ultrasonography (US):
  - No ionizing radiation
  - Good for detecting structural abnormalities
  - In childhood scars are often small and frequently missed on US
- Tc^{99}-dimercaptosuccinic acid (DMSA):
  - Useful for detection of tubular uptake defects, dysplastic lesions and scarring
  - Small dose of ionizing radiation
  - Timing: DMSA scan soon after acute infection may show areas of reduced uptake that are not permanent, therefore delay DMSA scan for 2–3 months post acute UTI
- Micturating cystourethrogram (MCUG) direct contrast study:
  - To show reflux as well as bladder and urethral anatomy
  - Requires insertion of a bladder catheter
  - Ionizing radiation to the gonads
- MCUG direct radioisotope study (outdated, no indication):
  - Lower radiation dose than contrast MCUG
  - Requires the insertion of a bladder catheter
  - Grading of reflux not possible
  - No anatomical features demonstrated
- Indirect radioisotope study MAG3 (mercaptoacetyltriglycine):
  - No bladder catheter is required but intravenous injection is necessary
  - Lower radiation dose than contrast MCUG
  - Partial renal function and urodynamic information
  - No or very limited anatomical information (does not detect reflux)
- Abdominal X-ray:
  - Useful for localization of stones in selective cases (e.g. *Proteus* infection) or where there is a suggestive history
  - Spinal defects may be identified and constipation demonstrated.

> **BOX 39.10 International grading of vesico-ureteric reflux**
>
> I Into ureter only
>
> II Into ureter, pelvis and calyces with no dilatation
>
> III With mild to moderate dilatation; slight or no blunting of fornices
>
> IV With moderate dilatation of ureter and/or renal pelvis and/or tortuosity of ureter; obliteration of sharp angle of fornices
>
> V Gross dilatation and tortuosity; no papillary impression visible in calyces

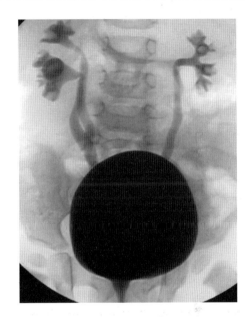

Fig. 39.2 Vesico-ureteric reflux on micturating cystourethrogram (duplex on right side)

It is important to acknowledge that there is no single test that answers all the essential questions in a child who has had a UTI. The specific tests used will depend on a variety of factors.

Vesico-ureteric reflux (VUR) (Box 39.10 and Fig. 39.2)

VUR is the retrograde flow of urine from the bladder into the upper urinary tract. It is usually congenital. VUR is a major risk factor for progressive renal damage associated with UTI. The incidence of VUR is in the order of 1% in infants and is increased in certain risk groups. There is good evidence that VUR is a genetic disorder, although disease-causing mutations have not been detected thus far.

VUR is thought to predispose to renal damage by facilitating passage of bacteria from the bladder to the upper urinary tract. An immunological and inflammatory reaction is caused by renal infection, leading to renal

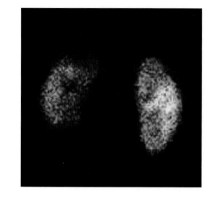

Fig. 39.3 Unilateral uptake defect ('scar') seen on DMSA

injury and scarring. Extensive renal scarring causes reduced renal function, reduced renal growth, renal failure, hypertension and increased incidence of pregnancy-related hypertension. Whilst these sequelae may occur in childhood, patients frequently do not present until many years or decades later. Some babies born with VUR have associated dysplastic or hypoplastic renal malformations, a complex called CAKUT (Congenital Anomalies of the Kidney and Urinary Tract), all of which may impair renal function. Therefore when a child being investigated following a UTI is found to have abnormalities on DMSA scan it may be difficult to distinguish whether this is scarring caused by UTI or a congenital renal abnormality or both (Fig. 39.3).

The risk of scarring following a UTI varies with age, but the precise details of this are not clear. In clinical situations it is often very difficult to know at what age an individual child acquired the scars. Young children appear to be at most risk.

It is thought that children with VUR should be protected from scarring until they outgrow their reflux, rather than up to an arbitrary age.

The child with evidence of scarring diagnosed at any age

When scarring is first detected it is not possible to determine at what age that scar occurred. Thus it is logical to need to know whether there is still VUR present, with the intention of trying to prevent further damage from UTI in those with VUR. It is important to understand that DMSA uptake defects are not specific for scars. Uptake defects may point towards dysplastic elements in CAKUT.

Management of VUR (Boxes 39.11 and 39.12)

Historically, both medical and surgical management strategies for VUR have been introduced without controlled studies documenting long-term benefit.

Resolution of VUR with time

Resolution of VUR over time with medical treatment is related to the grade of VUR and the age of the patient. In general a lower grade of reflux has a better chance of spontaneous resolution. In children with grade I or II reflux there is resolution in about 80–90% after 5 years. Bilateral grade IV and V reflux have the lowest chance, with spontaneous resolution in less than 20% of patients after 5 years.

Medical management

Since it is known that in the vast majority of cases VUR will resolve with time, the aim in medical management of VUR, with prophylactic antibiotics, is to prevent recurrent (or sometimes first) UTI and consequent renal scarring, whilst waiting for resolution of VUR.

Breakthrough infections may be problematic and may be due to non-compliance or true bacterial resistance. Cefalclor, cefalexin, trimethoprim or nitrofurantoin are frequently used for prophylaxis.

Surgical management

There are two main forms of surgical treatment of VUR:

- *Endoscopic subureteric injection (STING).* Injection of tissue-augmenting substances is done under general anaesthetic and requires only a short stay (or treatment as a day case) in hospital. The success rate in abolition of VUR varies with the centre, the material used, the timing of re-evaluation and test used in re-examination. The longevity of the treatment and need for repeat are not fully known.
- *Reimplantation.* Surgical success in curing VUR with reimplantation is high (> 95% overall). This is, however, a major operation requiring a stay of several days in hospital, with the associated risks and costs.

Two large multicentre prospective trials of medical versus surgical treatment for children with severe VUR do not show superiority of either treatment. Breakthrough infection, despite medical treatment or because of non-compliance, remains a commonly used factor for consideration of surgical treatment, as does deterioration of DMSA appearance.

Hypertension

Persistent systemic hypertension is an important risk factor for heart failure, myocardial infarction and stroke in adult life. There is increasing evidence that 'essential' hypertension is genetically determined; however, the detection rate during childhood is low. Obesity in childhood is an increasing problem and will be associated with an increasing number at risk of hypertension. The kidney has a very important role in hypertension, both as the 'villain', as in essential hypertension and primary renal disease, and as the 'victim', as demonstrated in the destruction of the kidney in malignant hypertension and the rapid progression of chronic renal insufficiency in the face of poor blood pressure (BP) control.

Accurate measurement is important and there are various methods for measuring BP in children. The mercury or aneroid sphygmomanometer, used with stethoscope or Doppler, is generally considered the gold standard. Automated methods are often used for ease and rapidity, but not all have been validated for use in children and in practice they may not be appropriately maintained and calibrated. Therefore BP should always be rechecked by another more reliable method when thought to be abnormal. Twenty-four-hour ambulatory BP monitoring or home BP monitoring may be useful to overcome the problem of 'white coat hypertension' to monitor borderline cases or monitor therapy. The cuff size used should be no less than two-thirds of the length of the upper arm from antecubital fossa to shoulder and it should also be large enough to encircle the arm. In effect the biggest cuff that will still allow the elbow to bend.

Defining normal blood pressure and hypertension

Definition of normality is difficult. There is a steady increase in blood pressure with age and no significant sex difference. The Second Task Force on Blood Pressure Control in Children has compiled charts of normal ranges for children from birth to 17 years.

 http://ww.nhlbi.nih.gov/guidelines/
hypertension/child_tbl.pdf

Normal ranges by child's height

Since BP is a continuous variable, any definition of hypertension is arbitrary and there are no universally accepted definitions. It is important to exclude errors in measurement. The most common are use of an incorrectly sized cuff, poor technique, use of unvalidated equipment and inappropriate interpretation (failing to use appropriate nomograms for age, height and sex). Reactive rises due to anxiety or pain are common pitfalls. Some conditions cause short-lived rises in blood pressure in otherwise normal children (e.g. hypovolaemia, raised intracranial pressure, drug therapy (e.g. steroids) and iatrogenic intravenous fluid overload). Even when errors have been excluded it is important that BP is measured repeatedly. Children with a systolic BP 15 mmHg or more above the 95th percentile can be considered to be severely hypertensive. For neonates, repeated systolic BP measurements above 90 mmHg at term and above 80 mmHg preterm are hypertensive.

Primary (essential) hypertension is rare during childhood but is the leading diagnosis of hypertension in adults. Hypertension is secondary in more than 80% of children and in two thirds it is of renal origin. Adequate control is not easy, therefore, the diagnosis of the exact underlying cause is important for choosing the optimal drug combinations. Because of the instability, patients with chronic renal failure or a transplant must have tightly controlled blood pressure.

Some specific renal causes of hypertension

Hypertension complicates chronic renal failure and transplantation, most often due to salt and water retention, usually with stimulation of the renin–angiotensin system. By the time children are in end-stage renal failure most will be hypertensive. In patients on dialysis hypertension is usually related to salt and water overload. In transplant patients early hypertension is often related to acute volume expansion and later may be associated with chronic allograft nephropathy, immunosuppressive therapy, rejection or renal artery stenosis.

Renovascular hypertension

This accounts for about 5–10% of severe childhood hypertension, usually due to renal artery stenosis with fibromuscular dysplasia. It is often found in relatively young children and may be associated with:

- A history of neonatal umbilical arterial catheter
- Idiopathic hypercalcaemia (Williams-Beuren syndrome)
- Neurofibromatosis
- Marfan syndrome

Experienced Doppler ultrasound has become a sensitive and highly specific method if the correct parameters are measured. A combination with captopril scintigraphy improves the diagnostic accuracy. Angiography may be confirmative and offer intervention therapy. Surgical treatment is nowadays indicated only in special situations.

Reflux nephropathy

This tends to be picked up in children after the age of 5 years. At least 5–10% of patients with renal scars develop hypertension. Treatment is usually medical but nephrectomy is highly effective where there is unilateral severe scarring and renal function on the affected side is below 10–15%.

Other renal causes

- Chronic glomerulonephritis
- Renal damage after haemolytic uraemic syndrome (HUS)
- Autosomal recessive polycystic kidney disease (ARPKD) in almost all cases
- Autosomal dominant polycystic kidney disease (ADPKD) rarely during childhood.

Important cardiovascular causes

- Coarctation of the aorta
- Renal artery stenosis
- Mid aortic syndrome.

Hypertension may also be a feature of endocrine disease, drug therapy, substance abuse and heavy metal poisoning.

Problem-orientated topic:

hypertension ● ● ● ● ●

A family move and register with a new primary care physician. At initial consultation Andelica, a 13-year-old girl, is found to have a systolic blood pressure of 150 mmHg. She is rushed to the paediatric unit where her blood pressure is found to be 160 mmHg systolic.

Q1. How would you assess Andelica?
Q2. What is your management?

Q1. How would you assess Andelica?

Aims
- Identify causes of secondary hypertension; severe hypertension needs aggressive investigation.
- Exclude primary (essential) hypertension.

History
Many cases in childhood are detected as an incidental finding on examination for another reason. In severe hypertension secondary to renal disease the presentation may be congestive cardiac failure. Hypertension should always be excluded as an explanation for recurrent headache (about one-tenth of children with hypertension will present with neurological symptoms and complications).

The following should be explored:
- Past medical history:
  - UTI
  - Systemic disease
  - Trauma
  - Neonatal intensive care (umbilical catheter)
- Family history
- Growth/weight/puberty
- Medications:
  - Prescription
  - Non-prescription
  - Oral contraceptives
  - Anabolic steroids
  - Diet pills
  - Substance abuse
- Review of systems:
  - Headache
  - Nosebleed
  - Rash.

Physical examination
Assessment of the child with suspected hypertension requires a full cardiac and neurological examination.

The abdomen should be examined for possible masses. The following should also be assessed:
- Pulses and BP in all four limbs
- Signs of systemic disease
- Stigmata of syndromes associated with hypertension, e.g. Williams, neurofibromatosis etc.
- Evidence of end-organ damage, e.g. fundi
- Bruits: carotid and renal
- Signs of endocrinopathy.

Investigations

These are done in stages. The initial general stage should include:
- Serum biochemistry profile
- Full blood count (FBC)
- Peripheral plasma renin and aldosterone levels – resting
- Urinalysis and microscopy
- Urine catecholamine and metabolites, neuron-specific enolase (NSE)
- Chest X-ray (CXR)
- Abdominal ultrasound
- Electrocardiogram (ECG)
- Echocardiography.

Supplementary investigations to identify a particular diagnosis may include:
- MCUG or renal DMSA scan
- MRI angiography
- Plasma catecholamines
- Isotope scan for phaeochromocytoma (MIBG)
- Other endocrine tests including steroid profiles.

Q2. What is your management?

- Treatment of underlying cause
- Weight reduction
- Salt intake reduction
- Lifestyle changes, e.g. exercise.

Medication

In the child with mild hypertension (> 95th percentile) drug therapy is usually not indicated. Appropriate advice on diet, reducing salt intake, avoidance of smoking and regular exercise is usually sufficient, with follow-up measurements of BP.

Severe hypertension as in Andelica's case should be considered a medical emergency and patients should be referred to specialist units. In severe hypertension it is important to reduce BP slowly; precipitous drops are hazardous and may particularly affect vision.

In the longer term the aim should be to maintain the BP at or below the 90th percentile for age, sex and height, or lower if there is continuing renal disease. The choices are:

- Diuretics
- Calcium channel blockers
- Angiotensin-converting enzyme (ACE) inhibitors
- Beta-blockers
- Vasodilators.

Glomerular disease

All glomerular diseases are characterized by proteinuria with or without haematuria. Children may present with a chance finding of proteinuria, with proteinuria associated with other symptoms and signs, or with oedema. However, not all children with proteinuria have glomerular disease. Transient proteinuria is also associated with febrile illnesses, UTI, surgery and trauma. There is also a physiological rise in protein excretion with upright posture and physical exercise. Ideally the first or second urine in the morning after rising should be used to test for proteinuria. Proteinuria in association with oedema, oliguria or hypertension should always be taken seriously and the child must be seen urgently.

Glomerular disease can cause a wide spectrum of clinical pictures:
- Nephrotic syndrome
- Acute glomerulonephritis
- Rapidly progressive glomerulonephritis
- Chronic progressive glomerulonephritis
- Asymptomatic proteinuria/haematuria.

The final diagnosis is often dependent on histology of renal biopsy. The findings may be due to a primary renal disease (most common in childhood) or secondary to a systemic illness (rare in early childhood but increasingly found towards adulthood).

Nephrotic syndrome

Idiopathic nephrotic syndrome in childhood is defined by proteinuria > 40 mg/m^2/hour and hypoalbuminaemia < 2.5 g/dl. The aetiology is unknown. The clinical picture is characterized by the sudden onset of proteinuria, oedema and hypoalbuminaemia, together with hyperlipidaemia. It is more common in boys. Most young children with nephrotic syndrome will have 'minimal change' on renal biopsy. The likelihood of this varies with age of presentation (Fig. 39.4).

The term minimal change is a histological diagnosis and refers to the relative lack of findings on light microscopy of renal biopsy. Most cases of minimal change disease will respond to steroid therapy, and for that reason, children who fit the typical clinical picture should be started on steroids. The long-term prognosis of steroid-sensitive nephrotic syndrome (SSNS) is excellent.

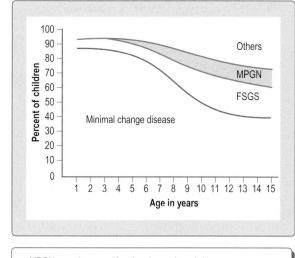

MPGN, membranoproliferative glomerulonephritis;
FSGS, focal and segmental glomerulosclerosis

Fig. 39.4 'Smoothed' representation of the distribution of the major causes of childhood nephrotic syndrome by age.
Based on pooled data from the International Study of Kidney Disease in Childhood and patients investigated at Guy's Hospital, London (n = 566).
Adapted from Postlethwaite RJ (2003) Clinical paediatric nephrology, 2nd edn. Elsevier Science Ltd, with permission.

Proteinuria in nephrotic syndrome

Glomerular filtrate is formed by ultrafiltration of plasma across the glomerular capillary wall, which is negatively charged. This wall has three layers: the endothelium, the basement membrane and an outer epithelium consisting of podocytes with interdigitating foot processes. Serum albumin is negatively charged and there is evidence for a barrier to passage of albumin by electrical charge, as well as a sieve-like size-specific barrier. Recent data give evidence that the intact podocyte function and the formation of the slit diaphragm are essential components for preventing proteinuria. On renal biopsy in minimal change, whilst there are minimal histological changes on light microscopy, there are changes to the appearance of the foot processes on electron microscopy. The underlying cause for loss of podocyte stability and proper function remains the subject of extensive research.

Oedema in nephrotic syndrome

Oedema is the central clinical feature in nephrotic syndrome. Its formation is related to changes to the balance of factors affecting the movement of water and small solutes between the intravascular and extravascular compartments.

The Starling equation tells us that oedema can result from an increase in capillary intravascular hydrostatic pressure or from decrease in capillary oncotic pressure. Since plasma protein (mainly albumin) is the main contributor to intravascular oncotic pressure, loss of urinary albumin, causing hypoalbuminaemia, will lead to a shift of fluid from the plasma to the interstitium. This results in contraction of the circulating volume leading to physiological responses such as activation of the renin–angiotensin–aldosterone system; release of arginine vasopressin (AVP); inhibition of atrial natriuretic peptide (ANP); and increased proximal tubular salt and water reabsorption, resulting in salt and water retention.

Problem-orientated topic:

oedema   ○ ○ ○ ○ ○

Jovana, a 4-year-old, has had generalized oedema for 2 days and is found to have proteinuria on stick testing. A diagnosis of nephrotic syndrome is suspected.

Q1. Is this likely to be minimal change disease?
Q2. What complications may be expected?
Q3. What investigations are appropriate at initial presentation?
Q4. What are the indications for consideration of renal biopsy?
Q5. What management is necessary?

Q1. Is this likely to be minimal change disease?

Clinical features suggestive of minimal change disease are:
- Age over 1 year and under 10 years
- Rapid onset of oedema (days rather than months)
- Heavy proteinuria +++/++++ on stick testing.

Q2. What complications may be expected?

Acute complications
- Discomfort or even skin breakdown related to extreme oedema
- Hypoalbuminuria, leading to intravascular hypovolaemia
- Acute renal failure secondary to hypovolaemia
- Hypercoagulability leading to vascular thrombosis (aggravated by hypovolaemia)
- Infection, especially peritonitis.

- Change in facial appearance and body shape
- Weight gain
- Poor growth
- Striae
- Acne
- Behavioural changes
- Adrenal suppression
- Infections (i.e. chickenpox)
- Reduction in bone mineral density
- Proximal myopathy

Assessment of hypovolaemia in an oedematous child is difficult. It may be suggested by:
- Cold periphery
- Delayed capillary refill
- Reduced jugular venous pressure (JVP)
- Abdominal pain
- Low urinary sodium and high urinary osmolality.

N.B. Abdominal pain in an oedematous child with nephrotic syndrome may be a symptom of peritonitis and should be taken seriously.

Chronic complications
- Steroid and other medication side effects (Box 39.13).

Q3. What investigations are appropriate at initial presentation?

- Serum urea, electrolytes, creatinine, albumin, total protein, calcium, phosphate, lipid profile, complement C3c and C4, antistreptolysin O titre (ASOT), antinuclear antibody (ANA), autoantibody screen
- Hepatitis B and C and varicella serology
- Complete blood count (CBC)
- Urine: stick test and microscopy; albumin (or protein):creatinine ratio; sodium, osmolality and creatinine.

Q4. What are the indications for consideration of renal biopsy?

Discuss these with the referral centre:
- Age under 1 year or over 10 years
- Gradual onset of oedema
- Macroscopic haematuria
- Hypertension
- Rash or other features of systemic disease
- Low complement C3c or C4
- Failure of response to steroids by 4 weeks.

Q5. What management is necessary?

- *Prednis(ol)one*: the International Study of Kidney Disease in Children (ISKDC) recommendations are 4 weeks of 60 mg/m^2 followed by 4 weeks of 40 mg/m^2 on alternate days for initial presentation. There is evidence from recent data that prolonging therapy from 4 weeks to 6 weeks for the initial, daily and subsequent alternate day treatments is beneficial.
- *Penicillin*: prophylactic to prevent pneumococcal peritonitis (especially when there is ascites).
- *Dietary sodium and fluid restriction*: without salt restriction, fluid restriction may be very difficult
- *Albumin infusion*: in symptomatic hypovolaemia.

Assessment of intravascular fluid volume and urine output is essential in the safe treatment of children presenting with acute oedema. Infusion of 20% albumin to restore oncotic pressure and treat hypovolaemia is often appropriate but can be hazardous in children whose GFR is so reduced they are in established renal failure.

Most children with SSNS will have more than one episode and some will go on to frequent relapses. Those having repeated courses of high-dose steroids or requiring long-term continuous steroids (> 0.5 mg/kg/day) or with clinical evidence of steroid toxicity should be considered for second-line therapy using agents such as levamisole (no longer available on the European market), cyclophosphamide or ciclosporin/tacrolimus (tacrolimus has no European market authorization for nephrotic syndrome). Initiation of such treatments is usually done in conjunction or discussion with a tertiary paediatric nephrology centre.

The children who do not have SSNS will turn out to have a variety of different histological findings on renal biopsy and generally have a less satisfactory response to treatments and a worse long-term prognosis. A small number will turn out to have minimal change disease but have a late (4–8-week) response to steroids or, extremely rarely, are steroid-resistant.

Glomerulonephritis

Problem-orientated topic:

haematuria ●●●●●

A 14-year-old boy, Lazar, develops haematuria and is sent by his primary care physician to the paediatric assessment unit. On questioning he admits to some pain on passing urine and also admits this has happened three times in the last year and

Continued overleaf

on each occasion has lasted for a few days before clearing.

Q1. What is the most likely diagnosis? What is the differential diagnosis?

Q2. What investigations would you order?

Q3. How would you decide if Lazar needs referral to a specialist centre?

Q1. What is the most likely diagnosis? What is the differential diagnosis?

Acute glomerulonephritis refers to diseases characterized by the acute onset of haematuria, proteinuria, oedema and often hypertension. There are a wide variety of underlying causes and the prognosis is often related to the underlying diagnosis.

Some children with glomerulonephritis may have a strong nephrotic element to their presentation. Diagnosis is usually histological. In Europe, IgA nephritis is probably more common than post-infectious or post-streptococcal nephritis since the decline in streptococcal infections in recent years.

Q2. What investigations would you order?

- *Blood* CBC: urea, electrolytes, creatinine, albumin, protein, calcium, phosphate, immunoglobulins, complement C3c and C4, ANA, antineutrophil cytoplasmic antibody (ANCA), anti-double-stranded DNA, anti-glomerular basement membrane (GBM) antibodies, autoantibody screen, ASOT, hepatitis B and C status
- *Urine*: sodium, osmolality, creatinine; stix; microscopy for red cell morphology, casts (and to exclude infection); albumin (or protein):creatinine ratio
- *Throat swab.*
- Almost all children will require renal biopsy if post-streptococcus GN is unlikely

Q3. How would you decide if Lazar needs referral to a specialist centre?

Features suggesting serious pathology include:
- Elevated or rising serum creatinine
- Oliguria
- Heavy proteinuria
- Persistent proteinuria
- Severe hypertension
- Severe oedema.

BOX 39.14 Stone formation

Complex interaction of several factors:
- Urinary concentration of stone-forming chemicals
- Urine flow rate
- Urine pH
- Balance of promoter and inhibitor factors for crystallization, e.g. citrate, magnesium, pyrophosphate
- Presence of foreign body
- Presence of infection
- Anatomical factors causing urinary stasis.
  Principles of treatment need to address these factors.

Urinary tract stones (Box 39.14)

Urolithiasis is a stone in the urinary tract whereas nephrocalcinosis implies an increase in the calcium content of the kidney.

The incidence and composition of stones vary with geographical region. In the UK incidence is around 2 children/million population (cf. 2 adults/thousand population). It is much higher in other parts of the world: for example, the Middle and Far East, North Africa. Factors such as climate, race, diet, fluid intake, dehydration, infections and socioeconomic status may be important. In European children more than half of cases are infective in origin and are frequently related to *Proteus* urine infection. The most common cause of metabolic stones in the West is hypercalciuria.

Clinical features may be non-specific, especially in younger children. About half will have abdominal, flank or back pain. A few will pass a stone and it is vital that such stones are retrieved and analysed chemically. Microscopic haematuria is usually present and renal stones should be part of the differential diagnosis of any child with haematuria.

Clinical approach
- History and examination, including careful attention to family history, dietary history, growth and blood pressure
- Urinalysis and urine microscopy
- Ultrasound
- Radiology (Ca content determines 'visibility' on abdominal X-ray)
- Serum biochemistry, including urea and electrolytes, ionized calcium, phosphate, magnesium, bicarbonate, chloride, parathyroid hormone (PTH)

- Urine biochemistry, including calcium, magnesium, oxalate, glycolate, glycerate, urate, urine amino acid anaylsis for cystinuria, citrate and urinary pH.

Causes of stone formation

See Box 39.15.

Management

Medical treatment depends on the underlying condition. Avoidance of dehydration is often important and dietary manipulation may be necessary in some conditions.

Surgical treatment may be required and techniques include ureteroscopy, extracorporeal shock-wave lithotripsy, percutaneous nephrolithotomy and open surgery.

Renal tubular disorders

Renal tubular disorders may be congenital or acquired. Since the renal tubule is responsible for the reabsorption of water and electrolytes in the glomerular ultrafiltrate, disorders may lead to profound electrolyte and volume disturbance. Most children with genetic tubular disorders present in infancy with non-specific symptoms like failure to thrive or poor feeding.

Bartter syndrome

The main problem is tubular loss of sodium and chloride and secondarily excess loss of potassium in the distal tubule associated with hyper-reninaemia and hyperaldosteronism. In all forms there is hypokalaemia, hyponatraemia and alkalosis with increased urinary chloride excretion. Different mutations may cause Bartter syndrome. Inheritance is autosomal recessive.

Fanconi syndrome

In Fanconi syndrome there is a generalized failure of proximal tubular reabsorption of sodium, bicarbonate, phosphate, glucose and amino acids, and in addition reabsorptive processes in the distal nephron are overloaded.

Causes

- Genetic:
  - Mitochondrial disorders
  - Cystinosis
  - Lowe syndrome
  - Wilson disease
  - Galactosaemia
- Acquired:
  - Drugs:
    - Aminoglycosides
    - Ifosfamide
  - Renal disorders:
    - Recovery phase of acute tubular necrosis
    - Early post-renal transplant
    - Acute interstitial nephritis
  - Other:
    - Heavy metal poisoning.

Cystinosis

Cystinosis is an autosomal recessive disorder in which there is excess accumulation of intracellular cystine because of a defect of lysosomal cystine transport. This particularly affects proximal tubule cells, leading to Fanconi syndrome. Treatment with Cystagon may prevent cystine accumulation and disease progression, otherwise renal failure and endocrinopathy are inevitable.

Nephrogenic diabetes insipidus (NDI)

NDI is a disorder in which the kidney fails to respond to the hormone AVP, leading to failure of urinary concentration. The congenital form is most severe and results from genetic defects in the AVP receptor. It is inherited in an X-linked manner and affected boys present in the newborn period with dehydration, poor growth and irritability. Mutations in the aquaporine gene cause an autosomal less severe disease.

Polycystic kidney disease

The use of the term polycystic implies specific diagnoses that should not be confused with the wide spectrum of other cystic kidney diseases that exist. These include glomerulocystic kidney disease, medullary cystic disease and cystic dysplasia. Multicystic dysplastic kidney is the extreme end of the dysplasia spectrum and implies a non-functioning kidney with no connection to the ureter. Cystic kidneys are an important component of a number of syndromes.

Polycystic kidney disease is an inherited disorder. In the autosomal recessive form (ARPKD), which was also called infantile polycystic kidney disease, the kidneys are large and are often easily palpated. There may be an antenatal diagnosis and there may be oligohydramnios and pulmonary hypoplasia, so some affected babies do not survive the neonatal period. Progression to renal failure frequently occurs in early childhood. Hepatic fibrosis is invariably present but early on may not be evident clinically or on ultrasound. Management is supportive with aggressive control of hypertension and management of renal failure and eventually renal and/or liver transplant.

Autosomal dominant polycystic kidney disease (ADPKD) may be detected antenatally, in the neonatal period or in early childhood but it is more likely to present in later childhood or in adulthood. Those presenting very early in life are thought to have a more severe outcome and some may progress to end-stage renal failure in childhood. Others may preserve renal function for many decades, though eventual progression into renal failure is a significant likelihood. Control of hypertension is a major factor influencing progression of disease as well as cardiovascular morbidity and mortality. This is an important issue in discussion and decisions regarding screening asymptomatic family members for the condition.

Urinary tract dilatation

Dilatation of the urinary tract is usually detected on ultrasound. This may be done as a follow-up of anoma-lies found on antenatal screening or when ultrasound is performed during investigation for urinary tract problems like UTI. Occasionally urinary tract obstruction may present acutely with pain or infection.

Hydronephrosis describes dilatation of the collecting system of the kidney and hydroureter describes dilatation of the ureter, but neither term implies obstruction.

There is no clear definition or test for obstruction, and diagnosis requires clinical and functional assessment as well as imaging.

Causes of a dilated urinary tract
- Obstruction:
    - e.g. stone in ureter
    - Posterior urethral valves
    - Pelvo-ureteric-junction obstruction
    - Neuropathic bladder
- VUR
- Non-obstructed and non-refluxing.

Rarely, reflux and obstruction can occur together in duplex system.

Dilated upper urinary tract presenting in the neonatal period is discussed on p. 750.

Acute renal failure

Acute renal failure (ARF) can result from a wide variety of causes. ARF should be suspected in any patient who is oliguric, though it may be picked up on 'routine' biochemistry of an unwell child.

In childhood, ARF may be seen with a high, normal or low urine output. On serum biochemistry an increase in urea and creatinine is seen and there is an inability of the kidney to regulate fluid and electrolytes appropriately. Beyond the newborn period, haemolytic uraemic syndrome (HUS) is the most frequent condition causing ARF. ARF may also occur in isolation — for example, in intrinsic renal disease like glomerulonephritis — or may coexist or result from other disorders — for example, in multi-organ failure in an intensive care situation.

Causes of ARF
- *Prerenal*: hypovolaemia secondary to gastroenteritis, haemorrhage, burns, septic shock, nephrotic syndrome, cardiac failure
- *Intrarenal*: HUS, acute tubular necrosis (ATN), ischaemia, nephrotoxic agents, acute glomerulonephritis, pyelonephritis, acute interstitial nephritis, cortical or medullary necrosis, bilateral renal artery thrombosis, infiltration by neoplastic disease
- *Postrenal*: bladder outflow obstruction — urethral valves, blocked catheter, bilateral ureteric

obstruction, bilateral stones, unilateral obstruction of a single kidney, neurogenic bladder, tumours, trauma (bleeding and clot).

Assessment of volume status is critical to initial treatment strategies. It is important to assess systolic BP together with intravascular volume, either directly with central venous pressure measurements, or indirectly by JVP, core peripheral temperature difference and capillary refill. Urinary urea and electrolytes and creatinine measurements are very useful tools in assessing whether renal failure is prerenal or established intrarenal. In hypovolaemia the urinary sodium and fractional excretion of sodium (Na) are usually low (urine Na < 20 mmol/l, fractional excretion of sodium < 1%) and the urine osmolality may be high.

In the case of suspected intrarenal disease, where there is no clear cause of ATN and no diagnosis of HUS, then a renal biopsy is often required. In the initial stages it is important to establish the diagnosis and identify and manage any life-threatening abnormalities. More complex investigations may take longer to establish the underlying cause, which may be multifactorial. It should be remembered that some children presenting in ARF actually have acute on chronic failure and may have had undiagnosed renal impairment for some time.

Life-threatening emergencies in ARF
- Hyperkalaemia (Box 39.16)
- Shock
- Metabolic acidosis
- Severe arterial hypertension
- Fluid overload/pulmonary oedema.

Children who are intravascularly hypovolaemic should be given a bolus of 20 ml/kg of 0.9% saline (except when hypovolaemia is due to haemorrhage, when it makes sense to infuse blood, or when nephrotic, when 20% albumin is used). This should be repeated

---

BOX 39.16 Treatment of life-threatening hyperkalaemia

1. Stabilize the myocardium: i.v. calcium gluconate
2. Shift potassium into cells from extracellular compartment:
   - Salbutamol via nebulizer or i.v.
   - Sodium bicarbonate i.v.
   - Glucose plus insulin i.v.
3. Remove potassium from body:
   - Ion exchange resins
   - Dialysis/haemofiltration

BOX 39.17 Practical tip: renal failure

Once adequate volume status is established, prescribe fluid intake volume as:

Insensible losses* + urine output + ongoing fluid losses

*(under normal conditions insensible losses are about 400 ml/m^2/day)

---

until circulatory volume has been restored, but if a urine output has not been established with good volume status and intravenous furosemide, then fluid restriction related to current urine output should be commenced (Box 39.17).

Indications for renal replacement therapy (RRT)
Indications for institution of RRT (haemo- or peritoneal dialysis or haemofiltration) are complex and there is no set of measurements or biochemical values that indicate RRT should commence. In general the underlying cause, clinical condition, speed of progression of ARF, response to treatments, access availability and setting will influence decisions to start RRT. RRT in children should only be performed in specialist settings, and discussions with specialist centres or better, referral, should take place at an early stage regarding any child whose renal function is deteriorating.

Henoch–Schönlein purpura (HSP)

This condition is discussed in detail on page 623.

Renal involvement is common, with microscopic or macroscopic haematuria or mild proteinuria in over 80% of cases. Generally these features resolve, but if proteinuria persists, nephrotic syndrome may result. Indicators of progressive renal disease are heavy proteinuria, oedema, hypertension and deteriorating renal function. Fewer than 1% of patients develop persistent renal disease and fewer than 0.1% severe renal disease. Initially important differential diagnoses of the vasculitic skin lesions of HSP are idiopathic thrombocytopenia and meningococcal disease.

Investigations
- CBC, inflammatory markers, immunoglobulins
- Urine microscopy and dipstick for red blood cells, white blood cells, casts or albumin
- Skin biopsy: rarely needed; will demonstrate a leucocytoclastic vasculitis
- Renal biopsy: similarly, may show IgA mesangial deposition and occasionally IgM, C3c and fibrin.

Haemolytic uraemic syndrome

HUS is the most common cause of ARF in childhood in Europe and North America. Most cases are associated with a diarrhoea prodrome (so-called 'D+ HUS'). HUS without diarrhoea has a large number of rare causes such as defects in the complement system and a worse prognosis. Most D+ HUS cases are associated with infection with verocytotoxin-producing *Escherichia coli*. The natural reservoir is farm animals, though outbreaks have been associated with a wide variety of foodstuffs.

Any age group can be affected but the disease is typically found in preschool children (and the elderly). They frequently have bloody diarrhoea several days to a couple of weeks before presenting with reduced urine output, pallor and malaise. There is microangiopathic haemolytic anaemia, thrombocytopenia and renal failure. The gastrointestinal disease may be severe. Neurological involvement carries a poor prognosis.

Diagnosis is by blood film and low platelet counts together with haemolytic anaemia and biochemical evidence of renal failure. If HUS is suspected but the initial blood film does not support the diagnosis, a film should be repeatedly examined over the next hours and days.

There is no specific effective treatment though many agents have been tried. Antibiotics should probably be avoided. The mainstay is supportive management with control of fluid and electrolyte disturbance, early dialysis and blood transfusion. Most children recover but there is still a significant mortality (reported 2–10%) and up to one-third of survivors, especially those who are 'diarrhoea negative', have some long-term renal sequelae in the form of ongoing renal impairment, proteinuria or hypertension.

Chronic renal failure

Chronic renal failure (CRF) may present in a wide variety of ways.

Presentation of CRF
- General or non-specific malaise
- Failure to thrive
- Short stature
- Rickets
- Anaemia/pallor
- Hypertension
- Bed wetting
- UTI
- Screening: sibling or antenatal
- Acute on chronic renal failure

- Congestive cardiac failure
- Pulmonary oedema.

Because of the wide range of presentations and causes a very detailed history and examination are essential to give clues towards further investigations. The history may help distinguish between ARF, when the child has been previously fit and well, and CRF, when the child may have been non-specifically unwell or have had problems with appetite or growth for many months or even years. There may have been specific urinary symptoms like polyuria, polydipsia, wetting or recurrent UTI.

Major causes of CRF
- Congenital abnormalities
- Hypoplasia/dysplasia
- CAKUT with reflux
- Glomerulonephritis
- Multisystem disease
- Inherited conditions.

Investigations
When a finding of impaired renal function is confirmed on initial blood biochemistry results, it is often not possible to estimate the chance of the kidney to recover. Therefore repeated biochemistry over days, weeks and months is important in determining both the chronicity of the condition and the actual level of renal function, once other factors like infection or hypertension are corrected.

Findings of non-haemolytic anaemia, small or dysplastic kidneys on ultrasound, X-ray evidence of renal osteodystrophy and end-organ damage from hypertension point towards chronic rather than acute renal failure.

Investigations in CRF may include:
- Urine microscopy and urinalysis
- Urine albumin:creatinine ratio
- Urine biochemistry, urea and electrolytes, creatinine, osmolality, calcium, phosphate, oxalate, cystine
- Blood biochemistry including liver function tests, bone biochemistry, bicarbonate, intact PTH, ferritin, lipid profile
- Renal tract ultrasound including Doppler ultrasound
- Chest X-ray
- X-ray of left hand and wrist
- Echocardiography
- MCUG
- Immunology parameters complement C3c and C4, ANCA, ANA, anti-GBM antibodies, autoantibodies, anti-double-stranded DNA antibodies
- Renal biopsy
- White cell cystine content.

Management

The first aim of management is to treat any underlying disorder and associated conditions, then to preserve and improve renal function to prevent a decline into end-stage renal failure for as long as adequate. Meticulous attention needs to be paid to maintaining nutrition and growth; controlling BP; treating fluid, electrolyte and acid–base imbalance; controlling renal osteodystrophy; and treating anaemia.

Indications for RRT

The indications for RRT are complex and dependent on a holistic view of the child, not specific biochemical values. In general RRT is started when the child becomes symptomatic from renal failure, with tiredness, anorexia and uncontrolled hypertension, or when blood biochemistry indicates harmful disturbances despite therapy and dietary restrictions.

End-stage renal failure and transplantation

Renal failure is a continuum from mild renal impairment through preterminal renal failure to the end stage. End-stage renal failure is when the need for RRT is imminent. The ultimate aim of therapy is renal transplantation because it places far less restriction on normal life and is associated with lower morbidity and mortality. Dialysis is generally considered as a therapy used before or between transplantation, except for those few individuals who are currently unable to be transplanted when dialysis is used as long-term therapy over many years and even decades. Transplantation before dialysis is common when the child is to receive a living donor kidney. Some children are not suitable for pre-emptive transplantation.

The choice of dialysis modality is individual to the child and family. Haemodialysis for children is based in a few specialist centres and therefore travel to and from the centre for a 3–5-hour session three times a week may be an issue. Fluid restriction is normally more severe when on haemodialysis, but the family is relieved of some stresses and responsibilities and the child retains some independence. Home peritoneal dialysis is usually done by machine overnight. This enables normal school attendance. There is a huge burden on the caregivers and the child is very dependent on them on a regular basis. In peritoneal dialysis sudden fluid and electrolyte shifts are avoided. Fluid and dietary restrictions are minimized. It is particularly suited to younger patients. Peritoneal dialysis is often the first choice of dialysis modality.

Successful renal transplantation offers the nearest to a normal lifestyle and is the preferred form of treatment for end-stage renal failure. Living donor kidneys have better graft survival figures than cadaveric. Immunosuppression medication needs to continue indefinitely and non-compliance with medication is a significant cause of graft failure in teenagers and young adults.

Cardiovascular system

LEARNING OUTCOMES

By the end of this chapter you should:
- Know the factors distinguishing an innocent and pathological murmur
- Be able to assess and manage the child in heart failure
- Be able to recognize the typical ECG appearance of the common arrhythmias and know the basic management of each
- Be able to recognize the historical and clinical features in the child with chest pain of cardiac origin
- Know the clinical features of the common cardiac conditions presenting in childhood
- Be able to recognize chest X-ray abnormalities associated with cardiac disease
- Refer to paediatric cardiologist when and if indicated.

MODULE SEVEN

Assessment

Congenital heart disease (CHD) is the most commonly occurring severe congenital abnormality. The prevalence is 0.8–0.9 per 1000 live births. For those with major CHD early and accurate diagnosis can be vitally important to morbidity and mortality. The presentation can vary from the asymptomatic child presenting with a murmur to the child who presents acutely unwell with cyanosis or heart failure.

History and physical examination

History

Key symptoms in the history to elicit when assessing a child for possible heart disease are as follows.

Infants
- Feeding difficulties: breathlessness, sweating or tiring with feeds
- Failure to thrive
- Episodes of central cyanosis.

The older child
- Breathlessness and fatigue with exertion
- Palpitations
- Chest pain
- Dizziness or syncope on exertion.

Physical examination
- An initial assessment of growth parameters is important since failure to thrive is a common presentation of CHD in infancy.

I Intensity: grade 1–6

II Timing — systolic, diastolic or continuous:
   – Systolic murmurs are classified as ejection systolic, pansystolic or late systolic
   – Diastolic murmurs should be classified as early or mid-diastolic

III Character: e.g. harsh, musical, vibratory, blowing

IV Area of maximal intensity

V Radiation: back, axilla, neck

- Is there central cyanosis? Assess the lips, tongue, mucous membranes and nail beds.
- Is the child in heart failure? The classical signs are tachycardia, tachypnoea and hepatomegaly.
- Check the pulses in all four limbs. Are they of normal, increased or decreased volume? Palpation of the femoral pulses is one of the most important points in the examination.
- Check the blood pressure in the right arm and also a leg blood pressure.
- Palpate the precordium: note the presence of any heaves or thrills, locate the apex beat.
- Finally auscultate the heart:
   – Assess the heart sounds. Is their intensity normal?
   – Is there normal splitting of the second heart sound?
   – Are there any additional heart sounds or clicks?

Any murmur should be evaluated according to the parameters in Box 40.1.

The specific clinical findings found in the more common congenital heart problems are described in later sections dealing with each in turn. Some lesions occur more commonly in association with certain syndromes (Table 40.1).

The electrocardiogram (ECG)

The ECG remains an important basic investigation in the assessment of any child suspected of having CHD. Consideration of the age of the patient is important in the interpretation of any ECG change. It is very difficult to remember normal values for all the ECG parameters at various ages, but the important ones are summarized in Box 40.2.

Congestive cardiac failure

Basic science

The cardiac output is governed by the equation:

Table 40.1 Congenital heart disease and syndromes

Syndrome	Associated defects
Down (trisomy 21)	Atrioventricular septal defect Ventricular septal defect Tetralogy of Fallot Atrial septal defect Patent ductus arteriosus
Edwards (trisomy 18)	Ventricular septal defect Atrial septal defect Double outlet right ventricle
Patau (trisomy 13)	Ventricular septal defect Atrial septal defect
Turner (XO)	Coarctation of aorta Aortic stenosis
Klinefelter (XXY)	Tetralogy of Fallot Ventricular septal defect Atrial septal defect Patent ductus arteriosus
22q11	Interrupted aortic arch Truncus arteriosus Tetralogy of Fallot Pulmonary atresia
Noonan	Pulmonary stenosis Atrial septal defect Hypertrophic cardiomyopathy
Marfan	Aortic root dilatation Dissecting aortic aneurysm Mitral valve prolapse and mitral regurgitation
Williams	Supravalvular aortic stenosis Pulmonary artery stenosis
Cri-du-chat	Ventricular septal defect Atrial septal defect Patent ductus arteriosus

$$\text{Cardiac output (l/min)} = \text{stroke volume (l)} \times \text{heart rate (bpm)}$$

The stroke volume is governed primarily by the preload, the myocardial contractility and the afterload (Table 40.2). In simple terms, the preload of a ventricle is the degree to which it is stretched prior to contraction, and the afterload is the vascular resistance against which it ejects.

The Frank–Starling law states that the energy of contraction is proportional to the initial length of the cardiac muscle fibre. There is therefore a close relationship between the ventricular end-diastolic volume and the stroke volume (Fig. 40.1).

Problem-orientated topic:

lethargy and breathlessness

Luka, an 8-week-old baby boy, presents to the primary care paediatrician's office with a history of decreased feeding over the

Continued overleaf

previous week. His parents report that they feel he is more lethargic this morning. Initial assessment reveals a respiratory rate of 60 breaths per minute, subcostal recession and intercostal indrawing. Oxygen saturations in room air are 94% and heart rate is 160 beats per minute. Capillary refill time is 3 seconds. The precordium is active and a harsh pansystolic murmur is audible. The liver is enlarged 3 cm below the right costal margin. Peripheral pulses are normal in volume. Luka has not gained weight since his last well baby check-up done in the paediatrician's office 10 days ago.

Q1. What is your differential diagnosis?

Q2. What investigations are you going to request?

Q3. What is your initial management plan?

BOX 40.2 A logical approach to reading the ECG

Must include analysis of the following parameters:

1. *Rhythm*. Is there sinus rhythm? In sinus rhythm a p wave should precede each QRS axis and the p wave axis should be normal, as indicated by the presence of an upright p wave in leads 2, 3 and aVF.
2. *Heart rate*. Is it within the normal range for age?
3. *P wave*. Axis and magnitude. Is there atrial enlargement? A p wave in any lead that is peaked and > 3 mm in magnitude is suggestive of right atrial enlargement. A bifid p wave in lead 2 is the traditional sign of left atrial enlargement but this can occasionally be observed in normal children.
4. *PR interval*. Is it shorter or longer than normal?
5. *QRS frontal axis*. In the newborn period the normal QRS axis is rightward; as the child grows, it becomes leftward, such that at age 1–3 years the 50th percentile is 60° and it remains at that level during the rest of childhood.
6. *QRS duration*. Is it prolonged?
7. *QT interval*. The important figure is the QTc, which is the QT interval corrected for heart rate. The upper limit of normal is 440 msec.
8. *T wave axis*. In the first few days of life the T wave is upright in lead V_1 but, in most cases, by days 5–7 the T wave axis has changed, so that the T wave becomes negative in this lead. Persistence of an upright T wave beyond 1 week of age is indicative of right ventricular hypertrophy. In the normal heart the T waves usually remain inverted until later childhood, when they again become upright.

BOX 40.2 A logical approach to reading the ECG (cont'd)

9. *Magnitude of R and S waves*. Is there evidence of hypertrophy of the right or left ventricle? In addition to an upright T wave the presence of a Q wave in V_1 is also an indicator of right ventricular hypertrophy. A frontal QRS axis of less than 30° is suggestive of left ventricular hypertrophy (LVH). In the newborn infant LVH is indicated by an SV_1 of > 19 mm or an RV_1 of > 11 mm.

Table 40.2 **Factors influencing stroke volume**

Factor	Affected by
Preload	Length of diastole
	Venous return
	Atrial systole
	Myocardial compliance
Myocardial contractility	Sympathetic nervous system
	Metabolic abnormalities
	Electrolyte imbalance
	Inotropic drugs
	Intrinsic myocardial dysfunction
Afterload	Aortic resistance
	Peripheral vascular resistance
	Haematocrit (blood viscosity)
	Vasodilator drugs

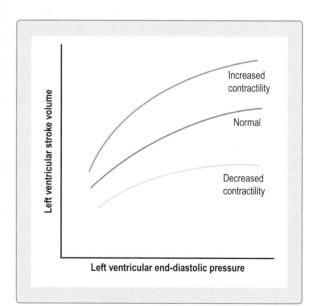

Fig. 40.1 The relationship between left ventricular end-diastolic volume and stroke volume.
As left ventricular end-diastolic pressure increases, stroke volume increases up to a critical point.

Q1. What is your differential diagnosis?

Luka's history and examination findings suggest that he has congestive cardiac failure (Box 40.3). He displays the typical triad of tachypnoea, tachycardia and hepatomegaly associated with heart failure. Heart failure occurs when the cardiac output can no longer meet the circulatory and metabolic needs of the body.

In Luka's case the most likely diagnosis is a congenital cardiac lesion causing a significant left-to-right shunt, such as a large ventricular septal defect (VSD).

The most common causes of heart failure in childhood are summarized in Box 40.4.

Q2. What investigations are you going to request?

- *Chest X-ray* (CXR): will usually show cardiomegaly and plethoric lung fields as a result of increased pulmonary blood flow or pulmonary venous congestion (Fig. 40.2).
- *ECG*: may demonstrate evidence of chamber enlargement.
- *Echocardiogram*: enables identification of the underlying cardiac lesion and provides information regarding ventricular function.

Q3. What is your initial management plan?

The initial management goal is to stabilize the patient by maximizing oxygen delivery to the tissues. This can be achieved by a combination of preload reduction, optimization of myocardial contractility and afterload reduction (Box 40.5). If this child is seen in the primary care setting he must be referred to a paediatric cardiologist or admitted to a paediatric department.

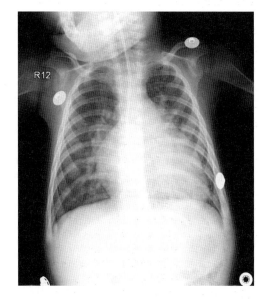

Fig. 40.2 Heart failure.
Chest X-ray showing cardiomegaly and pulmonary oedema due to a large ventricular septal defect.

BOX 40.5 Medical management of heart failure

Oxygen
- Judicious use if duct-dependent lesion suspected

Diuretics
- Result in preload reduction by inhibiting sodium and water reabsorption in the renal tubules
- Oral or i.v. furosemide (loop diuretic) often used in conjunction with a potassium-sparing diuretic (e.g. spironolactone or amiloride)

Inotropes
- Improve myocardial contractility
- Oral or i.v. digoxin: inhibits Na$^+$–K$^+$ adenosine triphosphatase in myocardium, which in turn increases intracellular Ca^{2+}. Patient is usually given loading doses followed by twice daily maintenance dose
- Beta-adrenergic agonists: i.v. infusion dopamine and/or dobutamine

Angiotensin-converting enzyme (ACE) inhibitors
- Result in afterload reduction by decreasing peripheral vascular resistance (inhibit conversion of angiotensin I to angiotensin II)
- May also produce venodilatation (and therefore preload reduction) and interfere with aldosterone production
- Oral captopril: commenced at low dose and built up in increments. Monitor for hypotension with dose increase, renal dysfunction and serum potassium

Box 40.5 summarizes management. Continual reassessment is important in the management of the child with heart failure. Further measures, such as ventilation and management in the intensive care setting, may be appropriate.

It is important to exclude concomitant aggravating factors, such as anaemia, and treat accordingly. Nutrition is also an important consideration and should be optimized with the addition of high-calorie supplements to feeds if necessary. Following medical stabilization, surgical or cardiac catheter intervention may be required to repair or palliate the underlying cardiac lesion.

Pathophysiology of left-to-right shunts

A congenital cardiac lesion that causes a left-to-right shunt essentially places a volume load on the heart. This results from a communication between the systemic and pulmonary circulations, which allows shunting of fully oxygenated blood back to the lungs. If we consider a VSD, there are two main factors that determine the magnitude of the left-to-right shunt and therefore the degree of volume loading:
- The size of the defect
- The pulmonary vascular resistance (PVR).

For a small VSD the degree of shunting is restricted by the size of the lesion. For a large VSD, the defect size could allow unrestrictive shunting, the degree of which is determined by the PVR. With a high PVR, such as occurs in the first weeks of life, there is minimal shunting and few symptoms. When the PVR falls at around 6–8 weeks of life, the magnitude of the left-to-right shunt increases and the symptoms of heart failure increase accordingly. It should be noted that it is the left heart that is volume-loaded in this scenario.

Ventricular septal defect

A VSD is a developmental defect in the interventricular septum, resulting in communication between the two ventricles. It is the most prevalent form of congenital heart defect, accounting for 30% of CHD. A VSD may occur as an isolated defect, or it may be a component of such anomalies as tetralogy of Fallot, coarctation of the aorta, transposition of the great arteries or complete atrioventricular septal defect. Broadly, VSDs may be classified as perimembranous, muscular or subarterial defects.

Clinical features
Symptoms and signs associated with an isolated VSD largely relate to the degree of left-to-right shunt. In those with a moderate to large VSD, at around 6–8 weeks of age when the PVR has fallen significantly, symptoms and signs of congestive cardiac failure become apparent. It should be noted that this change may occur earlier in preterm infants. An infant or child with a small VSD may well have normal growth and be free of symptoms, with suspicion raised by the presence of a murmur during routine examination.

Examination may reveal an active precordium, with a right ventricular heave and possibly a systolic thrill present at the left lower sternal border. Typically there is a pansystolic murmur that is harsh in character and loudest in this area. In the presence of a large left-to-right shunt there may be a mid-diastolic murmur over the apex from increased flow across the mitral valve.

Investigations
CXR may demonstrate cardiomegaly and increased pulmonary vascular markings, with the degree being directly related to the size of shunt. ECG may demonstrate evidence

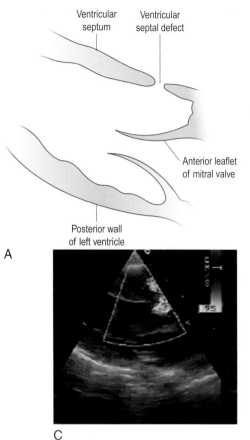

Posterior wall
of left ventricle

A

Ventricular
septum

Ventricular
septal defect

Anterior leaflet
of mitral valve

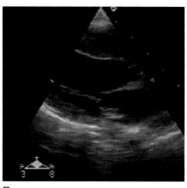

B

C

Fig. 40.3 Ventricular septal defect.
(A) Diagram showing locations;
(B) echocardiogram; (C) Colour
Doppler study showing left to right
shunting.

of chamber enlargement, typically of the left heart. Two-dimensional echocardiography allows diagnosis of the position and size of the VSD (Fig. 40.3). Colour and continuous wave Doppler interrogation allows assessment of the direction and magnitude of the flow across the defect.

Management

Initial management is directed towards medical treatment of symptomatic congestive cardiac failure and optimization of calorific intake. Early surgical closure of VSD is indicated when congestive cardiac failure/failure to thrive is unresponsive to medical therapy. Other indications include a Qp:Qs (ratio of pulmonary and systemic blood flow) greater than 2:1, when there is evidence of increasing PVR, and when closure will prevent the progression of associated aortic incompetence.

Pulmonary artery banding may be necessary in the infant with multiple VSDs or in the presence of associated anomalies. Transcatheter device closure of VSD may be possible in selected cases.

Children with a small VSD are usually asymptomatic and most do not require any active treatment. The defects tend to become smaller with time and the majority undergo spontaneous closure.

Complete atrioventricular septal defect

This is the congenital cardiac abnormality most commonly found in Down syndrome but it also occurs in otherwise healthy children. It is characterized by the presence of a common atrioventricular (AV) valve, a VSD and a defect in the ostium primum part of the atrial septum (Fig. 40.4).

As a result of the excessive pulmonary flow patients usually present with severe heart failure, failure to thrive and feeding difficulties. Early management involves medical anti-failure therapy with diuretics and angiotensin-converting enzyme (ACE) inhibitors in conjunction with maximizing calorie intake with the aid of nasogastric feeding. Since there is a significant risk of developing pulmonary vascular disease, especially in those with Down syndrome, early surgical repair is required. Surgical correction now has an operative mortality of approximately 5%. The most common problem post-surgery is residual left AV valve (mitral) regurgitation.

Left heart obstructive lesions

Where there is obstruction to normal blood flow there is an increased pressure load on the heart. In mild or

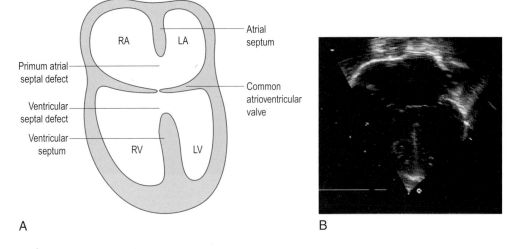

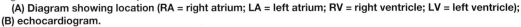

A

B

Fig. 40.4 Atrioventricular septal defect.
(A) Diagram showing location (RA = right atrium; LA = left atrium; RV = right ventricle; LV = left ventricle);
(B) echocardiogram.

moderate aortic stenosis there is compensatory left ventricular hypertrophy (LVH) and the cardiac output may be maintained with minimal symptoms of heart failure. However, with severe coarctation of aorta, critical aortic stenosis or hypoplastic left heart syndrome, infants can present within hours of birth with acute circulatory collapse.

Coarctation of aorta

This is the most common left heart obstructive lesion presenting with heart failure in childhood. Coarctation of the aorta is a narrowing that can occur at any point along the course of the aorta. It most frequently occurs in the thoracic aorta in the region of insertion of the ductus arteriosus. Coarctation accounts for 6–8% of live births with CHD and occurs more commonly in males, with a preponderance of 1.5–2:1. Coarctation may occur in isolation or it may be associated with other anomalies, with bicuspid aortic valve and VSD being the most common associations (see Table 40.3 below). An increased incidence of 15–20% occurs in Turner's syndrome.

Pathophysiology

It is hypothesized that coarctation results from decreased antegrade blood flow across the aortic valve in fetal life, as a result of an associated cardiac anomaly. Discrete coarctation most commonly occurs between the origin of the left subclavian artery and the insertion of the ductus arteriosus, and takes the form of an isthmal waist with the ductus open (Fig. 40.5). In the majority of cases, there is an extension of ductal tissue into this waist, such that when the ductal tissue constricts, the isthmal narrowing increases. Therefore, with ductal closure in neonatal life, there may be an

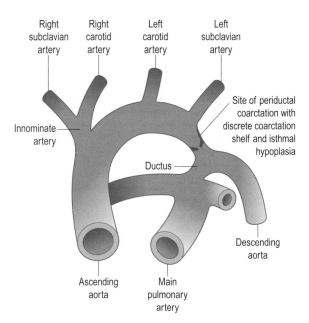

Fig. 40.5 Coarctation at site of ductus arteriosus remnant

acute increase in afterload on the left ventricle and the infant may rapidly decompensate. Where the increase in afterload is more gradual, compensatory ventricular hypertrophy results. Low blood pressure beyond the coarctation equates to decreased renal perfusion. This results in activation of the renin–angiotensin system in an attempt to improve renal perfusion pressure, causing hypertension proximal to the coarctation.

Presentation of coarctation

Clinical presentation can be largely considered as early (neonatal) or late presentation. The key features of early and late presentation are summarized in Table 40.3.

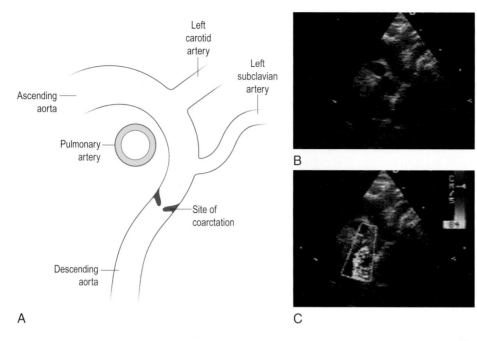

Fig. 40.6 **Severe periductal coarctation of the aorta.**
(A) Diagram showing locations; (B) echocardiogram; (C) colour Doppler study.

Table 40.3 **Possible presenting features of coarctation of the aorta**

	Early presentation	Late presentation
Symptoms	Poor feeding	Usually asymptomatic
	Dyspnoea	Headaches
	Lethargy	Epistaxis
		Calf claudication
Signs	Tachypnoea	Upper limb
	Increased work of	hypertension
	breathing	Diminished/absent
	Tachycardia	femoral pulses
	Prolonged capillary	Radiofemoral delay
	refill	Left ventricular impulse
	Active precordium	Systolic murmur
	Gallop rhythm	Continuous murmur
	Systolic murmur	(collaterals)
	Absent/diminished	
	femoral pulses	
	Hepatomegaly	

Investigations

In infants, a CXR frequently demonstrates cardiomegaly and pulmonary oedema (Fig. 40.2). In older children, the heart size may be normal, but more commonly there is cardiomegaly due to LVH. A pathognomonic sign, which may be seen on the chest radiograph of older children, is rib notching. This is rarely seen before 5 years of age and is due to enlargement of the intercostal arteries, with pressure erosion of the inferior border of the posterior ribs.

ECG in the neonate may reveal right ventricular hypertrophy due to increased in utero afterload but may be normal. Later, changes due to LVH with left ventricular strain may occur.

Diagnosis of coarctation in infancy is now almost always confirmed by echocardiography (Fig. 40.6). It allows evaluation of the aortic arch from the suprasternal notch view and assessment of the severity of coarctation. Using colour Doppler, a turbulent jet may be seen through the coarctation, and interrogation with continuous wave Doppler may demonstrate an increased velocity with typical 'sawtooth' pattern.

In neonatal presentation, echocardiography is useful to assess the size of the ductus arteriosus and response to prostaglandin therapy. It also allows delineation of intracardiac anatomy to look for possible associated anomalies.

In most cases of coarctation, particularly in the infant, clinical examination and echocardiography alone provide sufficient information to formulate a management plan. Cardiac catheterization is only necessary when echocardiographic findings are inconclusive. More commonly, it may be used in older children to provide further structural and haemodynamic information prior to catheter intervention in the form of balloon angioplasty. Magnetic resonance imaging (MRI) and computed tomogram (CT) angiography may be useful modalities in older patients or in post-operative patients.

Management

In neonatal presentation of coarctation, initial management focuses on medical stabilization prior to elective surgical repair. Ductal patency is maintained by administration of an intravenous infusion of prostaglandin E1. This allows possible partial reduction in the severity of coarctation and improves lower body perfusion, albeit with systemic venous blood. In children presenting beyond 2 weeks of age prostaglandin is unlikely to be effective. In the critically ill infant with coarctation and left ventricular failure ventilatory and inotropic support is often necessary to stabilize the child prior to surgery. It should be noted that drug pharmacokinetics may be altered due to renal hypoperfusion.

It is generally accepted that, for native coarctation in infancy, surgical repair is the best option. Surgical repair can take three forms:

- Resection of coarctation and end-to-end anastomosis
- Left subclavian flap repair
- Patch aortoplasty.

The particular technique employed depends on a number of factors, including location of the coarctation, aortic arch anatomy, associated problems such as transverse arch hypoplasia, and age and size at presentation.

In late presentation, the treatment of upper extremity hypertension, usually with β-blocker therapy, takes priority initially. Beyond 1 year of age, cardiac catheterization and balloon angioplasty of native coarctation may be considered as an alternative to surgical treatment.

Prognosis

For most children with coarctation the prognosis is good. About 10% of those requiring a procedure in infancy will require further treatment later in life.

The child with an asymptomatic murmur

(See also Ch. 23.)

Problem-orientated topic:

asymptomatic murmur ●●●●●

Petra, a 4-year-old girl, attends her primary care physician with an upper respiratory infection. She is a previously healthy girl with no cardiovascular symptoms. An incidental finding on examination is that she has a grade 3/6 ejection systolic murmur loudest at the lower left sternal edge. Both heart sounds are normal and on palpation the precordium is quiet. Pulses are normal in volume in all four limbs. Blood pressure in the right arm is 92/63 mmHg.

Q1. What is the differential diagnosis?

Q2. What features help differentiate between an innocent and a pathological murmur?

Q3. What are the relevant investigations?

Q4. When is a referral to a paediatric cardiologist indicated?

Q5. What advice would you give to the parents of a child with an innocent murmur?

Q1. What is the differential diagnosis?

The differential diagnosis is between an innocent or functional murmur and asymptomatic CHD.

Q2. What features help differentiate between an innocent and a pathological murmur?

Innocent murmurs are extremely common and the key features associated with them are summarized in Box 40.6.

In the attempt to differentiate those with CHD from those with innocent murmurs key features in history-taking are birth history, feeding patterns, growth, breathing difficulties and cyanosis.

Clinical assessment of the child with a murmur requires a full cardiovascular examination. This includes assessment of colour, heart and respiratory rates, and palpation of the precordium for heaves or thrills. Palpation of pulses in all four limbs and measurement of blood pressure is essential to rule out coarctation of aorta. On auscultation attention should first be focused on the heart sounds and then on the murmur. The murmur should be defined under the headings in Box 40.1 (p. 567).

Features suggesting that a murmur may be pathological are summarized in Box 40.7.

Very important congenital heart conditions such as aortic stenosis and hypertrophic cardiomyopathy may be asymptomatic in childhood and present as a

---

BOX 40.6 Clinical characteristics of an innocent murmur

- No symptoms
- Normal heart sounds
- No added sounds
- No thrills/heaves
- Intensity grade 3 or less
- Musical or vibratory quality
- Intensity changes with posture

- Presence of symptoms
- Cyanosis
- Diastolic murmur
- Abnormal heart sounds
- Abnormal heaves or thrills
- Presence of added sounds or clicks
- Abnormally strong or weak pulses

- Small ventricular septal defect
- Atrial septal defect
- Pulmonary valve stenosis
- Small patent ductus arteriosus
- Aortic valve stenosis
- Coarctation of aorta
- Hypertrophic cardiomyopathy

murmur. Recognition of such conditions is, however, vitally important since both are known causes of sudden death in young people, particularly during exertion. The common conditions presenting as an asymptomatic murmur are summarized in Box 40.8. Each of these conditions is described in more detail under the relevant headings in this chapter.

Innocent murmurs

By far the most commonly occurring innocent murmur is the Stills murmur, often first detected at the routine preschool examination. The classical Stills murmur is ejection systolic, has a musical or vibratory quality, and diminishes in intensity when the child sits upright. It is usually loudest at the lower left sternal edge. Venous hums are also very common in the preschool and school-age groups. A venous hum is a continuous noise, heard when the child is sitting upright. The murmur is created by blood returning through the great veins to the heart and it can be made to disappear by laying the child flat or applying gentle pressure over the great veins in the neck.

The pulmonary flow murmur is heard over the base of the heart and is more common in adolescents, particularly girls. It is distinguished from valvular pulmonary stenosis by the absence of an ejection click. It also alters with posture and may decrease in intensity or disappear with a Valsalva manoeuvre. Finally it is common in young healthy children to be able to hear a bruit over the carotid arteries in the neck. These murmurs are caused by the flow from aorta into the head and neck vessels, and in contrast to the murmur of aortic stenosis, the carotid bruit is louder over the neck than over the precordium.

Q3. What are the relevant investigations?

In many cases it is clear after clinical examination that the murmur is highly likely to be innocent. In practice most paediatricians assessing a child with a heart murmur will request an ECG and CXR. The ECG may be helpful in identifying an abnormal axis or evidence of atrial or ventricular enlargement (Table 40.1).

The main parameters to be assessed on the CXR are:
- Shape of the cardiac silhouette
- The cardiothoracic ratio: below 55% is considered to be normal
- Pulmonary vascularity: normal/increased/decreased.

It should be noted that a normal ECG and CXR does not preclude the presence of a congenital cardiac abnormality.

The gold standard investigation for the evaluation of cardiac structure and function in children is echocardiography performed best under the guidance of a paediatric cardiologist who has already examined the patient.

Q4. When is a referral to a paediatric cardiologist indicated?

If there is uncertainty after clinical examination that the murmur is innocent or there is any abnormality on the ECG or CXR, then referral to a paediatric cardiologist is indicated so that a definitive diagnosis can be obtained. Children with a family history of inheritable cardiac conditions such as hypertrophic obstructive cardiomyopathy (HOCM) should also be referred.

In many cases an experienced paediatric cardiologist will be able to confirm on clinical examination that the murmur is innocent. In the remainder echocardiography is necessary either to rule out or confirm pathology. It is crucial that someone skilled in paediatric echo-cardiography performs this investigation.

Q5. What advice would you give to the parents of a child with an innocent murmur?

For those children with an innocent murmur it is extremely important that a very clear message is given to the parents that their child's heart is normal. It should be made clear that the child should have no restrictions with regard to physical activity and that antibiotic prophylaxis for dental treatment is not necessary. The best way to reinforce the message that there are no ongoing concerns is to discharge the child from further follow-up. The child should be seen regularly over the years by the primary care physician for health supervision visits.

Pathological lesions presenting as a murmur in childhood

Atrial septal defect (ASD)

The majority of children with an isolated secundum ASD will not present until school age. They may be found to have a murmur on routine examination or may have symptoms of dyspnoea or fatigue on exertion. These symptoms become more prominent as the child gets older. Some may have been more prone to respiratory infections and misdiagnosed as asthmatic. Increasingly infants having echocardiography for other reasons are found to have small ASDs and the long-term significance of these is unclear.

Clinical features

If there is a significant left-to-right shunt through the ASD there is usually a palpable left parasternal impulse. The classical finding is fixed splitting of the second heart sound due to delayed emptying of the dilated right ventricle. An ejection systolic murmur is audible in the pulmonary area due to the increased flow across the pulmonary valve. In those with a large ASD a mid-diastolic murmur due to increased flow across the tricuspid valve may be heard.

Investigations

CXR will indicate cardiomegaly, with a prominent main pulmonary artery and increased pulmonary vascularity.

The ECG will usually show sinus rhythm with evidence of right atrial enlargement in about 50% of cases. In the majority there will be an 'RSR' (incomplete right bundle branch block) pattern due to the right ventricular diastolic volume overload.

The diagnosis is confirmed by echocardiography. This allows measurement of the size and location of the defect, and assessment of the degree of right atrial and right ventricular enlargement. The addition of colour Doppler imaging quantifies the direction and magnitude of shunting and also helps with excluding any associated anomaly of pulmonary venous drainage.

Management

For significant ASDs closure is indicated to prevent long-term complications. Closure is commonly performed around the age of 4–5 years but can be carried out earlier if there is evidence of heart failure. In the modern era the choice is between surgical and device closure at cardiac catheterization. Small to moderate secundum ASDs can often be closed by interventional catheter techniques, avoiding the need for surgery. Large secundum ASDs, sinus venosus ASDs and defects in the primum area of the atrial septum require surgical closure.

Both surgical and device closure have a very low mortality and patients with secundum ASD have an excellent long-term prognosis if corrected in childhood.

Sinus venosus ASD

This type of defect accounts for 5–10% of all ASDs. The defect usually lies posterior to the fossa ovalis and the superior vena cava overrides its upper margin. It is commonly associated with anomalous connection of the right upper pulmonary veins to either the right atrium or the superior vena cava.

Ostium primum ASD (partial ASD)

In this condition the defect lies antero-inferiorly to the fossa ovalis and is always associated with an abnormal mitral valve with a variable degree of mitral regurgitation. The degree of left-to-right shunting may be large and patients may present with heart failure in infancy, particularly if there is significant mitral regurgitation. Correction requires patch closure of the primum defect and, in most cases, repair of the 'cleft' in the anterior septal leaflet of the mitral valve also.

Pulmonary stenosis

Pulmonary valvular stenosis may occur as an isolated abnormality or as part of more complex abnormalities such as tetralogy of Fallot. Patients with Noonan syndrome commonly have a dysplastic stenotic pulmonary valve.

Clinical features

Those with mild or moderate pulmonary valve stenosis (PS) are often asymptomatic and the diagnosis is only made after a murmur has been detected on routine examination. At the other end of the spectrum those with critical PS may present with cyanosis in the neonatal period.

In children with PS palpation of the precordium may reveal a right ventricular systolic impulse and a palpable thrill. On auscultation the characteristic finding is an ejection click audible over the pulmonary area. There is also an ejection systolic murmur loudest over the upper left sternal border but radiating widely, particularly through to the back. In infants with critical PS and heart failure a second pansystolic murmur of tricuspid regurgitation is often audible.

Investigations

In mild or moderate PS the ECG may be normal. In severe PS there will be evidence of right ventricular hypertrophy. The most striking feature on CXR is prominent pulmonary artery conus caused by post-stenotic dilatation in the main pulmonary artery. In infants with critical PS there is generally very marked cardiomegaly with mainly right atrial enlargement secondary to tricuspid regurgitation. The diagnosis is easily made by echocardiography. The pulmonary valve leaflets appear thickened and doming with poor mobility, and the pulmonary valve annulus is often small. In those with critical PS the right ventricle will appear very hypertrophied with a small cavity and there will be tricuspid regurgitation with right atrial dilatation. Colour Doppler will demonstrate turbulent flow across the valve with increased velocity, and continuous wave Doppler allows accurate measurement of the peak systolic gradient across the valve.

Management
In infants and older children the preferred mode of treatment is now balloon pulmonary valvuloplasty performed at cardiac catheterization. In this group a Doppler gradient across the pulmonary valve of 60 mmHg or greater is often used as the cutoff point for intervention. The dysplastic pulmonary valve in patients with Noonan syndrome is usually also associated with a narrowed valve annulus and is less likely to have a good result from valvuloplasty.

In neonates with critical pulmonary stenosis, where pulmonary blood flow is ductus-dependent, initial management is to maintain patency of the ductus using a prostaglandin infusion. To relieve the obstruction the choice is between surgical pulmonary valvotomy and balloon pulmonary valvuloplasty. If there is hypoplasia of the right ventricle with a small main pulmonary artery it may be necessary to augment pulmonary blood flow with a Blalock–Taussig shunt.

For the vast majority of patients with PS the long-term prognosis is excellent. Some may need pulmonary valve replacement in adult life because of pulmonary regurgitation.

Small ventricular septal defect (VSD)

The typical finding in a small VSD is a blowing pansystolic murmur, usually loudest at the lower left sternal edge. There may be an associated thrill. The patient will be asymptomatic and will not require any treatment but antibiotic prophylaxis against infective endocarditis is important.

Patent ductus arteriosus (PDA)

PDA is the most common congenital heart lesion found in the newborn period, accounting for about 10% of all CHD in babies born at term. In the majority of newborns there is complete functional closure of the ductus within 72 hours of birth.

The most common clinical situation in which persistent patency of the ductus is important is in the ventilator-dependent premature infant with lung disease of prematurity. This is discussed in detail on page 713. In the older child the presentation may be with failure to thrive, with breathlessness on exertion or with the incidental finding of a murmur.

Clinical features
The severity of symptoms is related to the magnitude of left-to-right shunting from aorta to pulmonary artery. A large PDA will in most cases lead to symptoms of breathlessness and often an increased tendency to respiratory infection. There may be gradual onset of heart failure due to volume overload of the left heart.

In the presence of a significant PDA the peripheral pulses will be increased in volume and may be bounding. The child may be tachycardic and tachypnoeic at rest with the precordium active. In the newborn period the murmur is usually ejection systolic, and with a moderate to large PDA there may be multiple ejection clicks. In the infant or older child the classical continuous machinery murmur is easily audible. Very rarely with a large ductus, if the pulmonary vascular resistance remains high, the continuous murmur may never appear. This group are at risk of developing early irreversible pulmonary vascular disease.

Investigations
CXR will show cardiomegaly and increased pulmonary flow. Echocardiography will readily identify whether the ductus is patent and also establish its size. Colour Doppler will indicate the direction of shunting, which in the absence of pulmonary hypertension should be left-to-right (Fig. 40.7). Dilatation of the left atrium and left ventricle is an indicator of significant left-to-right shunting.

Management
Management of PDA in the premature ventilator-dependent infant is dealt with elsewhere (p. 713). In older children, when ductal patency has been established, the commonly accepted management is to proceed to closure. With a moderate to large PDA the indication for closure is to prevent the risk of developing pulmonary vascular disease. The indication for closure of the small PDA is the prevention of infective endocarditis. If the PDA is very large surgical ligation remains the treatment of choice. Surgical closure is performed through a left thoracotomy incision. For small to moderate PDA device occlusion at cardiac catheterization is usually possible. Both treatment options have a low morbidity

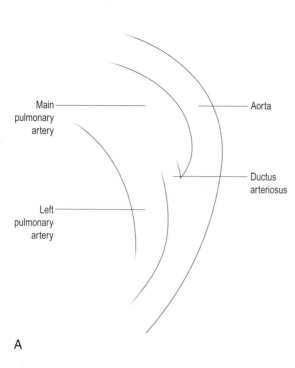

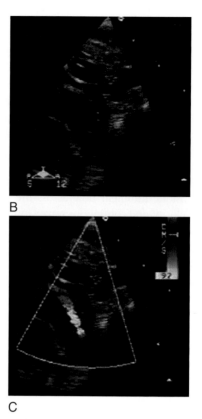

Main
pulmonary
artery

Aorta

Ductus
arteriosus

Left
pulmonary
artery

A

B

C

Fig. 40.7 Patent ductus arteriosus (PDA).
(a) Moderate PDA; (b) echocardiogram; (c) Doppler study.

and mortality. Occlusion devices may be in the form of coils or 'plugs'.

Aortic stenosis

Aortic stenosis accounts for about 5% of CHD diagnosed in childhood. The stenosis is most commonly valvular but subvalvular obstruction and more rarely supravalvular obstruction can occur. In valvular aortic stenosis the valve is often bicuspid with thickened leaflets and commissural fusion. Subvalvular obstruction is caused in most cases by a discrete fibromuscular ring. Supravalvular aortic stenosis is more common in children with Williams syndrome.

Clinical features

Children are often asymptomatic, even in the presence of severe stenosis. When symptoms do occur there may be a history of fatigue and/or chest pain with exertion. The first presentation may be with an episode of collapse during exercise, and aortic stenosis is a recognized cause of sudden death in young people.

With moderate to severe aortic stenosis there may be a palpable left ventricular heave and a thrill. The thrill is easily palpable in the suprasternal notch as well as over the aortic area. In valvular aortic stenosis an ejection click is audible. The murmur is harsh and, although loudest in the aortic area, radiates widely down to the apex and up into the neck. If there is mixed aortic valve disease with aortic regurgitation a diastolic murmur will also be audible. In severe aortic stenosis all pulses will be of reduced volume and blood pressure measurement will reveal a reduced pulse pressure.

Investigations

In severe aortic stenosis the ECG will usually show evidence of left ventricular hypertrophy but correlation between ECG change and the valve gradient is not good. The appearance of a left ventricular 'strain' pattern with ST depression and T wave inversion in the left precordial leads is an important indicator of the need for intervention to relieve the obstruction.

The diagnosis is easily confirmed by two-dimensional echocardiography. Imaging will clarify the level of obstruction (subvalvular, valvular or supravalvular) and its mechanism. The degree of left ventricular hypertrophy can be determined from wall thickness measurements and an ejection or shortening fraction calculated as a measure of left ventricular function. Colour Doppler also helps to clarify the level of the obstruction and quantify any associated aortic regurgitation. Continuous wave Doppler measurement estimates the transvalvular gradient.

Management

All patients, even those with mild obstruction, require endocarditis prophylaxis. Those with moderate or severe stenosis should not participate in competitive sport.

In the ill neonate with severe aortic stenosis the treatment of choice is still surgical aortic valvotomy. In the older child balloon aortic valvuloplasty performed at cardiac catheterization can be an effective and less invasive means of relieving the stenosis. The decision to intervene with surgery or valvuloplasty in childhood aortic stenosis can be difficult and intervention may be necessary in the asymptomatic child. In children a Doppler gradient of greater than 70 mmHg or a mean gradient of greater than 35 mmHg is often used as a level above which intervention needs to be considered. The ECG changes of ST depression or T wave inversion are further evidence of the need for treatment. Subvalvular aortic stenosis is potentially a much more dangerous lesion because of its dynamic nature, and in this condition surgery is indicated for even moderate degrees of obstruction.

Prognosis

Children with aortic stenosis require life-long follow-up. Since the valve is intrinsically abnormal a significant percentage of those who require surgery or valvuloplasty in childhood will go on to require further treatment. As the patient gets older aortic regurgitation may be the dominant problem, and valve replacement with a prosthetic valve is required in approximately 35% within 15–20 years of the original procedure. Those with a prosthetic valve require long-term anticoagulation.

Cyanotic heart disease

This usually presents in the neonatal period and is discussed in Chapter 46.

Chest pain in childhood

(See also Ch. 23.)

Problem-orientated topic:

chest pain ● ● ● ● ● ●

A 12-year-old boy, Karlo, has complained intermittently of chest pain over the past 4 months. He describes a left-sided pain occurring mainly with exercise but sometimes also at rest. Each episode lasts less than 5 minutes.

Q1. What points in the history help distinguish cardiac from non-cardiac chest pain?

Q2. What should you look for on clinical examination?

Q3. What is the differential diagnosis?

Q4. What investigations are appropriate?

Q1. What points in the history help distinguish cardiac from non-cardiac chest pain?

It is important to identify factors that bring on the pain:
- Is it related to exercise?
- What are the location, intensity and duration?
- Does it get worse with deep inspiration?
- Does it stop the child from doing any activity when it comes on?
- Is there any association with breathlessness, palpitations or dizziness?
- Is the pain associated with eating?
- Has there been any chest trauma?

It is also important to elucidate:
- Any history of wheezing, since exercise-induced asthma is a relatively frequent cause of chest pain in childhood
- A good social and family history, possible psychogenic factors influencing the child's symptoms, particularly recent stresses at school or at home.

Information gathered from previous encounters in the course of acute care or well child visits must be reviewed. Brief, infrequently occurring chest pain occurring over months or years in an otherwise well child is unlikely to have a serious aetiology. On the other hand, pain that is constant or frequently occurs with exercise and interferes with the child's activities needs to be taken more seriously. Cardiac pain due to ischaemia is often crushing in nature and associated with sweating, nausea, dyspnoea or syncope.

Q2. What should you look for on clinical examination?

As for any illness with an unknown aetiology, a complete physical examination should be performed. This should include a detailed cardiovascular examination, including measurement of blood pressure. On examination palpation for any signs of tenderness, particularly over the costochondral junctions, may reveal the diagnosis of costochondritis. In those with a musculoskeletal cause the pain may be increased in certain positions or activities and often is made worse by deep inspirations.

An active precordium, abnormal pulses or presence of a murmur will point towards a cardiac cause of the pain that needs to be further investigated. Auscultation

- Idiopathic
- Musculoskeletal
- Pulmonary
- Psychological
- Gastrointestinal
- Cardiac
- Mediastinal tumors
- Vaso-occlusive crisis (sickle cell disease)
- Herpes zoster
- Ingestion (cocaine, tobacco, amphetamines)

BOX 40.10 Cardiac causes of chest pain in childhood

- Left ventricular outflow tract obstruction: aortic valve stenosis, subaortic stenosis, hypertrophic obstructive cardiomyopathy
- Coronary artery stenosis: post-Kawasaki disease or Takayasu arteritis
- Anomalous origin of coronary arteries
- Tachyarrhythmias
- Inflammatory: myocarditis, pericarditis, rheumatic carditis, dissecting aortic aneurysm (Marfan syndrome)
- Mitral valve prolapse
- Coronary vasospasm
- Pulmonary hypertension

of the lungs may reveal evidence of infection or bronchospasm. Abdominal examination may reveal epigastric tenderness, suggesting a gastrointestinal cause.

Q3. What is the differential diagnosis?

The most common causes of chest pain in childhood are summarized in Box 40.9.

In the majority of children who complain of chest pain the cause will be non-cardiac. It does, however, provoke a lot of parental anxiety, particularly in young people who are participating in sport. It may not be possible to identify a clear cause and many cases are idiopathic, but in such cases both patient and parents need to be reassured that there is no cause for concern. Those in whom the cause is idiopathic will often describe sharp pain of very short duration occurring either at rest or during exercise. The cardiac causes of chest pain are summarized in Box 40.10.

Q4. What investigations are appropriate?

If the history is not suggestive of serious pathology and a thorough physical examination is normal, then further investigation is usually not indicated. In the remainder the investigations are guided by particular causes of concern from the history or clinical examination. For those with a possible cardiac aetiology ECG and echocardiography are mandatory. If possible an ECG should be obtained during an episode. The most useful investigation for those old enough to cooperate is a treadmill exercise test during which there is ECG and blood pressure measurement. A normal exercise test provides reassurance in many cases and in the remainder may more clearly help with the differential diagnosis between musculoskeletal and cardiac pain if the symptoms are reproduced during the test. If necessary, a chest X-ray, blood tests and urine toxicology screening may also need to be performed. However, if these investigations are deemed necessary it would be appropriate to refer the patient to a paediatric cardiologist.

Arrhythmias

Problem-orientated topic:

palpitations

Nika, a 12-year-old girl, presents to the accident and emergency department with a history of her 'heart beating strongly and very fast'. This feeling started while she was watching television and has continued for over an hour. She states that this has never happened before. She appears nervous but well. Colour is pink and there is no evidence of respiratory distress. Pulse is very fast and difficult to count. Capillary refill time is less than 2 seconds. Her rhythm strip is shown in Figure 40.8.

Q1. What does the rhythm strip demonstrate and what is the most likely diagnosis?

Q2. How are you going to manage this patient?

Q3. What are the long-term treatment options?

Q1. What does the rhythm strip demonstrate and what is the most likely diagnosis?

The rhythm strip demonstrates a narrow complex tachycardia with a rate of 240 beats per minute. The most likely diagnosis is of a supraventricular tachycardia (SVT) or, more specifically, an atrioventricular re-entry

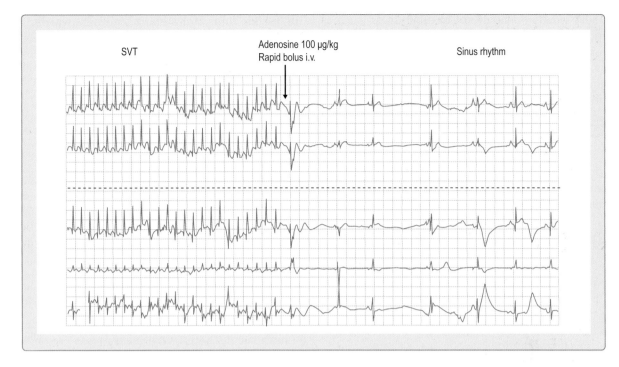

Fig. 40.8. Nika's rhythm strip demonstrating conversion from SVT to sinus rhythm following administration of intravenous adenosine (arrow head)

BOX 40.11 Factors distinguishing sinus tachycardia from supraventricular tachycardia

Sinus tachycardia

- May have history of preceding systemic illness
- Heart rate rarely exceeds 200 bpm
- P waves upright in leads II, III and aVF (may be difficult to identify at fast rates)
- Beat-to-beat variability can be seen
- Heart rate gradually slows with treatment (e.g. fluid resuscitation)

Supraventricular tachycardia

- Previously well with no preceding systemic upset
- May report sudden onset
- May have had similar previous episodes, which terminated abruptly
- Heart rate generally above 220 bpm (may be lower if on treatment)
- P waves may be absent: negative in leads II, III and aVF if present
- No beat-to-beat variability in SVT
- Rate abruptly changes following intervention

tachycardia. It can sometimes be difficult to differentiate sinus tachycardia from SVT, particularly at a heart rate around 200 bpm. In such cases, a 12-lead ECG should be performed. Box 40.11 sets out factors that help make this distinction.

Q2. How are you going to manage this patient?

After assessment of airway, breathing and circulation, it is clear that Nika is not in shock. It is reasonable to attempt manoeuvres, which result in vagal stimulation and may terminate the arrhythmia (e.g. Valsalva manoeuvre, one-sided carotid sinus massage). In a neonate or infant application of an ice pack to the face is an appropriate vagal manoeuvre but this should not be performed in older children.

It is important that Nika is put on a heart monitor from which the rhythm is archived and retrievable, or which is printing during such interventions, so that any change in rhythm can be analysed and documented.

If vagal manoeuvres fail, the treatment of choice is intravenous adenosine, at an initial dose of 50 µg/kg, which should be administered rapidly through a large-bore cannula in a large proximal vein and flushed through with normal saline (Fig. 40.8). Adenosine has a short half-life of a few seconds and works by blocking the AV node. Nika should be warned before administration that she will feel unpleasant for a short time following the injection. Again, continuous ECG monitoring should be in place. Further doses of adenosine at 100 µg/kg and then 250 µg/kg should be administered if the arrhythmia is not terminated.

If Nika remains in SVT following adenosine, it is important that she is discussed with a paediatric cardiologist, who may suggest synchronous DC cardioversion under sedation/anaesthesia, or other drugs (such as propranolol, flecainide, amiodarone or digoxin). After initial stabilization a paediatric cardiologist should evaluate the child with a significant dysrhythmia and co-manage the patient in collaboration with the primary care paediatrician.

🌐 http://www.aplsonline.com

Nika should have an echocardiogram to look for evidence of any CHD, although the majority of children presenting with SVT will have a structurally normal heart.

Q3. What are the long-term treatment options?

Nika should commence regular prophylaxis to prevent further episodes of SVT. This is usually in the form of a β-blocking drug. Some patients who have infrequent, self-terminating episodes of SVT may choose not to be on regular medication.

In recurrent or resistant SVT, identification of the accessory pathway by electrophysiological mapping in the cardiac catheter laboratory, along with its ablation, may be considered.

Supraventricular tachycardia (SVT)

SVT is the most common arrhythmia seen in children (Fig. 40.8). It commonly results from the presence of an accessory pathway between the atria and the ventricles, with normal electrical conduction across the AV node and retrograde conduction across the abnormal pathway. The best-known example of this phenomenon is Wolff–Parkinson–White syndrome. During sinus rhythm, antegrade conduction across the pathway may be possible and results in ventricular pre-excitation, with classical ECG findings of a delta wave and short PR interval.

About half of all cases of SVT in childhood present in infancy, with presentation ranging from a history of irritability or poor feeding, to presenting in extremis with heart failure. Older children tend to present earlier as they can vocalize symptoms and rarely present in heart failure.

Problem-orientated topic:

syncope ● ● ● ● ●

Andelko, a 10-year-old boy, is referred to outpatients with a history of syncope. This occurred most recently after playing football with his friends, when he fainted, lost consciousness briefly and complained of 'feeling funny' for a short time afterwards. Further questioning reveals that this has occurred on several other occasions, and he is awaiting an outpatient EEG for investigation of possible seizures. His cardiovascular examination is unremarkable. His 12-lead ECG is shown in Figure 40.9.

Q1. What abnormality does the ECG demonstrate?

Q2. What may have caused Andelko's episodes of syncope?

Q3. What is your further management?

Q1. What abnormality does the ECG demonstrate?

The QT interval appears prolonged, and when corrected for heart rate ($QTc = QT/\sqrt{R\!-\!R}$ interval) is 0.5 seconds. The causes of a prolonged QT interval are listed in Box 40.12.

The most likely cause in this scenario is congenital long QT syndrome. This condition is inherited and results from a mutation in the genes controlling the sodium and potassium channels in the myocardial cell wall.

BOX 40.12 Causes of an abnormal QT interval

Shortened QT interval
- Hypoxia
- Hypercalcaemia
- Digoxin
- Short QT syndrome

Prolonged QT interval
- Congenital long QT syndrome
- Hypocalcaemia
- Hypothermia
- Head injury
- Amiodarone
- Sotalol
- Tricyclic antidepressants

Q2. What may have caused Andelko's episodes of syncope?

The syncope could have resulted from episodes of arrhythmia, in particular ventricular tachycardia. Episodes of collapse in children with long QT syndrome are typically precipitated by activities or events that produce an increase in catecholamine levels.

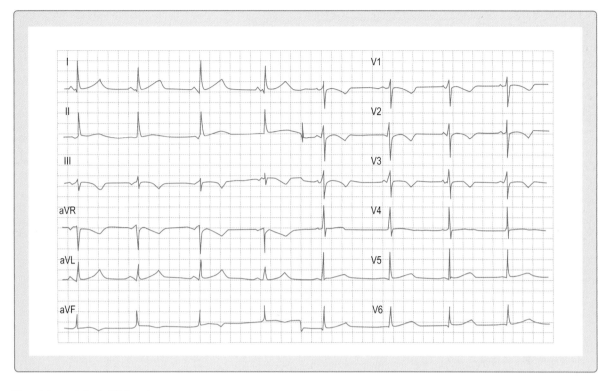

Fig. 40.9 Andelko's ECG strip

Q3. What is your further management?

If in the initial evaluation the symptoms suggest cardiac involvement, the primary care paediatrician should consider referral to a paediatric cardiologist. Given Andelko's history he should be commenced on a β-blocking agent, such as propranolol. A 24-hour ambulatory ECG recording should be arranged and analysed. Genetic screening should be arranged for Andelko, as an increasing number of genetic mutations are being identified, which help confirm the diagnosis and guide treatment. First-degree relatives should receive ECG and genetic screening. Avoidance of competitive sport and swimming should be advised.

Ventricular tachycardia (VT)

VT is defined as a series of three or more premature ventricular contractions. It typically has a rate of over 120 beats per minute and the QRS morphology is wide (Fig. 40.10).

VT is relatively uncommon in childhood. In the management of a child with VT it is important to consider possible underlying causes (Box 40.13).

This is potentially a very dangerous arrhythmia because of the possibility of its degenerating into ventricular fibrillation. If the patient is not clinically shocked then intravenous administration of amiodarone in a dose of 5 mg/kg given over 30 minutes is an appropriate initial treatment. In the clinically shocked patient DC cardioversion under sedation or anaesthesia should be undertaken. For treatment algorithms refer to APLS guidelines.

Inflammations and infections

Infective endocarditis

Infectious endocarditis is rare in childhood but remains a potential cause of serious morbidity and mortality. The vast majority of those affected will have underlying structural heart disease as a result of either congenital or rheumatic heart disease. With increasing survival following surgery for CHD the population potentially at risk is increasing. The lesions most commonly complicated by endocarditis are VSDs, aortic stenosis or incompetence, tetralogy of Fallot and PDA. An increasing group is those with artificial conduits or

---

BOX 40.13 Causes of ventricular tachycardia

- Congenital heart disease
- Previous cardiac surgery
- Congenital long QT syndrome
- Drugs (e.g. tricyclic antidepressants, cisapride, erythromycin)
- Electrolyte imbalance (e.g. hyperkalaemia)

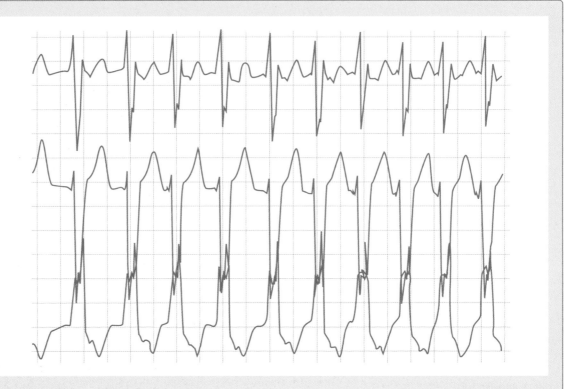

Fig. 40.10 **Ventricular tachycardia.**

> **BOX 40.14 Clinical features associated with endocarditis**
>
> - Fever
> - Heart murmur (N.B. new or changing murmur)
> - General malaise (myalgia, arthralgia)
> - Heart failure
> - Splenomegaly
> - Microscopic haematuria
> - Petechiae
> - Embolic phenomena: neurological or pulmonary
> - Osler nodes, Janeway lesions, splinter haemorrhages

prosthetic valves. Endocarditis can occur in those with structurally normal hearts: for example, those with indwelling central venous lines or intravenous drug users.

In most series streptococci (*Strep. viridans* more than enterococci) are the most common causative organism, with staphylococci (*Staph. aureus* and *Staph. epidermidis*) being the second largest group. In the paediatric age group 80% of cases are due to these two organism groups.

The clinical features of the illness depend on the virulence of the organism and host resistance. The most useful clinical features are summarized in Box 40.14.

Isolation of the infecting organism from blood culture is crucially important in making the diagnosis and guiding appropriate antimicrobial therapy. Two or three blood cultures over a 24-hour period are usually adequate. Diagnostic difficulty can arise in patients partially treated with antibiotics prior to a diagnosis of endocarditis being considered. *Candida* infection should be considered in those with negative blood cultures.

In most cases transthoracic echocardiography will demonstrate the vegetations attached to affected valves and will also help quantify any associated valve regurgitation (Fig. 40.11). Transoesophageal echocardiography may be necessary where the transthoracic images are inadequate.

Management

Treatment is required for a minimum of 4 weeks and is usually continued for 6.

For *Strep. viridans* a combination of penicillin and gentamicin given intravenously is effective. For *Strep. faecalis* a combination of amoxicillin and gentamicin is used. Flucloxacillin and gentamicin is the first-choice therapy for staphylococcal infection. *Candida* infection is difficult to treat and may require a combination of amphotericin and flucytosine. It may prove impossible to eradicate infection on a

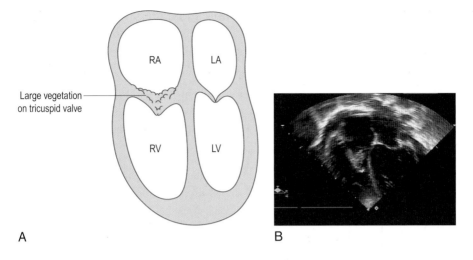

Fig. 40.11 Infective endocarditis.
(A) Diagram of infective endocarditis and large vegetations on the tricuspid valve (RA = right atrium; LA = left atrium; RV = right ventricle; LV = left ventricle); (B) echocardiogram.

prosthetic valve, patch, homograft or pacemaker with antimicrobial therapy alone and surgical exploration may be necessary.

Prophylaxis

Bacteraemia can occur in relation to dental or surgical procedures. It has been estimated that extraction of an abscessed tooth produces bacteraemia in up to 80% of cases. Streptococci form part of the normal flora of the mouth and are the usual cause of endocarditis following dental procedures. The most important prophylactic measure is good oral hygiene. In addition to extraction antibiotic prophylaxis is also indicated for scaling, major root fillings and orthodontic procedures. Prophylaxis should be given less than 1 hour prior to the procedure. Other procedures for which prophylaxis is indicated include:

- Tonsillectomy and adenoidectomy
- Appendicectomy
- Bronchoscopy
- Endotracheal intubation
- Urethral catheterization.

Rheumatic fever

Rheumatic fever is the most common cause of acquired heart disease in children and young adults world-wide. It is an inflammatory disease involving the joints and heart, and less frequently the central nervous system, skin and subcutaneous tissues. It arises as a complication of group A streptococcal infection. There is a 2–3-week latent period between the upper respiratory tract infection and the onset of rheumatic fever. The peak incidence is in children aged 5–15 years and there may be a genetic influence as

family clustering occurs. The incidence is strikingly higher in people living in overcrowded conditions. Current theories suggest that the inflammatory process is mediated by an immunological reaction precipitated by the streptococcal infection.

Pathology

In the early stages there is an acute inflammatory exudative reaction. This lasts 2–3 weeks and involves the myocardium, valves and pericardium. This is followed by a proliferative phase, during which Aschoff bodies form. This pathognomonic lesion consists of a perivascular infiltrate of large cells with polymorphous nuclei and basophilic cytoplasm arranged in a rosette around an avascular centre of fibrinoid. Subsequently fibrotic scarring occurs in the region of the Aschoff bodies.

Rheumatic carditis

Mitral valve involvement is the most common, with aortic valve involvement second. The tricuspid valve is infrequently involved and the pulmonary valve only very rarely. Valve lesions begin as small verrucae composed of fibrin and blood cells along the borders of the valves. Particularly with the mitral valve, this may progress to some loss of valve tissue and shortening and thickening of the chordae tendinae. With persistent inflammation fibrosis and calcification occur. Chronic mitral regurgitation leads to left atrial dilatation, which may in turn lead to atrial fibrillation. There is also the risk of endocarditis.

Clinical features

The diagnostic criteria of Duckett Jones, drawn up in 1944 (Box 40.15), are still used to guide the diagnosis

Major manifestations
- Carditis
- Polyarthritis
- Chorea
- Erythema marginatum
- Subcutaneous nodules
- Leucocytosis

Minor manifestations
- Clinical:
  - Fever
  - Arthralgia
  - Previous rheumatic fever or rheumatic heart disease
- Laboratory:
  - Acute phase reactants: elevated erythrocyte sedimentation rate (ESR) and/or C-reactive protein (CRP)
  - Prolonged PR interval

of rheumatic fever. The presence of two major criteria or one major plus two minor criteria indicates a high probability of acute rheumatic fever, if supported by evidence of recent group A streptococcal infection.

Supporting evidence of streptococcal infection includes:
- Increased antistreptolysin O titre (ASOT)
- Positive throat culture for group A streptococcus
- Recent scarlet fever.

Joint symptoms are the most common feature, occurring in 75%. Typically there is a migratory polyarthritis. The joint symptoms disappear in 3–4 weeks. Carditis occurs in 40–50% of initial attacks. Tachycardia disproportionate to fever is a typical finding. The most distinctive sign of rheumatic carditis is a new distinctive murmur. This is most commonly the blowing pansystolic apical murmur of mitral regurgitation. With aortic valve involvement the early diastolic murmur of aortic regurgitation may be heard. Other signs of carditis are finding a pericardial rub or evidence of congestive cardiac failure. Sydenham chorea occurs in about 15% of patients. Subcutaneous nodules are found in 5–10% and erythema marginatum in less than 5%.

Laboratory findings
ESR and CRP are elevated. Around 80% will have an elevated ASOT. Values of > 300 are abnormal. A moderate normochromic normocytic anaemia is common.

The ECG will demonstrate a prolonged PR interval in one-third of patients. Flattened T waves occur with myocarditis and elevated ST segments are found in pericarditis.

Management
- Eradicate streptococcal infection with oral or intramuscular penicillin.
- Bed rest is recommended for the period of carditis.
- Prescribe salicylates, initially aspirin 75–100 mg/kg/day.
- Give prednisolone (2 mg/kg/day) if there is evidence of carditis. This dose is continued for 2–3 weeks, followed by gradual withdrawal over a further 2–3 weeks. As the steroid is withdrawn, salicylate is introduced to prevent clinical rebound. Salicylate should be continued for at least 4–6 weeks.
- Give diuretics in heart failure.
- Digoxin can be used with careful monitoring of levels.

Prognosis
Cardiac involvement is the major factor determining morbidity in acute rheumatic fever. Around 75% of patients with congestive heart failure during the initial attack will have evidence of chronic valvular disease after 10 years. The 10-year mortality rate is approximately 4%.

Prevention
Prophylaxis needs to be continued through childhood and adolescence. Lifetime prophylaxis is recommended in patients with rheumatic valvular disease. Oral penicillin may cause the emergence of resistant alpha-streptococci in the oral cavity.

Myocarditis

Myocarditis is an inflammatory disorder of the myocardium, causing necrosis of myocytes. It is most commonly caused by a viral infection, such as Coxsackie B or adenovirus. Other infective agents have been implicated, including meningococcus, *Mycoplasma*, *Diphtheria*, *Toxoplasma*, and rickettsiae. Rarely, myocarditis may be caused by drugs, toxins or autoimmune disease. An autoimmune response to the initial viral insult may play a part in disease progression and this may have a genetic basis. Myocarditis can occur at any age, including the newborn period. As many cases are subclinical, incidence is difficult to determine.

Clinical features
Presentation varies widely from acute collapse to a subclinical picture. History may reveal a recent respiratory or gastrointestinal infection. There may be symptoms and signs of congestive cardiac failure (Box 40.3). Older children may complain of chest pain (from myocardial ischaemia or concurrent pericarditis) or palpitations.

Investigations

CXR may reveal cardiomegaly and pulmonary oedema. ECG abnormalities include resting tachycardia, low-voltage QRS, ST segment changes, Q waves and arrhythmia, including atrioventricular conduction disturbances. Two-dimensional echocardiography demonstrates a dilated and poorly contracting left ventricle, with reduced ejection fraction. Mitral regurgitation due to a dilated mitral valve annulus may be demonstrated and a pericardial effusion may be present. ESR, CRP and cardiac enzyme levels are usually elevated. Evidence of an infective agent should be sought, including blood culture, acute and convalescent viral serology, and throat swab and faeces for viral culture.

Management

Management is largely supportive, with some patients requiring intensive care, including intubation, ventilation, inotropic support, afterload reducing agents and prompt treatment of arrhythmia. There is no specific treatment for the disease process, with the use of steroid and immunosuppressive therapy remaining controversial. Many children will recover completely but some may progress to chronic dilated cardiomyopathy. Heart transplantation may be necessary.

Cardiomyopathy

Cardiomyopathy is a disease of the myocardium. Cardiomyopathies may be primary, but increasingly secondary causes are being identified.

Cardiomyopathies are broadly divided into the following categories:

- *Dilated cardiomyopathy*. The most common cardiomyopathy in childhood; characterized by ventricular dilatation and reduced systolic ventricular function.
- *Hypertrophic cardiomyopathy*. Characterized by asymmetric septal hypertrophy leading to left ventricular outflow tract obstruction in the more severe cases.
- *Restrictive cardiomyopathy*. Rare in childhood; characterized by abnormal diastolic ventricular function and atrial dilatation.

Pulmonary hypertension

Pulmonary hypertension is defined as a pulmonary artery systolic pressure greater than 30 mmHg or a pulmonary artery mean pressure greater than 20 mmHg.

Primary pulmonary hypertension (PPH)

PPH is a rare disorder of unknown aetiology. Incidence in the general population is 1–2 per million,

---

> **BOX 40.16 Diagnostic classification of pulmonary hypertension (World Health Organization 1998)**
>
> - Pulmonary arterial hypertension:
>   Primary pulmonary hypertension:
>   - Pulmonary hypertension associated with:
>   Collagen vascular diseases
>   Portal hypertension
>   Congenital systemic to pulmonary shunts
>   Drugs/toxins
>   HIV infection
>   Persistent pulmonary hypertension of newborn (PPHN)
> - Pulmonary venous hypertension
> - Pulmonary hypertension associated with disorders of respiratory system and/or hypoxaemia
> - Pulmonary hypertension due to chronic thrombosis and/or embolic disease
> - Pulmonary hypertension due to disorders affecting pulmonary vasculature

with onset in childhood rare. While there is a female preponderance in adulthood (1.7:1), prior to puberty incidence is equal between genders. The majority of cases are sporadic but familial forms may account for 10%. For a diagnosis of PPH to be made, other causes of pulmonary hypertension must be excluded (Box 40.16). PPH is caused by precapillary obstruction of the pulmonary vascular bed, as a result of intimal and medial proliferation in the arteriolar wall.

Secondary pulmonary hypertension

Secondary pulmonary hypertension is more common in childhood and is largely a consequence of pulmonary or cardiac disorders. Chronic hypoxaemia may occur in the setting of severe asthma, cystic fibrosis, interstitial lung disease or obstructive sleep apnoea. This causes pulmonary vasoconstriction through a variety of mechanisms (Fig. 40.12). Cardiac conditions may result in pulmonary hypertension because of volume and/or pressure overload on the pulmonary vasculature. This can occur from any left-to-right shunt, such as a VSD. Where pulmonary vasculature changes are severe and pulmonary arterial pressures are suprasystemic, reversal of the shunt from right to left may occur. This is termed Eisenmenger syndrome. Left heart problems, such as mitral stenosis, aortic stenosis, cor triatrium or left ventricular dysfunction, may result in left atrial hypertension and hence pulmonary venous hypertension. This results in pulmonary arterial hypertension, with intimal proliferation of pulmonary vessel walls occurring over time. Pulmonary veno-

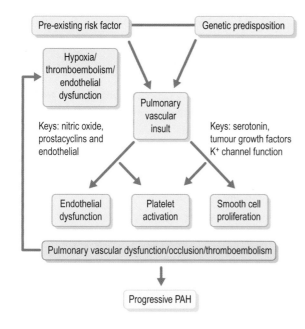

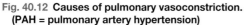

Fig. 40.12 Causes of pulmonary vasoconstriction. (PAH = pulmonary artery hypertension)

Table 40.4 Medical management of pulmonary hypertension	
Treatment	**Effect**
Oxygen	May provide symptomatic improvement
Calcium channel blockers	E.g. nifedipine. Systemic and pulmonary vasodilator. Prescribed in 'responders' (i.e. demonstrating acute reversibility of pulmonary vascular resistance in the catheter laboratory in response to a pulmonary vasodilator, such as inhaled nitric oxide)
Prostacyclin analogues	Epoprostenol: potent pulmonary vasodilator and inhibitor of platelet aggregation. Given by continuous i.v. infusion via a central line. May cause systemic hypotension Nebulized iloprost is an alternative but due to short half-life requires regular administration Oral (beraprost) and subcutaneous (treprostinil) analogues available
Inhaled nitric oxide	Potent and selective pulmonary vasodilator requiring continuous inhalation. May be given in the intensive care setting
Sildenafil	Oral phosphodiesterase-5 inhibitor. Results in increased cyclic guanosine monophosphate (GMP) levels and therefore an increase in endogenous endothelial nitric oxide production
Bosentan	Oral dual endothelin receptor antagonist. Competitively binds to endothelin-1 receptors ET_A and ET_B. Reduces smooth muscle cell proliferation

BOX 40.17 Symptoms and signs of secondary pulmonary hypertension

Symptoms
- Fatigue
- Exertional dyspnoea
- Syncope
- Chest pain
- Headaches

Signs
- Right ventricular heave
- Loud P2 (may be palpable)
- Pansystolic murmur (tricuspid regurgitation)
- Hepatomegaly
- Peripheral oedema
- Elevated jugular venous pulse (older children)

occlusive disease is a rare cause of pulmonary hypertension. Obliteration of the pulmonary vascular bed, such as can occur in connective tissue disorders or chronic pulmonary emboli, can result in progressive pulmonary hypertension.

Clinical features

In cases of secondary pulmonary hypertension, presenting features will be dominated by the underlying primary disease (Box 40.17).

Investigations

ECG demonstrates evidence of right axis deviation and right ventricular hypertrophy. CXR may demon-strate cardiomegaly, with prominent main and branch pulmonary arteries and paucity ('pruning') of the peripheral pulmonary vascular markings. Echocardiogram shows a hypertrophied right ventricle with reduced function. Pulmonary arterial pressure may be indirectly assessed by Doppler interrogation of any regurgitant jets. It may also identify a CHD as a cause of secondary pulmonary hypertension. Cardiac catheterization may be considered for direct measurement of pulmonary arterial pressures, to look for secondary causes and to assess for reversibility of pulmonary hypertension, which can aid treatment options. Other investigations to look for secondary causes may be necessary.

Management and prognosis

In cases of secondary pulmonary hypertension, management is largely targeted at the underlying cause. Medical treatment options are summarized in Table 40.4. Blade septostomy may improve prognosis. In end-stage disease, lung or heart–lung transplant should be considered. If PPH is untreated, most children will die within 1 year of diagnosis.

Bernadette S. O'Connor   Michael D. Shields   Maximilian Zach

CHAPTER

41

Respiratory paediatrics

LEARNING OUTCOMES

By the end of this chapter you should:

- Be able to identify the different respiratory noises and know their causes and significance
- Understand the role of pulmonary function testing and radiological imaging in investigating respiratory disorders
- Know how to diagnose the common and important respiratory disorders of childhood
- Know how to assess the severity of the common respiratory conditions
- Be able to outline a management plan for the common respiratory conditions
- Understand the important underlying problems that are associated with poor control of chronic respiratory disorders such as asthma and cystic fibrosis.

MODULE SEVEN

Approach to respiratory disease

Disorders of the respiratory system make up a substantial part of a general paediatrician's workload. Acute respiratory tract infections are frequent in childhood and range from the trivial to the serious and the life-threatening. Infections may be limited to the upper respiratory tract (e.g. head cold, pharyngitis/tonsillitis, otitis media and croup) or may also involve the lower respiratory tract (e.g. bronchiolitis, pneumonia, tuberculosis). Common chronic disorders include asthma and cystic fibrosis.

Typical signs of respiratory disease may be subtle or absent in the young child.

History (see also Ch. 5)

It is important to establish at an early stage what the parent/child's primary concern is. The main reasons for parents seeking medical attention are:
- Cough
- Noisy breathing
- Recurrent chest infections
- Shortness of breath.

The history is of particular importance for the diagnosis of episodic disorders such as the most common forms of asthma, since the child might be free of symptoms when seen by the doctor. It is important to determine the onset, duration and severity of that problem, the particular triggers or relievers of the symptoms, and the impact on the child's life.

In children who present with some form of noisy breathing, accurately identifying what the noise is and its timing in the respiratory cycle is helpful in arriving at a diagnosis and in particular establishing the location of the problem. If the noise is not currently present, make sure you understand what the parent is describing. You may have to try and make the noise yourself.

Following this, specific questions within the conventional history will shed further light on the problem.

Examination

Examination may need to be repeated several times, especially during an evolving illness where signs may initially be absent or very subtle.

While attention is paid to the respiratory examination, it is important to determine whether there are features suggestive of an underlying chronic disease (Table 41.1). General features to look for include:

- Failure to thrive: plot height and weight against percentile
- Scoliosis
- Ear, nose and throat: signs of allergic rhinitis, allergic salute
- Signs of atopic eczema.

Noisy breathing

Can you define and describe the following noises? Do you understand how each noise is produced?

Table 41.1 Signs to consider in respiratory disease

Examination	Clinical features to consider
Inspection	Finger clubbing (Fig. 41.1): suggestive of suppurative lung diseases Cyanosis Chest deformity: possible chronic condition (Figs 41.2 and 41.3) Effort of breathing/signs of respiratory distress
Palpation	Chest expansion reduced Hepatomegaly
Percussion	Reduced percussion note (may be omitted in the smaller child)
Auscultation	Breath sounds Crepitations Wheeze Cardiac murmurs
Sputum inspection	Volume Colour
Growth chart	Weight and height plotted

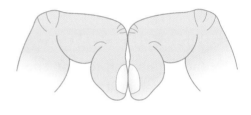
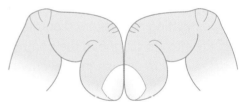

Fig. 41.1 Clubbing (loss of angle at the nail bed)

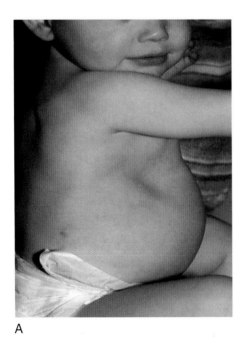

A

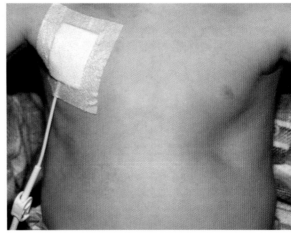

B

Fig. 41.2 **A toddler who had a long history of breathlessness and indrawing.**
(A) Side view; (B) front view. Note the valley that has been created where the diaphragm is attached to the ribs anteriorly and how the ribs distal to this then point outwards (marked Harrison's sulci).

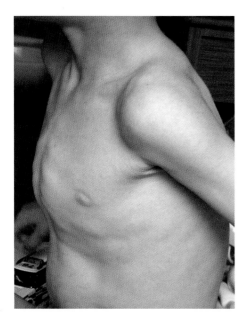

Fig. 41.3 Over-inflated 'barrel-shaped' chest

- Snoring
- Stridor
- Congestion/rattly breathing
- Grunting
- Wheezing
- Cough.

See Box 41.1 for a description of the common respiratory noises.

Shortness of breath (Dyspnoea)

When parents report that a young child experiences 'shortness of breath' this is likely to be based on their opinion of the child's appearance. This is probably correct when the child is overtly wheezing and has recession:

- Obese children report and appear to have 'shortness of breath' that is most likely due to deconditioning. In these children it can be difficult to exclude asthma.
- Parents of children with a spasmodic cough or children who are having difficulty expectorating phlegm often report that the child has 'shortness of breath'.
- 'Tightness in the chest' will cause the sensation of 'shortness of breath' and is a feature of asthma, even if audible wheezing is not heard.
- The lungs may be stiff, e.g. pneumonia.

Rarer causes of 'shortness of breath' include:
- Pulmonary hypertension
- Interstitial lung diseases
- Advanced chronic lung disease.

In these conditions the shortness of breath may be manifest initially with exercise, when the child becomes hypoxic.

Investigations

Lung function testing (Box 41.2)

Assessment of a child's respiratory rate may be considered as the most simple lung function test since practically all respiratory disorders manifest in the form of an increased breathing frequency. It is important not to forget that blood gas analysis (pH, $PaCO_2$, PaO_2) and O_2 saturation monitoring are important measures of lung function.

The most common lung function tests are spirometry (volume-time-curve of a forced expiratory vital capacity manoeuvre) and the maximum expiratory flow-volume-curve (p. 595). More complicated lung function tests will involve the measurement of lung volumes via body box plethysmography and determination of gas transfer (transfer factor) to detect gas transfer abnormalities across the alveoli to capillaries in the pulmonary circulation. Conventional lung function tests require an active cooperation of the patient and therefore, can only be used from school age on. Special techniques can assess lung function in infants and toddlers but these are only available in highly specialized institutions.

Chest imaging

Radiological imaging of the chest is an integral part of the diagnosis and follow-up of many respiratory diseases.

Plain chest X-ray

The plain chest X-ray is usually the initial study in the diagnostic work-up. Some general patterns occur but with overlap (Table 41.2). Always ask if the defect is localized or generalized (symmetrical versus asymmetrical).

Ultrasound scan (USS)

USS is especially useful for studying pleural disease, as air in the lung prevents penetration of the ultrasound beam; for example, in a child with a unilateral 'white lung' it might not be clear how large an effusion is relative to underlying intraparenchymal consolidation. Pleural effusions can be measured and the presence of loculations and debris determined. USS is also useful for observing diaphragmatic function.

Computed tomography (CT)

CT can give high-quality detailed images of the intrathoracic structures. The radiation dose needs to be kept to a minimum.

BOX 41.1 Description of the common respiratory noises

Snoring
- Rough inspiratory vibratory noise due to airflow obstruction in the pharyngeal region
- Occurs during sleep when muscle tone lax

Stridor
- Harsh crowing inspiratory sound due to airflow obstruction of the larynx or upper trachea
- The extrathoracic airways tend to collapse in inspiration therefore stridor is predominantly inspiratory

Congested or 'rattly' breathing
- Mucus is allowed to lie in the hypopharynx, trachea and large bronchi and the child 'breathes through' these secretions
- Parents say that they can feel the infant's chest to be 'rattly' and have the impression that a good cough would clear the problem
- Causes:
  - Transient mucus hypersecretion, e.g. with viral upper respiratory tract infection
  - Persistent mucus hypersecretion, e.g. with early asthma or cystic fibrosis

Grunting
- An end-expiratory noise that occurs when an infant breathes out against a partially closed glottis
- Produces an end-expiratory break and thus provides a positive end-expiratory pressure that prevents the bronchioles and alveoli from collapsing

Wheezing
- A musical high-pitched expiratory noise heard audibly or by auscultation
- Can be described to parents as a 'whistling noise in the chest when your child breathes out'
- Produced by intrathoracic airway narrowing causing turbulent airflow and therefore wheezing is predominantly expiratory

Cough
- The sudden forceful expulsion of air with the aim of:
  - Generating high-velocity airflow to expel material from the airway
  - In certain situations, squeezing the lung parenchyma and moving material (mucus/pus) further up the airway so that it can be expelled with further coughing

BOX 41.2 Use of lung function tests

Diagnostic
- To determine if and to what extent a child has an obstructive or restrictive lung disorder
- Single measure may confirm diagnosis but is rarely diagnostic
- Serial measurements are more useful

Measuring morbidity
- Baseline values
- Disease progression

Monitoring response
- Short-term response, e.g. bronchodilator responsiveness
- Long-term response, e.g. cystic fibrosis therapy

Bronchoscopy

Bronchoscopy can be via either a rigid or a flexible bronchoscope. This allows direct observation and access to the airways.

Rigid bronchoscopes allow good ventilation through the bronchoscope during the procedure and are best for removal of foreign bodies and larger tissue biopsies.

Flexible bronchoscopy requires the child to breathe around the bronchoscope. It is best for visualization of more difficult areas and allows samples to be obtained from different areas of the lung (bronchoalveolar lavage (BAL), brushings, mucosal biopsy).

Indications include:
- Visualizing anatomy, e.g. stridor, fixed wheeze, persistent atelectasis
- Obtaining BAL samples for microbiology or cytology
- Biopsy
- Therapeutic removal of mucus plugs and foreign bodies.

Table 41.2 Patterns in chest imaging

Pattern	Pathology

Hyperinflation
  Depressed diaphragms
  Narrow cardiothymic shadow/elongated heart
  Horizontal spread ribs
  Separation of vessels
	Symmetrical
	  Hyperinflation alone or associated with generalized and irregular opacities/areas of collapse
	  Causes: bronchiolitis, asthma, cystic fibrosis or other chronic suppurative lung disease, neonatal chronic lung disease
	Asymmetrical (Fig. 41.4)
	  Foreign body
	  Partial airways obstruction (unilateral 'ball valve' effect)
	  Localized lobar collapse
	  Hypoplastic lung with compensatory emphysema
	  Congenital lobar emphysema

Air space disease	Consolidation
	  Fluid, pus or blood is in the alveolar spaces
	  Characterized by fluffy opacities that have irregular margins and coalesce
	  Air bronchograms are produced by the contrast between the adjacent airspace disease with alveolar consolidation with a patent airway standing out in contrast
	  Distribution: lobar (Fig. 41.5), often with sharply defined margins along a fissure (suggest lobar pneumonia), or generalized and patchy (suggests bronchopneumonia, Fig. 41.6)
	Pulmonary oedema
	  'Bat's wing' distribution of shadowing extending from hilum
	  Look for fluid in fissures and interlobular septa
	Collapse
	  Produces a similar density as consolidation but without air bronchograms
	  Look for displacement of horizontal fissure
	  If large may show compensatory hyperinflation
	  ± Mediastinal shift (Fig. 41.7)
	Bronchiectasis
	  Thickened dilated bronchial walls
	  Cross-sectional appearance: ring shadows or white round shadows if plugged
	  Longitudinal appearance: 'tram lines' (Fig. 41.8)

Pleural disease	Pleural fluid accumulates below the diaphragmatic surface of the lung causing:
	  In upright position:
	    Blunting of the lateral costophrenic angle
	    Meniscus formation; increases superiorly (Fig. 41.9)
	    Lung compression or mediastinal shift
	  In supine position:
	    Fluid gravitates posteriorly
	    If large the whole lung will be white
	    ± Associated mediastinal shift

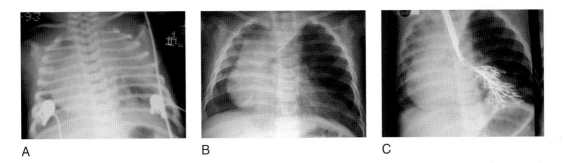

A   B   C

Fig. 41.4 Patterns in chest imaging.
(A) Unilateral hyperinflation: chest X-rays of a neonate with respiratory distress. (B) Once the delayed clearance of lung fluid had occurred the left upper lobe became massively over-inflated, herniating to the right and compressing the left lower lobe. Reduced air entry was heard on the left side. (C) A bronchogram confirmed no ventilation or perfusion to the left upper lobe. This child had a congenital left upper lobar emphysema, which was acting as a space-occupying lesion.

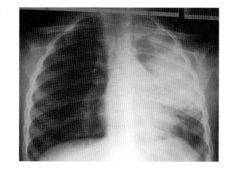

Fig. 41.5 Dense lobar consolidation in the left upper lobe

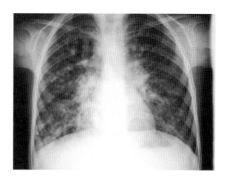

Fig. 41.6 Bronchopneumonia.
Bilateral fluffy shadows that are more confluent near the heart border. There is perihilar lymphadenopathy. This child had a late presentation of cystic fibrosis.

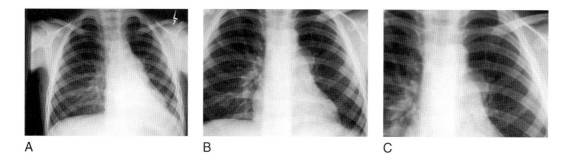

A   B   C

Fig. 41.7 Three chest X-rays from a boy whose wheezing and cough were being treated unsuccessfully with asthma therapy.
(A) There is left lower lobe collapse. Note the sharp line running behind the heart to the left costophrenic angle, and the absence of a visible left diaphragm. (B) After physiotherapy the left lower lobe has almost completely re-expanded (the left diaphragm is becoming visible) and the bronchogenic cyst at the left hilar region can be better visualized. (C) Focuses on the left hilar region; a bronchogenic cyst was compressing the left lower lobe bronchus.

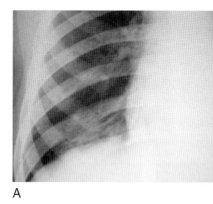
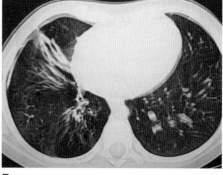

A   B

Fig. 41.8 Localized bronchiectasis (tramlines) in the right mid-zone.
(A) Chest X-ray; (B) high-resolution CT confirming localization of disease. A retained inhaled foreign body should be ruled out in localized bronchiectasis.

Pulmonary function testing (PFT)

Physiology of PFT

In normal breathing inspiration is an active process that begins with the contraction of the diaphragm, the intercostal muscles functioning to fix the chest wall. If greater work of breathing is required the accessory muscles (which are normally inactive during quiet respiration) are recruited. These include the scalene and sternocleidomastoid muscles. However, the diaphragm is the most important muscle used in inspiration.

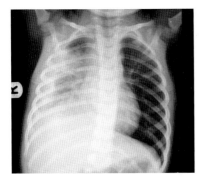

Fig. 41.9 Chest X-ray of an infant with a right-sided pleural effusion

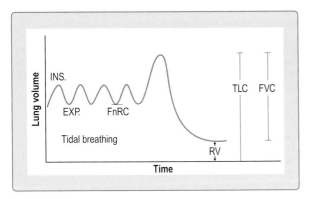

Fig. 41.10 Lung volume analysis.
The left hand aspect shows the volume (y axis) against time (x axis) of a child during normal tidal breathing. Remember inspiration is active and expiration is passive. The passive end-expiratory 'resting point' or trough occurs when the forces of elastic recoil of the lung balance the chest wall expansive forces and no airflow is occurring. This point is referred to as the functional residual capacity (FnRC). (RV = residual volume; TLC = total lung capacity; FVC = forced vital capacity)

Exhalation is usually a passive process. When the lungs are stretched, e.g. full of air after a maximal inspiration, the elastic recoil pressure of the lung outplays the natural tendency of the chest wall to expand.

The child is asked to inspire to total lung capacity (TLC) and then to do a maximal forced expiration manoeuvre to residual volume (RV). A visual incentive may be used to encourage the child to keep blowing out maximally until airflow has ceased. The forced vital capacity (FVC) is the volume of air shifted with this manoeuvre. From the FVC plot we can measure the volume exhaled at given time points. Most frequently used is the volume exhaled at 1 second or forced expiratory volume in 1 second (FEV_1) (Fig. 41.10).

Figure 41.11 shows a volume–time (V–T) and a flow–volume (F–V) curve of a forced expiratory vital capacity manoeuvre. Flow is volume moved (inspired or expired) per unit of time (seconds).

During forced expiration the rate of airflow rises rapidly to a maximum. As the lung volume decreases,

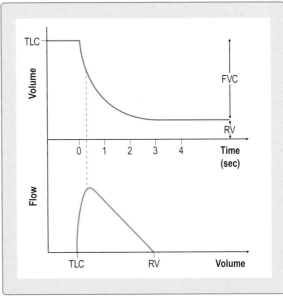

Fig. 41.11 Volume–time and flow–volume curves.
The flow–volume (F–V) curve is derived from the same forced expiratory manoeuvre used to show the volume–time curve, with volume on the upper y axis versus time (x axis), and flow on the lower y axis versus volume (x-axis).

the intrathoracic airways narrow and the expiratory airflow progressively falls until no further airflow is occurring.

The F–V-curve is used to measure forced expiratory flow rates at different points of the FVC (usually 50% and 25% of remaining FVC). 'Normal' is usually taken to be greater than the 2.5 percentile, i.e. 97.5% of healthy well children will be above this value after adjustment is made for age, height, gender and race.

Peak expiratory flow rate (PEFR)

The child gives a short sharp blow into a mini-handheld PEFR meter.

Advantages

- Cheap and easily available.
- Can be used at home to monitor airway calibre that varies over time. The normal diurnal variation (airways narrower in the morning and wider in the afternoon) is increased in asthmatics. The finding of exaggerated diurnal variability ('shark's teeth' pattern, Fig. 41.12) that improves with trial of asthma treatment is helpful diagnostically.
- In the occasional asthmatic child, recording PEFR twice daily can give an early warning of impending deterioration before significant symptoms have started.

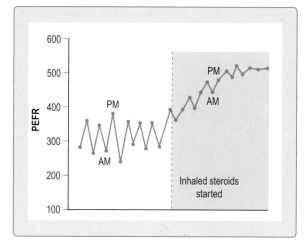

Fig. 41.12 **Peak expiratory flow rate (PEFR) showing 'shark's teeth' pattern**

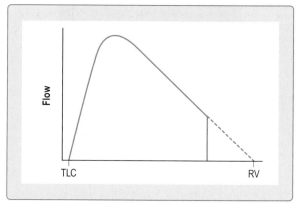

Fig. 41.13 **The F–V loop from a 'short blow', where the flow can be seen abruptly dropping to the zero line.**
Unless the child has blown for longer than 1 second the FEV_1 and the FVC will be almost equal and all that can be claimed is that the FEV_1 is at least that which was recorded. Clearly the FVC and all flow measurements will be inaccurate.

When using PEFR monitoring it is important to find out the maximum PEFR for the child. This may require a short course of intense anti-asthma therapy. Serial monitoring compares day-to-day values against the child's 'personal best' recording.

Disadvantages

- Some asthmatic children learn to 'check blast' into the PEFR meter in order to achieve high results. This illustrates that PEFR is measuring large airways calibre and that reduction in PEFR is a relatively late indicator of airways obstruction.
- Some children/parents invent the results that are recorded on diary cards.
- Overall, chronic asthma management using PEFR measurement action plans has not been shown to be superior to symptom-based plans.

Spirometry

Children over 5 or 6 years can generally perform spirometry, including F–V curves, FEV_1 and FVC manoeuvres.

When performing spirometry, first check if the spirogram is technically adequate. Common technical problems in children performing F–V loops include:

- Failure to blow to flow cessation, i.e. a short blow (Fig. 41.13).
- Double blow, when the child does a second blow into spirometer.
- The child who takes a submaximal inspiration and does not blow from TLC. This can be difficult to spot on the F–V loop, as the curves with and without a good inspiration will look similar.

- Younger children who take several attempts to optimize their technique but often start to tire after a further 2–3 attempts, with a deterioration in performance.
- The process can make some children cough.

Bronchodilator responsiveness (BDR)

Finding out if there is BDR is helpful confirmatory evidence that a child is likely to benefit from bronchodilators and is a feature of asthma (p. 604).

Problem-orientated topic:

respiratory function testing

Sebastian is an 8 year old. His paediatrician is not sure whether his respiratory symptoms indicate asthma. He tries to get Sebastian to blow into his new spirometer, which has a visual incentive. His FEV_1 is below normal at 63% predicted for his height (134 cm) and age (8 years).

Sebastian is given salbutamol (100 µg/puff, six puffs) via a small-volume holding chamber and 25 minutes later Sebastian performs another spirometry manoeuvre (Table 41.3).

Before interpretation check that both F–V loops (Fig. 41.14) are technically satisfactory and that Sebastian has blown out until there is no further flow.

Continued overleaf

Q1. Do these tests suggest that Sebastian's test is technically satisfactory?

Q2. How do you interpret the findings on these loops?

Table 41.3 Sebastian's spirometry results

	Before (% predicted)	After (% predicted)
FEV_1	1.10 (63%)	1.51 (86%)
FVC	2.00 (96%)	2.11 (101%)

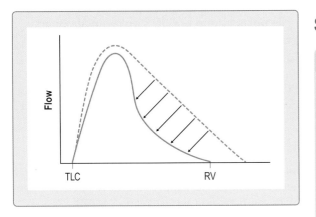

Fig. 41.14 Sebastian's F–V loops

Q1. Do these tests suggest that Sebastian's test is technically satisfactory?

Sebastian has blown out to flow limitation as the FV loop reaches baseline without a sudden drop. Looking at the two F–V loops, the dashed post-bronchodilator trace shows much less sagging (concavity), suggesting better flow at low lung volumes.

Q2. How do you interpret the findings on these loops?

There has been a significant increase in both FEV_1 and FVC, suggesting BDR. Generally an increase of > 10–15% in FEV_1 or FVC is taken as indicating BDR.

Tests of bronchial hyper-reactivity (BHR)

Often children attending clinics with a history in keeping with asthma have normal lung function and the question arises: does the patient have 'twitchy airways' or BHR? To answer this, bronchoprovocation tests are used. The typical challenge agents used are methacholine, histamine and adenosine. The concentration at which the FEV_1 falls by 20% is recorded. The lower the dose or concentration, the greater the BHR. The asthmatic typically responds to challenge at a lower than normal dose.

Exercise can also be used as the 'challenge'. This is mostly carried out on a treadmill but can be done using free running. Patients with asthma often have an exaggerated drop in lung function after exercise. FEV_1 should be measured before and 15 mins after cessation of exercise. A drop in $FEV_1 > 15\%$ suggests a positive test. Another non-pharmacological bronchial challenge test is the hyperventilation of cold and dry air according to a standardized protocol. In this case BHR is indicated by a drop in $FEV_1 > 9\%$.

Stridor

Problem-orientated topic:

acute stridor (part I) ● ● ● ● ○

Julian is a 14-month-old baby who presents at 1 a.m. He has a 1-day history of a runny nose and had developed a barking cough the previous evening. He is brought to the accident and emergency department because he is making an inspiratory crowing noise and has difficulty breathing.

He is assessed as having a loud inspiratory stridor when upset, which decreases in intensity but is still present at rest. His saturations are 95% in room air, with a respiratory rate of 40 breaths per minute, with some subcostal recession. He has good air entry on auscultation, with a heart rate of 90 beats per minute.

Q1. What is the differential diagnosis?

Q2. What is your assessment of the severity of Julian's condition?

Q3. What is your initial management plan?

Q1. What is the differential diagnosis?

The most likely diagnosis of acute stridor in a toddler is laryngotracheobronchitis (croup) (Box 41.3).

Q2. What is your assessment of the severity of Julian's condition? (Box 41.4 and Table 41.4)

Overall Julian is active and has good air entry and no signs of hypoxaemia, suggesting that the airways obstruction is currently not severe.

- Laryngotracheobronchitis (croup)
- Epiglottitis
- Bacterial tracheitis
- Foreign body
- Angioedema

BOX 41.4 Assessment for severity of stridor

Timing?
- The most prominent phase of the respiratory noise should be inspiratory
- An additional expiratory noise indicates more severe or intrathoracic airways obstruction

Work of breathing?
- Increased respiratory rate
- Sternal (supra- and sub-)recession
- Intercostal recessions

How effective is the breathing?
- Chest expansion
- Breath sounds for air entry

Is there adequate oxygenation?
- Is heart rate increased?
- Pallor, cyanosis
- O_2 saturation
- Activity levels

However, he has stridor at rest associated with some increased working of breathing (indrawing), indicating that the airways obstruction is not mild. He has mild to moderately severe airways obstruction.

Q3. What is your initial management plan?

You decide Julian's condition is severe enough to give budesonide via nebulizer. You assess him 30 mins after treatment and feel that he no longer has stridor at rest. You therefore allow him to be discharged home.

Problem-orientated topic:

acute stridor (part II) ● ● ● ● ●

Unfortunately, Julian reattends 2 days later, with similar symptoms. The stridor is loud with an expiratory component. His respiratory rate is 60 breaths per minute, with subcostal and intercostal retraction. His saturations are 90% on room air, heart rate is 120 bpm, capillary refill time is > 3 seconds and temperature 38°C.

Q1. What is your plan/diagnosis?

Q1. What is your plan/diagnosis?

Julian has had an acute deterioration and is unwell. He needs an immediate supply of oxygen and assessment of airway, breathing and circulation (ABC).

The differential diagnosis is between severe croup, epiglottitis and bacterial tracheitis. Ways of differentiating between these diagnoses are shown in Table 41.5.

He needs admission and further assessment by paediatric intensive care. After a further worsening of Julian's condition, the decision is made to intubate in order to secure the airway. Purulent exudates are noted during intubation, confirming the diagnosis of bacterial tracheitis. Following intubation, swab cultures via endotracheal tube and blood cultures are taken to confirm the organism.

Intravenous antibiotics are given to cover *Staphylococcus aureus* and *Haemophilus*.

Laryngotracheobronchitis ('croup')

(See also Ch. 23.)

Croup is an acute clinical syndrome that usually starts with a runny nose, followed by a barking cough

Table 41.4 Assessment and evaluation of croup

Croup	Assessment	Treatment
Mild	Active, well child, barking cough, stridor with agitation, minimal signs of increased work of breathing	Nil
Moderate	Stridor at rest, some signs of increased work of breathing	Oral or rectal steroid and/or nebulized budesonide
Severe	Stridor at rest, marked increased work of breathing (indrawing), increased respiratory and heart rate, agitation and pallor. As airways obstruction becomes very serious, the stridor becomes quieter but sounds 'tighter', agitation eventually turning into exhaustion	Oxygen to maintain O_2 saturation > 92% Nebulized adrenaline (epinephrine) may buy time, followed by oral (alternatively rectal, nebulized, i.v.) steroid Intubation and ventilation may be required

Table 41.5 Croup, epiglottitis and tracheitis: differential diagnosis

Typical features	Croup	Epiglottitis	Bacterial tracheitis
Prodrome	URTI	Nil/mild URTI	URTI
Age	6 mths–3 yrs	1–8 yrs	6 mths–8 yrs
Onset	Slow (1–2 days)	Rapid (2–8 hr)	Variable
Barking cough	Yes	No	Yes
Hoarseness	Yes	No	Yes
Loud stridor	Yes	No, usually soft noise	Yes
Drooling	No	Yes	No
Dysphagia	No	Yes	No
'Toxic appearance'	No	Yes	Yes
Ability to lie flat	Yes	No	Yes
Microbiology	Viral: Parainfluenza 1,3 RSV	*Haemophilus influenzae* B	*Staph. aureus* *Haemophilus influenzae*

(URTI = upper respiratory tract infection; RSV = respiratory syncytial virus)

and hoarse voice. Acute stridor often starts in the early hours of the morning. Children are usually between 6 months and 5 years.

Peak incidence is in autumn, often with a second peak in spring. Parainfluenza virus accounts for 75% of cases (especially type 1,3), with other respiratory viruses (respiratory syncytial virus (RSV), influenza, metapneumovirus, adenovirus) causing the remainder.

The illness resolves within 3 days but occasionally symptoms persist. Some children need to be hospitalized and very few require intubation and ventilation.

Acute spasmodic (recurrent) croup

This does not have signs of a preceding head cold; children are afebrile and awake suddenly with acute stridor during the night. Recurrences typically occur on the subsequent 2–3 nights. This syndrome occurs in children of the same age as in infectious croup, during the same seasons, and similar viruses can be isolated. Some would therefore say that they are not different conditions. However, children with recurrent spasmodic croup often have a strong atopic or asthmatic family background.

Bacterial tracheitis

The infection causes purulent secretions and mucosal necrosis. The child has a croupy cough but also looks toxic, febrile and ill. Some regard it as a bacterial superinfection after viral croup. Since routine immunization against *Haemophilus influenzae* was introduced, bacterial tracheitis is probably now more common than epiglottitis.

Epiglottitis

This presents with fever and a toxic look, which comes on over 4–6 hours. Patients have a quieter muffled stridor and often sit up, extending their neck slightly to maintain maximal airway patency. They do not like swallowing and therefore saliva pools in the mouth and drooling occurs. The epiglottis is inflamed and 'cherry red' with swollen arythenoids. Children with epiglottitis do not like being disturbed. Initial management is shown in Box 41.5. Epiglottiits is usually treated by intubation and i.v. antibiotics.

Problem-orientated topic:

persistent stridor ● ● ● ● ●

Hannah, a 2-month-old baby, has had persistent noisy breathing (which the physician believes to be stridor) from the first week of life. The stridor was initially intermittent and only occurred with crying or when she was lying supine, but has now become persistent and more severe. Hannah has some indrawing at rest, and you note that she sleeps with her neck extended. Her weight has dropped to the second centile.

Q1. What are the causes of persistent stridor in an infant?

Q2. Why is Hannah not thriving?

Q3. What investigations are indicated?

Do not

- Examine the throat
- Lay the child flat
- Order a lateral X-ray of the neck
- Upset the child by trying to gain intravenous access or place an oxygen mask

Do

- Call the airway team
- Stay with the child
- Allow the child to sit on mother's knee
- Measure O_2 saturation if possible
- Give O_2 therapy if absolutely needed and only if well tolerated

Q1. What are the causes of persistent stridor in an infant?

- Laryngomalacia
- Subglottic stenosis (congenital or acquired: usually preterm baby who was intubated)
- Subglottic web
- Subglottic haemangioma
- Vascular ring
- Glottic cyst
- Vocal cord paralysis.

Q2. Why is Hannah not thriving?

Hannah has signs of significant airways obstruction. The poor weight gain is likely to be due to energy expended with the extra work required for breathing. In addition, some children with congenital laryngomalacia (the most common cause of chronic stridor in an infant) have swallowing difficulties and gastro-oesophageal reflux, making it difficult to get adequate calories into the child.

Q3. What investigations are indicated?

Endoscopy of the airway will confirm the diagnosis. This should be performed in all who have significant stridor and especially those with stridor that progressively becomes more severe. They need to have a progressive lesion (such as an expanding haemangioma) ruled out.

Laryngomalacia

The stridor results from collapse of the supraglottic structures inwards during inspiration. Typically, stridor begins during the first 2 weeks of life and becomes more obvious by 2–6 months. It increases with activity, with lying supine or with respiratory tract infections. Over time (by 2 years) the stridor will usually disappear. The diagnosis is confirmed by flexible laryngoscopy/bronchoscopy.

Expectant observation and parental reassurance are required for the majority. Stridor can be associated with gastro-oesophageal reflux, which may need to be treated. Laryngomalacia will become more severe with a concomitant viral respiratory tract infection but with progressive stridor an expanding lesion (such as an expanding haemangioma) needs to be ruled out.

Other causes of stridor

Subglottic stenosis

This may be congenital but is more often acquired. Always suspect subglottic stenosis in a preterm baby that was intubated for a considerable time. If severe, repeated dilations or a tracheostomy may be required.

Haemangioma

Subglottic haemangiomas often enlarge in the first few months of life and are therefore associated with progressive development of increasingly severe stridor. Improvement occurs over the next few years.

Vocal cord paralysis

Bilateral recurrent laryngeal nerve palsy is associated with bilateral adducted vocal cords, causing stridor that can be severe. It may occur in infants with spina bifida and the Arnold–Chiari malformation.

Vascular compressions

These include vascular rings, such as the double aortic arch (Fig. 41.15), or aberrant origins of the subclavian arteries causing the subclavian artery to cross anterior to the trachea, resulting in some degree of pulsatile anterior compression of the trachea. As the resulting stenosis is intrathoracic, the respiratory noise produced is expiratory rather than inspiratory.

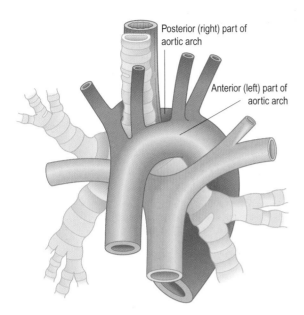

Posterior (right) part of aortic arch

Anterior (left) part of aortic arch

Fig. 41.15 Double aortic arch.
The ascending aorta divides into two, with the posterior (right) part passing behind and trapping the trachea and oesophagus before rejoining the descending aorta. There may therefore be swallowing difficulties and a barium swallow will show a fixed posterior indentation. The anatomy can be better defined using echocardiography but usually angiography (contrast or MRI) is required.

Problem-orientated topic:

snoring and obstructive sleep apnoea (OSA)

Simon, an 8-year-old boy with Down syndrome, has been noted by his teachers to have become unduly sleepy in his class. His parents describe loud snoring associated with rib recession after he has gone to sleep and they get very worried when the snoring stops and he appears to have stopped breathing. He is very restless at night.

Q1. What is the differential diagnosis of Simon's problem?

Q2. What are the risk factors for obstructive sleep apnoea?

Q3. What is the physiological sequence of an episode of OSA?

Q4. What are the long-term risks involved?

Q5. What investigations would you order?

Q6. What are the principles of management?

Q1. What is the differential diagnosis of Simon's problem?

Obstructive sleep apnoea syndrome (OSAS)

OSAS occurs when a child who snores experiences periods of complete obstruction, initially associated with increased respiratory efforts but followed by apnoea. These episodes can be associated with significant hypoxia and hypercarbia.

Primary snoring

Many children snore, which is due to partial obstruction of the nasal airways or pharynx.

Central apnoea/hypoventilation

This is defined as an elevated $PaCO_2$ due to a decreased central nervous system ventilatory drive. It is usually associated with hypoxaemia. Children fail to breathe normally, despite having normal airways, lungs, respiratory muscles and chest wall:

- *Congenital hypoventilation syndrome.* In this rare disorder children have intact voluntary control of breathing and are well when awake. They lack automatic breathing control and therefore hypoventilate when asleep. To remain alive these children need nocturnal ventilatory support.
- *Secondary central hypoventilation:*
  - Conditions associated with raised intracranial pressure (e.g. brain tumour in the hypothalamic region)
  - Rare neurological conditions, some with hypothalamic and endocrine dysfunction.

N.B. Children with Prader–Willi syndrome may have both OSAS (due to associated obesity) and central hypoventilation. It is also important not to blame OSAS for daytime somnolence when the cause is inadequate sleep. Increasingly we observe children who watch television or play computer or video games in their bedrooms into the early hours and become sleep-deprived.

Q2. What are the risk factors for obstructive sleep apnoea?

- Small and floppy airway relative to large tongue or adenotonsillar hypertrophy
- Relatively hypotonia, as in Down syndrome
- Pierre Robin syndrome
- Obesity, e.g. Prader–Willi syndrome.

Q3. What is the physiological sequence of an episode of OSA?

- *Loud snoring.* This is due to upper airways obstruction.
- *Complete obstruction.* Snoring stops attempts to breathe against complete obstruction.
- *Apnoea.* Stops breathing completely
- *Arousal.* PaO_2 falls and $PaCO_2$ rises, stimulating an arousal response and improved muscle tone with re-establishment of breathing.

Q4. What are the long-term risks involved?

- Poor-quality sleep and feeling unrefreshed in morning
- Sleepy by day:
  - Reduced school performance
  - Deterioration in behaviour
- Pulmonary hypertension if prolonged hypoxaemia.

Q5. What investigations would you order?

- Full clinical and ENT examination
- Overnight continuous recording of:
  - O_2 saturation
  - Respiratory movements
  - Airflow at nose/mouth
  - Heart rate.

In some studies this was regarded as adequate for OSAS screening, but other studies have suggested a high false negative rate compared with full polysomnography. A video of the snoring (obstructed breathing) and subsequent apnoea is helpful.

In polysomnography, electroencephalography, sleep staging, end-tidal CO_2, electro-oculograms, submental electromyography, and thoracic and abdominal movements are additionally measured.

Q6. What are the principles of management?

- Adenotonsillectomy
- Trial of nasal corticosteroids
- Nasal continuous positive airway pressure (CPAP)
- Uvulopalatopharyngoplasty
- Rarely, tracheotomy
- Weight loss for obese children.

Wheeze

Problem-orientated topic:

wheeze and lethargy ● ● ● ● ●

Over Christmas, 3-month-old Maximilian attends the accident and emergency department after 3 days of being generally unwell at home. His mother is anxious, as he has been breathing noisily for a few days but has now become sleepy and will not take his feeds. He has otherwise been a well child.

Maximilian is assessed to be lethargic but maintaining his colour; his respiratory rate is 80 breaths per minute, and he has a hyperexpanded chest and intercostal recession. There is an audible wheeze but predominantly widespread crepitations on auscultation.

Q1. What is the likely clinical diagnosis of Maximilian's illness?

Q2. What is your initial management?

Q3. What are the risk factors for more severe acute disease and can this disorder be prevented in high-risk infants?

Q1. What is the likely clinical diagnosis of Maximilian's illness?

Wheezing needs to be clearly defined, as parents may not have the same idea as you of what wheeze is. Specific details recorded from the history include timing and duration of wheeze episodes, precipitants such as dust, pollen, recent viral infection and seasonality, and other associated symptoms such as cough or shortness of breath.

Causes of wheezing in infants and preschool children

- Acute bronchiolitis (the most likely cause in Maximilian)
- Post-bronchiolitis recurrent wheezing
- Asthma:
  - True atopic asthma
  - Recurrent viral-induced wheeze
- Bronchopulmonary dysplasia
- Recurrent pulmonary aspiration
- Congenital bronchial stenosis, vascular rings, bronchogenic cysts
- Tracheobronchomalacia
- Inhaled foreign body
- Conditions causing chronic suppurative lung disease, e.g. cystic fibrosis
- Primary ciliary dyskinesia
- Immune deficiencies.

Q2. What is your initial management?

- ABC
- Assessment of breathing
- Further evaluation of history.

Subsequent management is largely supportive (Box 11.6).

Q3. What are the risk factors for more severe acute disease and can this disorder be prevented in high-risk infants?

Risk factors

- Prematurity, especially if there is neonatal chronic lung disease, congenital heart disease, immune deficiency and cystic fibrosis.

Prevention

- High-risk babies can be protected by giving a monoclonal antibody (palivizumab) to RSV to try to prevent infection.
- In hospital prevention measures to stop cross-infection are important. Sensible measures include cohort segregation of cases, strict hand washing, and the wearing of face masks and gowns.

Acute bronchiolitis

This is discussed in Chapter 23.

BOX 41.6 Management of acute bronchiolitis

Humidified oxygen
- Aim for O_2 saturation > 92%

Maintenance of clear airway
- Gentle nasopharyngeal suction
- Decongestant nose drops

Hydration
- May require nasogastric or i.v. fluids
- Take care not to overload the circulation, as bronchiolitis may be associated with inappropriate antidiuretic hormone (ADH) secretion

Apnoea
- Infants under 6 weeks may have seemingly milder disease but this may still be complicated by apnoeic episodes
- Prematurity or cardiac disease increases risk of severe disease
- May require paediatric intensive care unit (PICU) and ventilation

Nebulizer therapy
- Nebulized adrenaline (epinephrine) may benefit a few children
- May be considered but discontinue if no response
- Overall no specific treatment, including adrenaline, bronchodilators and corticosteroids, has been shown conclusively to be beneficial in all cases

Asthma

Problem-orientated topic:

asthma

Alexander is a 4-year-old boy who has been referred by his primary care physician. He has suffered frequent wheezing episodes in winter associated with head colds. Alexander also experiences day-to-day symptoms of cough and is breathless with exercise. Last month he was up all night wheezing after having a 'pillow fight' with his sister.

Alexander's mother has asthma and hay fever and his older sister had frequent wheezing episodes in infancy in addition to eczema. Alexander has mild eczema.

Alexander is diagnosed as having asthma and started on regular inhaled corticosteroids with salbutamol for relief medication.

Continued overleaf

Q1. What are the typical patterns of asthma in young children?

Q2. What issues need reviewing when a child does not seem to respond to anti-asthma therapy?

Q3. What are the principles of pharmacological management of chronic asthma?

Q1. What are the typical patterns of asthma in young children?

See Box 41.7. Note the flow chart in the British Thoracic Society/Scottish Intercollegiate Guidelines Network (BTS/SIGN) Guidelines for Asthma Management (see URL below).

Alexander is seen at the asthma clinic several months later. Mum reports that he still has day-to-day exercise wheezing and breathlessness and is up at night with cough on 2–3 nights per week. Mum feels the salbutamol gives him good relief but is not sure of the preventive 'steroid' inhaler (beclomethasone 100 μg twice daily).

BOX 41.7 Asthma patterns

Episodic viral-associated wheezing
- Episodes are more frequent in winter months
- Almost always associated with head colds
- Usually completely asymptomatic between episodes
- Evidence suggests that, for the majority of these children, the response to regular anti-inflammatory therapy is poor

Classic atopic asthma
- May have an atopic background (allergies or eczema)
- Positive family history of atopy and asthma
- Day-to-day symptoms triggered with exercise or occurring at night when no head cold
- Should respond well to regular anti-inflammatory asthma therapy

Cough variant asthma
- Nocturnal and/or exercise-induced cough when free from head colds
- Wheezing may just simply never have been heard
- A personal or family history of other atopic disorders is a helpful supporting finding
- Child responds rapidly to anti-asthma medication
- Symptoms relapse when therapy withdrawn

BOX 41.8 Review of management

Non-compliance
- Lack of knowledge that inhaled corticosteroids need to be taken regularly even when well
- Forgetting/chaotic family lifestyle
- Hidden health beliefs, e.g. fear of dependency on inhalers or fear of side-effects

Poor inhaler technique
- Check at each visit
- Remember a fighting crying child is unlikely to receive much medication administered via a spacer and face mask. Crying is predominantly expiratory. The face mask should have a seal against the child's face
- Choose a suitable age-appropriate inhaler device

Ongoing trigger factors
- Aero-allergens
- Environmental tobacco smoke

Concomitant disease
- Allergic rhinosinusitis
- Gastro-oesophageal reflux

Is asthma the correct diagnosis?
- Before stepping-up medication review whether the diagnosis of asthma is correct

Q2. What issues need review when a child does not seem to respond to anti-asthma therapy?

See Box 41.8.

Q3. What are the principles of pharmacological management of chronic asthma?

- Control symptoms
- Prevent exacerbations
- Achieve best possible pulmonary function
- Minimize side-effects.

Asthma management should follow a stepwise approach. Start at the step most appropriate to initial severity to achieve early control and maintain control by stepping treatment up and down according to symptoms.

http://www.sign.ac.uk/guidelines/published/#Respiratory

BTS/SIGN Guidelines for Asthma Management: full text version p. 8, Fig. 2 for flow chart for diagnosis of asthma in children, specific link to figure given

Problem-orientated topic:

acute exacerbation of asthma (part I)

A year later, Alexander is brought to the accident and emergency room by ambulance. He has had an upper respiratory tract infection for 2 days and has become increasingly wheezy and short of breath. His parents gave him some salbutamol using his inhaler and spacer device, but it only produced a slight and short-lived improvement.

In the emergency room he is pale, cyanosed, agitated and in marked respiratory distress and only gasps out single words at a time. His heart rate is 160/min and respiratory rate 60/min.

Q1. What immediate actions are needed in the accident and emergency department?

Q2. What are the features of severe and life-threatening asthma?

Q3. What tests are indicated if there is no improvement or if Alexander deteriorates?

Q1. What immediate actions are needed in the accident and emergency department?

Assessment of ABC is mandatory.

Airway

Alexander's upper airway appears patent; he can speak single words and is breathing, and there is audible expiratory wheeze.

Breathing

- Check respiratory rate.
- Assess work of breathing: marked indrawing (suprasternal, subcostal recession).
- Assess efficacy of breathing: pallor, cyanosis and agitation along with tachycardia suggest that Alexander is hypoxic.

You have identified a problem with breathing. Therefore:

- Check O_2 saturation with pulsed oximetry.
- Give O_2: enough to bring O_2 saturation > 92% and preferably > 94%.

Circulation

- Heart rate
- Capillary refill time
- Blood pressure.

Pulsus paradoxus occurs in acute severe asthma but is not always present.

Q2. What are the features of severe and life-threatening asthma?

According to guidelines Alexander has had a severe exacerbation of asthma. He is therefore given a nebulized β_2-agonist (3 nebulizations in the first hour), along with supplemental oxygen and prednisolone orally.

N.B. If a patient is unable to take steroid orally, then an i.v. line should be inserted and steroids given systemically.

http://www.sign.ac.uk/guidelines/fulltext/63/annex5.html

This refers to flow chart for the assessment of severity of acute asthma

Q3. What tests are indicated if there is no improvement or if Alexander deteriorates?

See Box 41.9.

When frequent bronchodilator therapy has not produced the desired response, additional therapy includes:

- I.v. aminophylline
- I.v. salbutamol
- I.v. magnesium.

A paediatric intensivist should also assess Alexander.

BOX 41.9 Investigations in severe asthma

Arterial blood gases

- A normal $PaCO_2$ in a child with very severe asthma is an ominous sign since in mild/moderately acute asthma the hyperventilation is associated with a low $PaCO_2$
- An elevated $PaCO_2$ is associated with exhaustion (Fig. 41.16)

Chest X-ray

- Performing a CXR is *not* usually a priority but should be done if a pneumothorax is suspected

PEFR or FEV_1

- This is an objective measure of airflow obstruction in children with acute asthma but it is difficult to teach a child to perform the test correctly during an acute severe attack

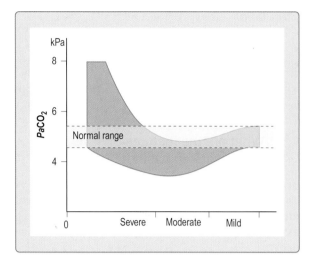

Fig. 41.16 In an asthmatic child with marked breathlessness the finding of a normal $PaCO_2$ should *not* be reassuring but taken as an indication of severe airways obstruction

Q1. **Before Alexander is discharged home what should be checked?**

See Box 41.10.

Other causes of expiratory noise

Tracheomalacia and tracheal stenosis are rare disorders and may occur with or without vascular compression of the trachea. In most cases they manifest with an expiratory noise that resembles a wheeze. In some textbooks this noise is referred to by the term 'expiratory stridor' but 'monophonic expiratory wheeze' might be more appropriate.

Vascular compressions include vascular rings, such as the double aortic arch (Fig. 41.15), or aberrant origins of the subclavian arteries causing the subclavian artery to cross anterior to the trachea, resulting in some degree of pulsatile anterior compression of the trachea. When the vascular ring includes the oesophagus in addition to the trachea, the child will show an exaggerated expiratory noise and some respiratory difficulty when swallowing food.

Cough

Q1. **What are the causes of a chronic productive (moist or wet) cough and what are the key investigations for each cause?**

See Table 41.6.

Julia has a moist/wet or productive cough suggesting a condition causing a chronic endobronchial infection,

---

BOX 41.10 Asthma information given to parents and child prior to discharge

All advice, verbal and written, should be documented in the patient's hospital notes.

Advice on reducing asthma triggers at home
- Environmental tobacco smoke exposure
- Anti-house dust mite measures
- Consideration given to removing pets

Advice on when to take medications
- Understanding importance of taking preventive anti-inflammatory therapy regularly

Advice on how to take medications
- 'Inhaler technique': it is not adequate to show a child/parent how to use an inhaler. Technique should be checked and shown to be satisfactory

Action plan for 'acute asthma attack'
- Recognizing severity and treatment of an exacerbation

Table 41.6 Causes of cough

Causes of productive cough	Investigations
Cystic fibrosis (CF)	Sweat test, CF gene phenotyping
Primary immune deficiency	IgGs, IgG subclasses, functional antibody response to tetanus, pneumococcus or *Haemophilus influenzae* vaccination
Primary ciliary dyskinesia	Saccharine test and nasal nitric oxide can be used as screening tests. Epithelial brushing for electron microscopy or cilial beat frequency should be obtained from nasal or bronchial mucosa when free from infection
Retained foreign body	History of sudden onset of symptoms, localized disease on CXR/high-resolution CT. Diagnostic and therapeutic test is rigid bronchoscopy
Recurrent aspiration	Observation of feeding, videofluoroscopy, barium swallow, milk scan and 24-hr pH studies

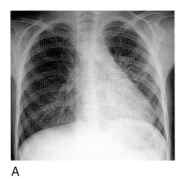

A

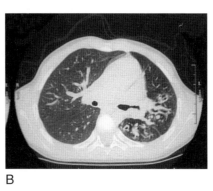

B

Fig. 41.17 Julia's investigations. (A) Chest X-ray. The left mid-zone and lower lobe show cylindrical bronchiectasis. Ring shadows can be seen. (B) CT scan.

and serious underlying conditions need to be excluded. It is important to obtain sputum for culture and order a CXR; high-resolution CT is likely to indicate cylindrical bronchiectasis.

Figure 41.17 shows her CXR and CT scan. This appearance followed an acute pneumonia with residual crackles heard in the left lung on follow-up. No foreign body was detected at bronchoscopy.

Q2. How will you treat Julia?

Short term
- Antibiotics and intensive physiotherapy to clear infection.

Long term
- Advise regular chest physiotherapy with postural drainage.
- Aim to control infections:
  - Sputum culture should be routinely monitored.
  - Antibiotics, oral or intravenous, are dictated by sputum culture and sensitivities.
  - Give an annual influenza vaccination.

Bronchiectasis

This is irreversible abnormal dilatation of the bronchial tree and represents a common end stage of a number of different processes.

Mechanisms
- Chronic endobronchial infections: progressive bronchial wall damage and dilatation
- Obstruction of the airway.

Causes
- Widespread disease:
  - Cystic fibrosis
  - Immune deficiencies
  - Primary ciliary dyskinesia
  - Recurrent pulmonary aspiration.
- Localized disease:
  - Retained inhaled foreign body
  - Infection in a congenital lung malformation
  - Local airways compression, e.g. tuberculosis, enlarged lymph node and active infection.

Clinical features
- Cough and copious purulent sputum
- Poor growth
- Crackles with or without wheeze, especially during infections
- Finger clubbing
- Severe extensive disease: dyspnoea, hypoxaemia.

Investigations
- Pulmonary function tests:
  - Obstructive/restrictive or mixed pattern
- CXR:
  - Bronchial wall thickening
  - Tramlining: parallel shadows of thickened dilated bronchial walls
  - Ring shadows: cross-sectional view of thickened dilated bronchial wall
- High-resolution CT:
  - Better than CXR for gauging the extent of disease and determining whether it is localized.

Management

- Order chest physiotherapy for bronchial drainage.
- Aim to control infections.
- Sputum culture should be routinely monitored.
- Antibiotics, oral or intravenous, are dictated by sputum culture and sensitivities.
- Give annual influenza vaccination.
- Order local surgery for local severe disease.
- Advise a transplant for end-stage disease.

Problem-orientated topic:

chronic cough (part II)

Earlier in life Julia was given a tentative diagnosis of asthma based on prolonged coughing following head colds. At this stage her primary care physician considered that Julia was otherwise well. She was growing along the 25th centile.

Q1. What are the other causes of problem coughing in an otherwise previously healthy child?

BOX 41.11 Causes of problem coughing in an otherwise healthy child

Specific infections causing cough

- Pertussis and pertussis-like syndromes, parapertussis, *Chlamydia/Mycoplasma* and viral infections
- Recurrent viral bronchitis and prolonged postviral cough
- Children with these conditions seem to have heightened 'cough receptor sensitivity' and the coughing is typically very troublesome and irritating for the child

Isolated cough with no other respiratory symptoms

- Cough variant asthma: atopic background, reversible airflow obstruction (history of recurrent wheezing, objective bronchodilator responsiveness or fall in FEV_1 after challenge)
- Clear-cut response to anti-asthma therapy with relapse when therapy withdrawn
- Postnasal drip
- Gastro-oesophageal reflux (rarely)
- Psychogenic cough: usually a dry habit cough or a bizarre honking cough that does not irritate the child (but does irritate parents and teachers). These coughs abate when the child is asleep or distracted

---

Q1. **What are the other causes of problem coughing in an otherwise previously healthy child?**

See Box 41.11. Other rare causes of chronic cough are interstitial lung diseases, such as the pulmonary fibrosis that can occur with connective tissue diseases.

Key points regarding cough are summarized in Box 41.12.

BOX 41.12 Key points: cough

- Parental reporting of cough frequency and severity does not correlate well with objective cough audiotapes, especially at night
- Parental and doctor characterization of cough as wet (moist with phlegm production) versus dry is generally correct and this classification is important
- Children < 5 years do not cough up phlegm/sputum but rather swallow it
- Cough receptors are concentrated in the larynx and upper tracheobronchial tree and coughing is a natural protective mechanism
- Many children with persistent isolated, postviral or recurrent viral coughing have heightened 'cough receptor sensitivity'
- Cough is a symptom not a disorder and treatment therefore should be targeted at the cause
- Short-term symptomatic relief of coughing associated with an URTI has *not* been proven to be effective

Cystic fibrosis (CF)

Problem-orientated topic:

cystic fibrosis (part I)

Katharina is the second child of non-consangineous parents. She was born after an uncomplicated pregnancy by normal delivery at term +5. Birth weight was 3.1 kg. She has an older brother who is 2 years old and well. There is no significant family history.

She was discharged well at 48 hours. Mum felt Katharina was a hungry baby compared to her older brother but was generally pleased with her progress. She had her routine heel prick blood test carried out on day 5 of life.

About a week later mum is called to say that the blood spot test for cystic fibrosis was high. She phones her doctor for some advice.

Q1. What advice would you give her?

Q1. What advice would you give her?

CF screening tests for raised immunoreactive trypsinogen (IRT) in the dried blood spot. If the test is positive or borderline a second test will be performed to confirm. If the second test is positive the child will be referred for a sweat test (Box 41.13).

BOX 41.13 The quantitative pilocarpine ionotrophoresis sweat test

- Remains the gold standard for confirming the diagnosis of CF
- Must be done in a specialized laboratory used to dealing with this test to decrease inaccuracies
- A minimum of 100 mg of sweat must be collected

Positive test	Cl$^-$ > 60 mmol/l
Borderline test	Cl$^-$ 40–60 mmol/l
Negative test	Cl$^-$ < 40 mmol/l

Problem-orientated topic:

cystic fibrosis (part II)

Katharina is subsequently sent for a sweat test. Her results are: sweat volume 153 µl, chloride 110 mmol/l and sodium 103 mmol/l.

Following her sweat test Katharina and her parents are admitted to the ward for initial assessment and to meet the CF team. Katharina is then seen at clinic. Retrospectively, mum feels that Katharina probably has not put much weight on since she was born. She notes that the baby has always been a bit chesty but just thought that she had caught her brother's head cold. Mum is upset about the results but does not know much about CF and is concerned that her baby will die very young.

Q1. What information and advice will you give this family?

Q2. What further investigations might be necessary?

Q3. What is your initial management plan?

Q1. What information and advice will you give this family?

Specific information regarding CF is tailored to the parents' needs at the time. Some wish to receive all the information at once, while others prefer to digest it more slowly. It is important that they are given written information, with the ability to come back with questions as required.

Some units have their own parent sheets, while others distribute the information pack from the Cystic Fibrosis Trust. An overview is given in Box 41.14.

BOX 41.14 Key points: cystic fibrosis

Presentation

- Classic presentation of recurrent chest infections, bulky, greasy, difficult-to-flush stools and malnutrition
- Spectrum of disease can be very wide, however, from classic CF presenting in early years to relatively asymptomatic patients who present later: e.g. adult males diagnosed on molecular genetic testing when seeking infertility treatment

Incidence

- Varies across Europe
- 1/25 people in UK are carriers; 1/2500 infants have CF

Life expectancy

- Current mean life expectancy is 31 years, compared with 5 years in 1960

Pathophysiology

- Impairment of cystic fibrosis transmembrane regulator (CFTR) function causes reduced fluid production and enhanced sodium resorption through the airways epithelium. This results in increased fluid absorption, leading to decreased airway surface liquid and impaired ciliary clearance. In addition there is an increased susceptibility of the airway epithelium to bacterial binding and this leads to chronic bacterial infection.

Genetics

- Autosomal recessive disorder, defect on chromosome 7
- Now over 1000 different mutations of CFTR responsible for CF
- Most common mutation is ΔF508; others include G551d, R117H, 621 +1 (G > T), G542X
- Mutations have been classified depending on the action that the mutation has on the production and/or transport of CFTR to the apical membrane of the cell

http://www.cftrust.org.uk

This links to Cystic Fibrosis Trust in the UK.

Q2. What further investigations might be necessary?

See Box 41.15.

A full history and examination of the child is needed, in particular growth parameters (weight, height, head circumference).

BOX 41.15 Baseline investigations in cystic fibrosis

- Sputum/cough swab:
  - Microbiology
- Chest X-ray
- Blood investigations:
  - DNA for genotyping
  - Full blood count
  - Urea and electrolytes
  - Liver function tests
  - Coagulation screen
  - Immunoglobulins
  - Vitamin A, D and E levels
- Faecal elastase:
  - ?Pancreatic insufficiency

Q3. What is your initial management plan?

See Box 41.16. From the time of diagnosis CF needs a multidisciplinary approach to care. The family will require support from all health professionals, and will also need to be reviewed by a social worker to help with application for benefits and allowances. If possible children should also be seen in their homes after diagnosis by a specialist CF nurse to maintain support and education.

Problem-orientated topic:

deterioration in a child with CF ● ● ●

Katharina was started on the standard CF regimen, with support and education for the family from social worker and CF community nurse.

Over the next few months Katharina remains well. She gains weight and is developing well. Her parents are coming to terms with her diagnosis and treatment but still find it difficult at times. Unfortunately Katharina develops a cough so her mum brings her to clinic for some advice. She has a fruity cough

---

BOX 41.16 Specific medical management of cystic fibrosis

Respiratory management
- 90% morbidity in CF is a result of chronic pulmonary sepsis and its complications
- Much of therapy is aimed at prevention of lung damage and early treatment of infection to minimize lung damage secondary to inflammation

Prevention of infection
- All regular immunizations
- Additional vaccine such as pneumovax and influenza; consider palivizumab for RSV protection
- Good infection control policy to prevent cross-infection
- Attempts to eradicate bacterial invaders after first signs of colonization

Physiotherapy
- Learnt at an early stage
- Multiple techniques that are adapted to patient age and severity of disease
- Reduces airways obstruction by improving clearance of secretions

- Decreases severity of infection by clearance of infected material
- Maintains respiratory function and exercise tolerance

Nutritional/gastrointestinal
- Direct link between pulmonary health and the patient's nutritional status
- Increased energy requirements due to increased demand and increased losses:
  - High-energy diet
- Malabsorption of fat:
  - > 90% patients require exocrine pancreatic supplements, e.g. Creon (pancrelipase) Vitamin A, D and E supplements
- Increased loss of salt:
  - Salt supplementation
- Close monitoring of weight, particularly in the younger child, to ensure growth and development:
  - Intervention with oral calorie supplements and use of enteral feeding via nasogastric tube or gastrostomy may be required in some patients

and crepitations are heard on auscultation. Her weight has also dropped slightly since her last visit. She has a CXR and sputum is sent for culture and sensitivities. Katharina's chest X-ray shows a right lower lobe consolidation.

She is commenced on oral antibiotic initially and is reviewed 1 week later. She is still unwell and her recent sputum has grown *Pseudomonas aeruginosa* for the first time.

Q1. What respiratory pathogens are found in the CF lung?
Q2. What is your respiratory management?
Q3. What other treatment may aid resolution of the right upper lobe consolidation?

Q1. What respiratory pathogens are found in the CF lung?

- *Staphylococcus aureus*
- *Haemophilus influenzae*
- *Pseudomonas aeruginosa*
- *Burkholderia cepacia*
- *Stenotrophomonas maltophilia*.

Q2. What is your respiratory management plan?

See Box 41.17.

Katharina's right lower lobe collapse/consolidation was slow to improve, so Katharina had a bronchoscopy and bronchial washout.

BOX 41.17 Management of cystic fibrosis exacerbations

Acute exacerbations
- Oral antibiotics or, depending on severity of exacerbation, i.v. antibiotics for 10–14 days, based on most recently colonized organisms

1st isolate *Pseudomonas*
- Aggressive treatment of 1st isolate can lead to eradication of *Pseudomonas* and delay the onset of chronic infection. Different CF centres adhere to different eradication protocols

Chronic *Pseudomonas*
- Reduce bacterial load and minimize lung damage
- Regular elective i.v. antibiotics and/or regular nebulized colomycin ± tobramycin

Q3. What other treatment may aid resolution of the right upper lobe consolidation?

Dedicated chest physiotherapy is the mainstay of treatment. Mucolytics such as Dnase (dornase alfa) or hypertonic saline may aid breakdown of the mucus plugging, allowing physiotherapy to clear it more easily. Both reduce sputum viscosity and therefore improve its clearance.

Problem-orientated topic:

CF and acute cough

Lara is 14 years old and was diagnosed with cystic fibrosis by routine neonatal screening. She is homozygous for the DF508 gene and has been chronically colonized with *Pseudomonas aeruginosa* since she was 9 years old. She is generally well but usually requires intravenous antibiotics 1–2 times a year. Her mother phones for an urgent appointment, as she is concerned that Lara is coughing and more tired than usual.

Lara arrives at clinic and is annoyed at her mum for bringing her. She does not want to miss more school as she has exams next month. She claims she feels well but her mother argues that Lara is coughing more, especially at night, and would be more productive with physiotherapy. She also says Lara comes home from school very tired and has to lie down to rest. Her weight has dropped just over 1 kg since her last visit 6 weeks ago.

Q1. What areas would you cover during this consultation?
Q2. What is your management plan?
Q3. What other diagnoses would you consider?

Q1. What areas would you cover during this consultation?

History
- School work
- Exercise tolerance
- Compliance

Table 41.7 Differential diagnosis of acute cough in cystic fibrosis

Diagnosis	Investigations
CF-related diabetes	Glucose tolerance test (GTT)
Allergic bronchopulmonary aspergillosis (ABPA)	ABPA work-up: Full blood count (eosinophilia) Skin prick test *Aspergillus* antigen Serum IgE Specific *Aspergillus* IgE/IgG Sputum for *Aspergillus*
Atypical infections	Sputum for atypical mycobacteria

- Nutrition/appetite
- Cough/amount of sputum production.

Investigations
- Lung function tests
- Sputum for culture.

Lara's previously stable lung function with FEV_1 around 95% predicted has dropped to 83% predicted. On assessment the physiotherapist feels the girl's chest was more productive than usual and has sent a good sputum sample to the laboratory, dirty-green in colour.

Q2. What is your management plan?

You send Lara home with a course of oral ciproxin to commence immediately and arrange for her to reattend next week for review. At this second appointment her chest is a lot worse, with FEV_1 now 70% predicted, and her weight has dropped a further 0.5 kg. You arrange for Lara to be admitted for intravenous antibiotics.

Lara's sputum grew mucoid *Pseudomonas* at the last clinic and her antibiotics were chosen from best sensitivities. However, after 7 days on antibiotics her FEV_1 is still only 75% predicted.

Q3. What other diagnoses would you consider?

See Table 41.7.
Lara's GTT result was:
- Baseline glucose: 4.2 mmol/l
- Blood glucose 2 hours after glucose challenge: 15 mmol/l.

The diagnosis is CF-related diabetes. This and other complications of CF are shown in Table 41.8.

Lung infections

> **Problem-orientated topic:**
>
> **lower respiratory tract infection**
>
> Felix, a 2-month-old boy, has been lethargic and not interested in feeding for 24 hours

Table 41.8 Complications of cystic fibrosis

Complication	Presentation/diagnosis	Treatment
Constipation/distal intestinal obstruction syndrome (DIOS)	Meconium ileus equivalent	Osmotic laxatives, hydration Gastrograffin orally
CF-related diabetes	Exclude in all patients with poor weight gain ± unexplained poor lung function Distinct from types 1 and 2 diabetes mellitus Polyuria and polydipsa are rare presentation Oral glucose tolerance test is gold standard for diagnosis	Involve diabetic team Dietician Insulin regimen tailored to individual lifestyle and eating patterns No evidence of benefit of oral hypoglycaemics
Liver	Abnormal bile flow and inspissated secretions. Leads to focal biliary cirrhosis Screened by annual liver function tests and ultrasound	Ursodeoxycholic acid Taurine: monitor response 6-monthly
Arthropathy	Up to 10% of children with CF Age 13–20 years Episodic pain and swelling of large joints Ciproxin-induced arthropathy separate problem	Spontaneous resolution Non-steroidal benefit Remember renal toxicity with non-steroidal anti-inflammatory drugs and aminoglycosides
Osteoporosis	10–20% of adolescents/adults Low vitamin D and K levels Use of inhaled and oral steroids Poor exercise Diagnosed via dual-energy X-ray absorptiometry (DEXA) scan	Increased calcium intake Vitamin D Bisphosphonates
Other respiratory complications	Pneumothorax Haemoptysis Allergic bronchopulmonary aspergillosis	

Table 41.9 Investigations in respiratory tract infection

Investigation	Bacterial	Viral

Chest X-ray (specificity is poor for predicting viral versus bacterial disease but can be useful)	Lobar/segmental pneumonia
	  Inflammation localized to one or more lobes or segments that are completely consolidated
	  Generally indicates bacterial infection
	  Pneumatoceles suggest *Staph. aureus* or anaerobic infection
		Bronchopneumonia
		  Inflammation of the lung, centred around the bronchioles, mucopurulent secretions block or obstruct small airways
		  Patchy infiltrates of adjacent lobules
		  Generally indicates viral infection

Sputum/nasal pharyngeal aspirate	Microbe identification Cultures Sensitivity of organism to guide antibiotic treatment	Rapid antigen diagnostic tests (immunofluorescence for RSV, polymerase chain reaction (PCR) for many respiratory viruses)
White cell count	Bacterial infections typically elevated, e.g. 15 000–40 000/mm^3, with granulocyte predominance	Viral infections typically normal or mildly elevated and usually < 20 000/mm^3 with lymphocyte predominance
Blood cultures	Blood cultures are rarely positive (10–30% cases) but are worth obtaining in sick children	
Serology	Requires paired samples (acute and convalescent), looking for a fourfold rise in specific antibody titres Cold agglutinins are positive in 50% of *Mycoplasma* cases but this test is not specific	
Inflammatory markers	Erythrocyte sedimentation rate (ESR) and C-reactive protein (CRP) levels tend to be higher in bacterial infections but neither test is specific enough to rule out a bacterial cause	

and has had a 'runny nose'. On examination, he is pale, febrile (temperature 39°C) and limp, and has rapid shallow breathing (respiratory rate 80/min) with minimal nasal flaring and retractions. He has grunting respirations. His heart rate is 180/min.

Q1. What is the likely diagnosis?
Q2. What is your assessment?
Q3. What investigations should be done?
Q4. What are the principles of management?

Q1. What is the likely diagnosis?

Acute pneumonia is an inflammation of the lung parenchyma. It usually presents with fever (children often have had a preceding URTI), tachypnoea, cough, grunting respiration, nasal flaring and recession. Crackles typically are auscultated and in older children there may be reduced intensity of breath sounds.

The most common cause of pneumonia in children is viral. Bacterial infection occurs in approximately 10–30%.

Q2. What is your assessment?

- Felix is very sick. Therefore use the ABC approach, including assessment of capillary refill time.
- He has an infection: elevated temperature and lethargy after an URTI ('runny nose').

- His work of breathing is increased but there is no respiratory noise that points to an airways obstruction.
- The grunting respirations and tachypnoea suggest pneumonia. (N.B. Sometimes infants in shock can have grunty respirations with tachypnoea.)
- His work of breathing is likely to be inadequate; tachycardia, pallor and lethargy suggest hypoxia. However, these findings may be contributed to by the fever and sepsis.

Q3. What investigations should be done?

See Table 41.9.

Q4. What are the principles of management?

Mildly ill
- Oral antibiotic (e.g. amoxicillin) at home
- In an older child consider a macrolide antibiotic to cover *Mycoplasma*.

Hospitalized child
- O$_2$ therapy
- Maintenance of hydration
- Intravenous antibiotics, e.g. cefuroxime.

http://www.brit-thoracic.org.uk/iqs/bts_guidelines_pneumonia_html

BTS 2002 Guidelines for the Management of Community Acquired Pneumonia in Childhood. Thorax 57: suppl 1

Table 41.10 Common organisms causing pneumonia

Age	Bacteria	Viruses	Others
Neonate	Group B streptococcus *Staphylococcus aureus* *Staph. epidermidis* *Escherichia coli*	CMV Herpes virus Enterovirus	*Mycoplasma hominis* *Ureaplasma urealyticum*
1–4 months	*Staph. aureus* *Haemophilus influenzae* *Strep. pneumoniae*	RSV Influenza CMV Parainfluenza	*Chlamydia trachomatis* *U. urealyticum*
< 5 years	*Strep. pneumoniae* *Staph. aureus* *H. influenzae* Group A streptococci	RSV Adenovirus Influenza	
> 5 years	*S. pneumoniae* *H. influenzae*	Influenza	*Mycoplasma pneumoniae* *Chlamydia pneumoniae* *Legionella pneumoniae*
Special cases Immunocompromised patients	In addition to those listed above: *Pneumocystis carinii* Enteric Gram negatives	CMV RSV Parainfluenza, influenza	Fungi *Aspergillus* *Histoplasma* Mycobacteria
Cystic fibrosis	*Staph. aureus* *Pseudomonas aeruginosa* *Burkholderia cepacia* *Stenotrophomonas maltophilia*		*Aspergillus*

(CMV = cytomegalovirus; RSV = respiratory syncytial virus)

Problem-orientated topic:

deteriorating pneumonia ●●●●●

Florian is a 6-year-old boy who attended his doctor's practice with a short history of fever, dry cough and mild tachypnoea. His doctor prescribed oral amoxicillin and referred him to the local accident and emergency department for a CXR. This showed a small area of dense consolidation in the left lower zone.

Three days later Florian reattends the emergency room looking much sicker. He is febrile and toxic-looking, and has increased tachypnoea (respiratory rate 65/min) and grunty respirations. He appears to have developed a scoliosis and is avoiding movement of the left side of his chest due to pain. His trachea and apex beat are displaced to the right and there is reduced intensity of breath sounds and stony dullness to percussion on the left.

Q1. What are the common organisms causing pneumonia?

Q2. What complication of pneumonia is likely to have occurred in Florian?

Q1. What are the common organisms causing pneumonia?

See Table 41.10. Remember, respiratory viruses are probably more common than bacteria as causes of pneumonia and include RSV, parainfluenza, influenza A and B, and adenovirus. Always consider *Tuberculosis* as a possible organism.

Q2. What complication of pneumonia is likely to have occurred in Florian?

He has developed a parapneumonic pleural effusion or an empyema. The features that suggest this complication are:

- Continuing fever and increasing 'toxicity' despite 3 days of oral antibiotic
- Mediastinal shift to left (deviation of trachea and apex beat)
- Stony dullness and reduced breath sounds on the right.

Florian's X-ray shows pleural fluid. Ultrasound scan is now important to determine the location and extent of this pleural fluid and whether it is loculated.

Principles of management of pleural fluid/empyema

- Pleural drainage
- Intravenous antibiotics.

BOX 41.18 Differential diagnosis of recurrent pneumonia

Genetic disorders
- Cystic fibrosis
- Sickle cell disease

Immune disorders/deficiencies
- Bruton agammaglobulinaemia
- IgG subclass deficiencies
- Severe combined immunodeficiency disease (SCID)
- AIDS

Leucocyte disorders
- Chronic granulomatous disease
- Hyperimmunoglobulin E syndrome
- Leucocyte adhesion defect

Ciliary disorders
- Immotile cilia syndrome

Anatomical disorders
- Sequestration
- Bronchial cyst
- Lobar emphysema
- Oesophageal reflux
- Recurrent aspiration
- Foreign body
- Tracheoesophageal fistula
- Bronchiectasis

 http://www.brit-thoracic.org.uk/iqs/bts_guidelines_pleurainfchild_html

BTS 2005 Pleural Infection in Children Guideline. Thorax 60: suppl 1

Recurrent lung infections

When a child presents with recurrent lung infections (Box 41.18) ascertain the following.

Have there been frequent upper respiratory viral infections?

This becomes especially noticeable if the child becomes febrile or lethargic, has a chesty cough and is given antibiotics with each head cold. Some children with early asthma give this history, i.e. viral triggered cough and wheeze episodes.

Is there a serious underlying cause?

Local abnormality associated with recurrent local infections
- Retained inhaled foreign body
- Sequestered lobe (an area of lung tissue that is not connected to the normal airways and has its own arterial blood supply, often from the descending aorta)
- Bronchial cyst.

Disorder eventually leading to chronic suppurative lung disease

Look for signs of chronic respiratory disease (finger clubbing, chest over-inflation) or chronic infection elsewhere (chronic ear infections with discharge).

Further reading

Lakhanpaul M, Atkinson M, Stephenson T 2004 Community-acquired pneumonia in children: a clinical update. Archives of Disease in Childhood, Education and Practice Edition 89: ep29–ep34

Rossi UG, Owens CM 2005 The radiology of chronic lung disease in children. Archives of Disease in Childhood 90:601–607

Smyth R 2005 Diagnosis and management of cystic fibrosis. Archives of Disease in Childhood, Education and Practice Edition 90: ep1–ep6

For more detailed information on specific topics refer to relevant chapter in: Taussig LM, Landau LJ eds. 2008 Paediatric Respiratory Medicine, 2nd edn, Mosby, Philadelphia

Agostino Nocerino   Edward Michael Richards

42

Blood and reticulo-endothelial disorders

LEARNING OUTCOMES

By the end of this chapter you should:
- Know the basic scientific principles of blood clotting
- Know the common causes of disease in children who present with anaemia, bruising, thrombocytopenia or pancytopenia
- Know the risks of blood transfusion
- Know the causes and risks of asplenism.

Introduction

The practice of haematology encompasses a close relationship between the clinical assessment and management of patients and the appropriate use of the laboratory. The haematology multidisciplinary team includes not only medical, nursing and allied professions but also the laboratory scientists in the haematology department. The fun of the topic is that, despite the advances in basic science, an individual haematologist can see the patient, undertake diagnostic procedures, interpret the results themselves and inform the patient of the diagnosis, often within a few hours of their presentation. The aims of this chapter are to introduce a rational approach to addressing common presentations of haematological disorders in order to formulate diagnostic algorithms and therefore appropriate use of laboratory facilities. It will also introduce basic principles of management.

A general principle in all paediatric haematology is the need to refer to age-specific normal ranges.

Anaemia

Problem-orientated topic:

pallor ● ● ● ● ●

Adamos, a 3-year-old boy whose family originate from Cyprus, presents to his primary care physician with a cough. The physician notices pallor and checks a complete blood count (CBC). The results indicate haemoglobin of 7.5 g/dl (normal range 11.5–13.5), mean corpuscular volume (MCV) of 64 fl (75–87), platelet count 550×10^9/l (150–450) and white cell count 4.5×10^9/l (5–17).

Q1. What are the potential causes of this anaemia?

Q2. What critical features would you elicit in the history?

Q3. What investigations would you request?

Q4. What management would you instigate?

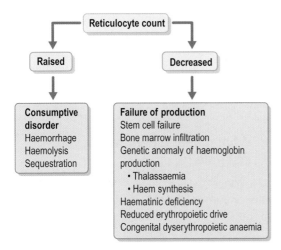

Fig. 42.1 Diagnostic algorithm of anaemia based on the reticulocyte count

Q1. What are the potential causes of this anaemia?

There are multiple causes of childhood anaemia. A rational approach to the diagnosis of any cytopenia involves the consideration of causes of a reduced rate of production and increased rate of either consumption or sequestration. The marker of the rate of red cell production is the reticulocyte, a red cell that retains ribonucleic acid permitting identification using special stains. Increased reticulocyte numbers infer an increased rate of bone marrow red cell production and vice versa. A diagnostic algorithm of anaemia using the reticulocyte count is outlined in Figure 42.1. The alternative pragmatic approach is use of the red cell size, represented by the mean corpuscular volume (MCV; Fig. 42.2). At birth, severe anaemia requiring treatment generally reflects haemorrhage (fetomaternal transfusion, placental abrup-tion or twin-to-twin); however, haemolysis, secondary to either enzymopathies or fetomaternal incompatibility and α-thalassaemia, may present during the neonatal period.

The most frequent cause of childhood anaemia is iron deficiency, which in turn is most commonly caused by inadequate dietary intake; alternative causes are chronic blood losses, malabsorption (coeliac disease), parasitic infections. The diagnosis is most commonly seen in those ethnic populations in whom the incidence of thalassaemia is greatest, this being the principal alternative diagnosis. The most urgent need is to exclude ongoing haemorrhage that may be life-threatening, such as with a Meckel diverticulum or pulmonary haemosiderosis. Chronically inadequate iron intake or thalassaemia trait does not constitute a medical emergency.

Q2. What critical features would you elicit in the history?

- Is the child failing to thrive?
- Ethnic origin:
  - Mediterranean, Middle East, Indian subcontinent, south-east Asia
- Family history of anaemia, coagulation disorders, consanguinity
- Dietetic assessment of iron intake
- Evidence of blood loss:
  - Gastrointestinal tract (parasitic infestation, Meckel's diverticulum, peptic ulceration)
  - Menstruation
  - Urinary (including paroxysmal nocturnal haemoglobinuria)
  - Pulmonary haemosiderosis
- Evidence of malabsorption/enteritis/bowel resection
- Drug intake associated with high gastric pH.

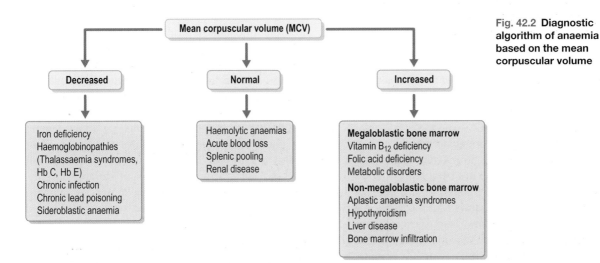

Fig. 42.2 Diagnostic algorithm of anaemia based on the mean corpuscular volume

Clinical signs

- Anaemia, jaundice
- Angular cheilosis (ulceration of angle of lips), smooth shiny appearance of tongue, koilonychia (spoon-shaped nails rare in childhood)
- Signs of malabsorption:
  - Failure to thrive, clubbing, abdominal distension
- Signs of gastrointestinal blood loss:
  - Telengiectasia, oral ulceration
- Facial appearance:
  - Frontal or parietal bossing.

Q3. What investigations would you request?

- Blood film and red cell indices:
  - Iron deficiency leads to hypochromia, microcytosis, anisocytosis (increased range of red cell sizes) and poikilocytosis (variation of shapes), including pencil cells and target cells.
  - Mixed iron/folate/B_{12} deficiency will produce a dimorphic population of red cells, one with a high MCV, one with a low MCV. The mean MCV may be misleadingly normal.
- Reticulocyte count: reduced in iron deficiency
- Frequent elevation of platelet count
- Measures of iron deficiency:
  - Serum ferritin: reduced in iron deficiency but elevated in inflammatory conditions, therefore may be falsely normal.
  - Zinc protoporphyrin: elevated in iron deficiency, also affected by inflammation
  - Percentage hypochromic red cells: increased in iron deficiency.
- Thalassaemia screen:
  - Elevation of HbA_2 is diagnostic of β-thalassaemia trait.
  - May be reduced into normal range by coexistent iron deficiency.
  - Rare forms of β-thalassaemia are associated with normal levels of HbA_2.
  - No confirmatory test for α-thalassaemia other than polymerase chain reaction (PCR)-based mutation screening.
- Therapeutic trial of iron replacement:
  - Laboratory investigations may identify iron deficiency but may not be able to exclude the coexistence of thalassaemia trait, notably α-thalassaemia trait. Prolonged iron replacement may lead to excess iron loading in children who have a diagnosis of thalassaemia trait, but a short therapeutic trial of iron for 3–6 months with close monitoring of haemoglobin is a reasonable diagnostic and therapeutic approach.
- Bone marrow (in selected cases) for assessment of marrow iron stores and exclusion of congenital sideroblastic anaemia.

Q4. What management would you instigate?

- Give dietetic advice.
- Give oral iron supplementation for at least 6 months:
  - Predicted response is 1 g/dl increment after each week of initial replacement
  - If inadequate, consider:
    Poor compliance (stool colour is dark when iron is being taken orally)
    Alternative/additional diagnosis
    Blood loss/malabsorption.
- Stop supplementation after 6 months.
- If there is further progressive anaemia, investigate for blood loss including gastrointestinal tract imaging.

Does chronic iron deficiency matter?

The effects of anaemia are well recognized as leading to weakness, fatigue, palpitations and lightheadedness. Less common effects of iron deficiency are the epithelial changes seen in the mouth and pica, the consumption of non-nutritive substances including soil and clay. Chronic iron deficiency can also impair growth and intellectual development. Studies of the effect of iron replacement on cognitive development have yielded disparate results.

Thalassaemia

Thalassaemia is a recessively inherited anaemia caused by abnormal imbalanced production of the globin chains within the haemoglobin molecule. It predominantly affects populations centred on the Mediterranean, the Middle East, the Indian subcontinent and South-East Asia. However, all ethnic groups may be affected. The thalassaemia syndromes are caused by underlying gene defects that are generally deletions of varying length. The nature of the deletion correlates with the resultant clinical phenotype. They all result in microcytic red cells and hypochromic anaemia of variable severity. The clinical phenotype is variable; thalassaemia major is a fatal disease if not managed with regular blood transfusions, thalassaemia intermedia is characterized by anaemia that may not require intervention, and thalassaemia trait is an asymptomatic carrier state.

Alpha-thalassaemia

Alpha-thalassaemia results in reduced production of α-chains, the resulting excess of β-chains causing red cell instability and haemolysis. The haemoglobin molecules present at birth contain α-chains, so that α-thalassaemia syndromes are present at delivery. Each individual has four α-genes; the clinical phenotype correlates with the number of gene deletions (Box 42.1).

Beta-thalassaemia

Beta-thalassaemia results in reduced production of β-chains, the resulting excess of α-chains causing red cell instability and haemolysis. Beta-thalassaemia syndromes only present at the age of 6 months, at the time of the major haemoglobin switch from HbF to HbA. Beta-thalassaemia major presents with a severe anaemia and a compensatory increase in the rate of erythropoiesis. Children present with failure to thrive, splenomegaly and expansion of the bone marrow space, resulting in skeletal anomalies including osteoporosis. Children not transfused die within the first few years of life. Diagnosis is based on quantitation of the different classes of haemoglobin. Initial treatment consists of red cell transfusion. This has a dual role: first, to abolish the symptoms and sequelae of anaemia, and second, to suppress endogenous erythropoiesis, so preventing bone marrow expansion and the skeletal and splenic consequences. The options for longer-term management are continuation of a hypertransfusion programme or allogeneic stem cell transplantation from a tissue type-matched sibling donor. Frequent red cell transfusions are complicated by tissue iron loading, which can result in multi-organ toxicity affecting the heart, liver, pancreas and endocrine organs. Prevention of such toxicity necessitates a chelation regimen currently involving subcutaneous infusions of desferrioxamine. Alternative oral iron chelators will hopefully soon be available.

Thalassaemia trait

The most common presentation of this disorder is thalassaemia trait or a silent carrier status, characterized by a mild microcytic anaemia often mistaken for and coexisting with iron deficiency. Beta-thalassaemia trait is identified by the presence of an elevated concentration of HbA_2; however, there is no simple test for α-thalassaemia, which is generally a diagnosis of exclusion. Thalassaemia trait has no clinical consequences for the individual; however, it is important to provide counselling that iron replacement is only indicated if iron deficiency has been confirmed. Genetic counselling is also important, given the recessive inheritance.

http://www.bcshguidelines.com

Transfusion guidelines for neonates and older children

Sickle cell disease

Sickling disorders are those in which red cells adopt a shape change in environments of low oxygen concentration to become a crescent or boat shape similar to the shape of the blade on a sickle. This shape results in red cells becoming lodged in small capillaries, leading to obstruction to blood flow, tissue ischaemia and further sickling. The most frequent disorders characterized by sickling are homozygous HbSS, compound heterozygous HbSC and coinheritance of HbS and β-thalassaemia trait. Sickle cell disease is seen most commonly in black Africans, Afro-Americans and Afro-Caribbeans but is also seen in the Mediterranean area (Balkans, Central Greece, Sicily), Middle East and parts of India. The abnormal haemoglobin molecules result from structural abnormalities of the globin chains resultant on gene mutations. Diagnosis is based on electrophoresis of haemoglobin, in which structural variants move at different speeds along an electrical gradient. Newer techniques are suitable for population screening programmes.

Sickle cell disease constitutes a chronic haemolytic anaemia complicated by acute crises. Vaso-occlusive events cause painful crises most frequently in bones, lungs (chest syndrome) and the spleen. A crisis involving the brain may result in a stroke. In young children dactylitis (infarcts of the small bones of the hand) may lead to digits of variable length. Sequestration crises represent sickling within organs and the pooling of blood with severe exacerbation of anaemia.

A severe chest syndrome is the most common cause of death; hepatic or splenic sequestration may require urgent blood transfusion. Other crises include aplastic crises and priapism. Splenic infarction consequent on sickling leads to an increased risk of overwhelming sepsis from encapsulated microorganisms. To protect against this, patients are immunized against encapsulated organisms and receive life-long antibiotic (penicillin, where available) prophylaxis. The universal neonatal haemoglobinopathy screening programme is centred around an early diagnosis of sickle cell disease and early introduction of prophylactic antibiotics. Chronic complications of sickle cell disease include proliferative retinopathy, avascular necrosis of the hips and ulcers of the lower limbs. Long term transfusion regimens, hydroxyurea or stem cell transplantation have to be considered for severe cases.

For further information, see Appendix.

http://www.bcshguidelines.com

Guidelines for the management of the acute painful crisis in sickle cell disease

http://www.rcpch.ac.uk/doc.aspx?id_Resource=4204

NHS — Sickle Cell Disease in Childhood Detailed guidance
Standards and guidelines for clinical care

Haemolytic anaemia

Haemolysis describes the destruction of circulating red cells at a pathologically increased rate. The potential causes of haemolysis are either intrinsic to the red cell or extrinsic (Table 42.1). The cardinal clinical features of haemolysis include anaemia, jaundice, gallstones and splenomegaly. Investigations reveal a raised level of bilirubin (predominantly unconjugated), reduced concentration of serum haptoglobin and increased urinary urobilinogen. There may be red cell morphological changes, including spherocytes. Intravascular haemolysis is also characterized by haemoglobinaemia and haemosiderinuria. A healthy bone marrow will respond by a compensatory increased rate of red cell production, evidenced by a raised reticulocyte count. Clinically there will be pallor and jaundice. There may be associated splenomegaly reflecting the principal site of red cell destruction.

Principles of management are supplementation of folic acid, avoidance of precipitants of acute crises and occasionally red cell transfusion, splenectomy and cholecystectomy. Specific disease states will require specific treatment.

Spherocytosis

The normal shape of a red cell is a biconcave disc; spherocytes are abnormal spherically shaped red cells. They are formed either as a consequence of immune-mediated red cell destruction or as an inherited defect of red cell membrane. The binding of immunoglobulin antibodies to the red cell membrane may result in an increased rate of haemolysis. Macrophages in the reticulo-endothelial system bind the Fc fragment of the immunoglobulin molecule and remove small areas of the membrane. As the area of available membrane is reduced, the red cell adopts the shape in which the maximum volume is enclosed by the minimum surface area. This shape is a sphere. The alternative mechanism leading to an increased number of spherocytes is the inheritance of a defect of different proteins of the cytoskeleton of the red cell membrane which causes the red cell to adopt a spherical shape. The spherical shape itself leads to premature red cell breakdown. This inherited condition is known as hereditary spherocytosis and is inherited both in an autosomal dominant and recessive fashion. It is characterized by a low-grade

Table 42.1 Causes of haemolysis

	Intrinsic to red cell	Extrinsic to red cell

Congenital	Haemoglobin defects:
	  Haemoglobinopathy
	  Thalassaemia
	Red cell enzyme defects:
	  Glucose-6-phosphate
	  dehydrogenase
	  Pyruvate kinase
	Red cell membrane defects:
	  Hereditary
	  spherocytosis
	  Hereditary
	  elliptocytosis
		Nil

Acquired	Paroxysmal nocturnal haemoglobinuria (increased red cell lysis by complement)	Immune:
		  Autoimmune:
		    Cold
		    Warm
		  Alloimmune:
		    HDN
		    Transfusion reaction
		  Drug-mediated
		Red cell fragmentation:
		  Microangiopathic:
		    TTP
		    HUS
		    DIC
		  Cardiac valve grafts
		  Infections:
		    Malaria
		    Clostridium
		    Meningococcus
		  Burns

(HDN = haemolytic disease of the newborn; TTP = thrombotic thrombocytopenic purpura; HUS = haemolytic uraemic syndrome; DIC = disseminated intravascular coagulation)

jaundice and moderate splenomegaly. Gallstones are common. Viral infections may precipitate an acute haemolytic crisis or an aplastic crisis in which the rate of erythropoiesis is reduced. Folate deficiency may also lead to a failure of erythropoiesis. Chronic haemolysis may lead to a failure to thrive with an increase in school non-attendance.

Management consists of appropriate counselling, supplementation of folic acid, and occasional red cell transfusions in the event of significant anaemia, especially in the neonatal period and following an aplastic crisis. The disease may be moderated by splenectomy, which may be indicated in patients with brisk haemolysis and gallstones.

http://www.bcshguidelines.com

Guidelines for the diagnosis and management of hereditary spherocytosis

Transfusion of blood products

Blood products may be donated as whole blood, which undergoes subsequent processing into individual components, or cell separator techniques can be utilized to collect specific cellular components or plasma from donors. The transfusion of blood products should be guided by haematological investigations and not done on the basis of non-substantiated clinical need. Individual components, either alone or in combination, should be used rather than whole blood. Cellular components include red cells, platelets and occasionally white cells. Plasma components include fresh frozen plasma, cryoprecipitate and cryosupernatant. The indications for use of these products can be found elsewhere. The transfusion of blood products constitutes one of the most dangerous aspects of patient care (Box 42.2). General principles of transfusion include avoidance, if at all possible, documentation of the indication for use in the clinical notes and the limitation of donor exposure. Scrupulous attention must be paid to the administrative aspects of requesting blood products for patients since most transfusion errors are consequent on documentation errors.

Coagulation disorders

Basic science

A rational approach to diagnosis requires some understanding of the normal process of coagulation, which for ease can be considered to consist of primary and secondary haemostasis. A breach of the endothelial lining of the blood vessel will lead to the release of von Willebrand factor. This large multimeric molecule binds to circulating platelets via specific membrane receptors and

---

BOX 42.2 Adverse effects of transfusion*

Immediate
- Febrile transfusion reaction:
  - White cell antibodies
  - Plasma protein antibodies
- Haemolytic transfusion reaction:
  - ABO-incompatible blood
- Bacterial infection
- Volume overload
- Air embolism
- Transfusion-associated lung injury (TRALI)

Delayed
- Haemolytic transfusion reaction:
  - Red cell antigens other than ABO
- Post-transfusion purpura
- Pathogen transmission (viruses, possibly variant Creutzfeldt–Jakob disease (vCJD))
- Graft versus host disease
- Transfusion haemosiderosis

* Most transfusion errors are consequent on administrative mistakes

---

draws the platelets to the breach in the blood vessel wall, creating a structure of cells across the blood vessel defect akin to a dam of pebbles across a stream. The creation of this dam constitutes primary haemostasis. Secondary haemostasis is the process of sealing the gaps between the platelets. The process of coagulation involves the sequential activation of enzymes to produce a crucial enzyme known as thrombin. Thrombin leads to the cleavage of fibrinogen to form fibrin, which is the cement that binds the platelets together. Ten enzymes are crucial to this process and deficiencies of eight are associated with a clinically significant increased risk of haemorrhage. The balance of haemostasis is ensured by the parallel control system of natural anticoagulants in the blood, principally antithrombin, protein C and protein S. Inherited deficiencies of the anticoagulants lead to an increased risk of thrombosis, a condition known as thrombophilia. Finally, recannulation of thrombosed blood vessels is undertaken by a process called fibrinolysis, the active enzyme being plasmin.

A rational approach to a child with excess bleeding or bruising

It is important to approach a child who presents with symptoms of excess haemorrhage in a systematic fashion (Fig. 42.3). It is necessary to determine whether the symptoms represent a congenital or acquired condition and to consider each part of the haemostatic system in the analysis of the cause.

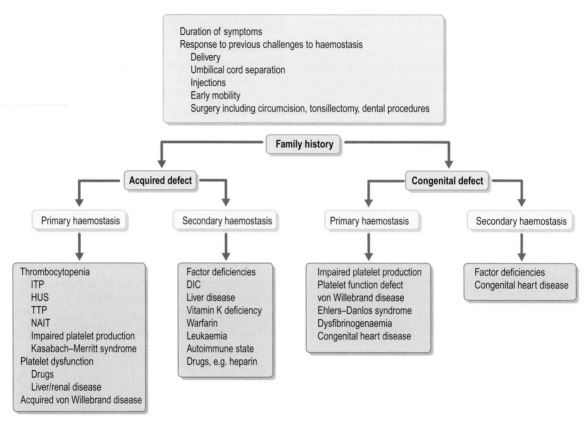

Fig. 42.3 **Diagnostic algorithm for a patient with increased bleeding tendency**
(ITP = idiopathic thrombocytopenic purpura; HUS = haemolytic uraemic syndrome; TTP = thrombotic thrombocytopenic purpura; NAIT = neonatal alloimmune thrombocytopenia; DIC = disseminated intravascular coagulation)

There are distinct patterns of bleeding in defects of primary and secondary haemostasis. Defects of primary haemostasis lead to bruising and petechiae as well as mucosal haemorrhage, including epistaxis, oral haemorrhage, gastrointestinal haemorrhage and increased menstrual losses. Defects of secondary haemostasis cause deep-sited bleeding in joints, muscles, internal organs and the central nervous system. Some disorders may lead to both types of bleeding, including type III von Willebrand disease.

Aspects of the history in delineating specific congenital defects include prolonged umbilical stump bleeding associated with factor XIII deficiency or fibrinogen deficiency and the association of factor XI deficiency with Ashkenazi Jewish descent. A thorough family history is essential in defining autosomal dominant, recessive and X-linked pedigrees. Assessment of acquired causes includes evidence of current organ dysfunction, recent viral infections and the ingestion of drugs. Examination should elicit current signs, including petechiae, bruising, oral haemorrhage, arthropathy and fundal bleeds, signs of concurrent illness, dysmorphism and signs of increased skin and joint laxity.

A rational algorithm for investigation is essential but beyond the scope of this chapter. Important tests include the following:

Defects of primary haemostasis

- Complete blood count (CBC)
- Platelet morphology
- Prothrombin time (PT)
- Activated partial thromboplastin time (APTT)
- Fibrinogen
- Von Willebrand screen
- Assessment of platelet function:
  - Platelet aggregometry
  - Platelet nucleotide analysis
  - Platelet surface glycoprotein expression.

Defects of secondary haemostasis

- FBC
- PT
- APTT
- Fibrinogen

- Assays of specific coagulation factors: sequence of analysis will follow pattern of PT/APTT abnormalities
- Factor XIII assay
- α_2-antiplasmin assay.

Idiopathic thrombocytopenic purpura

Problem-orientated topic:

spontaneous bruising ● ● ● ● ●

Kyrenia, a previously healthy 13-year-old girl, presents with a month-long history of fatigue and a week of spontaneous bruising and heavy menstrual loss. Examination is unremarkable other than bruises and petechiae. A CBC reveals haemoglobin of 10.1 g/dl (12–16), MCV of 78 fl (78–95), platelet count 13×10^9/l (150–450) and white cell count 4.5×10^9/l (4.5–13), of which neutrophils are 3.1×10^9/l and lymphocytes 0.9×10^9/l.

Q1. What do you consider Kyrenia's most probable diagnoses?

Q2. What investigations would you request?

Q3. What treatment would you offer?

Q1. What do you consider Kyrenia's most probable diagnoses?

Childhood idiopathic thrombocytopenic purpura (ITP) has an incidence of between 4.0 and 5.3 per 100 000. The typical presentation is a rapid onset of bruising and petechiae in an otherwise well child. This reflects an impairment of primary haemostasis. There is frequently an association with a previous viral infection or immunization in a younger child; this is less frequent in an older child, in whom association with other autoimmune diseases is more frequent. Additional signs or symptoms should raise the possibility of an alternative diagnosis, such as acute leukaemia, evolving marrow aplasia or thrombocytopenia in association with disorders such as systemic lupus erythematosus (SLE) or the antiphospholipid syndrome.

Q2. What investigations would you request?

Diagnosis is one of exclusion of other disorders and can in general be made by careful clinical assessment, an FBC and review of the blood film by an experienced morphologist. The most feared misdiagnosis is that of acute lymphoblastic leukaemia (p. 775), which has an annual incidence similar to that of ITP. This fear has encouraged the early assessment of bone marrow morphology; however, current advice is to delay such an invasive investigation until a time at which the course of ITP in an individual patient is atypical or prolonged or prior to the use of corticosteroids.

Patients with chronic ITP should be investigated to exclude other immune dysregulation disorders, such as autoimmune disorders like SLE, immune deficiency states and the rare condition, autoimmune lymphoproliferative syndrome.

Q3. What treatment would you offer?

The natural history in 80% cases of ITP is spontaneous resolution within 6–8 weeks. Patients have chronic ITP if disease duration exceeds 6 months. Intracranial haemorrhage occurs with a frequency of approximately 0.1–0.5% and is most frequent in children with chronic disease. The initial management of newly presenting children is reassurance, observation and provision of routes of rapid access to advice or support. Management should be guided by the patient's clinical condition and not solely the platelet count. In the event of significant haemorrhage in excess of petechiae and bruising, treatment options to elevate the platelet count include the use of corticosteroids, intravenous immunoglobulin or anti-D immunoglobulin (in patients who are red cell rhesus-D positive). Transfusion of platelets should only be considered in the event of life-threatening haemorrhage since they will be consumed as rapidly as endogenously produced platelets. None of the above measures will alter the underlying natural course of the disorder. The management of chronic ITP is highly specialized and should be performed in a regional centre. Treatment options include chronic immunosuppression and splenectomy.

http://www.bcshguidelines.com

Guidelines for the investigation and management of ITP in adults and children and in pregnancy

Henoch–Schönlein purpura

The diagnosis of Henoch–Schönlein purpura (HSP) relies on the recognition of a group of clinical signs, namely:
- A characteristic rash
- Arthralgia
- Periarticular oedema
- Abdominal pain
- Glomerulonephritis.

The peak incidence is between the ages of 3 and 10 years; boys are affected more frequently than girls. HSP is often preceded by a history of an upper respiratory tract infection; hence the incidence is greatest during winter. The clinical features may appear simultaneously over a short time period or there may be a gradual onset over weeks or months. Low-grade fever and fatigue occur in excess of half of affected children.

Clinical features
- *Rash*. This begins as pinkish maculopapules that initially blanch on pressure and progress to purpura. The purpura may be palpable and evolve from red to purple to rusty brown before fading. The rash can appear in crops over 3–10 days and may be episodic, occurring at intervals that vary from a few days to 4 months. The rash may recur rarely several years after the initial presentation. The classic localization of the rash is a symmetrical distribution on the buttocks, extensor surfaces of the arms and legs and the ankles. The trunk is spared unless lesions are induced by trauma. There may be local angioedema, especially in dependent areas such as below the waist and over the buttocks (or the back and scalp of an infant). Oedema may also occur in areas of tissue distensability, such as the eyelids, lips, scrotum or the dorsal surfaces of the hands and feet.
- *Arthritis*. This is present in excess of two-thirds of children, affecting predominantly the knees and ankles. There may be effusions that resolve after a few days without residual deformity or joint damage.
- *Abdominal symptoms*. Inflammation of the vascular supply to the gut may lead to intermittent colicky abdominal pain. Diarrhoea is well recognized and there may be passage of blood rectally and haematemesis. The symptoms may mimic an abdominal emergency. Intussusception may occur, which can be complicated by complete obstruction or infarction with bowel perforation.
- *Renal involvement*. Renal involvement is common; microscopic or macroscopic haematuria or mild proteinuria is present in more than 80% of cases (p. 559).
- *Other complications*. These include hepatosplenomegaly, lymphadenopathy and rarely testicular torsion. Central nervous system involvement may precipitate fits, paralysis or a coma. Other rare complications include rheumatoid-like nodules, cardiac and eye involvement, mononeuropathies, pancreatitis and pulmonary and intramuscular haemorrhage.

Differential diagnosis
The rash of Henoch-Schönlein purpura is very typical, and the diagnosis is usually straightforward. However, at the very beginning of the disease, some confusion may arise in the differential diagnosis with ITP and meningococcal disease. Patients with ITP will have thrombocytopenia. Meningococcal disease may be difficult to exclude initially but a more benign clinical course and negative microbiology will exclude it. HSP may occur in association with other systemic disorders such as autoimmune disorders, vasculitides, familial Mediterranean fever or inflammatory bowel disease. Similar but distinct presentations occur with polyarteritis nodosa, meningococcal disease, purpura fulminans, Kawasaki disease and systemic onset juvenile rheumatoid arthritis.

Investigations
There may be an elevated platelet and white cell number and an elevated erythrocyte sedimentation rate (ESR). Immune complexes are often present and levels of IgA and IgM may be increased. Renal involvement is demonstrated by red blood cells, white blood cells, casts or albumin in the urine. A skin biopsy demonstrates a leucocytoclastic vasculitis, and renal biopsy may show IgA mesangial deposition and occasionally IgM, C3 and fibrin.

Management
This is generally supportive, with adequate analgesia and hydration. Management of an acute abdominal crisis may require surgical or radiological reduction of an intussusception. However, steroids may have a role in improving both gastrointestinal and central nervous system complications. Management of renal complications may include the use of immunosuppressive drugs and require long-term follow-up.

Haemophilia

Haemophilia describes an increased tendency to bleed consequent on a failure of secondary haemostasis. The term 'haemophilia' is reserved to deficiencies of factor VIII (1:5000–10 000 males) and factor IX (1:35 000–50 000 males), known respectively as Haemophilia A and B. Haemophilia A and B are inherited in an X-linked fashion. Deficiency of factor XI is sometimes referred to as Haemophilia C. Deficiencies of coagulation factors I, II, V, VII, X and XIII can also result in an increased bleeding diathesis. The severity of the clinical phenotype is correlated with the plasma concentration of the deficient factor (Table 42.2). Untreated severe haemophilia A or B is characterized by chronic arthropathy consequent on repeated haemarthroses (joint bleeds). However, life-threatening haemorrhage can follow

Table 42.2 Classification of haemophilia A and B

Plasma concentration of coagulation factor (IU/dl)	Severity of haemophilia	Clinical symptoms
< 1	Severe	Spontaneous bleeding into joints, muscles or other internal organs
1–5	Moderate	Bleeding episodes following minor trauma
5–50	Mild	Bleeding episodes following significant trauma
50–150	Normal individual	Nil

minor surgery in patients in whom haemophilia has not been considered, whether that is mild, moderate or severe. The results of diagnostic tests are described in Table 42.3.

The initial presentation with haemophilia will depend on the challenges to haemostasis sustained by the individual patient and the severity of the disease. Severe haemophilia is associated with a risk of intracranial haemorrhage following delivery. It may cause excess bruising in a toddler raising concerns of non-accidental injury, a haemarthrosis in a 1-year-old boy or excess bleeding following minor surgery such as dental extraction many years later.

Haemophilia care encompasses education, avoidance of drugs that impair haemostasis and activities associated with a high risk of trauma. The expectations of modern care are a normal life expectancy and joint integrity and a life of normal activities undertaken with caution. Treatment for an individual minor bleed involves local measures and antifibrinolytic agents but for significant bleeds elevation of the level of the deficient factor is required. This is achieved by infusion of vials of the relevant factor concentrate via the intravenous route in a dose that is proportional to the weight of the individual. For patients with mild haemophilia A, administration of DDAVP desmopressin may elevate the levels of von Willebrand factor and factor VIII to therapeutic levels. DDAVP is ineffectual in haemophilia B and should be used with caution in children under the age of 2 years.

Haemophilia treatment has progressed from treatment of an established bleed, so-called on-demand therapy, to prophylactic administration of concentrate to prevent bleeds. The most significant complication of haemophilia treatment has been the transmission of plasma bone infections including HIV and hepatitis B and C. This risk has now been virtually eliminated by the use of recombinant products, infection screening and viral inactivation. The remaining complication of coagulation factor replacement is inhibitor development, alloantibodies that bind to and destroy the exogenously administered coagulation factor. Genetic counselling is essential in any inherited disorder and carrier identification of female members of the family can be offered in the majority of cases. However, 30% of new patients with haemophilia A or B have no previous family history since they represent new mutations.

Von Willebrand disease

This is the most common inherited bleeding disorder, which according to some series affects 1:100 of the population. It is characterized by a deficiency of von Willebrand factor (vWf). The clinical features reflect the roles of vWf: namely in the adherence of platelets to the endothelium, in primary haemostasis, and in protecting circulating factor VIII, a role in secondary haemostasis. The deficiency of vWf may be quantitative (type 1, mild; type 3, severe) or qualitative (type 2, in which the function of the molecule is impaired).

The symptoms of type 1 disease are typical of the features of failure of primary haemostasis. The symptoms of type 3 disease combine those of primary haemostatic defects with deep-seated haemorrhage more commonly associated with defects of secondary haemostasis. Type 2 von Willebrand disease usually presents with symptoms similar to those of type 1 disease but a particular disorder, type 2b von Willebrand disease, is associated with thrombocytopenia. The symptoms of types 1 and 2 von Willebrand disease are relatively mild. Treatment consists of conservative measures and DDAVP desmopressin infusions when normal haemostasis is required. Type 3 and some subtypes of type 2 require infusion of intact vWf in the form of specific factor VIII concentrates. The clinical phenotype of von Willebrand disease is influenced by multiple genetic influences but type 1 disease follows an autosomal dominant inheritance. Type 3 disease results from the coinheritance of two vWf genetic defects which may present as type 1 disease in the parents; it is effectively inherited as an autosomal recessive disorder.

Table 42.3 Investigation of haemophilia, von Willebrand disease and vitamin K deficiency

Investigation	Haemophilia A	von Willebrand disease	Vitamin K deficiency
Prothrombin time	Normal	Normal	Prolonged
Activated partial thromboplastin time	Prolonged	Prolonged/normal	Prolonged
Factor VIII	Reduced	Reduced/normal	Normal
vW factor antigen	Normal	Reduced	Normal
Platelet aggregation	Normal	Reduced with ristocetin	Normal

Table 42.4 Classification of haemorrhagic disease of the newborn

	Early	Classical	Late
Age of onset	Days 1 or 2 Rarely up to day 5	Days 2–7 Rarely up to 1 month	2–12 weeks

Risk factors	Maternal ingestion of drugs during pregnancy
	Anticonvulsants
	Coumarin anticoagulants
	Anti-tuberculosis treatment
		Failure to administer vitamin K at birth	Failure to administer vitamin K at birth
			Breastfeeding
			Impaired vitamin K absorption:
			  Liver disease
			  GI malabsorption

Features	May not be prevented by vitamin K at birth	Haemorrhage may be intracranial, gastrointestinal or in other internal organ	Haemorrhage may be intracranial, gastrointestinal or in other internal organ

http://www.nhlbi.nih.gov/guidelines/vwd/index.htm

Vitamin K-deficient bleeding

Four of the coagulation factors — namely, factors II, VII, IX, X — and two of the anticoagulant factors, proteins C and S, require vitamin K to modify the precursor molecules and render them fully functional. Vitamin K is necessary for the post-translational gamma-carboxylation of these molecules. The principal effect of vitamin K deficiency is an increased risk of bleeding, as is seen in haemorrhagic disease of the newborn (HDN, p. 727), following the use of coumarin anticoagulants such as warfarin, and in certain malnourished children. However, if warfarin anticoagulation is initiated without concurrent heparin, the initial deficiency of protein C can lead to the thrombotic complication, purpura fulminans.

There is considerable evidence that the newborn infant is deficient in vitamin K; however, only a minority of neonates have clotting abnormalities at birth as a consequence. Vitamin K deficiency is intensified in the first few days of life unless the baby receives an exogenous source of vitamin K either by specific injection or as a dose by mouth or by inclusion in cow's milk or formula feeds. Breast milk contains little vitamin K.

The differentiation of haemorrhagic disease of the newborn (HDN) from other bleeding disorders is shown in Table 42.4.

A deficiency of the vitamin K-dependent coagulation factors will prolong the PT and APTT. Further evidence of vitamin K deficiency can be obtained from increased levels of proteins produced in the absence of vitamin K (PIVKA). The prevention of HDN by administration of vitamin K at birth is well established. This established efficacy justifies its use despite the previously suggested risks of haemolysis and leukaemia. Emergency treatment of vitamin K deficiency consists of intravenous administration of vitamin K. If life-threatening bleeding is recognized, immediate replacement of the deficient factors will be required, ideally with a coagulation factor concentrate of factors II, VII, IX and X. If no such concentrate is available fresh frozen plasma may be used, although the concentration of coagulation factors is insufficient for complete reversal of the haemorrhagic state.

Asplenism

The spleen serves as an efficient filter of red blood cells as they pass through large pools of blood, where they encounter macrophages and other immune effector cells. During their passage through this organ abnormal red cells may be removed by virtue of their senescence, abnormal membrane caused by binding of immunoglobulin, abnormal membrane structure, haemoglobin or cytoplasmic enzymes. The spleen also plays an important role in the immune system, allowing antigen-presenting cells to be exposed to circulating antigens and allowing macrophages to remove blood-borne bacteria, especially encapsulated organisms. The absence of the spleen will result in an increased risk of overwhelming bacterial sepsis, especially secondary to *Streptococcus pneumoniae*, *Haemophilus influenzae* type b and *Neisseria meningitidis*. The patient is also at risk of increased levels of parasitic infection with *Plasmodium* and *Babesia*.

Impaired splenic function can be seen on examination of the peripheral blood film. Red cells with abnormal morphology may circulate and red cell inclusions, including Howell–Jolly bodies (nuclear fragments), are frequently seen. There is an associated elevated platelet and white cell count (predominantly a monocytosis and lymphocytosis) in the peripheral blood.

Causes of a hyposplenic state are listed below. The clinical importance is the protection against overwhelming post-splenectomy sepsis with appropriate immunizations and penicillin prophylaxis.

Causes of asplenia
- Neonatal period, especially in premature infants
- Congenital absence or hypoplasia (associated with situs invertus and cardiac anomalies)
- Congenital polysplenism

- Surgical splenectomy
- Splenic infarction (sickling disorders and splenic torsion)
- Splenic atrophy (associated with coeliac disease, dermatitis herpetiformis, ulcerative colitis, Crohn disease, tropical sprue, autoimmune disorders including SLE, graft versus host disease and splenic irradiation
- Splenic infiltration with malignancy or sarcoidosis.

Causes of splenomegaly
- Haematological:
  - Chronic myeloid leukaemia
  - Juvenile myelomonocytic leukaemia
  - Acute leukaemia
  - Lymphoma
  - Thalassaemia major or intermedia
  - Sickle cell anaemia (before infarction in HbSS)
  - Haemolytic anaemia
  - Megaloblastic anaemia
- Portal hypertension
- Storage diseases:
  - Gaucher
  - Niemann–Pick
  - Histiocytosis X
- Systemic diseases:
  - Sarcoidosis
  - Collagen vascular disease, SLE, juvenile idiopathic arthritis
- Acute infections:
  - Bacterial: septicaemia, bacterial endocarditis, typhoid
  - Viral: infectious mononucleosis, cytomegalovirus and others
  - Protozoal: malaria, leishmaniasis, toxoplasmosis
- Chronic infections:
  - Tuberculosis, brucellosis
  - Tropical: malaria, leishmaniasis, schistosomiasis.

Causes of hepatomegaly
- Infection:
  - Congenital, hepatitis A, B and C, infectious mononucleosis, septicaemia, malaria
- Inflammation:
  - Hepatitis secondary to toxins, autoimmune disorders

- Infiltration:
  - Primary tumours:
    Hepatoblastoma
    Hepatocellular carcinoma
  - Secondary tumours:
    Leukaemia
    Lymphoma
    Haemophagocytic lymphohistiocytosis
- Liver disease:
  - Neonatal liver disease
  - Chronic liver disease
  - Autosomal dominant polycystic liver/kidney disease
  - Alpha$_1$-antitrypsin deficiency
- Storage disorders:
  - Lipid, e.g. Gaucher, Niemann–Pick
  - Mucopolysaccharidoses, e.g. Hurler syndrome
  - Glycogen
- Haematological:
  - Sickle cell anaemia, thalassaemia
  - Leukaemia, lymphoma
- Cardiovascular:
  - Right heart failure, tricuspid regurgitation.

Bone marrow failure

Marrow failure presents with a reduced number of circulating peripheral blood cell numbers. The pathology frequently affects one cell line before the others so that a single cytopenia may be the initial presentation. The symptoms will depend on the nature of the cytopenia with pallor, fatigue and reduced exercise tolerance reflecting anaemia, atypical bacterial infections reflecting neutropenia, and bleeding and bruising reflecting thrombocytopenia. Bone marrow failure may reflect abnormalities of the stem cell, either deficiency (aplasia) or abnormal maturation (dysplasia); absence of the raw materials for haemopoiesis, including iron, vitamin B$_{12}$ and folic acid, and hypopituitarism; and infiltration of the bone marrow by abnormal cells such as leukaemia or neuroblastoma or bone as in osteopetrosis (Table 42.5).

Table 42.5 Causes of pancytopenia

Disease category	Specific disorders	Associated features

Marrow aplasia	Congenital:
	  Fanconi anaemia
	  Dyskeratosis congenita
	  Shwachman–Diamond syndrome
	  Reticular dysgenesis
	  Amegakaryocytic thrombocytopenia
	Acquired:
	  Idiopathic
	  Drugs:
	    Predictable
	    Idiosyncratic
	  Viruses
		Congenital disorders are associated with somatic anomalies
		Fanconi anaemia: short stature, hyperpigmentation, abnormal radii and thumbs, renal anomalies
		Dyskeratosis congenita: dystrophic nails, leucoplakia of mucous membranes
		Shwachman–Diamond syndrome: exocrine pancreatic insufficiency

Myelodysplasia	Stem cell disorder characterized by atypical cellular maturation and morphology	Rarely seen in childhood Frequent associated cytogenetic abnormalities

Haematinic deficiency	Megaloblastic anaemia:
	  Vitamin B_{12} deficiency
	  Folic acid deficiency
	Predominant feature is macrocytic anaemia with atypical peripheral blood morphology
	Leucopenia and thrombocytopenia in B_{12} deficiency
	Hypercellular marrow
	Atypical marrow morphology
		Vitamin B_{12} deficiency:
		  Causes: inadequate dietary intake or malabsorption, including pernicious anaemia
		  Associated neuropathy
		Folic acid deficiency:
		  Causes: inadequate dietary intake or malabsorption, increased use as in haemolysis and pregnancy

Bone marrow infiltrate	Malignant:
	  Leukaemia
	  Metastatic solid tumours including:
	    Neuroblastoma
	    Rhabdomyosarcoma
	Other:
	  Osteopetrosis
	  Haemophagocytosis
	  Myelofibrosis
	  Storage disorders
		Clinical features dependent on primary disorder
		Leucoerythroblastic peripheral blood film with evidence of immature cellular forms circulating in peripheral blood

Further reading

British Committee for Standards in Haematology: General Haematology Task Force 2003 Guidelines for the investigation and management of idiopathic thrombocytopenic purpura in adults, children and in pregnancy. British Journal of Haematology 120(4):574

British Committee for Standards in Haematology: General Haematology Task Force 2003 Guidelines for the management of the acute painful crisis in sickle cell disease. British Journal of Haematology 120(5):744

Cunningham MJ 2008. Review. Update on thalassemia: clinical care and complications. Pediatr Clin North Am. 55(2):447–460

De Mattia D et al 2000 Review. Acute childhood idiopathic thrombocytopenic purpura: AIEOP consensus guidelines for diagnosis and treatment. Haematologica 85(4):420–424

George JN et al 1966 Review. Idiopathic thrombocytopenic purpura: a practice guideline developed by explicit methods for the American Society of Hematology. Blood. 88(1):3–40

Khair K, Liesner R 2006 Review. Bruising and bleeding in infants and children — a practical approach. Br J Haematol. 133(3):221–231

Mannucci PM 2004. Review. Treatment of von Willebrand's Disease. N Engl J Med. 351(7):683–694

Orkin SH, Nathan DG, Ginsburg D et al 2009 Nathan and Oski's Haematology of infancy and childhood, 7th edn. WB Saunders, Philadelphia

Van Winckel M et al 2009 Vitamin K, an update for the paediatrician. Eur J Pediatr. 2009 168(2):127–134

Zipurski, A 1999 Review: prevention of vitamin K deficiency bleeding in newborns. British Journal of Haematology 104:430–437

Noura Al-Aufi   Huda Al-Hussamy   Julia Clark
José Lopes dos Santos   Sachin Mannikar

CHAPTER

43

Immunology and infectious disease

LEARNING OUTCOMES

By the end of this chapter you should:

- Know the body's basic immune mechanisms
- Understand some basic principles of immunology
- Know the principles of allergy
- Know how to investigate and manage recurrent infection
- Understand the prevention and management of HIV/AIDS
- Understand the investigation of fever with rash
- Understand the investigation and management of prolonged fever
- Know how to investigate a child with suspected tuberculosis
- Understand the management of meningitis and septicaemia
- Understand the investigation and management of allergy.

MODULE SEVEN

Basic science

The immune system relies on the interaction of many different parts. Different pathogens stimulate and are controlled by different arms of this system, yet at the same time all components depend on each other, working as a team. The body has both innate and adaptive responses to pathogens (Box 43.1) and the component parts are discussed here. Different defence mechanisms are provoked by different pathogens (Table 43.1).

Phagocytes

Phagocytes are 'eating cells'. They include neutrophils (or polymorphonuclear cells) and the mononuclear

phagocyte system (monocytes in blood, macrophages in tissues). Neutrophils are critical for immunity to bacteria and fungi. Phagocytosis of extracellular pathogens is followed by their destruction by superoxides, proteases etc. within the neutrophil phagosomes. Macrophages also phagocytose and are important in T-cell activation, taking up and presenting antigens to T cells.

Antibodies (from B cells)

Immunoglobulins are γ-globulins of differing size that play important roles in humoral and cellular defence mechanisms; they are present in varying amounts through childhood. They participate in complement-dependent and independent opsonization, bactericidal activity, virus and toxin neutralization, and the

BOX 43.1 Innate and adaptive responses

Innate (natural immunity)

First line; no memory

- Phagoctyes
- Natural killer (NK) cells
- Dendritic cells
- Mast cells
- Cytokines
- Complement
- Acute phase proteins (C-reactive protein, CRP)

Adaptive

Second line; specific; memory

- T cells
- B cells
- Antibodies
- Cytokines

Humoral

- B cells, producing antibody

Cellular

- NK cells
- T cells
- CD4 (T-helper)
- CD8 (T-cytotoxic)

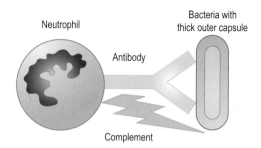

Fig. 43.1 **Antibodies and complement**

formation of immune complexes. IgM is produced early in infection, then interaction with CD4 cells by the binding of CD40 ligand to CD40 on B cells produces immunoglobulin class switching to IgA, IgG or IgE.

Complement

Complement attracts neutrophils to pathogens, helps attach pathogen to phagocyte (opsonization), enhances degranulation of mast cells (hence inflammation), and aids killing by cell lysis.

Antibodies and complement are particularly important for immunity to bacteria with thick carbohydrate capsules (e.g. *Streptococcus pneumoniae*, *Haemophilus influenzae*, *Neisseria meningitidis*). This is because the thick capsule prevents direct phagocytosis of the bacteria. Antibodies and complement act as a link (e.g. opsonin) between the bacteria and the neutrophil (Fig. 43.1).

T cells

T lymphocytes are the key orchestrators of the immune system (Fig. 43.2). They interact directly with cells via major histocompatibility complex (MHC) molecules

Table 43.1 **Defence mechanisms by pathogen**

	Pathogen	Mechanism
Intracellular pathogens	Viruses *Salmonella* Mycobacteria *Listeria* Fungi	T cells Natural killer (NK) cells Macrophages
Extracellular pathogens	Polysaccharide bacteria	Neutrophils Complement Antibodies

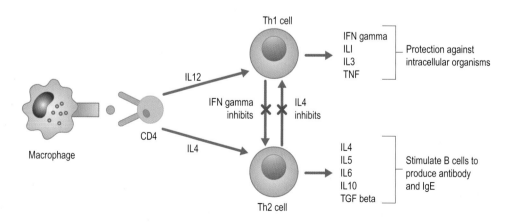

Fig. 43.2 **Th1/Th2 responses**
(IL = interleukin; IFN = interferon; TNF = tumour necrosis factor; TGF-β = transforming growth factor-β)

on the surface of cell targets. CD4 cells help control intracellular pathogens and help B-cell responses; CD8 cells kill infected cells. CD4 cells produce different cytokine responses depending on the stimulus. Th1 responses are proinflammatory, producing interferon-gamma (IFN-γ), tumour necrosis factor-alpha (TNF-α) and interleukin 2 (IL-2); they activate and recruit macrophages and help CD8 responses, hence intra-cellular killing.

Th2 responses produce IL-4, 5 and 6 and promote B-cell proliferation and differentiation to IgA, IgE and IgG2, as well as eosinophil recruitment. These are important in improving defence of mucosal surfaces, eradication of parasites and polysaccharide antigen responses.

Natural killer (NK) cells

These kill 'self-cells' infected with a virus.

Recurrent infection

Problem-orientated topic:

recurrent infections

Alexio, a 10-month-old boy, presents acutely unwell with a short history of cough and fever. He has a respiratory rate of 60 breaths per minute, is using accessory muscles showing marked subcostal recession, and has an SaO_2 of 94% in air. He is thin and has some oral thrush. His chest X-ray (Fig. 43.3) shows bilateral interstitial shadowing.

Mum says Alexio has been in hospital on two or three occasions before and has had antibiotics, but has never really been back to normal. The history is vague and this is clearly a large chaotic family that includes three other older children who are well. Hospital notes show Alexio was admitted at the age of 7 months with an acute parotid abscess that responded rapidly to intravenous antibiotics, and again at 9 months with a left lower lobe pneumonia; this required oxygen and again responded to antibiotics, but it took about 5 days for his fever to settle and to start to improve. The boy seems to have gained little weight since then.

Q1. What is the differential diagnosis of Alexio's problem?

Q2. What, if any, underlying disorders will you want to look for? How will you seek them?

Q3. What other family and social history would be useful?

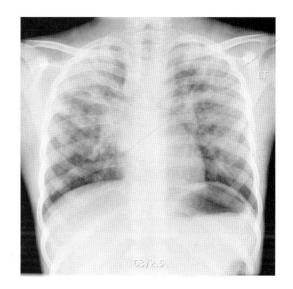

Fig. 43.3 Bilateral interstitial shadowing

Q1. What is the differential diagnosis of Alexio's problem?

In thinking of underlying causes of recurrent infection, the type of infection is important. Viral and fungal infections suggest problems with T-cell function, whereas bacterial infections may indicate humoral, neutrophil or complement defects. This boy has had two previous invasive bacterial infections, but now has candida and a pneumonitic chest X-ray picture, suggestive in this context of virus or *Pneumocystis carinii (jirovecii)* pneumonia (PCP). You would thus be thinking mainly of T-cell defects, though antibody and neutrophil problems could have been considered after the first two apparently bacterial infections (see Table 43.2 below).

Q2. What, if any, underlying disorders will you want to look for? How will you seek them?

See Table 43.2.

Table 43.2 Immune deficiencies

Type	Disease	Family history	Features
T-cell defect (always ask about consanguinity)	HIV (see text)	Maternal infection almost certain — antenatal screening completed?	
	Severe combined immune deficiency	Previous miscarriages or early infant deaths	Initial low lymphocyte counts — < 2.5 Absent T- and B-cell function Infections in first few months of life with viral, bacterial or fungal pathogens Death if untreated by bone marrow transplantation
	CD40 ligand deficiency (Hyper-IgM)	X-linked — previous infants or maternal male relatives	B cells produce IgM but unable to switch to IgG, IgA Neutropenia
	Di George syndrome	Microdeletion at chromosome 22q11.2	Congenital heart defect (tetralogy of Fallot), immunodeficiency (T-cell disorder) and hypocalcaemia Dysmorphic face, palatal abnormalities, autoimmune phenomena, renal anomalies, neuropsychiatric disorders and short stature
	Wiskott–Aldrich syndrome	X-linked: previous infants or maternal male relatives	Recurrent infection due to combined immunodeficiency, eczema, thrombocytopenia with small platelet volume Autoimmune haemolytic anaemia and malignancy increase with age
	Ataxia telangiectasia	Most cases are sporadic	Developmental delay, cerebellar ataxia, oculomotor apraxia, choreoathetosis, dystonias, progressive spinal muscular atrophy, progressive neurological deterioration T-cell lymphopenia/dysfunction/secondary poor antibody responses
	Common variable immune deficiency (CVID)	Some are AR, AD, XLR	Combined T- and B-cell deficiency Low serum level of IgG, IgA and possibly IgM Recurrent pyogenic infections of upper and lower respiratory tracts, persistent diarrhoea (*Giardia lamblia*) High incidence of autoimmune disorders Common genetic basis for CVID and selective IgA deficiency High risk of malignancy (lymphoma and GI carcinomas)
B cell defects	Selective IgA deficiency	Most cases occur sporadically but AR, AD or multifactorial pattern may occur Family history of CVID	Serum IgA low, other Ig levels normal The most common type of primary immune deficiency Usually asymptomatic but might be associated with recurrent sinopulmonary infections, allergy, GI disease, neurological disease, autoimmunity and malignancy
	X-linked agammaglobulinaemia (XLA, Bruton disease) See text	X-linked disease, family history of affected boys Maternal asymptomatic carrier New mutations common	Very low or absent IgG, IgM, IgA and IgE Recurrent otitis media, pneumonia and sinusitis before the age of 1 year with extracellular encapsulated bacteria, recurrent attacks of diarrhoea (*Giardia, Campylobacter*), chronic pulmonary disease, paucity of lymph nodes
Neutrophil defects	Severe congenital neutropenia (including Kostmann syndrome)	?AD form	Recurrent mouth ulcers and pyogenic infections (sinopulmonary and abscesses)
	Chronic granulomatous disease (see text)	X-linked form (similar problems in maternal male cousins) AR Mother may have symptoms of SLE	Symptoms suggestive of inflammatory bowel disease Previous abscesses, recurrent bacterial infections, fungal infections Clinical features indicative of cystic fibrosis (CF) but sweat test and CF mutation screen normal
	Shwachman–Diamond syndrome	AR	Neutropenia, pancreatic insufficiency, anaemia Recurrent bacterial infections, symptoms of malabsorption Short stature

(AR = autosomal recessive; AD = autosomal dominant; XLR = X-linked recessive; SLE = systemic lupus erythematosus)

BOX 43.2 Summary: transmission of HIV

You cannot contract HIV from:

- Kissing
- Touching
- Hugging
- Sneezing
- Coughing
- Toilet seats
- Cups, cutlery, sharing food

Q3. What other family and social history would be useful?

See Table 43.2.

Human immunodeficiency virus (HIV)

HIV is an enveloped RNA virus. There are two types: HIV-1 and HIV-2. HIV-1 is the most prevalent and therefore the most important. Up to 40% of the population are HIV-positive in some African countries. In 2006, 2.3 million children under the age of 15 years were living with HIV/AIDS and 380 000 died of AIDS worldwide. (See p. 511 for HIV in developing countries.)

Transmission (Box 43.2)

- Vertical: main route in children. Average risk of transmission is around 25%. Risk increases with:
  - Higher maternal HIV viral load
  - The presence of maternal sexually transmitted infections (STIs) or chorioamnionitis
  - Prolonged rupture of membranes
  - Prematurity
  - Breastfeeding
  - Risk of blood-to-blood contact, such as vaginal delivery or interventions (e.g. fetal scalp electrodes)
- Blood-to-blood: intravenous drug use, infected transfusions or contaminated injections
- Sexual contact: infected semen, vaginal secretions, oral sex (rarely).

Principles of prevention of mother-to-child transmission (MTCT) of HIV

- Provide good maternal antenatal care.
- Low maternal viral load: start maternal highly active antiretroviral therapy (HAART) in pregnancy, aiming for viral load < 50.
- Treat maternal STIs.
- Give intravenous AZT (zidovudine) to the mother just before and during delivery.
- Prescribe oral AZT for the baby for the first 4–6 weeks of life.

- Perform elective caesarean section (although vaginal delivery may be considered by some where all other risk factors are very good, i.e. viral load < 50, mother well).
- Avoid prolonged rupture of membranes.
- Bottle-feed the baby.

Diagnosis of HIV in an infant born to an HIV-positive mother

HIV antibody (IgG) is placentally transferred and so does not indicate neonatal infection, reflecting maternal status only.

HIV proviral DNA polymerase chain reaction (PCR) detects viral DNA and is a specific and sensitive marker of infection. However, at birth PCR is less sensitive, as infection may have only just been acquired and the viral load is very low. By 3 months sensitivity is > 99%. HIV infection is unlikely when there has been any of:

- Two negative PCRs, one after 3 months
- Two negative antibody tests if < 12 months
- One negative antibody test after 18 months.

Presentation

HIV infects and affects CD4 cells as well as macrophages and neuronal and glial cells, and steadily decreases CD4 counts. Hence opportunistic infections that require T-cell help for control are the hallmark of progressive infection, with falling CD4 counts. Clinical presentations of HIV disease in children are shown in Box 43.3. HIV itself can cause encephalopathy and failure to thrive (FTT). Untreated, about one-fifth of children progress rapidly to severe infection and death in the first few years of life; others progress more slowly and a few do not present with clinical features until their early teens.

BOX 43.3 Clinical presentations of paediatric HIV disease

- *Pneumocystis carinii* (*jirovecii*) pneumonia (PCP)
- *Candida* oesophagitis
- Cytomegalovirus (CMV)
- Atypical mycobacteria
- Cryptosporidiosis
- Toxoplasmosis
- Cryptococcal meningitis
- Recurrent bacterial infections
- Parotitis/parotid swelling
- HIV encephalopathy
- Neoplasms
- Wasting/failure to thrive (FTT)
- Lymphocytic interstitial pneumonitis (LIP)

Acquired immune deficiency syndrome (AIDS) is essentially HIV disease rather than infection. CD4 counts have decreased such that illness as either opportunistic infection or effects of HIV itself is found. Hence the CD4 count, as well as the amount of virus in the blood (HIV viral load), is important in disease progression. However, CD4 counts vary by age, with a peak for infants under 1 year; they have less variation when expressed as a percentage of total T-cell count.

The US Centers for Disease Control (CDC) have produced a classification for symptoms/signs and immune suppression using CD4 counts and percentages. Clinical categories range from N (non-symptomatic) to A (mildly symptomatic), B (moderately symptomatic) and C (severely symptomatic). Immune categories are simply no immunosuppression (CD4 > 25%), mild immunosuppression (15–25%) and severe immunosuppression (< 15%).

http://www.aidsmap.com/en/docs/289A9ABC-1D62-467E-924E-6B9D79789327.asp

Revised classification system for HIV infection in children less than 13 years of age

http://www.ctu.mrc.ac.uk/penta/
http://www.ctu.mrc.ac.uk/penta/hppmcs/calcProb.htm

A risk calculator for disease progression and death

Management

Treatment depends on combinations of at least two, and preferably three, elements of antiretroviral therapy (HAART). The aim is to decrease viral replication to an undetectable level and hence to increase CD4 count.

Combinations are chosen from three main categories: nucleoside transcriptase inhibitors, non-nucleoside transcriptase inhibitors and protease inhibitors.

Treatment decisions are made on viral load, CD4 percentage (count in older children and adults), and disease category as defined by CDC.

http://www.AIDSinfo.nih.gov
http://www.bhiva.org/chiva/

For information on HIV infection

Primary T cell defects

Children with primary immunodeficiencies of T lymphocytes may present with unusual or severe viral infections, unusual autoinflammatory disorders (which, although often triggered by infections, particularly viruses, frequently result from bystander damage of neural tissue) and also an increased propensity to primary lymphoma/lymphoproliferative disease (LPD). With LPD there is often an increased susceptibility to lymphotrophic herpes virus infections (e.g. Epstein–Barr virus, EBV).

Chronic granulomatous disorder (CGD)

This is a rare inherited immunodeficiency disorder of defective phagocytes. Incidence is about 1 in a million, with the male:female ratio being 4:1. About 80% are X-linked recessive; the rest are autosomal recessive.

Basic science

The underlying defect lies within phagocytes (neutrophils, monocytes, eosinophils and macrophages), which lack microbiocidal reactive oxidant superoxide anion, which is important for killing bacteria and fungi. This results in recurrent life-threatening bacterial and fungal infections and granuloma formation. Granulomas are a result of exuberant anomalous chronic inflammatory response to frequent infections; hence the name of the condition. Infections are commonly caused by catalase-producing microorganisms like *Staphylococcus*, *Serratia*, *Aspergillus*, *Burkholderia* and *Nocardia*.

Clinical features

Presentation is usually with unusual infections by 2 years of age (suppurative lymphadenitis, osteomyelitis, pneumonia, recurrent soft tissue infections, brain abscess, sepsis and hepatosplenomegaly with or without a liver abscess).

Granulomas can be symptomatic if they are causing gastrointestinal or genitourinary obstruction. Gastrointestinal symptoms are often prominent and inflammatory bowel disease with diarrhoea and FTT can be the sole presentation.

Maternal carriers may have features of autoimmune disease, including SLE.

Prenatal diagnosis for siblings of affected individuals could be achieved by DNA analysis, obtained by either chorionic villus biopsy or fetal blood sampling.

Diagnosis and significance

Diagnosis is based on observation of a pattern of recurrent atypical infections and tests to demonstrate the defective oxidative function in neutrophils:

1. *Nitro-blue tetrazolium (NBT) reduction.* This is used as a screening test and demonstrates oxidase activity of leucocytes during phagocytosis.
2. *Dihydroflavonol-4-reductase (DHR) reduction.* This is a flow cytometry test and shows fluorescent rhodamine in the presence of oxidative burst.

   These two tests also help in detecting carriers for CGD.
3. *Genetic tests.* Direct genetic tests can detect mutations and help find the nature of the genetic inheritance (XLR vs. AR).

Management

Early diagnosis, aggressive and prompt treatment of infection with prolonged high doses of antibiotics, aggressive search for an infectious agent, and antimicrobial and antifungal prophylaxis together with IFN-γ form the cornerstone of management. Haematopoietic stem cell transplant, from a human leucocyte antigen (HLA)-matched donor, is curative.

Prognosis

Overall prognosis has improved over the last 2 decades. Mortality rates are highest in childhood because of infections. However, most patients now live up to 20–25 years, with a mortality rate of 2–5% each year.

X-linked agammaglobulinaemia (XLA, Bruton disease)

Basic science

B cells fail to develop from B-cell precursors; hence immunoglobulin is not produced. A defective gene (*btk*) on the X chromosome codes for tyrosine kinase, which is essential for B-cell maturation.

Presentation

As maternal antibody (> 6 months) wanes, bacterial infections become common. Recurrent respiratory and ear infections are typical, with meningitis, bone and joint infections often seen, as are FTT and chronic diarrhoea. Chronic lung infection may lead to bronchiectasis. Interestingly, enteroviral infection may cause a chronic meningo-encephalitis. There is sometimes an association with growth hormone deficiency.

Management

Treatment is with immunoglobulin: either intravenous or subcutaneous. Immunoglobulin levels should be maintained well within the normal range, and prompt and prolonged antibiotic treatment should be given for infections.

Live oral polio vaccine should not be given, as virus may fail to clear.

Fever and rash

Causative organisms

Viruses

Viruses are very small (10–400 nm), have a simple acellular organization consisting of one or more molecules of DNA or RNA enclosed in a coat of protein, and are obligate intracellular parasites (Box 43.4). The

---

BOX 43.4 Virus classification	
The DNA viruses	
Herpesviridae family	Varicella zoster virus (VZV), Herpes simplex virus (HSV), Human herpes virus 6 (HHV 6), Cytomegalovirus (CMV), Epstein–Barr virus (EBV)
Adenoviridae	Adenovirus
Poxviridae	Molluscum
Parvoviridae	Erythrovirus 19 (parvovirus B19)
Hepadnaviridae	Hepatitis B virus (HBV)
The RNA viruses	
Astroviridae	Astrovirus
Caliciviridae	Small round structured virus (SRSV), norovirus (Norwalk virus)
Picornaviruses	Poliovirus, Coxsackie A and B, rhinovirus, hepatitis A virus (HAV), echovirus
Paramyxoviridae	Measles virus, mumps virus, respiratory syncytial virus (RSV), parainfluenza virus
Orthomyxoviridae	Influenza virus
Retroviridae	Retrovirus, human immunodeficiency virus (HIV)
Filoviridae	Ebola virus
Reoviridae	Rotavirus
Flaviviridae	Dengue virus, hepatitis C virus (HCV), Japanese encephalitis (JE) virus

---

genome (DNA or RNA) codes for the few proteins necessary for replication.

Bacteria

Staphylococci

- Staphylococci live on the skin and mucous membranes (nose) of humans.
- *Staphylococcus aureus* is an important pathogen but can be a skin commensal, as can *Staph. epidermidis*.
- *Staph. aureus* is a Gram-positive β-haemolytic facultative coagulase- and catalase-positive coccus. It may occur singly or be grouped in pairs, short chains or grape-like clusters.

Diseases caused by staphylococci include:
- *Skin infections*: abscess, impetigo, cellulitis
- *Invasive infections*: septicaemia, osteomyelitis, pyelonephritis

- *Toxin-mediated infections*: food poisoning, toxic shock, staphylococcal scalded skin syndrome.

Streptococci

- Streptococci that cause human disease are usually facultative anaerobes, are Gram-positive cocci, either spherical or ovoid in shape, and tend to form chains with each other.
- They are classified into subtypes based on sugar chains expressed on their outer shell (Lancefield group) and their behaviour when grown in the laboratory (α- or β-haemolysis).
- Most streptococci important in rashes or skin infections belong to the Lancefield groups A (*Streptococcus pyogenes*), C and G, and are β-haemolytic.
- *Strep. pneumoniae* (pneumococci) are important bacteria in sepsis, pneumonia and meningitis but rarely cause skin rashes. Pneumococci are α-haemolytic and do not belong to the Lancefield groups.
- Group B streptococci (also known as *Strep. agalactiae*) are important pathogens in the neonate.

Superantigens

Superantigens are proteins (toxins) that bind non-specifically to T-cell receptors (TCR) and MCH class II molecules on antigen-presenting cells (APCs), bypassing the normal peptide groove and hence activating large numbers of T-lymphocytes. Between 5% and 30% of the entire T-cell population may be activated (Fig. 43.4).

Superantigens lead to a massive release of cytokines, especially TNF-α, IL-1 and IL-6. These cytokines are responsible for a capillary leak syndrome and account for many of the clinical signs of toxic shock syndrome (TSS).

Problem-orientated topic:

fever and rash ● ● ● ● ●

Rodrigo, a 4-year-old boy, is seen in the accident and emergency department. He has been unwell for the preceding 4 days, being pyrexial with headaches, aches and swollen glands, and is sleepy and tired most of the time. He has lost some weight and missed nursery school. An antibiotic (amoxicillin) was prescribed by his primary care physician yesterday and a fine rash developed afterwards. On examination there is an erythematous non-itchy maculopapular rash all over his body, his temperature is

39°C and large swollen bilateral posterior cervical lymph nodes are palpable, as is a 3 cm spleen.

Q1. What are the most likely diagnoses?

Q1. What are the most likely diagnoses?

Clearly there are many causes of fever and rash in childhood to be considered when confronted with a history as outlined above. Viruses are most common, but some bacteria such as *Strep. pyogenes* (group A streptococcus), *Staph. aureus* or *Mycoplasma* cause erythematous rashes, as do inflammatory processes such as Kawasaki disease.

Rodrigo's symptoms could be due to:
- Infection
- Inflammation: Kawasaki disease (p. 642), juvenile idiopathic arthritis (p. 451)
- Autoimmune disorders (p. 639)
- Malignancy (Ch. 50)
- Drugs: especially antibiotics (Ch. 10).

Infective causes are summarized in Tables 43.3 and 43.4. Rarer causes include meningococcal sepsis, Lyme disease (common in the New Forest and Scotland) and leptospirosis.

Infectious mononucleosis (glandular fever; Epstein–Barr virus, EBV)

Incubation period is 30–50 days. Respiratory transmission is through saliva, coughing and sneezing.

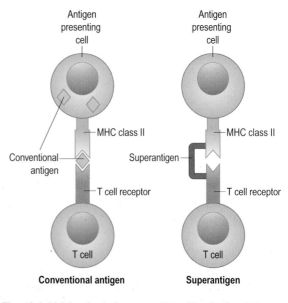

Fig. 43.4 **Mechanism of superantigen T-cell stimulation (MHC = major histocompatibility complex)**

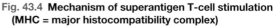

Table 43.3 Other viral causes of fever and rash

Disease	Virus	Clinical features
Adenovirus	Adenovirus	Different serotypes cause either GI (40, 41) or respiratory disease Fever, purulent conjunctivitis, erythematous rash, respiratory symptoms Associated with bronchiolitis obliterans
Cytomegalovirus (CMV)	CMV	Can cause glandular fever-like illness
Erythema infectiosum (slapped cheek/Fifth disease)	Erythrovirus 19 (parvovirus B19)	Fever, sore throat, GI symptoms, lymphadenopathy, bright erythematous macular rash on face (slapped cheek), lacy reticular rash spreading to rest of the body Complications include arthropathy and marrow aplasia
Roseola infantum (exanthema subitum/Sixth disease)	Human herpes virus 6 (or 7)	Infants, young children High fever for 3–6 days; fever drops and child is better then small red/pink flat raised lesions appear on trunk then extremities Associated with febrile convulsions
Herpangina	Coxsackie virus (A1–10, 16, 22), enterovirus	Fever with small vesicles or ulcers on the posterior oropharynx, cervical lymphadenopathy, anorexia and sometimes macular, papular or vesicular rash
Hand, foot and mouth disease	Coxsackie virus (A16), enterovirus	Fever, blisters to the mouth, tongue, hands and feet Resolves spontaneously, rarely severe
Gingivostomatitis	Herpes simplex virus	

Table 43.4 Other non-viral infective causes of fever and rash

Disease	Pathogen	Clinical features
Scarlet fever	Group A streptococcus (*Strep. pyogenes*)	Throat infection with streptococci producing exotoxin Tonsillitis with an erythematous fine punctate rash, which characteristically has a sandpaper texture, initially on the trunk but spreading rapidly Other features are glossal inflammation with prominent papillae, a strawberry tongue and circumoral pallor, with rash sparing the skin around the mouth There is often desquamation of the fingers and toes on resolution
Staphylococcal scalded skin syndrome	*Staph. aureus*	Caused by exotoxins in young children, particularly neonates and immunocompromised individuals Initially fever, irritability and widespread redness of skin; within 24–48 hr fluid-filled blisters form Rash spreads all over the body and the top layer of skin peels off in sheets, leaving exposed moist red and tender area (Nikolsky sign) Fluid and pain management essential

Clinical features

These include fever, fatigue, 'flu-like symptoms, sore throat, swollen tonsils, enlarged lymph nodes (cervical, epitrochlear), palatal petechiae, maculopapular rash, eyelid oedema and hepatosplenomegaly. A florid erythematous macular rash is often seen after ampicillin/amoxicillin has been given.

Complications

Complications include chronic fatigue, 0.1–0.5% splenic rupture, hepatitis, jaundice, anaemia, meningoencephalitis and Guillain–Barré syndrome.

Diagnosis

Diagnosis is by Monospot and Paul–Bunnell reaction (detects heterophile antibody, not sensitive), EBV IgM (or early antigen IgG) antibody titre, EBV PCR and viral culture from throat swab.

Management

Treatment is non-specific and is based on supportive medical care, e.g. analgesia. Steroids and aciclovir are of limited use. Treatment may be surgical in case of organ rupture.

Chickenpox (varicella)

See Ch. 23.

Toxic shock syndrome (TSS)

This is a 'superantigen' disease with fever, hypotension, rash, vomiting and multi-organ failure from toxin-producing *Staph. aureus* or *Strep. pyogenes*. Delay in recognizing the early signs of TSS is associated with increased morbidity and mortality, which may be as high as 15%.

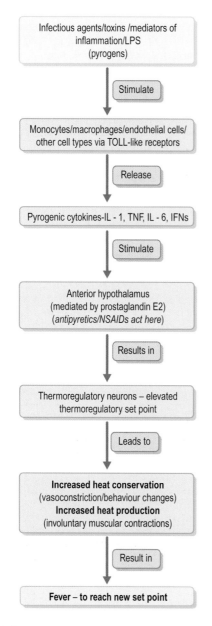

Fig. 43.5 Pathophysiology of fever
(LPS = lipopolysaccharide; IL = interleukin; TNF = tumour necrosis factor; IFN = interferon; NSAIDs = non-steroidal anti-inflammatory drugs)

http://www.emedicine.com/MED/topic2292.htm

Information and case definitions for TSS

Prolonged fever: pyrexia of unknown origin

Basic science of fever (Fig. 43.5)

- Fever is 'a state of elevated core temperature, which is often, but not necessarily, part of the defensive responses of multicellular organisms (host) to the invasion of live (microorganisms) or inanimate matter recognized as pathogenic or alien by its host'.
- Thermoregulation is controlled by a centre within the hypothalamus. Normal body temperature is around 37°C but varies with age, time of day (increasing in the late afternoon) and activity.
- Core temperature is best measured rectally; oral measurement is an alternative. Axillary and tympanic measurement are other possibilities but temperature here may be variable and is usually 0.5–1°C lower than rectal temperature.
- High temperature may inhibit viral replication and virulence, and enhance phagocytosis, interferon production and leucocyte migration.

Problem-orientated topic:

prolonged fever ● ● ● ● ●

An 11-year-old boy, Martim, presents to the casualty department with a 10-week history of intermittent fever, night sweats, lethargy, muscle aches and pains, anorexia and possibly some weight loss, though this is not obvious. He has had no cough and is not breathless but feels he does get out of breath playing football.

He is an asylum seeker recently arrived from the Congo and is one of six children ranging from 2 to 16 years old. Mum is a single parent, is pregnant again (now 30 weeks) and thus has had a recent HIV test, which is negative; the rest of the family are well. Martim was immunized as a baby and has a BCG scar.

On examination his height is on the 25th centile for age and his weight is on the 9th centile. He is pale, is not jaundiced or clubbed, has cervical lymphadenopathy but none elsewhere, has a temperature of 38°C but does not look unwell. He has some scattered crepitations over all lung fields, and a liver edge and spleen tip can be felt.

Q1. What differential diagnoses can you think of?

Q2. How will you investigate these?

Table 43.5 Investigations and their significance in prolonged fever

History/examination	Possible diagnoses	Investigations
Travel abroad	Tuberculosis	Mantoux test; ≥ 10 mm induration
	Typhoid	Stool culture, blood culture
	Legionella infection	Urinary antigen, serology
	Brucellosis	Serology
	Viral haemorrhagic fever	Viral detection, serology
Mosquito bites abroad	Malaria	Thick and thin blood films
	Arbovirus infection: yellow fever, dengue	Viral detection, serology
Animal exposure	Toxoplasmosis	Serology
	Leptospirosis	Urinary antigen, serology
	Q fever (*Coxiella*)	Serology
	Cat scratch disease	Serology (*Bartonella henselae*)
Conjunctivitis	Kawasaki disease	Serology to exclude other diagnoses
	Measles	Measles IgM
	Adenovirus infection	Serology (blood PCR)
Rigors, high swinging fever	Septicaemia	Blood culture and PCR
	Malaria	Thick and thin blood films
	Brucellosis	Serology
	Abscess	Pus aspiration; microscopy and culture
GI symptoms	*Giardia, Salmonella, Campylobacter* infection	Stool culture
	Inflammatory bowel disease	Barium enema, white cell scan
	Appendicitis, abscess	Ultrasound scan
Sore throat	Glandular fever	Serology (EBV IgM)
	CMV	Serology
	Tonsillitis	Throat swab (ASOT)
Lymphadenopathy	Glandular fever, CMV	Serology
	Tonsillitis	Throat swab (ASOT)
	Cat scratch disease	Serology (*Bartonella henselae*)
	Mycobacterial infection	Mantoux, IFN-γ blood test, tissue TB culture
	Toxoplasmosis, toxocariasis	Serology
	Hodgkin disease	Tissue histology
	Malignancy	Blood film, bone marrow, tissue histology
Respiratory	Pneumonia	CXR
	TB	CXR, Mantoux, IFN-γ blood test
ESR > 100	TB	CXR, Mantoux, IFN-γ blood test, autoantibodies
	Kawasaki	Blood film, bone marrow, tissue histology
	Autoimmune (JIA)	
	Malignancy	

(PCR = polymerase chain reaction; EBV = Epstein–Barr virus; CMV = cytomegalovirus; ASOT = antistreptolysin titre; IFN = interferon; TB = tuberculosis; ESR= erythrocyte sedimentation rate; CXR = chest X-ray; JIA = juvenile idiopathic arthritis)

Q1. What differential diagnoses can you think of?

- History is vital: fever pattern, when started, travel, immunization status (Table 43.5)
- Family history: genetic background (periodic fevers)
- Symptoms: pain to localize infection (bones, GI, respiratory)
- Signs: foci of infection
- If in doubt: admit patient to document fevers and pattern
- Do not start antibiotics until the patient is assessed.

Fever without focus and prolonged fever is often referred to as 'pyrexia (or fever) of unknown origin' (PUO). This is usually defined as fever over 38°C for more than 3 weeks with no cause identified even after 1 week's hospital assessment.

A fever continuing for more than 3 weeks is unusual in children. Causes are:
- Infective
- Malignant
- Autoimmune (Fig. 33.2)
- Factitious
- Undiagnosed.

Q2. How will you investigate these?

See Table 43.5.

Tuberculosis

Basic science

- TB is caused by *Mycobacterium tuberculosis* (MTB) and rarely by *M. bovis*.
- MTB is usually inhaled and so first lodges and begins to multiply in the lungs (known as the Ghon or primary focus).
- Bacilli are then carried to regional lymph nodes, where non-specific immunity controls infection and prevents dissemination. After a period of 4–8 weeks, cell-mediated immunity either:
    - Eradicates the infection
    - *Or* walls it off to an asymptomatic focus (latent TB infection)
    - *Or* fails to control it and mycobacteria replicate to produce TB disease.
- The primary focus and the infected regional lymph node together make the primary complex.
- During the formation of this primary complex and for some months later, bacilli may escape intermittently into the blood stream and may lodge anywhere in the body, but particularly in the central nervous system, bones or kidneys.
- If circumstances favour the organism rather than the host — for example, in a young child or if nutrition is poor — then haematogenous disease occurs either as a localized lesion or multiple lesions (miliary disease).

Transmission

- TB is spread by airborne particles that contain *M. tuberculosis*.
- These particles are expelled when a person with infectious TB coughs or sneezes.
- Higher infectivity is associated with cavitatory disease, laryngeal TB and frequent cough.
- Children rarely form cavities and have poor tussive force; they are therefore rarely infectious.
- Close contact is the most important risk factor for acquiring infection.
- Persons with latent TB infection but no disease are not infectious.

Natural history of TB infection (Fig. 43.6)

Primary infection before 2 years of age may progress to serious disease (including miliary or disseminated) within the first 12 months without significant prior symptoms. Primary infection between 2 and 10 years of age generally produces significant symptoms but rarely progresses to serious disease. Primary infection after 10 years of age often produces adult-type disease.

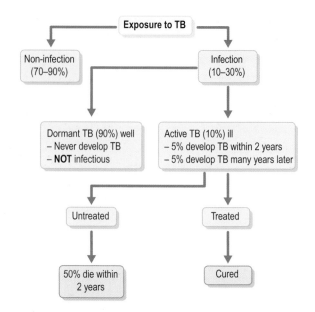

Fig. 43.6 **The natural history of tuberculosis infection**

Clinical features of TB

- May be non-specific, especially in young children
- Fever
- FTT or weight loss
- Lethargy
- Poor feeding
- Cough
- Night sweats
- Lymphadenopathy
- Pleural effusion
- Hepatosplenomegaly
- History of headache, vomiting and drowsiness lasting several weeks
- Erythema nodosum
- Phlyctenular conjunctivitis
- Choroidal tubercles.

Diagnosis of TB in children

TB should be suspected when two of the following are present and is likely when three are present:
- Positive Mantoux test (Box 43.5)
- Clinical findings compatible with TB
- History of contact with TB
- Suggestive CXR
- Positive histological findings from a tissue biopsy.

Positive culture of MTB from secretions or tissue biopsy on its own confirms the diagnosis.

BOX 43.5 Skill: Mantoux test

Perform and read an intradermal Mantoux test.

Table 43.6 Investigations and their significance in tuberculosis

Investigation	Significance
Mantoux	Skin test identifies tuberculin sensitivity Positive in TB, BCG and non-tuberculous mycobacterial infection Infection with TB usually taken as ≥ 6 mm without BCG, ≥ 15 mm with prior BCG using 2TU Mantoux (Danish SSI)
IFN-γ stimulation test (Quantiferon Gold or T SPOT TB)	Identifies an immune response to MTB (independent of BCG status), hence prior infection with MTB Does not distinguish latent infection from TB disease
CXR	Identifies focal lesions and mediastinal lymphadenopathy
Sputum, induced sputum, BAL	Respiratory specimens suitable for identification and culture of mycobacteria
Gastric aspirate	Early morning aspiration of gastric contents may identify swallowed acid-fast bacilli 30% yield
TB smear	The older Ziehl–Neelsen stain is now being superseded by auramine stains in TB reference labs, giving higher sensitivity for smear-positive diagnoses
TB culture	Developments have also progressed in TB culture with rapid liquid culture and gene probes decreasing time to positive culture result from 6 weeks to 2–3 weeks
PCR	The sensitivity of PCR for detecting *M. tuberculosis* in CSF of patients with TBM is reported in recent studies as between 33% and 93%
Contact tracing	If no known TB contact, then screening close contacts may be helpful diagnostically, as finding active pulmonary TB suggests the diagnosis in the child
ESR, CRP	Often elevated, but non-specific markers of inflammation

(BCG = Bacille Calmette–Guérin; MTB = *Mycobacterium tuberculosis*; IFN = interferon; BAL = bronchoalveolar lavage; PCR = polymerase chain reaction; ESR = erythrocyte sedimentation rate; CRP = C-reactive protein)

Investigations
See Table 43.6.

Management
See Box 43.6.

http://www.nice.org.uk/page.aspx?o=CG033N
ICEguideline

Guideline on tuberculosis

BOX 43.6 Principles of management of tuberculosis

- NICE guidelines (2005) suggest quadruple therapy:
  - Isoniazid
  - Rifampicin
  - Pyrazinamide
  - Ethambutol
  for adults and children as standard *unless* they are Caucasian, with no travel or high-risk behaviour, in which case initial therapy is triple (minus ethambutol)
- 6 months of treatment includes 2 months of triple or quadruple and 4 months of isoniazid only. TB meningitis requires 12 months in total
- Treatment must be taken regularly; if there is doubt about compliance, it can be directly observed (DOT)
- Contact tracing is central to the control of TB
- Prevention: BCG vaccination for neonates at high risk of TB

Malaria

There are four species of the protozoan parasite *Plasmodium*: *falciparum, vivax, ovale* and *malariae*:

- Human reservoir, transmitted by the bite of the female *Anopheles* mosquito
- Imported to European countries after travel to tropics or subtropics
- *P. falciparum* more likely in travellers from Africa, *P. vivax* in those from South Asia
- First symptoms usually 10 days to 4 weeks after transmission.

The life cycle of the parasite in the human phase is shown in Figure 43.7.

Clinical features
- Fever
- Influenza-like symptoms: headache, myalgia, rigors, cough, diarrhoea, vomiting
- Splenomegaly, thrombocytopenia, anaemia, jaundice, but these may be absent
- Decreased conscious level
- Seizures
- Shock.

Diagnosis and investigations
- Microscopy of thick and thin blood films: three films 12 hours apart
- Rapid diagnostic tests: dipsticks for malaria antigen
- Full blood count

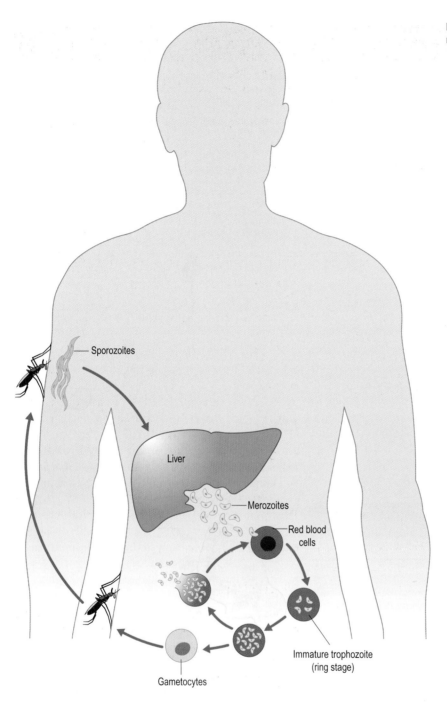

Fig. 43.7 **Human stages of the malaria parasite**

Sporozoites

Liver

Merozoites

Red blood cells

Immature trophozoite (ring stage)

Gametocytes

- Urea and electrolytes
- Liver function tests
- Blood glucose.

Management

- Depends on type and severity.
- Check glucose-6-phosphate dehydrogenase (G6PD) status.
- *P. vivax, ovale, malariae*:
  - Oral chloroquine for 3 days then oral primaquine for 14–21 days.
- *P. falciparum*:
  - Oral proguanil with atovaquone (Malarone)/ mefloquine/artemether with lumefantrine
  - Oral or intravenous quinine.

Prevention is better than cure. Advise prophylaxis and avoidance of mosquito bites (cover up with clothes, use impregnated mosquito nets) when travel is planned to endemic areas.

Kawasaki disease (KD)

This is an acute, self-limiting vasculitis occurring predominantly in infants and young children.

Aetiology

- Infectious agent (young age, winter seasonality, epidemicity) but still no specific organism identified
- Superantigen-mediated (vβ4 and vβ8 family expansion)
- Immune perturbation: marked cytokine cascade and endothelial cell activation.

Clinical features

There is a sudden-onset high spiking fever, with malaise and irritability (Box 43.7).

KD is also associated with other non-specific features, such as arthritis, nausea, vomiting, diarrhoea, abdominal pain, extreme irritability, aseptic meningitis and urethritis.

Coronary artery aneurysms are the most serious complication, with possible long-term morbidity and mortality.

Investigations

See Box 43.8.

Management

- Aspirin 80–100 mg/kg/day in four divided doses
- IV Ig infusion 2 g/kg in a single infusion
- Aspirin reduced to 3–5 mg/kg/day after fever settled for > 48 hours and continued until absence of coronary abnormalities by 6–8 weeks after the onset is confirmed.

Severe infection

Septicaemia

Structural components of microorganisms such as lipopolysaccharide (LPS, endotoxin) in Gram-negative bacteria and the cell wall fragments (teichoic acid) of Gram-positive bacteria or the exotoxins synthesized by them have been shown to be potent activators of a wide range of cells. These include monocytes/macrophages, neutrophils and endothelial cells. These cells release proinflammatory mediators that activate complement and coagulation, hence producing endothelial damage and capillary leak.

Inflammation is essential for host defence. Unfortunately excessive inflammatory reactions, as occur in septic shock, are detrimental. This is illustrated in Figure 43.8.

Meningitis

Meningitis is an inflammation of the meninges, the membranes that cover the brain and spinal cord. This inflammation is usually caused by bacteria, viruses or fungi (Table 43.7).

Access to the CNS is gained by:

- The blood stream (the most common mode of spread)
- A retrograde neuronal pathway (some viruses)
- Direct contiguous spread, e.g. sinusitis, otitis media, congenital malformations, trauma.

Bacteria are frequent nasopharyngeal colonizers of young children and this is a prerequisite for invasion. Host factors such as local secretory immunity (IgA), integument lesions (picked nose!) and intercurrent viral infections, as well as microbial 'virulence' where certain strains attach to mucosa more strongly, all contribute to bacterial invasion. Once in the blood stream bacteria disseminate and may attach to cerebral endothelium or

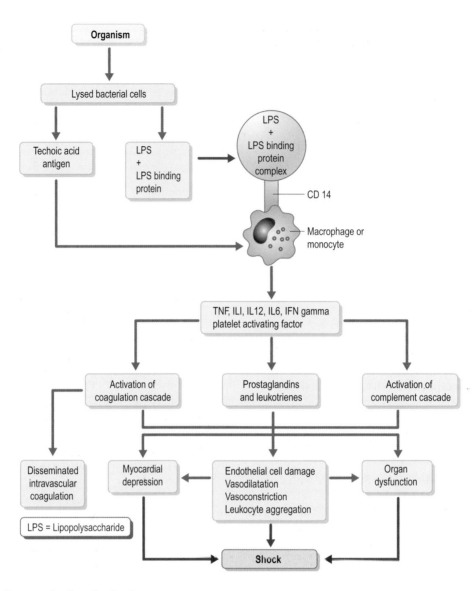

**Fig. 43.8 Pathogenesis of septic shock
(LPS = lipopolysaccharide)**

choroid plexus. The systemic inflammatory response includes IL-1 and TNF secretion, stimulating vascular endothelial cells and breaking down the tight junctions within the blood–brain barrier (BBB), making this permeable to larger molecules such as white cells, IgG and organisms. Once breached, white cells, inflammatory cells, organisms within the CSF and resident microglia continue the cytokine cascade with platelet activating factor (PAF), complement, prostaglandin and leuco-trienes. This continues to make the BBB permeable and increases vasculitis, oedema, CSF outflow and intracranial pressure.

This systemic inflammatory response accounts for many of the clinical symptoms and signs, and acute and long-term neurological morbidity and mortality.

Actual neuronal injury and death are also primarily due to an immunological response.

Brain oedema contributes to high intracranial pressure; consequently low cerebral blood flow occurs, resulting in anaerobic metabolism and low CSF glucose, which also stems from decreased glucose transport into the spinal fluid.

Aseptic meningitis

Aseptic meningitis is a non-pyogenic cellular response, which may be caused by many different aetiological agents. The most common cause are viruses such as enteroviruses, CMV, EBV, VZV, HSV 1 and 2, HHV6, mumps and measles.

Table 43.7 Characteristics of the three most common bacterial agents

Bacterial agent	Description
Streptococcus pneumoniae	Gram-positive coccus, common colonizer of the human nasopharynx (20–40% of healthy children) The most common overall cause of invasive bacterial sepsis, meningitis and pneumonia Conjugate vaccines covering seven to thirteen serotypes effective in young children
Neisseria meningitidis	Gram-negative diplococcus, carried in the nasopharynx of otherwise healthy individuals Groups A, B, C, W135 and Y most frequently pathogenic, with B and C most common in Europe Polysaccharide vaccine available for A, C, W135, Y, and a conjugate C vaccine for young children is now in the primary immunization schedule People with deficiencies in terminal complement components are at risk of recurrent infection
Haemophilus influenzae type B	Small Gram-negative coccobacillus, normal flora in the upper respiratory tract Before the introduction of the HiB vaccine it was the most common cause of invasive bacterial disease, meningitis and epiglottitis in children under 5 years. Since HiB vaccine introduced, carriage rates have decreased

Problem-orientated topic:

acute fever, no focus ●●●●●

Tatiana, a 9-month-old girl, presents to casualty with a history of fever, vomiting and loose stools over the last 3 days. She had a brief convulsion just before arrival at the hospital in the form of a generalized clonic seizure with uprolling of the eyes, which settled spontaneously. Mum feels that the child has not been herself for the last few days and seems irritable most of the time.

On examination Tatiana is febrile at 39°C, drowsy and irritable but had appropriate reactions on being handled, is mildly dehydrated and has cool peripheries. Her throat is slightly inflamed.

Q1. What are the most important differential diagnoses?

Q2. What examination findings and observations would you like to establish immediately?

Q3. Management will depend on cause. What is the management of these conditions?

Q1. What are the most important differential diagnoses?

This little girl appears acutely unwell with a fever but no obvious source of infection is described. Clearly you will be most concerned about bacterial infection causing septic shock and meningitis. However, a young child requires careful assessment then investigation for an initially unapparent focus.

Q2. What examination findings and observations would you like to establish immediately?

Look for a focus:
- Ears: otitis media, mastoiditis
- Throat: tonsillitis, epiglottitis, glandular fever, quinsy
- Mouth: hand, foot, mouth (Coxsackie), gingivostomatitis (herpes simplex), membrane (diphtheria)
- Skin: impetigo, cellulitis, abscess
- Chest: bronchiolitis, upper respiratory tract infection, pneumonia, influenza
- Abdomen: appendicitis, perforation, abscess
- Bone or joint: osteomyelitis, septic arthritis
- Blood: septicaemia, toxic shock, acute viraemia
- Renal: urinary tract infection, pyelonephritis
- Gastrointestinal tract: gastroenteritis, viral or bacterial
- Central nervous system: meningitis, encephalitis, brain abscess.

Clinical features
- Fever, headache, neck stiffness, photophobia, nausea, vomiting and signs of cerebral dysfunction (e.g. lethargy, confusion, coma)
- Cranial nerves palsies, focal neurological signs, seizures and papilloedema.

Symptoms depend on the age of the patient; younger children may not have meningism (Box 43.9).

Investigations in acute fever with no apparent focus
See Table 43.8.

Investigations in suspected meningitis
Brain computed tomography (CT) or magnetic resonance imagining (MRI) is indicated if there are focal

BOX 43.9 Detecting signs of meningeal irritation

Kernig sign

- In a supine patient, flex the hip to 90° while the knee is flexed at 90°. An attempt to extend the knee further produces pain in the hamstrings and resistance to further extension

Brudzinski sign

- Passively flex the neck while the patient is in a supine position with extremities extended. This manoeuvre produces flexion of the hips in patients with meningeal irritation

Neck stiffness

- Resistance to passive neck flexion

BOX 43.10 Findings and their significance in septicaemia and septic shock

Fever	Increasing
Tachycardia	severity
Tachypnoea	Decreasing intravascular
Cool peripheries (toe: core temperature > 3°C)	volume
	Acidosis
Prolonged capillary refill (> 3 seconds)	Electrolyte and glucose loss
Poor urine output	Disseminated
Irritability, restlessness, confusion	intravascular coagulation
	Multi-organ failure
Deteriorating conscious level	
Hypoxia	
Hypotension (late sign)	

neurological signs, signs of raised intracranial pressure (ICP) or prolonged fever. These are helpful in the detection of CNS complications of bacterial meningitis, such as hydrocephalus, cerebral infarct, brain abscess, subdural empyema and venous sinus thrombosis.

Diagnosis is only definitively made by lumbar puncture (Ch. 12). Findings are interpreted in Table 43.9.

Q3. Management will depend on cause. What is the management of these conditions?

General management

- Airway.
- Breathing.

- Circulation: fluid resuscitation where there are signs of capillary leak and decreased intravascular volume (sepsis; Box 43.10).
- Dexamethasone: improves neurological outcome when given before or with first dose of antibiotics in *H. influenzae* B and *Strep. pneumoniae* meningitis. Neurological outcome in meningococcal meningitis is generally good and the benefit of dexamethasone is not proven. Its use in meningococcal meningitis is therefore still debated; some experts recommend it, some do not.
- Antibiotics (Table 43.10).

Table 43.8 Investigations and their significance in acute fever with no apparent focus

Investigation	Significance
Urine dipstick/microscopy	Nitrites, leucocytes; white cells, organisms seen — urinary tract infection
CXR	Consolidation, collapse, effusion — lower respiratory tract infection
Neutrophil count	Raised in bacterial infection, low in severe sepsis
Lymphocyte count	Raised or 'atypical' in viral infection
Platelet count	Raised in longstanding inflammation, low in severe sepsis
CRP	Raised suggests bacterial infection or adenovirus
ESR	Raised suggests bacterial infection or inflammation
Blood culture	Bacteria or fungi grown from blood
PCR	Detection of bacterial or viral genomic material in blood indicates infection (*Strep. pneumoniae*, *N. meningitidis*, herpes simplex virus, enterovirus)
Immunofluorescence or PCR of nasopharyngeal secretions (or sputum)	Detection of respiratory tract viruses, e.g. respiratory syncytial virus, influenza A and B, adenovirus, indicates infection
Culture of nasopharyngeal secretions (or sputum)	Detection of bacteria or fungi — may be infection or commensal
Serology	Detection of IgM or four-fold rise in IgG on paired samples suggests infection
Lumbar puncture	Glucose, protein, cells, organisms seen or cultured — meningitis

Table 43.9 Lumbar puncture and its significance

Condition	Leucocytes (mm³)	Protein (g/l)	Glucose (mmol/l)	Comments
Normal	< 5 ≥ 75% lymphocytes	0.2–0.45	> 5 (or 75% serum glucose)	
Acute bacterial meningitis	100–10 000 or more; usually 300–2000 PMNs predominate	1–5	Decreased, usually < 4 (or < 66% serum glucose)	Organisms may be seen on Gram stain and recovered by culture Latex agglutination of CSF may be positive
Partially treated bacterial meningitis	5–10 000 PMNs usual but mononuclear cells may predominate if pretreated for extended period of time	1–5	Normal or decreased	Organisms may be seen on Gram stain Latex agglutination of CSF may be positive Pretreatment may render CSF sterile
Viral meningitis or meningo-encephalitis	Rarely > 1000 cells PMNs early but mononuclear cells predominate through most of the course	0.5–2.0	Generally normal; may be decreased to < 4 in some viral diseases, particularly mumps (15–20% of cases)	Herpes simplex virus (HSV) encephalitis is suggested by focal seizures or by focal findings on CT, MRI or EEG HSV and enteroviruses may be detected by PCR of CSF
Brain abscess	5–200 CSF lymphocytes may predominate If abscess ruptures into ventricle, PMNs predominate and cell count may reach > 100 000	0.75–5	Normal unless abscess ruptures into ventricular system	No organisms on smear or culture unless abscess ruptures into ventricular system

(PMNs = polymorphonuclear leucocytes)

Table 43.10 Antibiotics and suggested duration of therapy for acute bacterial meningitis

Patient	Medication	Organism	Days of treatment
Neonate	Cefotaxime/ceftriaxone + Amoxicillin ± Gentamicin	Group B streptococcus (GBS) Escherichia coli Listeria monocytogenes	14 21 21
Infant (1–3 months)	Cefotaxime/ceftriaxone ± Amoxicillin	GBS E. coli Strep. pneumoniae H. influenzae B N. meningitidis	14 21 10–14 7–10 7
Child	Cefotaxime/ceftriaxone ± Dexamethasone	Strep. pneumoniae H. influenzae B N. meningitidis	10–14 7–10 7
Resistant pneumococcus possible	Cefotaxime/ceftriaxone + Vancomycin/rifampicin		10–14
HSV suspected	Aciclovir		21

Chemoprophylaxis

Prevention of secondary cases by eradication of nasal carriage is effective for infections with HiB and *N. meningitidis*. Rifampicin is offered to the index case and:

- All close contacts with *N. meningitidis*: rifampicin 10 mg/kg/day × 2 days or a single injection of ceftriaxone
- Only those contacts under 5 years for HiB: rifampicin 20 mg/kg/day × 4 days.

Complications

- Extent depends on the infecting pathogen. HiB and *Strep. pneumoniae* have poorer neurological outcome than does *N. meningitidis*.

- Early complications include seizures, the development of venous sinus thrombosis, subdural empyema and brain abscess, obstructive hydrocephalus, cerebral infarction and brain parenchymal damage, cranial nerve palsies.
- Later complications include visual and hearing impairment (p. 436) and motor deficits; cerebral palsy, learning disabilities, mental retardation, cortical blindness, continued seizures.

http://www.meningitis.org

Go to health professionals then doctors in training

Herpes simplex virus (HSV) encephalitis

HSV is the most common treatable cause of encephalitis in Europe, causing direct inflammation of brain tissue.

Presentations of HSV infection
- Neonatal: skin, eye, mouth; encephalitis; disseminated
- Acute encephalitis
- Mild/subacute encephalitis
- Psychiatric syndromes
- Brainstem encephalitis
- Aseptic meningitis
- Benign recurrent meningitis
- Myelitis.

Diagnosis
- Clinical presentation
- CT: diffuse oedema initially, atrophy, parenchymal calcification or cystic encephalomalacia
- MRI: frontobasal and temporal lesions can be seen as hypointense lesions on T1 weighted images and hyperintense on T2 early in disease
- EEG: periodic high-voltage spike/wave activity and slow wave complexes
- CSF: white cell count 5–500, protein < 0.5, HSV PCR (for 1 and 2)
- HSV IgG, IgA, IgM (CSF and blood)
- Viral culture.

Management
Treatment is with aciclovir:
- 0–3 months 20 mg/kg/dose t.d.s.
- 3 months–12 years: 50 mg/m^2 every 8 hours
  There is no evidence for the use of steroids.

Tonsillitis (see also p. 440)

Fever, sore throat, cervical lymphadenopathy and enlarged inflamed tonsils often with exudates may be caused by:
- Adenovirus
- Enterovirus
- EBV
- Group A streptococcus (GAS) (*Strep. pyogenes*)
- *Corynebacterium diphtheriae.*

Clinical examination cannot distinguish viral from bacterial causes. In primary care most sore throats are self-limiting and do not need antibiotics or throat swabs. Paracetamol or ibuprofen provides symptomatic relief. Those with severe symptoms and signs do improve more quickly with antibiotics, as do those with proven GAS infection. Penicillin V, amoxicillin (or erythromycin) for 10 days is suggested.

Complications of bacterial (GAS) tonsillitis include:
- Cervical abscess
- Scarlet fever: pharyngitis, erythematous 'sandpaper' rash, strawberry tongue
- Rheumatic fever: following tonsillitis.

Influenza

- Caused by an RNA virus. Influenza A and B circulate within Europe. The antigenic structure changes slightly each year; hence new vaccines are produced each year.
- Respiratory pathogen: fever, headache, aches and pains, coryza, sore throat, cough.
- Can cause myositis, pneumonia or sepsis, especially in infants.
- Secondary bacterial infection common: otitis media, pneumonia.
- Diagnosis by antigen detection (immunofluorescence or immunochromatography) or viral nucleic acid detection (PCR) in nasopharyngeal secretions, virus culture or serology.
- Zanamivir and oseltamivir decrease severity and duration of symptoms from influenza A or B by 1 day. Oseltamivir is 60–90% effective in preventing illness from influenza when used prophylactically.

Allergy

Basic science

Atopy

Atopy nowadays describes a hereditary predisposition to produce IgE antibody against common environmental allergens in a type 1 hypersensitivity reaction (Fig. 43.9). In sensitized individuals contact with allergen may result in respiratory, cardiovascular, mucocutaneous and gastrointestinal manifestations, and when severe can be life-threatening (anaphylaxis).

Anaphylactoid reactions are identical to anaphylaxis other than not being IgE-mediated, e.g. reactions to radio contrast media, non-steroidal anti-inflammatory drugs (NSAIDs) etc.

Immunological responses to allergens

Central to an allergic response is T-cell differentiation (Th2) to cells that produce appropriate stimulatory cytokines (IL-4) and promote class switching of antigen-specific B cells for the production of IgE.

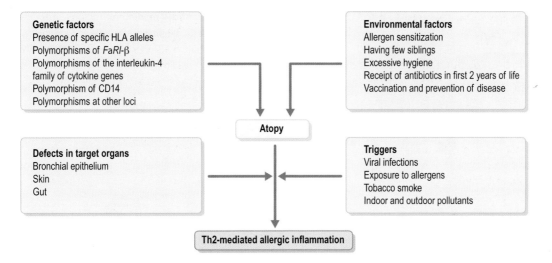

Genetic factors
Presence of specific HLA alleles
Polymorphisms of *FaRl*-β
Polymorphisms of the interleukin-4
family of cytokine genes
Polymorphism of CD14
Polymorphisms at other loci

Environmental factors
Allergen sensitization
Having few siblings
Excessive hygiene
Receipt of antibiotics in first 2 years of life
Vaccination and prevention of disease

Atopy

Defects in target organs
Bronchial epithelium
Skin
Gut

Triggers
Viral infections
Exposure to allergens
Tobacco smoke
Indoor and outdoor pollutants

Th2-mediated allergic inflammation

Fig. 43.9 Factors influencing the development of atopy
(HLA = human leucocyte antigen)

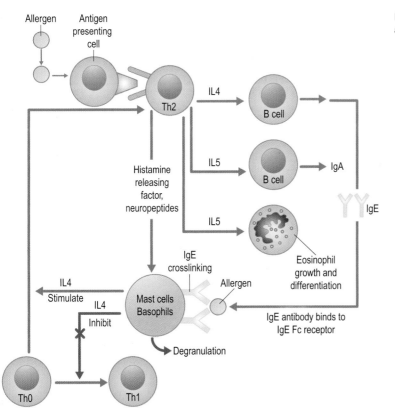

Fig. 43.10 Immunological response to allergens
(IL = interleukin)

When an allergen is encountered by an antigen-presenting cell (APC), it is taken up and carried from the periphery to T cells in the local lymph node. Depending on the amount of antigen, interaction of T cell with APC, relative production of IL-4, IL-12, IFN-γ and the presence of CpG (cytidine-phosphate-guanosine) repeats in the microbial DNA, differentiation to Th1 or Th2 occurs. Allergen is then presented to this Th2 cell via an allergen-specific B cell and this is stimulated to produce IgE antibody (Fig. 43.10).

These IgE-specific antibodies bind to IgE receptors on the surface of mast cells. On re-exposure to the same allergen, it will bind to two adjacent IgE molecules on the mast cell and basophils (cross-linking), leading to its degranulation and the release of pharmacological mediators inducing vasodilatation and inflammation (Fig. 43.11).

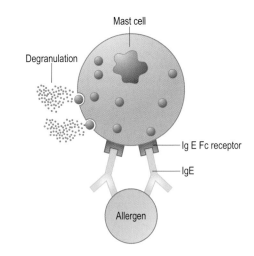

Fig. 43.11 **Type 1 hypersensitivity**

Cells and mediators

Mast cells

Mast cells are found mainly in the epithelial tissue of the respiratory and gastrointestinal tract, and of skin. They include preformed substances stored in granules of mast cells and basophils (histamine, tryptase, heparin, chymase and cytokines), or newly synthesized mediators, like derivatives of arachidonic acid metabolism (prostaglandins and leucotrienes). These are released on stimulation. They precipitate:

- Smooth muscle contraction
- Vasodilatation
- Increased vascular permeability
- Mucus hypersecretion.

Histamine is considered to be the prime mediator of anaphylactic shock through its binding to receptors.

Eosinophils

Eosinophilia is usually present in atopy. Granules contain proteins mediating:

- Damage to epithelial cells
- Degranulation of basophil and mast cells
- Airway hyper-responsiveness
- Blocking of muscarinic receptors, increasing acetylcholine and resulting in airway hyper-reaction.

Effects of mast cell mediators

See Table 43.11.

Late phase response

On exposure to allergens atopic people develop immediate hypersensitivity, which may, depending on the amount of allergen, be followed by a late phase reaction after 6–9 hours.

Eosinophils and neutrophils accumulate, then CD4 and basophils infiltrate. Depending on the target organ

Table 43.11 **Mast cell mediators**

Physiological effect	Clinical presentation	Potential complication

Capillary leak	Urticaria
	Angioedema
	    Cutaneous
	    Laryngeal
	Hypotension
		Respiratory arrest
		Shock

Mucosal oedema	Laryngeal oedema Asthma Rhinitis	Respiratory arrest Respiratory arrest
Smooth muscle contraction	Asthma Abdominal pain	Respiratory arrest

Table 43.12 **Immunological response**

Immediate type	Delayed type
Skin wheal and flare within minutes	Within hours
Nose sneezing, running nose	Sustained blockage
Chest wheezing	Further wheezing

involved, a late phase reaction can be provoked by a mast cell or T cell. If skin is involved mast cells provoke both immediate and late phases, while when lungs are involved T cells are responsible (Table 43.12).

Allergic rhinitis

Clinical features include sneezing, nasal congestion, stuffiness, rhinorrhoea, cough, itching of the nose, eyes and throat, sinus pressure and epistaxis. Rhinitis is induced by specific allergy, often pollen (seasonal rhinitis; hay fever), animals or house dust mite.

Symptoms and signs include large pale turbinates, nasal polyps, allergic salute, eosinophils in nasal smear, blood eosinophilia, raised IgE, and a positive blood IgE or skin prick test to allergen.

Management includes avoidance of allergens if known, oral and nasal antihistamines, nasal steroids, cromoglicate and oral steroids. Immunotherapy may be offered in specialist allergy centres and can be useful to control symptoms and to prevent progression to asthma.

Allergic asthma (see also pages 277–80)

In European children, the prevalence of asthma symptoms ranges from 5–21%. It is clinically characterized by recurrent wheezing, (sometimes persistent) cough and dyspnoea, totally or partially reversible by bronchodilator treatment. Most asthmatic children are atopic and most likely have eosinophilic inflammation and underlying bronchial hyperreactivity. Allergy plays a significant role both as a trigger of symptoms and as a predisposing factor for other triggers such as viral infections and physical exercise.

Long-term treatment includes allergen avoidance, bronchial anti-inflammatory treatment (inhaled steroids, cromones, inhibitors of leukotriene receptors), bronchodilators (short-acting β_2 agonists as rescue and sometimes long-acting β_2 agonists) and also allergen immunotherapy in selected cases. Many children outgrow their asthma, particularly in milder cases. With adequate management, most asthmatic children may lead a normal life, including participation in competitive sports at high level.

Problem-orientated topic:

atopy ● ● ● ● ●

Admon is a 6-year-old boy who has been referred by his primary care physician to the children's outpatient clinic with a history of recurrent episodes of 'nettle rash' (hives), which seem to appear after some meals and settle with antihistamine.

On reviewing his medical records it is noticed that he was admitted last year because of an acute attack of respiratory distress associated with difficulty breathing and cough but no rash. His chest examination on that admission revealed rhonchi bilaterally and diminished breath sounds; the CXR showed hyperinflation but no evidence of infection. He was treated with bronchodilators, oxygen and short-course steroids and made a good recovery.

He had eczema as a baby, but this has improved over the last few years and now he is troubled only with patches on flexor areas of his limbs.

Q1. How would you assess the cause of the rash?
Q2. What family and social history might be relevant?
Q3. What treatment could you offer?
Q4. How will you advise Admon and his parents about how to manage his diet?

Q1. How would you assess the cause of the rash?

Urticaria is a cutaneous vascular reaction characterized by sudden but transient appearance of erythematous wheals, often itchy. These usually disappear in 20 minutes to 3 hours but may continue for up to 48 hours. They are often described as nettle rash. Recurrent

Table 43.13 Urticaria

Type	Precipitant
Infectious	Follows infection; streptococci, Epstein–Barr virus, hepatitis A, B and C, enteroviruses, adenoviruses
Sting bites	Bee, wasp, scorpion, spider
Drugs and food	Peanuts, nuts, milk, eggs, wheat, fish Antibiotics
Physical	Cold, heat, pressure, sunlight or vibration
Papular	In contact with fleas or mites; usually toddlers; resolves in 6–12 months
Secondary to underlying systemic disease	Connective tissue, autoimmune, thyroid or coeliac disease
Idiopathic	Unknown precipitant; frequent

episodes for > 6 weeks indicate 'chronic urticaria' and may be associated with angioedema: local soft tissue swelling, most often of the face, eyelids, hands or feet.

Urticaria is caused by extravasation of plasma into the dermis, while angioedema is subcutaneous oedema resulting in deep swelling. Immunologically, it may be IgE-mediated (drugs/food/insect venom) but can also be non-IgE-mediated (infection, physical) (Table 43.13).

Q2. What family and social history might be relevant?

Children with IgE-mediated diseases are 'atopic'. There is often a family history of atopy. If one parent is atopic, the risk to the child is roughly 25%; if both parents are atopic, the risk rises to 50%. Atopic diseases include atopic dermatitis, asthma, hay fever and allergic rhinitis, urticaria and food allergies.

Q3. What treatment could you offer?

- Establishing the precipitant, if possible
- Avoidance of the allergens where possible
- Antihistamine as required for acute treatment or regularly for prevention (second generation long-acting); may use higher doses
- Steroids: local or systemic depending on the severity of the disease
- Chronic urticaria: combination of H_1-blockers with H_2-blockers or leucotriene antagonists may help.

Q4. How will you advise Admon and his parents about how to manage his diet?

Food allergy

The terms shown in Box 43.11 need to be considered and understood.

Adverse reactions to food consist of any abnormal reaction resulting from eating or swallowing even a tiny amount of a particular food (Fig. 43.12).

BOX 43.11 Food allergy: terminology

Food intolerance
- Non-allergic food hypersensitivities include any physiological response such as metabolic disorders, e.g. lactose intolerance, coeliac disease, dietary protein enterocolitis

Food allergy
- Adverse immunological response usually due to IgE, occasionally non-IgE-mediated immune mechanisms

Toxic
- Toxic or pharmacological contaminants inherent in a food

Food aversion
- Where patients are convinced that they are allergic to food but when challenged with food no reactions appear

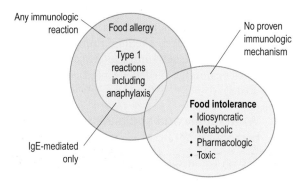

Fig. 43.12 **Adverse food reactions**

BOX 43.12 Major food allergens

In infants
- Milk
- Egg
- Peanut
- Soya

In pre-school children
- Milk
- Egg
- Peanut
- Soya
- Wheat
- Tree nut
- Fish
- Shellfish

In school children, adolescents and adults
- Peanut
- Tree nut
- Fish
- Shellfish

Table 43.14 **Food allergens**

Food	Prevalence	Allergen
Milk	2.5–7.5%	Bos d3, Bos d5
Egg	1.3%	Gal d1, Gal d2, Gal d3
Peanut	0.8%	Arah1, Arah 2, Arah 3
Fish	0.1%	Gad c1
Tree nut	0.2%	

The major food allergens are water-soluble glycoproteins, are generally resistant to proteolysis and are heat-stable (Box 43.12 and Table 43.14). Sensitization to food allergens occurs in the gastrointestinal tract, or in the respiratory tract with inhalant allergens.

Food allergy is a world-wide problem and like other atopic disorders it appears to be on the increase. It remains a leading cause of anaphylaxis treated in emergency departments and the public has become increasingly aware of the problem. Around 6% of infants and children experience food allergy reaction in the first 3 years of life, and 33% of children with moderate to severe atopic disorders have IgE-mediated food allergy.

Most infants and young children outgrow milk (90%) and egg (75%) allergy by 2–4 years. Around 20% of young children with a peanut allergy within the first 5 years of life may outgrow this; however, older children tend to be allergic for life.

Occasionally there may be cross-reactions:
- Peanuts: soybeans, green beans and peas
- Wheat: rye
- Cow's milk: goat's milk, soya (30–50% cross reactivity)
- Kiwi fruit: avocado, banana, raw potato, chestnut, latex
- Pollen: hazelnuts, green apples, peaches and almonds.

Clinical features of food allergies
See Table 43.15.

Diagnosis
History is most important and should cover:
- Food suspected to have provoked the reaction
- Quantity of the food ingested
- Length of time between ingestion and development of symptoms
- Description of the symptoms provoked
- Similar symptoms developed on other occasions when the food was eaten
- Other factors, e.g. exercise
- Length of time since the last reaction.

Investigations should include:

- Skin prick test (Box 43.13)
- Allergen-specific IgE
- Food elimination
- Food challenge.

Management of food allergy

- Food allergen avoidance: advice from a dietitian may be necessary
- Medication:
  - Antihistamine
  - Adrenaline (epinephrine) autoinjector (Epipen or Anapen) *with training* in management of anaphylaxis
  - For reactions involving respiratory involvement: α-agonist effect causes peripheral vasoconstriction, while β-agonist effect causes bronchodilatation
  - Oral corticosteroid
- Optimization of asthma control
- Management plan outlining indications for above
- 'Medic Alert' identification
- School support and education
- Psychological support may be necessary in special cases.

Anaphylaxis

Anaphylaxis is a severe life-threatening allergic reaction. Symptoms can include urticaria, swelling (especially of the lips and face), difficulty breathing (because of either swelling in the throat or an asthmatic reaction), vomiting, diarrhoea, cramping, and in anaphylactic shock, a fall in blood pressure, circulatory collapse and death.

Causes

See Box 43.14.

Investigations

Diagnosis of anaphylaxis in acute settings is based on a brief directed history of presenting symptoms and

Table 43.15 Clinical features of food allergies

Type	IgE-mediated	Cell-mediated	Mixed IgE-mediated
Gastrointestinal	Oral allergy syndrome, GI anaphylaxis	Food protein-induced enterocolitis (cow's milk protein intolerance), proctocolitis, enteropathy syndrome, coeliac disease	Allergic eosinophilic oesophagitis, allergic eosinophilic gastroenteritis
Cutaneous	Urticaria, angioedema, morbilliform rashes, flushing	Contact dermatitis, dermatitis	
Respiratory	Acute rhinoconjunctivitis, bronchospasm		
Generalized	Anaphylactic shock		

BOX 43.16 Anaphylaxis is a clinical diagnosis; diagnose the presence or likely presence rapidly

If facilities for full treatment are not immediately available:

1. Ask for help and place the patient in a recumbent position and elevate the lower extremities.

2. **GIVE EPINEPHRINE, if available.** *Adrenaline (epinephrine) is the most important drug for anaphylaxis* and should be given intramuscularly as soon as possible if the child had a previous severe reaction, has difficult breathing or appears unconscious. Dose: 0.01 ml/kg of 1 : 1000 aqueous solution, to a maximum of 0.3–0.5 ml (subcutaneous or intramuscularly only). (Epipen/Anapen Júnior — 0.15 mg, up to 6 years or 20 kgs; Epipen/Anapen 0.3 mg over 6 years or 20 kgs). If necessary, repeat every 15 minutes, up to two doses.

3. Assess and support breathing. An inhaled β_2 agonist agent, like salbutamol, may be needed to treat bronchospasm. Use the child's own inhaler if available and the patient is cooperative. Mouth to mouth breathing and chest compression may be necessary.

4. Give an anti-histamine and a corticosteroid if available and feasible (see below)

In the hospital, clinic or the ambulance:

1. Give epinephrine if not given before or repeat doses if necessary

2. Assess and maintain the airway. An oropharyngeal airway device may be needed to keep the airways patent. Provide 100% oxygen. Give an inhaled β_2 agonist if necessary.

3. Assess circulation (heart rate, capillary refill and blood pressure). Fluids — 20 ml/kg of normal saline (0.9% saline), 5% human albumin solution or Ringer lactate solution — may be used as fluid resuscitation to treat hypotension.

4. Give an antihistamine once the emergency measures described above have been carried out. (0.2 mg/kg of intravenous chlorpheniramine; in countries where not available, intravenous clemastine 0.0125 mg/kg may be given after 4 years of age, although more experience is desirable). For mild reactions, an oral anti-histamine may be suitable (chlorpheniramine, loratadine, desloratadine, cetirizine, levocetirizine, ebastine). Syrups and oral dispersible tablets are more quickly absorbed and may be easier to give to children than ordinary tablets.

5. Administer a corticosteroid to reduce the risk of protracted or recurring anaphylaxis. (Hydrocortisone 4 mg/kg or approximately 250 mg intravenously, Methyl prednisolone or prednisolone 1 to 2 mg/kg, Dexamethasone, 0.15 to 0.7 mg/kg. Further doses could be repeated 6-hourly. If the child's clinical condition permits it, oral methyl prednisolone, prednisolone or prednisone can also be used.

6. In refractory cases not responding to adrenaline because a ß-adrenergic blocker is complicating management, glucagon, 1 mg intravenously as a bolus, may be useful. A continuous infusion of glucagon, 1–5 mg/hour, may be given if required.

7. Severe cases may need transfer to the intensive care unit, while less severe cases may need a period of observation before discharge

8. All children with anaphylactic reactions should be referred to a paediatrician or an allergologist for an outpatient clinic assessment, education, further investigations and follow-up.

---

evaluation to focus on manifestations that are likely to be life-threatening. History should include questions regarding common causative factors (Box 43.14) and past history of atopy and anaphylaxis, and ruling out conditions that may mimic anaphylaxis (Box 43.15).

The only immediate test that is useful at the time of reaction is mast cell tryptase. It is only raised transiently; therefore blood should be taken when it peaks at about an hour after the onset of reaction.

Principles of management (see Box 43.16)

An important aspect of treatment is prevention of further events, which includes education of the patient regarding strategies for allergen avoidance and being aware of cross-reacting allergens, particularly nuts and drugs.

Adrenaline (epinephrine) autoinjector pen training for the patient, parent and school is also important for success of future treatment.

Patients prone to anaphylaxis should also receive information on wearing 'Medic Alert' bracelets.

http://www.resus.org.uk/pages/anafig2.pdf

Anaphylaxis, guidance for first responders

Further reading

Maitland K et al 2005 Management of severe malaria in children: proposed guidelines for the United Kingdom. British Medical Journal 331:337–343

For use of adrenaline see Drug and Therapeutics Bulletin 2003; 41(3):21–24

The child in hospital

MODULE EIGHT

Michael J. Marsh   Jean-Christophe Mercier

Care of the critically ill child

LEARNING OUTCOMES

By the end of this chapter you should:

- Understand the basis of physiological control of the circulation and organ perfusion
- Understand circulatory responses to insults
- Understand the factors influencing blood pressure and cardiac output
- Understand the causes and management of the acute respiratory distress syndrome.

You should also:

- Know how to recognize a severely ill child
- Know the principles of cardiopulmonary management and be able to perform this effectively
- Know the causes and management of coma
- Know the causes and management of shock
- Have attended a life support course such as Advanced Paediatric Life Support (APLS), Paediatric Advanced Life Support (PALS) etc.

MODULE EIGHT

Basic science

Control of the circulation

The circulation is vital for providing tissues with the nutrients they need and for taking away their waste products so that they may function optimally. In order to understand the control of the circulation it is first important to remind ourselves of some fundamental basic facts about its physical characteristics.

The flow of blood (Q) in the circulation is dependent on two factors:

- Pressure difference (ΔP)
- Resistance (R).

They are related by Ohm's Law:

$$Q = \Delta P / R$$

From this it is clear that a pressure drop across a blood vessel is required for forward flow and that the lower the resistance, the higher the flow.

The most important determining factor in vessel resistance is the radius (r) of that vessel. This is described by Poiseuille's Law:

$$Q = \pi \Delta P r^4 / 8 \eta l$$

Simplified, this expresses the fact that blood flow is proportional to the radius of the vessel to the power of 4. When we look at the vasculature we see that the arterioles have a very muscular wall that enables them to change diameter and they therefore provide a very powerful method of controlling blood flow.

In order to assess circulation the measurement of arterial pressure is crucial, as it is this pressure gradient to a negligible venous pressure that enables forward flow and tissue perfusion. The elastic nature of arteries reduces the pressure changes that would occur between systole and diastole and enables continuous flow. The pressure difference between systole and diastole is known as the pulse pressure. The blood pressure changes from the aortic root to the arterioles and therefore the concept of a single measurement that represents the driving force of the arterial tree is known as the mean pressure. This is not simply the average of the systolic and diastolic pressures but can be approximated by the formula:

Mean pressure = diastolic pressure + ⅓ pulse pressure

The characteristic of veins is that they are normally partially collapsed and are therefore able to distend (compliance) and act as a store for up to 60% of the circulating volume. This can be very useful when there is acute loss of blood but can be a disadvantage when the right side of the heart is not working effectively. Because of their low resistance they require very little pressure difference to enable venous return. They also make use of non-cardiac pumps such as skeletal muscle and the negative intrathoracic pressure effect of respiration to improve venous return and subsequently cardiac output.

Local control of blood flow by tissues

Tissues control their own circulation in order to achieve metabolic demands. The mechanism behind this can be divided into acute and chronic types.

Acute

- *Vasodilator theory*. When tissue metabolism increases, blood, oxygen and nutrient supply reduces. A vasodilator substance (lactic acid, CO_2, K^+, adenosine) is released by tissues, causing dilatation of the arterioles.
- *Oxygen demand theory*. Tissue is very sensitive to oxygen supply and when levels decrease it is thought that precapillary sphincters relax and encourage blood supply.
- *Autoregulation*. Tissues respond to a sudden change in blood pressure to enable continuous blood flow. This may be partly explained by the above-mentioned metabolic theories. It may also be explained by the response of the vessel to sudden stretch, which is to contract and, in the absence of stretch, to relax (myogenic theory).

Chronic

The body adapts to long-term changes in circulation by altering tissue vascularity, so that if metabolic demand increases in a particular tissue, so does the vascularity. Many angiogenic factors have been found to enable this, such as endothelial cell growth factor and fibroblast growth factor.

Neural control of blood flow in tissues

The sympathetic part of the autonomic nervous system plays a powerful role in the acute regulation of the circulation. This is done through specific fibres that innervate the heart and blood vessels. The sympathetic fibres secrete noradrenaline (norepinephrine), which causes vasoconstriction of both arterioles and veins as well as increasing heart rate and contractility.

The parasympathetic fibres play less of a role through fibres that innervate blood vessels of the head and body viscera and the heart. These fibres secrete acetylcholine, which causes vasodilatation and reduction in heart rate.

Blood pressure regulation

Acute

We have seen how the body goes to extraordinary lengths to maintain blood pressure in order to provide tissues with the nutrients they require. There have to be feedback mechanisms to enable coordination of these systems. The most acute of these are the baroreceptors. Located in the carotid sinus and aortic arch, they respond to stretch and send impulses to the vasomotor centre in the brainstem, which controls autonomic stimulation. They provide excellent acute control but reset themselves to the new blood pressure if it is sustained for more than 1–2 days. As well as these baroreceptors, there are chemoreceptors that exist in the carotid body and aortic arch, which respond to oxygen lack, CO_2 and acid excess. They also stimulate the vasomotor response to increase arterial pressure. The vasomotor centre itself is an intensely powerful controller of blood pressure and the strongest response is seen when it is subjected to ischaemia (i.e. cerebral ischaemia) itself. The stimulus is so strong that other organs and tissues in the body are potentially sacrificed. It may also be influenced by higher centres in the brain, as is seen in the rise in temperature that leads to vasodilatation.

Intermediate

Three mechanisms exist for intermediate control:
- *Transcapillary volume shift.* As blood pressure rises, fluid moves into the extracellular space and vice versa. The extracellular space thus provides a fluid reserve for the vascular system.
- *Vascular stress relaxation.* As the veins are stretched they expand slowly, absorbing any change in pressure over 10–60 minutes. Thus when the pressure falls the veins are able to return the pressure to normal over a similar time frame.
- *Renin–angiotensin system.* This is the more familiar method by which the kidneys start to regulate blood pressure. The juxtaglomerular cells of the kidney secrete an enzyme, renin, in response to a fall in blood pressure. Renin then converts angiotensinogen to angiotensin I in the plasma. Angiotensin I is converted to angiotensin II in the lung; this is a powerful vasoconstrictor and directly causes the kidney to retain salt and water. Angiotensin II also stimulates the adrenals to secrete aldosterone, causing more salt and water retention.

Long-term

The kidney regulates the fluid balance in the body, responding to changes in blood pressure by varying urine output. This mechanism is mediated by two hormones:
- *Aldosterone.* This hormone is secreted in the adrenal cortex in response to angiotensin II and III, leading to salt and water retention. Aldosterone takes 2–3 hours to be stimulated and almost a week to reach peak effect.
- *Antidiuretic hormone (ADH).* Secreted in the hypothalamus in response to reduced atrial stretch receptor response, this hormone then acts on the kidney to promote water reabsorption. In high concentrations it also causes strong vasoconstriction; hence its other name of vasopressin. The atrial stretch receptor is now known to produce a hormone called atrial natriuretic peptide, which promotes salt and water excretion and counteracts the effects of aldosterone and ADH.

Cardiac output

An understanding of the concept of cardiac output is essential to understanding the control of the circulation, for it is the cardiac output that ensures a sustainable blood pressure and therefore tissue perfusion. It can be described in different ways:

Cardiac output = heart rate × stroke volume
Cardiac output = arterial pressure/total peripheral resistance

Different methods also exist to measure it. The Fick method uses the principle that by looking at the oxygen consumption (O_2/min) of a particular organ and then measuring the venous (O_2ven) and arterial (O_2art) oxygen concentrations, one can estimate the cardiac output (CO):

$$CO = \frac{O_2/min}{O_2art - O_2ven}$$

The heart needs to be able to respond to the changing demands of the body, whether they are physiological or pathological. Control of cardiac output can be divided into intracardiac and extracardiac mechanisms.

Intracardiac mechanisms

These rely on the physical properties of the cardiac muscle. When this muscle is stretched, it responds with a more forceful contraction up until a certain point. This relationship is well described by the Frank–Starling curve. It plays particular importance in ensuring that the left and right ventricles perform equally and fluid does not accumulate in the lungs.

Extracardiac mechanisms

These rely on the autonomic nervous system, as already described. The sympathetic system increases rate and contractility, thus increasing output, and the parasympathetic reduces the heart rate.

It is quickly apparent that the body has many ways of controlling the circulation, which on initial inspection seem quite complex. However, by applying basic principles, one can see that they are all working towards the same goal, that of tissue perfusion. In the approach to the care of the critically ill child it is therefore important that there is an appreciation of the circulatory status and methods by which it may be supported.

Recognition and management of the seriously ill child

All paediatric senior house officers should have attended APLS, PALS or a similar course.

In this section an introduction will be given describing the importance of a structured approach to the seriously ill child. The outcome of cardiac arrest in children is poor; therefore, in order to reduce both morbidity and mortality, it is essential that early recognition is achieved and appropriate action taken. The primary assessment systematically looks at respiratory, cardiovascular and neurological status and addresses problems as they are found. A secondary assessment is then performed, looking at each system in turn and instituting emergency treatment.

Primary assessment

- A (Airway):
  - Look for chest movement
  - Listen for additional sounds, e.g. wheeze, stridor etc.
  - Feel for breath
- B (Breathing):
  - Effort, e.g. rate, accessory muscles
  - Efficacy, e.g. oxygen saturations
  - Effect, e.g. heart rate, skin colour, conscious level (*N.B. Severe respiratory distress may present with little sign of increased effort due to exhaustion. This is a preterminal sign and requires prompt intervention.*)
- C (Circulation):
  - Heart rate
  - Pulse volume
  - Capillary refill time (CRT)
  - Blood pressure (*N.B. Hypotension is a preterminal sign.*)
- D (Disability):
  - Level of consciousness (AVPU/Glasgow Coma Score, p. 664)
  - Posture
  - Pupils
  - Blood glucose.

It is essential that appropriate resuscitation is carried out during the primary survey before proceeding to a secondary assessment.

Secondary assessment

This aims to take a focused history and institute further emergency treatment whilst developing a differential diagnosis. It requires a full physical examination from head to toe. If there is any clinical deterioration during this procedure, then the primary assessment must be repeated.

Monitoring and post-resuscitation management

As part of your recognition and management of critically ill children, whatever the underlying diagnosis, you need to make optimal use of the monitoring equipment available to you in the hospital environment. It is important to keep the principles in Box 44.1 in mind at all times.

Outside of the intensive care unit, the high-dependency unit or the emergency department, the following physiological variables should be assessed regularly:

- Respiratory rate
- Heart rate
- Non-invasive blood pressure (NIBP)
- Oxygen saturations
- Electrocardiogram (ECG)
- Temperature.

At the time of initial assessment of a critically ill child it is important to take note of each of these variables and relate them to the standardized airway, breathing, circulation (ABC) approach of resuscitation guidelines.

Clinical observations form an integral part of the assessment (Box 44.2), along with the information yielded from the monitoring equipment. Therefore, whilst assessing 'airway' and 'breathing' using the respiratory rate, you should look at the respiratory

---

BOX 44.1 Principles when using equipment

- Be familiar with the equipment available where you work
- Have basic troubleshooting skills for common equipment
- Always remember that a machine/monitor can give incorrect information
- Be aware that you are more likely to question abnormal results, e.g. accept 'normal BP' on non-invasive blood pressure monitoring, when it is reading falsely high
- Equipment should be fit for its purpose
- Trends are generally more important/useful than spot measurement
- Equipment will not work if it is not plugged in, switched on and connected to the patient
- The most common mistake made is to use the incorrect cuff when measuring non-invasive blood pressure (NIBP)

effort, effectiveness of breathing, signs of increased
work of breathing and respiratory distress, as well as
effect of respiration (resulting oxygen saturation).

The key skill is to relate the initial observations and
subsequent trends to normal age-appropriate values
(Table 44.1) and to know where to access a reference
chart rapidly.

After initial assessment, resuscitation and emergency
treatment it is important to keep noting the observations
and thinking in terms of the underlying trends, e.g. a
respiratory rate that settles or steadily rises. The fail-
safe measure is to make sure that there is a way to
have the regularly documented observations available
for review. If they are displayed electronically, keep
checking; if they are charted, keep reviewing. You must
constantly ask the question:

- Are things getting better/responding to treatments?
  or
- Are things deteriorating and do I need to escalate
  treatment and ensure senior involvement?

These principles, together with experience and
knowledge, can be combined with the systematic
resuscitation training courses (APLS/EPLS/neonatal
life support (NLS)) to help clinicians improve their
clinical skills and enable them not only to recognize
but also to treat the critically ill child safely and
effectively (Boxes 44.3 and 44.4).

Acute respiratory distress syndrome

In 1967 Ashbaugh described the clinical syndrome
of acute respiratory distress syndrome (ARDS). This
is an acute clinical condition of hypoxic respiratory
failure rather than a collection of discrete diseases
characterized by severe hypoxaemia, tachypnoea and
diffuse bilateral pulmonary infiltrates seen on chest
X-ray. Though with the advent of modern intensive
care it became recognized as a serious problem with a

high mortality, morbidity and considerable healthcare
costs, there was a lack of information as to definition
and incidence. In 1992 the American–European
consensus conference produced a clearer definition
and devised the term 'acute lung injury' (ALI) (Table
44.2). Hypoxaemia is defined using Pa/FiO_2 ratio,
the illness must be acute and there must be no left
atrial hypertension (low pulmonary capillary wedge

Table 44.1   Age-appropriate normal values for common physiological variables

	Newborn	1 month–1 year	2–5 years	5–12 years	Adolescence
Respiratory rate	40–60	30–40	25–30	20–24	15–20
Heart rate	100–180	100–140	80–110	70–100	60–90
Systolic BP	60–80	70–100	90–110	90–115	105–130
Diastolic BP	20–60	50–65	55–65	55–70	65–80

Table 44.2 American–European Consensus Definitions

	ALI	ARDS
Pa/FiO_2 ratio	39.5 kPa (300 mmHg)	< 26.7 kPa (200 mmHg)
Chest X-ray	Bilateral infiltrates	Bilateral infiltrates
Pulmonary capillary wedge pressure	< 18 mmHg	< 18 mmHg

pressure, PCWP) to exclude hypoxaemia due to pulmonary oedema from heart failure. The incidence of ALI increases with age from 16 per 100 000 person-year for those 15–19 years of age. ARDS and ALI incidence has been estimated to 12.8 cases per 100 000 children-year in a US county, whilst it accounts for about 5% of admissions to paediatric intensive care units (PICU) in the UK, and about 1.5% in China.

Pathophysiology

ALI and ARDS are caused by an acute inflammatory reaction in the lungs that is complex and follows either a direct injury to the lungs or an indirect 'non-pulmonary' injury (Box 44.5). The exact process varies depending on the underlying cause; in common there is damage and injury to the alveolar unit at the endothelium, interstitium and epithelium. For the sake of simplicity it is useful to summarize the current knowledge of both conditions as one clinical entity.

BOX 44.5 Conditions associated with or leading to ALI and ARDS

Direct: pulmonary
- Pneumonia
- Aspiration
- Lung contusion
- Inhalation injury
- Near-drowning
- Emboli

Indirect: non-pulmonary
- Sepsis
- Massive transfusion
- Pancreatitis
- Trauma
- Traumatic brain injury
- Post-cardiopulmonary bypass

Endothelium

The endothelium is undoubtedly pivotal to the process and may be damaged and generally activated in a variety of ways. Swollen injured endothelial cells release proinflammatory cytokines, including interleukin (IL)-8. Neutrophils become activated and attracted to the endothelium, passing through the endothelial cell junctions, where gaps have developed into the inter-stitium. The activated endothelium has important functions, including the control of inflammation and coagulation, regulation of local blood flow and control of cell and fluid migration.

Interstitium

The interstitium becomes swollen with a combination of oedematous fluid leaking from the vascular space and increased activated inflammatory cells, particularly migrating neutrophils. These neutrophils are active and produce a range of highly active substances, including proteases such as neutrophil elastase. Fibroblasts also become activated and secrete IL-8 and procollagen into the interstitial space. All of these disrupt the integrity and disturb the normal close relationship of the endothelium to the alveolar space, thus impairing gas exchange.

Epithelium

Type I pneumocytes form the majority of the alveolar surface as a layer of thin cells in close proximity to the basement membrane. In health type II pneumocytes produce and release surfactant that forms a monolayer, facilitating gas exchange. In ARDS and ALI there is accumulation of protein-rich oedema fluid in the alveolar space (pulmonary oedema), and there is necrosis and apoptosis of type I cells and proliferation of type II cells. There is an increase in alveolar macrophages that are activated by migration inhibition factor (MIF). Macrophages release both pro- and anti-inflammatory cytokines, including IL-8, IL-6, IL-10 and IL-1 and growth factors TGF-α. It is thought that macrophages amplify inflammation as well as playing a role in resolution of lung injury via a variety of processes, including binding and internalizing proteases, modulating repair process via transforming growth factor (TGF-α), which stimulates endothelial growth and fibrosis. Neutrophil numbers are massively increased in the alveolar space and, once activated, release leucotrienes, reactive oxidants, proteases and platelet activating factor (PAF). As a result of the inflammation and protein-rich oedema fluid there is inactivation of surfactant and severe impairment of gas exchange.

Prognosis

In adults the mortality has steadily fallen over the last 20 years but is still in the region of 30–40%. In relation to age, mortality has increased from 24% in patients from 15 to 19 years of age to 60% in patients 85 years of age or older. In children, mortality is also relatively high, but varies both with the severity of lung injury (ALI or ARDS) and the level of supportive care (18% in a US state, 6% in British PICUs, but 64% in China). In the childhood population mortality is also relatively high and in British paediatric intensive care units (PICUs) it is in the region of 6%.

Table 44.3 **The adapted Glasgow Coma Score**

Activity	Best response	Score
Eye opening	Spontaneous	4
	To verbal stimuli	3
	To pain	2
	None	1
Verbal	Orientated	5
	Confused	4
	Inappropriate words	3
	Non-specific sounds	2
	None	1
Motor	Follows commands	6
	Localizes pain	5
	Withdraws in response to pain	4
	Flexion in response to pain	3
	Extension in response to pain	2
	None	1

Maximum score 15
Minimum score 3
Score ≤ 8 indicates coma needing intubation

BOX 44.10 AVPU Scale

- *A*wake
- Responds to *v*oice
- Responds to *p*ain
- *U*nresponsive
- Pupil size and reaction

BOX 44.11 Rapid neurological assessment

- Assess conscious level: AVPU or GCS
- Posture
- Pupil size + pupil reaction

BOX 44.12 Key levels indicating need for intubation

- P or lower on AVPU scale
- ≤ 8 on GCS

Q3. What is the differential diagnosis and what key questions in the history will help you make the diagnosis?

See Box 44.13.

Q4. What key investigations will make the diagnosis?

The key investigations are those that will help you identify the treatable causes rapidly whilst also looking

BOX 44.13 Differential diagnosis of coma

Hypoxic and ischaemic
- Out-of-hospital arrest
- Other event

Vascular
- Sudden-onset headache
- Abrupt loss of consciousness

Traumatic
- Episode of trauma
- Non-accidental injury — suspect

Toxic or poisoning
- Assess drug history, bizarre behaviour

Metabolic
- Polyuria and polydipsia
- Odour in diabetic ketoacidosis

Infective
- Signs and symptoms of infection

Post-ictal
- Seizures

Space-occupying lesion
- Symptoms of early morning headache

BOX 44.14 Key investigations

- Blood glucose: hypo- or hyperglycaemia
- Toxicology
- Blood cultures ± lumbar puncture (*Caution: do not perform if ↑ intracranial pressure*)
- Neuroimaging
- CT scan
- MR scan (MR angiography (MRA) or MR venography (MRV) if evidence of intracranial blood and suspicion of arteriovenous malformation)
- Cerebral angiogram in selected cases

for signs of raised intracranial pressure (ICP) that should be managed (Box 44.14).

Head injury

Severe traumatic brain injury (STBI) represents a major cause of childhood deaths. The majority of cases are accidental and therefore by definition are preventable. All paediatricians have a duty to encourage road safety and public education to try to decrease incidence and hence morbidity and mortality (Ch. 17). STBI accounts for 15% of deaths of 1–15-year-olds and 25% in 5–15-year-olds;

BOX 44.15 Modes of injury

Road traffic accidents (RTAs)

- Pedestrian
- Cyclist
- Motor vehicle accident: passenger/driver

Falls

- Toddlers:
  - Domestic
  - Low-impact falls inside
  - Falls from open windows
- Older child:
  - Falls from trees, walls, buildings whilst playing outside

Impact injuries

- Sport

Penetrating

- Gunshot
- Other

BOX 44.17 Principles of management in severe traumatic brain injury

Assess severity of injury: rapid neurological assessment

- GCS + pupils *or*
- AVPU + pupils
- Note mechanism of injury and RTA speed impact:
  < 50 km/h 80% survival
  > 60–70 km/h 80% mortality

Prevent secondary injury

- Avoid and prevent hypoxia: airway and breathing
- Avoid and prevent ischaemia: hypotension and ↑ ICP

Goals

- Rapid and appropriate resuscitation
- Adequate ventilation
- Adequate circulation
- Ensure urgent evacuation of haematoma

---

along with malignancies, represents the major cause of deaths in teenagers.

The mode of injury (Box 44.15) has a significant influence on the morbidity and mortality, reflecting the force involved in the head injury. For example, the mortality is higher in pedestrian road traffic accidents (RTAs) compared to passenger RTAs. Penetrating injuries are relatively rare in Europe compared to some American cities.

Primary brain injury

During the episode of trauma a large amount of energy is transmitted through the head, including the brain and all its supporting and connective tissues. This produces four main types of injury:

- Cerebral laceration
- Cerebral contusion
- Dural tear
- Diffuse axonal injury.

The pattern and severity (Box 44.16) depend on the forces and the part of the head involved.

Management is outlined in Boxes 44.17, 44.18 and 44.19.

BOX 44.16 Definition of severity of traumatic brain injury using the Glasgow Coma Score (GCS)

GCS 13–15	Mild
GCS 9–12	Moderate
GCS 3–8	Severe

BOX 44.18 Initial treatment on presentation

- ABC + oxygen with cervical spine immobilization
- Avoid hypoxia:
  - Intubate if GCS < 8 /AVPU/rapidly falling GCS
  - Aim to maintain oxygen saturations > 96% (equates to PaO_2 10 kPa or 75 Torr)
  - Ventilate to control $PaCO_2$: measure blood gas correlate end-tidal CO_2
- Avoid ischaemia:
  - Aim for adequate CPP by increasing MAP:
    Volume expansion
    Inotrope or vasoconstrictor
  - Assume ICP 20 mmHg
  - Aim for CPP:
    Infant > 50
    Child > 60
    Teenager > 70
  - Reduce ICP:
    Sedation
    Control $PaCO_2$
    Paralysis
    Cool?

Physiological basis for intracranial pressure (ICP) and cerebral perfusion pressure (CPP): Monro–Kellie Principle (Box 44.20)

The head can be thought of as a 'rigid box' with a fixed potential volume that is made up of the brain, cerebrospinal fluid (CSF), arterial and venous blood and the respective vessels (Fig. 44.1A). Following trauma to the head there can be expansion of the brain volume due to cerebral oedema or there can be 'new

BOX 44.19 Neuroprotection

Standard

- Maintain $PaO_2 > 10$ kPa (75 Torr)
- Control $PaCO_2$ 4.5–5.0 kPa (33–35 Torr)
- Paralyse and sedate as necessary
- Maintain CPP
- Control ICP
- Head up 30° in midline
- Maintain normothermia (> 36°C)

Unproven

- Moderate hypothermia (32–33°C)
- Decompressive craniectomy

BOX 44.20

CPP = MAP – ICP

(CPP = cerebral perfusion pressure; MAP = mean arterial pressure; ICP = intracranial pressure)

matter' that occupies space, e.g. expanding haematoma. There is a limited capacity for compensation for the cerebral oedema or expanding clot by decreasing the amount of CSF or venous blood (Fig. 44.1B). Even whilst this compensation occurs there will be some increase in the ICP towards 20 mmHg. When the capacity to compensate fails, the system becomes non-compliant and further small increases in volume will produce large rapid rises in pressure (Fig. 44.1C). Understanding this helps you appreciate the need for rapid appropriate action, including the rationale for osmotic diuretics and the need to perform definitive surgery within 4–6 hours of injury to remove expanding haematomas. Untreated, either uncal herniation or herniation through the foramen magnum will occur, resulting in brainstem compression and ultimately brain death.

Indications for a CT scan

- ↓ Ventricular size
- Effacement of sulci
- Effacement of basal cistern
- Mass.

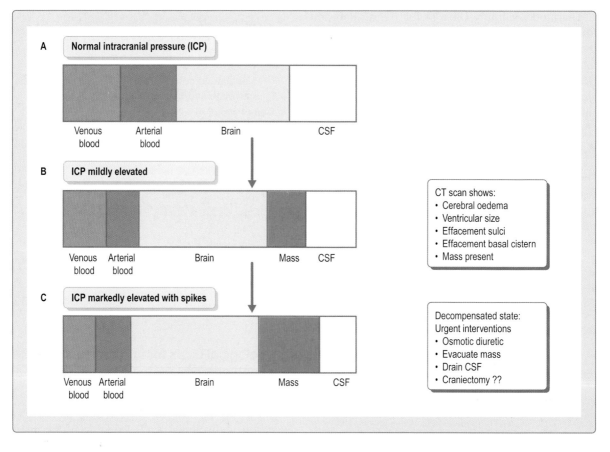

Fig. 44.1 Diagrammatic representation of intracranial volume: relative contribution of each component shown for three situations (Monro–Kellie Principle).
(A) Normal intracranial pressure (ICP); (B) ICP mildly elevated; (C) ICP markedly elevated with spikes. (CSF = cerebrospinal fluid)

Intracranial haemorrhage: non-neonatal

The presentation of intracranial haemorrhage outside the neonatal period depends on the underlying diagnosis. The prognosis is also influenced by this diagnosis, though intracranial haemorrhage, whatever the cause, carries a significant risk of mortality, especially if the child requires intensive care at the time of initial bleed.

The clinical history will in the majority of cases enable you to make a diagnosis rapidly (Box 44.21). In accidental trauma there is rarely any doubt about the diagnosis, but in the case of non-accidental injury (NAI, p. 499) there may be all the classical pointers to the diagnosis, including clear evidence of trauma, absent or inconsistent history, evidence of previous traumatic injuries and even retinal haemorrhages.

The presentation can vary from acute catastrophic loss of consciousness through to a much less acute gradual non-specific neurodegeneration (Box 44.22).

With a simple combination of clinical history and examination, along with initial radiological investigation (CT scan in the majority and MRI in a minority), a diagnosis of intracranial haemorrhage can be reached and the likely cause established. Subsequent investigation as listed in Box 44.23 will usually confirm the cause confidently.

BOX 44.21 Differential diagnosis of intracranial haemorrhage (non-neonatal)

- Trauma:
  - Accidental
  - NAI
- Arteriovenous malformation
- Bleeding disorder:
  - Inherited
  - Anticoagulant treatment
- Acute leukaemia
- Tumour
- Thrombosis
- Infection

BOX 44.22 Modes of presentation

- Acute loss of consciousness
- Gradual-onset coma
- Status epilepticus
- Acute focal neurology
- Acute severe headaches
- Progressive neurological deterioration

BOX 44.23 Investigations of suspected or proven intracranial haemorrhage

Trauma
- CT scan
- Additional appropriate X-rays

NAI
- CT scan
- Skeletal survey
- Expert fundoscopy
- Clotting screen
- Serum copper

AVM
- If suspected on CT scan proceed to cerebral angiography ± MRA or MRV

Inherited bleeding disorder
- Clotting screen
- Platelets
- Specific factor assays as directed by paediatric haematologist

Anticoagulant therapy
- International normalized ratio (INR)
- Seek expert advice rapidly

Acute leukaemia
- White cell count
- Blood film
- Bone marrow aspirate and trephine

Tumour
- Enhanced CT scan

Thrombosis
- MRA, MRV

Infection
- *Do not* carry out lumbar puncture in a hurry

Purpura

Problem-orientated topic:

purpura ● ● ● ● ●

Noah, an 8-year-old boy, is referred urgently to the paediatric emergency department. He has been unwell for 12 hours with a fever, vomiting, malaise and muscle aches. Examination reveals a widespread petechial rash with a few purpuric areas. He is alert and cooperative but has a tachycardia of 150 beats per minute and a respiratory rate of

Continued overleaf

20 breaths per minute. Initial assessment of ABC is undertaken.

Q1. What is the most likely diagnosis and what immediate treatments should be given?

Q2. What is the differential diagnosis?

Q3. What clinical signs and laboratory investigations inform the prognosis?

Q4. What is the prognosis?

Q1. What is the most likely diagnosis and what immediate treatments should be given?

The clinical history is highly suggestive of meningococcal septicaemia and therefore the priority is to start appropriate high-dose antibiotics immediately; do not delay whilst trying to confirm diagnosis. The antibiotic can be either intravenous cefotaxime 50 mg/kg or ceftriaxone 80 mg/kg; blood should be taken first for culture and a meningococcal polymerase chain reaction (PCR). Once vascular access is secured and the antibiotics have been given, Noah should be reassessed so his early treatment can be planned.

http://www.meningitis.org

Meningitis Trust

Q2. What is the differential diagnosis?

See Box 44.24.

Q3. What clinical signs and laboratory investigations inform the prognosis?

80

See Box 44.25.

Q4. What is the prognosis?

The prognosis of meningococcal septicaemia has steadily improved over the last 15 years. Now the reported mortality from most PICUs is less than 10% and is usually in the region of 5%. The reasons for this are undoubtedly multiple and reflect increased public awareness, early and prompt management by physicians, including prehospital antibiotics, improved recognition and resuscitation in hospitals and, to some extent, introduction of early and aggressive intensive care management.

Meningococcaemia

Pathogenesis

Neisseria meningitidis is a Gram-negative diplococcus that is carried in the nasopharynx of 2–5% of the population.

BOX 44.24 Differential diagnosis of purpura

Acute onset with fever and systemic symptoms
- Meningococcal septicaemia
- Viral illness
- Disseminated intravascular coagulation of septic origin
- Acute leukaemia

Less acute onset/absent fever
- Immune thrombocytopenia
- Idiopathic thrombocytopenia
- Thrombotic thrombocytopenia
- Protein C deficiency
- Drugs:
  - Under-production
  - Decreased survival

BOX 44.25 Signs of severe disease suggesting poor prognosis at presentation

- Short history
- Absence of meningism
- Widespread rash at presentation
- Rash that continues to spread despite treatment
- Shock (decompensated > compensated)
- Hyperpyrexia $\geq 40°C$
- Low white cell count $< 10 \times 10^9$
- Low platelet count $< 150 \times 10^9$

Group B is the most common serotype. Groups A, C, Y and W now have vaccines, although group C is the only one routinely given. Group A is less common but has caused significant outbreaks in the past and in Africa. Children usually acquire the organism from colonized adults and the majority develop a bactericidal response. A concurrent viral infection may predispose to mucosal penetration and subsequent bacteraemia.

Septicaemia

Systemic inflammatory response syndrome (SIRS) describes the sequence of events that occurs following infection with meningococcus. It may be defined as:
- Temperature $> 38°C$
- White cell count $> 20\ 000$
- Tachycardia
- Tachypnoea (reduced $PaCO_2$)
  in association with an infective cause.

Clinical features

With the increased awareness of the general public and other health professionals meningococcaemia is being recognized and treatment instituted earlier in its course. It only takes a brief period of working in any PICU, however, to realize how devastating the disease can be. Clinical presentation has classically been divided into acute, subacute and chronic. The acute form is the most dramatic; a child may be sitting up talking to his or her parents one minute and be ventilated on intensive cardiovascular support the next!

Initial symptoms may well be of non-specific fever and malaise, but the presence of a purpuric or morbilliform rash sometimes with leg pain with inability to walk should alert the clinician to the potential diagnosis. Trying to predict which child is going to need full intensive care and which will just require a course of antibiotics has been the subject of much research, and the effect of the infection on the child is most likely to be partly a genetic-mediated response. Continual clinical reassessment of the child is vital, paying particular attention to the cardiovascular system. Features that should alert the clinician include:

- Spreading purpuric rash
- Poor perfusion
- Low blood pressure
- Reduced pulse volume
- Respiratory distress
- Low platelet and neutrophil count
- Abnormal clotting.

The subacute form takes the form of a classical rash that is then accompanied by a localized infection, e.g. meningitis. The chronic form may present with non-specific symptoms and may well be picked up incidentally on cultures.

Investigations

Culture of blood, purpuric lesions and CSF may well identify the organism; however, the early use of antibiotics out of hospital has reduced the success rate. PCR of the blood and CSF or alternatively of skin elements has provided an accurate way of identifying meningococcal DNA and the type responsible. It should therefore be performed in all suspected cases.

Management

Early use of antibiotics is essential in eradicating the organism and currently high-dose cefotaxime is often the drug of choice in suspected septicaemia.

Aggressive resuscitation is important if there is haemodynamic compromise. Often large volumes of fluid are required (up to 200 ml/kg!) and therefore early intubation is recommended to support diaphragmatic function and control using appropriate levels of PEEP and the almost inevitable pulmonary oedema that follows. Inotropes are often required, with dopamine and dobutamine being used initially, the advantage being they can be given peripherally. Once central access has been obtained these drugs may be changed

for noradrenaline (norepinephrine) and adrenaline (epinephrine) if further support is required. Attention should also be paid to the correction of coagulopathy and electrolyte disturbances, particularly calcium and magnesium. Once initial stabilization has occurred, rapid referral to paediatric intensive care should be arranged for further management.

Public health must be informed of all suspected cases and the patient and close family contacts should be treated with prophylactic antibiotics for invasive disease and nasal carriage.

Prognosis

The mortality of septic shock secondary to meningococcaemia is 20–40%, often within the first 12 hours. If there is coexistent meningitis present the outcome is better, and if there is just meningitis alone mortality is less than 10%. Unfortunately, due to the severe nature of the acute form of presentation, children are still losing limb extremities from vascular occlusion.

Raised intracranial pressure

Problem-orientated topic:

headaches and loss of consciousness

Jade, a 15-year-old girl, is referred to clinic with a history of headaches worsening over a 3-month period whilst she has been studying for her final examinations at school. Her father, who found her unconscious in her bedroom where she was doing her homework, brings her into the paediatric emergency department. Initial assessment reveals a GCS of 8.

Q1. What immediate care should be given?

Q2. What is the differential diagnosis?

Q3. What signs suggest the presence of raised ICP?

Q4. What specific emergency medical treatments can be instituted if raised ICP is suspected?

Q1. What immediate care should be given?

The fact that the GCS is 8 means that the child needs to be urgently intubated. Whilst preparations for this are being made, the ABC should be formally assessed and a rapid neurological assessment should be carried out (p. 664).

Q2. What is the differential diagnosis?

The differential diagnosis is the same as in the coma vignette (p. 663) but in this case the clinical history strongly suggests the possibility of a space-occupying lesion. Once Jade has been intubated and sedated, an urgent CT scan should be organized to confirm or refute this diagnosis. If there is a tumour or other space-occupying lesion the acute loss of consciousness suggests raised ICP, either as a direct mass effect from the lesion or from acute hydrocephalus. These need to be identified to facilitate timely surgical intervention and prevent coning.

Q3. What signs suggest the presence of raised ICP?

Signs of raised ICP (Box 44.26) include:
- Pupils unequal or unreactive
- Hypertension
- Bradycardia (relative)
- Abnormal posture
- Focal neurology
- Abnormal respiratory pattern.

In any patient with a decreased level of consciousness the possibility of raised ICP should be raised; however, most children with decreased level of consciousness do not have raised ICP. The combination of signs and symptoms listed is enough to initiate full management as described.

BOX 44.26 Warning: papilloedema in raised intracranial pressure

Papilloedema is a late sign of raised ICP. Do not be reassured by its absence.

Q4. What specific emergency medical treatments can be instituted if raised ICP is suspected?

See Box 44.27.

Caution. Once the patient is intubated, a formal blood gas should be measured to determine the $PaCO_2$. This should be correlated to an end-tidal CO_2 measurement, allowing you to adjust the ventilation constantly to avoid hyperventilation, which can induce ischaemia, and hypoventilation, which may lead to increased cerebral blood flow and exacerbation of raised ICP.

Steroids are not included in the treatment of raised ICP as there is limited evidence of beneficial effects in most causes. They may have a role if the primary diagnosis is meningitis or tumour. In tumours, to combat cerebral oedema the drug of choice is dexamethasone. The usual paediatric therapy consists of an initial loading dose of 1–2 mg/kg once, orally, i.v. or i.m., followed by a maintenance dose of 1–1.5 mg/kg/day given in split doses

---

BOX 44.27 Management of raised ICP

- ABC + oxygen
- Sedated: analgesia + hypnotic
- Ventilate
- Normocapnia ($PaCO_2$ 4.5 kPa (40 Torr))
- 30° head up in midline
- Osmotic diuretic:
  - 0.25–0.5 g/kg mannitol
  - 2–5 ml/kg 3% saline

---

every 4–6 hours for 5 days, then reduced over 5 days, then discontinued. The maximum dose is 16 mg/day. In cases of meningitis, dexamethasone should be started at the same time as the first dose of antibiotic. In children older than 2 months, the dose should be 0.6 mg/kg/day i.v. every 6 hours during the first 4 days of antibiotic treatment.

All the treatments of a raised ICP are aimed at trying to decrease or limit cerebral oedema and acutely dropping the ICP by creating more space (Monro–Kellie Principle, p. 666).

Encephalopathy

Acute encephalopathy may be described as a sudden onset of diffuse brain dysfunction with or without an associated change in level of consciousness. Whilst it is not a diagnosis in itself it is the manifestation of a significant abnormality and must be recognized and managed in a systematic way to improve outcome.

Causes

The causes of acute encephalopathy can seem endless but may be simply classified:
- Hypoxic–ischaemic
- Infectious
- Haemorrhagic
- Metabolic
- Toxic
- Epileptic.

The hypoxic–ischaemic injury to the brain can result from many clinical situations. The combination of hypoxia leading to anaerobic metabolism and ischaemia leading to accumulation of toxic metabolites results in neuronal cell death and raised ICP. If unchecked, this leads to further ischaemia because of poor cerebral perfusion, then worsening coma and death.

Infectious encephalopathy is caused by organisms able to invade the central nervous system and may result in encephalitis, cerebral oedema, ventriculitis and abscess formation.

Haemorrhagic causes may be accidental or non-accidental and will be discussed elsewhere.

Any buildup of toxic metabolites will cause an impairment of neurological function, be it from a significant electrolyte disturbance, endocrine dysfunction, organ failure or the more uncommon inborn errors of metabolism. One must also remember those toxins that have been ingested deliberately or accidentally.

Seizures may be the manifestation of an encephalopathy as well as the cause. It is therefore important to recognize whether they are new in onset or longstanding.

Management

The initial resuscitation should involve stabilizing the airway, breathing and circulation whilst making an assessment of conscious level (GCS/AVPU). One of the major decisions that needs to be made early is the need for artificial ventilation. The advantages of airway protection and controlling gas exchange are obvious but artificial ventilation also reduces the ability to monitor conscious level and results in other parameters being monitored, e.g. pupils, heart rate, blood pressure etc.

Once the patient has been stabilized, the management can be further divided as follows.

Neuroprotection

To prevent further damage being done to the brain and allow any recovery, it is important that certain factors are addressed:

- *Treatment of infection.* Until a confirmed microbiological diagnosis has been made patients should be started on high-dose antibiotic and antiviral treatment. Specimens must be taken to identify the cause and ideally should include CSF, but raised ICP must first be excluded because of the risk of coning. PCR is now routinely done for both bacterial and viral (herpes simplex) causes.
- *Seizure control.* Unless effectively controlled, seizures result in further hypoxia and ischaemia. Seizure control should be part of the initial resuscitation but looking for further seizure activity is also vital. This can be done clinically but it is not always obvious when the patient is paralysed and sedated. One therefore relies on electroencephalography (EEG) and the cerebral function activity monitor (CFAM) to identify seizure activity. Whilst brief seizures may be managed with benzodiazepines (e.g. lorazepam), prolonged seizure activity often requires intravenous anticonvulsants (e.g. phenytoin) or barbiturate infusions (e.g. phenobarbital, thiopental). APLS has produced recognized protocols for the management of status epilepticus.

http://www.aplsonline.com

American Academy of Pediatrics APLS learning resources

- *Intracranial pressure.* As the head is a closed box, the blood supply to the brain can be compromised if the brain swells. Unless this is looked for and monitored, the patient with increasing ICP will subsequently present with brainstem herniation, by which time it is often too late. All patients with encephalopathy must therefore have some neuroimaging to make an assessment of ICP. Consideration must also be given as to whether a monitoring device is necessary. The advantage of this device is that an accurate assessment of cerebral perfusion pressure (CPP) can be obtained:

$$CPP = MAP - ICP$$

The control of CPP is paramount in order to prevent cerebral ischaemia and normal values change with age (infant > 50, child > 60, adolescent > 70 mmHg). Whilst many factors influence CPP, changes in cerebral blood flow will be paramount. As can be remembered the basic science principle is that the flow through a vessel is dependent on the pressure difference and diameter. The diameter of cerebral blood vessels is affected by the $PaCO_2$, low levels causing vasoconstriction and high levels vasodilatation. The pressure difference is dependent on arterial pressure and therefore it is important to maintain blood pressure often to supranormal levels, with inotropes if necessary.

Diagnostic investigations

The sequence of investigation will obviously be dictated by the clinical history and examination but some of the baseline tests that should be considered in all cases are listed in Box 44.28.

Further investigation must be guided by specialist input from a multidisciplinary team. Treatment is then aimed at trying to correct the underlying cause if possible or prevent further damage from being caused.

> **BOX 44.28 Urine and blood (± gastric aspirate) toxicology**
>
> - Full blood count, liver and renal function, laboratory glucose
> - Blood, urine and CSF culture, viral serology
> - Urine amino and organic acids, plasma amino acids, ammonia, lactate (urine should be kept on ice or in the refrigerator before being sent to the Lab)
> - Neuroimaging and EEG

Shock

Problem-orientated topic:

septic shock ● ● ● ● ●

Léa, a 3-year-old girl, is referred to hospital by her primary care physician with a 12-hour

Continued overleaf

history of fever, vomiting and muscle aches. She is seen on the paediatric admission unit, where examination reveals that she is pale, awake and responsive, but pyrexial at 39.5°C, with a respiratory rate of 40, heart rate of 170 and a capillary refill time (CRT) of 7 seconds.

Q1. What is Léa's physiological state?

Q2. What important clinical measurement should be taken?

Q3. What immediate treatment should be given and what tests should be performed?

Q1. What is Léa's physiological state?

All resuscitation courses teach you how to recognize and treat failure of the respiratory system, cardiovascular system, a combination of these two and neurological failure. The logic of this is to ensure that you rapidly recognize the life-threatening problem and immediately institute the most appropriate treatment without being distracted by concerns as to the primary underlying diagnosis.

Respiratory failure continues to be the most common reason for children to present with a life-threatening illness, and the outcome following a cardiac arrest remains poor, with less than 10% survival for out-of-hospital arrest and 20–30% for in-hospital arrest.

Using an ABC approach, this child can be classified as being shocked; with the fever this will be due to sepsis. The cardiac output (Box 44.29) is inadequate and compensatory mechanisms to increase it have occurred; the heart rate has increased to maintain cardiac output and systemic vascular resistance has increased in order to maintain blood pressure.

Q2. What important clinical measurement should be taken?

The key clinical measurement that must be recorded is the blood pressure. Without this information you are unable to classify the shock as compensated or decompensated. A key clinical measurement is the colour and temperature of extremities. If the capillary filling time is prolonged and the extremities cold, shock is likely associated with vasoconstriction, and the child should benefit from both fluids and inodilators (e.g. adrenaline (epinephrine) and milrinone). If, however, capillary filling pressure is rapid and the extremities warm, shock is likely to be associated with vasodilation, and the child should benefit from both fluids and inopressors (e.g. noradrenaline). This is vitally important as, once compensatory mechanisms have failed and the blood pressure is falling, the condition can progress rapidly to irreversible shock and cardiorespiratory arrest with a high probability of death.

Q3. What immediate treatment should be given and what tests should be performed?

The principles of management of shock include:
- Administering 100% oxygen; ensuring adequate airway and ventilation
- Securing vascular access × 2 — intra-osseous if necessary
- Blood for culture, blood count and glucose
- Intravenous cefotaxime or ceftriaxone if there is sepsis
- Volume resuscitation as bolus:
  - 10–20 ml/kg colloid or 0.9% saline
  - Reassess and repeat depending on response
- Monitor heart rate, oxygen saturations and urine output (insert catheter).

Observe closely for response and deterioration. Once 40–60 ml/kg fluid resuscitation has been administered and if still signs of shock, then:
- Elective intubation and ventilation:
  - Use most appropriate team
  - Seek expert advice
- Continue fluid resuscitation
- Consider vasoactive infusions:
  - Start dopamine or dobutamine (can be peripheral initially)
  - Adrenaline (epinephrine) if poor response
- Central line access and arterial line
- Look for and treat hypoglycaemia, hypocalcaemia ± acidosis (if poor response)
- Pass nasogastric tube and urinary catheter, if not already done
- Transfer to intensive care unit.

BOX 44.29 Cardiac output = heart rate × stroke volume

Compensates when inadequate:
- Increased heart rate
- Increased systemic vascular resistance
- Increased stroke volume (not in younger children)

Problem-orientated topic:

non-septic shock

Camille, a 4-month-old girl presents to the local paediatric department. She has had poor weight gain for 6 weeks and has been off her feeds for 3 days; she is pale and tachypnoeic at 60 breaths per minute. She is apyrexial, examination of her chest reveals widespread crackles, her heart rate is 190 per minute with a CRT of > 5 seconds and her systolic blood pressure is 50 mmHg.

Q1. What clinical investigation will help make a diagnosis?
Q2. What are the common causes of cardiogenic shock in infancy?
Q3. How should Camille be managed?

Q1. What clinical investigation will help make a diagnosis?

This child has decompensated shock and, though sepsis is always a concern in young children, the history is more chronic and there is nothing to suggest sepsis strongly. In this situation the picture is highly suggestive of cardiogenic shock; therefore, at the same time as instituting appropriate general management for a shocked child, you should also arrange an urgent chest X-ray and ECG (echocardiogram if available), as these help confirm the diagnosis.

An enlarged heart supports cardiogenic shock and if this is present you are likely to need to give vasoactive agents earlier and to be cautious with fluid resuscitation. The ECG should identify arrhythmias such as supraventricular tachyarrhythmias (p. 582) or a predisposing conduction pathway such as Wolff–Parkinson–White syndrome.

Q2. What are the common causes of cardiogenic shock in infancy?

The more common causes of cardiogenic shock in infancy include:
- Cardiomyopathy:
  - Dilated
  - Hypertrophic
  - Restrictive
- Myocarditis:
  - Infective
  - Autoimmune, e.g. Kawasaki disease
- Arrhythmia
- Congenital heart disease:
  - Obstructive left heart lesion, e.g. aortic stenosis, hypoplastic left heart syndrome, coarctation
  - Other complex heart disease.

Q3. How should Camille be managed?

Cardiogenic shock in an infant should be referred to the local PICU and the paediatric cardiologist will play a central role in the acute and long-term management. Echocardiography will enable you to place the child in one of the diagnostic groups and direct further investigation and treatment.

Apparent life-threatening events (ALTEs)

See also page 756.

See also page 756.

Problem-orientated topic:

a collapsed and pale infant

Mathis, a 4-month-old boy, is rushed into the emergency department after mum found him pale and unresponsive in his cot. The ambulance crew report that he responded to rescue breaths and has a heart rate of 170/min.

Q1. What is an apparent life-threatening event?
Q2. What is the initial assessment of Mathis?
Q3. What are the possible causes?
Q4. What is the prognosis?

Q1. What is an apparent life-threatening event?

An apparent life-threatening event is said to have occurred when an infant has one or more episodes in which there is a combination of cyanosis, marked pallor, apnoea, bradycardia and hyper- or hypotonia. The frequency of presentation to hospital is approximately 1–2/1000 births.

The control of respiration changes during different aspects of sleep. In rapid eye movement (REM) sleep there is loss of postural tone and subsequently increased upper airway resistance. The thermoregulatory system has a marked impact on respiratory drive; decreasing temperature increases minute ventilation. In quiet sleep (QS), however, respiratory effort is controlled by chemoreceptor input and the autonomic nervous system. During the first 6 months of life up to 60% of sleep is REM, falling to 30% by 1 year. Hence temperature control is essential during the first year of life.

Q2. What is the initial assessment of Mathis?

Initial management should be geared to making a primary assessment of the child and, if the patient is presenting acutely, checking a blood glucose and blood gas. A thorough history is essential in order to identify any particular aetiology. Carers must be allowed the chance to describe fully the sequence of events leading up to, during and after the episode. Particular attention should be paid to the relationship to feeds, position in the cot, temperature, family history and associated disorders.

Q3. What are the possible causes?

Recognized causes include:
- Gastro-oesophageal reflux (p. 533)
- Infection (e.g. bronchiolitis, p. 603; meningitis, p. 643)
- Seizures (p. 370)
- Cardiac disorders (e.g. arrhythmias, p. 582)
- Metabolic (e.g. medium-chain acyl CoA dehydrogenase deficiency, MCAD)
- Overheating
- Idiopathic (apnoea of infancy).

Up to half of infants with ALTE have no identified cause and it is therefore important that advice is given to carers on trying to avoid further episodes and on how to respond if faced with a similar circumstance.

Q4. What is the prognosis?

The neurodevelopmental outcome obviously depends on the initial severity of presentation, and the risk of recurrence depends on the cause. If there is any associated seizure activity post presentation, this is a bad prognostic factor. Of the 'idiopathic' group with less severe presentation, the majority have no neurological sequelae.

Cardiopulmonary arrest

Problem-orientated topic:

near-drowning ● ● ● ● ●

Sarah, a 6-year-old girl, is on the way to the paediatric emergency department after being found face down in the swimming pool. The ambulance crew phone ahead to say that she is making no respiratory effort and they cannot feel a pulse.

Q1. What is the initial management of this child?
Q2. What further information do you require?
Q3. What is the likely outcome?

Q1. What is the initial management of this child?

When managing cardiopulmonary arrest it is vital that help is called for straight away. As has been described, a primary survey of airway, breathing and circulation is essential, as is the continuation of basic life support once cardiopulmonary arrest is confirmed. With all potential trauma, particular attention must be paid to ensuring cervical spine immobilization. The subsequent management depends upon the arrest rhythm identified and following the protocols as detailed in APLS.

Q2. What further information do you require?

In the management of cardiopulmonary arrest, especially out of hospital, it is important to try to ascertain how long it was before basic life support was commenced and for how long resuscitation has continued. This will guide the duration of further resuscitation efforts and give some idea of outcome. As in this case, the patient may well be cold and it is important to measure the core temperature and actively rewarm if this is $< 30°C$. It is also important to measure the blood glucose and obtain a blood gas so that any metabolic or electrolyte derangements can be corrected.

Q3. What is the likely outcome?

Despite all the improvements in basic and advanced paediatric life support, the outcome of paediatric cardiac arrest is very poor and particularly so when this occurs out of hospital. Survival of out-of-hospital arrests is almost non-existent.

The floppy infant

See also page 381.

Problem-orientated topic:

a pale floppy infant ○ ○ ○ ○ ○

A 2-month-old boy, Lucas, is referred to the paediatric assessment unit by his primary care physician, who is concerned that all is not quite right. On the child's arrival, the nurse calls you straight away as he is pale and floppy.

Q1. What is the first diagnosis to consider?
Q2. What further information will help make this diagnosis?
Q3. What alternative diagnoses should be considered?

Q1. What is the first diagnosis to consider?

When faced with an ill-looking infant, the reflex response tends to be to manage as sepsis. In the majority of cases this will be correct but it must be remembered that other treatable causes do exist.

Q2. What further information will help make this diagnosis?

In order to make the diagnosis of sepsis supportive information should be obtained from the history, such as symptoms of tiredness, irritability, vomiting and fever over a few days. Examination may well reveal a tachycardia, tachypnoea and poor peripheral perfusion. Whilst investigations such as cultures can be very useful in confirming the diagnosis they can take 1–2 days and the full blood count and C-reactive protein are not always helpful. A pragmatic approach tends to be to treat for possible sepsis whilst awaiting cultures and considering other diagnoses.

Q3. What alternative diagnoses should be considered?

Other possible causes of apparent sepsis in an infant can be approached in a systematic way:
- Cardiovascular:
  - Congenital heart disease
  - Arrhythmias
  - Myocarditis and pericarditis
- Gastrointestinal:
  - Severe dehydration
  - Pyloric stenosis
  - Intussusception
- Metabolic:
  - Electrolyte abnormalities
  - Inborn errors
  - Hypoglycaemia
- Endocrine:
  - Congenital adrenal hyperplasia

- Neurological:
  - Intracranial haemorrhage (consider NAI).

Spinal muscular atrophy

Spinal muscular atrophy (SMA) covers a spectrum of inherited neuromuscular diseases caused by degeneration of the anterior horn cells. Separation according to diagnostic groups is in part based on the age of presentation/onset of symptoms (Box 44.30). Diagnostic groups are still clinical and the disease is not classified on a genetic basis.

Clinical features
- Unexplained 'flatness' at birth
- Poor respiratory effort
- Recurrent apnoeas
- ALTE: hypoxic–ischaemic brain injury
- Chest infection
- Floppy/generalized muscle weakness
- Feeding difficulties.

Management
- Non-invasive ventilation
- Intubation and ventilation
- Tracheotomy and long-term support
- Palliative care.

There are marked differences in treatments offered at different centres. Until recently in the UK only palliative care was offered; ventilatory support was not offered with a prediction of death within 2 years. In Japan children with SMA type I have routinely been treated with ventilatory support and the morality of the Western European practice is questioned.

Ethical and legal considerations
Principles based on 'best interests' should be used:
- Disparity of offered treatments; contrast:
  - Duchenne muscular dystrophy
  - Spinal cord injury
  - Hypoplastic left heart syndrome

- Imbalance of opinions:
  - Medical
  - Family
- Non-invasive ventilation:
  - Increases survival
  - Significant cost of home ventilation

  - Internet's powerful effect on family expectations.

 http://www.mda.org/disease/sma1.aspx

Further information about spinal muscular atrophy type 1

Neena Modi   Tom Stiris   Sabita Uthaya

CHAPTER

45

Neonatology I: Problems of the prenatal and perinatal period

LEARNING OUTCOMES

By the end of this chapter you should:

- Be able to recognize high-risk obstetric situations and anticipate likely problems in the newborn
- Be able to obtain and understand the importance of a comprehensive clinical history
- Understand the fundamentals of physiological support in the newborn
- Understand the relevance of informing and involving parents
- Be familiar with standard definitions in neonatal medicine
- Ensure that you are trained in newborn resuscitation
- Ensure that you are able to examine a newborn infant objectively.

MODULE EIGHT

Fetal physiology, growth and development

(See also Chs 22 and 47.)

Growth and development of the placenta

The placenta is a metabolically active organ and is an important determinant of the growth and wellbeing of the fetus. It regulates two-way transport between mother and fetus. Disruption of placental development results in a range of problems, including intrauterine growth restriction (IUGR) and death, and may lead to preterm birth.

Placentation begins with the implantation of the blastocyst in the decidua, the uterine mucosal lining. Following contact with the endometrium, the blastocyst becomes surrounded by an outer layer known as the syncytiotrophoblast and an inner layer of cytotrophoblast.

The trophoblast differentiates into villous or extravillous trophoblast. Extravillous trophoblast invades the maternal tissues and modifies the maternal spiral arteries to accommodate the increase in blood flow to the implantation site. The villous trophoblast comes into contact with maternal blood in the intervillous space and is involved in transport across the placenta. Beginning at around day 18 post conception and carrying on to term, placental blood vessels form by vasculogenesis inside the placental villi, leading to the tertiary villi that make up the villous trees of the placenta until the end of pregnancy. Terminal villi are responsible for gas and nutrient exchange.

Uteroplacental insufficiency results from defective extravillous invasion and failure to modify the maternal spiral arteries.

Fetal growth and development

The most rapid growth rate occurs during fetal life, followed closely by that in the postnatal period.

Assessment of fetal growth

The clinical assessment of uterine size correlates poorly with fetal growth. Fetal size is best measured using ultrasound. Standard measurements are fetal biparietal diameter, abdominal circumference and head to abdominal circumference ratios. Fetal weight may also be estimated with good accuracy. Measurements are plotted on population-based centile charts that may be used for monitoring fetal growth over time.

The term small for gestational age (SGA) is used to describe a baby whose birth weight lies below the 10th centile for gestational age. The term intrauterine growth restriction (IUGR) is applied to an infant in whom there has been a decline in growth velocity in utero.

Fetal growth restriction is considered 'symmetrical' when head size and weight are proportionately reduced or 'asymmetrical' when weight is affected to a greater extent than head size. Symmetrical growth restriction arises when growth declines early in pregnancy, while third-trimester restriction leads to 'head sparing' and disproportionate growth.

Aberrant fetal growth

IUGR results from limitation of fetal growth by one or more pathological processes. These include congenital infections, chromosomal abnormalities and 'uteroplacental insufficiency', in which failure of the extravillous trophoblast invasion results in high uteroplacental resistance and reduced uterine artery blood flow. High uteroplacental resistance is indicated by abnormal Doppler waveforms in the fetal umbilical arteries with absent or reversed end-diastolic flow. Intrauterine growth may also be constrained by poor maternal health or small maternal size.

Fetal macrosomia is a term used to describe a fetus growing above the 90th centile. The most common cause is poorly controlled maternal diabetes and the finding of macrosomia may be an indication to investigate the mother. Alternatively, a constitutionally large fetus is a possibility. Shoulder dystocia is a potential problem and must be anticipated to avoid complications during delivery.

The perinatal outcome of infants with growth restriction secondary to problems of placentation tends to be poorer than in infants where placental function has been normal. The management of pregnancies where there is abnormal placental function is based on close surveillance with longitudinal assessment of fetal growth and Doppler waveforms. The aim is to plan the optimal time for delivery by balancing the risks of prematurity with those of fetal demise and compromise in an unfavourable uterine environment. If there is evidence of decompensation, delivery by caesarean section after administration of antenatal steroids is indicated if the infant is at a gestational age less than 32 weeks. Where uncertainty exists over management, early delivery has been shown in a randomized controlled trial to make no difference to overall perinatal mortality when compared with delayed delivery. However, neurodevelopmental morbidity was greater in the more premature infants who were delivered early. Where the infant is above 34 weeks' gestation, the risks of prematurity are outweighed by those of delayed delivery. Assessment of fetal wellbeing is summarized in Table 45.1.

The effect of labour and delivery on the neonate

The overwhelming majority of newborns are born healthy and at term. The outcomes of pregnancy can be summarized in the rates of stillbirth and perinatal, neonatal and infant mortality (Table 45.2). It is important to recognize the factors that contribute to variations in these rates over time, between countries and between different areas and populations within countries. The legal definition of viability differs, but in many countries was reduced from 28 to 24 weeks' gestational age.

Care during labour and delivery can have profound effects on infant wellbeing. Labour that is delayed or complicated and births that are unsupervised or supervised by unskilled attendants characterize maternal care in many parts of the world and lead to high rates of mortality and morbidity. With improvements in obstetric care, rates of birth trauma, asphyxia, infection and congenital malformations decline and the proportion of mortality and morbidity attributable to preterm birth increases.

Table 45.1 Assessment of fetal wellbeing

Method	What it involves	Comments
Fetal movements	Maternal counting of movements over a given time	Decrease in fetal movements is associated with increased mortality and fetal compromise
Liquor volume assessment	Clinical assessment by palpation verified by ultrasound assessment of deepest liquor pool or amniotic fluid index	Oligohydramnios is a sign of placental insufficiency and polyhydramnios is associated with high perinatal loss rate
Doppler studies	Umbilical artery Doppler measurement of resistance to blood flow	Reversed and absent end-diastolic flow indicate impaired placental function
Antenatal cardiotocography	Fetal heart rate record	Of value when combined with other measures
Biophysical profiles	Ultrasound scanning for fetal movements, fetal muscular tone, fetal breathing movements, amniotic fluid volume, fetal heart rate record. Combination of all to produce single score	Time-consuming and superseded by Doppler studies

Table 45.2 Stillbirth and perinatal, neonatal and infant mortality rates

Rate	Definition
Stillbirth	The number of babies born without signs of life after 24 weeks' gestation per 1000 total (live and still) births
Perinatal mortality	The number of stillbirths and deaths within the first 7 days of postnatal life per 1000 total (live and still) births
Early neonatal mortality	The number of deaths within the first 7 days of postnatal life per 1000 live births
Late neonatal mortality	The number of deaths between 8 and 28 days of postnatal life per 1000 live births
Neonatal mortality	The number of deaths up to 28 days of postnatal life per 1000 live births
Post-neonatal mortality	The number of deaths from 28 days to 1 year per 1000 live births
Infant mortality	The number of deaths in the first year per 1000 live births

Infants with IUGR tolerate labour and delivery less well than appropriately grown infants. However, the evidence to support the routine delivery of IUGR infants by caesarean section is not conclusive.

Birth trauma

Fractures may occur at the time of birth. They are seen more often with large babies. They may involve any long bones but are most commonly seen involving the clavicle. Clavicular fractures do not require treatment, unlike those involving the femur and humerus. The infant may present with a swollen and tender limb and avoid voluntary movement of the particular limb.

Brachial plexus injuries

These are described in association with shoulder dystocia when the head is delivered and traction is applied in order to deliver the rest of the body, in cases of breech delivery when attempting to deliver the head following delivery of the trunk, and also in the absence of a history of difficult delivery. The resulting paralysis is dependent on which nerve roots are involved. Erb palsy involves a lesion of C5–6 with denervation of the deltoid, supraspinatus, biceps and brachioradialis. The infant holds the arm with the shoulder internally

> **BOX 45.1 Causes of hypovolaemic shock in the perinatal period**
>
> - Maternal antepartum haemorrhage (placenta praevia, abruption placenta, uterine rupture)
> - Feto–maternal or feto–fetal haemorrhage
> - Ruptured vasa praevia
> - Traumatic delivery resulting in haemorrhage (subcapsular haematoma of the liver, intraventricular haemorrhage, subdural haemorrhage, subaponeurotic haemorrhage, extensive bruising)
> - Early cord clamping
> - Cord accidents

rotated, and the forearm pronated with extension of the elbow and flexion of the wrist (the 'waiter's tip position'). In this condition the Moro reflex is asymmetrical. In the majority of cases there is recovery of function but this may take several months.

Shock

Hypovolaemic shock now rarely results from traumatic delivery (Box 45.1). The hallmark of neonatal shock is profound pallor. The peripheral pulses are weak and thready but the baby, especially if mature, may have a weak cry and show respiratory movements.

The immediate management of hypovolaemic shock is shown in Box 45.2.

BOX 45.2 Management of hypovolaemic shock

- Manage airway and respiration as required
- Commence chest compressions if indicated
- Insert umbilical venous catheter immediately
- Take blood for an urgent haematocrit and blood gas analysis, but do not wait for the results
- Administer a bolus of 20 ml/kg normal saline if blood not immediately available
- Use emergency O negative blood (usually stored on labour ward), 20 ml/kg
- Request a Kleihauer test on the mother to detect the presence of fetal blood in the maternal circulation

---

Asphyxia

See page 722.

Infection

See page 733.

High-risk pregnancy and its outcome

A pregnancy is described as high-risk if there are maternal or fetal conditions that pose a threat to the health of the fetus and/or the mother (Box 45.3).

Once a pregnancy is identified as high-risk, close monitoring of the fetus and the mother is required. The parents need to be counselled on the plan of management and possible outcomes. If appropriate, termination of pregnancy may be offered. Management plans should be made jointly by obstetricians, neonatologists and other appropriate specialists such as surgeons and geneticists. The plan of management will include treatment of the mother, the timing of delivery, the mode and place of delivery and the subsequent management of the infant. If indicated, the need for a paediatrician to be present at the time of delivery or to be informed of the birth once it has occurred should be clearly documented. Good communication between the various professionals involved is vital.

Following delivery further management must be discussed with a senior colleague, even if a plan has been made antenatally. The baby must be examined carefully to confirm antenatal assessments (Table 45.3).

BOX 45.3 High-risk conditions

Maternal high-risk conditions

- Extremes of age
- Chronic illness (e.g. hypertension, heart disease, diabetes, thyroid disease, renal disease)
- Infections (e.g. human immunodeficiency virus, HIV)
- Drugs (recreational and therapeutic; alcohol abuse)
- Poor past obstetric history
- Obstetric complications (pre-eclampsia, placenta praevia, obstetric cholestasis)
- Significant oligohydramnios or polyhydramnios

Fetal high-risk conditions

- Multiple pregnancy
- Twin-to-twin transfusion syndrome
- Congenital malformations
- Chromosomal abnormalities
- IUGR
- Hydrops fetalis

Management of threatened preterm delivery (Box 45.4)

The aim of managing threatened preterm delivery is to allow adequate time for the administration of antenatal steroids to the mother while balancing the risks of delayed delivery with those of prematurity. Tocolytics are only indicated in preterm labour between 25 and 34 weeks of gestation. The reason for using tocolytics is to allow sufficient time for the administration of antenatal steroids and not to delay delivery indefinitely.

Immediate or early delivery may be indicated if the risks of continuing pregnancy outweigh the risks of prematurity, as may be the case, for example, with frank chorioamnionitis. Alternatively, allowing the pregnancy to continue may place the health of the mother at risk, as in severe pre-eclampsia.

Twin pregnancy

The twinning rate in the last two decades has risen largely as a result of the new reproductive technologies. Twins have a higher perinatal mortality rate than singletons. This is due to the higher rate of prematurity and growth restriction. Growth restriction in twins occurs after the second trimester.

Types of twinning

Two sperm fertilizing two ova produce dizygotic twins. Separate amnions, chorions and placentas are formed

Table 45.3 Characterizing the newborn baby

Description	Definition	Comments
Low birth weight baby Very low birth weight baby Extremely low birth weight baby	A baby weighing less than 2.5 kg at birth A baby weighing less than 1.5 kg at birth A baby weighing less than 1.0 kg at birth	Low birth weight may be attributable to preterm delivery or IUGR 15.5% of births worldwide are of low birth weight (16.5% in developing countries vs 7% in developed regions) LBW in Europe ~6.4% (6.5% in northern Europe; 6.4% eastern Europe; 5.9% southern Europe; 6.7 western Europe) About 1.5% of births in Europe are of very low birth weight
Preterm baby	A baby born before 37 completed weeks after the first day of the last menstrual period	In Europe approximately 1 in 5 (20%) preterm babies is born below 32–33 weeks' gestation
Small for gestational age (SGA) baby Large for gestational age (LGA) baby Intrauterine growth restriction (IUGR)	A baby whose birth weight is less than the 10th centile for gestational age A baby whose birth weight is greater than the 90th centile for gestational age The slowing of fetal growth velocity	The 10th and 90th centiles for gestational age differ between boys and girls and between different ethnic groups SGA and LGA are statistical terms; a baby may have suffered IUGR and still have a birth weight above the 10th centile Third-trimester IUGR results in a characteristic clinical phenotype: asymmetric growth, scaphoid abdomen, reduced subcutaneous adipose tissue

BOX 45.4 Paediatrician checklist in the event of threatened preterm delivery

- Get a good history and establish the gestation accurately
- Alert colleagues
- If delivery is extremely preterm, a senior doctor must speak with the parents. They must be counselled on what to expect in terms of outcome, as well as on what will happen at delivery. In cases of borderline viability their views on resuscitation must be sought
- Invite parents to visit the neonatal unit, if time permits
- Check the resuscitaire and equipment
- Ensure the delivery room is warm
- Ensure that the various members of the team know their role

in dizygotic twins. The placentas in dizygotic twins may fuse if the implantation sites are close to each other.

Monozygotic twins develop when a single fertilized ovum splits during the first 2 weeks after conception. Monozygotic twins also are called identical twins. An early splitting (i.e. within the first 2 days after fertilization) of monozygotic twins produces separate chorions and amnions (dichorionic/diamniotic). Dichorionic twins have different placentas but these may be separate or fused. Approximately 30% of monozygotic twins have dichorionic/diamniotic placentas.

Later splitting (i.e. during days 3–8 after fertilization) results in monochorionic/diamniotic placentation.

Approximately 70% of monozygotic twins are mono-chorionic/diamniotic. If splitting occurs even later (i.e. during days 9–12 after fertilization), then monochorionic/ monoamniotic placentation occurs. If twinning occurs beyond 12 days after fertilization, then the monozygotic pair only partially split, resulting in conjoined twins.

Twin-to-twin transfusion syndrome (TTTS)

This occurs in 15% of monochorionic twin pregnancies. If untreated, the mortality is high and results in significant neurodevelopmental impairment. TTTS results when there is unbalanced transfusion from a net donor twin to a net recipient twin via placental arteriovenous anastomoses in the absence of bidirectional superficial anastomoses. The diagnosis is made on serial ultrasounds. The characteristic picture is that of a recipient twin with hypervolaemia, polyhydramnios, cardiac enlargement and/or failure, abnormal umbilical venous Doppler waveforms and, in terminal cases, fetal hydrops. The donor twin tends to be 'stuck' with oligohydramnios, oliguria, growth restriction and abnormal umbilical arterial Doppler waveforms.

Although traditionally weight and haemoglobin discordance were used to diagnose TTTS, this is unreliable and should no longer be used. The diagnosis rests on the finding of arteriovenous anastomoses, the fetal observations described above and the presence or absence of compensatory arterio-arterial anastomoses.

There is a high incidence of prematurity in TTTS. Premature TTTS twins tend to do worse than those without TTTS. The donor twin is more likely to die in utero. When one twin dies, although there is improvement in TTTS, the surviving twin has a high risk of death and long-term neurological morbidity. This is irrespective of which twin has died.

Postnatally, the main problems following TTTS are growth restriction and renal impairment in the donor and cardiac dysfunction in the recipient. Management of the condition during pregnancy depends on the severity. Various methods that exist include serial amnioreduction, selective laser ablation, selective feticide and septostomy.

Management of antenatally detected congenital malformations

With advances in ultrasound technology, the diagnosis of structural abnormalities in the fetus has improved. Additionally, the availability of invasive procedures such as chorionic villus sampling, and biochemical and DNA analysis has made antenatal diagnosis more accurate, allowing for better counselling of parents (Box 45.5).

BOX 45.5 Antenatal detection of congenital malformation

Use of ultrasound for antenatal diagnosis
- Neurological conditions (neural tube defects, hydrocephalus)
- Cardiac defects (congenital heart disease)
- Gastrointestinal malformations (congenital diaphragmatic hernia, anterior abdominal wall defects)
- Renal tract anomalies (hydronephrosis, multicystic kidneys)
- 'Soft' markers of aneuploidy (choroid plexus cysts, increased nuchal translucency)
- Skeletal dysplasias

Use of invasive procedures
- Chorionic villus sampling, after 10 weeks of gestation (genetic diagnosis)
- Amniocentesis, 14–16 weeks (karyotyping)
- Fetal blood sampling

Physiological adaptations at birth

During fetal life there is high pulmonary vascular resistance and a low-resistance placental component of the systemic communication. Owing to this and the presence of a patent ductus arteriosus, only a small amount of blood flows into the pulmonary circulation.

At birth two events occur that alter this pattern. Firstly, the umbilical cord is clamped and secondly the lungs fill with air. When the umbilical cord is clamped, venous return to the right atrium from the placenta is reduced. This has the effect of closing the foramen ovale due to the resultant low right atrial pressure, coupled with the rise in left atrial pressure secondary to increased pulmonary venous return. Additionally, the ductus venosus closes due to the reduced umbilical venous return.

The second event, lung aeration, results in decreased pulmonary vascular resistance. This is mediated by the mechanical effects of ventilation, raised arterial oxygen tension and lowered arterial carbon dioxide tension.

Other endogenous factors also contribute towards regulating pulmonary vascular resistance. Nitric oxide and prostaglandin I_2 (PGI_2) both reduce pulmonary vascular resistance. PGI_2 production increases after birth as a result of pulmonary tissue stretch. Bradykinin increases PGI_2 as well as nitric oxide production. Nitric oxide acts by causing smooth muscle cell relaxation.

Factors that increase pulmonary vascular resistance and interfere with the adaptation process after birth include acidosis, hypoxia, under-inflation of the lung, pulmonary hypoplasia and ventricular dysfunction.

Problem-orientated topic:

assessment at birth ● ● ● ● ●

Linnea, a 25-year-old healthy primigravida, delivers a newborn boy weighing 1.8 kg. The baby cries at birth and appears lusty and vigorous. The midwife dries and wraps him, gives him to his mother and calls you to see him.

Q1. What immediate assessment should be made?
Q2. What are the causes of low birth weight?
Q3. To what problems are low-birth weight babies vulnerable?
Q4. What investigations do you carry out and what management do you initiate?

Q1. What immediate assessment should be made?

The principles of newborn care at delivery are the same in every setting and for every baby. The World Health Organization publication, 'Pregnancy, Childbirth, Postpartum and Newborn Care', contains clear guidance.

http://www.who.int/reproductive-health/
publications/pcpnc/pcpnc.pdf

Large PDF WHO publication on pregnancy, perinatal
and post-partum care

Immediate assessment should indicate whether a newborn baby is in need of assistance. If the baby is pink, lusty, vigorous and breathing regularly, no respiratory intervention is necessary. The baby should be kept warm and allowed to stay in skin-to-skin contact with his or her mother.

Oxygen should not be given as a matter of routine but only if indicated by cyanosis. Accumulating evidence suggests that air resuscitation is safe and effective.

Immediate assessment will also indicate whether the baby is preterm. A full examination should be performed. Where there is uncertainty a formal estimate of gestational age can be made using a structured system such as the Dubowitz or Parkin assessments.

Clinical history

It is vital that a thorough and complete history is obtained on any baby either on the postnatal ward prior to carrying out a newborn examination, or on the neonatal unit if he or she has required admission (Box 45.6). This is best obtained by speaking to the parents rather than looking at someone else's notes!

> **BOX 45.6 Clinical history**
>
> - Maternal history: medical, social
> - Family history: including history of consanguinity
> - Previous obstetric history
> - Antenatal history: including results of screening, ultrasounds, medications, admissions and illnesses, antenatal steroids
> - Labour: onset, duration of each stage, analgesia, meconium-stained liquor, complications
> - Delivery: mode, anaesthetic, resuscitation

Q2. What are the causes of low birth weight?

Maternal associates
- Younger and older age
- Poor socioeconomic status
- Certain ethnic groups
- Small mother
- Maternal illnesses (essential hypertension, pre-eclampsia, renal disease)
- Alcohol/drug abuse/smoking
- Multiple pregnancy.

Fetal associates
- Constitutionally small
- Chromosomal anomaly

- Metabolic disorders
- Congenital infection
- Exposure to toxins early in pregnancy (drugs, alcohol).

Q3. To what problems are low-birth weight babies vulnerable?

IUGR babies are at risk of:
- Hypothermia
- Hypoglycaemia
- Polycythaemia
- Neutropenia
- Thrombocytopenia
- Infection
- Enteral intolerance
- Necrotizing enterocolitis.

Q4. What investigations do you carry out and what management do you initiate?

- Confirm gestational age and carry out a clinical assessment of gestational age if dates are uncertain.
- Obtain a karyotype if the baby has dysmorphic features or congenital abnormalities.
- Consider screening for congenital infection.
- Initiate early, regular and frequent feeds.
- Monitor temperature and blood glucose levels.
- Check a free-flowing venous haematocrit.

Principles of homeostatic support in very immature sick newborns

> **Problem-orientated topic:**
>
> **preterm delivery** ● ● ● ● ●
>
> You are called to the delivery suite where Thea, a 17-year-old primigravida, is in advanced preterm labour. A baby believed to be 25 weeks' gestational age is delivered as you arrive. You successfully resuscitate the baby and arrange transfer to the neonatal unit.
>
> Q1. What are the problems the infant is likely to face in the subsequent 48 hours?
>
> Q2. How would you attempt to prevent or ameliorate these?

Q1. What are the problems the infant is likely to face in the subsequent 48 hours?

- Thermoregulation
- Fluid and electrolyte balance
- Avoidance of hypo- and hyperglycaemia
- Establishment of feeds (Ch. 4)
- Lung diseases (Ch. 46)
- Intracranial lesions (Ch. 47)
- Infection (Ch. 47).

Q2. How would you attempt to prevent or ameliorate these?

The following are described below:
- Thermoregulation
- Fluid and electrolyte balance
- Glucose homeostasis
- Acid–base balance.

Thermoregulation (Box 45.7)

Newborn infants, particularly if born preterm, differ from adults and older children in their ability to maintain body temperature. Their large surface area to body weight ratio results in heat loss that is greater relative to heat production. Infants also lack the behavioural and physiological responses to warm and cold environments that older age groups possess. Heat production is dependent on basal metabolic rate. Babies are incapable of shivering in response to cold. Catecholamine release during cooling leads to heat production, through the activation of 'brown adipose tissue'. This is metabolically distinct from white adipose tissue. Brown adipose tissue is found in many depots within the body. The main areas are the perirenal, interscapular, cervical and peri-aortic depots. These sites account for 90% of the total stores. Premature infants lack the ability to recruit brown adipose tissue for heat generation. This, coupled with their large surface area to volume ratio and propensity for heat loss, places them at higher risk of hypothermia.

Infants who become cold are more likely to die and suffer morbidities. Hypothermia can exacerbate surfactant depletion, oxygen uptake and hypoglycaemia

BOX 45.7 Definition of mild, moderate and severe hypothermia

Normal	36.5–37.5°C
Mild	36.0–36.4°C
Moderate	32.0–35.9°C
Severe	< 32.0°C

BOX 45.8 Heat loss

Convection
- Loss of heat to the surrounding air, determined by the difference in temperature between the baby and the surrounding air
- Avoiding draughty rooms helps prevent loss of heat by this means

Conduction
- Loss of heat to surfaces that the infant is in contact with
- Ensuring the baby is wrapped in warm towels avoids heat loss in this way

Radiation
- Loss of heat to the surrounding surfaces
- Using double-walled incubators protects against radiation heat loss; radiant warmers may be used to keep babies warm

Evaporation
- Evaporation of water through the skin and respiratory tract
- This is especially a problem with extremely premature infants whose skin is thin and whose stratum corneum is not keratinized; this results in large transepidermal water loss
- Each ml of water that evaporates from the skin is accompanied by the loss of 560 calories of heat, and so it is also difficult to keep a baby with a high transepidermal water loss warm

and lead to the increased utilization of calorific reserves and tissue acidosis. Temperature control is therefore extremely important in newborn babies (Boxes 45.8 and 45.9).

Measurement of temperature

Temperature measured in the rectum, axilla and skin over the abdomen reflects the core temperature. Rectal temperature may be measured using either a mercury thermometer or a flexible thermocouple. If the former is used, it is inserted to 3 cm in a term infant and 2 cm in a preterm infant. If the latter is used, the probe is inserted to 5 cm. The normal rectal temperature varies between 36.5 and 37.5°C.

Fluid and electrolyte balance

Postnatal alterations in body water compartments

Disturbances in electrolyte and water balance are not uncommon in newborn infants. Loss of body

- A warm, draught-free delivery room (at least 25°C)
- A warm surface to receive, dry and wrap baby
- Immediate drying
- Mother–infant skin-to-skin contact
- Putting a warm cap on baby's head
- Covering baby and mother together
- Delayed washing and bathing
- Do not remove vernix
- Warm transport incubator if transfer to the neonatal unit is anticipated
- Babies < 29 weeks or with estimated birth weight of < 1000 g may be placed in a plastic bag up to the neck without prior drying, and covering the head but not the face. This prevents heat loss through evaporation, a major contribution to hypothermia

water is an integral part of the physiology of postnatal adaptation and the transition from an aqueous intra-uterine environment to a gaseous environment. The postnatal loss of body water derives principally from the extracellular compartment and this accounts for the major part of postnatal weight loss. As sodium is the principal electrolyte in extracellular fluid, negative sodium balance is the physiological norm during the period of postnatal adaptation. The timing of the loss of extracellular fluid is closely linked to cardiopulmonary adaptation and is delayed in infants with respiratory distress syndrome.

Water balance

In very immature babies the principal determinant of water balance in the first days after birth is the magnitude of insensible water loss. Every effort should be made to reduce this to a minimum. Water should be provided in an intake sufficient to allow the excretion of a relatively small initial renal solute load and to maintain tonicity in the face of initially high, but rapidly falling, transepidermal losses. Skin maturation, unlike the maturation of renal function, is accelerated by birth. After 32 weeks' gestation water loss through the skin has fallen to around 12 ml/kg/day. Extremely immature preterm babies, in whom minimum urine osmolality is of the order of 90 mosm/kg, will be able to achieve a maximum urine flow rate of around 7 ml/kg/hr.

Sodium balance

Preterm neonates have a limited ability to excrete and retain a sodium load. In neonates, a smaller proportion of filtered sodium is absorbed in the proximal tubule and a correspondingly larger proportion delivered distally. Distal tubular sodium reabsorption is regulated via the renin–angiotensin–aldosterone system (RAAS). Poor sodium retention is due to impaired reabsorption at the proximal tubule, resulting in a higher distal sodium delivery, and to limited aldosterone responsiveness at the distal tubule. Intestinal absorption is also limited. Sodium is not lost through the skin because babies born below 36 weeks' gestation do not sweat, though this develops within the first 2 weeks after birth. Both preterm and full-term neonates have a limited capacity to excrete a sodium load. This is because acute sodium loading results in only a blunted fall in RAAS activity and a limited natriuretic response. Excessive sodium administration in the immediate postnatal period will delay the postnatal loss of extracellular fluid, including loss of pulmonary interstitial fluid, and exacerbate respiratory distress.

Management of neonatal fluid balance is outlined in Box 45.10.

Glucose homeostasis

Neonatal glucose metabolism

During fetal life glucose is transported across the placenta by a process of facilitated diffusion. The fetal brain is able to utilize ketones in addition to glucose. Glucose is the predominant energy source for the fetus and only negligible amounts of fetal glucose are produced, if any. At birth, the constant supply of glucose is interrupted and the newborn has to make adaptations to mobilize glucose and other substrates in order to meet its energy requirements.

At birth there is an increase in adrenaline (epinephrine), noradrenaline (norepinephrine) and glucagon, whereas the concentration of insulin decreases. The level of glucose falls and reaches its nadir at 1 hour of postnatal age, followed by a gradual rise at 2–4 hours of age. The result of the hormonal surges is that glycogen and fatty acid levels rise. Adipose tissue stored in the third trimester is a protective mechanism against postnatal decline in glucose concentration. The insulin/glucagon molar ratio is high in the fetus at term and then declines rapidly after birth, promoting glycogenolysis and gluconeogenesis.

Prevention and anticipation of hypoglycaemia (Box 45.11)

Hypoglycaemia is defined as a blood glucose < 2.6 mmol/l. Severe hypoglycaemia (blood glucose < 1.5 mmol/l) is a potentially serious condition and should be treated immediately. Good practice centres

BOX 45.10 Ten steps to successful management of neonatal fluid balance during intensive care

1. Minimize insensible water loss through adequate humidification of inspired gases, maintenance of high ambient humidity and meticulous skin care

2. What is the infant's estimated transepidermal water loss? Base your estimate on gestational age, postnatal age and ambient humidity

3. Calculate initial fluid requirement as 'estimated insensible water loss PLUS allowance for urine output'

4. Avoid or minimize parenteral sodium intake until the period of postnatal contraction of the extracellular fluid compartment is over; this is marked by stabilization of postnatal weight loss

5. Optimize renal perfusion; monitor core–peripheral temperature gap, capillary refill time and blood pressure; provide volume and/or inotrope support as necessary

6. Review regularly; monitor urine output and serum sodium, potassium and creatinine

7. Urine output should be > 1 ml/kg/hr; if not, administer a fluid challenge followed by a single dose of furosemide 2 mg/kg

8. If the serum sodium falls below 134 mmol/l, decrease the intravenous volume administered; if the serum sodium rises above 142 mmol/l, increase intravenous intake

9. The blood urea is of little value in the assessment of renal function in the newborn as it is influenced by numerous non-renal factors

10. Successful management is marked by steady fall in serum creatinine, stable electrolytes and weight gain of around 12–16 g/kg/day after the period of initial weight loss

Box 45.11 Risk factors for hypoglycaemia

- Small for gestational age
- Postmaturity
- Infant of diabetic mother
- Prematurity
- Severe rhesus alloimmunization
- Polycythaemia
- Seizures
- Septicaemia
- Hypothermia
- Hypoxic–ischaemic encephalopathy
- Maternal therapy with tolbutamide or β-blockers
- Inborn errors of metabolism:
  - Glycogen storage disease (type 1)
  - Galactosaemia
  - Fructose 1–6 diphosphatase deficiency
  - Hereditary fructose intolerance
  - Adrenocortical deficiency
  - Proprionic acidaemia
  - Fatty acid oxidation defects, e.g. medium-chain acyl CoA dehydrogenase deficiency (MCAD)
- Beckwith–Wiedemann syndrome
- Primary islet cell disorders (hyperinsulinism)
  - Hyperplasia
  - Adenoma
  - Persistent hyperinsulinaemic hypoglycaemia of infancy
- Pituitary insufficiency

on the anticipation and prevention of hypoglycaemia and the early establishment of enteral feeds. Healthy well-grown term infants do not require screening for hypoglycaemia. Persistent hypoglycaemia, especially in the presence of symptoms (floppiness, jitteriness, poor feeding and lethargy, rarely seizures and coma), must be treated as an emergency, as it is associated with adverse neurological outcome. Infants who are symptomatic need admission to the neonatal unit and further investigation. Always remember that a baby who is sleepy and feeding poorly may have an infection or be hypothermic or hypoglycaemic and that these conditions may coexist.

Prevention of hypoglycaemia

Infants at risk of hypoglycaemia should be identified and a plan of management drawn up. At-risk infants should be fed within 1 hour of birth and the blood glucose checked at 3–4 hours of age before the second feed. There is no need for a blood glucose measurement before this time. The baby with a blood glucose measurement < 3 mmol/l at 3–4 hours of age should be fed every 3 hours until the prefeed blood glucose is at least 3 mmol/l on two consecutive occasions.

If the blood glucose remains low and the baby remains asymptomatic, increase the feed frequency and volume. Breastfed babies can have formula top-ups either by cup or by nasogastric tube. If the glucose measurement is < 2.6 mmol/l, check a true blood glucose using a blood gas machine or send a sample to the laboratory in a fluoride oxalate tube.

If the true whole blood glucose concentration is < 2.6 mmol/l, close surveillance should be maintained and intervention is recommended if whole blood glucose remains below this level despite frequent appropriate volume feeds or if abnormal clinical signs develop.

Admit the baby if frequency of feeds needs to be increased to 2-hourly. Continue feeding with breast milk whenever it is available, as there is evidence that breast milk helps in the earlier achievement of a normal blood glucose level. If additional milk is required, use a preterm formula. Early referral to a specialist centre is indicated in cases of hyperinsulinaemic hypoglycaemia.

Management of infants with intravenous glucose

- Any baby who has persistent symptoms, is not tolerating enteral feeds, or is unable to maintain normoglycaemia with appropriate enteral feeds alone should be commenced on an intravenous infusion of 10% glucose.
- Babies on i.v. glucose should still receive breast or enteral feeds, if appropriate.
- Normal neonatal hepatic production rate of glucose is between 4 and 6 mg/kg/min.
- Large volumes of enteral feed may not be tolerated.
- I.v. bolus 3 ml/kg 10% glucose should only be given if whole blood glucose measured on blood gas machine is < 1.5 mmol/l and the baby has not responded to previous treatment or there are severe symptoms. Always increase the concentration of glucose infusion as well.
- If the blood glucose is not maintained, increase the concentration of glucose rather than the volume. A central line will be necessary if glucose concentrations exceeding 15% are required.
- Consider glucagon early (see below).
- Discuss all babies with persistent hypoglycaemia with a senior colleague.

Management of persistent hypoglycaemia

(Boxes 45.12 and 45.13)

- If a baby requires glucose infusion rates of greater than 8 mg/kg/min, insert a central line (long line/ umbilical venous catheter).
- If the baby remains hypoglycaemic despite increasing glucose infusion rate to 12 mg/kg/min, draw blood at the time baby is hypoglycaemic for:
  - Blood glucose
  - Insulin
  - Cortisol
  - Growth hormone.
- The presence of insulin in the face of hypoglycaemia is indicative of hyperinsulinism. Urine will be found to be negative for ketones. Consider the diagnosis of hyperinsulinism if a history of maternal diabetes is not forthcoming. This will require early referral to a specialist centre for further management.

BOX 45.12 Emergency treatment of hypoglycaemia

If the baby has major clinical signs (convulsions, coma) or the blood glucose (BG) is < 1.0 mmol/l:

- Take a sample for confirmatory BG but do not wait for result
- Give an intravenous bolus of 3 ml/kg 10% glucose followed by an infusion of at least 3 ml/ kg/hr
- Hypoglycaemia may need to be treated with glucagon (100 μg/kg given intramuscularly or intravenously) if there is difficulty in securing intravenous access in the presence of clinical signs or there is persistent hypoglycaemia despite increasing the glucose infusion rate
- Check BG hourly until > 2.0 mmol/l

BOX 45.13 Investigation of severe or persistent hypoglycaemia

Conditions
- See Box 45.12

Blood
- pH, lactate, ketone bodies, fatty acids, insulin, glucagon, catecholamines, cortisol, growth hormone, amino acid profile

Urine
- Organic acid profile

Acid–base balance

Blood gas measurements are frequently made in neonatal medicine . During aerobic metabolism carbon dioxide is produced. In the presence of carbonic anhydrase CO_2 combines with H_2O to form carbonic acid, which in turn dissociates to form HCO_3^- and H^+. CO_2 is excreted through the lungs and H^+ through the kidneys.

$$CO_2 + H_2O \longleftrightarrow H_2CO_3 \longleftrightarrow H^+ + HCO_3^-$$

The regulation of acid–base balance involves buffers, respiratory function and renal function. In the proximal renal tubular cells H^+ ions are actively pumped into the tubular lumen and combine with filtered bicarbonate to form carbonic acid, which dissociates to water and CO_2. The CO_2 then diffuses back into the tubular cell to repeat the cycle. The net effect is that for each hydrogen ion excreted, one bicarbonate ion is retained, so that bicarbonate reserves are continuously regenerated.

A metabolic acidosis is due to an increase in acid or a decrease in base. The most common cause of metabolic acidosis in neonatal intensive care is tissue hypoxia leading to lactic acidosis. Metabolic acidosis occurs with sepsis, renal failure, amino acid intolerance during parenteral nutrition and in inborn errors of metabolism. A metabolic acidosis is marked by a low pH, PCO_2 and bicarbonate and a high negative base excess. If respiratory compensation occurs, the pH normalizes as the PCO_2 falls.

A respiratory acidosis is characterized by a high PCO_2. Sodium bicarbonate will exacerbate the condition and further raise the PCO_2. As renal compensation occurs, the plasma bicarbonate will rise.

The most common cause of a metabolic alkalosis is excessive administration of bicarbonate or loss of gastric acid with vomiting or in nasogastric aspirates. A respiratory alkalosis results from over-ventilation, whether iatrogenically during mechanical ventilation or spontaneously in neurologically damaged infants.

The correct management of disordered acid–base balance should always begin with consideration of the cause.

Congenital malformations

Examination of the newborn

(This is described in more detail in Chapter 8.)

Aims

The purpose of the first routine postnatal check, usually done on day 1–2, is to:

- Identify any antenatal issues that may be relevant for the infant's health
- Identify any abnormalities in the baby
- Identify abnormalities where early referral impacts on outcome (cataracts, hips, cleft palate)
- Deal with parental concerns/questions
- Investigate/refer any abnormalities found.

How to examine a newborn

- Adopt a top-to-toe approach.
- Follow the sequence: look, feel, listen, measure.
- Check general appearance (dysmorphic features, skin).
- Plot anthropometric indices (weight, head circumference, length).
- Neurological:
  - Check movements, tone, reflexes, posture, alertness, visual orientation.
- Cardiovascular:
  - Look at the precordium, look for cyanosis; feel apex beat and femoral pulses; listen for murmurs.
- Abdominal:
  - Examine liver, spleen, kidneys, testes, genitalia.

- Inspect anus and establish patency.
- Respiratory:
  - Look for recession, indrawing, nasal flaring, cyanosis; listen for air entry, stridor, wheeze; measure respiratory rate.
- Eyes:
  - Seek red reflexes, colobomas, squint; check the orbit.
- Examine the palate (soft and hard).
- Hip examination:
  - Are hips stable, subluxable or dislocated? Are hips relocatable if dislocated?
- Musculoskeletal:
  - Look for talipes, brachial plexus injury, fractures, spine.

Problem-orientated topic:

abdominal masses ● ● ● ● ●

Whilst carrying out first-day checks on the postnatal ward you discover a baby has bilateral masses on abdominal examination. The baby appears well and the parents are anxious to go home.

Q1. What is your differential diagnosis?

Q2. What do you do?

Q1. What is your differential diagnosis?

- Renal dysplasia (multicystic kidney diseases)
- Polycystic kidney disease
- Hydronephrosis (dilatation of the renal pelvis due to functional or anatomical obstruction along the urinary tract); if bilateral, may be indicative of posterior urethral valves in a male
- Tumours.

Q2. What do you do?

Bilateral abdominal masses are suggestive of a renal abnormality. Examine the baby carefully for any other abnormalities. Explain to the parents what you have found and the need for further tests. Discuss with a senior colleague. Request an urgent renal ultrasound. Monitor urine output and check baseline serum creatinine and electrolytes.

Care of the parents (Box 45.14)

The arrival of a new baby is an emotional time for parents and can be extremely stressful if the baby is

BOX 45.14 **Care of the parents**

- Courtesy is important: take the trouble to establish the names of the parents at the first meeting
- Take a clinical history from the parents, not from someone else's notes!
- Social factors are relevant to newborn health and wellbeing: take a social history, politely but meticulously
- Avoid jargon
- Listen to parents' concerns but do not be tempted to make promises you cannot keep ('I'm sure he'll be fine')
- If you cannot answer a question, say so and explain that you will find out or ask someone more senior to speak to them
- Document a summary of your discussion

unwell. A neonatal unit can be a bewildering place. Information must be obtained from parents and imparted to them. Introduce yourself and explain that you are one of a large team of staff who may be involved in the care of their baby. Take a careful clinical history as soon as possible. Social factors are relevant to newborn health and wellbeing. It is wise to take an objective social history as a matter of admission routine. Explain what their baby's problem is in simple terms and describe what is being done. Make it clear that this is the first of many discussions. No matter how busy, staff must keep parents informed.

Supporting parents of a sick newborn baby

Parents have greatly differing needs. They may require practical, emotional and financial support. A parent may be an unsupported teenager or a senior healthcare professional. A parent may attempt to cope by staying away from the hospital or by attempting to control every detail of his or her baby's care.

Explain the working practices of the unit and provide written information. A careful social history obtained at the outset will help direct support as appropriate. Nursing and medical staff are inevitably most closely involved but additional support may be drawn from social workers, psychologists, counsellors, religious advisors, support and self-help groups, primary care physicians, relatives and friends.

It can be difficult to retain information, especially in a stressful situation, and information may have to be given to parents repeatedly. It can be helpful to begin each update by asking parents to tell you what they were last told. Documentation and team debriefings are important to ensure that information is shared.

Many sick newborn babies require prolonged hospitalization. Parents have to live through lengthy uncertainty while continuing to deal with the ongoing requirements of daily life. This can take its toll and staff may find themselves used as 'punch-bags'. Staff, particularly if junior or inexperienced, may have to be supported themselves. They should be made aware of normal human responses when confronted with bad news and the progression from denial to anger and ultimately to acceptance.

Every parent wants to know what the future holds for his or her baby. A prognosis may be clear-cut or uncertain, very good or very poor. It can be easy for staff to forget that what may seem obvious to them — for example, that the prognosis for physiological jaundice is excellent — may not be obvious to a parent. A guarded prognosis can be difficult to impart and should be undertaken by a consultant.

Assessment of home care

An introduction to parenting skills is usually included in antenatal and postnatal classes. For the majority of parents with healthy mature babies, this, along with the support they receive from family and friends, is sufficient. Maternity units try to provide access to breastfeeding counsellors, who are skilled at supporting new mothers and offering practical advice. Every mother–baby dyad is different and helping a new mother gain confidence in caring for her baby is an important part of the professional role. All parents need information on how to minimize the risks of sudden infant death and on immunization schedules.

If a baby has special requirements or is going home after a long period of hospitalization, or if parents have difficulties of their own to contend with, extra assessment and support are likely to be necessary. Parents will need training if their baby has specific requirements. This may be in nasogastric tube or gastrostomy feeding, in physiotherapy exercises, in the management of convulsions, or in feeding technique and positioning for gastro-oesophageal reflux. If a baby requires continuing oxygen therapy, a home visit by the community support team is necessary to assess pushchair access with heavy cylinders, installation of suction equipment and general suitability. Single parents or very young parents may need early support from their health visitor. Terminal care at home will require multidisciplinary input. Families with social difficulties will require the assistance of a social worker.

A good family and social history on admission will indicate areas where extra help may prove necessary.

MODULE EIGHT

Regular ongoing discussions with parents and a team approach with good communication will identify needs as they arise. As discharge approaches, a checklist of requirements should be drawn up.

Bereavement

Death may occur suddenly and unexpectedly or after a prolonged and difficult period of intensive care. The care of parents does not stop with the death of a baby. A senior member of the medical staff, usually a consultant, should explain the process of the post-mortem examination and ask for parental permission to perform this. Most hospitals or neonatal units are able to call upon the services of a bereavement support coordinator, who is able to explain the death registration procedure to parents and help them make arrangements for the funeral or cremation. Parents often form close bonds with staff, particularly if their baby has spent many weeks in hospital. Many parents appreciate staff attending the funeral. They may be comforted by being able to talk to staff about their baby, particularly as friends and relatives may find this difficult to do. After a period of about 4–6 weeks, an appointment is usually made with a consultant and nurse. This provides an opportunity to discuss unresolved questions, explain autopsy findings and come to terms with what has happened.

Further reading

Dubowitz LMS, Dubowitz V, Mercuri E, editors. (1999) The Neurological Assessment of the Preterm & Full-Term Newborn Infant. Clinics in Developmental Medicine No. 148. London: MacKeith Press

Ravindra Bhat   Anne Greenough   Marta Thió

Neonatology II: Respiratory and cardiac disorders

LEARNING OUTCOMES

By the end of this chapter you should:

● Know how to diagnose the common and important causes of respiratory distress in term and prematurely born babies

● Understand the basic science of respiratory disorders in the neonate and how this relates to their presentation and management

● Know how to diagnose common cardiac disorders presenting in the neonatal period

● Know how to manage common neonatal respiratory and cardiac disorders

● Be able to interpret arterial blood gas measurements appropriately

● Be able to recognize the chest radiograph abnormalities of common neonatal respiratory disorders.

Neonatal respiratory disorders

Basic science

Fetal lung fluid

- In fetal life, the lung is filled with liquid, increasing from 4 to 6 ml/kg body weight at mid-gestation to about 20 ml/kg near term.
- Compared to either amniotic fluid or plasma, lung liquid has a high chloride but a low bicarbonate and protein concentration.
- The secondary active transport of chloride ions from the interstitial space into the lung is the main force for lung liquid secretion, sodium ions and water following passively down electrical and osmotic gradients.
- The presence of lung liquid is essential for normal lung development; chronic drainage results in pulmonary hypoplasia.

- During labour and delivery, the concentration of adrenaline (epinephrine) increases, the chloride pump responsible for lung liquid secretion is inhibited and lung liquid secretion ceases.
- Lung liquid resorption commences as the raised adrenaline levels stimulate sodium channels on the apical surface of the pulmonary epithelium, via which fetal lung liquid absorption occurs.
- Thyroid hormone and cortisol are necessary for maturation of the normal response of the fetal lung to adrenaline. Exposure to postnatal oxygen tensions increases sodium transport across the pulmonary epithelium.
- Although some liquid is squeezed out under the high vaginal pressure during the second stage of labour, the majority is absorbed into the pulmonary lymphatics and capillaries.
- Delayed lung liquid clearance, as occurs following delivery without labour, results in transient tachypnoea of the newborn (TTN) or 'wet lungs'.

Surfactant

Surfactant synthesis increases with increasing gestational age and, as respiratory distress syndrome (RDS) is due to surfactant deficiency, the incidence is inversely related to maturity at birth.

Surfactant composition

- Surfactant is a complex mixture of phospholipids; 70–80% is phosphatidylcholine (PC) and 5–10% is phosphatidylglycerol (PG).
- Approximately 60% of the PC is formed from saturated fatty acids; the primary saturated fatty acid is palmitic acid and the largest component of the phospholipids is dipalmitoyl phosphatidylcholine (DPPC).
- Surfactant proteins (SP-A, B, C and D) constitute 5–10% of surfactant by weight.

Surfactant function

- Surface tension reduction
- Stability of the alveoli and prevention of atelectasis
- Prevention of transudation of fluid.

Surfactant proteins' function

- SP-B is essential for surfactant surface activity.
- SP-C enhances surface absorption and spreading of phospholipids.
- SP-A and SP-D are collectins and, as such, have important roles in the host defence against infection. They target the carbohydrate structures of invading microorganisms.

Lung hypoplasia

Primary pulmonary hypoplasia usually occurs with other associated anomalies, particularly of the renal and urological tract. Some apparently idiopathic cases may have a genetic basis. Secondary pulmonary hypoplasia is more common and occurs if there has been reduced amniotic fluid or intrathoracic space or inadequate fetal breathing movements:

- The timing of onset of the oligohydramnios in pregnancies complicated by ruptured membranes is critical; pulmonary hypoplasia occurs only if the onset is prior to 26 weeks of gestation but is not an invariable consequence.
- Reduction in amniotic fluid production occurs in fetal renal anomalies — for example, Potter syndrome and uteroplacental insufficiency.
- Reduction in intrathoracic space — for example, in small chest syndromes (e.g. asphyxiating thoracic dystrophy or Jeune syndrome), cystic adenomatoid malformation/sequestration of the lung, congenital diaphragmatic hernia (CDH) and pleural effusions — can result in pulmonary hypoplasia due to compression. In fetuses that are hydropic due to

rhesus isoimmunization, pulmonary hypoplasia is a consequence of the pleural effusions but there is also an immune mechanism.

- In neurological or neuromuscular diseases that present in utero — for example, Werdnig–Hoffmann disease and myotonic dystrophy inherited from the mother — impaired fetal breathing movements result in abnormal lung growth.
- Infants with trisomy 18 or 21 are at increased risk of pulmonary hypoplasia.

Problem-orientated topic:

a premature infant with respiratory distress from birth

A male infant, Dimitry, is born by spontaneous vaginal delivery at 28 weeks of gestation weighing 0.946 kg; antenatal steroids were not given. The membranes ruptured at 22 weeks of gestation. Dimitry has poor respiratory effort at birth and is therefore intubated and transported to the neonatal unit, supported by mechanical ventilation. An umbilical arterial catheter is inserted and the first blood gas demonstrates pH 7.15, $PaCO_2$ 8 kPa (60 mmHg) and PaO_2 6 kPa (45 mmHg); at this time the baby is receiving 80% oxygen and peak inspiratory pressure (PIP) and positive end-expiratory pressure (PEEP) of 20/5 cm H_2O and ventilating at a rate of 60/min. (PEEP is usually set at ≥5 cm H_2O to allow for lung recruitment and prevent atelectasis in a premature baby with surfactant deficiency)

Q1. Does the baby have RDS?

Q2. What further information would help you to be sure?

Q3. What differentials should be considered when a prematurely born infant develops respiratory difficulties at birth and has an ongoing respiratory support requirement?

Q4. Are any of the differentials likely here?

Q5. How would this influence your management?

Q1. Does the baby have RDS?

Dimitry has been born very prematurely and antenatal steroids were not given. The arterial blood gases are compatible with severe RDS.

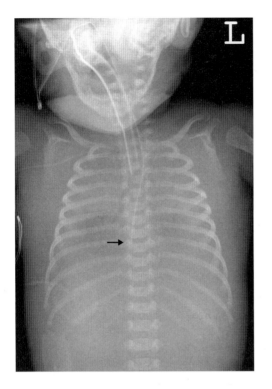

Fig. 46.1 Severe respiratory distress syndrome: 'a white-out'.
Note the infant is ventilated and the nasogastric tube is misplaced, the tip being in the oesophagus (arrow).

Table 46.1 Lung function abnormalities in neonatal respiratory disorders

	Compliance	Resistance	Lung volume
Respiratory distress syndrome (RDS) (severe)	↓↓	Normal	↓↓
Transient tachypnoea of the newborn (TTN)	↓	Normal	↓
Pulmonary hypoplasia	↓↓	Normal	↓↓
Meconium aspiration syndrome (MAS)	↓	↑	↑↓
Bronchopulmonary dysplasia (BPD)	↓	↑	↑↓

BOX 46.1 Differential diagnosis of a baby born prematurely with respiratory difficulties from birth

- Respiratory distress syndrome
- Infection: congenital pneumonia/group B streptococci
- Transient tachypnoea of the newborn
- Air leak
- Coexistent pulmonary hypertension
- Pulmonary hypoplasia

Q2. What further information would help you to be sure?

A chest radiograph in an infant with RDS shows a symmetrical picture of reticulogranular shadowing and air bronchograms to the outer thirds of the lung fields (Fig. 46.1), but importantly does not exclude infection due to group B streptococcus (GBS). A radiograph is essential to exclude other causes of respiratory distress, in this case pulmonary hypoplasia in particular, given that the infant was born following prolonged and premature rupture of the membranes.

Lung function measurements would demonstrate an infant with RDS as having non-compliant lungs and a low functional residual capacity (lung volume); similar results, however, would also be found in an infant with pulmonary hypoplasia (Table 46.1).

Pulmonary maturity can be assessed by measurement of lecithin to sphingomyelin (L:S) ratio in amniotic fluid or in fluid from the baby's pharynx or stomach, but such tests are not part of routine clinical practice.

An echocardiograph examination would be necessary to determine whether the infant has pulmonary hypertension as a cause of the high supplementary oxygen requirements.

Q3. What differentials should be considered when a prematurely born infant develops respiratory difficulties at birth and has an ongoing respiratory support requirement?

In any prematurely born baby who develops respiratory difficulties, infection must be considered (Box 46.1).

Q4. Are any of the differentials likely here?

- The mother has gone into preterm labour at 28 weeks of gestation and infection is a cause of preterm labour; hence infection must be considered as a possible or contributory cause to this infant's respiratory distress.
- The infant has a raised carbon dioxide level and thus has lung disease, but it is possible that the infant has coexisting pulmonary hypertension. Pulmonary hypertension is common in infants with RDS, affected infants often having a poor response to exogenous surfactant therapy. Pulmonary hypertension is more common in infants who have had birth depression.
- The infant was born following preterm and prolonged rupture of the membranes and

pulmonary hypoplasia is more likely in such infants.

- Air leak and other congenital abnormalities would be excluded by the chest radiograph appearance.
- The infant was born following labour and had a vaginal delivery, making transient tachypnoea of the newborn unlikely.

Q5. How would this influence your management?

- In addition to his respiratory support being optimized, Dimitry should receive treatment with a natural surfactant.
- Antibiotics should be given.
- If the infant's oxygen requirement was out of proportion to the severity of lung disease, after optimizing lung recruitment by either increasing the PEEP level or transferring him to high-frequency oscillation and increasing the mean airway pressure, pulmonary hypertension should be considered and an echocardiograph examination undertaken.

Respiratory distress syndrome (RDS)

Approximately 1% of infants develop RDS. Many factors influence the development of RDS (Box 46.2).

Clinical features

- Infants with RDS present within 4 hours of birth; they are tachypnoeic (respiratory rate > 60 breaths/

BOX 46.2 Factors influencing the development of respiratory distress syndrome

Positive
- Cortisol
- Thyroxine
- Beta-adrenergic drugs
- Epidermal growth factor
- Prolactin?

Negative
- Prematurity
- Male gender
- Ethnicity (Caucasian)
- Genetic predisposition
- Insulin
- Hypoxia
- Hypothermia
- Acidosis
- Hypotension

---

min) and have intercostal and subcostal indrawing, sternal retraction, nasal flaring and an expiratory grunt.
- In the absence of surfactant therapy, the dyspnoea worsens over the first 24–36 hours after birth, due to the disappearance of the small quantities of surfactant present in an infant with RDS and the inhibitory effect of plasma proteins on surfactant, which leak on to the alveolar surface in the early oedematous stage of lung damage.
- At approximately 36–48 hours of age, endogenous surfactant synthesis commences and the infant's respiratory status improves; this is associated with a spontaneous diuresis.
- Nowadays, the classical presentation is unusual, as exogenous surfactant is given and relatively mature infants so treated are frequently in room air by 48 hours of age.

Chest radiograph appearance

- There is symmetrical diffuse atelactasis resulting in fine granular opacification in both lung fields and on air bronchogram the air-filled bronchi stand out against the atelectatic lungs.
- If the disease is severe, there may be 'white-out', the lungs appearing so opaque that it is not possible to distinguish between the lung field and the cardiothymic silhouette (Fig. 46.1).
- If the radiograph is taken in the first 4 hours, interpretation may be difficult because of retention of fetal lung fluid.

Assessment of lung maturity

- Antenatally, fetal lung maturity can be assessed by sampling amniotic fluid because, as the fluid secreted by the fetal lung moves out into the amniotic fluid, it carries with it surfactant.
- As the lung matures, the amount of DPPC (lecithin, L) in the amniotic fluid increases, but the amount of sphingomyelin (S) remains unchanged throughout gestation; thus lung maturity can be assessed from the ratio of lecithin to sphingomyelin (L:S ratio).
- An L:S ratio greater than 2.0 is usually associated with lung maturity and in 95% of cases will predict the absence of RDS. However, a mature L:S ratio can be associated with RDS in the infants of diabetic mothers or those with rhesus disease, as in such cases the abnormality is deficiency of phosphatidyglycerol.
- The lower the L:S ratio, the more likely the infant is to develop RDS, but an L:S ratio less than 2.0 predicts RDS with an accuracy of only 54%.

Differential diagnosis

- It is impossible to differentiate severe early-onset septicaemia from RDS.
- Infants with RDS may have coexistent pulmonary hypertension, their oxygen requirement will be out of proportion to their chest radiograph appearance and they frequently have a poor response to surfactant therapy.
- Respiratory distress presenting after 4–6 hours of age is usually due to pneumonia.
- Consider air leak (tension pneumothorax etc.).

Preventative strategies

Antenatal corticosteroids (Box 46.3) may be used:

- Antenatal steroids mature the fetal lung, inducing the enzymes for surfactant phospholipid synthesis and the genes for the surfactant proteins.
- Randomized trials have demonstrated that treatment with antenatal corticosteroids is associated with an overall reduction in neonatal death (relative risk (RR) 0.69, 95% confidence interval (CI) 0.58 to 0.81), RDS (RR 0.66, 95% CI 0.59 to 0.73), cerebroventricular haemorrhage (RR 0.54, 95% CI 0.43 to 0.69), necrotizing enterocolitis (RR 0.46, 95% CI 0.29 to 0.74), respiratory support, intensive care admissions (RR 0.80, 95% CI 0.65 to 0.99) and systemic infections in the first 48 hours of life (RR 0.56, 95% CI 0.38 to 0.85).
- Benefit is maximal in infants delivered between 24 and 168 hours (7 days) of maternal therapy

---

BOX 46.3 Guidelines for antenatal steroid usage

- Should be considered for all women at risk of preterm labour between 23–24 and 36 weeks
- Both dexamethasone (four 6 mg doses 12 hours apart) and betamethasone (two 12 mg doses 24 hours apart) have been shown to be effective. Dexamethasone has been shown to be associated with less intraventricular haemorrhage, although perhaps a higher rate of NICU admission (seen in only one trial). In an observational study, betamethasone was associated with a lower occurrence of cystic periventricular leucomalacia
- Corticosteroids should be given unless immediate delivery is anticipated
- In the absence of chorioamnionitis, antenatal corticosteroids are recommended in pregnancies complicated by preterm and prolonged rupture of the membranes and in other complicated pregnancies, unless there is evidence that corticosteroids will have an adverse effect on the mother

---

being started; a smaller benefit is seen in infants whose mothers have received less than 24 hours of treatment.
- Randomized controlled trials have given conflicting results. Overall, a small benefit regarding postnatal lung function has been observed, but this is associated with restricted growth including the brain; therefore, repeated courses are not recommended.

Other antenatal strategies include the following:

- Thyrotrophin-releasing hormone (TRH), unlike T_4 (thyroxine), T_3 (tri-iodothyronine) or thyroid-stimulating hormone (TSH), crosses the placenta. However, meta-analysis of the results of randomized trials examining the efficacy of antenatal administration of TRH has demonstrated that it does not reduce the risk of neonatal respiratory distress or bronchopulmonary dysplasia (BPD), but may have adverse effects.
- The effect of antenatal β-mimetics appears to be small.
- Benefit from ambroxol has been reported but this is not a consistent finding.

Management

Practice differs in the labour suite as to whether preterm babies at risk of RDS are placed immediately on nasal continuous positive airway pressure (CPAP) or intubated and given surfactant. Once surfactant is given, again practice varies, some clinicians immediately extubating the infant on to nasal CPAP while others keep the infant intubated until further assessment takes place on the neonatal intensive care unit (NICU). Others will delay giving surfactant until the infant is on the NICU.

Surfactant therapy is as follows:

- Commercially available surfactant preparations are described as 'natural' (derived from animals' lungs) or synthetic surfactants.
- Meta-analysis of data from randomized trials demonstrated that administration of natural rather than synthetic surfactant was associated with reductions in mortality and pneumothorax.
- Surfactant is usually given prophylactically, within the first hour of birth, as such a policy is associated with significant reductions in neonatal mortality, BPD and death, and in pneumothorax.
- Surfactant given as 'rescue' therapy — that is, to infants with established RDS — results in reductions in pneumothorax, mortality and the combined outcome of mortality and BPD.
- Although beneficial effects are seen after a single dose of surfactant, better results are obtained with more than one dose. Many clinicians usually now give two doses of a natural surfactant.

- Not all babies respond to surfactant, including those with a patent ductus arteriosus (PDA), cardiogenic shock, pulmonary hypertension or an air leak; failure to respond marks out a group of babies with a poorer prognosis.

Mortality and morbidity
- Overall the mortality from RDS is between 10 and 15%; the mortality rate is inversely proportional to gestational age.
- Acute complications of RDS include air leaks, PDA and pulmonary haemorrhage. Infants with RDS may suffer an intracerebral haemorrhage or periventricular leucomalacia, both conditions increasing the risk of adverse neurodevelopmental outcome.
- BPD, defined as oxygen dependency beyond 36 weeks' postmenstrual age, can develop in up to 50% of infants born prior to 29 weeks of gestation.

Types of respiratory support
- *Warm humidified supplementary oxygen.* This may be all that infants with mild RDS require.
- *Continuous positive airway pressure (CPAP).* This prevents atelectasis and can improve oxygenation.
- *Conventional mechanical ventilators.* These deliver intermittent positive pressure inflations and positive end-expiratory pressure (PEEP). The ventilator inflations are delivered at a preset rate.
- *Patient-triggered ventilation (PTV).* This can be delivered as assist/control (A/C); that is, every spontaneous breath can trigger a positive pressure inflation at preset peak and PEEP levels and as synchronous intermittent mandatory ventilation (SIMV) in which only a predetermined number of positive pressure inflations can be triggered regardless of the number of spontaneous breaths that exceed the critical trigger level.
- *High-frequency jet ventilation (HFJV).* High-velocity 'bullets' of gas are fired at rates of 200–600 per minute and this entrains gas down the endotracheal tube.
- *High-frequency oscillatory ventilation (HFOV).* Small tidal volumes are usually delivered at frequencies between 10 and 15 Hz.

During conventional mechanical ventilation:
- Oxygenation is controlled by the inspired oxygen concentration and the mean airway pressure (MAP).
- The MAP is controlled by the PIP, inspiratory time (Ti) and PEEP. Increased PEEP is the most effective method of increasing oxygenation.

Table 46.2 Adjustments to ventilator settings according to blood gas values

PaO_2 result	$PaCO_2$ result	Suggested changes in ventilation
Low PaO_2	Normal $PaCO_2$	↑ FiO_2 ↑ MAP by ↑ PEEP (not ↑ PIP, which will ↓ $PaCO_2$)
Low PaO_2	High $PaCO_2$	↑ PIP (which will increase MAP and increase delivered volume)
Normal PaO_2	High $PaCO_2$	Keep MAP constant ↓ PEEP or ↑ rate

(MAP = mean arterial pressure; PEEP = positive end-expiratory pressure; PIP = peak inspiratory pressure)

- Carbon dioxide elimination is controlled by the minute ventilation (= tidal volume × rate); tidal volume is determined by the difference between PIP and PEEP.
- Ventilator settings should be altered according to the blood gas abnormality (Table 46.2).

Transient tachypnoea of the newborn (TTN)

TTN occurs in between 4 and 6 per 1000 term-born infants. TTN may be more common in prematurely born infants but coexisting RDS may mask the presentation.

Pathogenesis
TTN is more common in infants who are born by caesarean section without labour, in male infants and in those with a family history of asthma.

Clinical features
Infants with TTN are tachypnoeic with respiratory rates of up to 100–120 breaths/min, but rarely grunt. Peripheral oedema is often present and affected babies lose weight more slowly than controls. There is usually only a mild hypoxia and rarely a marked respiratory or metabolic acidosis.

Chest radiograph appearance
There is hyperinflation and prominent perihilar vascular markings due to engorgement of the periarterial lymphatics, oedema of the interlobar septae and fluid in the fissures.

Management
- Supplementary oxygen may be required, but rarely high concentrations of oxygen or even mechanical ventilation are needed.
- Intravenous antibiotics should be administered until infection has been excluded.

- Prolonged rupture of the membranes
- Premature labour
- Organisms present in the vagina
- Chorioamnionitis
- Prolonged labour
- Frequent pelvic examinations in labour
- Mothers who, despite having GBS in their vagina, have little or no circulating anti-GBS immunoglobulin
- Food, especially dairy products, contaminated with *Listeria monocytogenes* by infected farm animals

- Nasogastric tube feeds should be withheld until the respiratory rate settles.
- Diuretics are not of benefit.

Mortality and morbidity

- TTN is self-limiting and affected infants have usually made a complete recovery within a few days of birth.
- Complications are rare, but air leaks may occur if the infant has required CPAP or mechanical ventilation.
- Infants who have had TTN are more likely to wheeze at follow-up.

Pneumonia

Early-onset pneumonia

Early-onset pneumonia (Box 46.4) is acquired transplacentally or during labour or delivery:

- Transplacentally acquired organisms include *Listeria monocytogenes*, *Mycobacterium tuberculosis*, *Treponema pallidum*, rubella virus, cytomegalovirus (CMV), herpes simplex virus (HSV), adenovirus and influenza A virus.
- In ascending infection causing pneumonia, 60–70% of cases are due to *Streptococcus agalactiae* (group B streptococcus, GBS). *Escherichia coli* (*E. coli*) is the second most common cause of early neonatal sepsis.
- Other organisms that cause ascending infection include *Haemophilus influenzae*, *Strep. pneumoniae*, *Listeria monocytogenes*, *Klebsiella pneumoniae*, *Candida albicans*, adenovirus, CMV, HSV and echovirus.

Clinical features

- Infants with transplacentally acquired infection present at birth and those infected with organisms

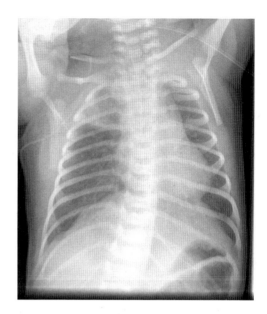

Fig. 46.2 **Lobar pneumonia with right upper lobe changes**

acquired from the birth canal present within the first 48 hours after birth.
- The infant typically suffers progressive respiratory distress and has signs of systemic sepsis, which develop within a few hours of birth. There may be fever or hypothermia, or non-specific signs such as poor feeding and irritability.
- Infants with congenitally acquired listerial infection are often extremely ill at birth with severe pneumonia and hepatomegaly. Diarrhoea and an erythematous skin rash may occur. Characteristically, affected infants have small pinkish-grey cutaneous granulomas; these granulomas are widespread in lung, liver and nervous system.

Chest radiograph appearance

The appearance is varied; there can be lobar (Fig. 46.2) or segmental consolidation, atelectasis or diffuse haziness or opacification (Fig. 46.3). Pleural effusions may occur, particularly if the pneumonia is the result of bacterial or fungal infection. Abscess or pneumatoceles occur with staphylococcal or coliform pneumonia.

Management

- Initial treatment for early-onset pneumonia should be a combination of ampicillin or benzylpenicillin and an aminoglycoside. Modification to that regimen may be necessary once the culture results are known:
  - *H. influenzae* with ampicillin resistance is emerging and cefotaxime should be added.
  - Cefotaxime and ceftriaxone are used for *E. coli* sepsis.
  - For *Listeria*, the most effective antibiotic therapy is ampicillin plus gentamicin; *Listeria* is resistant to all third-generation cephalosporins.

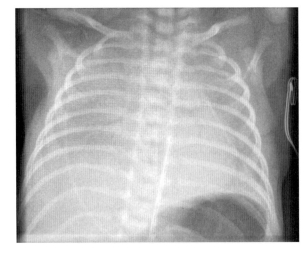

Fig. 46.3 Diffuse group B streptococcal pneumonia with changes mimicking respiratory distress syndrome

- Antibiotic therapy should continue for at least 10 days, and for 3 weeks if the pneumonia is due to *Staphylococcus aureus*.
- Long-term intravenous therapy should be given if there is abscess formation.
- Empyemas should be drained and intravenous antibiotics administered for at least 2 weeks.
- It is important to prevent vertical transmission of GBS by giving intrapartum antibiotic prophylaxis (penicillin or ampicillin) to women identified by screening in pregnancy as carrying GBS and/or having risk factors:
  - A previous infant with GBS disease
  - GBS in the maternal urine during pregnancy
  - Preterm labour
  - Ruptured membranes for more than 18 hours prior to delivery
  - Intrapartum fever.

Late-onset pneumonia

- The most commonly responsible bacteria are coagulase-negative staphylococci, *Staph. aureus* and Gram-negative bacilli, including *Klebsiella, E. coli* and *Pseudomonas*.
- Viruses can also cause late-onset pneumonia, including respiratory syncytial virus (RSV), influenza virus, parainfluenza virus, adenovirus and rhinovirus.
- Fungal infections can occur in infants who have had prolonged exposure to antibiotics, particularly third-generation cephalosporins.

Clinical features

There is an increasing requirement for ventilatory support and/or supplementary oxygen.

Management

- Initial antibiotic treatment should be guided by local microbiological data.
- If the infant is already on antibiotics, the regimen should usually be changed and the spectrum of cover broadened. Samples for septic screening should be taken before that change, to better adjust antibiotic treatment once results are available.

Pulmonary hypoplasia

Clinical features

- Infants with mild pulmonary hypoplasia may be apparently asymptomatic but on inspection are tachypnoeic.
- Those more severely affected require ventilatory support from birth.
- Infants with pulmonary hypoplasia have small-volume, non-compliant lungs and their chest wall is disproportionately small with respect to the abdomen.
- Infants with secondary pulmonary hypoplasia may have associated congenital anomalies: for example, diaphragmatic hernia/eventration, an anterior abdominal wall defect, a dislocated hip and/or talipes. They may also have the features of neuromuscular diseases such as Werdnig–Hoffmann disease or congenital dystrophia myotonica.

Diagnosis

- On the chest radiograph, the ribs may appear crowded with a low thoracic to abdominal ratio and a classically bell-shaped chest, but the lung fields are clear unless there is coexisting RDS.
- Pneumothorax or other forms of air leak are frequently present.

Differential diagnosis

The 'dry lung syndrome' has been described following oligohydramnios due to premature rupture of the membranes and is likely to be due to functional compression. Affected infants are difficult to resuscitate, requiring high peak inflating pressures; the requirement for high pressures may continue for 48 hours but then the infants make a spontaneous recovery, indicating that they have no structural abnormality.

Pathology

Pulmonary hypoplasia is diagnosed if the lung weight to body weight ratio is less than 0.015 in infants born before 28 weeks of gestation and less than 0.012 in infants born after 28 weeks of gestation; in addition there is a radial alveolar count of less than 4%.

Management

Antenatal measures are as follows:

- Pleural effusions can be chronically drained by thoraco-amniotic shunts, which will facilitate ease of resuscitation.
- In utero surgery has been undertaken for infants with CDH but this has been problematic. The efficacy of reversible tracheal 'obstruction' is being investigated in cases predicted to be at high risk of fatal pulmonary hypoplasia.

Postnatal measures are as follows:
- The minimum ventilator pressures compatible with acceptable gases should be used, as these infants are at high risk of air leaks.
- Low-pressure, fast-rate ventilation or high-frequency oscillatory ventilation (HFOV) can be helpful in some infants, but extra-corporeal membranous oxygenation (ECMO) would usually be contraindicated as the infants do not have a reversible condition.
- Pulmonary vasodilators can be useful if there is coexisting pulmonary hypertension.
- Home oxygen therapy allows early discharge, but parents need to be counselled that supplementary oxygen may be required for many months.
- Every attempt should be made to reduce further compromise to the lungs; hand hygiene education and full immunization are essential, and RSV prophylaxis should be considered.

Mortality and morbidity
- Infants with Potter syndrome (renal agenesis, large low-set ears, prominent epicanthic folds and a flattened nose) and postural limb defects die in the neonatal period.
- There is also 100% mortality rate in infants with the oligohydramnios syndrome (pulmonary hypoplasia, abnormal facies and limb abnormalities) due to prolonged rupture of the membranes. In less severely affected infants, the perinatal mortality rate is approximately 50% if membrane rupture occurs between 15 and 28 weeks.
- Infants with pulmonary hypoplasia who remain on high-pressure ventilation and high inspired oxygen concentrations at the end of the first week are in an extremely bad prognostic group, rarely surviving to discharge; those that do survive require home oxygen therapy and many die in the first 2 years following infection.
- Infants born following oligohydramnios can suffer limb abnormalities due to the compression, the reported incidence varying from 27 to 80%.
- Neurological or developmental deficits are common, being reported in 28% of infants born after preterm rupture of the membranes prior to 26 weeks of gestation.

Problem-orientated topic:

a term baby with respiratory distress from birth ● ● ● ● ●

A female infant (birth weight 4.1 kg) is delivered at 42 weeks of gestation by emergency caesarean section for fetal distress. The infant is covered with meconium, makes no respiratory effort at birth and has a heart rate of 40 beats/min. The infant is intubated and no meconium is seen below the cords. The infant responds rapidly to positive pressure inflations and is extubated at 5 minutes. At 1 hour, however, the infant is still tachypnoeic and is then noted to have an oxygen saturation of 80% in air.

Q1. Does the baby have meconium aspiration syndrome (MAS)?

Q2. What further information would help you to be sure?

Q3. What differentials should be considered?

Q4. Are any of the differentials likely and, if so, how would this influence your management?

Q1. Does the baby have meconium aspiration syndrome (MAS)?

The baby was born post-term and MAS is more common in post-mature babies. In addition, she has fetal distress and is covered in meconium at delivery. There is, however, no meconium below the vocal cords when the infant is intubated.

Q2. What further information would help you to be sure?

The chest radiograph in MAS demonstrates widespread patchy infiltration and over-expansion (Fig. 46.4); small pleural effusions occur in approximately 20% of patients. A radiograph facilitates exclusion or diagnosis of other causes of respiratory distress such as air leak, infection or a congenital abnormality (e.g. a diaphragmatic hernia or cystic adenomatoid malformation). It also demonstrates whether an infant has RDS, which would be very uncommon in a mature infant; when it does occur, there is often a family history. Acute respiratory distress syndrome (ARDS) is more likely than RDS and occurs in infants who have suffered birth depression.

In this case, there is no patchy infiltrate but bilateral pneumothoraces.

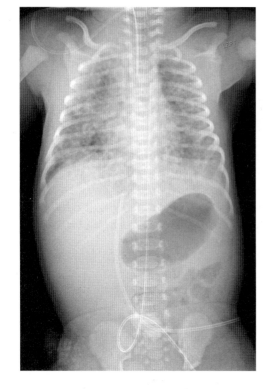

Fig. 46.4 Meconium aspiration syndrome with diffuse bilateral patchy infiltrates

---

BOX 46.5 Causes of respiratory distress from birth in a term infant

- Meconium aspiration syndrome
- Congenital pneumonia/sepsis
- Transient tachypnoea of the newborn
- Air leak
- Respiratory distress syndrome
- Acute respiratory distress syndrome
- Congenital abnormalities

Q3. What differentials should be considered?

In any baby with respiratory problems, infection must be considered (Box 46.5).

Q4. Are any of the differentials likely and, if so, how would this influence your management?

- In the absence of any rapid reliable diagnostic test for infection, any infant with respiratory distress should receive intravenous antibiotics until blood culture results are available at 48 hours.
- This infant required positive pressure resuscitation and this increases the risk of air leak; whether an

air leak requires intervention, such as a drainage procedure, is determined by the size of the air leak and the magnitude of the infant's respiratory distress.
- This infant's respiratory status deteriorated and she required 60% supplementary oxygen to maintain appropriate oxygen saturation levels. The bilateral pneumothoraces were drained by placement of chest tubes and underwater-sealed drains.

Meconium aspiration syndrome (MAS)

- Meconium staining of the amniotic fluid occurs in 8–20% of pregnancies.
- Five percent of babies born through meconium-stained amniotic fluid develop MAS.
- Meconium aspiration is a disease of term or post-term babies; if meconium staining of the liquor occurs in a preterm pregnancy, it suggests infection.

Pathophysiology

Prolonged severe fetal hypoxia can stimulate fetal breathing with inhalation of amniotic fluid containing meconium or the inhalation occurs perinatally if the airway contains meconium-stained amniotic fluid. Meconium inhalation causes a number of problems:

- Meconium is irritant and inflammatory cells and mediators are released in response to the presence of the meconium in the airways. An inflammatory pneumonitis with alveolar collapse develops.
- The pulmonary artery pressure is increased, as the inflammatory response results in release of substances that cause vasoconstriction.
- Although meconium is initially sterile, because of its organic nature, its presence in the airway predisposes to pulmonary infection, particularly with *E. coli*. In addition, as meconium may inhibit phagocytosis and the neutrophil oxidative burst, bacteria can grow in meconium-stained amniotic fluid.
- Meconium (particularly the chloroform-soluble phase: free fatty acids, triglycerides and cholesterol) inhibits surfactant function and production in a concentration-dependent manner.
- Meconium is sticky and composed of inspissated fetal intestinal secretions. When it is inhaled it creates a ball valve mechanism in the airways; air can be sucked in but cannot be exhaled. The result is gas trapping and lung over-distension, predisposing to air leaks.

Clinical features

- Infants with MAS are tachypnoeic and have intercostal and subcostal recession.

- They are frequently hypoxic due to ventilation–perfusion mismatch and pulmonary hypertension.
- The meconium in the airways causes widespread crackles and, due to air trapping, affected infants have an over-distended chest.
- In mild cases recovery may occur within 24 hours.
- Infants who require ventilation are frequently still symptomatic at 2 weeks of age and may remain oxygen-dependent beyond the neonatal period.

Chest radiograph appearance
- Early radiographs demonstrate widespread patchy infiltration and over-expansion (Fig. 46.4); small pleural effusions occur in approximately 20% of patients.
- In severe cases, by 72 hours of age the appearance is of diffuse and homogeneous opacification of both lung fields because of pneumonitis and interstitial oedema.
- In severe cases the chest radiograph appearance may merge into the pattern seen in BPD.

Management
- Broad-spectrum antibiotics, such as penicillin and gentamicin, should be given.
- Sufficient supplementary oxygen should be given to maintain the arterial oxygen saturation levels at 95% or arterial oxygen level greater than 10 kPa (75 mmHg). Warmed humidified oxygen should be delivered into a head box, even if the infant requires an oxygen concentration of up to 80%, providing there is no respiratory acidosis.
- CPAP may improve oxygenation but will increase the risk of pneumothorax and thus is not recommended in MAS.
- Intubation and ventilation are indicated if the $PaCO_2$ rises above 8 kPa (60 mmHg), particularly if the infant is hypoxic. If, however, the infant has hypoxic–ischaemic encephalopathy more rigid control of the blood gases is required.
- Babies with MAS can be very difficult to ventilate; theoretically, a long expiratory time and a low level of PEEP should be used, but elevation of PEEP may be necessary to improve oxygenation.
- A neuromuscular blocking agent should be considered, as infants with MAS often 'fight' the ventilator, thus increasing their risk of an air leak.
- In infants with severe disease and pulmonary hypertension, HFOV, particularly if used with nitric oxide, can improve oxygenation and reduce the need for ECMO.
- Meta-analysis of the results of two randomized trials demonstrated that surfactant administration also reduces the risk of requiring ECMO. Administering the surfactant by dilute surfactant

lavage may be particularly effective in improving gas exchange.

Preventative strategies
- A meta-analysis of the results of four randomized trials showed no significant benefit of routine endotracheal intubation and suctioning at birth over routine resuscitation, including oropharyngeal suctioning of vigorous term meconium-stained babies.
- On the evidence to date, intubation and suctioning should be restricted to newborns who are depressed: that is, they have a heart rate less than 100 beats/min, poor respiratory effort and poor tone.
- Compression of the neonatal thorax is not recommended, as it is unlikely to prevent gasping and can stimulate respiratory efforts.
- Aspiration of the stomach is frequently undertaken to prevent subsequent inhalation following vomiting or reflux of previously swallowed meconium.

Mortality and morbidity
- Mortality rates are between 4 and 12%; the majority of deaths are from respiratory failure, pulmonary hypertension or air leaks.
- Fifty percent of babies who require mechanical ventilation because of MAS suffer an air leak.
- Bronchopulmonary dysplasia is a rare complication of MAS.
- Neurological sequelae occur in infants with coexisting HIE.
- Lung function abnormalities, including increased bronchial hyper-reactivity, have been reported and up to 40% of those who have had severe MAS go on to develop asthma at school age.

Pulmonary hypertension of the newborn

Clinical features
- Infants with persistent pulmonary hypertension of the newborn (PPHN) usually present within 12 hours of birth.
- Affected infants are cyanosed but have only mild respiratory distress, unless they have an underlying disorder such as GBS infection or CDH.

Diagnosis
- Hypoxaemia is disproportionately severe for the radiological abnormalities.
- There is a right-to-left ductal shunt with a lower level of oxygenation in the distal aortic blood

(obtained from an umbilical artery catheter) compared to the preductal blood (obtained from the right radial artery).

- The echocardiograph demonstrates a structurally normal heart.

Chest radiograph appearance

The chest radiograph changes may be minimal in primary pulmonary hypertension and in secondary pulmonary hypertension the appearance is that of the underlying lung disease.

Investigations

- The response to ventilation with 100% oxygen can help to distinguish between PPHN and cyanotic heart disease; in some infants with pulmonary hypertension, the arterial oxygen level will increase to above 13 kPa (97.5 mmHg), whereas in cyanotic congenital heart disease it will not rise above 5–6 kPa (37.5–45 mmHg).
- Not all neonates with pulmonary hypertension, however, especially those with sepsis or a CDH, have a large improvement in oxygenation in response to 100% oxygen.
- Echocardiography is important, not only to establish the diagnosis but also to exclude cyanotic congenital heart disease.

Management

- It is easy to precipitate severe hypoxaemia in infants with pulmonary hypertension; thus minimal handling is important.
- Aggressive therapy should be used to achieve an appropriate systemic blood pressure, as the size of the right-to-left shunt is in part dependent on the systemic blood pressure.
- To maximize oxygen transport to the tissues, the haemoglobin level should be kept greater than 13 g/dl (packed cell volume (PCV) 40%). If the infant is polycythaemic (central PCV greater than 70%), a dilutional exchange transfusion should be undertaken.
- Broad-spectrum antibiotic cover should be given. Infants should be ventilated if their PaO_2 is less than 5–6 kPa (37–45 mmHg) in 70% oxygen. Hyperventilation to reduce the $PaCO_2$ to 2.6–3.5 kPa (20–26 mmHg) is no longer recommended, as this has adverse effects.
- Alkalosis can promote pulmonary vasodilatation, but prolonged alkalosis should be avoided as this increases the hypoxic reactivity of the pulmonary vasculature.
- ECMO is an effective rescue therapy for infants with pulmonary hypertension.
- A number of vasodilator drugs have been used to treat pulmonary hypertension in the neonate.

- Epoprostenol (prostacyclin) is not a specific vasodilator; its administration can result in systemic hypotension and it is not always effective. Tolazoline, another systemic and pulmonary vasodilator which had been used for this pathology, also causes system hypotension and many other adverse effects. It is currently off the market in many European countries.
- Magnesium sulphate administration also can improve oxygenation, but levels must be carefully monitored, as hypermagnesaemia can cause hyporeflexia, hypotension and calcium and potassium disturbances.
- Inhaled nitric oxide (NO) is a specific pulmonary vasodilator. When NO is inhaled, it diffuses across the capillary membrane and activates guanylate cyclase in the pulmonary arteriolar smooth muscle; the resulting increase in cyclic guanosine monophosphate (cGMP) causes smooth muscle relaxation. NO then binds rapidly to haemoglobin; once bound, it is inactivated and therefore produces no systemic effects.
- In term infants 5 ppm of iNO appears as effective as higher doses.
- In term-born babies, meta-analysis of the results of randomized trials demonstrated that inhaled NO results in an improvement in oxygenation and a reduction in the combined outcome of death or need for ECMO; the effect is due to a reduction in the need for ECMO.
- Inhaled NO works best if given in association with a volume recruitment ventilation strategy.
- No significant long-term benefits of inhaled NO have been demonstrated in babies with CDH and its use in preterm infants remains experimental.
- NO does have side-effects related to nitrogen dioxide and methaemoglobin formation and its administration has been associated with an increased bleeding time.
- Promising oral drugs include Sildenafil and Bosentan.

  Sildenafil is a 5-phosphodiesterase (PDE5) inhibitor. PDE5, a cGMP-specific inactivator, is expressed in smooth muscle cells, vascular endothelium, and platelets. Inhibition of PDE5 increases intracellular cGMP levels, promotes alveolar growth and angiogenesis, and attenuates inflammation and airway reactivity in animal models. It also improves pulmonary vascular physiology in infants with persistent pulmonary hypertension, which may lead to prevention of right ventricular hypertrophy.

  Bosentan is a dual endothelin-1 receptor antagonist and has only anecdotally been used and reported.

Mortality

The mortality rates are between 10 and 20% in infants who require ECMO because of primary pulmonary hypertension or pulmonary hypertension complicating RDS or MAS. In babies with GBS sepsis, the mortality rate ranges from 10 to 50%.

Problem-orientated topic:

respiratory deterioration in an older premature infant

A 26-week gestation infant, Larisa, has been ventilator- and oxygen-dependent since birth. At 3 weeks of age she develops gradually increasing respiratory support requirements.

Q1. Does the infant have bronchopulmonary dysplasia?

Q2. What is the most likely cause of the infant's condition?

Q3. What is the differential diagnosis of the deterioration?

Q4. What further information would help you to be sure?

Q1. Does the infant have bronchopulmonary dysplasia?

Bronchopulmonary dysplasia (BPD) is diagnosed in an infant with or without ventilator dependence who is chronically oxygen-dependent beyond at least 28 days after birth. As Larisa is only 3 weeks old, she does not yet fit the definition of BPD but is at high risk of developing the condition.

Q2. What is the most likely cause of the infant's condition?

Ventilator-dependent prematurely born infants are at increased risk of nosocomial infection and this is a frequent cause of deterioration in such babies. Organisms isolated from the endotracheal tube may not be responsible for the infection and could reflect colonization only. Viral infections should also be considered as a cause of the deterioration and the appropriate samples sent to the laboratory, including a nasopharyngeal aspirate to exclude RSV and other respiratory viruses.

Q3. What is the differential diagnosis of the deterioration?

- Infection
- PDA
- Gastro-oesophageal reflux with aspiration.

Q4. What further information would help you to be sure?

- A new or worsening PDA murmur would suggest this to be the cause of the deterioration; this should then be investigated by an echo examination.
- A chest radiograph demonstrating new abnormalities would be suggestive of infection.
- If there were abnormalities in the right upper lobe on the chest radiograph, this would be suggestive of aspiration, particularly if there was a history of obtaining milk on suctioning. A pH study would determine if there was acid reflux.

Bronchopulmonary dysplasia (BPD)

Northway et al (1967) originally described four stages of BPD, based on a sequence of chest radiograph changes. A more functional definition has been recommended at a workshop sponsored by the National Institutes of Health (NIH):

- Infants are considered to have BPD if oxygen-dependent for at least 28 days.
- They are then classified as suffering from mild, moderate or severe BPD according to their respiratory support requirement at a later date:
  - Mild BPD if they were breathing air
  - Moderate BPD if they required less than 30% supplementary oxygen
  - Severe BPD if they needed more than 30% oxygen and/or intermittent positive pressure ventilation (IPPV) or CPAP.
- Immature infants (less than 32 weeks of gestational age) are assessed at 36 weeks post-menstrual age (PMA) or at discharge home, whichever comes first.
- Infants born at 32 weeks of gestation or more are assessed at 56 days' postnatal age (8 weeks) or discharge home, whichever comes first.

Pathogenesis

- There is an inverse relationship between the incidence of BPD and gestational age.
- BPD most commonly occurs in prematurely born infants who have had RDS, but can occur in immature infants who had no initial lung disease.
- Infants born at term may also develop BPD, particularly if they suffered severe initial lung disease, as evidenced by a requirement for ECMO.
- BPD was originally ascribed to oxygen toxicity. Oxygen toxicity is caused by the increased production of cytotoxic oxygen free radicals, which overwhelm the antioxidant defences. Prematurely born infants are particularly vulnerable, as they have incomplete development of their pulmonary

antioxidant enzyme systems and low levels of antioxidants, such as vitamins C and E.

- Baro- or volutrauma is incriminated and there is an inverse relationship between hypocarbia during mechanical ventilation and BPD development. Volutrauma may occur at resuscitation if rapid lung expansion is attempted.
- Pulmonary interstitial emphysema (PIE) has been associated with a high incidence of BPD; respiratory function is compromised by air dissection into false air spaces.
- Fluid overload may explain the association of PDA and BPD, as it causes congestive heart failure and hence deterioration in lung function. The association of PDA and an increased risk of BPD is potentiated by infection, particularly if temporally related.
- Antenatal infection, chorioamnionitis and postnatal infection may predispose to BPD development.
- BPD has been associated with persisting surfactant abnormalities; the L:S ratio increases slowly in BPD infants and there is late appearance of PG. Abnormalities related to surfactant proteins, particularly SP-A, have also been associated with BPD.

Pathophysiology

During the acute phase of lung injury, a host response is initiated that persists in infants who develop BPD:

- Proinflammatory cytokines (interleukins (IL) IL-1, IL-6 and soluble intercellular adhesion molecule (ICAM)-1) are demonstrated in the lung lavage from day 1, reaching a peak in the second week. ICAM-1 is a glycoprotein that allows cell-to-cell contact.
- Direct contact between activated cells leads to further production of proinflammatory cytokines and other mediators.
- IL-1β activity also increases during the first week, inducing the release of inflammatory mediators, activating inflammatory cells and upregulating adhesion molecules on endothelial cells.
- There is release of the α-chemokine, IL-8, which induces neutrophil chemotaxis, and the β-chemokine macrophage inflammatory protein (MIP)-1-α, which is chemotactic for monocytes and macrophages.
- The activated neutrophils mediate endothelial cytotoxicity, inhibit phosphatidylcholine synthesis and release elastase. There are also raised levels of collagenase and phospholipase A2.
- Inactivation of α-1-antiprotease by oxidative modification further compromises the protease–antiprotease imbalance.

- Leukotrienes, present in high levels in the lungs of infants developing BPD, cause bronchoconstriction, vasoconstriction, oedema, neutrophil chemotaxis and mucus production in the lung.
- The inflammatory infiltration is associated with loss of endothelial, basement membrane and interstitial sulphated glycoaminoglycans, which are important in restricting albumin flux and inhibiting fibrosis.
- Tumour necrosis factor-alpha (TNF-α) activity increases late; TNF-α and IL-6 induce fibroblast and collagen production and cause pulmonary fibrosis in animal models.

Clinical features

- The majority of cases have been dependent on oxygen supplementation and often mechanical ventilation since birth. Some, however, may have had minimal or no initial respiratory distress, but then deteriorate and become chronically oxygen-dependent.
- Infants with BPD frequently fail to thrive. Feeding difficulties and aspiration are common, due to bulbar dysfunction or gastro-oesophageal reflux.
- They are at high risk of deterioration related to recurrent respiratory infections. Copious endotracheal secretions, persistent atelectasis, lobar hyperinflation and tracheomalacia and/or bronchomalacia are common.
- The most severely affected infants develop right heart failure, and cor pulmonale develops in those who are chronically hypoxaemic.
- Osteopenia is common and fractures may occur.

Chest radiograph appearance

- Infants with the most severe BPD have hyper-expansion, streaks of abnormal density (Fig. 46.5), areas of emphysema and cystic abnormalities more marked at the lung bases; this picture is consistent with 'Northway BPD type IV'.
- The majority of prematurely born infants have non-specific abnormalities, which include small-volume hazy lung fields.

Computed tomography (CT)

CT scans at follow-up, rather than chest radiographs, give more detailed information. Common findings on CT are multifocal areas of hyperaeration, and linear and triangular subpleural opacities.

Pathology

- Histological examination of the lungs demonstrates areas of emphysema, which may coalesce into larger cystic areas surrounded by areas of atelectasis.

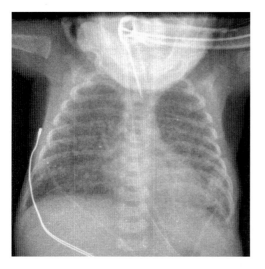

Fig. 46.5 Bronchopulmonary dysplasia with diffuse fibrotic shadows

- Florid obliterative bronchiolitis occurs, particularly if high peak inflating pressures have been used. This results in occlusion of the airway lumen and distal pulmonary collapse.
- In older infants, there is airway injury, smooth muscle hypertrophy, squamous metaplasia of the respiratory epithelium, glandular hyperplasia, fibrosis alternating with areas of emphysema and hypertrophy of the pulmonary arterial smooth muscle.
- In 'new' BPD there is dilated distal gas exchange structures, decreased alveolarization, minimal small airway injury and less prominent inflammation and fibrosis. As a consequence, it has been proposed that the 'new' BPD is not primarily the injury/repair paradigm of traditional BPD, but rather a maldevelopment sequence resulting from interference/interruption of normal developmental signalling for terminal maturation and alveolarization of the lungs of very preterm infants.

Management

- The peak inspiratory pressures and inspired oxygen concentrations should be kept to the minimum compatible with appropriate blood gases (a PaO_2 of 6.7–9.3 kPa (50–70 mmHg) and no evidence of a respiratory acidosis (pH < 7.20)).
- Results of recent randomized trials have demonstrated that there is no overall advantage in keeping oxygen saturation levels above 92%, but in infants with evidence of pulmonary hypertension the oxygen saturation level should be maintained at 95% at least.

- After the first week, increasing the PEEP level to 6 cmH_2O can improve oxygenation without adversely affecting CO_2 elimination, but this strategy may not be successful in infants with severe 'cystic' BPD.
- Inhaled NO can improve oxygenation in infants with developing or established BPD; randomized trials are required to determine whether inhaled NO will improve long-term outcome.
- Certain infants, despite appropriate respiratory support, suddenly become grey, pale, sweaty and cyanosed, frequently associated with poor chest wall expansion. These episodes seem to occur in agitated infants and sedation can help to reduce the number of episodes, but if they are very frequent and troublesome it may be necessary to paralyse affected infants.
- Infants with BPD may require prolonged ventilation, and tracheostomy should be considered for infants who remain fully ventilated after 3 months of age.
- Frequent attempts should be made to wean the infant from the ventilator.
- Methylxanthines may be useful to hasten weaning but have only been of proven value in infants less than 1 month old.
- No long-term positive effects of bronchodilator administration to infants on the neonatal unit have been demonstrated and their use should be restricted to infants whose respiratory status is compromised by reversible airways obstruction.
- The timing of administration of systemic corticosteroids influences the impact of their efficacy and they have numerous side-effects:
  - Commenced < 7 days, corticosteroids facilitate extubation and reduce the risk of chronic lung disease and patent ductus arteriosus, but cause short-term adverse effects including gastrointestinal bleeding, intestinal perforation, hyperglycaemia, hypertension, hypertrophic cardiomyopathy and growth failure. Long-term follow-up studies report an increased risk of abnormal neurological examination and cerebral palsy.
  - Initiated > 7 days of age suggests that late therapy may reduce neonatal mortality without significantly increasing the risk of adverse long-term neurodevelopmental outcomes, but long-term results are limited. It appears prudent to reserve the use of late corticosteroids to infants who cannot be weaned from mechanical ventilation and to minimize the dose and duration of any course of treatment.

– Inhaled compared to systemic administration of corticosteroids has a slower onset of action and a smaller magnitude of effect; inhaled steroid therapy initiated in the first 2 weeks after birth results in a reduction in requirement for rescue systemic steroids and facilitates extubation.

- Chest infections occur frequently in infants with BPD and should be treated with antibiotics or antiviral therapy as appropriate.
- Infants with severe BPD will not usually tolerate more than 150 ml/kg/24 hr. If their weight gain is greater than 20 g/kg/24 hr on such a regimen, this may indicate heart failure and regular diuretics should be considered. If chronic diuretic therapy is given, acid–base balance, chloride and calcium levels must be carefully monitored and regular renal ultrasounds performed to check for the development of nephrocalcinosis.
- Meta-analysis of randomized trials has demonstrated that chronic administration of diuretics results in no long-term benefits and can result in side-effects; thus diuretics should be reserved for infants with acute fluid overload or who are in incipient heart failure.
- Infants with BPD require a calorie intake approximately 20–40% greater than age-matched infants without respiratory embarrassment. Energy requirements above 150 kcal/kg are rare and usually associated with malabsorption. Large-volume, enterally administered feeds are poorly tolerated and restriction to 120 ml/kg/day, using either a concentrated preterm feed or calorie supplementation, is preferable. A milk fortifier may be needed if the infant is receiving human milk.
- Parental support is essential as affected infants have prolonged admissions.
- Routine immunizations should be given once BPD infants reach 2 months of age, but a killed polio vaccine should be used if they are still on the NICU. Immunization against influenza should also be considered, especially for infants receiving home oxygen therapy. Immunoprophylaxis against RSV should be given for infants discharged home on supplementary oxygen and considered for other BPD infants.
- Home oxygen therapy should be considered for infants who have no medical problem other than their increased inspired oxygen requirement or, if there is appropriate community support, tube feeding.

Mortality and morbidity

- Mortality is usually caused by intercurrent infection, cor pulmonale or respiratory failure.

- BPD infants may require many months, if not years, of supplementary oxygen at home.
- BPD infants suffer frequent respiratory deteriorations and require on average two rehospitalizations in the first 2 years. Rehospitalization is more likely in those who require supplementary oxygen at home and/or have an RSV infection.
- Pulmonary function abnormalities in the first year are common and include a high airways resistance, low dynamic pulmonary compliance, reduced functional residual capacity and abnormal gas exchange. Lung function usually improves with age but may still be abnormal, with reduced exercise tolerance and increased airway hyper-reactivity, in school-age children.
- Infants with severe BPD suffer growth failure and, although growth accelerates as respiratory symptoms improve, those with severe BPD may still be of small stature as adults.
- Poor developmental outcome is more common in those requiring a prolonged hospitalization.

Apnoea

Apnoea is a common problem in prematurely born infants and the incidence is inversely related to gestational age. There are three types of apnoea:

- *Central.* There is total cessation of inspiratory efforts with no evidence of obstruction.
- *Obstructed.* Infants have chest wall movement but no nasal airflow, as they try to breathe against an obstructed airway.
- *Mixed.* Obstructed respiratory efforts are usually followed by central apnoeas.

Infants may also have periodic breathing: regular cycles of breathing of 10–18 seconds' duration interrupted by pauses in respiratory activity of at least 3 seconds in duration, that pattern occurring for at least 2 minutes.

Causes

- Immaturity of the respiratory centre
- Intracranial bleed
- Hydrocephalus
- Infection
- Anaemia
- Metabolic disturbances
- Temperature instability
- Medications, e.g. opiates.

Management

- Stimulation
- CPAP, which may be of benefit in infants who have frequent troublesome apnoeas

- Severe refractory apnoea: intubation and ventilation
- Pharmacological treatment:
  - Caffeine, preferred to theophylline as it has a higher therapeutic index and is 'once a day'
  - Doxapram, a respiratory stimulant, has been used for treatment of refractory cases but it is difficult to monitor levels. It is currently unavailable in many European countries.

Air leaks

Pneumothorax

Pathogenesis

- Spontaneous pneumothoraces occur immediately after birth due to the high transpulmonary pressure swings generated by the first spontaneous breaths.
- Pneumothoraces more usually occur as a complication of respiratory disease or a congenital malformation, particularly if there is uneven ventilation, alveolar over-distension and air trapping and the infant is receiving ventilatory support.
- Approximately 5–10% of ventilated babies develop air leaks; they are particularly likely to occur in babies who 'fight' the ventilator and actively exhale during ventilator inflation (active expiration).
- Rarely, pneumothoraces occur as a result of a direct injury to the lung: for example, by perforation by suction catheters or introducers passed through the endotracheal tube or by central venous catheter placement.

Clinical features

- Small pneumothoraces may be asymptomatic.
- Large pneumothoraces are associated with dramatic deterioration and marked respiratory distress, desaturation, pallor and shock.
- A tension pneumothorax results in a shift of the mediastinum and abdominal distension due to displacement of the diaphragm.
- Pneumothorax can aggravate intracerebral haemorrhage in preterm infants.

Chest radiograph appearance

- A large pneumothorax is associated with absent lung markings and a collapsed lung on the ipsilateral side.
- If the pneumothorax is under tension, there will also be eversion of the diaphragm, bulging intercostal spaces and mediastinal shift (Fig. 46.6).
- A small pneumothorax, however, may only be recognized by a difference in radiolucency between the two lung fields (Fig. 46.7).

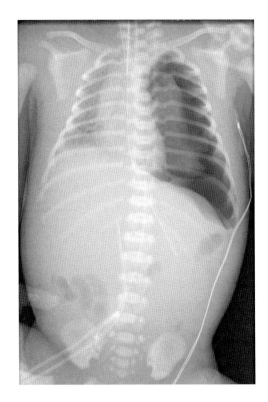

Fig. 46.6 Tension left-sided pneumothorax with mediastinal displacement and eversion of the ipsilateral diaphragm

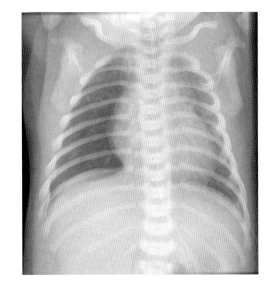

Fig. 46.7 Small right-sided pneumothorax demonstrated by the discrepancy in the translucency of the lung fields and a small rim of basal free air

- A lateral chest radiograph (Fig. 46.8) can be useful to demonstrate the free air and to identify whether the tip of the chest drain is optimally placed.

Differential diagnosis

Unusually the appearance of either lobar emphysema or cystic adenomatoid malformation of the lung may

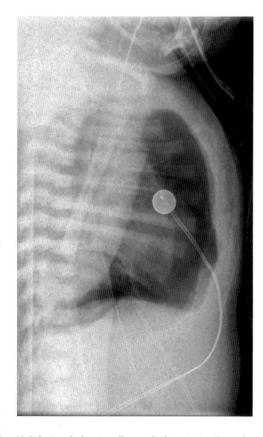

Fig. 46.8 Lateral chest radiograph demonstrating a large pneumothorax

resemble a pneumothorax. In a preterm infant with a thin chest wall, transillumination with an intense beam from a fibreoptic light will demonstrate an abnormal air collection by an increased transmission of light, but pulmonary interstitial emphysema can give a similar appearance.

Management
- Asymptomatic pneumothoraces do not require treatment, but the infant should be monitored until the pneumothorax has resolved.
- Nursing an infant with a pneumothorax in an inspired oxygen concentration of 100% favours resorption of the extra-alveolar gas, but this strategy should not be used in infants at risk of retinopathy of prematurity.
- If the infant is symptomatic or has a tension pneumothorax, the pneumothorax must be drained. If the infant is in extremis and there is no time for insertion of a chest drain, emergency aspiration should be undertaken with a butterfly needle (18-gauge).
- A chest tube (French gauge 8–14, depending on patient's weight) should be inserted under local anaesthesia through either the second intercostal space just lateral to the mid-clavicular line or the fourth–fifth space in the mid-axillary line.

The tip of the chest tube should be retrosternal to achieve the most effective drainage. A lateral chest radiograph should be obtained to determine whether the drain has been positioned correctly.
- Once inserted, the tube should be connected to an underwater seal drain with suction of 5–10 cmH$_2$O. Heimlich valves are useful during transport but, as they can become blocked, they should not be used for long-term drainage. The chest drain can be removed 24 hours after there is no further bubbling of air into the water seal.
- Complications of chest drains include traumatization of the lung, the thoracic duct resulting in a chylothorax, cardiac tamponade due to a haemorrhagic pericardial effusion and phrenic nerve injury.

Preventative strategies
- Neuromuscular blocking agents can be given to stop infants breathing out of phase with the ventilator (active expiration or asynchrony).
- Analgesics and/or sedatives are also given to try to suppress respiratory activity but have not been demonstrated in randomized trials to reduce the pneumothorax rate.
- An alternative approach is to use a form of ventilatory support that encourages the infant to breathe synchronously with the ventilator: that is, inspiration and inflation coinciding. Use of a faster (60/min) rather than a slower (30–40/min) ventilator rate and rescue high-frequency oscillation, but not patient-triggered ventilation, has been associated with a lower pneumothorax rate.
- Surfactant administration is associated with a lower risk of pneumothorax development.

Pulmonary interstitial emphysema (PIE)

The incidence of PIE is inversely related to birth weight. It occurs in neonates with respiratory distress supported by positive-pressure ventilation and exposed to high-peak inspiratory pressures and/or malpositioned endotracheal tubes. PIE commonly involves both lungs but may be lobar in distribution. It frequently occurs with either a pneumothorax or a pneumomediastinum.

Pathogenesis
In surfactant-deficient infants, rupture of the small airways can occur distal to the termination of the fascial sheath; gas then dissects into the interstitium and becomes trapped within the perivascular sheaths of the lung, resulting in PIE. The trapped gas reduces pulmonary perfusion by compressing the vessels and interfering with ventilation; as a result, affected infants are profoundly hypoxaemic and hypercarbic.

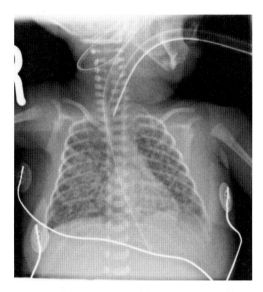

Fig. 46.9 **Diffuse pulmonary interstitial emphysema**

Chest radiograph appearance

The chest radiograph demonstrates hyperinflation and a characteristic cystic appearance (Fig. 46.9).

Management

If the PIE is localized:
- The infant should be nursed in the lateral decubitus position with the affected lung dependent and hence under-ventilated; this promotes partial or complete atelectasis.
- Selective bronchial intubation to bypass the affected lung for 24–48 hours may also be associated with resolution of the PIE.
- If the PIE persists and compresses adjacent normal lung parenchyma despite such manoeuvres, resection of the affected area may be necessary to alleviate respiratory distress.

If the infant has widespread PIE:
- The ventilator pressures should be reduced to the minimum compatible with acceptable gases.
- Transfer to high-frequency jet, flow interruption or oscillatory ventilation may improve gas exchange.
- If the infant is in extremis, linear pleurotomies, scarifing the lung through the chest wall to create an artificial pneumothorax, may help to decompress the PIE.

Mortality and morbidity

The mortality from diffuse PIE is high and survivors frequently develop BPD.

Pneumomediastinum

Pneumomediastinum occurs in approximately 2.5 per 1000 live births. An isolated pneumomediastinum rarely causes severe symptoms, but pneumomedi-astinum usually occurs with multiple air leaks in severely ill ventilated babies.

Chest radiograph appearance

On the chest radiograph, a pneumomediastinum appears as a halo of air adjacent to the borders of the heart, and on lateral view there is marked retrosternal hyperlucency. The mediastinal gas may elevate the thymus away from the pericardium, resulting in a crescentic configuration resembling a spinnaker sail.

Management

An isolated pneumomediastinum usually requires no treatment. Drainage of a pneumomediastinum is difficult; multiple needling and tube drainage may be required, as the gas is in multiple independent lobules.

Acute respiratory distress syndrome (ARDS) (see also p. 661)

Pathogenesis

ARDS can occur following asphyxia, shock, sepsis or MAS. Asphyxia results in damage to the myocardium and the associated severe metabolic acidaemia in depressed myocardial contractility; this leads to heart failure and pulmonary oedema. Asphyxia also damages the pulmonary blood vessels and ARDS develops if there is a large leak of protein-rich fluid on to the alveoli.

Clinical features

ARDS is a disease of term babies. In the first hours after birth affected infants usually present with tachypnoea (respiratory rate of at least 100/min) rather than with retraction or grunting. Respiration is stimulated by the metabolic acidaemia, by damage to the central nervous system and/or by pulmonary oedema. Infants with ARDS are severely hypoxaemic.

Chest radiograph appearance

This demonstrates diffuse pulmonary infiltrates and in severe cases there will be a 'white-out'.

Management

- Surfactant administration can improve oxygenation in ARDS and is most effective if administered early and in larger doses than used in RDS.
- In adults and children with ARDS, prone positioning has been shown to improve oxygenation.
- A high level of PEEP should be used in an attempt to restore the functional residual capacity to normal values; this will also increase the MAP level and hence oxygenation.
- High-volume strategy HFOV can also improve oxygenation, particularly in those patients who had a positive response to PEEP elevation.

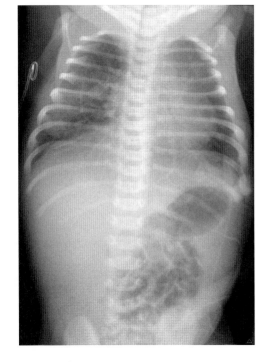

Fig. 46.10 Congenital cystic adenomatoid malformation. Note the delayed lung fluid clearance on the right and displacement of the mediastinum to the left.

- Fluid intake should initially be restricted to 40 ml/kg/24 hrs, and if heart failure is present, furosemide should be administered.
- Broad-spectrum antibiotics should be administered, but aminoglycoside levels should be monitored for toxicity.
- ECMO may be indicated for non-respondent cases.

Mortality and morbidity

The mortality of ARDS is high, particularly in infants who develop secondary infection or do not respond to elevation of their PEEP level. Air leaks and infection are commonly seen in infants with ARDS.

Other congenital anomalies of the lung

- Pulmonary agenesis
- Sequestration
- Congenital cystic adenomatoid malformation of the lung (CCAM, Fig. 46.10)
- Congenital lung cysts
- Congenital lobar emphysema
- Immotile cilia syndrome
- Congenital pulmonary lymphangiectasia
- Alveolar capillary dysplasia.

BOX 46.6 Causes of upper airway obstruction

Nasal
- Choanal atresia:
  - Unilateral or bilateral
  - Associated with other congenital anomalies, e.g. CHARGE syndrome (*c*oloboma, *h*eart defects, *a*tresia of the choanae, *r*etardation of growth and/or development, *g*enital and/or urinary abnormalities, *e*ar abnormalities and deafness)

Pharyngeal
- Microglossia
- Micrognathia
- Craniofacial syndromes, e.g. Pierre Robin, Crouzon syndrome, hemifacial microsomia

Laryngeal
- Polyps
- Cysts
- Vocal cord palsy
- Laryngomalacia

Diaphragmatic abnormalities

Congenital diaphragmatic hernia (CDH) is described on page 743; other anomalies include eventration and paralysis.

Upper airway obstruction

There can be nasal, pharyngeal or laryngeal obstruction (Box 46.6).

Clinical features
- If the obstruction is partial, the only sign may be tachypnoea.
- Infants more severely affected will be obviously working hard to breathe against the obstruction and have a respiratory acidosis.
- Stridor occurring immediately after birth should raise the suspicion of a laryngeal lesion.
- Infants with complete upper airway obstruction will have severe respiratory failure, which will be fatal if unrelieved.

Investigations
- ENT opinion
- CT scan: choanal atresia
- Chest radiograph or a penetrated filtered (Cincinnati) view: laryngotracheobronchial lesions
- MRI: extrinsic laryngeal lesions
- Laryngoscopy
- Rigid laryngotracheobronchoscopy.

Management

- Nasal causes of obstruction are relieved by an oral airway.
- Surgical intervention is required for choanal atresia.
- If the tongue is causing the obstruction because it is too large or displaced posteriorly, the infant should be nursed prone.
- Laryngeal obstruction is relieved by intubation but not by an oral airway.
- Vocal cord palsy resulting from a birth injury usually resolves spontaneously.
- Bilateral cord lesions associated with a neurological lesion do not respond spontaneously and a tracheostomy and feeding gastrostomy will be required.
- Subglottic oedema requires pre-extubation corticosteroids and adrenaline (epinephrine) nebulizers.
- Subglottic stenosis may require a cricoid split or laryngeal reconstruction using rib cartilage.
- Laryngomalacia usually resolves over 12–24 months.

Pulmonary haemorrhage

Pulmonary haemorrhage is a severe form of pulmonary oedema, where there has also been leakage of red cells giving haemorrhagic pulmonary oedema. Pulmonary haemorrhage can occur:

- At birth, following severe birth depression
- Most commonly in very low birth weight infants who have heart failure secondary to elevated pulmonary blood flow because of a PDA
- If a synthetic surfactant is given, particularly if used prophylactically
- In infants with:
  - Heart failure
  - Sepsis
  - Fluid overload
  - Clotting abnormalities
  - Intrauterine growth retardation.

Clinical features

- If the pulmonary haemorrhage is large, the infant will deteriorate suddenly with copious bloody secretions appearing from the airway.
- Spontaneously breathing infants are dyspnoeic and cyanosed; those who are ventilated will desaturate.
- The infant may be hypotensive due to blood loss and heart failure.
- On examination, the infant may be limp and unresponsive with reduced air entry and widespread crackles in the lungs.

Chest radiograph appearance

- If severe, there will be a 'white-out' with air bronchograms.

- Less commonly there is a lobar pattern of consolidation.

Management

- Infants should be intubated and ventilated; high peak pressures may be required. A high PEEP level should be used to help redistribute fluid back into the interstitial space.
- Broad-spectrum antibiotics should be used.
- Neuromuscular blockade should be given until the haemorrhage has stopped.
- Blood transfusions may be required.
- The infant should be fluid-restricted.
- There is some evidence to suggest a single dose of surfactant may improve oxygenation.

Mortality and morbidity

- The mortality may be as high as 40%.
- High-pressure ventilation puts the infant at increased risk of BPD.
- The incidence of cerebral bleeds is doubled.

Neonatal cardiac disorders

The common disorders are listed in Box 46.7.

Problem-orientated topic:

a prematurely born infant who cannot be weaned from the ventilator ● ● ● ●

A female infant, Svetlana, is born at 24 weeks of gestation and with a birth weight of 0.55 kg following spontaneous-onset labour. She has been ventilated since birth. After 2 weeks of mechanical ventilation, attempts to wean the baby from ventilation fail. On examination Svetlana is hypotensive, with a wide pulse pressure. She has an active precordium and a systolic murmur of grade 3/6, with maximum intensity in the left second intercostal space. Her peripheral pulses are easily palpable.

Q1. Does the baby have a patent ductus arteriosus?

Q2. What are the other possible causes of failure to wean this baby from the ventilator?

Q3. What would you expect the chest radiograph to demonstrate?

Q4. How would you confirm your diagnosis and what would you expect to find?

Q5. What is the appropriate management?

Acyanotic heart disease

- Lesions with systemic outflow obstruction:
  - Coarctation of aorta
  - Severe aortic stenosis
- Lesions with left-to-right shunt:
  - Ventricular septal defect (VSD)
  - Atrial septal defect (ASD)
  - Atrioventricular septal defect (AVSD)
  - Patent ductus arteriosus (PDA)

Cyanotic heart disease

- With pulmonary oligaemia:
  - Tetralogy of Fallot
  - Pulmonary atresia with or without septal defects
  - Tricuspid atresia with pulmonary stenosis
  - Ebstein anomaly
  - Double-outlet right ventricle with pulmonary stenosis
  - Persistent pulmonary hypertension of the newborn (PPHN)
- With pulmonary plethora:
  - Double-outlet right ventricle without pulmonary stenosis
  - Transposition of great arteries with large VSD
  - Truncus arteriosus
  - Single ventricle

Lesions presenting with heart failure

- AVSD
- Total anomalous pulmonary venous return
- Duct-dependent left ventricular outflow tract obstruction
- Hypoplastic left heart syndrome

Lesions with systemic outflow obstruction

- Coarctation of aorta
- Aortic arch anomalies

Lesions with left-to-right shunt

- VSD
- ASD
- PDA
- Rhythm disturbances:
  - Supraventricular tachycardias
  - Congenital complete heart block
- Cardiac muscle dysfunction:
  - Cardiomyopathy
  - Pompe disease
  - Asymmetric septal hypertrophy (infant of diabetic mother)
  - Viral myocarditis
  - Severe perinatal asphyxia

Q1. Does the baby have a patent ductus arteriosus (PDA)?

- Yes, she does. Infants with a haemodynamically significant PDA have tachycardia, bounding pulses, an active precordium and a murmur, although this might be absent.
- The typical ductal murmur is systolic in about 75% of cases, but can be continuous and is best heard at the upper left sternal edge, under the clavicle.
- As the pulmonary vascular resistance falls, the left-to-right shunt through the ductus increases and the peripheral pulses become bounding. This reflects the widened pulse pressure due to the 'steal' of blood being shunted from the high-pressure systemic circulation into the lower-pressure pulmonary circulation.

Q2. What are the other possible causes of failure to wean this baby from the ventilator?

- Svetlana may have an increased work of breathing related to either residual lung disease or pulmonary congestion secondary to another cardiac lesion. The latter is unlikely, as the murmur has appeared only at 2 weeks of age.
- The baby may also have weakness of her respiratory muscles related to extreme prematurity and/or prolonged ventilation.

Q3. What would you expect the chest radiograph to demonstrate?

The radiograph would show cardiomegaly and increased pulmonary vascularity. There may be additional residual lung disease or evidence of evolving BPD.

Q4. How would you confirm your diagnosis and what would you expect to find?

Echocardiography would confirm typical findings of a PDA (see below) and exclude other cardiac lesions.

Q5. What is the appropriate management?

- Initial treatment is fluid restriction.
- Diuretics may be needed if the infant is in heart failure, but theoretically furosemide might promote ductal patency via its effect on renal prostaglandin synthesis.

- Closure of the PDA can be attempted by using prostaglandin inhibitors such as indometacin or ibuprofen.
- Surgical ligation of the duct is indicated if medical management fails and it is not possible to wean the baby from the ventilator.

Patent ductus arteriosus (PDA)
(see also p. 577)

- In fetal life, blood is shunted from the right heart via the pulmonary artery through the ductus arteriosus to the aorta and the lungs are 'bypassed'.
- At birth, the ductus arteriosus begins to constrict with the onset of breathing.
- In the majority of infants, the ductus arteriosus has closed by 24 hours of age and in 90% will have closed by 60 hours of age.
- Ductal closure is delayed in infants with pulmonary hypertension and respiratory failure as a consequence of acidosis or persistence of low oxygen tensions; in such circumstances prostaglandin E_2 levels remain high.
- The incidence of PDA is inversely related to gestational age, reflecting the association between maturity at birth and RDS.

Clinical features
- Infants with a haemodynamically significant PDA have tachycardia, bounding pulses, an active precordium and a murmur, although the latter might be absent.
- The typical ductal murmur is systolic (in about 75% of cases), but can be continuous and is best heard at the upper left sternal edge, under the clavicle.
- As the pulmonary vascular resistance falls, the left-to-right shunt through the ductus increases and the peripheral pulses become bounding, reflecting the widened pulse pressure due to the 'steal' of blood being shunted from the high-pressure systemic circulation into the lower-pressure pulmonary circulation.
- The left-to-right shunt means higher blood flow in the lungs and affected infants are tachypnoeic with crackles at the lung bases.
- The increased pulmonary blood flow results in a decrease in lung compliance, and thus a PDA can present as failure of improvement in an infant with RDS or an acute deterioration necessitating an increase in respiratory support.

Chest radiograph appearance
The chest radiograph demonstrates cardiomegaly, pulmonary plethora and a wide angle between the left and right main bronchi due to left atrial dilation.

Investigations
- Typical echocardiographic findings of a moderate to large left-to-right ductal shunt are bowing of the interatrial septum to the right with enlargement of the left atrium and ventricle, and left atrium enlargement with a left atrial:aortic root (LA:Ao) ratio greater than 1.4:1 and an increased ductal diameter (usually 2–3 mm).
- Colour Doppler examination reveals a continuous flare in the main pulmonary artery from the arterial duct.
- The size of the shunt can be determined from the ductal size on colour Doppler examination and the LA:Ao ratio; if the shunt is large, diastolic flow in the descending aorta is reversed throughout diastole.

Management
- Initial management of an infant with a PDA usually includes fluid restriction.
- Diuretics may be needed if the infant is in heart failure, but theoretically furosemide might promote ductal patency via its effect on renal prostaglandin synthesis.
- If there is no improvement following fluid restriction for 24 hours and there are no contraindications, such as poor renal function or a low platelet count, a prostaglandin inhibitor (indometacin or ibuprofen) can be given.
- Ductal closure is achieved with indomethacin treatment in 48 hours in approximately 70% of infants.
- Surgical ligation of the duct is indicated if medical management fails and it is not possible to wean the baby from the ventilator.

Morbidity
- BPD is significantly increased in infants who have had a PDA, particularly if they have also suffered nosocomial infection.
- If there is a large PDA, there is a diastolic steal and retrograde diastolic flow in the cerebral circulation, the descending aorta and renal and mesenteric blood vessels. This compromises gastrointestinal blood flow and hence the incidence of necrotizing enterocolitis is increased in infants who have had a PDA.

Problem-orientated topic:

a baby born at term with cyanosis

A male infant, birth weight 3.3 kg and born at term, is noticed to be blue soon after birth.

Continued overleaf

He is the first child of unrelated parents. The mother recently flew in from Africa and has not received any antenatal care. Examination reveals the baby to be centrally cyanosed, but without signs of respiratory distress or dysmorphic features. The apical impulse is in the left fourth intercostal space and there is no increased precordial activity. The first and second heart sounds are normal and there are no murmurs. The femoral pulses are felt and there is no discrepancy in the four limb blood pressures. The baby has oxygen saturation levels of 80% in all four limbs.

Q1. Does this infant have cyanotic congenital heart disease?

Q2. What are the differential diagnoses?

Q3. What investigations would you undertake to make the diagnosis?

Q4. How should this infant be managed?

Q1. Does this infant have cyanotic congenital heart disease?

Yes, the infant has an atrioventricular septal defect (AVSD). The mother has had no antenatal care, so any major cardiac abnormality will not have been detected during the pregnancy.

Q2. What are the differential diagnoses?

- Persistent pulmonary hypertension of the newborn (PPHN) should be considered, but is unlikely given the similar saturation levels in all four limbs.
- The lack of respiratory distress also makes a primary respiratory disease unlikely.
- Rarely, infants with a myopathy or spinal muscular atrophy can present with cyanosis, but are also usually floppy.
- Babies with methaemoglobinaemia have normal arterial oxygen tensions despite central cyanosis.
- The lack of dysmorphic features makes an underlying syndrome (Table 46.3) unlikely.

Q3. What investigations would you undertake to make the diagnosis?

- An arterial blood gas from pre- and post-ductal arteries should be taken or a pre- and post-ductal pulse oximeter should be placed; similarity in the PaO_2 or in pulse oximetry will exclude pulmonary hypertension and a normal CO_2 level significant respiratory disease.

Table 46.3 Examples of syndromes with associated cardiac conditions

Syndrome	Cardiac condition
CHARGE	VSD, AVSD, ASD
CATCH 22	Aortic arch anomalies and tetralogy of Fallot
Down	AVSD, VSD
Noonan	Valvular pulmonary stenosis
Turner	Coarctation of aorta
Williams	Supravalvular aortic stenosis

(ASD = atrial septal defect; AVSD = atrioventricular septal defect; CATCH 22 = cardiac defects, abnormal facies, thymic hypoplasia, cleft palate, hypocalcaemia, variable deletion on chromosome 22; CHARGE = coloboma, heart defects, atresia of the choanae, retardation of growth and/or development, genital and/or urinary abnormalities, ear abnormalities and deafness; VSD = ventricular septal defect)

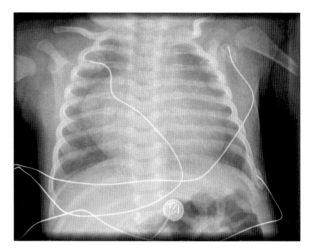

Fig. 46.11 Atrioventricular septal defect. Note the large heart.

- Chest radiograph (Fig. 46.11) and 12-lead ECG will give further clues to the aetiology of cyanosis in this infant (Box 46.8 and Table 46.4 below).
- Echocardiography will confirm the exact nature of cardiac defect.

Q4. How should this infant be managed?

- A hyperoxia test should be done, with the infant breathing 100% oxygen via a face mask for 15 minutes.
- A further post-ductal arterial blood gas should then be obtained. If the PaO_2 has risen above 33 kPa (245 mmHg), congenital heart disease is extremely unlikely and primary pulmonary hypertension is the most likely cause of central cyanosis.
- If the PaO_2 fails to rise above 5 kPa (around 40 mm Hg), cyanotic congenital heart disease is more likely. A prostin infusion should be started after consultation with the regional paediatric cardiology unit prior to transfer for possible surgical intervention (Box 46.8).

BOX 46.8 Surgical procedures for congenital heart disease

Balloon atrial septostomy (Rashkind procedure)

- Creates an interatrial opening to allow mixing of blood in the atria
- Used for transposition of the great arteries, tricuspid atresia

Palliative systemic to pulmonary artery shunts

- Use systemic arterial flow to improve pulmonary blood flow in cardiac lesions with impaired pulmonary perfusion
- Used for tetralogy of Fallot, hypoplastic right heart, tricuspid atresia
  - Modified Blalock–Taussig shunt (subclavian and ipsilateral pulmonary artery anastomosis)
  - Waterston–Cooley shunt (ascending aorta and right pulmonary artery)
  - Potts shunt (descending aorta and left pulmonary artery anastomosis)

Palliative cavopulmonary shunt (Glenn shunt)

- Anastomosis of the superior vena cava to the right pulmonary artery
- An intermediate procedure in patients awaiting Fontan procedure, which allows systemic venous flow to go directly into the pulmonary circulation

Hybrid palliation

- Atrial septostomy to create adequate intra-atrial mixing, branch pulmonary artery banding to protect the distal pulmonary vascular bed and stenting of the PDA to maintain systemic blood flow
- Used as an alternative approach to the stage 1 Norwood procedure for the hypoplastic left heart syndrome (HLHS) and as a bridge to cardiac transplantation in babies with severe HLHS.

Jatene procedure

- Arterial switch procedure where the arteries are switched back to their appropriate ventricles (right ventricle to pulmonary artery and left ventricle to aorta with re-implantation of coronary arteries).
- Used for transposition of the great arteries.

Fontan procedure

- Redirection of the flow from the inferior vena cava to the right pulmonary artery with functionally univentricular heart
- Used in tricuspid atresia, hypoplastic left heart syndrome

Norwood procedure

- Stage 1: anastomosis of proximal main pulmonary artery to aorta with aortic arch reconstruction and transection and patch closure of distal main pulmonary artery (MPA), modified Blalock–Taussig shunt and creating atrial septal defect (ASD)
- Stage 2: bidirectional redirection of the flow from the inferior vena cava to the right pulmonary artery (Glenn shunt and modified Fontan)
- Stage 3: total cavopulmonary connection (Fontan)

Ross procedure

- Pulmonary root autograft for aortic stenosis

Cyanotic congenital heart disease

- Cyanosis in congenital heart disease (Table 46.4) is caused by either an obstruction to the pulmonary blood flow or mixing of the pulmonary venous and systemic venous returns in the heart or major arterial trunks with a right-to-left shunt or abnormal arterial connections.
- Infants with PPHN have right-to-left shunts at the level of the ductus arteriosus and the foramen ovale.
- PPHN was previously called persistent fetal circulation but that term is inaccurate, as the high-flow, low-resistance circuit through the placenta present in the fetal circulation is missing.
- Pulmonary hypertension in the neonate may also be secondary to a number of conditions, including severe intrapartum asphyxia, infection, pulmonary hypoplasia, drug therapy (for example, the use of prostaglandin synthetase inhibitors before delivery), congenital heart disease or over-ventilation.
- The neonatal pulmonary vasculature is extremely sensitive to changes in pH, PaO_2 and $PaCO_2$. A rise in the haematocrit can also cause pulmonary hypertension.
- When pulmonary hypertension occurs due to failure of the normal decrease in pulmonary vascular resistance after birth, affected infants have a normal arteriolar number and muscularization.
- In other conditions, there are varying degrees of vascular remodelling and a decreased arteriolar number.
- Following chronic hypoxia in utero, excessive muscularization of the pulmonary arterioles is found and muscle extends into the normally muscle-free intra-acinar arteries; such changes are seen in extremely small for dates infants.
- The pulmonary hypertension seen in infants with CDH or in other conditions associated with pulmonary hypoplasia is due to a reduction in the number of intralobar arteries and increased muscularity of the arteries.
- PPHN may also be due to alveolar capillary dysplasia with congenital misalignment of the pulmonary veins.

Clinical features

Cyanotic heart disease presents with cyanosis and in addition with a murmur, heart failure or shock:

Table 46.4 Cyanotic congenital heart diseases (CHD)

CHD	Clinical presentation	Age at presentation	Examination	Chest radiograph	ECG	Management
Transposition of great arteries	Cyanosis in the first week Degree of cyanosis is variable: can be very severe, or very mild and may be missed	Around 48–72 hours of age but can also present at birth Usually when duct is closing	Single second sound No murmurs	Normal or increased pulmonary blood flow Narrow mediastinum and cardiac silhouette showing 'egg on side' appearance	May be normal Right ventricular hypertrophy	Prostaglandin infusion Balloon atrial septostomy Arterial switch operation
Tetralogy of Fallot	Mild cyanosis in the newborn Degree of cyanosis depends upon degree of right ventricular outflow tract (RVOT) obstruction	Variable depending upon degree of pulmonary stenosis May be symptom-free until 6 months of age	Single second sound Ejection systolic murmur in the second space	Pulmonary oligaemia Upturned apex giving boot-shaped appearance	Right ventricular hypertrophy Right axis deviation	Primary repair of RVOT at 3–4 months of age if anatomy is favourable Palliative shunt (Blalock–Taussig) may be needed in the meantime
Tricuspid atresia	Severe cyanosis since birth Associated tachypnoea	Usually in the first 2 weeks of life	Single second sound Systolic murmur in lower left sternal border	Normal or slightly enlarged Decreased pulmonary blood flow	Left ventricular hypertrophy Left axis deviation	Prostaglandin infusion and balloon atrial septostomy for neonates with severe cyanosis Palliative shunt (Blalock–Taussig) followed by Fontan procedure
Total anomalous venous return with obstruction	Symptoms of heart failure Marked respiratory distress Cyanosis variable	Usually in the first week of life	No murmurs Wide fixed splitting of second heart sound Hepatomegaly	Pulmonary venous congestion/pulmonary oedema with small cardiac size Snowman appearance in supradiaphragmatic obstruction	Right ventricular hypertrophy	Surgical correction of pulmonary venous drainage
Truncus arteriosus	Cyanosis and heart failure in the first few weeks	First 2 weeks of life	Continuous ejection systolic murmur Single second sound	Cardiomegaly Increased pulmonary vascularity	Combined ventricular hypertrophy	Surgical repair
Ebstein anomaly	Cyanosis and heart failure in the first week of life	First week	Characteristic triple or quadruple rhythm with soft systolic murmur on lower left sternal edge	Extreme cardiomegaly in severe cases Mild cases have normal-sized heart	Right bundle branch block and right atrial enlargement First degree AV block may be present	Surgical repair of tricuspid valve

- A murmur in the pulmonary area suggests the presence of pulmonary stenosis and makes the diagnosis of Fallot tetralogy more likely, whereas the absence of a murmur suggests transposition of the great arteries.
- Cyanotic heart diseases with normal or increased pulmonary circulation, transposition of great arteries, single-chamber lesions (univentricular heart) and total anomalous pulmonary venous return and truncus arteriosus present with a combination of heart failure and cyanosis. If there is associated pulmonary stenosis, however, this is protective against heart failure and affected infants present with cyanosis alone.
- Infants with severe pulmonary obstruction present with severe cyanosis and shock when the ductus arteriosus closes; in such infants patency of the ductus arteriosus is vital for blood to reach the pulmonary circulation.

Chest radiograph appearance

The shape of the heart may give a clue to the underlying heart lesion:

- A boot-shaped heart is said to be characteristic of tetralogy of Fallot.
- An egg-shaped heart with a narrow mediastinum is characteristic of transposition of the great arteries.
- A snowman or figure of eight appearance is characteristic of supracardiac total anomalous pulmonary venous return.
- A scimitar appearance over the right lower lung field is sometimes seen in infradiaphragmatic anomalous pulmonary venous return.
- The presence of a small heart and increased pulmonary vascularity can be a feature of obstructed pulmonary venous return.
- Lesions associated with pulmonary oligaemia include tetralogy of Fallot, pulmonary atresia, various forms of single ventricle with pulmonary stenosis and tricuspid atresia.
- Pulmonary plethora can occur in transposition of the great arteries, single-chamber lesions (univentricular heart), total anomalous pulmonary venous return and truncus arteriosus.

Electrocardiogram appearance

A superior axis on the ECG is seen if there is an AVSD or tricuspid atresia. A conduction abnormality is commonly associated with Ebstein anomaly.

Acyanotic congenital heart disease

Common acyanotic congenital heart diseases are listed in Table 46.5.

BOX 46.9 Causes of heart failure in the newborn according to age at presentation

At birth
- Severe hypoplastic left heart syndrome
- Severe tricuspid and pulmonary insufficiency
- Large systemic arteriovenous fistula

The first week
- Transposition of great arteries
- Hypoplastic left heart syndrome
- Total anomalous pulmonary venous return
- Critical aortic and pulmonary stenosis

Between 7 and 28 days
- Coarctation of aorta
- Critical aortic stenosis
- AVSD with large left-to-right shunt and low pulmonary vascular resistance

Clinical features

The presentation depends on whether the lesion produces predominantly volume overload or pressure overload:

Lesions causing volume overload tend to remain asymptomatic in the neonatal period unless severe:

- Left to right shunt lesions such as atrial septal defect (ASD), ventricular septal defect (VSD) and patent ductus arteriosus (PDA)
- Regurgitant lesions like congenital mitral regurgitation and cardiomyopathy.

Lesions causing pressure overload tend to present with symptoms of heart failure (Box 46.9) or shock with decreased peripheral perfusion:

- Lesions with outflow tract obstruction such as coarctation of aorta, aortic arch anomalies and valvular pulmonary stenosis.

Neonatal arrhythmias

Supraventricular tachycardia (SVT)

Clinical features

This is the most common symptomatic arrhythmia in the neonatal period. Affected infants can present antenatally with hydrops fetalis or postnatally with heart failure. The heart rate is usually faster than 200 beats/min.

Pathogenesis

SVT in neonates is usually due to an accessory atrioventricular pathway. It can be associated with underlying structural heart disease such as Ebstein's anomaly, tricuspid atresia or corrected transposition of great arteries.

Neonatology II: Respiratory and cardiac disorders

Table 46.5 Common acyanotic congenital heart diseases

CHD	Clinical presentation	Age at presentation	Examination	Chest radiograph	ECG	Management
Ventricular septal defect (VSD) (p. 570)	Usually asymptomatic in the neonatal period	Infancy	Pansystolic murmur in the lower left sternal edge	Cardiomegaly and increased pulmonary vascularity if large left-to-right shunt	Normal or left ventricular hypertrophy	Small VSDs close spontaneously Large VSDs need closure
Atrial septal defect (ASD) (p. 576)	Asymptomatic	Childhood	Ejection systolic murmur with wide fixed split second heart sound	Normal or enlarged heart Increased pulmonary vascularity	Right axis deviation and right bundle branch block	Closure surgical or catheter
Atrioventricular septal defect (AVSD) (p. 571)	Symptoms of heart failure usually after 4 weeks of age Cyanosis	Usually after 4 weeks of age	Hyperdynamic precordium Pansystolic murmur	Cardiomegaly with increased pulmonary vascularity	Left axis deviation or superior QRS axis Biventricular hypertrophy	Pulmonary artery banding Surgical closure
Coarctation of the aorta (p. 572)	Symptoms of heart failure Poorly felt femoral pulses on routine examination	Usually symptomatic after 1 week of age	Ejection systolic murmur at upper left sternal border with radiation to interscapular area Discrepancy in upper and lower limb BP	Cardiomegaly and pulmonary venous congestion	Right ventricular hypertrophy with right bundle branch block	Prostaglandin infusion as emergency Repair of coarctation
Hypoplastic left heart syndrome	Shock and heart failure	Usually within 72 hours of age	Loud and single second heart sound No murmurs	Pulmonary venous congestion Cardiomegaly	Right ventricular hypertrophy	Prostaglandin infusion Balloon atrial septostomy Staged repair using Norwood-type procedure Palliative care

Investigations

The ECG shows narrow QRS complexes, with a heart rate in the range of 180–300 beats/min. The P wave is often difficult to see, but when present usually has an abnormal axis or morphology.

Management

SVT usually responds to intravenous adenosine. Infants who are in shock may need DC cardioversion with 1–2 joules/kg. It is important to liaise with the regional cardiology team with regard to choice of maintenance treatment.

Congenital complete heart block

Clinical features

Affected fetuses may be detected by the presence of bradycardia at routine ultrasound examination or during labour. Neonates with congenital heart block can be asymptomatic or present with heart failure or Stokes–Adams attacks. Infants may have underlying congenital heart disease such as septal defects. It is important to exclude maternal systemic lupus erythematosus or collagen vascular disease.

Management

In symptomatic infants or in those with heart rates of less than 40 beats/min, artificial pacing may be needed. Isoprenaline infusion is used occasionally in infants to raise the heart rate temporarily in an acute situation.

Approach to a neonate with a suspected cardiac problem

History

- Family history of congenital heart disease
- Exposure to intrauterine infections or teratogens
- Symptoms of heart failure: difficulty to manage sucking while feeding, forehead sweating and tachypnoea, increased precordial activity.

Examination

- General examination to look for any evidence of dysmorphism
- Evidence of cyanosis?
- Peripheral pulses, femoral pulses, brachial femoral delay
- Signs of heart failure: hepatomegaly and intercostal and subcostal recessions
- Precordial activity
- Auscultation of the heart and heart sounds and determining the presence of murmurs

- Blood pressure in all four limbs
- Pre- and post-ductal oximetry.

Investigations

- Chest radiograph:
  - Size and shape of the heart
  - Vascularity of lung fields
  - Exclusion of any primary or coexistent respiratory problem (important)
  - Anomalies of ribs and vertebrae.
- Electrocardiogram:
  - ECG is important, particularly if there are ischaemic and rhythm disturbances of the heart.
- Echocardiography:
  - This is mandatory in a neonate with a suspected congenital cardiac problem.
- Cardiac catheterization:
  - Used for either diagnosis and treatment of specific cases (valvulotomy, valvuloplasty, placement of devices)
- Multislice CT scan (three dimensional imaging), cardiovascular MRI:
  - These new techniques give anatomical and functional information, and may sometimes substitute catheterization studies.

Management

- It is important to liaise with a paediatric cardiac centre regarding the management of all infants with suspected serious congenital cardiac problems to facilitate stabilization and transfer of such infants.
- Apply the basic principles of stabilization of the airway, breathing and circulation.
- It is essential to keep the duct patent in conditions suspected of being duct-dependent; this is achieved by a continuous infusion of prostaglandins (5–10 ng/kg/min).
- Management of heart failure depends upon the underlying aetiology and includes strategies to improve preload and afterload and increase cardiac contractility.
- Many cardiac disorders require surgical intervention (Table 46.5).

References and further reading

Aghajafari F, Murphy K, Matthews S et al 2002 Repeated doses of antenatal corticosteroids in animals: a systemic review. American Journal of Obstetrics and Gynaecology 186(4):843–849

Barrington KJ, Finer NN 2007 Inhaled nitric oxide for respiratory failure in preterm infants. Cochrane Database Syst Rev. Jul 18;(3):CD000509

Baud O, Foix-L'Helias L, Kaminski M et al 1999 Antenatal glucocorticosteroid treatment and cystic periventricular leukomalacia in very premature infants. New England Journal of Medicine 341:1190–1196

Brownfoot FC, Crowther CA, Middleton P 2008 Different corticosteroids and regimens for accelerating fetal lung maturation for women at risk of preterm birth. Cochrane Database Syst Rev. Oct 8;(4):CD006764

Cooke L, Steer P, Woodgate D 2004 Indomethacin for asymptomatic patent ductus arteriosus in preterm infants (Cochrane Review). In: Cochrane Library, issue 3

Costeloe K, Hennessy E, Gibson AT et al for the Epicure Study Group 2000 The EPICure study: outcomes to discharge from hospital for infants born at the threshold of viability. Pediatrics 106:659–671

Crowther CA, Alfirevic Z, Haslann RR 2004 Thyrotropin-releasing hormone added to corticosteroids for women at risk of preterm birth for preventing neonatal respiratory disease (Cochrane Review) In: Cochrane Library, issue 3

El Shahed AI, Dargaville P, Ohlsson A, Soll RF 2007 Surfactant for meconium aspiration syndrome in full term/near term infants. Cochrane Database Syst Rev. Jul 18;(3):CD002054

Greenough A 2002 Update on modalities of mechanical ventilators. Archives of Disease in Childhood, Fetal and Neonatal Edition 87:F3–6

Greenough A, Milner AD, Dimitriou G 2004 Synchronised mechanical ventilation for respiratory support in newborn infants (Cochrane Review). In: Cochrane Library, issue 3

Halliday HL 2004 Endotracheal intubation at birth for preventing morbidity and mortality in vigorous, meconium-stained infants born at term (Cochrane Review) In: Cochrane Library, issue 3

Halliday HL, Ehrenkranz RA, Doyle LW 2009 Early (< 8 days) postnatal corticosteroids for preventing chronic lung disease in preterm infants. Cochrane Database Syst Rev. Jan 21;(1): CD001146.

Halliday HL, Ehrenkranz RA, Doyle LW 2009 Late (> 7 days) postnatal corticosteroids for chronic lung disease in preterm infants. Cochrane Database Syst Rev. Jan 21;(1):CD001145.

Lewis V, Whitelaw A 2004 Furosemide for transient tachypnoea of the newborn (Cochrane Review). In: Cochrane Library, issue 3

Newnham JP, Jobe AH 2009 Should we be prescribing repeated courses of antenatal steroids? Semin Fetal Neonatl Med 14:157–163

Northway WHJ, Rosan RC, Porter DY 1967 Pulmonary disease following respiratory therapy of hyaline membrane disease: bronchopulmonary dysplasia. New Eng J Med 276: 357–368

Ohlsson A, Walia R, Shah S 2004 Ibuprofen for the treatment of a patent ductus arteriosus in preterm and/or low birthweight infants (Cochrane Review). In: Cochrane Library, issue 3

Roberts D, Dalziel S 2006 Antenatal corticosteroids for accelerating fetal lung maturation for women at risk of preterm birth. Cochrane Database Syst Rev. Jul 19;3: CD004454.

Soll RF, Blanco F 2004 Natural surfactant extract versus synthetic surfactant for neonatal respiratory distress syndrome (Cochrane Review). In: Cochrane Library, issue 3

Soll RF, Morley CJ 2004 Prophylactic versus selective use of surfactant for preventing morbidity and mortality in preterm infants (Cochrane Review). In: Cochrane Library, issue 3

UK Collaborative ECMO Trial Group 1996 UK collaborative randomized trial of neonatal extracorporeal membrane oxygenation. Lancet 348:75–82

Wiswell T, Knight GR, Finer NN et al 2002 A multicentre randomized controlled trial comparing Surfaxin (Lucinactant) lavage with standard care for treatment of meconium aspiration syndrome. Pediatrics 109:1081–1087

CHAPTER

47

Neonatology III: Neurology, haematology, metabolism and sepsis

LEARNING OUTCOMES

By the end of this chapter you should:

- Be able to describe the features of neonatal encephalopathy
- Be able to explain the mechanisms of brain injury in full-term and preterm infants
- Know how to initiate the management of neonatal encephalopathy
- Know the common causes and management of neonatal anaemia and thrombocytopenia
- Be able to discuss the differential diagnosis, investigation and management of haemolysis and jaundice in the newborn
- Have an understanding of glucose and calcium metabolism in the newborn
- Have an understanding of the pathophysiology of sepsis and its presentation in the newborn.

MODULE EIGHT

Neurology

Basic science

Brain development

During intrauterine and early neonatal life the baby's brain is developing extremely fast. At 20 weeks the brain is almost completely smooth, and although neuronal formation is complete myelination has not begun, nor has glial cell differentiation (Fig. 47.1). In the second and third trimester the rapid pace of development continues, with the formation of sulci and gyri and continued organization of the central nervous system (CNS). Interference with the normal process of development can occur and modern neuroimaging has made the diagnosis of such disorders much easier

(examples are schizencephaly, polymicrogyria and lissencephaly).

Cerebral blood flow

Cerebral blood flow (CBF) is relatively low in the newborn compared to later in life and the major determinant of CBF is blood pressure. Other factors that affect CBF are carbon dioxide concentration and intracranial pressure (ICP). Babies are not as good as older children at 'autoregulating' CBF; autoregulation means that CBF is kept constant over a range of blood pressure, thus protecting the brain from fluctuations in blood pressure. The concept of loss of autoregulation is important in understanding why brain injury occurs when there is cerebral oedema (ICP) and in preterm brain injury

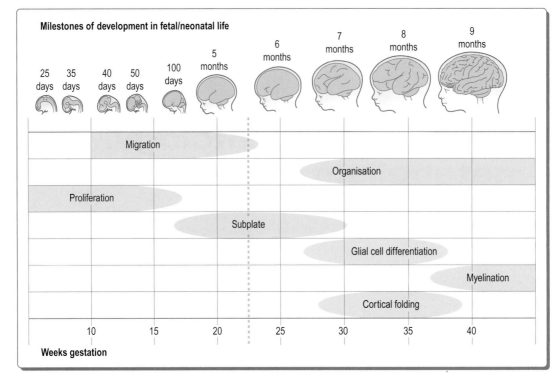

Fig. 47.1 **Milestones of development in relation to the neonatal intensive care unit (NICU)**

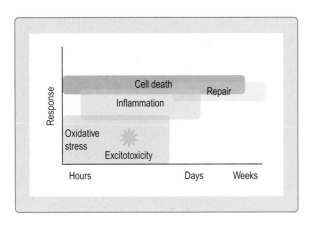

Fig. 47.2 **Mechanisms of brain injury in the term neonate**
(From: Ferriero 2004 DM Neonatal brain injury. New England Journal of Medicine 351:1985–1995)

(lost autoregulation, fluctuating blood pressure, and high carbon dioxide levels in respiratory failure).

Mechanisms of neonatal brain injury

A reduction in CBF and brain energy supply sufficient to cause damage initially causes some cell death but the damaging process continues long after CBF is restored (Fig. 47.2). The key processes in ongoing damage are:

- Oxidative stress
- Apoptosis
- Excitotoxicity
- Cytokine damage.

Some cells appear to commit cell suicide ('apoptosis') because of upregulation of genetic triggers; others are damaged by excitotoxicity due to glutamate release, or die from free radical oxidative stress or from cytokine release as a consequence of inflammation. Understanding of the ongoing process of cell death and damage has led to an understanding of a 'therapeutic window' lasting some hours immediately after the injury. There is hope that appropriate intervention during this window can ameliorate some of the ongoing damage, and currently there is much interest in brain cooling as an intervention in full-term infants.

Problem-orientated topic:

abnormal movements

Jakub, a 2-day-old baby of an 18-year-old single primiparous woman who works in a nightclub, is noticed to make repetitive jerky movements of his arms and to be slightly blue. The whole episode lasts less than 1 minute. Jakub was born by ventouse and had previously been feeding well from the breast.

Continued overleaf

Q1. What other information from the history would be helpful?

Q2. What emergency investigations are indicated?

Q3. What management are you going to arrange?

Q1. What other information from the history would be helpful?

Babies with encephalopathy are characteristically lethargic and floppy, with a reduced level of spontaneous activity at first. They then become irritable, with seizures, which are the hallmark of the disease. Babies who have seizures without encephalopathy are likely to have suffered a stroke. The most common cause of an early neonatal encephalopathy with seizures in a term baby is hypoxic–ischaemic encephalopathy (Box 47.1). Neonatal encephalopathy is a serious condition, occurring in 1–6 per 1000 births at term. The mortality is around 15%, and 25% of survivors will suffer significant neurological disability.

Q2. What emergency investigations are indicated?

See Box 47.2.

Q3. What management are you going to arrange?

- Admit the baby to the intensive care unit; establish monitoring.
- Get urgent glucose and blood gas.
- Establish intravenous and ventilatory support, if required.
- Arrange first-line investigations, including lumbar puncture (LP), promptly.
- Consider initiating treatment with a loading dose of phenobarbital if seizures quickly recur or if a single seizure is very prolonged (rare in the newborn).
- Restrict fluid in babies thought to have HIE but maintain glucose levels.
- Explain seizure to the parents but do not try to prognosticate too early; the prognosis varies considerably according to the cause and accurate prognosis requires information from EEG and MRI.

Preterm brain injury

Germinal matrix-intraventricular haemorrhage

The preterm brain is particularly vulnerable to injury because autoregulation of CBF is often impaired,

---

BOX 47.1 Differential diagnosis of neonatal seizures

Hypoxic–ischaemic encephalopathy
- Seizures within 24 hours of birth, history of fetal distress and birth depression, often with early metabolic acidosis
- Baby is encephalopathic; altered CNS state

Focal infarction (stroke)
- Seizures often occur on day 2 or 3 and can be focal
- Baby usually still feeding and alert between seizures — not encephalopathic

Meningitis
- There may be a history of prolonged membrane rupture or of maternal pyrexia in labour
- Fontanelle often full; baby systemically ill
- Remember to ask about maternal genital herpes

Neonatal abstinence syndrome
- History of maternal drug use, including methadone programmes
- Babies often sleep poorly, feed avidly and scratch their faces

Withdrawal from maternal medication
- E.g. selective serotonin reuptake inhibitors (SSRIs)
- Take a good history of maternal therapeutic drug use in all cases of neonatal seizure

Hypoglycaemia
- There can be a history of poor feeding or maternal diabetes
- Diagnosis depends on performing urgent glucose estimation on all babies with seizure

Inborn error of metabolism
- Worsening metabolic acidosis and seizures difficult to control
- Diagnosis depends on careful investigation

Intracranial haemorrhage (subdural or intraparenchymal)
- More common after instrumental delivery, particularly if multiple attempts or failed instrumental delivery
- Baby may be pale and may not have received vitamin K prophylaxis
- This is the most common cause of seizure in preterm babies

Full blood count

- Anaemia, thrombocytopenia in intracranial haemorrhage (ICH)
- Thrombocytopenia in hypoxic–ischaemic encephalopathy (HIE), alloimmune thrombocytopenic purpura

Urea and electrolytes

- Glucose is an emergency investigation
- Occasionally hyponatraemia or hypernatraemia or hypocalcaemia can cause seizures

Blood culture

- Helpful in identifying organism in meningitis, usually positive

Blood gas

- Early metabolic acidosis in HIE
- Worsening in inborn errors of metabolism, in which case check the ammonia and lactate

Lumbar puncture

- Essential investigation to diagnose meningitis
- Contraindicated if very low platelet count or severe respiratory compromise
- If cerebrospinal fluid (CSF) white cell count is elevated (more than 30) but no organisms are seen on Gram stain, think of viral meningitis; ask for polymerase chain reaction (PCR) to be carried out and give aciclovir until result available

Electroencephalography (EEG) or cerebral function monitor (CFM) trace

- EEG helpful in confirming diagnosis of seizure and in assessing response to treatment
- Background EEG helpful in determining prognosis in HIE
- CFM not as reliable but can be a useful cotside monitor

Ultrasound brain scan

- First-line imaging investigation for all babies with seizure

Magnetic resonance imaging (MRI)

- Second-line imaging choice in all babies except those with suspected ICH who require CT
- Useful to determine extent of disease and assist with prognosis
- Essential if ultrasound normal and stroke suspected

Grade 1	Germinal matrix haemorrhage
Grade II	Intraventricular haemorrhage with no ventricular enlargement
Grade III	Intraventricular haemorrhage with ventricular enlargement
Grade IV	Haemorrhagic periventricular infarction or intraparenchymal lesion; bleeding into the parenchyma of the brain

associated illness causes changes in CBF and blood pressure, and the developing brain contains the germinal matrix, which is situated over the head of the caudate nucleus in the floor of the lateral ventricle. The germinal matrix has thin-walled vessels and is often the site of bleeding. Blood clot in the germinal matrix can obstruct the draining vein of the adjacent brain parenchyma, leading to further damage from haemorrhagic venous infarction. This pattern of bleeding is called germinal matrix-intraventricular haemorrhage (GMH-IVH). Bleeding into the substance of the brain is often called haemorrhagic periventricular infarction (HPI) or intraparenchymal lesion (IPL). Older books use the Papile classification for IVH (Box 47.3), but more modern thinking is that this implies a hierarchy that does not exist and fails to take into account the fact that some lesions in the parenchyma of the brain can be ischaemic.

Periventricular leucomalacia

In addition to bleeding into the parenchyma of the brain, preterm babies are vulnerable to injury to the area in which white matter will form. This tends to occur in the periventricular area and is termed periventricular leucomalacia (PVL). In preterm babies the predominant cell type in this area of the brain is the oligodendrocyte precursor. These cells eventually mature and make myelin, which begins to form at around term. The oligodendrocyte precursor cell is exquisitely vulnerable to damage from free radicals and cytokines. Areas of damaged cells remain demyelinated in the long term, and babies with extensive white matter injury usually have cerebral palsy as a result. MRI reveals far more white matter damage in groups of preterm babies than was previously suspected with ultrasound diagnosis alone, and the importance of subtle changes in the white matter remains to be determined. There is concern that even subtle white matter injury leads to altered connectivity in the brain, with effects on the cortical and central grey matter. This may be the reason why short attention span and learning difficulties are commonly seen in very preterm survivors.

Key points: preterm brain injury

- Preterm brain injury is usually diagnosed with ultrasound screening in the nursery in a baby with no clinical signs. Occasionally presentation may be with anaemia, seizures and a tense fontanelle.
- GMH-IVH is tightly linked with gestational age (large haemorrhages are more common in very preterm babies, particularly below 28 weeks of gestation).
- Hypercarbia, acidosis and bruising are associated with GMH-IVH.
- PVL is less tightly linked with gestational age than GMH-IVH but is rare after 34 weeks.
- Hypocarbia and maternal chorioamnionitis are associated with PVL.
- Severe PVL that is cystic is associated with the development of cerebral palsy.
- Subtle white matter damage is very common in preterm babies but can only be diagnosed with MRI; early research suggests that this may be linked to the neurocognitive and behavioural problems that are common in preterm survivors who do not have cerebral palsy.

Hydrocephalus

The occipito-frontal head circumference should be measured in all babies at birth, and should be measured again whenever a baby presents with an illness. Measuring the infant's head is also part of child health surveillance. The measurements should be plotted on a centile chart; any deviation from the expected trajectory along the centile line established at birth should be taken seriously. A baby with an enlarging head requires investigation, initially with a cranial ultrasound scan, although CT or MRI should be performed if the diagnosis is not quickly apparent.

Not all babies with enlarging heads have raised CSF pressure due to hydrocephalus. Other diagnoses are important, such as subdural haematoma and benign enlargement of the subarachnoid space. Babies tolerate raised ICP better than adults because the skull is not fused, but eventually signs will develop. These include sunsetting of the eyes, bulging fontanelle, prominent scalp veins and vomiting. Neurosurgical help should be sought but in an emergency CSF can be drained via an LP or a ventricular tap.

Neonatal abstinence syndrome

Neonatal abstinence syndrome can present at any time in the first 2 weeks of life, but in general signs are present in the first 2–3 days and include irritability, tremor, vomiting, diarrhoea, sweating and fever. The drugs of abuse most likely to be followed by neonatal abstinence syndrome are opioids, including methadone. Babies are often snuffly and scratch their faces. Seizures can occur but should be avoided by early diagnosis and effective treatment. Assessment of the severity of neonatal abstinence syndrome can be made with a scoring system and there are a number in common use around the UK. These vary in complexity and only one (the Finnegan chart) has been shown to reduce treatment duration when compared to subjective assessment alone. None of the charts has been validated against a population of normal babies. Treatment is usually started with an oral opioid, usually morphine up to a total daily dose of 0.5 mg/kg, and few would now consider treatment with sedative agents alone to be adequate. Treatment is often required for around a month, occasionally longer.

Haematology

Basic science

The production of blood cells and platelets from a stem cell line is referred to as haematopoiesis and the cells produced are known as haematopoietic cells (Fig. 47.3). The 'mother' of all stem cells is, of course, the fertilized oöcyte, but stem cells are defined as cells that can self-renew and can differentiate into one or more of the 200 cell types found in the body. There is currently great interest in harvesting stem cells from umbilical cord blood for use in bone marrow transplantation, which is a rich source of haematopoietic stem cells.

In older children and adults haematopoiesis takes place in the bone marrow, but in the fetus the process begins as early as the sixth week of pregnancy, in the liver. The liver remains an important site of haematopoiesis until term. Haematopoiesis is under the control of cytokines; red blood cell production is stimulated by erythropoietin, white cells by different colony stimulating factors (e.g. granulocyte colony stimulating factor, G-CSF) and platelets by thrombopoietin. The production of red cells and haemoglobin falls dramatically after birth, probably because of the sudden increase in tissue oxygenation. Production gradually increases so that by 3 months a healthy baby can produce around 2 ml of red cells each day. However, the reduced capacity for formation in the early weeks, combined with a shortened red cell survival and a need for frequent blood tests, leads to anaemia in preterm babies. In fetal life the predominant haemoglobin is haemoglobin F, which has a greater affinity for oxygen than haemoglobin A.

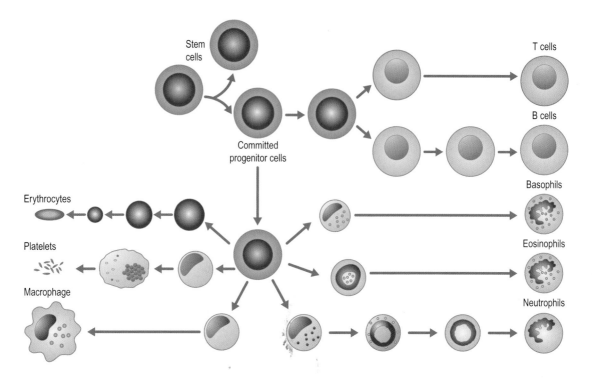

Fig. 47.3 **Haematopoiesis**

Production of haemoglobin A remains at low levels until after 30–32 weeks of pregnancy, and forms about 20–25% of total haemoglobin at term.

Anaemia

Problem-orientated topic:

pallor ● ● ● ● ●

Tereza is born by emergency caesarean section at term. Her mother, a 35-year-old physician, presented to the hospital because she noticed that Tereza had not moved at all that day. A cardiotocograph (CTG) has shown reduced baseline variability with decelerations. At surgery, there is meconium-stained liquor. Tereza weighs 3.5 kg and has Apgar scores of 3[1] and 6[5]. She responds to bag and mask resuscitation but is admitted to the nursery because she is noticed to be pale and is grunting slightly. Her haemoglobin is 8 g/dl.

Q1. Is Tereza significantly anaemic? What is the expected haemoglobin for a baby of this age?

Q2. What are the most likely causes of the anaemia and how can this be investigated?

Q3. What is the appropriate management for Tereza and what is the prognosis?

Q1. **Is Tereza significantly anaemic? What is the expected haemoglobin for a baby of this age?**

The normal haemoglobin at birth is high compared to adult life at 15–23 g/dl, and any baby with a haemoglobin of less than 14 g/dl on a properly taken sample should be considered to have anaemia. Not all such babies will need a blood transfusion, but all such babies certainly deserve investigation into the cause. The haemoglobin level falls over the first few weeks of life in all babies, reaching a nadir of around 10 g/dl at about 2 months. Preterm babies have a more rapid and steeper fall.

Q2. **What are the most likely causes of the anaemia and how can this be investigated?**

There are three main groups of disorders that cause neonatal anaemia, and some babies have more than one problem at the same time. The groups are:
- Impaired red cell production
- Increased red cell destruction (haemolysis)

Maternal Kleihauer test

- Shows the presence of fetal red cells in the maternal circulation
- Important to diagnose fetomaternal haemorrhage as a cause of neonatal anaemia
- Often a history of reduced fetal movements and there can be CTG abnormalities
- Baby pale right from the start of life

Full blood count including reticulocyte count and film

- Low white cell count and platelet count combined with anaemia suggest a marrow problem
- Low reticulocyte count also suggests a primary failure of red cell production due to inherited disorder or congenital viral infection
- Elevated reticulocyte count suggests haemolysis
- Red cells may be seen to be an abnormal shape on blood film, e.g. spherocytosis

Blood group and Coombs test

- Positive Coombs test suggests alloimmune haemolytic anaemia due to blood group incompatibility between mother and fetus, e.g. ABO incompatibility, although the test is not always sufficiently sensitive
- Non-immune haemolysis is usually due to red cell membrane disorders, red cell enzyme deficiency or a haemoglobinopathy (e.g. thalassaemia)

Liver function tests

- Elevated unconjugated bilirubin level supports haemolysis
- Family history
- Some cases of congenital anaemia (e.g. Diamond–Blackfan anaemia in some families) are autosomal dominant
- Spherocytosis is also an inherited disorder with a history of intermittent aplastic crises in affected family members
- Ask about splenectomy in family members

- Blood loss.
  Investigations are described in Box 47.4.

Q3. What is the appropriate management for Tereza and what is the prognosis?

Consideration should be given to blood transfusion when a term baby is found to be significantly anaemic shortly after birth and in preterm babies who are ill with more modest anaemia. The appropriate blood product is leucocyte-depleted cytomegalovirus (CMV)-negative concentrated red cells, ideally from a cross-matched satellite pack. Irradiation is often used to ameliorate the risk of graft versus host disease, and is important for top-up or exchange transfusion in babies who received blood products in utero. Preterm babies need iron and folate supplementation. Erythropoietin can be used to treat the anaemia of prematurity, although the reduction in transfusion requirements has not been impressive.

Vitamin K deficiency bleeding

Newborn babies have low levels of vitamin K-dependent procoagulant factors, and continued vitamin K deficiency can lead to vitamin K deficiency bleeding (VKDB), sometimes termed haemorrhagic disease of the newborn. Vitamin K supplementation prevents most cases of VKDB. There is a very early form that occurs in mothers receiving medication that interferes with vitamin K metabolism, e.g. phenytoin, which requires maternal vitamin K administration in addition to neonatal supplementation. Originally, vitamin K was mainly given by intramuscular injection but since 1992 there has been controversy about the route of administration. The debate was generated by a study showing a link between intramuscular vitamin K and later childhood malignancy, and in spite of the fact that seven of nine further studies on the same topic have failed to confirm the link, the debate continues to rage. Oral vitamin K preparations are available and have not been shown to be linked to later malignancy, but there is concern about unpredictable absorption and parental compliance with the multiple oral doses that are thought to be required to prevent late-onset VKDB. With no vitamin K prophylaxis at all, the incidence of late-onset VKDB is about 7 in 100 000 births. The American Academy of Pediatrics in their policy statement on the use of vitamin K in the newborn (Pediatrics 2003;112:191–2) has endorsed the universal supplementation of vitamin K using the intramuscular (IM) route. Although oral administration of vitamin K has been shown to have efficacy similar to that of parenteral vitamin K in the prevention of early VKDB, several countries whose policies promote the use of orally administered vitamin K (even with multiple-dose regimens) have reported a resurgence of late VKDB (1.2 to 1.8 per 100 000 live births compared with rates of approximately 2 to 4 per 100 000 in those receiving incomplete oral prophylaxis and with no reported cases after IM administration). In favour of the oral efficacy of vitamin K, current practice in the Netherlands to administer small daily oral doses may decrease the risk of late VKDB and approach the efficacy of the parenteral route; however, this needs to be studied further.

VKDB is much more common in breastfed babies because there are very low amounts of vitamin K in breast milk, and it has also been suggested that the gut bacterial flora of breastfed babies produces less vitamin K than that of formula-fed infants.

VKDB can be categorized as follows.

Early

- Presents within 24 hours of birth.
- Uncommon now with modern standards of obstetric care.
- Most likely to occur in babies born to mothers taking drugs such as anticonvulsants during pregnancy.
- Sites of bleeding and bruising involve areas related to birth trauma (e.g. cephalhaematoma)
- May present with melaena or intracranial haemorrhage.

Classic

- 40–50% of cases of VKDB.
- Presents between 1 and 7 days following birth.
- Primarily occurs in breastfed babies and those born to mothers taking procoagulant medications.
- Typically presents with bleeding from the cord stump.
- May also present with melaena, haematemesis or bleeding from the oral or nasal mucous membranes.
- Does not usually involve intracranial haemorrhage.

Late

- Mainly occurs in breastfed babies.
- May also occur as a complication in babies with conditions causing cholestasis, such as α_1-antitrypsin deficiency, and in babies with malabsorptive conditions such as cystic fibrosis.
- Infants who are treated with long-term broad-spectrum antibiotics may also be at risk because of reduction in bacteria that produce vitamin K.
- Classically presents with signs of sudden intracranial haemorrhage.

Diagnosis

The diagnosis is based on a prolongation of the prothrombin time. The platelet count is normal and so is the fibrinogen level; the baby does not have disseminated intravascular coagulation (DIC). In severe cases the partial thromboplastin time is also prolonged.

Management

Treatment is with vitamin K, either orally or intravenously, depending on the severity of the situation. The prothrombin time rapidly corrects to normal once vitamin K is given. Fresh frozen plasma may also be required for babies with severe or continuing haemorrhage or intracranial haemorrhage.

Bleeding in the neonatal period is not always due to VKDB, and other causes to consider are:

- Trauma, including non-accidental
- DIC
- Inherited coagulation disorders, e.g. haemophilia
- Platelet problems (see below)
- Gastrointestinal pathology, e.g. necrotizing enterocolitis (NEC).

Haemolysis in the newborn

Haemolysis is a relatively common cause of neonatal anaemia. The diagnosis of haemolysis is suggested by anaemia, unconjugated hyperbilirubinaemia and a high reticulocyte count. The Coombs test may be positive, suggesting a diagnosis of immune haemolytic disease. The main causes of haemolysis are:

- Haemolytic disease of the newborn (HDN), immune haemolytic anaemia
- Red cell membrane disorders
- Red cell enzymopathies
- Haemoglobinopathies.

The most common cause of Coombs-positive haemolysis is HDN due to the transplacental passage of IgG antibodies against rhesus antigens or antigens of the Duffy (F^y) or Kell blood group systems. HDN can also be caused by antibodies to the ABO system, in which case it mainly occurs in babies born to mothers who are blood group O and whose babies are blood group A or B. Haemolysis due to anti-A is more common than that due to anti B.

In modern obstetric practice mothers with rhesus antibodies are usually detected during pregnancy and carefully monitored. The timing of delivery is a matter for discussion and requires cooperation between obstetric and neonatal staff with input from specialists in transfusion medicine (in case fresh blood for an exchange transfusion is required). Fetal transfusion has revolutionized the management of severely rhesus-affected babies, so that hydrops is now rare. Further, the use of anti-D immunoglobulin given to rhesus-negative mothers in pregnancy and after the birth of a rhesus-positive baby (and at other times such as external cephalic version when fetomaternal haemorrhage could cause sensitization) has reduced the number of affected women substantially.

The treatment of severe haemolysis is with exchange transfusion, which corrects the anaemia and washes out the bilirubin. Babies with mild haemolysis can be managed with phototherapy initially and a 'top-up' transfusion, if required, later on. Folic acid must be given to all babies with haemolysis.

Glucose-6-phosphate dehydrogenase (G6PD) deficiency

This red cell enzyme disorder can present in the neonatal period, usually with marked jaundice but not with anaemia. G6PD deficiency is X-linked and hence is rare, but not unknown, in female babies. The disorder has a high prevalence in central Africa, the Middle East, tropical and subtropical areas of Asia and the Mediterranean. The geographical distribution mirrors, to some extent, that of malaria and G6PD deficiency is associated with a reduced susceptibility to malaria. Not all babies with G6PD develop marked hyperbilirubinaemia but many do and kernicterus can occur. Current thinking is that the combination of G6PD deficiency and Gilbert syndrome is the explanation for the very severe hyperbilirubinaemia seen in some babies. Once the diagnosis is made, parents must be counselled about foods and medicines that can trigger acute haemolysis. Examples are antimalarial drugs, broad beans (fava beans) and sulphonamide antibiotics (e.g. Septrin). Most people with G6PD deficiency do not have chronic haemolysis and do not require folic acid.

Hydrops

Hydrops describes the condition that occurs when the fetus has excess body water, with massive subcutaneous oedema often accompanied by pleural and peritoneal effusions. Hydrops is not a diagnosis but is the end result of a number of disorders. The condition is serious, with a high mortality, and it is important to try to make a specific diagnosis in order to counsel parents about the likely outcome for future pregnancies.

Hydrops can be caused by fetal anaemia, in which case it does not usually develop in fetal life unless the fetal haemoglobin is less than 5 g/dl, and it is often around 3 g/dl. HDN due to rhesus immune disease can cause hydrops, and ABO incompatibility can be severe enough to cause hydrops in very rare cases. In the past, rhesus iso-immunization was the most common cause of hydrops, which is often classified into 'immune' and 'non-immune' categories as a result.

Other important causes of anaemia causing hydrops are erythrovirus 19 (parvovirus B19) infection. Alpha-thalassaemia major can also cause hydrops and predominantly affects families of South-East Asian origin. Both parents of a baby with α-thalassaemia major will be carriers of the gene (localized to chromosome 16) and will have hypochromic microcytic anaemia themselves.

The broad diagnostic categories of disorders that can cause hydrops are:

- Haemolytic disease of the newborn (rhesus iso-immunization)
- Cardiac disease causing raised central venous pressure
- Intrathoracic space-occupying lesions interfering with lymphatic drainage
- Liver and gut disorders
- Congenital infection
- Metabolic disorders
- Chromosomal disorders, e.g. trisomy 13, 18, 21
- Fetal anaemia
- Syndromes, e.g. Noonan
- Placental abnormalities
- Maternal indometacin therapy.

The delivery of a baby with hydrops is an emergency, and intubation can be difficult because of oedema. An attempt should be made to resuscitate the baby and aspiration of pleural or peritoneal fluid may make resuscitation easier. Investigations should be set in train as soon as possible to investigate the cause because the baby may die early in spite of full intensive care.

Thrombocytopenia

The normal platelet count in the newborn is the same as that in adults: above $150 \times 10^9/l$. Thrombocytopenia is a common problem in the newborn period, particularly in sick preterm babies receiving intensive care when it is often an indicator of sepsis.

Many of the possible causes of thrombocytopenia are very rare, but for practical purposes there are only a few conditions that must be remembered and understood.

Early-onset (< 72 hours) thrombocytopenia

This is common in growth-restricted babies who have been subjected to placental insufficiency causing a degree of chronic intrauterine hypoxia. These babies have reduced numbers of progenitor cells, but the condition gradually resolves over a period of time. The thrombocytopenia is not usually very severe but on occasion platelet transfusions are required.

Babies who do not have intrauterine growth restriction (IUGR) but who are found to have early-onset thrombocytopenia may have the condition of neonatal alloimmune thrombocytopenia (NAITP). This is the platelet equivalent of HDN and occurs when a mother forms antibodies against her baby's platelets as a result of exposure during pregnancy (usually a platelet group HPA 1a-negative mother with a HPA 1a-positive baby). The condition can cause severe thrombocytopenia with platelet counts below $30 \times 10^9/l$, and the baby may present with petechiae, or intracranial haemorrhage in about 10% of untreated cases. Treatment is with compatible platelet transfusion if available or random platelet transfusion together with intravenous immunoglobulin.

Autoimmune thrombocytopenia

Caused by the placental transfer of platelet antibodies from a mother with idiopathic thrombocytopenic purpura (ITP) or conditions such as systemic lupus erythematosus, autoimmune thrombocytopenia may also occur in the neonate. The risk of intracranial haemorrhage is about 1%. In babies with platelet counts below 30×10^9/l, who are otherwise well, the current advised treatment is a platelet transfusion.

Late-onset thrombocytopenia

This is often associated with systemic disease, either late-onset sepsis or NEC. Thrombocytopenia can also be a clue to congenital infection with CMV, *Toxoplasma* or rubella.

Platelet transfusions are indicated if the platelet count is below 30×10^9/l in an asymptomatic baby, and below 50×10^9/l in a baby who has a bleeding problem ($< 100 \times 10^9$/l if there is major haemorrhage). The main risk of thrombocytopenia is intracranial haemorrhage.

Metabolism

Neonatal jaundice

Basic science of bilirubin metabolism

Bilirubin is produced as a breakdown product of haemoglobin. During the breakdown process the iron is reused and a molecule of carbon monoxide is excreted. Carbon monoxide can be measured in breath and the concentration is an index of bilirubin formation. Bilirubin is transported to the liver in the plasma, largely bound to albumin. This form of bilirubin is termed 'unconjugated' or 'indirect' bilirubin (the term indirect comes from the way the laboratory tests are used). There it is taken up by the hepatic conjugating system, forming 'conjugated' or 'direct' bilirubin. Conjugated bilirubin is water-soluble and is excreted into bile. Bile travels in the bile ducts to the small bowel and bilirubin undergoes further metabolism in the gastrointestinal tract. Some bilirubin in the small bowel is deconjugated again by an enzyme, β-glucuronidase, and it can be reabsorbed from the lumen of the small bowel. This adds to the load of unconjugated bilirubin. This 'enterohepatic recirculation' of bilirubin is a particular problem in

babies who are not fully fed or whose bowel is not yet colonized by normal flora. In fetal life unconjugated bilirubin can easily cross the placenta for disposal by the maternal liver, and maternal liver disease can lead to high bilirubin levels at birth.

Jaundice (including biliary atresia)

Jaundice is extremely common in newborn babies and 60% of all white-skinned babies are visibly jaundiced in the first week of life. The key problems in neonatal jaundice are in determining when jaundice is a sign of more serious disease and in the prevention of kernicterus. Kernicterus occurs when unconjugated bilirubin crosses the blood–brain barrier. Once inside the brain bilirubin is toxic to the deep grey matter, the globus pallidus in particular. Children who survive acute bilirubin encephalopathy only to develop kernicterus are usually profoundly disabled by athetoid cerebral palsy and sensorineural deafness. Kernicterus can be prevented by avoiding high levels of unconjugated bilirubin, using phototherapy and exchange transfusion.

http://www.pickonline.org

Hyperbilirubinaemia. A US website for parents of children brain-damaged by bilirubin, including videos showing the long-term effects

Phototherapy works by providing photons of light energy in a wavelength likely to be absorbed by the bilirubin molecule, which enters an excited state. About 80% of the time the bilirubin molecule loses the excess energy and returns to normal, but about 20% of the time a photochemical reaction occurs; these reactions include configurational and structural isomerization, and photo-oxidation. The photoproducts (which include lumirubin) are thought to be more water-soluble than unconjugated bilirubin and hence more rapidly excreted in bile. The rate of bilirubin decline is proportional to the dose of phototherapy, and in babies with severe jaundice it is important to expose as much skin as possible to light of an appropriate spectrum and to use adequate irradiance (more bulbs, well maintained).

Haematological causes of neonatal jaundice are common and usually related to haemolysis (see above). They include:
- Immune haemolysis (HDN): rhesus, ABO, Duffy or Kell incompatibility with maternal antibodies
- Red cell membrane disorders, e.g. spherocytosis
- Red cell enzyme disorders, e.g. G6PD deficiency
- Haemoglobinopathy (rare)
- Infection causing haemolysis, e.g. CMV, toxoplasmosis, syphilis.

late-onset jaundice

Lucie is a 15-day-old baby who was born at 37 weeks' gestation and who required respiratory support for 3 days. She was slow to establish feeds but is now on full feeds of breast milk, partly through a nasogastric tube. She was first noted to be jaundiced at 7 days and the levels of bilirubin are slowly rising.

Q1. What is the definition of late neonatal jaundice?
Q2. What is the main differential diagnosis?
Q3. How would you assess this child?

BOX 47.5 Causes of late unconjugated hyperbilirubinaemia

- Breast milk jaundice
- Haemolysis:
  - Blood group incompatibilities (ABO and rhesus)
  - Spherocytosis
  - G6PD deficiency
- Increased enterohepatic circulation:
  - Pyloric stenosis
  - Bowel obstruction
- Endocrine/metabolic:
  - Hypothyroidism
  - Hypopituitarism
  - Hypoadrenalism
  - Galactosaemia
  - Sepsis:
    Systemic
    Urinary

Q1. What is the definition of late neonatal jaundice?

Prolonged or late neonatal jaundice can be defined as visible jaundice — serum bilirubin > 85 μmol/l — persisting or occurring at 14 days of age in full-term babies and at 21 days in preterm infants.

Q2. What is the main differential diagnosis?

The most common cause of prolonged jaundice in full-term infants is benign and attributable to breastfeeding; up to 9% of breastfeeding infants are still jaundiced at 28 days of age. However, late-occurring jaundice can be an important sign of a number of relatively rare conditions, the long-term outcome of which may be favourably influenced by early diagnosis. These include congenital biliary atresia, congenital hypothyroidism and galactosaemia. Late jaundice can also be a sign of acute illness, such as urinary infection or septicaemia, or of persisting haemolysis.

In preterm infants the most common cause of conjugated hyperbilirubinaemia is parenteral nutrition.

Q3. How would you assess this child?

In assessing infants with late jaundice the following are important questions to address:
- Is the baby unwell?
- Is the urine dark and/or are the stools pale?
- Is the serum/plasma conjugated bilirubin concentration raised (> 15% of the total)?

A list of causes of prolonged/late jaundice is shown in Boxes 47.5 and 47.6.

Galactosaemia

Galactosaemia is an extremely rare disease with a frequency of approximately 1:30 000–60 000 in Europe and is a recessive genetic disorder. It is due to deficiency of the enzyme galactose-1-uridyl transferase, an enzyme involved in the conversion of galactose into glucose (galactose is derived from lactose, milk sugar, which is broken down to galactose and glucose). Classically, babies present towards the end of the first week with vomiting, diarrhoea, failure to thrive and jaundice. They may present with signs of VKDB due to the liver disease. There is an association with sepsis, most commonly an *Escherichia coli* urinary tract infection that can cause septicaemia. Cataracts often form very early on and, if not recognized and treated, lead to visual impairment from amblyopia.

The diagnosis can be suspected if there are reducing substances present in the urine, but this test is not sensitive or specific and must be confirmed by the analysis of erythrocyte galactose-1-phosphate uridyl transferase. Affected babies must be given a lactose-free diet, best achieved in infancy by using soy milk. Unfortunately the IQ is often permanently affected by the time a diagnosis is made and treatment begun, even though the liver disease recovers and the cataracts can be treated (or may regress somewhat). In the long term osteoporosis is a complication and dietary calcium supplementation is required. Young women with galactosaemia require hormone replacement therapy.

A screening test on the blood sample currently collected for phenylketonuria screening would be possible but is not considered cost-effective at present.

BOX 47.6 Causes of conjugated hyperbilirubinaemia

Cholestasis
- Biliary atresia
- Choledochal cyst
- 'Inspissated bile' syndrome (following haemolysis)
- Congenital bile duct hypoplasia (Alagille syndrome)
- Gallstones

Neonatal hepatitis syndrome
- Idiopathic neonatal hepatitis syndrome
- Intrauterine infections (e.g. 'TORCH' infections — *to*xoplasmosis, *r*ubella, *c*ytomegalovirus, *h*erpes simplex)
- Alpha$_1$-antitrypsin deficiency

Metabolic
- Total parenteral nutrition (TPN)
- Hypothyroidism
- Cystic fibrosis
- Abnormalities of carbohydrate metabolism, e.g. galactosaemia, fructosaemia
- Abnormalities of bile acid metabolism
- Abnormalities of lipid metabolism, e.g. Niemann–Pick type C
- Abnormalities of amino-acid metabolism, e.g. tyrosinaemia
- Congenital peroxisomal disorders, e.g. Zellweger syndrome
- Hypopituitarism
- Sepsis
- Urinary tract infection

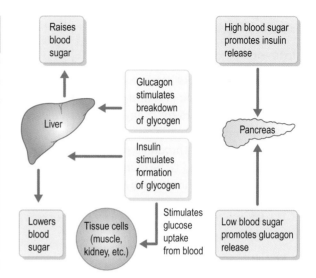

Fig. 47.4 **Regulation of glucose**

Hypoglycaemia (see also p. 685)

Basic science of glucose metabolism

Healthy adults maintain serum glucose levels within a very tight range of 3.5–7 mmol/l during fasting or after meals, and they do this on a diet in which the main energy sources are fat- and sugar-based. Maintenance of serum glucose depends on a feedback loop involving the liver, the pancreas and the process of glycogenolysis (the breakdown of glycogen stores to make glucose) (Fig. 47.4). Gluconeogenesis is the process involved in the production of glucose from precursors such as amino acids, lactate, and glycerol derived from lipolysis. The fetus cannot make glucose from glycogen, and is wholly dependent on a supply of glucose via the placenta. The fetus does make glycogen, and the liver stores at term are sufficient for about 10–12 hours of fasting. At birth, the fetus is disconnected from the continuous supply of glucose and has to adapt quickly to the

fast-feed cycle; glucose levels fall and there is a surge of glucagon and a fall in insulin levels. It takes more than a few hours for the newborn baby to switch on gluconeogenesis. During the inevitable fasting phase of the first few days of life (the volume of colostrum is very small, about 7 ml per feed) the baby's brain can use ketone bodies as an alternative fuel. There is a brisk ketogenic response in the normal baby, and the neonatal brain can extract and use ketones much more efficiently than the adult brain. There is a suggestion that formula feeding interferes with the ketogenic response, and this thinking is behind much of the current advice regarding initiation of breastfeeding.

Definition of hypoglycaemia

In recent years the tolerance for low blood sugar in newborn infants has increased so that it is now accepted that low blood sugar levels of < 2.6 mmol/l should be treated. Studies have suggested that blood sugar values below this are associated with poorer neurodevelopmental outcome and acute deterioration in neurological function measured by evoked potentials.

Causes of neonatal hypoglycaemia

See Box 47.7.

Hypocalcaemia, metabolic bone disease and vitamin D-deficient rickets

The serum ionized calcium level falls in the first 24 hours of life, as calcium continues to be taken up into newly forming bone, even though there is a cessation in the calcium supplied via the placenta and a postnatal

Transient

- Developmental lags in gluconeogenesis and ketogenesis
- Transient hyperinsulinism; infants of diabetic mothers
- Reduced glycogen stores: IUGR, HIE

Persistent

- Hyperinsulinism:
  - Idiopathic hyperinsulinism
  - Potassium–adenosine triphosphate (ATP) channel
  - Beckwith–Wiedemann syndrome
- Counter-regulatory hormone deficiency:
  - Panhypopituitarism
  - Isolated growth hormone deficiency
  - Cortisol deficiency
- Glycogenolysis disorders:
  - Debrancher deficiency
- Gluconeogenesis disorders:
  - G6PD deficiency
  - Pyruvate carboxylase deficiency
- Fatty acid oxidation disorders

surge in calcitonin. The failure to calcify newly forming bone adequately eventually causes rickets.

The definition of hypocalcaemia thus varies according to postnatal age, with a lower limit of normal during the first day. Total serum calcium should fall in the range 2.18–2.48 mmol/l (ionized 0.81–1.41) on the first day, and rise to 2.26–2.69 (ionized 1–1.5) by the end of the first week of life.

Signs of hypocalcaemia include:

- Irritability, twitching
- Seizures
- Lethargy
- Feed intolerance, vomiting.

Early hypocalcaemia is common in preterm babies, infants of diabetic mothers, babies whose mothers had poor vitamin D status during pregnancy (often immigrant mothers), and babies stressed by perinatal hypoxia.

Persistent hypocalcaemia suggests hypoparathyroidism, and a baby who is hypocalcaemic and who also has cardiac disease should be checked for Di George syndrome by examining the chromosomes for the characteristic 22q11 deletion. There are a number of other rare genetic causes of hypoparathyroidism such as HDR syndrome (*h*ypoparathyroidism, *d*eafness and *r*enal dysplasia).

The newborn baby has a store of vitamin D, which reflects the vitamin D status of the mother. Preterm babies fed unsupplemented human milk may develop borderline vitamin D levels. Vitamin D supplementation improves calcium absorption and retention, although there is no evidence that massive doses (above 1000 IU per day) or administration of the active metabolite are of benefit. There is an argument for supplementation of all pregnant mothers and newborn babies in countries where sunlight is limited. In the British Isles, sunlight exposure is often not adequate for vitamin D manufacture, and in this situation dietary sources become essential. Rickets and vitamin D deficiency are a particular problem in immigrant families in the UK and northern Europe at the present time. Dietary sources of vitamin D in infancy have been shown to be marginal, and poor diet combined with indoor living, atmospheric pollution and increased use of sunscreen has been responsible for the resurgence of simple vitamin D deficiency rickets in recent years. The American Academy of Pediatrics has recently revised its vitamin supplementation policy to advise that all breastfed infants, and those on mixed feeding receiving less than 500 ml of formula daily, should be given 200 IU of vitamin D daily.

Rickets presents with the signs of hypocalcaemia and the bony changes are diagnostic. X-rays show cupping, fraying and splaying of the metaphysis of a long bone, and the changes are often best seen at the wrist. The skull bones are softened, termed craniotabes. Hypocalcaemia can present with seizures in the neonatal period. Rickets is most often due to simple dietary deficiency, but rarely can be due to a non-functioning vitamin D receptor (vitamin D-resistant rickets), renal disease or familial forms of hypophosphataemic rickets.

Preterm babies are at risk of developing metabolic bone disease, which can progress to rickets if left untreated, because the dietary supply of calcium and phosphate is insufficient to meet their needs. These babies usually have a low serum phosphate with a high alkaline phosphatase and their bones are demineralized on X-ray. Fractures can occur, particularly rib fractures.

The emergency treatment of symptomatic hypocalcaemia is with intravenous 10% calcium gluconate, given over 30–60 minutes. Babies can then be started on oral calcium and calciferol whilst confirmation of the diagnosis is sought with X-rays. Phosphate supplementation is not required, except for preterm babies. When a diagnosis of rickets is made in a baby who was born at term, of normal weight, evidence of osteomalacia should be sought in the mother, whose vitamin D status is likely to be marginal, and the other children in the family should be investigated for rickets.

Sepsis

Basic science

Babies are particularly vulnerable to infection for many reasons, including:

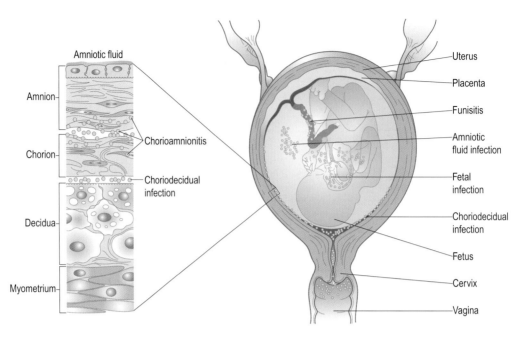

Fig. 47.5 Potential sites of bacterial infection within the uterus.
(From: Goldenberg RL et al 2000 New England Journal of Medicine 342:1500–1507)

- There is reduced skin integrity.
- There is frequent damage to the respiratory epithelium from oxygen or ventilation.
- There is an immature response to organisms in the gastrointestinal tract.
- The neonatal neutrophil pool in the marrow is easily exhausted and the neutrophils are poor at migrating and ingesting opsonized pathogens.
- T and B cells are immature and are naïve with respect to foreign antigens and pathogens.

An understanding of the way in which the body reacts to pathogens is important and there has been an explosion of knowledge in the last 20 years. The inflammatory response includes a 'cytokine cascade'. Cells such as macrophages, when stimulated, release tumour necrosis factor and interleukin (IL)-1. These molecules trigger a cascade that includes other interleukins, platelet activating factor, prostaglandins and leukotrienes. There is upregulation of the adhesion molecules such as selectin and this helps leucocytes to roll along the endothelium directed by a chemotactic gradient, in order that they can reach the area of invasion.

Occasionally there is an over-zealous response, resulting in the 'systemic inflammatory response syndrome' (SIRS). This is responsible for the clinical features of septic shock: hypotension, thrombosis, pulmonary oedema with increased vascular permeability and multiple organ failure. SIRS is the reason why some babies with NEC and early-onset group B streptococcal (GBS) disease die very rapidly in spite of antibiotic therapy and full intensive care support.

There is increasing interest in the fetal inflammatory response syndrome too; infection is a common trigger for preterm delivery. Chorioamnionitis occurs when the maternal polymorphs gather under the chorionic plate, attracted there from the intervillous space (Fig. 47.5). Eventually they may invade it and cross to the amnion and the amniotic fluid. Chorionic vasculitis and funisitis are thought to be fetal inflammatory responses, and are associated with a 'cytokinaemia'; babies whose placenta showed funisitis have high levels of interleukins in cord blood, for example. There is a relationship between the fetal inflammatory response syndrome and later cerebral palsy, which is present for both chorioamnionitis and funisitis but is weaker for the former.

Problem-orientated topic:

early neonatal collapse ● ● ● ●

Jan is born by emergency caesarean section for failed induction, at term, weighing 2.5 kg. He is in good condition with a normal cord pH. The membranes were ruptured for 11.5 hours. Jan is noted to be grunting from the age of an hour; he is intubated because of rising oxygen requirements and given surfactant and antibiotics. Two hours later Jan has a cardiac arrest.

Q1. What are the most likely causes of the cardiac arrest?

Q2. How would you investigate this child?

Q3. Is any other management indicated?

Q1. What are the most likely causes of the cardiac arrest?

See Box 47.8.

Q2. How would you investigate this child?

See Box 47.9.

Q3. Is any other management indicated?

Babies with shock from any cause, particularly septic shock, have a high mortality and need full intensive care support and monitoring with aggressive treatment as soon as the condition is recognized. Assessment of acid–base and cardiovascular status is urgent, and ventilatory support is required whilst an attempt is made to elucidate the cause and offer specific treatment. Milk feeds should be stopped in case of inborn error of metabolism and because an ill baby

---

BOX 47.8 Differential diagnosis of shock early in life

- Sepsis: particularly early-onset GBS disease
- Congenital heart disease, ductal-dependent, with closure of the ductus: e.g. hypoplastic aortic arch, coarctation of the aorta, hypoplastic left heart syndrome (p. 717)
- Arrhythmia: e.g. supraventricular tachycardia (SVT; usually babies cope well for many hours); ventricular tachycardia (VT; very rare in babies, suggests a myocarditis) (p. 717)
- Inborn error of metabolism (Ch. 34)
- Blood loss: e.g. massive subgaleal haematoma, ruptured liver, splenic rupture, intracranial haemorrhage with raised ICP
- Tension pneumothorax (p. 707): especially in an intubated and ventilated baby or a baby who required resuscitation or needling of the chest
- Cardiac tamponade: especially if there is a central venous line in place
- Gut perforation: think of this in a small preterm baby, particularly with NEC, but gastric and ileal perforation can occur due to ischaemic hypoperfusion; milk curd bezoars are rare causes of perforation but are reported

---

BOX 47.9 Investigations for neonatal shock and their significance

- Electrocardiogram (ECG) monitoring, blood gas, blood pressure, saturation monitoring: to assess the need for inotropic support, volume replacement and cardiac rhythm
- Chest and abdominal X-ray: to exclude pneumothorax and to check the heart size and position; look for free air in the peritoneal cavity
- Blood culture, urine culture and surface swabs: to attempt to identify the organism in sepsis, not a rapid test
- Full blood count: a low white cell count or a very high one suggests infection. Babies do not mount a specific neutrophil response to bacterial sepsis. The platelet count often falls in sepsis or NEC
- C-reactive protein (CRP): the normal value varies between laboratories but is usually less than 1 mg/dl. Serial measurements are more valuable than a single estimate, and the CRP may take 48 hours to rise in response to sepsis. A normal value in the acute situation does not exclude sepsis
- IL-6: not yet available clinically, but more likely than CRP to be elevated early in the presence of infection
- Urea and electrolytes, lactate, ammonia: clues to inborn errors of metabolism
- Echocardiography: to detect congenital heart disease
- Cranial ultrasound scan: to detect intracranial bleeding but not a good technique for detection of subdural collections and will not diagnose subgaleal bleeding either. For this, careful clinical examination and serial head circumference measurements are helpful

---

will not absorb feeds, which may cause vomiting and aspiration.

Group B streptococcal (GBS) infection

GBS is a common vaginal commensal, which causes serious early-onset disease in about 1 per 2000 births. Risk factors for early-onset GBS disease include:

- Prematurity
- Heavy vaginal carriage
- Prolonged membrane rupture (more than 18 hours)
- Maternal pyrexia
- Previous affected baby (mother has no antibodies, usually against type III GBS).

Management

Intrapartum antibiotic prophylaxis is a proven effective treatment that can interrupt the vertical transmission of GBS infection from mother to baby. Intravenous penicillin 3 g should be given as soon as possible after the onset of labour and 1.5 g 4-hourly until delivery in women whose babies are at high risk of acquiring early-onset GBS disease. Women who are allergic to penicillin should receive clindamycin 900 mg intravenously 8-hourly. The current guidelines for intrapartum antibiotic prophylaxis adopt a risk factor-based approach; screening for GBS carriage at 35 weeks has been adopted in some countries.

🌐 **http://www.gbss.org.uk**

Group B streptococcus support group; an excellent source of information, including leaflets for parents

🌐 **http://www.nsc.nhs.uk**

UK national screening committee

🌐 **http://www.rcog.org.uk**

The Royal College of Obstetricians comprehensive guideline on GBS, which is endorsed by the Royal College of Paediatrics and Child Health and the Royal College of Midwives in the UK

Most babies with early-onset GBS disease present soon after birth and virtually all present within 12 hours. Signs include raised respiratory rate, grunting, apnoea, poor feeding and mottling, and the disease can progress very rapidly to shock and death. The mortality is still around 10%.

Septicaemia

Apart from GBS, babies can acquire a bacteraemia from any one of hundreds of potential pathogens. Sepsis in the neonate is usually categorized as 'early-onset' and 'late-onset':

Early-onset:
- Presents by about 48 hours of age
- Is caused by organisms acquired from the birth canal or occasionally transplacentally, e.g. GBS, *E. coli, Listeria monocytogenes*

Late-onset:
- Presents after 48 hours of age
- Is usually caused by organisms acquired from the environment or nosocomially, e.g. coagulase-negative staphylococci (CONS), *Staphylococcus aureus, E. coli, Klebsiella,*

Enterobacter, Serratia, Citrobacter, Acinetobacter, Pseudomonas, Candida spp and other fungi, or viruses.

Exceptions to this pattern of acquisition and presentation include:
- Late-onset GBS
- Herpes simplex infection
- *Chlamydia* infection
- Congenital candidal and other fungal infections.

Infections caused by these organisms may be acquired at birth but present later. Anaerobic bacteria may also be a cause of sepsis, usually in association with bowel pathology.

It is important to remember viral infections including herpes virus, not least because aciclovir can be a life-saving treatment. Think of congenital candidiasis in preterm babies whose mothers have a history of chronic vaginal thrush and who had cervical cerclage, or who became pregnant with an intrauterine device fitted.

Babies with septicaemia usually present with non-specific signs such as poor feeding, mottling, lethargy, floppiness, apnoea and temperature instability. There may be tachypnoea and tachycardia. Quite often there is an ileus, with feed intolerance, dilated loops and abdominal distension, and these signs can be present even when the diagnosis is not NEC.

Treatment of septicaemia depends on accurate identification of the organism and appropriate use of antibiotics.

Meningitis

Think of meningitis in babies with signs of sepsis who are irritable. A full fontanelle and seizures are late signs, and meningitis should be diagnosed with LP before this stage is reached. LP is an essential tool in the diagnosis of meningitis, but it is known that in about 15% of cases the blood culture does not yield the organism.

The normal white cell count in neonatal CSF is higher than at other times of life, and in general counts of up to 30 per mm^3 are considered to be within the normal range. Differential white cell counts in CSF do not help to distinguish bacterial from viral meningitis in the newborn. If there is a high white cell count and no organisms are seen on Gram stain in CSF from a baby who has not received antibiotic treatment, think of viral meningitis and start aciclovir whilst awaiting PCR for herpes virus.

Meningitis carries a significant risk of brain damage and treatment must be carefully monitored. Brain imaging is important in order to detect ventriculomegaly and abscess (fortunately rare), and EEG can help in prognostication.

Eye infection

Sticky eyes are common in babies but serious eye infections are rare. The management depends on the organism, and an attempt should be made to identify *Chlamydia* because this may be 'masked' by treatment with topical chloramphenicol and requires systemic treatment with erythromycin (plus tetracycline eye drops) in order to treat any associated pneumonia. Staphylococcal infections are the most common. Mild infections can be treated by cleaning with sterile saline, but if cultures are positive and discharge persists, topical antibiotics should be used. Chloramphenicol or neomycin eye drops are suitable. Gonococcal ophthalmia remains rare but, because the corneal damage can occur very quickly, it is important to consider this as a diagnosis, particularly when there is a profuse purulent discharge very early in life. The current recommended treatment is with intravenous ceftriaxone; the baby and mother must be isolated.

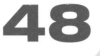
David M. Burge   Melanie Drewett   Eleanor J. Molloy

Neonatology IV: Disorders requiring surgical intervention

LEARNING OUTCOMES

By the end of this chapter you should:

● Be able to understand the ways in which serious congenital anomalies may present
● Know how to manage babies suspected as having these conditions prior to and during transfer to a surgical centre
● Be aware of surgical complications that may occur in preterm babies
● Know when to refer babies with minor surgical conditions.

Introduction

Babies who require surgical referral in the neonatal period usually have one of the following three problems:
• A serious congenital anomaly
• An acquired surgical complication of prematurity
• A minor anomaly detected on routine examination.

Congenital anomalies are now often detected antenatally and delivery is planned at a regional surgical centre (e.g. gastroschisis, congenital diaphragmatic her-

nia). However, some conditions (e.g. most forms of congenital intestinal obstruction, oesophageal atresia) are rarely diagnosed antenatally and will be detected when symptoms develop postnatally. Antenatal counselling with up-to-date outcome data that are region-specific is important. There is a large variation in termination of pregnancy in Europe (e.g. it is illegal in Ireland), which has a great impact on incidence and outcomes of various congenital anomalies. The correct early management of many of these conditions will influence morbidity and sometimes mortality.

Intestinal obstruction

Embryology

The intestine develops as a single tube from mouth to anus. At about 5 weeks of gestation the gut herniates through the umbilicus before returning to the abdominal cavity at about 10 weeks. As it returns it rotates so that the stomach lies on the left, the duodenum starts on the right, looping round to the duodenojejunal (DJ) flexure on the left, the caecum is in the right iliac fossa and the colon extends from this point up the left side, across the upper abdomen and down the right side to the rectum. If this process fails to occur correctly, malrotation will exist.

The blood supply to the stomach and duodenum arises from the coeliac axis. The entire small bowel and right colon are supplied by the superior mesenteric artery and the remainder of the colon by the inferior mesenteric artery. Intestinal atresia occurs as a result of an antenatal ischaemic event. Innervation of the gut is thought to occur by migration of ganglion cells from neural crest tissue. Failure of this migration results in Hirschsprung disease.

Problem-orientated topic:

intestinal obstruction

A well term male infant of 3.2 kg starts feeds on day 1 but develops bile-stained vomiting on day 2. The baby has not passed meconium. On examination the abdomen is distended but not tender.

Q1. What three specific clinical features are likely to be present?

Q2. How would you initially assess a baby with possible intestinal obstruction?

Q3. How should a baby with suspected intestinal obstruction be managed?

Q4. What are the possible causes of intestinal obstruction?

Q1. What three specific clinical features are likely to be present?

Intestinal obstruction is usually associated with three key features:

- Bile-stained vomiting
- Abdominal distension
- Failure to pass stool or flatus.

However, some of these features may be absent in specific causes of neonatal obstruction:

- Bile vomiting is absent in the one-third of babies with duodenal atresia in whom the atresia is proximal to the bile duct insertion.
- Distension may be absent in high intestinal obstruction (malrotation, duodenal atresia).
- Meconium may be passed by some babies with intestinal atresia if the atresia formed after the colon was filled with meconium.

Bilious vomiting

Bile is produced by the liver, is stored in the gallbladder and drains into the duodenum via the common bile duct (CBD). Bile is a golden-yellow/green colour but turns dark green on contact with gastric acid. Bile is not usually seen in gastric aspirate or vomit unless the intestine is obstructed beyond the point of entry of the CBD into the duodenum.

Mechanical obstruction to the lumen of the gut may be associated with impairment of the gut blood supply (e.g. volvulus, incarcerated hernia), which may progress to ischaemia, gut necrosis, peritonitis and death. Thus bile vomiting may be a warning sign of an impending catastrophe and should be assumed to be due to mechanical obstruction until proved otherwise.

Intestinal secretions

Considerable volumes of gastrointestinal secretions are produced each day. In the presence of obstruction fluid will accumulate within the gut lumen, which can affect fluid and electrolyte balance and cause intravascular volume depletion.

Passage of meconium

Around 98% of term babies pass meconium within 24 hours of delivery. Delay in passing meconium may occur with any of the causes of mechanical intestinal obstruction but may also be present if bowel function is altered, as may occur in many medical conditions (see below). It is important to rule out cystic fibrosis in any infant with a meconium plug or severe constipation in infancy. Preterm babies, especially if very growth-retarded, may not pass meconium for 10 days or more, during which time they may develop significant abdominal distension.

Q2. How would you initially assess a baby with possible intestinal obstruction?

- Initially ensure the infant is clinically stable and establish intravenous access.
- Assess the baby's general wellbeing; consider sepsis, metabolic causes and hypothyroidism.
- Assess the abdomen: most babies with a functional disorder will have a soft abdomen despite distension. Tenderness is a worrying sign and may require surgical review.

- Nil by mouth
- Adequate-sized NGT (e.g. 8 Fr in term baby) on free drainage and hourly aspiration
- Establish i.v. access
- Assess hydration/perfusion
- Provide i.v. fluids:
  - Fluid resuscitation if required
  - Maintenance fluids
  - Nasogastric loss replacement ml for ml with normal saline + KCl

- Check hernial orifices.
- Check the anus is present.
- If mechanical obstruction is suspected, stimulate the rectum (e.g. glycerine suppository). If a plug passed or there is explosive decompression, discuss with surgeons.
- If distension persists in the absence of a cause, discuss with surgeons.
- Review maternal drug history.

Some babies have bilious vomiting that resolves and no cause is ever found but it is a clinical symptom that requires careful clinical evaluation.

Q3. How should a baby with suspected intestinal obstruction be managed?

Immediate management (Box 48.1) involves fluid resuscitation and strict attention to fluid and electrolyte balance. All enteral intake should be stopped and maintenance fluids given intravenously. A nasogastric tube (NGT) should be sited to prevent vomiting and aspiration. Gastric aspirates should be discarded but replaced by an equal volume of normal saline with potassium.

Q4. What are the possible causes of intestinal obstruction?

There are a number of causes of mechanical obstruction, some of which are described below. In some of these a precise diagnosis can be made by plain abdominal X-ray (AXR) or contrast radiology, but in many cases the precise diagnosis is not made until laparotomy.

Malrotation

This is the most dangerous cause of intestinal obstruction in the neonate because the position of the gut predisposes to midgut volvulus with subsequent ischaemia. The normally rotated gut is protected from volvulus because the base of the mesentery has a broad attachment from the DJ flexure to the caecum. In malrotation these two points lie side by side and the base of the mesentery is narrow and prone to twisting (volvulus; Fig. 48.1). If this occurs, the superior mesenteric artery may be occluded and the entire small intestine will become ischaemic; even if surgery takes place quickly, the whole of the gut may be lost.

Features of obstruction due to malrotation to note are:

- The abdomen is not usually distended.
- Bile vomiting may be intermittent.
- Blood may be passed rectally or found in the nasogastric aspirate.
- Although tenderness may be absent, volvulus may have already occurred, and by the time clinical features of an acute abdomen develop, the bowel may already be beyond salvage.
- Blood tests such as lactate and C-reactive protein (CRP) may initially be normal, even in the presence of gut ischaemia.
- The diagnosis is usually suggested by an abnormal AXR with a paucity of gas or an asymmetric gas pattern (Fig. 48.2) or by contrast study.

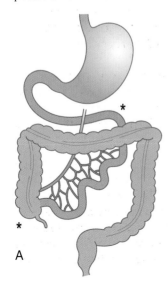
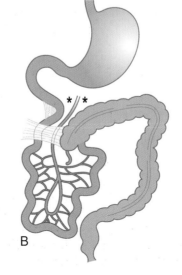

Fig. 48.1 Malrotation.
(A) Normal rotation; (B) typical malrotation. Note wide root of mesentery (indicated by *) in normal rotation compared to malrotation.

A   B

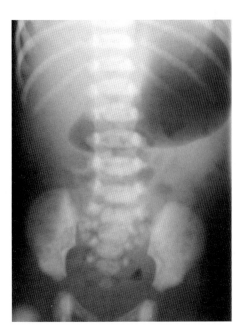

Fig. 48.2 Malrotation.
Note full stomach and duodenum but asymmetric gas pattern elsewhere.

If malrotation is suspected, the baby should:
- Be transferred immediately to a surgical centre
- Have an immediate barium meal to identify the position of the DJ flexure
- Have immediate laparotomy if malrotation is confirmed.

Volvulus with ischaemia is fortunately quite rare and in most cases obstruction is due to a loose twist or bands and can be corrected easily. Surgery involves mobilizing the duodenum to correct any band obstruction and widening the base of the mesentery to reduce the risk of volvulus in the future.

Duodenal atresia/stenosis

In this condition there is obstruction in the second or third part of the duodenum.
Duodenal atresia:
- May be diagnosed antenatally
- Approximately one third of such patients also have Down syndrome.
- Is not usually associated with abdominal distension (although there may be epigastric fullness)
- Is associated with non-bilious vomiting in about 30% of patients because the atresia has occurred above the point of entry of the bile duct into the duodenum.

The diagnosis is made on AXR with a typical 'double bubble' appearance produced by air filling the stomach and the dilated proximal duodenum (Fig. 48.3). The

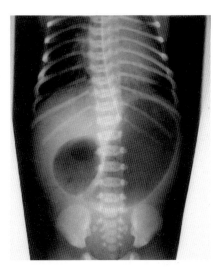

Fig. 48.3 Duodenal atresia 'double bubble'

presence of any air distal to the duodenum may indicate malrotation rather than atresia and urgent referral is indicated.

Corrective surgery is usually performed in the following 24–48 hours and involves an anastomosis to bypass the atresia (duodenoduodenostomy). Recovery of gut function postoperatively may be slow due to poor propulsion of feeds by the very dilated proximal duodenum. Long-term outcome is normal.

Small bowel atresia

Atresia is produced if a section of the intestine becomes ischaemic prenatally and this can occur at any stage, even in late pregnancy. Early atresia may be detected on prenatal scans. In late atresia the colon may have already filled with meconium and this may be passed postnatally, which may be confusing if a diagnosis of intestinal obstruction is being considered.

In babies with small bowel atresia:
- The abdomen becomes distended and dilated bowel loops may be visible. The more distal the atresia, the more distended the abdomen (Fig. 48.4).
- Contrast enema may be performed to try to distinguish obstruction caused by meconium ileus or meconium plugs (see below).
- Precise diagnosis may only be made at laparotomy.

Surgical correction usually involves primary anastomosis of the ends of the atresia. Subsequent recovery depends on how much, if any, intestine was lost at the time of the atresia formation. In most cases the amount lost is negligible. However, if a large amount of ileum has been lost, short bowel syndrome may occur and total parenteral nutrition (TPN) may be needed long-term. In the absence of short bowel syndrome long-term outlook is normal.

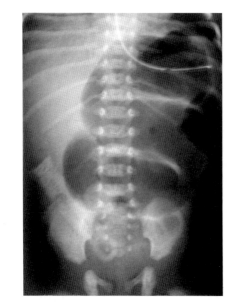

Fig. 48.4 Small bowel atresia (high).
Note only a few dilated loops with no gas beyond.

Meconium ileus

In this rare condition obstruction to the small intestine is caused by very sticky meconium. In almost all cases this is because the baby has cystic fibrosis. The diagnosis is usually only made by contrast enema or at laparotomy after transfer to a surgical centre.

Hirschsprung disease (HD)

In this condition ganglion cells, which are responsible for the promotion of peristalsis along the length of the gut, are absent from the rectum upwards for a variable distance but usually extending to the sigmoid colon. This results in a functional obstruction to the colon.

In babies with HD:
- Abdominal distension is present.
- Obstruction is usually relieved by the passage of meconium and flatus on rectal examination.
- Continued decompression is usually possible by colonic washouts.
- Severe sepsis may occur due to Hirschsprung enterocolitis.

HD is associated with trisomy 21 in 5–15% of patients. Mutations in the Ret-proto-oncogene have been associated with multiple endocrine neoplasia (MEN) type 2A and familial Hirschsprung disease. Other associations include Waardenburg syndrome, congenital deafness, malrotation, gastric diverticulum, and intestinal atresia. If HD is suspected, the baby should be transferred to a surgical centre. Here decompression is usually achieved with colonic washouts, and a rectal suction biopsy is taken to confirm the diagnosis. Subsequent management is usually by continued washouts in the community until definitive surgery is performed in the first few months of life, although some surgeons opt for temporary colostomy formation, an intervention that will be required if washouts fail to decompress the bowel.

Although most babies with HD are clinically well, albeit obstructed, some present with or develop enterocolitis. This is characterized by:
- An ill baby with signs of severe sepsis
- Abdominal distension ± erythema or tenderness
- Bilious vomiting
- Offensive watery stool.

This serious complication of HD requires:
- Broad-spectrum intravenous antibiotics
- Regular decompression with colonic washouts
- NGT, nil by mouth.

Emergency laparotomy with colostomy may be required if these measures fail.

Anorectal malformation

The absence of an anal opening will obviously cause intestinal obstruction. It is therefore important to check the anus in any baby with obstruction. Even if the anus is present stenosis may occur and can cause obstruction. The anal size should be assessed by rectal examination in term infants, when the anal canal should permit the passage of a small fingertip. If doubt exists in the preterm baby, specialist referral is indicated. Stenosis can usually be treated by dilatation, although surgery is sometimes required.

Meconium plug

In some babies with clinical intestinal obstruction rectal examination or washout results in the passage of a meconium plug. This usually takes the form of a solid lump of meconium, sometimes with a white inspissated tip, followed by the passage of additional plugs or normal meconium. Most of these babies are normal but this may be the presenting feature of Hirschsprung disease or meconium ileus. It is therefore essential that both conditions be excluded.

Obstructed inguinal hernia

See below.

Non-surgical causes of intestinal obstruction or delayed passage of meconium

- Normal transient delay (especially preterm babies)
- Sepsis

- Maternal diabetes, medications, narcotics
- Metabolic derangement: hypermagnesaemia, hypokalaemia, hypercalcaemia
- Hypothyroidism
- Congestive cardiac failure.

Diaphragmatic hernia

Problem-orientated topic:

respiratory distress at birth

A term baby develops respiratory distress 10 minutes after a normal vaginal delivery. On examination there is displacement of the trachea and cardiac apex beat to the right, there are reduced breath sounds on the left and the abdomen looks unusually flat.

Q1. What is the likely diagnosis?

Q2. What radiological investigations should be performed?

Q3. What immediate action should be undertaken?

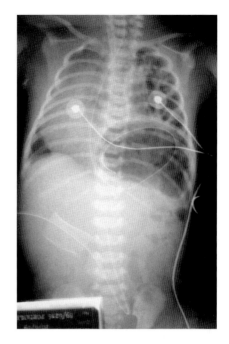

Fig. 48.5 **Left-sided congenital diaphragmatic hernia. Note stomach (with nasogastric tube) in chest, absence of bowel gas in abdomen and mediastinal shift to right.**

Q1. What is the likely diagnosis?

A space-occupying lesion in the fetal chest (e.g. liver or bowel, as in congenital diaphragmatic hernia) will often prevent normal lung development and produce pulmonary hypoplasia, the severity of which will depend on the timing of herniation. Alveolar insufficiency and pulmonary vascular abnormality, both of which are features of pulmonary hypoplasia, commonly cause persistent pulmonary hypertension of the newborn (PPHN), which is the major cause of respiratory complications and determines outcome.

It is important to exclude a tension pneumothorax using cold light transillumination of the chest. Congenital cystic adenomatoid malformation of the lung (CCAM) may also cause this clinical picture.

In babies with congenital diaphragmatic hernia (CDH) there will be:

- Respiratory distress: varies from none (in those with normal lungs) to profound (in those with severe pulmonary hypoplasia)
- Mediastinal shift (trachea and cardiac apex beat), usually to the right, as 80% of hernias are on the left side
- Scaphoid abdomen (because the gut is in the chest)
- Bowel sounds heard in the chest.

Q2. What radiological investigations should be performed?

- Diagnosis is made on chest and AXR (Fig. 48.5).
- Loops of gut ± stomach are seen in the chest.
- There is mediastinal shift to the opposite side.
- There will be an abnormal intestinal gas pattern on AXR. It is essential to perform an AXR, as a cystic lung may look very like a CDH on CXR but will have a normal gas pattern below the diaphragm.

Q3. What immediate action should be undertaken?

Immediate management includes:

- ABC: Airway, breathing and circulation. If the diagnosis is made antenatally elective intubation at birth and avoidance of bag and mask ventilation with rapid placement of NGT are recommended. Early transfer to a surgical facility is ideal as pulmonary hypertension may complicate delayed transfer. Gentle ventilation with permissive hypercapnia, use of high frequency oscillatory ventilation and nitric oxide are vital in current management.
- Gastric decompression with large NGT (8 Fr)
- Avoidance of bag and mask ventilation, as this may expand the stomach and compromise lung expansion

743

- Appropriate respiratory support and intensive care: many babies will require immediate intubation and ventilation, umbilical arterial and venous access etc. but some will have minimal problems.
- Nil by mouth, i.v. access and fluids
- Transfer to a neonatal surgical centre.

Subsequent management includes:
- *Respiratory support.* In severe cases the lungs are too small to support life and the baby will die within hours. At the other extreme the lungs may be fully developed and there may be no respiratory problems. In most there is a degree of hypoplasia resulting in PPHN (p. 701).
- *Assessment of other congenital anomalies*, e.g. echocardiography. These are present in about 40% of cases.
- *Surgical repair of the diaphragm.* This is usually delayed for at least 24–48 hours, even in babies with minimal respiratory problems.

Timing of surgery
Survival and severity of clinical problems are determined by the degree of pulmonary hypoplasia and not by the presence of the gut in the chest. Surgery is performed when respiratory status allows. Some babies will never become this stable and will die without surgery. In others surgery may be delayed for several days.

Prognosis
The mortality from CDH is 20–30% and is due to lung hypoplasia or other congenital anomalies.

Abdominal wall defects

Problem-orientated topic:

abdominal wall defects

An emergency caesarean section is about to take place on a 36 weeks' gestation pregnancy with an antenatal diagnosis of an abdominal wall defect. The mother is on holiday in your area and does not know the name of the condition diagnosed in her baby but remembers being told that the intestine was on the outside.

Q1. What are the possible diagnoses?
Q2. What action will be needed at the delivery?
Q3. How will the baby need to be supported before and during transfer for surgery?

Q1. What are the possible diagnoses?

At about 5 weeks of gestation, probably as a response to rapid liver enlargement, the intestine herniates out of the abdominal cavity, returning at about 10 weeks of gestation, at which time the umbilicus closes. Failure of development of lateral mesoderm is thought to result in exomphalos. In this condition the herniated viscera are contained within a semi-transparent sac, which may contain intestine alone or in combination with liver, depending on the size of the abdominal wall defect.

The embryology of gastroschisis is unclear but may be related to vascular changes at the umbilicus. The fetus initially has two vitelline veins; the left remains as the umbilical vein and the right obliterates. As the defect in gastroschisis is almost invariably to the right side of the umbilical ring, it has been suggested that abnormal obliteration of the right vitelline vein may result in the formation of gastroschisis.

The two primary conditions are exomphalos and gastroschisis (Figs 48.6 and 48.7). The features of these conditions are shown in Table 48.1. The major differences are the presence of a sac and the associated anomalies in babies with exomphalos. It is the latter that contributes to the increased mortality in exomphalos. In both conditions, if isolated, the survival rate is 95%.

Q2. What action will be needed at the delivery?

See Box 48.2.

Q3. How will the baby need to be supported before and during transfer for surgery?

- Large-bore NGT left on free drainage with hourly aspiration
- Replacement of gastric aspirates with i.v. normal saline with added potassium
- Regular assessment of circulation, e.g. capillary refill time, with further bolus fluid replacement as required
- Regular assessment of colour of the herniated viscera with repositioning or rewrapping if required.

Immediate transfer to a surgical centre should be arranged. During transfer further fluid boluses may be required and the viscera should be inspected regularly and repositioned as required to prevent venous engorgement or ischaemia.

In babies with exomphalos also be prepared for:
- *Lung hypoplasia*: some babies have severe respiratory problems.

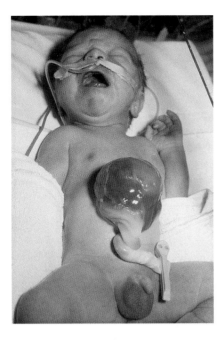

Fig. 48.6 **Exomphalos.**
Note sac covering gut.

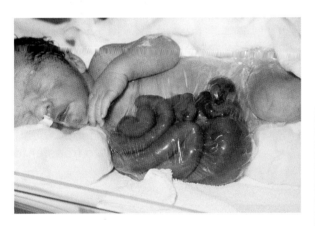

Fig. 48.7 **Gastroschisis.**
Note exposed gut without covering sac, Clingfilm wrap and towelling nappy under gut to support it in the midline.

Table 48.1 **Comparison of exomphalos and gastroschisis**

	Gastroschisis	Exomphalos
Anatomy	No sac Usually only gut out	Sac Gut ± liver, spleen etc.
Abnormal karyotype	No	May be trisomy 18/13
Associated anomalies	Gut atresia only (5%)	Cardiac, renal, pulmonary hypoplasia, Beckwith syndrome etc.
Postnatal outcome	95% survival	50–80% live-born survive 95% live-born survive if only abnormality

- *Beckwith–Wiedemann syndrome*: macroglossia, gigantism, exomphalos. Associated with hyperinsulinism and thus hypoglycaemia — watch the blood sugar.
- *Trisomy 18, 13 or 21*.
- *Associated anomalies*: cardiac anomalies are the most relevant (20%), therefore echocardiography is vital.

Surgery is required for both conditions but is more urgent in gastroschisis as the exposed bowel will lose heat and fluid rapidly. Intravenous feeding is usually required for babies with gastroschisis as the bowel takes several weeks to function normally. Long-term outcome is normal in the absence of associated anomalies.

Oesophageal atresia

Problem-orientated topic:

oesophageal atresia

You are called to see a 12-hour-old term baby who has been noticed by the staff on the postnatal ward to have excessive oropharyngeal secretions. Staff on the neonatal unit have been unable to pass an NGT more than a few centimetres.

Q1. What are the possible causes of failure to pass the NGT?

Q2. How would you distinguish these?

Q3. How should a baby with oesophageal atresia be managed prior to transfer to a surgical centre?

Q1. What are the possible causes of failure to pass the NGT? (Box 48.3)

The foregut begins development as a single tube from which the oesophagus and trachea form in the early weeks of gestation. The exact process is not understood but it is thought that failure of full separation of these

- Nasal obstruction:
  - Nasal oedema: common and resolves with time and/or decongestants
  - Choanal atresia
- Oesophageal atresia: with or without tracheo-oesophageal fistula

developing structures results in oesophageal atresia and tracheo-oesophageal fistula formation.

Choanal atresia

In this rare condition there is an obstruction at the back of the nose, at the level of the back of the hard palate, about 3–4 cm from the opening of the nostril. It is more commonly unilateral, so if passing the tube fails on one side, try the other. There is a solid feeling to the obstruction as the NGT hits the atresia. Due to respiratory problems bilateral atresia will usually require surgery in the first few weeks of life. Unilateral atresia does not require treatment in the neonatal period, with surgery being deferred until several years of age.

Oesophageal atresia (OA) and tracheo-oesophageal fistula (TOF) (Box 48.4)

The usual anatomy is:

- Oesophagus ending blindly in the upper chest (OA)
- Lower oesophagus connected to the lower trachea (TOF) but other anatomical varieties exist.

BOX 48.4 Clinical problems in oesophageal atresia with tracheo-oesophageal fistula

- Problems caused by atresia:
  - Failure to swallow saliva (mucousy baby)
  - Cyanosis and choking with feeds as milk spills over to the lungs
- Problems caused by the fistula:
  - Lung irritation from acid reflux to trachea
  - Gastric distension from air via trachea, especially if respiratory support is required
- Problems caused by associated malformations:
  - 50–70% have some other defects
  - VACTORL describes the most common combination of defects with EA (vertebral, anorectal, cardiac, tracheal, oesophageal, renal, limb)

Q2. How would you distinguish these?

To confirm the diagnosis of OA with TOF:

- Try to pass a large-bore (at least 8 Fr) naso- or orogastric tube. If successful, test aspirate with

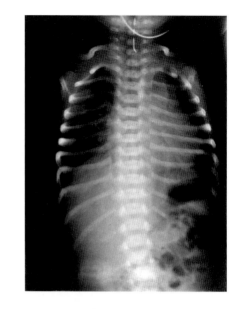

Fig. 48.8 **Chest and abdomen in a baby with oesophageal atresia and tracheo-oesophageal fistula.**
Note the tube arrested in the upper oesophagus and the air in the gut.

pH paper to confirm an acid reaction, as the tube could be coiled in the oesophagus.

- If the tube fails to pass, fix it as far as it will go and obtain CXR *and* AXR. This will show the tube in the upper chest, confirming atresia, and gas in the abdomen, confirming a fistula (Fig. 48.8). If the abdomen is gasless, there will be OA without TOF.

Q3. How should a baby with oesophageal atresia be managed prior to transfer to a surgical centre?

See Box 48.5.

BOX 48.5 Management of oesophageal atresia with tracheo-oesophageal fistula

- Remove the NGT and replace with a Replogle tube, if one is available. This is a 10 Fr sump suction catheter, which is connected to low-pressure continuous suction. Saline is flushed down the side-limb of the catheter every 15 minutes (or more often if necessary) to remove saliva from the oesophagus
- Nurse the baby head up to reduce flow of gastric acid into the trachea via the fistula. Prone position will further reduce the risk of reflux
- Establish i.v. access and commence maintenance fluids
- Notify regional surgical centre and arrange transfer, which should take place in the next few hours
- Continue above management during transfer

Respiratory management in OA with TOF

Most babies do not need respiratory support. Preterm babies, or those in whom the diagnosis has been delayed until after aspiration pneumonitis has already occurred, may develop respiratory distress. Positive pressure ventilation will result in ventilator gases passing down the fistula and inflating the stomach. This can cause abdominal distension and worsen respiration. In severe cases gastric perforation and death may occur. If respiratory support is required, immediate transfer to a surgical centre should be arranged for emergency ligation of the fistula.

Management at surgical centre

Echocardiography is performed to exclude cardiac defects. Primary repair is performed in the first 24–48 hours. OA often occurs in association with other anomalies. Because of this, routine screening of other systems is performed (echocardiography, renal ultrasound).

Outcome

Long-term outcome is variable, with respiratory and gastrointestinal complications being commonplace.

Rectal bleeding

Problem-orientated topic:

rectal bleeding

Jaden, a 4-day-old breastfed term baby, is noted to have passed dark red blood into his nappy. He appears alert, active and well perfused.

Q1. What are the possible causes of rectal bleeding?
Q2. How would you manage this baby?

Q1. What are the possible causes of rectal bleeding?

The colour of blood passed rectally will usually give a clue to the anatomical site of bleeding. Bright red blood is usually coming from the rectum or anus, dark red blood from the colon or terminal ileum, and melaena from the oesophagus, stomach or duodenum. If there is massive bleeding then upper intestinal blood may emerge still red from the rectum, but the baby would show signs of acute hypovolaemia.

Causes of rectal bleeding are:
- Idiopathic: in many babies no cause is found
- Consider gastroenteritis e.g. *Shigella*, *Salmonella*

- Milk allergy: due to cow's milk protein in formula milk or ingested by the mother and secreted in breast milk
- Haemorrhagic disease of the newborn (HDN, p. 728)
- Anorectal trauma
- Necrotizing enterocolitis (NEC, p. 748)
- Intestinal ischaemia: e.g. volvulus
- Intestinal malformation: e.g. haemangioma, duplication cyst
- Swallowed maternal blood, from delivery or from a cracked nipple (can be checked using the Apt test).

Q2. How would you manage this baby?

Assess the baby's general condition and abdomen. If the baby is haemodynamically unstable or if the abdomen is distended or tender:
- Establish i.v. access immediately
- Give a fluid bolus
- Cross-match blood
- Check clotting and vitamin K status
- Perform an AXR
- Inspect the anus for signs of trauma
- Check for an external haemangioma — this may be a marker for an internal one.
- Send stools for culture, sensitivity, microscopy and viruses such as rotavirus and enterovirus.

Practical points in management
- If the baby is systemically unwell or shocked, full resuscitation is required.
- If NEC is suspected on X-ray, stop enteral feeds and commence i.v. antibiotics.
- Treat vitamin K deficiency if HDN is proven.
- If the baby is well, wait. Most babies with milk allergy will stop bleeding either spontaneously or after change to milk devoid of cow's milk protein.

Scrotal swelling

Problem-orientated topic:

scrotal swelling

Liam, a male infant born at 28 weeks' gestation and now 5 weeks old, is found on routine examination to have a non-tender swelling in the left scrotum, which is not reducible.

Q1. What are the possible causes of this swelling?
Q2. How can these be differentiated?
Q3. What action is required?

Q1. What are the possible causes of this swelling?

The processus vaginalis is an outpouching of the peritoneum, which extends through the inguinal canal. It develops in early gestation and is involved in the process of testicular descent. Passage of peritoneal fluid down the patent processus vaginalis (PPV) results in a hydrocele. In most cases the PPV is very narrow and the fluid cannot be reduced back into the peritoneum by manual pressure. If the PPV is wide enough, intestine can pass down it; this is an indirect inguinal hernia.

The testis develops from the gonadal ridge on the posterior abdominal wall and descends to the internal inguinal ring by mid-gestation. Between 28 weeks and term the testis emerges into the PPV and descends into the scrotum. In approximately 5% of boys at term the testis has not fully descended but by 6 months of age this figure has reduced to 1.5%. Undescended testis is more common in preterm and low-birth weight babies.

Inguinal hernia

- 1–2% of term babies will develop an inguinal hernia.
  - In preterm babies under 1.5 kg the incidence rises to 20%.
- Boys are much more commonly affected than girls.

Hernias are usually reducible but may become irreducible, causing intestinal obstruction and ischaemia, a risk that seems to be greater in preterm babies than in older children. For this reason inguinal hernia repair is usually carried out before or soon after discharge from the neonatal unit.

In the case described the swelling is irreducible. If this is a hernia then:

- Signs of intestinal obstruction will develop.
- The swelling may become tender.
- It should not transilluminate (although this may be a difficult sign to elicit confidently).
- It should not be possible to get above the swelling — it should extend to the level of the inguinal canal.

Hydrocele

Hydroceles are common, affecting 10% of term babies. They are harmless and usually asymptomatic despite occasionally being very large. Hydroceles normally:

- Surround the testis
- Transilluminate
- Are usually confined to the scrotum.

Q2. How can these be differentiated?

The most common scrotal swelling is a hydrocele but it is important to exclude an inguinal hernia. Differentiation

Table 48.2 Comparison of features of inguinal hernia and hydrocele

Clinical feature	Groin/scrotal swelling	
	Hernia	Hydrocele
Reducible	✓	✗ (usually)
Intestinal obstruction	May be present	✗
Tenderness	May be present	✗
Can get above it to feel spermatic cord	✗	✓
Transilluminates	✗	✓

between the conditions can usually be made on clinical grounds:

- Check for signs of intestinal obstruction: vomiting, distension.
- Confirm that the swelling is not tender.
- Determine whether the swelling is discrete from the testis and that the testis is descended.
- Attempt transillumination of the swelling.

Features of hernia and hydrocele are compared in Table 48.2.

Testicular torsion

Neonatal torsion usually occurs as a late prenatal event and the infant is typically found to have a hard discoloured non-tender hemiscrotum. The testis in such cases cannot be salvaged by surgery but surgical referral is essential, as many surgeons will opt to fix the contralateral testis. Acute postnatal torsion can also occur and any infant with a tender testis should be referred for emergency surgical assessment.

Q3. What action is required?

If a hernia is suspected, then urgent surgical opinion should be sought. Once diagnosed, there is no need for repeated reduction.

A hydrocele requires no treatment. Spontaneous resolution will occur in most cases over several weeks or months.

Pneumoperitoneum/ necrotizing enterocolitis

Problem-orientated topic:

pneumoperitoneum/necrotizing enterocolitis

Krista, a 25-week gestation baby now 2 weeks old, is noted to have abdominal distension with bilious aspirates. A pneumoperitoneum is noted on abdominal X-ray.

Continued overleaf

Q1. What are the causes of pneumoperitoneum?

- Perforated NEC
- Spontaneous isolated intestinal perforation (SIP)
- In association with a pneumothorax.

The diagnosis of pneumoperitoneum is usually made easily on a supine AXR (Fig. 48.9), although sometimes a lateral decubitus X-ray of the abdomen is needed to show small air collections.

Q2. How would you differentiate between them?

Necrotizing enterocolitis (NEC)

Most babies do not require surgical referral but, in some, surgery will be life-saving. Surgical opinion should always be sought if there is a pneumoperitoneum or if clinical deterioration occurs despite maximal medical therapy.

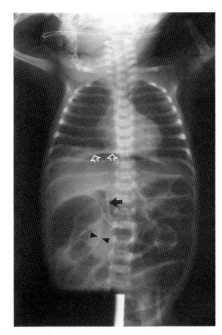

Fig. 48.9 Pneumoperitoneum.
  Air is visible below the diaphragm (open arrows), on either side of the bowel wall (black triangles) and outlining the falciform ligament (black arrow).

The diagnosis of NEC is usually made on the basis of a combination of clinical and radiological features.

Clinical features are:
- Bile-stained aspirate
- Abdominal distension
- Blood in the stool
- Sepsis.

Radiological features are:
- Intramural gas
- Thickened bowel loops/free fluid
- Portal gas
- Pneumoperitoneum.

The diagnosis of pneumoperitoneum with pneumothorax should be obvious from the chest X-ray.

The diagnosis of SIP is by exclusion of NEC, but the diagnosis is usually not confirmed until laparotomy. However, in the case of SIP there are usually no elevations of inflammatory markers such as CRP, white cells and immature-to-mature neutrophil ratio.

Q3. What are the management options?

When indicated, surgery involves a laparotomy with either resection and anastamosis or stoma formation. If there is a tense pneumoperitoneum compromising ventilation, insertion of a needle or peritoneal drain in the right iliac fossa prior to transfer may make transfer safer. Drain insertion should only be performed after discussion with a surgeon.

Spontaneous intestinal perforation

Perforation without NEC may occur and is most usually seen in very preterm babies in the first few days of life. Differentiation from perforated NEC may be difficult and the diagnosis is often not made until laparotomy. Occasional babies with isolated perforation can be managed by peritoneal drainage alone.

Pneumothorax and pneumoperitoneum

Air from a pneumothorax may track into the peritoneal cavity in the absence of intestinal perforation. Signs of abdominal sepsis will be absent.

Indications for surgery in NEC

- Intestinal perforation
- Failure of medical treatment:
  - Clinical deterioration: vital signs, abdominal mass, tenderness, erythema
  - Worsening laboratory results (platelets, electrolytes, acidosis, lactate)
- Stricture: usually presenting as obstruction some weeks after an episode of NEC and diagnosed by contrast radiology.

Bladder outflow obstruction

Problem-orientated topic:

bladder outflow obstruction

A male term infant is noted not to have passed urine at the age of 36 hours. On examination the abdomen is distended and a mass arising from the pelvis is palpable above the umbilicus.

Q1. What diagnoses should be considered?

Q2. What immediate investigations and intervention are required?

Q1. What diagnoses should be considered? (Box 48.6)

The failure to pass urine in the first day of life is not necessarily abnormal. Seven percent of healthy babies do not pass urine until the second day. However, the presence of an abdominal mass suggests an enlarged obstructed bladder, although other causes (e.g. abdominal teratoma) are possible.

Posterior urethral valves

Valves in the posterior urethra obstruct the flow of urine from the bladder. The degree of obstruction varies. Obstruction in fetal life may cause severe renal dysplasia, oligohydramnios and subsequent pulmonary hypoplasia (p. 698).

Clinical presentation in the neonate is very variable. At the worst end of the spectrum, babies may present with severe respiratory difficulty due to pulmonary hypoplasia and may die. Others with good lungs may present with failure to pass urine or have dribbling micturition, with abdominal distension due to an enlarged bladder and kidneys.

Q2. What immediate investigations and intervention are required?

- Prophylactic urinary antibiotics
- Urinary tract ultrasound
- Immediate referral to a paediatric urologist.

Key points

- Neonatal urea and electrolyte levels reflect maternal renal function in the first few hours of life and thus may be misleading.
- Bladder catheterization should not be performed without discussion with a paediatric urologist.
- Once the infant is catheterized, diuresis may be profound with rapid dehydration and hyponatraemia.

BOX 48.6 Causes of bladder outflow obstruction

Males
- Posterior urethral valves
- Prune belly syndrome (lax abdominal muscles, undescended testes, large bladder)
- Ureterocele

Females
- Ureterocele
- Cloacal anomaly (anorectal malformation, urogenital sinus)

Table 48.3 Some of the common surgical conditions diagnosed at the postnatal check

Condition	Refer to surgeon before discharge	Routine surgical outpatient appointment	Primary care services to refer if needed
Hypospadias		✓	
Undescended testis (uni- or bilateral)			✓
Impalpable testis (unilateral)			✓
Impalpable testes (bilateral)	✓		
Hydrocele			✓
Hernia: inguinal	✓		
Hernia: umbilical			✓
Accessory digit*		✓	
Pre-auricular skin tag*		✓	
Tongue tie with breastfeeding difficulty	Notify lactation nurse		
Request for religious circumcision			✓

* Refer to appropriate local surgeon. In some centres this may be plastic surgeon, ENT or paediatric surgeon.

Surgical management

Endoscopic obliteration of the valves is usually performed, followed by long-term nephro-urology care. Some patients eventually develop end-stage renal failure.

Surgical conditions detected at postnatal check

Table 48.3 lists some of the common surgical conditions diagnosed at the postnatal check and states what action is required, if any.

Hypospadias

This has three key features:
- *Abnormally sited urethral meatus*: anywhere from the underside of the glans to within the perineum
- *Chordee*: ventral curvature of the penis
- *Hooded foreskin*.

Surgery is not usually considered before 2 years of age. Routine outpatient surgical referral is required.

However, if the testes are not both descended, more urgent referral is indicated, as this may constitute an intersex anomaly.

Undescended testis

Assessment of testicular descent forms part of the routine newborn check. An undescended testis will be found in 5% of term babies and in most the testis is palpable in the inguinal area. Routine surgical referral is not necessary, as testicular examination forms part of the routine Community Child Surveillance 6-week examination; referral will be made if necessary at that time or subsequently after the 8-month check.

Tongue tie

This affects about 3% of babies. It is debated whether this condition requires any treatment in the newborn period. There is some evidence that it may prevent effective breastfeeding. Local protocols for management usually exist.

49

Injuries, poisoning and apparent life-threatening events

LEARNING OUTCOMES

By the end of this chapter you should:

- Understand the contribution that injuries make to childhood death and disability
- Know which children with head injuries should be referred to hospital and what the indications are for brain imaging
- Understand the management of the common causes of poisoning in children
- Know and understand the risk factors of SUDI and how to minimize risk
- Know and understand the mechanisms by which a child may present with apparent life-threatening episodes (ALTEs)
- Know the appropriate advice to give to parents whose baby has had an ALTE.

MODULE EIGHT

Injuries (see also Ch. 17)

Injury is a major cause of child death across the world, accounting for almost 40% of deaths in the age group 1–15 years (Table 49.1). Once children reach the age of 5 years, injuries are the biggest threat to their survival. Among those children who live in poverty, the burden of injury is highest. We need to create a Europe where children can learn, play and grow up without risks of death due to serious injury. In the developed world, road traffic accidents account for approximately 41% of all injury-related deaths. Taken together, traffic accidents, intentional injuries, drownings, falls, fires, poisonings and other injuries kill more than 200 000 children every year in developed countries. In developing countries, an estimated 1 million children under 15 die each year from injuries.

Deaths from injuries are just the tip of the iceberg. For every death there are 145 admissions to hospital and 1300 emergency department attendances due to injuries. Annually about 10% of children suffer an injury necessitating contact with the health services. Injuries make up 29% of emergency department visits for children aged 0–5 years.

In general, injury causation varies from country to country and even within countries from region to region, as injuries depend on living conditions and the surrounding environment, both indoors and outdoors. However, in all countries the vast majority of all children's injuries involve falls, with a smaller number relating to motor vehicle accidents, fires, drownings, foreign body ingestion and poisoning. A child's risk for specific causes of injury is linked to developmental age, with studies showing differences in rates by 3-monthly

Table 49.1 Causes of death in children and young people

Top three causes of death	0–1 year	1–4 years	4–15 years	15–24 years
1	Developmental and genetic problems present at birth	Injuries	Injuries	Injuries
2	Sudden unexplained death in infancy (SUDI; sudden infant death syndrome, SIDS)	Developmental and genetic problems present at birth	Cancer	Homicide
3	Prematurity/low birth weight	Cancer	Homicide	Suicide

intervals for children aged 0–3 years. Boys are 70% more likely to die by injury than girls.

Although it is true that child injury death rates have been falling for more than two decades, there is further room for improvement. Sweden has had intensive child protection programmes running for over 35 years and has the lowest child injury death rate of any country.

The burden of accidental injury is disproportionately heavy on the most disadvantaged. Children from the poorest families are more likely to die from injuries, to be admitted to hospital and to be admitted with more severe injuries. The likelihood of a child being injured or killed is associated with single parenthood, low maternal education, low maternal age at birth, poor housing, large family size, and parental drug or alcohol abuse.

Accident prevention programmes need to be multi-faceted and to include poverty reduction programmes. Accident prevention is discussed in detail in Chapter 17.

Head injury

Minor closed head injury is one of the most frequent reasons for visits to a hospital. Only 1 in 800 results in any serious complications. The National Institute of Clinical Excellence (NICE) has described algorithms for referral to hospital and investigation of head injuries. The most recent recommendations for referral to hospital for further assessment include any of the following:

- Glasgow Coma Scale (GCS) < 15 (p. 664) at any time since the injury
- Any loss of consciousness as a result of the injury
- Any focal neurological deficit since the injury
- Amnesia for events before or after the injury in children > 5 years
- Persistent headache since injury
- Any vomiting since injury
- Any seizure since injury
- Any previous neurosurgical interventions
- High-energy head injuries (e.g. being struck by a car, fall from a height)
- Suspicion of non-accidental injury (Ch. 36)
- Finding of irritability or altered behaviour since the injury

- Any suspicion of skull fracture or penetrating head injury:
  - Cerebrospinal fluid (CSF) from nose or ear
  - Black eye with no associated trauma around eyes
  - Bruising behind one or both ears
  - Visible trauma to scalp or skull.

If the child is sent home, a reliable caregiver should be in charge at home and be given an instruction sheet for observation and for when to return the child to hospital.

Investigations

Skull radiography has no role in the evaluation and management of head injury. If neuroimaging is considered necessary, then computed tomography (CT) or magnetic resonance (MR) brain imaging is required. NICE recommends that urgent CT brain imaging should be undertaken if any of the following features is present:

- GCS < 13 at any time since the injury
- GCS 13 or 14 at 2 hours after the injury
- Focal neurological deficit
- Suspected open or depressed skull fracture
- Any signs of basal skull fracture
- Post-traumatic seizure
- > 1 vomiting episode.

http://www.nice.org.uk

The GCS and the AVPU scales are described on page 664.

Head trauma may be due to child abuse or serious neglect by a parent or caregiver. In all cases a thorough history should be obtained of past injuries and of circumstances surrounding the present injury.

Road traffic accidents

While uncommon, motor vehicle accidents account for 40% of all fatal injuries in children. The child may be involved either as a passenger who is usually unrestrained or improperly restrained or as a pedestrian hit by oncoming traffic. Motor vehicle accidents are more common in underprivileged overcrowded areas with a lack of playground space. Adequate adult supervision is essential if children are outdoors, especially if there is access to passing traffic. Child safety in cars needs to be addressed. Legislation and enforcement of child passenger restraints in cars lead to an increase in observed use. Age-appropriate child passenger restraints lead to a decrease in death and injury. Keeping children facing rearward longer has been shown to increase protection by 3–5 times. Booster seats are very important in older children (6–11 years old). All cars should be fitted with correct backseat child restraints, carefully selected according to the child's weight, height and length. Seat belts are designed for people 1.52 m tall and over. Recommendations state that seat belts alone are inadequate until approximately 11 years of age.

Drowning

Drowning is ranked third overall as a cause of accidental death among children up to the age of 5. Incidence is closely related to climate, time of year and geographical zone. Toddlers account for the majority, with a second smaller peak incidence in adolescence. At all ages males are more at risk. Personal flotation devices for boating or other water recreational devices are a recommended preventive strategy as is legislation requiring isolation fencing with secure self-latching gates for all outdoor pools. Infantile drowning mainly occurs in the bath. Outdoor pools are the major sites of accidental drowning in toddlers. Children with epilepsy are up to four times as likely to suffer a drowning incident.

Immediate and effective cardiopulmonary resuscitation (CPR) is the largest determinant of outcome. Each minute that passes prior to implementation of CPR dramatically reduces survival and long-term outcome. Of near-drowning victims with cardiac arrest who received prehospital CPR, only 7–21% will be neurologically intact. Management is supportive, with attention to lung aspiration and hypothermia. Supervision of children around water is essential. Installation of pool fencing has been shown to be effective in preventing more than 50% of swimming pool drownings among young children.

Swallowed foreign body

Preschool children commonly swallow coins, toys and stones. The majority pass without complications. However, oesophageal hold-up requires urgent endoscopy. Sharp and long objects are the most likely to cause perforation. Abdominal pain and tenderness and failure of an object to progress radiologically in 24 hours are each independent indications for evaluation/endoscopy/surgical evaluation.

Poisoning

More than 50% of all poisonings occur in children 5 years or younger. Almost all are unintentional/accidental, with intentional poisoning becoming more common in the female adolescent. More than 85% of toxic exposures in children occur in the child's home, usually during the day and more commonly during school or public holidays. Most involve only a single substance. About 60% involve non-medicinal drug products, most commonly cosmetics, cleaning substances and hydrocarbons. Pharmaceutical products comprise the remainder, with analgesics, cough products, antibiotics and vitamins being the most common. More than 75% of paediatric poisoning exposures can be treated without direct medical intervention because either the product involved is not inherently toxic or the quantity involved is not sufficient to produce significant toxic effects. Death from acute poisoning in children less than 10 years has declined dramatically in the last decade. The two most important factors have been child-resistant containers and use of safer medicines. Secure storage of poisons is an effective means of preventing poisoning injury.

Management

Detailed history, if possible documenting magnitude of exposure, timing of exposure, progression of symptoms and medical history, is vital to determine risk. Consultation with a poison control centre may assist in identifying active components within a product and likely side-effects. If further management is required, it is generally divided into two parts:

- *General management.* Supportive care is given, with management of airway, breathing and circulation and avoidance of hypoglycaemia.
- *Specific management.* The American Academy of Toxicology and the European Association of Poisons Centres and Clinical Toxicologists have released statements that the routine administration of ipecac syrup or other cathartics is not endorsed. Neither do they support gastric lavage or whole-body lavage, except in extreme circumstances.

Administration of activated charcoal should be considered as soon as possible after emergency department presentation, unless the agent and quantity are known to be non-toxic, the agent is known not to adsorb to activated charcoal, or the delay has been so long that absorption is probably complete.

Antidotes are available for only a limited number of poisons. Enhancing excretion is useful for only a few toxins. Few drugs or toxins are removed by dialysis in sufficient amounts to justify the difficulties and risks of dialysis in children. Blood levels are important in the management of poisoning with paracetamol, salicylates and iron. For other intoxicants quantifying levels may help in confirming the diagnosis but will not alter treatment.

Paracetamol

Paracetamol is the most widely used childhood analgesic and antipyretic. Unintentional paracetamol overdose in children rarely causes illness or death. This may be due in part to the immature cytochrome P450 (CYP) enzyme system in children. Fasting is a risk factor, possibly because of depletion of hepatic glutathione reserves. Concomitant use of other drugs that induce CYP enzymes, such as antiepileptics (including carbamazepine, phenytoin, barbiturates etc.), has also been reported as a risk factor. The acute toxic dose in children is considered to be 200 mg/kg.

Anorexia, nausea, vomiting and diaphoresis are common in the first 24 hours. If a toxic dose was absorbed, overt hepatic failure develops over 24–48 hours, peaking at around 72–96 hours. In massive overdoses, coma and metabolic acidosis may occur prior to hepatic failure.

Damage generally occurs in hepatocytes, as they metabolize the paracetamol. However, acute renal failure may also occur. This is usually caused by either hepatorenal syndrome or multisystem organ failure. Acute renal failure may also be the primary clinical manifestation of toxicity. In these cases, it is possible that the toxic metabolite is produced more in the kidneys than in the liver. A blood level 4 hours post ingestion is taken and plotted on a nomogram to determine whether antidotal treatment is indicated. Liver function tests and prothrombin time should be followed daily in those with potentially toxic levels. After large acute overdose activated charcoal should be considered. In cases of definite toxicity N-acetylcysteine should be started as soon as possible and has benefit up to 24–36 hours after ingestion.

Tricyclic antidepressants (TCAs)

TCAs are an extremely toxic source of poisoning in young children. The lowest toxic dose in the literature is 6.7 mg/kg. Overdoses of TCAs can cause coma, seizures, hypotension, cardiac arrhythmias and cardiac arrest. Central nervous system (CNS) symptoms occur in children more frequently than do cardiovascular effects. Treatment is directed at rapid assessment, monitoring and support of vital functions, halting drug absorption, and treating CNS and cardiac toxic effects. All children should be monitored for a minimum of 6 hours and many require admission to a critical care unit. The mainstay of therapy is alkalinization. Intravenous administration of sodium bicarbonate is the preferred treatment for hypotension, shock and arrhythmias. Hypotension is a poor prognostic sign. Blood pH should be monitored and should be maintained between 7.45 and 7.55. More specific drug therapy, cardioversion or artificial pacing may be required for refractory arrhythmias. Before the child is discharged from the hospital, strategies to reduce the risk of future poisonings should be discussed with the child's family.

Smoke inhalation

Referral for assessent after smoke inhalation is common after home fires. Physical examination, looking for signs such as singed hair, facial burns and carbonaceous sputum, aids in determination of extent of exposure. If there is hoarseness, stridor, increasing respiratory distress or difficulty handling secretions, the airway should be directly visualized by bronchoscopy or laryngoscopy. Signs of impeding airway obstruction due to mucosal oedema are an indication for elective intubation. Signs of carbon monoxide poisoning include headache, confusion, irritability and visual changes. Management includes blood carboxyhaemoglobin level (HbCO), haemoglobin level, arterial pH and urinalysis for myoglobin. Treatment includes close observation and oxygen until the HbCO level falls below 5%. Hyperbaric oxygen should be considered if there is a history of coma or seizures, or persistent metabolic acidosis in the case of a pregnant woman or neonate or for an HbCO level greater than 25%.

http://www.eapcct.org/show.php?page=links

European Association of Poisons Centres

Sudden unexplained death in infancy (SUDI; sudden infant death syndrome, SIDS)

It is proposed to discuss ALTEs after an introduction on SUDI, despite there being no proven link between the two conditions, primarily because both are unexpected unpredictable events predominantly affecting well/healthy infants in the first 6 months of life. Both remain largely unexplained and ALTEs cause considerable parental anxiety and distress because of the frightening nature of the episode and the worry of a future SUDI occurring.

SUDI is the term used for the sudden unexpected death of a well infant occurring during the first year of life (80% during the overnight sleep), which remains unexplained after a thorough case investigation, including a complete autopsy, examination of the death scene and review of the clinical history. In developed countries SUDI is the most common cause of death after the neonatal period in children less than 1 year, with the peak incidence between 2 and 4 months of age. SUDI is an unexplained death after investigation and is a diagnosis of exclusion. It is possible that, in about 50% of cases, incomplete case/postmortem investigations have been performed and a cause of the child's death has been missed.

Epidemiological studies have identified the prone sleeping position and maternal smoking during pregnancy as increasing the risk of SUDI, and 'reduce the risk of SUDI' campaigns in most developed countries have led to a dramatic decrease in the use of the prone sleeping position and an associated reduction in SUDI incidence over the last two decades from 2 to 0.6 per 1000 live births in Ireland. This fall in SUDI rates has resulted in the number of SUDI deaths falling from about 150 to 45 per year in Ireland, with no diagnostic transfer, and the overall infant mortality rate falling by the same amount. Maternal smoking rates have declined only slightly over the past few years, leaving smoking in pregnancy as the major current SUDI risk factor in Western countries, with a clear dose–response effect evident (this includes the number of cigarettes smoked by the mother and the number of smokers in the infant's environment).

Since the recent dramatic reduction in SUDI rates other epidemiological factors increasing the risk of SUDI have been sought. Risk factors include:

- Social deprivation.
- Infant–parent cosleeping. Sharing an adult bed for the entire night is a well-recognized risk factor and sharing a sofa is especially dangerous.
- Maternal smoking (risk of cosleeping being especially pronounced in infants of smoking mothers).
- Infant soother use has recently been shown to have some protective effect if used every night.

Despite much research the underlying aetiology of SUDI remains unknown. It is known that SUDI infants are lighter, with a smaller head (brain) size, than gestational age-matched controls at birth. SUDI infants also have demonstrable histological differences, probably an in utero growth restriction effect, in many different organs from lungs, diaphragm and kidneys to decreased brain myelination and increased brainstem gliosis, especially in areas crucial to autonomic/homeostatic control. Consequently it seems likely that SUDI infants are vulnerable in situations where the brain's controlling/protective systems (autonomic system) are heavily down-regulated (as in quiet/deep sleep, which is more prevalent in the prone sleeping position or after sleep disturbance/deprivation), often with an added stress from mild intercurrent illness or environmental stress such as overheating.

In the rare cases of recurrence of SUDI in a family (6/1000 families with a previous SUDI), other genetic disorders (e.g. central hypoventilation syndrome, metabolic disorders), as well as infanticide, should be excluded.

Apparent life-threatening episodes (ALTEs) (see also p. 673)

In 1986 a National Institutes of Health (USA) consensus conference on infantile apnoea and home monitoring defined an ALTE as:

an episode that is frightening to the observer and that is characterized by some combination of apnoea (central or occasionally obstructive), colour change (usually cyanotic or pallid but occasionally erythematous or plethoric), marked change in muscle tone (usually marked limpness), choking or gagging.

Essentially, such a broad definition can include any unexpected frightening episode in an infant. Most typically, ALTE episodes occur in the first few months of life and are mostly reported during the day, as caregivers are present and the events are witnessed. Infants are usually well or only slightly unwell before and after the event.

Some babies are described as being groggy, floppy or quiet and not themselves for a few hours after the episode. The level of resuscitation required dictates the level of worry regarding the possibility of SUDI occurring in a future episode, and although the literature in this regard is conflicting and confusing, there seems to be only a slight, if any, increased risk of future SUDI in these infants. The source of this confusion is clearly shown in the data from the Irish National SUDI Register on the relationship between a prior ALTE/apnoea/lifeless episode and SUDI. The data show that apnoea/lifeless episodes were significantly more frequent among SUDI cases than among controls (12/334 (3.6%) SUDI cases vs 6/1419 (0.4%) controls OR 2.81; CI: 1.65–4.76) on univariate analysis. However, on multivariate analysis the odds ratio of 2.56 for subsequent SUDI was not significant when adjusted for maternal age, education, smoking, alcohol consumption, urinary infection during pregnancy, social deprivation, tog value of bedding, problems in the last 48 hours, absence of usual soother use, cosleeping and being placed prone in the last sleep. The validity of continuing to add in the number of variables included in a multivariate analysis until the variable ALTE becomes not significant is highly debatable. Consequently, different authors have published that there is either a slightly increased (doubling) or no increased risk of SUDI in infants who have suffered a previous ALTE, depending on what has been included in the multivariate model.

An ALTE is a common reason for admission of infants to hospital and poses a problem for paediatricians as to what constitutes an adequate diagnostic workup and also as to how these infants and their worried parents should be managed. A careful history of the event, including a detailed description of the precipitating circumstances, the infant's appearance, the amount of resuscitation employed by the caregiver and its duration, will usually provide the pointers as to what may be appropriate investigations. Awake-onset episodes, whether associated with an obvious precipitating event such as crying, vomiting or gagging, fit most neatly into the spectrum of cyanotic/pallid breath-holding or reflex anoxic seizure type of events (Ch. 24), usually attributed to immature autonomic/brainstem control. These are mostly benign, sometimes with a positive family history, and are difficult to treat effectively. The presence of anoxic seizures should be obvious from the sequence of events in the history, as reflex-induced seizures in infants are extremely rare.

Sleep-related episodes logically fit most neatly within the realm of SUDI, with down-regulated protective reflexes (arousal responses to hypoxia or nasal occlusion are much slower during sleep and worse again during deep sleep) allowing otherwise normal infants to drift into slightly dangerous situations. The frequency of poor physiological responses to noxious situations in infants can be gauged from a study of healthy 6-week old infants, conducted many years ago, where 40% were unable to establish an oral airway within 25 seconds of the onset of nasal occlusion during sleep. Given the poor/immature background physiology, it is not surprising that some infants allow themselves to drift into slightly dangerous/frightening situations and present as an ALTE.

Causes

In children with ALTEs the factors described below are often considered as a possible cause.

Gastro-oesophageal reflux (GOR)
(see also p. 534)
A recent systematic review of the causes of ALTEs in the published literature revealed a remarkable heterogeneity in the quality of the published literature and diagnostic labels attached to ALTE cases (McGovern & Smith 2004). The fact that, of an initial 2912 papers, only 8 studies involving 643 infants could be included in the systematic review speaks volumes as to the poor quality of this literature. Even among the 8 papers used in the review, the definition of ALTE varied between the studies, as did study methodology, making it difficult to draw firm conclusions. Notwithstanding these limitations, this literature review found the most common 'diagnoses' reported as 'causing' ALTEs were GOR in 227, followed by a seizure ($n = 83$), lower respiratory tract infection ($n = 58$) and unknown ($n = 169$). However, it is particularly important in this

situation to distinguish between the chance temporal association of two events (an ALTE and another extremely common event in infants, such as GOR) and a causal relationship.

Most infants exhibit intermittent GOR in the first few months of life, due to immaturity of the gastro-oesophageal sphincter (p. 534). Recent studies have found no evidence for acid reflux either causing or exacerbating episodes of apnoea or oxygen desaturations or ALTE or SUDI, but there is an increased incidence of respiratory problems. In addition, treating GOR has not been shown to prevent recurrences of ALTEs or apnoea. Also given that most infants occasionally reflux acid stomach contents, an infant who has a massive over-reaction to a common event implies poor central control.

Consequently there is little support in the literature for GOR as the cause of either ALTEs or SUDI, making it difficult to justify the use of diagnostic tests (none of which is either sensitive or specific) aimed at establishing the presence of GOR. Also, the use of the varied treatments employed in treating this non-condition, which is mostly a variation of normal immature physiological development, is difficult to justify. However, clinically we do occasionally see infants with severe and/or recurrent ALTEs with the most severe GOR, both probably indicating poor central controlling mechanisms, where using a thickened feed may be justified.

Seizures
Seizures are the second most frequently diagnosed 'cause' of ALTEs in the published literature, yet it is rare that an ALTE is proven to be caused by a massive synchronous cerebral electrical discharge, i.e. epilepsy. The vast majority of ALTEs attributed to a seizure are either cyanotic breath-holding or pallid syncopal episodes. Breath-holding attacks are familiar to most doctors as non-epileptic episodes occurring in some infants and young children as a consequence of either a physical or a psychological hurt (Ch. 24). Diagnosis is usually not difficult when a detailed history of the sequence of events, with a clear triggering event, is available. The sequence of events involves either crying or breath-holding that raises intrathoracic pressure (a Valsalva manoeuvre) sufficiently to disrupt venous return and consequent cardiac output, resulting in cerebral ischaemia, loss of consciousness and sometimes a brief hypoxic seizure. Epilepsy in the first 6 months of life is rare and occurs in the presence of major underlying brain problems, as seen in severe birth asphyxia or infantile spasms with hypsarrhythmia. The stark normality of ALTE infants, once recovered from the event, excludes such a possibility.

Pallid syncopal episodes, by contrast, are due to periods of asystole induced by a mildly unpleasant experience such as being placed in a bath. Such infants have been shown to develop periods of asystole of up to 32 seconds (normal is < 2 seconds) following vagal stimulation by eyeball compression. Pallid syncopal attacks tend to feature extreme pallor, total limpness, the appearance of death and perhaps a cold sweat with a rapid return to normality, presumably once the heart restarts and a circulation is restored. Again, a brief tonic–clonic seizure, secondary to cerebral ischaemia and not underlying epilepsy, is not unusual. Diagnosis of these conditions is largely by history, management is by parental reassurance as to the benign nature of the episodes, and treatment (with atropine) highly specialized and not to be undertaken by the enthusiastic amateur.

Respiratory infections

Respiratory tract infections are the third most common 'cause' of ALTEs in the published literature. The literature clearly supports the concept of infants having 'funny' episodes while incubating an infectious disease such as whooping cough or bronchiolitis, often before other overt signs of infection. Consequently the presence of an evolving infection must always be considered. Infants who are incubating an infection have been demonstrated to be physiologically different, not showing the normal sleep-induced fall in core body temperature, for example, for several days before overtly becoming infected.

However, a major problem with this literature is the tendency to diagnose a respiratory infection based on the presence of snuffles, mucousy noisy breathing or a wheeze, all of which are extremely common in the healthy infant population and are usually not due to an infection. Unfortunately there are no case control studies showing infections (respiratory or otherwise) to be more common in ALTE infants than in carefully matched controls; consequently we have to rely on an anecdotal literature of case reports.

Other causes

Rarer causes of ALTEs, mostly single case reports, include metabolic or developmental problems, cardiac conduction defects or upper airway obstruction during sleep. Again a careful history of the event, a detailed family history and a history of the infant's preceding health and development will usually give clues to an underlying problem requiring investigation. In recurring ALTEs (10% of the total) inflicted or fabricated episodes pose a diagnostic and management dilemma, often with parents demanding ever more extensive investigations for an infant in rude good health (Chs 21 and 36).

Management

Management of ALTEs is made difficult by the poor-quality conflicting literature and often by the huge parental anxiety engendered by the witnessing of the apparent near-death of their infant. Understandably, if a healthy infant nearly dies, with no apparent cause, then parents feel their babies are at a greater risk of SUDI than if this episode had not happened. However, the literature would say that the subsequent risk of SUDI is at most 2–3 times higher than the baseline SUDI risk. It is important to translate this into an actual risk for parents; in non-smoking Caucasian non-socially deprived families the baseline SUDI risk is about 1/8000, so doubling or trebling this is still a very low risk situation. Obviously for smoking parents the baseline SUDI risk ranges from 1/980 (smoker) to 1/400 (most socially disadvantaged and a smoker).

Parents should be reassured that these events are mostly the result of poor/immature physiology, with infants maturing out of the danger of recurrence in a matter of months. As a rough guide, 50% of ALTE infants will have a second episode, with 10% having recurring episodes. Also the fact that very few SUDI cases have a prior warning event (3.6%) and that the actual risk of SUDI is still very low should help parents cope. Emphasizing the known risk reduction measures for SUDI also helps, as does the fact that the baby has essentially survived the first episode and is inherently likely to survive a second, should one occur. Unfortunately the literature on physiological testing/sleep studies in ALTE infants generally supports the concept of immature underlying (especially sleep) physiology, without suggesting any way of influencing this or predicting recurrent episodes.

Paediatricians generally take a pragmatic approach to the use of cardiorespiratory monitors at home in ALTE infants, despite there being evidence that their use does not prevent the rare subsequent occurrence of SUDI. Monitors used in the home tend to give frequent false alarms and generate considerable parental anxiety and stress. However, if parents are already very distressed by the ALTE — for example, if they are taking turns to stay awake at night to watch the baby — then the use of a monitor can help them to cope better. Easy access to the unit issuing the monitor is essential if there are any issues or worries, and this is a service parents value and rarely overuse. All parents should be taught basic resuscitation, whilst being reminded that whatever they did the first time worked and would probably do so again. Medication use for documented apnoea, including caffeine or aminophylline, has no evidence base and generally medicalizes and complicates the management without any proven benefit; it is best avoided. 'Sleep studies' are often used for research investigation and generally add little to the diagnosis or management of the infant.

Reference

McGovern MC, Smith MBH 2004 Causes of apparent life-threatening events in infants: a systematic review. Archives of Disease in Childhood 89:1043–1048

Further reading

Carpenter RG, Irgens LM, Blair PS et al. 2004 Sudden unexplained infant death in twenty regions in Europe: case control study. Lancet 363:185–191

Committee on Injury, American Academic of Pediatrics 2005 Poison treatment in the home. Pediatrics 112:1182–1185

Matthews T 1992 The autonomic nervous system — a role in sudden infant death syndrome. Archives of Disease in Childhood 67:654–656

National Institutes of Health 1987 Consensus development conference on infantile apnoea and home monitoring. Pediatrics 79:292–299

Matthew Murray   James C. Nicholson   Giorgio Perilongo

Oncology and palliative care

LEARNING OUTCOMES

By the end of this chapter you should:

● Have an understanding of the aetiology and epidemiology of childhood cancer
● Have the knowledge to assess a patient presenting with a malignancy
● Be able to select appropriate investigations for such a patient
● Be able to recognize and institute initial management of common complications of cancer patients
● Understand the principles of different modalities used to treat cancer
● Be aware of the short- and long-term side-effects of chemotherapy and radiotherapy
● Be aware of the indications for stem cell or bone marrow transplantation
● Appreciate the issues involved in the care of a child with a life-limiting illness, including symptom control
● Understand the concept of the paediatric oncology multidisciplinary team.

You should also take this opportunity to ensure that:

● Your history from, and examination of, the patient enable you to make an accurate assessment/differential diagnosis
● You can interpret the results of a full blood count and peripheral film
● You can interpret electrolyte disturbances secondary to tumour lysis syndrome.

Aetiology and epidemiology of childhood cancer

Childhood cancer is rare and accounts for only 0.5% of all cancers. The overall risk of developing cancer in childhood is 1 in 600.

Malignancy is the most common cause of death in children in the 5–14-year age group and is second only to trauma and accidents between 15 and 19 years (Table 50.1).

Very little is known about the aetiology of most childhood cancers. Inherited predisposition accounts

Table 50.1 Most common causes of death by age (England and Wales 2002)

Age (years)	Cause of death
< 1	Congenital abnormalities Sudden unexplained death in infancy (SUDI; sudden infant death syndrome, SIDS) Infection
1–4	Congenital Trauma/accidents Cancer
5–14	Cancer Trauma/accidents Congenital
15–19	Trauma/accidents Cancer Congenital

for less than 5% of cases and environmental factors play a minor role compared with adults. Examples of inherited syndromes with a predisposition for cancer include familial Wilms tumour, Beckwith–Wiedemann (10% develop tumours, of which Wilms is most common) and neurofibromatosis-1 (NF-1, 40-fold greater risk of brain and spinal cord tumours than the general population).

Inherited predisposition to childhood cancer

Retinoblastoma is the most common example and provides a suitable model for understanding the principles of inherited predisposition, having been linked to a single gene locus. Familial retinoblastoma accounts for approximately 40% of cases and presentation is usually early (first year of life) and bilateral. Sporadic cases present later, are unilateral and are not associated with a positive family history. Survivors of familial retinoblastoma have a very high risk of developing second primary tumours, of which osteosarcoma is the most common.

These features of retinoblastoma were noted by Knudson and led him to propose the 'two-hit' mutational hypothesis in 1971. This states that two mutations are necessary in a cell for a tumour to develop. In hereditary cases the first mutation is germline, while the second is somatic. In sporadic cases two somatic mutations are required in the same cell for a tumour to develop.

Knudson's hypothesis was confirmed in the 1980s with the identification of the retinoblastoma tumour suppressor gene (*RB1*) on chromosome 13. Retinoblastoma results as a consequence of two mutations in the *RB1* gene within the somatic cells of the retina.

In comparison to retinoblastoma, familial clusters of other embryonal tumours are rare. For example, in Wilms tumour, inherited cases are thought to represent

only 1% of all cases. Beckwith–Wiedemann is the most common syndrome associated with Wilms tumour. Organomegaly, macroglossia, hemihypertophy, neonatal hypoglycaemia and exomphalos are characteristic features of this congenital fetal overgrowth syndrome. Around 10% of cases develop tumours, of which Wilms is the most common, and imprinting has been implicated as a causative mechanism. Patients with some forms of syndromes involving aniridia, genital abnormalities, nephritis and pseudohermaphroditism have up to a 50% risk of developing Wilms tumour due to gene alterations.

NF-1 is inherited as an autosomal dominant condition, although many cases are new mutations, and accounts for about 0.5% of all childhood cancers. As described earlier, NF-1 is associated with an increased risk of brain and spinal cord tumours. Optic nerve gliomas are the most common brain tumours seen, with a 1000-fold increased risk.

Molecular mechanisms for the development of malignancies

Molecular mechanisms for the development of malignances all relate to the alteration in structure or activity of genes that perform important regulatory functions of growth or differentiation of cells in the normal state. These may include:

- Mutation or deletion of a tumour suppressor gene. These genes code for proteins that have negative regulatory roles in the cell cycle. Complete loss of protein function is required to initiate the tumorigenic process and hence requires loss of both genomic copies.
- Activation of a 'proto-oncogene', which then becomes an oncogene, i.e. a tumour-promoting gene. This may occur through mutation or amplification.
- Translocation of a gene to a different locus may result in over-expression, as a result of juxtaposition with a 'promoter' region, or fusion with another gene that creates an oncogenic 'fusion product'.

Subsequent tumorigenesis is a multistep process involving the development of immortalization of cells, growth factor autonomy, inhibition of cell death pathways/apoptosis (programmed cell death), angiogenesis and the ability to invade local tissues/metastasize.

Tumour-specific acquired chromosomal abnormalities are seen in a wide range of solid and haematological malignancies. Whilst some of these appear to be random, others conform to recognized patterns with diagnostic or prognostic significance. The translocation t(9;22), resulting in the Philadelphia chromosome, was the first consistent cytogenetic abnormality to be described, occurring in chronic myeloid leukaemia (CML) and in some high-risk cases of acute lymphoblastic leukaemia (ALL).

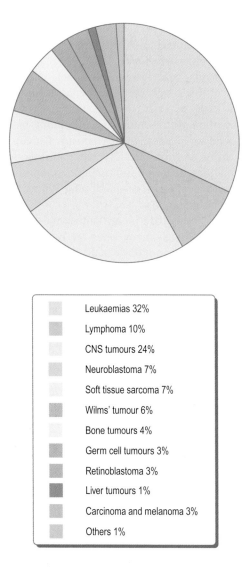

Leukaemias 32%

Lymphoma 10%

CNS tumours 24%

Neuroblastoma 7%

Soft tissue sarcoma 7%

Wilms' tumour 6%

Bone tumours 4%

Germ cell tumours 3%

Retinoblastoma 3%

Liver tumours 1%

Carcinoma and melanoma 3%

Others 1%

Fig. 50.1 Percentage of cases by diagnostic group, ages 0–14 years, Great Britain 1989–98
(Cancer Research UK 2004)

Types of malignancy

The most common childhood malignancy is leukaemia, accounting for one-third of cases, followed by brain and spinal tumours, which constitute one-quarter of cases (Fig. 50.1). All the other solid tumours account for 45% of cases, of which lymphoma, neuroblastoma, rhabdomyosarcoma and Wilms tumour are the most common extracranial solid tumours.

Principles of cancer therapy

Entry into trials and centralized treatment has been shown to be of direct benefit to patients. In most of the Western European countries children are now treated according to standardized protocols, many of which are co-ordinated by the International Society of Paediatric Oncology (SIOP).

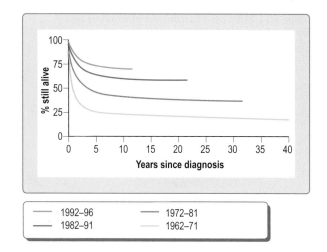

1992–96   1972–81
1982–91   1962–71

Fig. 50.2 Survival of childhood cancer patients diagnosed in the UK from 1962 to 1996
(Cancer Research UK 2004)

http://www.siop.nl
International Society of Paediatric Oncology

http://www.eurocare.it
European Cancer Register

Therapeutic strategies for childhood malignancies include chemotherapy, radiotherapy and surgery, alone or in combination. Chemotherapy forms the core of treatment for the majority and care is therefore usually coordinated by paediatric oncologists, working in designated centres. Geographical considerations dictate the provision of some treatment, including much of the supportive care, in local hospitals.

A multidisciplinary team approach is central to management and should include paediatric oncologists, haematologists, surgeons, neurosurgeons, radiation oncologists, specialist nurses for inpatient and outpatient care, outreach nurses, dieticians, play therapists, social workers, teachers and psychologists.

Prognosis

Overall cure rates for childhood cancer now exceed 70% in the developed world (Fig. 50.2). There is a wide variation between different tumour types. For example, localized Hodgkin disease is cured in well over 90% of cases, compared with around 20% in disseminated neuroblastoma. The current challenge facing oncologists is to develop and employ treatment strategies that minimize long-term side-effects of treatment without compromising cure.

Chemotherapy

Chemotherapy is the mainstay of treatment for most types of paediatric malignancy. Many cancers present

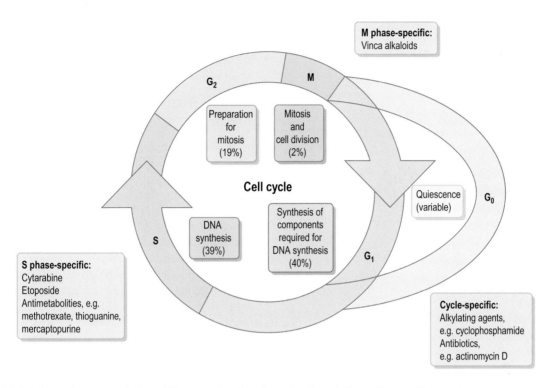

Fig. 50.3 Schematic representation of the normal cell cycle and action of chemotherapeutic agents

as localized tumour masses, but previous experience has shown that local treatment with surgery and/or radiotherapy alone is insufficient for cure and may result in later recurrences at distant sites. For this reason, most patients receive systemic treatment with chemotherapy as well as local therapy. This has resulted in a dramatic improvement in overall cure rates in the last 20–30 years.

Chemotherapy may be given as adjuvant treatment (following surgery), neoadjuvant treatment (before surgery) or both. Combination therapy is usually employed to increase efficacy, reduce development of resistance and limit single-organ toxicity. In order to act as effective chemotherapeutic agents, drugs must either block cell replication or induce cell death.

The cell cycle itself is divided into four active phases — G_1, S, G_2 and M — and a resting phase, G_0 (Fig. 50.3). After cell division, cells enter G_1 or 'gap' phase and then synthesize DNA (S phase) before a second gap phase, G_2. Cells subsequently enter M phase, where mitosis occurs, resulting in cell division.

In aggressive tumours, many cells are actively undergoing mitosis, giving rise to a high 'mitotic index' when sections of these tumours are examined under the microscope. These tumours are more likely to respond to chemotherapy than slow-growing, indolent tumours with a low mitotic index in which a large proportion of cells are in the G_0 resting phase.

Almost all current agents employed interfere with cell division further by:

- Damaging DNA
- Blocking DNA synthesis
- Interfering with DNA processing
- Disrupting mitosis.

The selectivity of cytotoxic drugs is dependent upon the fact that in malignancy a higher proportion of cells are undergoing division than in normal tissues. However, the difference between an effective treatment dose and a toxic one (the therapeutic index) is often quite small. Agents may be phase-specific (work at a particular phase of the cell cycle) or work through all phases (cycle-specific) (Fig. 50.3).

Most common short-term side-effects include vomiting, myelosuppression, alopecia and mucositis. Long-term effects on organ function (kidneys, gonads, hearing and heart) are variable (Box 50.1). Side-effects differ depending on the agents employed; examples of these are given below.

Administration of chemotherapy

Chemotherapy should only be given by fully trained individuals, aware of potential risks and complications, and working in centres fully equipped and accredited to support chemotherapy administration. Dosage is usually calculated according to surface area or by body weight in children less than 10 kg. Most chemotherapy

BOX 50.1 Side-effects of chemotherapy

Short-term
- Nausea and vomiting
- Alopecia
- Myelosuppression
- Mucositis, diarrhoea
- Hepatitis
- Haemorrhagic cystitis
- Nephrotoxicity/renal tubular leak
- Encephalopathy
- Radiation recall

Long-term
- Cardiotoxicity
- Pulmonary fibrosis
- Nephrotoxicity/renal tubular leak
- Infertility
- Hearing loss
- Secondary malignancy

is administered intravenously; central venous access is preferred. The risk of extravasation from peripheral veins is greatest with vinca alkaloids and anthracyclines. A number of agents are given orally as liquids or tablets, such as steroids, methotrexate and mercaptopurine in the 'maintenance' phase of leukaemia treatment. Certain drugs (e.g. ifosfamide, cisplatin and methotrexate) are given with concomitant intravenous fluids to minimize potential toxicity. Mesna is given with cyclophosphamide and ifosfamide to protect the bladder from haemorrhagic cystitis, and folinic acid 'rescue' is given with high-dose methotrexate; folinic acid is selectively taken up by normal cells and helps to minimize mucositis and other side-effects. The benefit of cardioprotective agents (given with anthracyclines) remains unproven.

Intrathecal chemotherapy

Intrathecal methotrexate (i.t. MTX) is used for treatment or prophylaxis of central nervous system (CNS) disease in leukaemia and non-Hodgkin lymphoma (NHL). Safety of arrangements for administration of intrathecal chemotherapy is paramount because of the catastrophic consequence of intrathecal administration of agents not suitable for this modality of administration (such as vincristine).

Monitoring for toxicity depends on the agents used and may include the following during or between courses:
- Full blood count (FBC)
- Electrolytes and liver function
- Glomerular filtration rate (GFR) measurement
- Hearing tests
- Echocardiogram.

High-dose (HD) therapy and stem cell transplant

This involves 'conditioning', which is the delivery of myelo-ablative doses of chemotherapy and/or total body irradiation to the patient. This is followed by rescue with haemopoietic stem cells, which may be autologous, derived from the patient him- or herself, or allogeneic, for which the donor may be a sibling, matched unrelated donor or occasionally haplo-identical from a parent.

Conventional bone marrow transplant (BMT), in which stem cells are harvested directly from the bone marrow, is usually used for allografts. Peripheral blood stem cell transplants (PBSCT) are favoured for autografts. Stem cells are harvested by leucopheresis from peripheral blood using granulocyte colony stimulating factor (G-CSF) to mobilize them from the bone marrow after priming with chemotherapy. After high-dose chemotherapy, these pluripotential stem cells from BMT or PBSCT are reinfused intravenously and subsequently repopulate the marrow. Advantages of PBSCT include less risk of tumour contamination from marrow affected by disease, more rapid engraftment (usually 2–4 weeks), less severe infections and avoidance of anaesthetic for harvesting.

Indications for use in childhood malignancy include selected high-risk and relapsed leukaemias (allograft), high-risk solid tumours, including metastatic neuroblastoma, high-risk Ewing sarcoma and relapsed tumours (autologous). The patient should be in remission prior to the procedure for it to be effective.

Causes of morbidity and mortality from stem cell transplant include graft failure, infection secondary to profound immune suppression, mucositis and veno-occlusive disease of the liver. Allografts carry greater risk, with approximately 10% procedure-related mortality. Graft versus host disease (GvHD) is a particular risk; it may affect any organ system but commonly skin and gastrointestinal system are involved. Ciclosporin A is given as prophylaxis and steroids may also be employed in treatment.

Radiotherapy

Radiotherapy is the clinical use of ionizing radiation to kill cancer cells. Dose and fractionation (number of treatments to deliver a total dose) vary according to the nature of the tumour and tolerance of the surrounding tissues. The target volume is determined by size and type of tumour and includes a safety margin. The aim is to deliver effective treatment to the target volume whilst sparing surrounding tissues.

Indications

Radiotherapy is indicated in selected cases of Hodgkin disease, neuroblastoma, Wilms tumour, soft tissue and Ewing sarcomas and most subgroups of CNS tumours.

Studies have shown only limited benefit in osteosarcoma, extracranial germ cell tumours and NHL. In leukaemia, radiotherapy is limited to treatment of the CNS, to testicular disease and to conditioning for BMT (total body irradiation, TBI). Radiotherapy is also used for symptom control in palliative care, e.g. bony metastases, spinal cord compression.

Preparation for radiotherapy includes:
- Planning, by combination of computed tomography (CT) and magnetic resonance imaging (MRI)
- Immobilization using masks/shells, tattoos as markers, sedation or general anaesthesia for youngest children
- Protection of surrounding tissues (e.g. gonads) using lead shields
- Involvement of play therapists, who have a central role in this process.

Side-effects

Toxicity of radiotherapy is potentiated by certain chemotherapy agents, e.g. actinomycin D or anthracyclines. This may give rise to the phenomenon of 'radiation recall' when these drugs are used after radiotherapy, causing further damage to the organ/tissues. Side-effects can be classified as acute or late and depend on the dose and site to which radiotherapy is given, as well as the age of the patient at the time of radiotherapy (Box 50.2). Late effects of chemotherapy may occur months or even years after treatment, and are usually progressive and irreversible.

Surgery

Surgical interventions for solid tumours

- *Biopsy only necessary to formulate the definitive diagnosis.* Chemotherapy and/or radiotherapy may be curative without further surgery, e.g. Hodgkin disease, NHL, rhabdomyosarcoma, germ cell tumours.
- *Resection, primary or following chemotherapy.* Completeness of excision influences subsequent need for adjunctive treatment (radiotherapy or chemotherapy), e.g. bone tumours, Wilms tumour, hepatoblastoma and most CNS tumours.

BOX 50.2 Common side-effects of radiotherapy

Acute
- Nausea and vomiting
- Cutaneous erythema/desquamation
- Diarrhoea
- Myelosuppression
- Pneumonitis
- Hepatitis

Late
- Cardiotoxicity
- Lung dysfunction
- Renal dysfunction
- Musculoskeletal hypoplasia/asymmetry
- Hypothyroidism
- Spinal growth
- Hypopituitarism
- Neuropsychological sequelae
- Cataracts
- Infertility
- Second primary tumours (~5%)

Supportive and emergency care

- Management of the acute abdomen in neutropenic patients (patients may develop neutropenic colitis, also known as typhlitis).
- Raised intracranial pressure (ICP) and spinal cord compression (urgent referral to neurosurgical centre).
- Most children receiving chemotherapy will require a tunnelled central venous line: either a 'Hickman' line or a 'Portacath'.

Problem-orientated topic:

neck mass ● ● ● ● ● ●

Nava, an 11-year-old girl, presents with a painless lump in the right side of her neck which was noticed 4 months ago. She has had two courses of antibiotics with no benefit. The lump was approximately the size of a broad bean when first noticed but has enlarged steadily, and a similar lump has appeared over the last 2 weeks on the left side. Nava has lost a little weight over the last few weeks but has had no other constitutional symptoms. Examination reveals a firm, non-tender mass measuring 4 cm by 3 cm in the right anterior cervical triangle and a 2 cm lump

Continued overleaf

in a similar position on the left side. Although she appears thin, there are no other positive findings on general examination.

Q1. What are the features pointing to a diagnosis of malignancy?

Q2. What other information from the history and examination would help in the differential diagnosis?

Q3. What is the differential diagnosis?

Q4. How should Nava be managed?

Q1. What are the features pointing to a diagnosis of malignancy?

Enlarged cervical nodes in children are very common; the differential diagnosis is wide and malignancies account for only a very small fraction of cases. However, delay in diagnosis may have serious adverse consequences, in terms of extent of disease, intensity of treatment required and ultimate prognosis, so it is important to investigate cases thoroughly if there are features suggesting the possibility of malignancy.

Suspicious features in this case are:
- Absence of symptoms or signs of infection to account for lymphadenopathy
- Weight loss
- Size and characteristics of nodes. Nodes > 2 cm in diameter are a cause for concern and warrant consideration for biopsy. This patient has nodes that are significantly bigger than this and are progressively enlarging. Although they are not described as fixed or rubbery, terms particularly associated with malignancy, they are firm and non-tender, both features consistent with a diagnosis of malignancy.

Q2. What other information from the history and examination would help in the differential diagnosis?

Age
Of the malignant causes, Hodgkin disease is more likely in older children, rarely occurring before the age of 5, whereas NHL and ALL are more likely to be seen in younger children. Disseminated neuroblastoma is unusual in children over 5 years old.

Systemic symptoms
These may help point towards the cause, whether infective or malignant. In particular, weight loss is a common finding in children with cancer and, when combined with fever and night sweats, is particularly associated with Hodgkin disease (B symptoms).

Rate of progression
A timescale of days to weeks is more suggestive of NHL or ALL, whilst Hodgkin disease tends to progress more slowly and the history may span many months.

Characteristics of nodes
In addition to size and presence or absence of tenderness, texture (firm, hard, craggy, rubbery, soft, fluctuant) and mobility (fixed, tethered, mobile) may be helpful.

Systemic examination
This may reveal evidence of a primary tumour or of pallor, bruising and/or petechiae, suggestive of pancytopenia. A child with advanced disease may look pale and non-specifically unwell. Presence of other palpable lymph nodes at all other stations and hepatosplenomegaly should be commented on. Supraclavicular lymphadenopathy is more likely to reflect an underlying malignant process.

Q3. What is the differential diagnosis?

Hodgkin disease and NHL may both present with cervical lymphadenopathy, as may ALL. Distant spread from other solid malignancies is less common but neuroblastoma should be considered and rhabdomyosarcoma and nasopharyngeal carcinoma are also recognized causes in childhood. Hodgkin disease is the most likely, given the age of the patient, the relatively slow progression and the lack of systemic disturbance that would be seen commonly with ALL or NHL.

Other possibilities to consider include bacterial infection, viral infection including cat scratch fever, toxoplasmosis, and rarely connective tissue disorders or Kawasaki disease. Atypical mycobacteria may produce large nodes in an otherwise well child that may be difficult to differentiate and will need (complete) excision biopsy (both to treat effectively and to exclude malignancy).

Q4. How should Nava be managed?

Initial investigations
These should look for evidence of mediastinal and intra-abdominal pathology, and exclude other causes of lymphadenopathy:
- Chest X-ray (CXR)
- Abdominal ultrasound
- Full blood count and film: not very discriminating diagnostically, but if pancytopenia is present, this points to bone marrow involvement as part of a malignant process
- Viral serology.

Biopsy

This should be arranged without waiting for all the results of other investigations in this patient, because of the size of the nodes. It should be an excision biopsy to maximize the yield of diagnostic material and minimize the need for second-look surgery in the case of atypical mycobacterial infection. If the history were of lymph nodes that were more borderline in size (e.g. 1.5–2 cm) and the above investigations did not suggest malignancy, it would be reasonable to treat the child with oral broad spectrum antibiotics and then proceed to biopsy if there had been no reduction.

Staging investigations

Further management, if malignancy is confirmed or considered highly likely, may include the following staging investigations:

- Bone marrow examination (aspirate and trephine)
- Lumbar puncture (if ALL or NHL)
- CT or MRI scan of chest and abdomen (not needed if ALL confirmed)
- Isotope scans (technetium or mIBG, meta-iodobenzylguanidine imaging), according to primary diagnosis
- Baseline fluorodeoxyglucose positron emission tomography (FDG-PET) scans may become routine, particularly for Hodgkin disease.

Baseline investigations and procedures

Baseline investigations and procedures prior to starting treatment, related to recognized toxicities of chemotherapy, varying according to diagnosis and regimen employed. They may include:

- Echocardiogram
- Lung function tests
- GFR or creatinine clearance
- Audiometry
- Sperm cryopreservation.

Problem-orientated topic:

respiratory compromise

Maor, a 9-year-old boy, has experienced episodes of wheezing for 3 weeks, steadily increasing in frequency and severity. He is now unable to sleep lying horizontally. He has been previously well with no hospital admissions, no history of asthma and no family history of atopy. His primary care physician has given him a trial of inhaled bronchodilators but these seem to have made little difference. On examination, he is a little pale with obvious dyspnoea, recession, marked expiratory wheeze throughout the chest and some small 'shotty' cervical lymph nodes, none more than 0.5 cm in diameter.

Q1. Why should this not be treated as asthma without further investigation?

Q2. What is the differential diagnosis?

Q3. What investigations should be performed?

Q4. What is your initial management of Maor?

Q1. Why should this not be treated as asthma without further investigation?

Any child presenting for the first time with wheeze, severe enough to need more than simple bronchodilators, warrants further investigation with a CXR, before being treated as asthmatic. Similarly, any marked change in pattern of wheeze in a known asthmatic should be investigated. Children with a mediastinal mass presenting with wheeze may have clinical signs that are atypical for asthma but this is not always so. These include evidence of compression of the superior vena cava (p. 773), protuberance of the chest wall secondary to the tumour mass, unilateral wheeze, effusion, pallor and petechiae. A trial of steroids for a presumptive diagnosis of asthma could be catastrophic in the event of malignancy, particularly lymphoblastic lymphoma or leukaemia (NHL or ALL), as life-threatening tumour lysis could be precipitated. Partial treatment of these conditions can also delay or prevent accurate diagnosis, and may impart a worse prognosis.

In this case, the history alone should raise suspicions. This boy has experienced rapid progression of his airway obstruction with poor response to bronchodilators, without a previous history of asthma. The presence of small lymph nodes (< 0.5 cm) is not in itself particularly helpful as they are extremely common in children and rarely significant.

Q2. What is the differential diagnosis?

Causes of mediastinal masses in children are shown in Table 50.2. In this case, the most likely cause is T cell NHL or ALL, based on the short history. Given this history, non-malignant causes are unlikely. Foreign body inhalation could present in this way, although the history would generally be much shorter — minutes or hours rather than days or weeks. Structural abnormalities are likely to have presented in infancy rather than this late in childhood. Heart failure may present in this way, after a viral illness causing a cardiomyopathy, but would be extremely rare.

Table 50.2 Differential diagnosis of mediastinal mass in childhood

	Anterior mediastinal	Posterior mediastinal
Malignant	T-cell NHL* ALL* Hodgkin disease* Malignant germ cell tumour	Neuroblastoma* Ganglioneuroblastoma Sarcoma
Benign	Teratoma Cystic hygroma Haemangioma Thymic cyst	Ganglioneuroma Schwann cell tumour Neurofibroma Bronchogenic cyst

* Most common malignant causes of mediastinal mass. (NHL = non-Hodgkin lymphoma; ALL = acute lymphoblastic leukaemia)

Q3. What investigations should be performed?

- CXR (preferably posterior–anterior and lateral) will be enough to demonstrate the presence of a mass causing these symptoms, together with any associated effusion.
- CT scan of chest and abdomen for staging may also provide useful additional information regarding compression of the airway if a general anaesthetic is being considered for subsequent procedures.
- Definitive 'tissue' diagnosis from one of the following:
  - FBC and film (may be sufficient if T cell ALL with high white cell count)
  - Bone marrow aspirate
  - Lumbar puncture (rarely positive but should be performed if possible)
  - Pleural tap
  - Biopsy of lymph node mass: via thoracotomy or mediastinoscopy if there are no significant peripheral lymph nodes
  - Serum tumour marker: α-fetoprotein (AFP) and human chorionic gonadotrophin (hCG) may be elevated in germ cell tumours, which arise in the midline and may rarely occur in the mediastinum.

If one of the above investigations provides the definitive diagnosis, then there will be no need to perform all of the others, the aim being to avoid the most invasive investigations.

Q4. What is your initial management of Maor?

The child should be nursed on a high-dependency unit. He may well need elective intubation and mechanical ventilation to protect the airway, with transfer to an intensive care unit. Good intravenous access should be secured, ideally centrally, such as via a femoral line.

The order of further investigations and management will be dictated by the condition of the child, who may be at risk of severe acute respiratory failure. Caution should be exercised in lying any such child flat in a scanner without full anaesthetic support present. Avoid any sedation for scans in such children, as this may result in loss of airway tone and subsequent respiratory arrest.

The aim should be to obtain definitive diagnostic material and proceed swiftly to definitive treatment. However, in the event that open procedures or general anaesthetic are considered too hazardous, treatment with chemotherapy may have to commence without tissue diagnosis.

Commencing chemotherapy

If ALL or NHL is confirmed, then treatment with oral steroids (prednisolone or dexamethasone), with or without vincristine, may be sufficient as initial treatment in the sickest cases. Hyperhydration should accompany treatment, together with allopurinol or recombinant urate oxidase to minimize the risk of severe tumour lysis syndrome (p. 771).

Monitoring

The response to chemotherapy may be dramatic in T-cell lymphoblastic disease and the attendant risk of tumour lysis high. Renal function and electrolytes should be monitored 4–6-hourly initially, and monitoring should include assessment of calcium, phosphate and uric acid. Alkalinization of urine to help clear urate should not be necessary with the availability of recombinant urate oxidase and may exacerbate hyperphosphataemia.

Problem-orientated topic:

abdominal mass

A 2-year-old boy, Akim, attends the primary care physician's office with his mother after she notices whilst bathing him that his abdomen appears distended. On reflection she admits that it may have been distended for 2 weeks but has become more obvious in the last 3 days. There is no other history of note.

Examination reveals a large firm mass in the right side of the abdomen. Blood pressure is 145/85 mmHg. Urinalysis reveals moderate protein only.

Continued overleaf

Q1. What are the two most likely diagnoses?

Q2. What else should you look for in your clinical evaluation?

Q3. What further investigations are warranted and why?

Q1. What are the two most likely diagnoses?

The two most likely diagnoses are right-sided Wilms tumour (nephroblastoma) and neuroblastoma. These tumours account for 6% and 7% of total paediatric malignancies respectively. The incidental finding of an abdominal mass without other symptoms makes a Wilms tumour the most likely diagnosis. The presence of significant hypertension can occur in both Wilms tumour and neuroblastoma but is very rare in any other paediatric abdominal tumour.

The tumour may be difficult to differentiate from hepatomegaly or a liver mass such as hepatoblastoma, although it should be possible on examination to palpate above a Wilms tumour or neuroblastoma. In addition primary liver tumours in paediatrics are very rare. Other rare causes of a malignant abdominal mass include B cell lymphoma and rhabdomyosarcoma, although the latter usually arises from within the pelvis.

Q2. What else should you look for in your clinical evaluation?

Wilms tumour is associated with a number of syndromes. The presence or absence of clinical signs of these syndromes should be documented: for example, hemihypertrophy, Beckwith–Wiedemann (macroglossia, umbilical defects, horizontal earlobe crease), WAGR syndrome (aniridia, Wilms, microcephaly, cryptorchidism).

In addition, evidence of metastatic disease should be sought. Most Wilms tumours present as localized disease. The most common site for metastases in Wilms is the lungs but this is usually asymptomatic. However, most children with neuroblastoma present with advanced disease, and symptoms and signs often come from sites of metastasis, e.g. 'panda' eyes due to periorbital infiltration, or from constitutional symptoms associated with advanced disease such as cachexia and generalized wasting.

Q3. What further investigations are warranted and why?

- *Urine catecholamines* (homovanillic acid, HVA; and vanillylmandelic acid, VMA): elevated in neuroblastoma. A single spot sample is sufficient, as levels are expressed as ratios with creatinine.
- *Ultrasound* of the abdomen: to confirm renal or adrenal mass. Calcification is strongly suggestive of neuroblastoma.
- *CXR*: staging for Wilms.
- *CT chest and abdomen*: further staging may demonstrate intra-abdominal lymphadenopathy more clearly than ultrasound.
- *ECG/echocardiogram*: patient is hypertensive and therefore evidence of heart strain should be sought. It is important to perform baseline investigations, as chemotherapy may include cardiotoxic agents.
- *Blood tests*, including CBC, clotting, urea and electrolytes, liver function tests, ferritin, lactate dehydrogenase (LDH) and neuron-specific enolase (NSE): NSE and ferritin are tumour markers for neuroblastoma.
- *Biopsy* to establish definitive diagnosis: ultrasound/CT-guided needle biopsy or open procedure (the definitive diagnosis of Wilms tumour can also be based on unequivocal radiological findings).
- *Further staging*: may be required, depending on the results of other investigations, e.g. bone scan and bone marrow aspirates/trephines in neuroblastoma.

Problem-orientated topic:

limb swelling

Noa, a 14-year-old girl, has a 4-month history of pain in her right lower leg. The pain can wake her at night. Over the last month she has noticed a swelling over her right shin. She is a keen gymnast and her parents have attributed her symptoms to 'growing pains', although they note she had a fall from parallel bars 6 months previously.

On examination, she appears well. There is a tender smooth 12 × 8 cm swelling over the medial aspect of the upper third of the right tibia. The rest of the examination is unremarkable.

Q1. What is the most likely diagnosis? What benign condition may this be confused with?

Q2. What would you expect to see on plain X-ray?

Q3. What other investigations would you perform?

Q1. What is the most likely diagnosis? What benign condition may this be confused with?

Osteosarcoma is most likely. Bone tumours account for 4% of all paediatric malignancies, of which osteosarcoma and Ewing sarcoma account for more than 90%. Both have a peak incidence at 12–14 years of age, classically presenting with pain and subsequent swelling over the affected area. Over 90% of osteosarcomas are located in the metaphysis (growth plate) of bone. Around 80% occur in the bones around the knee (i.e. distal femur, proximal tibia or fibula). In contrast, most Ewing sarcomas occur in the diaphysis (mid-shaft) of the bone and only about one-third occur in the femur, tibia and fibula collectively. Ewing sarcoma is more often associated with fever, soft tissue masses and nerve root pain. It may be difficult to distinguish Ewing sarcoma from chronic osteomyelitis on the basis of history, clinical examination and radiological findings.

The benign condition which this may be confused with is Osgood–Schlatter syndrome. This is apophysitis of the tibial tuberosity, occurring in children aged 10–14 years. It is usually bilateral. Pain is felt over the tibial tuberosity, just below the knee, and is worse with strenuous exercise. The tibial tuberosity is prominent and tender to palpation. Plain X-rays should be performed to exclude other pathology and demonstrate simple enlargement of the tibial tuberosity only. The condition is self-limiting and responds to rest and simple analgesics.

Significant diagnostic delay often occurs in such cases, as symptoms are attributed to 'growing pains'. The nature of the pain, being both unilateral and causing waking at night, is not consistent with this. It is also important not to be put off by a history of trauma; patients and families are frequently able to recall episodes of trauma in an attempt to explain symptoms that turn out to be presentations of malignancies.

Q2. What would you expect to see on plain X-ray?

Osteosarcomas have a classical appearance on X-ray of chaotic new bone formation, destruction of the cortex and cortical elevation. This is known as 'Codman's triad'.

In Ewing sarcoma bone destruction gives rise to a 'moth-eaten' appearance. Cortical thickening also usually occurs. However, new bone formation is rare, unlike in osteosarcoma, and in addition, the soft tissue component of Ewing sarcoma may be visualized on plain X-ray.

Q3. What other investigations would you perform?

- *MRI of the primary lesion*: to allow accurate planning for biopsy as well as a baseline to assess response to chemotherapy prior to definitive surgery

- *CXR and CT chest*: to look for evidence of pulmonary metastases (10% in osteosarcoma, 25% in Ewing sarcoma)
- *Technetium-labelled bone scan*: if suggestive of metastatic lesions then these should be confirmed with MRI
- *Bone marrow aspirates and trephines*: in Ewing sarcoma up to 10% of patients have bone marrow involvement at diagnosis.

Problem-orientated topic:

headache (see also p. 377) ● ● ● ●

A 6-year-old girl, Zivah, presents to the accident and emergency department with a 3-week history of morning headaches and intermittent vomiting, having previously been well. Her parents have noted that she appears more clumsy than usual and that she has been falling over. As a result, her parents report that her attendance at school recently has been poor.

On examination she is apyrexial. Blood pressure is 90/55 mmHg. Ataxia and past-pointing are demonstrated. On fundoscopy bilateral papilloedema is seen to be present.

Q1. What is the most likely cause for this presentation?

Q2. What other conditions should be considered?

Q3. What investigations should be arranged?

Q4. What are the initial aims of management?

Q5. After establishing the diagnosis, what general management options can be pursued?

Q1. What is the most likely cause for this presentation?

Headaches and vomiting are the classical symptoms of raised ICP. This is associated with cerebellar symptoms such as ataxia, nystagmus and past-pointing. It should be noted that the absence of papilloedema does not exclude raised ICP. The most likely diagnosis is a posterior fossa tumour. The most common tumours at this site are medulloblastoma or low-grade astrocytoma, but ependymoma is also seen. A long history points more to an astrocytoma than a medulloblastoma. However, an astrocytoma may have been present asymptomatically for some time before acutely presenting with a short history of raised ICP when the tumour reaches a critical size. Thus a short history per se cannot reliably distinguish between the two.

Q2. What other conditions should be considered?

Ataxia can occur following varicella infection but this would rarely present with headaches and papilloedema. Benign intracranial hypertension presents with headache, raised ICP and papilloedema but cerebellar symptoms would be uncommon. A cerebral abscess would be unlikely in a previously well child.

Q3. What investigations should be arranged?

- *CT head with contrast*: if MRI is not readily available. This will identify the tumour and the presence of any hydrocephalus and will dictate the urgency of referral to a neurosurgical centre.
- *MRI head and spine*: MRI head more clearly delineates the tumour than a CT head and allows for planning of surgery. As a medulloblastoma is the most likely diagnosis, given the history, we also need to image the spine to look for evidence of spinal metastases.
- *Lumbar puncture*: to look for evidence of microscopic tumour cells in CSF. This is usually performed 2–3 weeks post-operatively to allow any cellular debris from surgery to resolve. Even presence of microscopic disease, which is not visible on neuroimaging, imparts a poorer prognosis and is therefore important staging information to ascertain.

Q4. What are the initial aims of management?

- *Control raised ICP*. Raised ICP is caused by direct infiltration of the tumour itself or the compression of other brain structures. A rapidly growing tumour often has significant surrounding oedema and this may contribute to raised ICP. Steroids such as dexamethasone are used to reduce oedema and provide an improvement in symptoms. However, raised ICP may also be secondary to obstruction of CSF by the tumour. Urgent neurosurgery may be required for a CSF diversion procedure, e.g. extraventricular drain (EVD) or third ventriculostomy if raised ICP persists despite administration of steroids.

- *Control pain, seizures or electrolyte disturbances*. Seizures and electrolyte disturbances are more common with tumours of the cerebral hemispheres and suprasellar regions respectively.
- *Establish a tissue diagnosis*. In most cases attempt at complete excision is appropriate and associated with better outcome. Neurosurgery should be performed promptly but allowing for appropriate preoperative investigation and stabilization.

Q5. After establishing the diagnosis, what general management options can be pursued?

The subsequent management depends on histology and may range from surveillance imaging alone in completely resected astrocytomas, to further surgery if there is interval growth or symptoms from the tumour, and use of radiotherapy and/or chemotherapy. Radiotherapy-based strategies are avoided in young children, wherever possible, particularly in those less than 3 years of age, because of the impact on the developing brain. Chemotherapy regimens have a place alongside radiotherapy, particularly in medulloblastoma, and may be used in young children to spare toxicity of radiotherapy, by allowing dose or field reductions, or by delaying or avoiding it altogether.

Presentation of malignancy

The list shown in Table 50.3 is not exhaustive. A child presenting several times with the same problem and without a firm diagnosis should be investigated appropriately.

Paediatric oncology emergencies

Tumour lysis syndrome

This syndrome (Box 50.3) is caused by the rapid lysis of malignant cells on initiating chemotherapy, with subsequent release of intracellular contents, exceeding renal excretory capacity and physiological buffering mechanisms, and leading to risk of acute renal failure. It is mainly seen in 'bulky' disease such as high-count ALL and NHL (especially B cell); it may occur spontaneously or be precipitated by a single dose of steroids.

Prevention and close monitoring are the keys to management:
- Hyperhydration before and during initiation of therapy (e.g. 2.5% dextrose 0.45% saline) with no added potassium.

Table 50.3 Presentation of malignancy

Presenting complaint	Suspicious features and comments
Pancytopenia	• Pallor/lethargy due to low haemoglobin • Recurrent fever/infection due to low white count • Bruising and/or petechiae due to low platelets Occurs due to displacement of marrow by leukaemia or disseminated malignancy. Note that not all cell lines may be equally affected
Lymphadenopathy/unexplained mass	• Diameter greater than 2 cm • Progressive enlargement • Non-tender, rubbery, hard or fixed character • Supraclavicular or axillary location • Associated with other features, e.g. pallor or lethargy • Hepatosplenomegaly
Respiratory symptoms	• New episode or change in pattern of wheeze Suggestive of intrathoracic mass
Bone and joint pain and swelling	• Persistent back pain — rarely innocent in children May reflect bone marrow infiltration with leukaemia, metastases or a spinal tumour
Abdominal mass	• Progressive enlargement • Association with general malaise, e.g. neuroblastoma N.B. May be painless and isolated finding, e.g. Wilms tumour
Raised intracranial pressure	• Early morning headache • Vomiting • Ataxia • Papilloedema • III and VI cranial nerve palsies (false localizing signs)
Neurological signs	• Cranial nerve deficits • Cerebellar signs, including head tilt • Visual disturbances or abnormal eye movements • Abnormal gait • Motor or sensory signs • Behavioural disturbance • Deteriorating school performance or milestones • Increasing head circumference in infants
Endocrine or systemic disturbances	• Poor feeding or failure to thrive (diencephalic syndrome) • Diabetes insipidus • Growth hormone deficiency • Precocious puberty

---

BOX 50.3 Biochemical features of tumour lysis syndrome

- Hyperkalaemia
- Hyperuricaemia
- Hyperphosphataemia
- Hypocalcaemia
- Metabolic acidosis, if severe

- Ensure good renal output, with furosemide if necessary.
- Urate precipitation: reduced with allopurinol, or recombinant urate oxidase in high-risk cases.
- Hyperphosphataemia/hypocalcaemia: increase fluids, use haemofiltration in extreme cases.

- Hyperkalaemia: salbutamol, calcium resonium, dextrose/insulin, haemofiltration.

Hyperviscosity syndrome

This refers to symptoms caused by sludging of venous blood in various organ systems, which may ultimately lead to organ failure. Some of the most concerning symptoms relate to neurological effects which may include seizures, stroke, coma and death. It is particularly associated with high-count leukaemias (presenting peripheral white blood count > 200 × 10⁹/l). To treat/prevent, commence prompt leukaemia treatment: hydration, recombinant urate oxidase and chemotherapy. Transfuse slowly and only if essential for symptomatic anaemia, as this may exacerbate hyperviscosity. In severe cases, leucopheresis may relieve symptoms.

Superior vena cava (SVC) obstruction

This is caused by mediastinal masses (Table 50.2); airway obstruction may also occur. It may present with dyspnoea, chest discomfort, hoarseness or cough, and findings include plethora, facial swelling, engorgement of veins of the chest wall and venous dilatation of optic fundi. Sedation or anaesthesia for diagnostic purposes is hazardous and empirical treatment may therefore be based on imaging alone.

Acute abdomen

The most common cause in a child with an underlying malignancy is neutropenic enterocolitis or typhlitis, particularly associated with leukaemia, where bacterial invasion of bowel wall leads to inflammation, full-thickness infarction, perforation, sepsis and coagulopathy with high mortality. Symptoms may be masked by steroid use in ALL induction. Management includes prompt institution of antibiotics, resting of the bowel and close monitoring with surgical review. Most cases resolve with conservative management.

Raised intracranial pressure

Raised ICP is a neurosurgical emergency (p 669). High-dose dexamethasone should be commenced immediately to reduce associated oedema.

Spinal cord compression

This presents with back pain, abnormal gait, sensory loss, and bladder and bowel disturbance. Causes include neuroblastoma, sarcoma, lymphoma and CNS tumours (also infection, osteomyelitis and abscess). Multidisciplinary input is vital; urgent MRI and surgical decompression and biopsy must precede steroids to avoid tumour lysis under anaesthetic. Perform other essential diagnostic procedures (e.g. lumbar puncture, bone marrow examination) under the same anaesthetic if possible. Treatment depends on cause but may include subsequent steroids, radiotherapy and supportive bladder and bowel management.

Supportive care

All paediatric oncology treatment centres should have clear local guidelines for supportive management, which should be referred to for details. This section should not be regarded as a substitute for such guidelines.

Infection

Fever should be treated as an emergency, as immuno-compromised children may succumb to overwhelming sepsis within hours. Greatest risks are associated with count nadirs, usually 10 days into a course of chemotherapy. Central venous catheter (CVC) infection should be considered regardless of count, particularly with symptoms such as rigors, associated with line flushing.

Febrile neutropenia

Febrile neutropenia is usually defined as fever > 38°C and a neutrophil count < 1.0×10^9/l, resulting in increased risk of bacterial infection.

Causes of neutropenia
- Chemotherapy
- Spinal radiotherapy
- Bone marrow disease.

Organisms
- Skin or gut flora
- Greatest risk from Gram-negative organisms, including *Pseudomonas*
- Gram-positive organisms may be from a CVC.

Examination
Include inspection of the skin, mouth, intravenous line sites, surgical sites and perianal area.

Investigations
- FBC and differential, CRP
- Culture of blood, urine, stool
- Swabs of throat, nose, suspicious skin lesions or central line exit sites
- Plain CXR or abdominal X-ray if indicated by symptoms or signs.

Management
Broad-spectrum antibiotics should be commenced without delay as infection with Gram-negative bacilli may be fatal within hours. Choice of antibiotics will vary by institution and local resistance patterns but must include adequate cover for both Gram-negative (including *Pseudomonas*) and Gram-positive organisms, and for anaerobes in the presence of abdominal pain, diarrhoea or mucositis.

Viral infections in immunocompromised patients

If there has been varicella zoster (VZV) contact and the patient is non-immune, give prophylactic aciclovir or zoster immune globulin. Active chickenpox or shingles should be treated aggressively with intravenous aciclovir. Herpes simplex (HSV) may cause painful oral ulceration; treat early with aciclovir. Cytomegalovirus (CMV), adenovirus, respiratory syncytial virus (RSV) and adenovirus may all cause pneumonitis, associated with high morbidity and mortality, especially in BMT patients. Other antiviral therapy may be employed in these cases.

Fungal infections

Consider in prolonged febrile neutropenia and treat promptly. Clinical spectrum includes pulmonary aspergillosis, hepatic candidiasis and abscess formation. Risk is highest during intensive chemotherapy, such as reinduction for relapsed leukaemia and following BMT. Mortality remains high, although it is reduced by newer agents, e.g. liposomal amphotericin. Prophylaxis is used in high-risk treatment regimens.

Pneumocystis carinii (jirovecii) pneumonia (PCP)

Interstitial pneumonitis, associated with prolonged immunosuppression, presents with tachypnoea, dry cough and oxygen requirement. Co-trimoxazole prophylaxis is usual for patients on chemotherapy lasting over 6 months. Treatment involves high-dose co-trimoxazole and steroids in severe cases.

Haematological support

The usual threshold for blood transfusion is 8 g/dl but teenagers are often symptomatic at higher levels. Caution should be used if there is high-count leukaemia, long-standing anaemia or heart failure. Platelets should be maintained above $10 \times 10^9/l$ if the patient is well or $20 \times 10^9/l$ if febrile or for minor procedures (e.g. lumbar puncture), but higher for brain tumours, after significant bleeds or for major surgery. Thresholds may vary between institutions and should be overridden in the event of bruising or bleeding. Blood products should be leucodepleted to reduce viral transmission and incidence of reactions, which may be treated with antihistamine and/or steroid. Irradiated products are required in certain circumstances, such as following BMT and in patients with Hodgkin disease.

Renal toxicity

Glomerular or tubular toxicity may result from chemotherapy, antibiotics and antifungals, particularly in combination. Close attention should be paid to electrolytes, including magnesium and phosphate levels. Hypercalcaemia rarely complicates disseminated paediatric malignancies.

Nausea and vomiting

Chemotherapy varies in its emetogenicity, from oral antimetabolites and vincristine requiring no prophylaxis, to cisplatin and ifosfamide requiring multiple agents. Aim to prevent rather than treat severe symptoms:

- 5-hydroxytryptamine (5-HT) antagonists such as ondansetron are usually used as first line agents.
- However, metoclopramide or domperidone may be considered for chemotherapy with low-emetogenicity.
- Dexamethasone is a useful adjunct (avoid prior to diagnosis in presumed leukaemia or lymphoma)
- Cyclizine is useful, particularly for those with CNS tumours.
- Small doses of nabilone and chlorpromazine are reserved for very resistant cases.

Nutrition and mucositis

Good nutritional status is essential for recovery from chemotherapy, surgery and radiotherapy, but is compromised by the presence of malignancy, direct effects of treatment on appetite and taste, mucositis and infection. Mucositis may be caused by chemotherapy or radiotherapy and may cause significant pain and diarrhoea. Treatment includes analgesia, often with opiates, good oral hygiene and antiseptic mouthwashes to reduce infection. Nasogastric or gastrostomy feeding should be employed early; total parenteral nutrition (TPN) is used only when the enteral route is inadequate.

Table 50.4 summarizes management of common symptoms.

Palliative care

Palliative care is the active total care of patients whose disease is no longer curable and whose prognosis is limited. It needs to embrace physical, emotional, social and spiritual needs of children and their families.

Children with cancer constitute the largest paediatric group requiring palliative care and over one-quarter will die, mostly from progressive disease. Recognition of the appropriate time to stop active 'curative' treatment is always difficult and is compounded by differing views of family members and professionals. Palliative treatment may still involve chemotherapy, radiotherapy or surgery, as these may be effective for symptom control. Many families are willing to explore experimental treatments, as part of phase I or II studies, at a time when conventional treatment has no more to offer. Death from complications of treatment is more likely to be rapid, with limited opportunity for preparation.

In discussions with families, an honest and open approach is essential and careful consideration should be given to the needs and wishes of the child. It is important to emphasize that the focus of treatment is changing to quality of life and symptom control. Families should be discouraged from keeping the truth from older children through their desire to protect them, as this is likely to create problems of trust when the truth can no longer be hidden.

Table 50.4 Other common symptoms and examples of treatment

Symptoms	Treatment options
Nausea, vomiting	Domperidone, cyclizine (particularly for raised ICP), levomepromazine, haloperidol
Constipation	Laxatives when starting opioids Use less constipating opiates where possible
Bowel obstruction	Antispasmodics, stool softeners, octreotide reduces secretions and vomiting
Convulsions, cerebral irritation, terminal restlessness	Diazepam, midazolam
Spinal cord compression	Dexamethasone, radiotherapy, bladder and bowel management
Dyspnoea	Non-pharmacological measures (position, relaxation, play therapy, fan), opioids, benzodiazepines, oxygen, steroids
Excess secretions	Hyoscine, glycopyrronium
Anxiety, depression	Diazepam, levomepromazine or amitriptylline
Pruritus	Cimetidine if due to disease Antihistamine if opioid-induced
Haematological	Anaemia, haemorrhage, bruising; transfuse only for symptomatic improvement and quality of life Topical tranexamic acid or adrenaline (epinephrine) for troublesome mucosal bleeding

Organization of care

Few children will have their palliative care coordinated by a paediatrician specializing in palliative care. The role of the multidisciplinary team is vital and may include specialist nurses, social workers, psychologists and play therapists, with the medical lead taken by either a general or a specialist paediatrician. Most children die at home, through family preference, but some prefer to be in a hospice and a minority in a hospital ward setting.

 http://www.act.org.uk
Association for Children's Palliative Care

Symptom control

Symptoms will vary according to diagnosis and should be anticipated as far as possible, with the aim of correcting underlying causes, such as constipation and infection. Good communication and consideration of psychosocial and spiritual factors will contribute to good control, which may include pharmacological and non-pharmacological measures. See Table 50.4 for common symptoms.

Pain

- Stepwise progression is from paracetamol and non-steroidal drugs to opioids of increasing strength.
- Oral route is preferred; transdermal route employed for some agents.
- Subcutaneous infusion is used for the terminal phase, often in combination with antiemetics, sedatives or anticonvulsants.

- Combining different agents is more effective than escalating dose of single one.
- Adjuvants are additional drugs used in pain management. They include gabapentin for neuropathic pain, antispasmodics (hyoscine, glycopyrronium), muscle relaxants (diazepam) and steroids.

Specific malignancies

Leukaemia

Leukaemia is the most common malignancy of childhood. Approximately 80% of cases are acute lymphoblastic leukaemia and 20% acute myeloid leukaemia, other types being rare. The risk of developing leukaemia in Down syndrome is increased 30-fold compared with the general population.

Acute lymphoblastic leukaemia (ALL)

ALL has an annual incidence of about 1 in 25 000 children, with a peak age of 2–5 years. It results from malignant proliferation of 'pre-B' or T-cell lymphoid precursors. Mature B-cell ALL is a separate entity that is treated with more intensive chemotherapy, similar to B-cell NHL. The cause of ALL is unknown, but genetic predisposition and patterns of childhood infection may account for some cases.

Clinical features

Presentation is of short history (days/weeks) of symptoms reflecting pancytopenia, pain (bone marrow expansion) and lymphadenopathy (Table 50.3). Clinical examination should include testes in boys.

Investigations

These include bone marrow examination and CSF for cytospin to look for the presence of leukaemic cells (CNS involvement is rare). A CXR will exclude a concomitant mediastinal mass.

Management

Treatment involves remission induction, consolidation/CNS-directed therapy, and then prolonged maintenance with one or two intensive blocks during the first year.

Induction lasts for 4 weeks as an inpatient and the aim is to have a morphological remission (< 5% blasts) when the bone marrow is reassessed at day 28. The consolidation phase provides CNS prophylaxis and includes weekly doses of intrathecal methotrexate. Maintenance phase involves continuation treatment to a total of 2 or 3 years for girls or boys respectively. Oral chemotherapy includes daily 6-mercaptopurine (6-MP) and weekly methotrexate; doses are adjusted according to blood count, aiming for mild marrow suppression without prolonged neutropenia. Patients attend for monthly intravenous vincristine with a 5-day pulse of oral dexamethasone and 3-monthly intrathecal methotrexate. Intensive blocks of chemotherapy interrupt the first year of maintenance, with combinations of oral, intravenous and intrathecal chemotherapy.

Prognosis

Prognosis is improving steadily and overall survival is ~80% for standard-risk patients with current treatment. Adverse prognostic indicators are listed in Box 50.4.

The evaluation of minimal residual disease (MRD) using molecular techniques is now standard practice. This allows the detection of low levels of disease, undetectable by conventional morphology. This advance has resulted in trials evaluating the efficacy of treatments which are stratified according to MRD risk.

Relapsed ALL may be confined to bone marrow or involve extramedullary sites (mainly CNS, testes).

BOX 50.4 Adverse prognostic indicators in childhood leukaemia

- Male gender
- Age < 2 or > 10 years
- High white cell count (> 50 × 10^9/l) at diagnosis
- Unfavourable cytogenetics:
  - Philadelphia chromosome: t(9;22)
  - MLL gene rearrangements: e.g. t(4;11) in infants
  - AML1 amplification
- Poor response to induction treatment
- High levels of minimal residual disease at end of induction*

* See text.

Treatment involves intensive reinduction and consolidation for all, with a further 2 years of maintenance for low-risk and BMT for higher-risk cases. Cure rates are variable but highest in isolated extramedullary relapse more than 2 years off treatment.

Acute myeloid leukaemia (AML)

AML results from the malignant proliferation of myeloid or non-lymphoid precursors. It is subclassified by morphology, according to the 'FAB' (French, American, British) classification, M1 to M7, each with different behaviour and cytogenetics. Favourable prognosis is associated with translocations t(15;17), t(8;21) and inv(16), and poor prognosis with monosomy 7 or complex abnormalities. Mutations of the FLT3 gene are common in AML and associated with a worse prognosis.

Clinical features

This is similar to ALL. Lymphadenopathy is less prominent and intrathoracic and extramedullary disease are also less common than in ALL.

Management

Treatment differs fundamentally from that of ALL. Four or five courses of intensive myelosuppressive chemotherapy are usually given, with no prolonged maintenance therapy. High-risk cases, including those slow to respond, are transplanted in the first remission if an HLA compatible donor is available. The anti-CD33 monoclonal antibody gemtuzumab (trade name Mylotarg) has also been used, particularly in relapsed or resistant cases, with some success and is still being evaluated. Furthermore, therapy with FLT3 inhibitors are at the trial stage and offer future promise. Neither of these are standard therapy at present.

Prognosis

Prognosis has improved dramatically due to intensive treatment and supportive care, with overall survival more than 60%. Relapses may be salvaged with BMT.

Lymphoma

Lymphomas are malignant proliferations of lymphoid precursor cells at various stages of differentiation. However, non-Hodgkin lymphoma (NHL) and Hodgkin disease are distinct disease entities and differ in terms of natural history, presentation and management. Both are more common in males than females.

Non-Hodgkin lymphoma

Clinical features

Presentation varies according to site, including palpable lymphadenopathy, pain, obstruction or ascites from abdominal mass, respiratory symptoms or SVC obstruction from mediastinal mass, and pancytopenia (Table 50.3).

Investigations

Investigation includes bone marrow examination, lumbar puncture, imaging according to site, biopsy for histology with immunophenotyping and cytogenetics. The majority in childhood are high-grade tumours, divided according to histology, immunophenotype and cytogenetics:

- *Lymphoblastic* (90% T-cell, 10% pre-B): 30% of NHL cases. Most present with an anterior mediastinal mass. If there are > 25% blasts in bone marrow, then disease is regarded as ALL.
- *Mature B cell* (Burkitt or atypical Burkitt): 50% of cases occur in the abdomen, head and neck, bone marrow and CNS, and may grow very rapidly. Endemic or African Burkitt lymphoma is associated with early Epstein–Barr virus (EBV) infection and frequently affects the jaw, a site rarely involved in sporadic disease.
- *Anaplastic large cell lymphoma* (ALCL): < 20%.

Management

Lymphoblastic (T cell, pre-B cell) lymphoma is treated similarly to its ALL counterparts, treatment lasting up to 2 years.

Mature B cell disease and ALCL are treated with short series of dose-intensive chemotherapy, including significant doses of alkylating agents. The risk of tumour lysis is high.

Prognosis

More than 70% of children with NHL survive overall and over 90% of cases with localized disease survive with limited treatment. Relapse tends to occur early. Although the cure rate for primary NHL is high, salvage options are limited and few relapsed patients survive.

Hodgkin disease

Hodgkin disease is characterized by the presence of neoplastic Reed–Sternberg cells in a reactive lymph node infiltrate. It is much slower-growing than NHL and rare under 5 years, incidence rising with age. Some cases show evidence of previous EBV infection. Hodgkin disease is classified as classical or lymphocyte-predominant; the latter usually involves localized disease and has a better prognosis.

Clinical features

There is progressive painless lymph node enlargement, cervical in around 80%, mediastinal (often asymptomatic) in 60%. Dissemination to other organs occurs late. Fever, night sweats and weight loss constitute 'B' symptoms, which are more common in advanced stages.

Ann Arbor staging

Stage I   Single site
Stage II   > 1 site of disease, on one side of the diaphragm
Stage III > 1 site of disease, on both sides of the diaphragm
Stage IV   Disseminated disease.

Investigations

These are as for NHL, without lumbar puncture but including EBV serology.

Management

Stage I disease may be cured with either involved field radiotherapy or a short course of chemotherapy. All other stages require chemotherapy, which usually includes significant doses of anthracyclines and/or alkylating agents. The additional use of radiotherapy is subject to national and institutional variation, but is usually employed in bulky mediastinal and disseminated disease, as well as in resistant or relapsed cases, when further intensive chemotherapy is also indicated.

Prognosis

Overall survival at 5 years exceeds 90%, ranging from 70% for stage IV to 97% for stage I.

Late effects remain a significant concern, as both radiotherapy and the chemotherapy regimens carry risks (p. 764). The role of functional imaging with PET scans shows promise in Hodgkin disease and may help to identify good-risk disease requiring less toxic treatment.

CNS tumours

Brain tumours are the most common solid tumours, as they constitute 25% of childhood malignancies, but they represent a wide spectrum of histological subtypes with widely different features, management and outcome:

- Infratentorial tumours predominate (> 50%), usually associated with raised ICP, headaches, vomiting and cerebellar ataxia.
- Supratentorial tumours present with raised ICP and/or focal signs according to site, hypothalamic/pituitary dysfunction or visual impairment.
- Primary spinal tumours are very rare and are managed similarly to their intracranial counterparts; they may present with cord compression (p. 773).
- CNS metastases of extracranial tumours are rare in children.

Delay in diagnosis is common, as few cases present classically. For every childhood brain tumour there are around 5000 children with migraine.

Involvement of the multidisciplinary team is central to management and should involve neurosurgeons, paediatric oncologists, radiotherapists and endocrinologists.

Initial management

- Diagnostic imaging: CT provides essential information for emergency management of hydrocephalus. MRI provides better tumour definition combined with spinal imaging for staging.
- Raised ICP requires prompt management, particularly if onset is rapid: prompt referral and transfer to a paediatric neurosurgical unit, using dexamethasone to control oedema, and intensive care unit (ICU)/ventilation in severe cases.
- Initial surgery may involve CSF diversion only (third ventriculostomy or external ventricular drain to relieve hydrocephalus), or biopsy or complete resection, depending on location and likely diagnosis.
- Other investigations may include CSF cytology and tumour markers.
- Postoperative scan within 48 hours of surgery avoids confounding artefact from post-surgical change (haematoma/oedema).

Low-grade glioma (~45%)

Most have histological characteristics of pilocytic astrocytoma (grade I) and behave in an indolent fashion, with variable responses to treatment. Outcome depends on site, with cerebellar tumours usually cured by surgery alone. Unresectable cases that progress or are symptomatic, such as optic pathway or hypothalamic gliomas with diencephalic syndrome or threat to vision, are treated with chemotherapy. Radiotherapy may be employed in older children, except in NF-1-associated cases (~50%), in which the risks of second primary tumours and cerebrovascular complications are increased.

High-grade glioma (~10%)

These may be World Health Organization grade III or IV. They occur predominantly in older children and teenagers, and supratentorial sites predominate. They are usually incompletely resectable and cure is rarely achieved. Radiotherapy is the treatment of choice but responses are rarely sustained and chemotherapy is of limited benefit.

Brainstem glioma (< 5%)

Intrinsic pontine gliomas are usually diagnosed on characteristic MRI appearances alone. They are high-grade and inoperable, and their response to radiotherapy is variable and short-lived. Chemotherapy has failed to improve median survival of < 1 year. Tumours growing outwards from the brainstem (exophytic) may be low-grade and amenable to biopsy with less morbidity, and have a better outcome.

Primitive neuroectodermal tumours (PNETs) (~25%)

This is the most common group of malignant brain tumours of childhood, with peak incidence at 5 years. The majority occur in the cerebellum (where they are called medulloblastoma), and present with raised ICP and ataxia. Supratentorial PNETs, including pineoblastomas, have a worse prognosis. CSF-borne metastases occur in 10–15% of cases. Excision and craniospinal radiotherapy form the basis of treatment, but chemotherapy provides further benefit. About 70% of localized cases are cured but long-term morbidity from radiotherapy is significant, particularly in young patients.

Ependymoma (~10%)

Ependymomas usually arise in and around the ventricles, with presenting features according to site of origin but usually including obstructive hydrocephalus. Complete surgical excision confers the best outcome (> 70% survival, compared with < 50% for those in whom complete surgical excision is not possible) and involved field radiotherapy is then given. Chemotherapy may delay or occasionally remove the need for radiotherapy in younger patients.

Craniopharyngioma (5–10%)

Craniopharyngioma is a slow-growing midline benign epithelial tumour that arises in the suprasellar area from remnants of Rathke's pouch. Treatment involves complete resection in 80% and partial resection with focal radiotherapy in the remainder. Management of complications of the disease and its treatment — including damage to the hypothalamus, vision and behaviour — remains the greatest challenge, particularly as most become long-term survivors.

Neuroblastoma

Neuroblastoma is a malignant embryonal tumour derived from the neural crest and represents 7% of childhood malignancies. It has a median age of onset of 2 years with the majority of cases arising in the adrenal glands, abdomen or thorax, usually related to the sympathetic chain. Small numbers occur in the pelvis, neck and elsewhere. Disease is often advanced at diagnosis with metastases to bone, bone marrow, liver, and occasionally CNS and lungs. There is a wide spectrum of behaviour according to age of patient and disease stage.

Clinical features

Presentation is often non-specific, depending on site, spread and metabolic effects:

- Lymphadenopathy or palpable masses
- Compression of structures, including nerves (e.g. Horner syndrome, spinal cord), airway, veins, bowel
- Pancytopenia
- Bone pain, limp
- Sweating, pallor, watery diarrhoea and hypertension.

Investigations

Specific diagnostic tests include:

- Imaging of affected area for staging purposes (CT or MRI)
- Urine VMA/HVA creatinine ratios (urine catecholamines); raised in > 80% cases and may be used for monitoring of disease progress
- ^{131}I-mIBG uptake by primary tumour and metastases, in the majority; if negative for primary, ^{99}Tc bone scan is required
- Bilateral bone marrow aspirates/trephines (disease infiltration may be patchy)
- Biopsy of lesion
- Cytogenetic analysis of biopsy, bone marrow and blood.

Management

Treatment ranges from surgery only for resectable localized (stage 1) neuroblastoma to induction chemotherapy, surgery, high-dose chemotherapy with autologous stem cell rescue and radiotherapy in stage 4 (disseminated) and *MYCN*-positive stage 3 disease.

Infant neuroblastoma characteristically presents with disseminated disease restricted to bone marrow, liver and skin (stage 4S), which usually resolves spontaneously; chemotherapy is only required for life-threatening symptoms.

Prognosis

Disseminated neuroblastoma is only cured in 20–30%, despite intensive treatment. Survival in low-stage cases in infants is more than 90%. Adverse prognostic indicators are listed in Box 50.5.

Wilms tumour

Wilms tumour, or nephroblastoma, is an embryonal tumour of the kidney accounting for 6% of childhood malignancies. Around 75% of cases occur in patients less than 4 years.

Clinical features

Presentation is most commonly as a visible or palpable mass, often painless, in a well child. Haematuria and

---

> **BOX 50.5 Adverse prognostic indicators in neuroblastoma**
>
> - Age > 1 year
> - Stages 3 and 4
> - Raised tumour markers: ferritin, lactate dehydrogenase (LDH), neuron-specific enolase (NSE)
> - Unfavourable histology
> - Cytogenetic abnormalities: *MYCN* amplification, 17q gain, 1p loss

---

hypertension are found in one-third. Most tumours are localized at diagnosis but lung metastases may occur. Bilateral (stage 5) disease accounts for 10% of cases and is more likely to be associated with an inherited predisposition (p. 761).

Investigations

These include:

- Abdominal ultrasound
- CT scan of abdomen
- CXR or CT chest
- Urine catecholamines to exclude neuroblastoma (prior to anaesthetic)
- Full blood count and coagulation studies (a transient acquired von Willebrand-like syndrome is recognized in 1% of cases)
- Biopsy.

Management

Definitive surgery usually follows a short course of chemotherapy. Subsequent treatment depends on stage and histology, ranging from a short course of vincristine to 6 months of three- or four-drug anthracycline-based chemotherapy. Radiotherapy is required for incompletely resected disease and most cases with lung metastases. In bilateral disease (stage V), the aim is to maximize response to chemotherapy prior to performing nephron-sparing surgery to avoid the need for dialysis.

Prognosis

Overall survival ranges from ~70% for stage IV disease to > 95% in stage I. Follow-up should include regular CXR as well as abdominal ultrasound, as pulmonary relapse is more common than local recurrence.

Other renal tumours are rare in childhood. Mesoblastic nephroma occurs in infants and most cases can be cured with surgery alone. Clear cell sarcoma requires more intensive treatment than Wilms tumour, and malignant rhabdoid tumour carries a very poor prognosis.

Osteosarcoma and Ewing sarcoma

Bone tumours are rare in childhood, accounting for 4% of all paediatric malignancies.

Incidence increases with age, peaking in teenage years and early adulthood. The majority of cases are osteosarcoma or Ewing sarcoma, histologically distinct and with differing patterns of disease and response to treatment but with many common features. All cases should be referred to a specialist bone tumour centre for surgical management.

Clinical features

This is with pain, swelling, pathological fracture, and rarely overlying erythema. Osteosarcoma occurs mostly in long bones and around the knee in 80%. In Ewing sarcoma the axial (central) skeleton is involved more often and the pelvis is the most common site. Delay in diagnosis is a common feature. Metastases are more common at diagnosis in Ewing sarcoma (25%) than osteosarcoma (10%), and in lungs more commonly than bone, with bone marrow metastases in Ewing sarcoma only.

Investigations

Diagnostic investigations include:
- Plain X-rays of bony lesion
- MRI of primary site to define extent of tumour and aid surgical planning
- Definitive diagnosis requires biopsy, which should be carried out at a specialist centre where definitive surgery will be performed
- CT chest
- Isotope bone scan
- Bone marrow aspirates and trephines (bilateral): Ewing sarcoma only.

Management

Surgery, with the aim of limb preservation, is preceded and followed by chemotherapy in all cases. Prostheses are designed to allow lengthening as the patient grows. Radiotherapy is an effective adjunct and alternative to surgery, particularly in axial Ewing sarcoma, but its role in osteosarcoma is restricted mainly to palliation.

Prognosis

Overall survival for both groups is around 60%, but adverse outlook is associated with large primaries, axial sites, poor response to preoperative chemotherapy and metastatic disease.

Rhabdomyosarcoma

Rhabdomyosarcoma (RMS) is the most common soft tissue sarcoma in childhood and represents 6% of childhood malignancies. Most cases occur before the age of 10 years and are sporadic.

Clinical features

This depends on site, mostly bladder, pelvis, nasopharynx, parameningeal or paratestis, and may include palpable mass, pain or bladder outflow obstruction. Metastases are uncommon.

Investigations

Diagnosis and staging involve:
- Imaging of primary: ultrasound, followed by staging CT or MRI
- Biopsy: for histology and molecular cytogenetic analysis. Alveolar RMS is associated with adverse prognosis and is characterized by the presence of t(2;13) or t(1;13), which produce fusion products of *PAX* and *FKHR* genes
- Bone marrow examination
- Bone scan
- Lumbar puncture for parameningeal disease.

Management

Treatment involves 6–9 courses of combination chemotherapy. Some cases achieve complete remission with chemotherapy alone. Surgery for accessible sites (paratesticular, peripheral) occurs after three or six courses of chemotherapy. Radiotherapy is also required in cases with residual disease and for alveolar histology.

Prognosis

This depends on risk factors and ranges from around 10% for bony metastatic disease to over 70% for completely excised paratesticular tumours with favourable histology. The outcome for metastatic relapse and local recurrence within a previous radiotherapy field is extremely poor.

Rare tumours

Many other forms of cancer occur in children but all are very rare. They include:

Germ cell tumours	3% of childhood cancers
Retinoblastoma	3% of childhood cancers
Liver tumours	1% of childhood cancers
Histiocytosis	1:200 000 children
Chronic myeloid leukaemia	Very rare in childhood
Juvenile myelomonocytic leukaemia	Very rare in childhood

Appendix
Sickle cell disease

Sickle cell disease is an autosomal recessive inherited disorder caused by a single mutation in the β-haemoglobin chain (Glu6→Val) that produces a variant defined as HbS. As a consequence, upon deoxygenation the haemoglobin molecules aggregate and red cells acquire the shape of a sickle. It was first described in Afro-Americans, but whereas the average incidence of the gene among Afro-Americans is approximately 8%, its frequency is much higher across the middle third of Africa, where there are four major sickle haplotypes. The 'Benin' haplotype can be found in Algeria, Greece, Turkey and southwestern Saudi Arabia. The gene is also very common in India.

Clinically evident disease is due to homozygous HbS mutation (HbSS), while sickle cell trait is asymptomatic; the coinheritance of other haemoglobinopathies (HbC, β-thalassemia trait) causes sickle cell disease of varied severity (HbSC, HbSβ°, HbSβ+). The erythrocytes are maintained in the unsickled state while in the oxygenated environment of the arterial circulation; as the cell enters the capillary circulation, where the oxygen saturation rapidly decreases, the cell will sickle and will occlude the capillary. However, in normal conditions the erythrocytes tend to sickle only after the exit from the capillaries, and vascular occlusion does not occur.

Microvascular occlusion is more likely in the presence of increased numbers of HbSS red cells that contain polymerized HbS even in the event of arterial oxygen saturation, rapid deoxygenation, or prolongation of the transit time through the microcirculation (due to infections, inflammation).

The final event is a blockage of the blood flow, with consequent tissue hypoxia and damage, and acute sickle cell painful crisis.

1. The most frequently involved areas are lumbosacral spine, knee, femur, elbow, shoulder. The majority of painful episodes are of mild to moderate severity, and are usually treated at home with oral analgesics. A typically severe crisis reaches a peak within 2 or more days, with a severe, steady pain usually lasting 4–5 days that requires hospitalization for opiate analgesia.
2. Microvascular occlusion in the lungs causes acute chest syndrome (ACS), an important cause of death. In children, pulmonary crises are usually caused by bacterial pneumonia with pneumococcus, mycoplasma and other agents. In other cases, the precipitating event may be hypoventilation secondary to chest pain crisis. The incidence of ACS is age-dependent, with rates of 24.5 events per 100 patient-years in young children and decreasing to approximately 8.8 events per 100 patient-years in older adults.
   Oxygen therapy is indicated in all hypoxic patients as well as in those with clinical distress. Nebulized albuterol should be attempted in all patients initially, because benefit can be documented even in patients who do not have audible wheezing. Transfusions are often recommended for the treatment of acute lung disease.
3. Vaso-occlusion caused by red cells sickling can elicit other clinical pictures, according to the organ involved: acute abdominal pain, dactylitis of hands

and feet, priapism that is often recurrent ('stuttering priapism'), acute infarction of the brain.

4. Acute infarction of the brain can result in a severe stroke, with a 7% incidence in children with sickle cell disease. The underlying lesion is an intracranial arterial stenosis, due to chronic endothelial injury by sickle erythrocytes. For this reason, cranial Doppler ultrasonography can be helpful to children at risk for stroke lesions. In untreated patients the mortality rate is approximately 20%, and the risk of recurrence is 70%. Recurrences can be reduced to 10–15% by a chronic transfusion programme, but stroke is an indication for stem cell transplantation.

5. Chronic endothelial injury is the leading cause for chronic organ damage (cardiovascular system, renal system, eyes, skin)

6. Sickling causes splenic hypoperfusion, with recurrent infarctions, functional hyposplenia and increased risk of severe infections by capsulated bacteria. The enlarged spleens of young children with sickle cell disease are usually nonfunctional. In the past, infections were the most common cause of death. But active prevention with prophylactic antibiotics and vaccines and aggressive treatment of fever has dramatically reduced mortality.

7. Children with sickle cell disease may have sudden enlargement of the spleen with entrapment of a considerable amount of blood ('*splenic sequestration*'), one of the leading causes of death. Splenic sequestration is more common in younger children.

The newborn infant with sickle cell anaemia is generally not anaemic and is asymptomatic because of the protective effect of fetal haemoglobin. As β^S globin production increases and HbF decreases, the clinical syndrome of sickle cell anaemia emerges. Haemolytic anaemia, with a haemoglobin level of 7–10 g/dl and a reticulocytosis of 10–20%, is usually evident by 4 months of age. However, mortality due to bacterial sepsis or sequestration crisis is increased in infants with sickle cell disease after 2 or 3 months of age.

The clinical manifestations of sickle cell anaemia are extremely variable. Some patients are entirely asymptomatic, whereas other are constantly plagued by painful episodes; most patients fall between these extremes, and have relatively long asymptomatic periods punctuated by occasional clinical crises.

Options for treatment of children with a more severe course include hydroxyurea to increase intracellular concentration of HbF (that has a protective effect against sickling) and stem cell transplantation. Hydroxyurea reduces the incidence of acute vaso-occlusive episodes and chest syndrome increasing HbF production, a well known factor of protection against sickling. Stem cell transplantation offers a potential cure for sickle cell disease; however the risks must be balanced against the benefits. At this time, stem cell transplantation is recommended for children with neurologic or pulmonary complications.

Index

Echovirus, 697
ECMO (extracorporeal membrane oxygenation)
acute respiratory distress syndrome, 709
pulmonary hypertension of newborn, 702
Ectoderm, 368
Eczema, *348*, 354–5
chronic eruptions, 361
compliance/understanding, 354
diagnosis, 354
distribution, 353, *353*, 354
management, 354–5, *355*
presenting features, 354
prevalence, 354
Eczema herpeticum, 362, *362*
Edrophonium chloride test, 383
Education
attention deficit hyperactivity disorder (ADHD), 400
diabetes mellitus, 487–8, *488*
disabled children, 201–2
language difficulties, 407
Education, skills and training deprivation, 148
Education Code of Practice, 396
Education professionals, role in children's health, 159
Educational difficulties/problems
cerebral palsy, 404
and language disorders, 408
Edwards syndrome (trisomy 18), 95
and congenital heart disease, 567
EEG *see* Electroencephalogram (EEG)
Efficacy of studies, measurement of, 135, *136*
Egg intolerance, 323
Eighth cranial nerve, 51
Elastase, faecal pancreatic, 528–9
Electrocardiography (ECG), *124*, 567
abdominal masses, 769
coarctation of aorta, 573
congestive cardiac failure, 568, *569*
critically ill child, *661*
cyanotic heart disease, 717
murmurs, 575
neonatal shock, *735*
palpitations, 269
Electroencephalogram (EEG)
absence epilepsy, 301
autism, 410
febrile convulsions, 298
neonatal seizures, *724*
paroxysmal episodes, 299
Electrolytes
absorption, 530–1, *531*
balance in preterm infants, 684–5
imbalance, 548–50
Electromyography, *381*
Electroretinogram, 424
Eleventh cranial nerve, 51
Elimination half-life, 104, *104*
Embase, 132
Emetics, *533*
Emotional abuse, 232–3, *493*
assessment, 233
definition, 233

impact of, 231
management, 233
and neglect, 232
see also Neglect
Emotional and behavioural problems, *152*, 215–26
in adolescents, 216
consultation, *218*, 218–19
consultation skills, 217–19
diagnostic formulation, 219
factors influencing the development of, 216–17, *217*
management, 219
and obesity, 260
in preschool children, 216, 220–4
prevalence, 216
recurrent and unexplained symptoms, 225
in school-age children, 216, 224–6
sexual abuse, 235, 504
Emotional development, 20–1
Emotional environment, effect on growth, 241
Empathy, 66
Emphysema, pulmonary interstitial *see* Pulmonary interstitial emphysema (PIE)
Employment
deprivation, 148
and diabetes mellitus, 491
Empowerment, health promotion, 185
Empyema, 268, 615
Encephalitis, herpes simplex virus (HSV), 648
Encephaloceles, 10, 389–90
Encephalopathy
acquired immune deficiency syndrome (AIDS)-related, 385
causes of, 670–1
diagnostic investigations, 671, *671*
hypoxic-ischaemic, 723, *723*
inborn errors of metabolism, 460–2
management, 671
neonates, 723
neuroprotection, 671
portal hypertension, 545
raised intracranial pressure, 670–1
with seizures, 459
Encopresis, 226, 311
Endocarditis, infective *see* Infective endocarditis
Endocrine axis, *467*, 467–8
Endocrine disorders, 466–90
constipation, 310
failure to thrive, 254
malignancy, *772*
obesity, 262
short stature, 245
Endoscopic subureteric injection (STING), 554–5
Endoscopy, gastrointestinal, 528, *528*
Endothelium, acute respiratory distress syndrome, 662
Enema, contrast, *526*
Energy
deficiency, *459*
requirements of toddlers, 32
total daily intake, *487*

Entamoeba histolytica, 319
Enteral nutrition, 529, *530*
Enterocolitis
allergic, 542
infectious, 542
Enteropathy
malabsorption, 536
protein-losing, 537, *537*
Enuresis, 226, 331–4, 404
basic science of, 331–2
causes of, 332, *333*
clinical valuation, 333
guidelines for concern, *332*
investigations, *334*
referral, 333–4
Environmental factors
growth, 240, 241
hyperkinetic disorder, 398
Enzyme deficiencies, 386, *386*
Enzyme-linked immunosorbent assay (ELISA) tests, 527
Enzymes, 457, *458*
Eosinophilic pustulosis, *84*
Eosinophils, 650
Ependymoma, 770–1, 778
EPICURE study, 116
Epidemiology, 143–60
Epidermis, 347–8
Epidermolysis bullosa (EB), 362
Epididymo-orchitis, 322, 323, 343, *343*
Epiglottitis, 599
differential diagnosis, *599*
management, *600*
Epilepsy, 369–72
absence, 301–2
apparent life-threatening events, 757
causes of, *372*
cerebral palsy, 404
classification, 299
counselling, 301
cryptogenic, 299
definition, 299
diagnosis, 299
disability in, 204–5
epileptic syndromes *see* Epilepsy syndromes
idiopathic, 299
investigation, 299–300
and language disorders, 408
management, 300, *300*, 372
in primary care, 299–302
reasons for developing, 299
referral, 301
seizures, *296*, 299, *300*, 369–72
(*see also* Seizures)
symptomatic, 299
syncope, 270
Epilepsy syndromes, 300, *371*, 371–2
benign Rolandic, 371, *371*
childhood absence, 371
juvenile myoclonic, 371, *371*
West syndrome, 372, *372*
Epinephrine *see* Adrenaline (epinephrine)
Epiphora, 422
Episodic events, 369, *369*
Epistaxis, 286
Epithelium, acute respiratory distress syndrome, 662

Polyarthritis nodosa (PAN), 454
Polycystic renal disease, 561–2
  autosomal dominant, 562
  autosomal recessive, 562
Polydactyly, 75, 79
Polydipsia, 334
Polyethylene glycol, 310
Polymerase chain reaction (PCR), *641*
Polyploidy, 94
Polyps, 542
Polyuria, 334–6
  causes of, 335, *335*
  clinical evaluation, 335
  features, 334
  guidelines for concern, *335*
  investigations, 335–6, *336*
  referral, 336
Population, child, 144
Population paradox, 191
Portal hypertension, 545–6
  extrahepatic, 546
Portal vein thrombosis, 546
Port-wine stain, *75, 83,* 350, *350*
  Sturge-Weber syndrome, 374
Positive end-expiratory pressure (PEEP),
    696
  acute respiratory distress syndrome,
    709
  meconium aspiration syndrome, 701
Positive predictive value (PPV), 58,
    163–4
Positron emission tomography (PET),
    paroxysmal episodes, 300
Possetting, 84
  failure to thrive, 233
  see also Vomiting
Posterior fossa tumour, *377, 378,* 770–1
Post-mortem, 115
Postnatal check, 688
  common conditions is diagnosed at,
    750, 751
  see also Neonatal screening
Postnatal depression, 221–2
Post-neonatal death, *508*
Post-resuscitation management, 660–1
Post-transcriptional processing, 93
Post-translational modification, 93
Potter syndrome, 699
Poverty
  absolute, 146–7
  effect on health, 147
  government targets, *151,* 151–2
  health inequalities, *145*
  and malnutrition, 515
  measuring, 148
  relative, 147
PR interval, 269–70
Practical procedures, 118–23
  failing to complete, 119
  learning new, 118
  minimising distress, 119
  see also specific procedures
Practice nurses, role in children's health,
    160
Practice-based Learning and
    Improvement, 8
Prader-Willi syndrome (PWS), 99–100
  obstructive sleep apnoea syndrome,
    601

Pragmatics, 405, 406–7
Precocious puberty, 248
Precordial catch syndrome, 268
Precordium auscultation, 45
Predictive genetic test, 90
Prednisolone, 559
Pregnancy
  energy cost of, 26–7
  high-risk, 680, *680*
  history, 42
    newborn evaluation, 73
  low maternal weight gain in, 27
  nutrition in, 26–7
  screening in see Antenatal screening
  sexual abuse, 235, 504
  teenage see Teenage pregnancy
  termination see Termination of
    pregnancy
  twin see Twin pregnancy
Pregnancy-associated plasma protein-A
    (PAPP-A), 92
Prenatal testing, genetic disorders,
    92
Prepuce, 344
Preschool children
  crying, 220
  disabled, 201
  emotional abuse, 233
  emotional and behavioural problems
    in, 216, 220–4
  growth in, 241
  sleep problems, 220–2, *221*
  urinary tract infection, 550
  wheezing, 603
Prescribing for children, 107–8
Presenting complaint, 42
  history of, 42
Presymptomatic genetic test, 90
Preterm delivery
  homoeostatic support to newborns,
    683–8
  management of threatened, 680, *681*
Preterm infants
  acid-base balance, 687–8
  apnoea, 706
  brain injury, 723–5
  definition, *681*
  in developing countries, 513
  fluid and electrolyte balance, 684–5,
    686
  glucose homeostasis, 685–7, *686, 687*
  homoeostatic support in very sick,
    683–8
  respiratory deterioration in older, 703
  with respiratory distress from birth,
    692–4
  resuscitation, 116
  retinopathy of prematurity (ROP), 425
  thermoregulation, 684, *684, 685*
  viability and outcome, 116–17
Pre-test probability, 58
Prevalence, 154
Preventative healthcare, 158
Primary care physicians, writing to, 70–1
Primary healthcare team (PHCT), 202–3
Primitive neuroectodermal tumours
    (PNETs), 778
Primitive reflexes, *81*
Privacy, 66

Problem lists, 61, *62*
Procedures, practical see Practical
    procedures; *specific procedures*
Processus vaginalis (PV), 342, 747–8
  patent, 342, 748
Professionalism, 8
Prolactin (PRL), *28,* 468
Prolonged QT syndrome, 269–70
Prophylaxis
  group B streptococcal infection, 736
  infective endocarditis, 585
Propionibacterium acnes, 214
Propofol, 106
Proptosis, 421
Propylthiouracil, 476
Prosencephalon, 10
Prostacyclin analogues, *588*
Prostaglandin I$_2$ (PGI$_2$), 682
Protein
  absorption/malabsorption, 537, *537*
  malabsorption tests, 529
  synthesis, 93–4
Protein C, 621
Protein S, 621
Protein-losing enteropathy, 537, *537*
Proteinuria, *340,* 342
  glomerular disease, 557
  in nephrotic syndrome, 557–8
Proteus, 551
Proton pump inhibitors, 317, *535*
Protozoal gastroenteritis, 319
Proximal convoluted tubule, 330
Pruritus, *348,* 351–9
  diagnosis, 351, 354
  differential diagnosis, 352, *353*
  history, 352–4
  investigations, 351, 354
  referral, 351
  see also specific pruritic conditions
Pseudomonas infection
  cystic fibrosis, 611, *611*
  mastoiditis, 445
  urinary tract infection, 551
Pseudoseizures, 296
Psoriasis, 360–1
  compliance/understanding, 354
  distribution, 353, *353*
  guttate, *360*
  management, *361*
  skin abnormality in, 361
Psychogenic disorders, 269
Psychological development, 20–5
Psychological disorders, 404
Psychological distress, 331–2
Psychometric tests, 392, 399
Psychosis, acute, 417–18, *418*
Psychosocial factors
  hospital admission, 61–3
  short stature, 244, 246
Psychotherapy, eating disorders, 212
Ptosis
  eyelid, 421
  in the newborn, 75
Puberty
  assessment, 53–4, *54*
  delayed, *472,* 474, *474*
  disorders of, 471–4, *473*
  normal, 471
  normal variants, 472

813